187

Handbuch der experimentellen Pharmakologie
Handbook of Experimental Pharmacology

Heffter Heubner New Series

XXXIII

Add: Vol. 33. Catecholamines. Edited by H. Blaschko and E. Muscholl. 1972.

Add: BLASCHKO, H. and MUSCHOLL, E. editors

Catecholamines

By

H. Blaschko, F.E. Bloom, R.E. Coupland, U.S. v. Euler,
R.F. Furchgott, W. Haefely, J. Himms-Hagen, M. Holzbauer,
I.J. Kopin, H.W. Kosterlitz, G.M. Lees, E. Marley,
E. Muscholl, M. Sandler, D.F. Sharman, A.D. Smith, J.D. Stephenson,
L. Stjärne, H. Thoenen, U. Trendelenburg, J.H. Welsh, H. Winkler

Editors

H. Blaschko and E. Muscholl

With 167 Figures

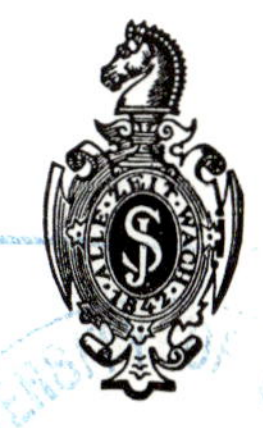

Springer-Verlag Berlin · Heidelberg · New York 1972

Professor Dr. H. Blaschko
University Department of Pharmacology
South Parks Road, Oxford, OX1 3QT/Great Britain

Professor Dr. E. Muscholl
Pharmakologisches Institut der Universität
Abt. für Neuropharmakologie
D—65 Mainz, Obere Zahlbacher Str. 67

ISBN 3-540-05517-7 Springer-Verlag Berlin · Heidelberg · New York
ISBN 0-387-05517-7 Springer-Verlag New York · Heidelberg · Berlin

Druck: Joh. Roth sel. Ww., München

List of Contributors

BLASCHKO, H., University Department of Pharmacology, South Parks Road, Oxford, OX1 3QT/Great Britain

BLOOM, F.E., Laboratory of Neuropharmacology, National Institute of Mental Health, Saint Elizabeths Hospital, Washington, D.C. 20032/USA

COUPLAND, R.E., Department of Human Morphology, The Medical School, University of Nottingham, Nottingham NG7 2RD/England

EULER, U.S. von, Department of Physiology, Karolinska Institutet, S—10401 Stockholm 60/Schweden

FURCHGOTT, R.F., Department of Pharmacology, Downstate Medical Center, 450 Clarkson Ave., Brooklyn, N.Y. 11203/USA

HAEFELY, W., Medizinische Forschungsabteilung, Hoffmann-La Roche AG, CH—4000 Basel/Schweiz

HIMMS-HAGEN, JEAN, Department of Biochemistry, University of Ottawa, Ottawa 2, Ontario, Canada

HOLZBAUER, MARGARETHE, Agricultural Research Council, Institute of Animal Physiology, Babraham, Cambridge CB2 4AT/England

KOPIN, IRWIN, J., Laboratory of Clinical Science, National Institute of Mental Health, Bethesda, Maryland 20014/USA

KOSTERLITZ, H.W., Department of Pharmacology, University Medical Buildings, Foresterhill, Aberdeen, AB9 2ZD/Scotland

LEES, G.M., Department of Pharmacology, University Medical Buildings, Foresterhill, Aberdeen, AB9 2ZD/Scotland

MARLEY, E., Institute of Psychiatry, University of London, Maudsley Hospital, de Crespigny Park, Denmark Hill, London SE5 8AF/England

MUSCHOLL, E., Pharmakologisches Institut der Universität, Abt. f. Neuropharmakologie, D—65 Mainz, Obere Zahlbacher Straße 67, Germany

SANDLER, MERTON, Bernhard Baron Memorial, Research Laboratories, Dept. of Chemical Pathology, Queen Charlotte's Maternity Hospital, Goldhawk Road, London, W6 0XG/England

SHARMAN, D.F., Agricultural Research Council, Institute of Animal Physiology, Babraham, Cambridge CB2 4AT/England

SMITH, A. DAVID, Department of Pharmacology, University of Oxford, Oxford OX1 3QT/England

STEPHENSON, J.D., Institute of Psychiatry, University of London, Maudsley Hospital, de Crespigny Park, Denmark Hill, London, SE5 8AF/England

Stjärne, L., Department of Physiology, Karolinska Institutet, S—10401 Stockholm 60/Schweden

Thoenen, H., Biozentrum der Universität Basel, Klingelbergstr. 70, CH—4056 Basel/Schweiz

Trendelenburg, U., Pharmakologisches Institut der Universität, D—87 Würzburg, Koellikerstr. 2, Germany

Welsh, J.H., Dover Road, Boothbay, Maine 04537/USA

Winkler, H., Pharmakologisches Institut der Universität, A—6020 Innsbruck/Österreich, Peter-Mayr-Str. 1

Contents

Chapter 7:

Chapter 11:

Chapter 16:

Factors Influencing the Concentration of Catecholamines at the Receptors.

Chapter 1

Introduction
Catecholamines 1922–1971

H. Blaschko

Adrenaline and related substances were discussed in the 1924 edition of Heffter's Handbook by Paul Trendelenburg. On 164 pages he described what was then known not only of adrenaline and its closest relatives but also of the sympathomimetic compounds such as tyramine and ephedrine.

When the present Editors of the Handbook entrusted us with the task of editing the present Volume it was decided to restrict it to adrenaline and the other naturally occurring catecholamines. The sympathomimetic amines in general will be discussed only in their relation to the catecholamines.

Since Trendelenburg completed his review this field has undergone an enormous expansion. There has been a wealth of new findings, and a succession of new ideas. The new theories that have been built into contemporary thought will be fully discussed in the succeeding contributions. But many of the hypotheses that have been put forward since 1924 have long been discarded and yet, they have often led to important observations that we still consider as valid.

The first page of Trendelenburg's chapter carries this footnote:

"die nach Ende 1922 erschienene Literatur ist nicht berücksichtigt."

One is surprised to find that there is no mention of Otto Loewi's early reports on the Accelerans substance (Loewi, 1921). In January 1922 there appeared Loewi's first review article in "Naturwissenschaften". On re-reading this article today, one understands why there is no reference to this work in Trendelenburg's chapter. The word adrenaline is not at all mentioned by Loewi. Trendelenburg briefly refers to the similarities between the effects of adrenaline and those of sympathetic stimulation, well known from earlier observations, and also to Elliott's (1904) hypothesis that the stimulation of the sympathetic fibres may cause a release of adrenaline.

The connection between adrenaline and the Accelerans substance was gradually brought out in Loewi's later publications. Cannon and his co-workers began to work on what they called sympathin; their first paper, on distant effects caused by sympathetic stimulation in Mammals, also appeared in 1921 (Cannon and Uridil, 1921). In 1933 Dale introduced the term *adrenergic* neurones and thus emphasised the relations between the transmitter and adrenaline. Cannon and his colleagues made a number of contributions which are of relevance to the pharmacology of the catecholamines. Through his own writings Cannon did much to make his readers aware of the functional unity of the sympathico-adrenal system and particularly of its physiological significance in preparing the body for muscular activity (see Cannon, 1928). For the peripheral adrenergic mechanisms this picture is still essentially valid; it also applies to much of our recent knowledge on the metabolic actions of the catecholamines.

In their work on the sympathetic transmitter Cannon's school made much use of structures rendered hypersensitive to catecholamines by denervation. These observations, and the resulting "Law of Denervation", led to much experimental work, some of which will be reviewed in this Volume.

For the further development of our ideas on the adrenergic transmitter Cannon's work on what he called sympathin was of great importance. The term "sympathin" has been found useful by later observers (see e.g. Vogt, 1954). Cannon and his colleagues discovered that the substance released upon sympathetic stimulation in Mammals, e.g. upon stimulation of the hepatic nerves, was not identical with adrenaline. Many of these observations are still valid but they were linked to a hypothesis on the nature of sympathin which is now obsolete (Cannon and Rosenblueth, 1937).

During the nineteen thirties the ideas on the chemical nature of sympathin, as distinct from adrenaline, were widely disregarded. In 1936, Otto Loewi produced weighty evidence in favour of the assumption that the Accelerans substance in the frog heart was adrenaline; the substance gave the fluorescence test described by Gaddum and Schild (1934) that allowed to distinguish between adrenaline and noradrenaline.

Cannon's theory was simplified by Z.M. Bacq, who suggested that the sympathin which exerted an action on distant tissue sensitized by denervation was not, as Cannon had suggested, a product of the interaction of the transmitter and the receptor on the effector cell (see Cannon and Rosenblueth, 1937) but the transmitter itself. In other words it seemed likely that the transmitter itself was not adrenaline, but a closely related substance. Bacq (1934) discussed a number of possible candidates for the transmitter, including noradrenaline; however, from a subsequent review (Bacq, 1935) one gets the impression that he favoured the idea that sympathin was a slightly oxidized derivative of adrenaline.

The idea, that noradrenaline might be the sympathetic transmitter, received support when a number of authors showed that the distant effects of stimulating the hepatic nerves were better reproduced by noradrenaline than by adrenaline (Stehle and Ellsworth, 1937; Melville, 1937; Greer et al., 1938).

A new approach to the problem of the nature of sympathin had its origin in enzymological studies. In 1939, it was shown that the enzyme L-DOPA decarboxylase, discovered by Holtz et al. (1938) in the guinea-pig kidney, had a very characteristic and restricted substrate specificity, and it was therefore proposed that this enzyme was the catalyst of one of the steps in the biosynthesis of adrenaline (Blaschko, 1939, 1942). What was of particular interest in the context of noradrenaline was the finding that N-methyl DOPA was not a substrate. One was therefore able to conclude that in the formation of adrenaline a primary amine like noradrenaline occurred as an intermediate.

The subsequent development of our present knowledge of catecholamine formation will be discussed by other contributors. The early observations by Holtz have been fully reviewed in recent years (Holtz and Palm, 1966), and we are fortunate to list U.S. von Euler among our contributors. It is chiefly his work that established the role of noradrenaline as transmitter in adrenergic neurones. The first observation on release of noradrenaline after stimulation of sympathetic nerves was made by Peart (1949) in Gaddum's laboratory.

The dual role of noradrenaline, as a precursor of adrenaline as well as a mediator was established when in 1949 Miss Bülbring demonstrated the formation of adrenaline from noradrenaline by chromaffin tissue. This reaction is brought about by the enzyme phenylethanolamine N-methyl transferase, discovered by Axelrod (see Axelrod, 1962).

The main pathway of catecholamine formation is shown below (see BLASCHKO, 1957 b):

HO⟨ring⟩—$CH_2.CH.NH_2$ (COOH) L-tyrosine

(1) ↓ Hydroxylation

HO, HO⟨ring⟩—$CH_2.CH.NH_2$ (COOH) L-dopa

(2) ↓ Decarboxylation

HO, HO⟨ring⟩—$CH_2.CH_2.NH_2$ dopamine

(3) ↓ Hydroxylation

HO, HO⟨ring⟩—$CHOH.CH_2.NH_2$ noradrenaline

(4) ↓ Methylation

HO, HO⟨ring⟩—$CHOH.CH_2.NH.CH_3$ adrenaline

The catalysts of the different steps will be described in this Volume. All the enzymes of the biosynthetic pathway are present in the adrenal medulla; this was first demonstrated for L-DOPA decarboxylase (LANGEMANN, 1951). Since Langemann's work the bovine adrenal medulla has often served as a convenient starting material for enzymological studies. One of the most important aspects of the recent work on these enzymes is the finding that the overall rate of biosynthesis depends upon the functional state of the adrenergic system. In chromaffin cells as well as in adrenergic neurones the new formation of catecholamines is governed by the amount of amine released. These relationships and the mechanisms by which this control is brought about will be fully discussed in the succeeding contributions.

For the pharmacologist the properties of L-DOPA decarboxylase have been particularly relevant. Its substrate specificity is important because this enzyme converts a pharmacologically inert amino acid into a biologically active sympathomimetic amine. An early study (BLASCHKO, 1950) discussed some of the specificity requirements of this enzyme. The inability to act upon N-methyl DOPA (and other N-methylamino acids) is accounted for by the fact that the enzyme contains pyridoxal-5-phosphate as a prosthetic group. The carbonyl group of this cofactor generally interacts only with a primary amino group. The general rules determining the interaction between phenolic hydroxyl groups and enzyme were also established: of the mono-phenolic amino acids only the meta- and the orthohomologues of tyrosine, but not tyrosine itself, were rapidly decarboxylated. Thus, in L-DOPA it must be the hydroxyl group in meta position that is chiefly involved in the enzyme-substrate interaction. Of great importance for the therapeutic applications was the study of compounds in which the α-hydrogen atom of L-DOPA (and related compounds) was replaced by a methyl group. (SOURKES et al., 1952). Originally studied as inhibitors of the decarboxylase these α-methylated amino-acids are now known to be slowly decarboxylated.

We have seen how our concepts of the dual role of noradrenaline as both precursor and chemical messenger have developed in parallel. A similar pattern can be discerned in the study of dopamine. In 1939 it was still uncertain if dopamine was the first sympathomimetic amine that made its appearance in the biosynthetic pathway. It was GOODALL (1951) who discovered dopamine in the adrenal medulla; in sympathetic nerves it was first found by SCHÜMANN (1956).

For some time, there was some reluctance to accept dopamine as the immediate precursor of noradrenaline, but the idea continued to be favoured by the biochemists (see BLASCHKO, 1954). It was the subsequent biochemical studies by which the positions of L-DOPA and dopamine in the biosynthetic pathway were at last established (DEMIS et al., 1955, 1956; HAGEN, 1956; HAGEN and WELCH, 1956; UDENFRIEND and WYNGAARDEN, 1956; GOODALL and KIRSHNER, 1957, 1958); this work has been reviewed some time ago (BLASCHKO, 1957b, 1959).

The discussion of a possible role of dopamine as a chemical messenger was taken up as soon as its role in the biosynthetic pathway had become clear. The development of our knowledge of dopamine as a transmitter substance is bound up with the study of the occurrence and distribution of the catecholamines in the central nervous system. In 1954, Miss VOGT described what she called brain sympathin. She showed that catecholamines occurred in the brain; noradrenaline was the main catecholamine present, and it occurred chiefly in the hypothalamus and the brain stem. This was the first hint that catecholamines might serve as mediator substances in neurones other than those situated in the peripheral autonomic system. A few years later dopamine was discovered in the brain (MONTAGU, 1957; WEIL-MALHERBE and BONE, 1957) and this discovery was followed by the finding that the latter amine was mainly present in the basal ganglia, unaccompanied by noradrenaline (BERTLER and ROSENGREN, 1959). Soon afterwards followed the important discovery that in the brains of Parkinsonian patients the amounts of dopamine present were abnormally low (EHRINGER and HORNYKIEWICZ, 1960).

These studies, which depended upon advances made in our knowledge of catecholamine formation, have led to therapeutic gains which have considerably extended the usefulness of the catechol compounds. Ehringer and Hornykiewicz's observations were soon followed by the application of L-DOPA for the relief of akinesia in Parkinsonism (BIRKMAYER and HORNYKIEWICZ, 1961; COTZIAS et al., 1967).

Another early application of biochemical ideas was in the treatment of arterial hypertension. There are obvious analogies in the use of L-DOPA in Parkinsonism and that of α-methyldopa in arterial hypertension (see SJOERDSMA, 1966). In both instances it is not the therapeutically active amine that is administered but a pharmacologically inert precursor. We rely on the body's own enzymes to produce the therapeutically effective molecular species. In treatment with L-DOPA, the amino acid is the precursor of what we believe to be the natural transmitter; in treatment with α-methyldopa the therapeutically active substance formed acts as a false transmitter. The concept of a "false transmitter" owes much to the work of Kopin and his colleagues (see KOPIN, 1968).

In the study of the role of the catecholamines in the central nervous system new morphological techniques have been of immense value. First and foremost we must here record the advent of fluorescence microscopy, first applied to the adrenal medulla (ERÄNKÖ, 1955), but particularly useful in studies of catecholaminergic neurones (FALCK et al., 1962). Ultrastructural studies on the catecholamines, both in chromaffin tissue and in neurones, will be fully dealt with in this Volume.

It is the combination of biochemical and morphological techniques that has helped in the fine localization of the catecholamines in the tissues. In 1953 methods were described for the isolation of the chromaffin granules by differential centrifugation (BLASCHKO and WELCH, 1953; HILLARP et al., 1953); some years later density-gradient centrifugation was introduced for the separation of the chromaffin granules from other cell organelles (BLASCHKO et al., 1957). VON EULER and HILLARP (1956) successfully applied similar techniques to the organelles that store noradrenaline in the adrenergic neurones. These observations have led to a much better understanding of biosynthesis and storage of the catecholamines; this work will be described in much detail in some of the subsequent chapters. Another gain that has followed from a study of the chemical composition of the storage organelles is in relation to the mechanism of liberation of the catecholamines. These aspects have been the subject of recent discussions (see BLOOM, IVERSEN and SCHMITT, editors, 1970; BLASCHKO and SMITH, editors, 1971); the present Volume will contribute fresh material to these arguments. The main outcome of the recent work is the recognition that the secretory activities of adrenergic structures are much wider than had previously been known (see DOUGLAS, 1968; BANKS and HELLE, 1965; BLASCHKO et al., 1967). The release of catecholamines, as hormones and as mediators, involves a mobilization also of macromolecules such as chromogranin or dopamine β-hydroxylase, although there are interesting differences in the quantitative relationships; these are fully discussed by SMITH and WINKLER in this Volume (see Chapter 13).

The importance of amine storage for the interpretation of drug action has only fully emerged since the early observations on the amine storage organelles were made. Reference has already been made to drugs that act as false transmitters; these drugs can act as transmitters because they can be taken up by the storage organelles. The relationship between reserpine and amine storage was not yet fully recognized when BEIN (1956) wrote the first comprehensive review on the *Rauwolfia* alkaloids. Release of 5-hydroxytryptamine by reserpine was first reported by PLETSCHER, SHORE and BRODIE in 1955; the depletion in noradrenaline of the cat's hypothalamus after administration by reserpine was described by HOLZBAUER and VOGT in 1956. Reserpine has proved a most useful research tool, not only in the analysis of the action of sympathomimetic amines (CARLSSON et al., 1957; BURN and RAND, 1958) but also in the discovery of the pharmacological applications of the amino acids (CARLSSON et al., 1957; BLASCHKO and CHRUSCIEL, 1960).

These relations will be fully covered by some of the contributors to this Volume.

The fate of catecholamines was unknown when PAUL TRENDELENBURG wrote his review almost 50 years ago. Today the main pathways of catecholamine catabolism are well known. We owe mainly to AXELROD (see AXELROD, 1966) our full understanding of these pathways.

The enzyme now known as monoamine oxidase (MAO) was discovered (HARE, 1928) as tyramine oxidase. Miss HARE states that she did not see any oxidation of adrenaline and it was only some years later that the action of MAO on adrenaline, noradrenaline and dopamine was established (BLASCHKO et al., 1937a, b). Although there seemed little doubt that the enzyme was active on the catechol compounds *in vivo* (see BLASCHKO, 1952), there were good reasons for the belief that other catalysts were at work. In a lecture, given in Switzerland in 1956, the situation was summarized as follows:

"...experience gained by the use of isotopically labelled amines makes it likely that some at least of the adrenaline and noradrenaline is metabolized by amine oxidase *in vivo*. However, this oxidation is a slow process, and it appears likely that other mechanisms of inactivation of these two amines will be found to play an important part. Here is a gap in our knowledge which remains to be filled." (BLASCHKO, 1957a).

Within a few months, ARMSTRONG, MCMILLAN and SHAW (1957) had described the occurrence of vanillylmandelic acid in human urine and its elevated excretion in phaeochromocytoma. This observation found its explanation when soon afterwards AXELROD (1957) (see also AXELROD and TOMCHIK, 1958) discovered the enzyme catechol-O-methyl transferase.

Catechol-O-methyl transferase and MAO are enzymes with greatly differing properties. Two properties of MAO seem to be particularly important, its intracellular localization and its close association with adrenergic neurones. The intracellular location of the oxidase gave early hints on amine uptake and the possibility that drugs could act as potentiators of the response to catecholamines by interfering with amine uptake (see BLASCHKO, 1954). It is the intraneuronal localization of the enzyme which has proved of great importance in recent studies.

The biochemists have made important contributions to the study of MAO. The enzyme acts on a host of sympathomimetic amines other than the naturally occurring catecholamines; many of these are compounds of use in drug therapy (see BLASCHKO, 1952; KAPELLER-ADLER, 1970; QUASTEL, 1970). It has been known for some time that the enzyme has a mainly mitochondrial distribution and more recently it was found that the oxidase is located in the outer mitochondrial membrane (SCHNAITMAN et al., 1967). MAO has since been used by many observers as a marker enzyme for the outer mitochondrial membrane.

These observations have still to be evaluated in regard to catecholamine turnover. They indicate that the ability to metabolise these amines is deeply seated in the cytoplasm (and axoplasm) and they make one suspect that the adrenergic neurones are by no means the only sites in which the amines have an intracellular existence. In other words, the location of MAO is closely connected with the problem, to be discussed elsewhere in this Volume, of catecholamine uptake, both neuronal and extra-neuronal.

In addition, the analysis of the fine localization of MAO has increased our understanding of the architecture of biological membranes: RACKER and PROCTOR (1970) have prepared "ghosts" of outer mitochondrial membranes from bovine kidney; subjected to sonication these ghosts can be depleted of MAO activity. When a purified preparation of MAO was added to such ghosts, the enzyme was again bound to the membranes. Such an observation suggests that the outer mitochondrial membrane possesses a specific binding site for the enzyme; the nature of this site is at present entirely unknown.

Another important advance is in the study of isoenzymes of MAO. It seems now certain that in many animal tissues MAO is not present as one homogeneous catalyst but as a mixture of several proteins, each with a different pattern of substrate and inhibitor specificities (YOUDIM and SANDLER, 1967; KIM and D'IORIO, 1968; JOHNSTON, 1968; COLLINS and YOUDIM, 1970). These differences are in the main relative and not absolute, but they have revived hopes that selective inhibitors may be found which might be particularly effective in suppressing the biological inactivation of one particular compound, without unduly inhibiting the oxidation of other amines.

The role of the MAO inhibitors has been discussed ever since Zeller et al. (1952) showed that iproniazid was an inhibitor of the enzyme. Whether the antidepressant agents which are inhibitors of the enzyme owe their activity to their enzyme-inhibitory action is at present under discussion. It seems difficult to see how inhibitors of MAO can fail to affect amine uptake; these inhibitors would be expected to increase the concentration of free intraneuronal amine and thus to decrease the concentration gradient in amines on the two sides of the axonal membrane. The similarities between the effects of MAO inhibitors and uptake inhibitors were discussed in relation to the mode of action of cocaine and related compounds many years ago (Blaschko, 1954).

The mechanism of action of MAO is still incompletely understood. It has always been assumed that oxidative deamination by the classical monoamine oxidase involved the hydrogen atoms at the α-carbon atom. This has been proved in elegant studies in which one or both α-hydrogen atoms were replaced by deuterium (Belleau et al., 1960, 1961). The pharmacological activity of the α-dideuterated form of tyramine was compared with that of tyramine itself. It was found that the α-dideuterated form had a more prolonged time course of action, indicating that the splitting of the carbon-deuterium bond occurred at a slower pace than that of the carbon-hydrogen bond. When the two stereoisomeric α-monodeuterated forms were tested it was found that one of the enantiomorphs was split slowly, like the dideuterated amine, whereas the other was split more rapidly, like ordinary tyramine. The more slowly oxidized isomer has the S-configuration, the more rapidly oxidized one the R-configuration. These observations represent one of the first instances in which a pharmacologically demonstrable isotope effect was studied.

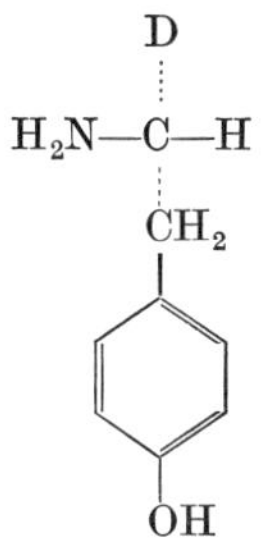

D
$H_2N—C—H$
CH_2
OH
R-configuration

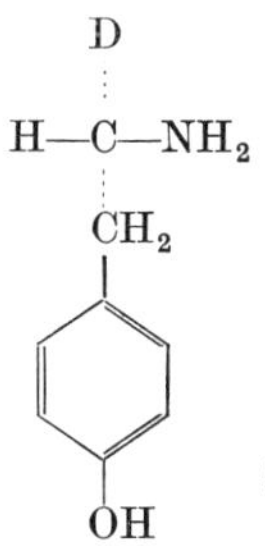

D
$H—C—NH_2$
CH_2
OH
S-configuration

Recent biochemical work has established that the classical intracellular MAO is a flavin enzyme (Erwin and Hellerman, 1967; Tipton, 1967, 1968). In addition to this enzyme there exist in Mammals enzymes which are also monoamine oxidases and which share certain substrates with the classical intracellular MAO. Chemically, however, they are quite distinct from the intracellular oxidase; they do probably not contain flavin. Much work has recently been carried out on this group which includes enzymes not related to the biological inactivation of amines — one of them appears to be active in the formation of both elastic and also collagen fibres (Partridge, 1966; Carnes, 1968). Most is known of the two amine oxidases of mammalian blood plasma (see Blaschko, 1962), the spermine oxidase of ruminant plasma (Hirsch, 1953) and benzylamine oxidase (Bergeret et al., 1957). Benzylamine oxidase is present in human blood plasma (McEwen, 1965).

(See also Note added in proof at the bottom of p. 15.)

The study of the biochemistry of the plasma enzymes has advanced prior to our understanding of their function. Both spermine oxidase (Yamada and Yasunobu, 1962) and benzylamine oxidase (Buffoni and Blaschko, 1964) have been crystallized. They are known to be copper-containing enzymes and the pig plasma enzyme is absent in animals reared on a diet deficient in copper (Blaschko et al., 1965). There is also evidence in favour of the presence of pyridoxal-5-phosphate in benzylamine oxidase (Blaschko and Buffoni, 1965).

In relation to catecholamine metabolism it seems worth pointing out that dopamine is rapidly oxidised by benzylamine oxidase (McEwen, 1965; Della Corte and Perrino, 1968).

Adrenaline, like all catechol compounds, is subject to "autoxidation" in aqueous solution. The oxidation is probably catalysed by trace impurities of metal. The same type of oxidation is brought about by a number of biological catalysts containing either copper (tyrosinase) or iron (the cytochrome system). This so-called phenolase type of oxidation leads to the formation of adrenochrome (Green and Richter, 1937).

Now that the metabolic fate of the catecholamines is fairly well understood it can be stated with some confidence that quantitatively the adrenochrome pathway of catecholamine catabolism can at best play a very minor role. This is puzzling, because of the widespread occurrence of catalysts like the cytochrome system of caeruloplasmin which will catalyse this type of oxidation.

It was Bacq (1949) who repeatedly stressed this kind of catabolism of the catecholamines. These ideas led to attempts to assign to adrenochrome some pathological significance, in particular in psychiatry, but no secure facts have been gained from these attempts. However, the possibility cannot be excluded that in some sites this type of reaction occurs. Axelrod (1964) has found it in homogenates of the parotid gland of the cat and some other Mammals (see also Suko et al., 1967 and Pichler et al., 1968).

The general conditions for the occurrence of the phenolase type of oxidation have been discussed some time ago (Blaschko and Levine, 1961). The fact, that in the formation of melanin an analogous reaction takes place, shows that there are sites where the oxidation of catechol compounds with the formation of a compound analogous to adrenochrome is possible.

This might be the place to mention relations between the occurrence of melanin and that of catecholamines. It used to be said that the melanin-forming cell and the chromaffin cell were related because both were able to convert L-tyrosine to L-DOPA. This is true, but in the two locations the conversion is brought about by two different catalysts, in chromaffin tissue (and in catecholamine-containing neurones) by tyrosine hydroxylase and in melanin cells by a "tyrosinase", a copper-containing enzyme (see Nagatsu et al., 1964).

We should remember these facts when the formation of melanin and catecholamines in, say, the *substantia nigra* are considered. We have to assume that either here too the L-DOPA is formed by two different pathways, or that, in contrast to other sites, it may arise here by a common pathway.

In the cholinergic system the early work on the mode of action of physostigmine showed at once that the enzymic degradation of the transmitter was of great importance in determining the time course of the response of the effector cell. We know today that in adrenergic systems breakdown by enzyme action is not the main factor that governs the concentration of free, extracellular amine and its removal. Uptake of amine has been recognised to play an important part. This will be amply documented by the contributors to this Volume. However, we must remember that enzymic degradation within the axoplasm (or cytoplasm) may facilitate uptake by keeping the intracellular concentration of free amine low (see e.g. GRAEFE and TRENDELENBURG, 1970).

One argument that was used against the very early speculations on humoral transmission of impulses in the sympathetic nervous system was that there were divergencies in the response to adrenaline and to sympathetic stimulation respectively. Some of these difficulties were resolved when noradrenaline was recognised as the adrenergic mediator in Mammals (see DALE, 1965). In addition, it became clear that not all postganglionic sympathetic fibres were adrenergic. Our knowledge of the cholinergic postganglionic sympathetic fibres has been much advanced in recent years, in relation to the "cholinergic link" hypothesis of BURN and RAND (1959). This topic will be fully discussed in the present Volume.

The literature on the sympathomimetic amines has taken such dimensions that it was clearly not possible to follow the example set by PAUL TRENDELENBURG and to include these substances within the compass of a single volume. In the actions of these compounds at least two components can be distinguished, firstly a direct action on the receptors in the effector cell, and secondly an indirect action, catecholamine release from stores (see BURN and RAND, 1958). The ability of the sympathomimetic amines to release the mediator will be discussed by U. TRENDELENBURG in this Volume.

There is an aspect of the new insight into the mode of action of the sympathomimetic amines that has not yet been fully exploited: the fact that many of these amines act mainly on the storage sites for noradrenaline means that the range of compounds with "receptor-activating" properties is smaller than was previously believed. One can hope that this may eventually lead to a better understanding of the amine-receptor interaction.

Most of what has been discussed so far has been in relation to the sites of formation, storage and liberation of the catecholamines. However, our knowledge of the actions of the catecholamines upon the effector organs, and the mechanism of these actions, has also been greatly advanced since 1922.

The receptor concept was not mentioned by PAUL TRENDELENBURG in 1924. Five years later, referring to Dale's analysis of the actions of ergotoxine, he writes: „Also kann mit ihm gefolgert werden, daß das Adrenalin an den Elementen angreift, die nach der Sympathicusdegeneration lebensfähig bleiben, aber durch Ergotoxin ausgeschaltet werden. Daß diese Elemente sich morphologisch von der Muskelzelle trennen lassen, ... ist eine unbewiesene Hypothese" (P. TRENDELENBURG, 1929). Incidentally, there is again no reference to the Accelerans substance in this book from 1929.

It should be recorded here that it is in one of the earlier volumes of this Handbook that A.J. CLARK (1937) introduced the term receptors into pharmacological use, building upon the earlier concepts of LANGLEY and EHRLICH.

As to the catecholamines, CLARK discusses the adrenaline receptors. He says, in relation to ergotoxine: "Hence, if the receptor theory of drug action be adopted, it is necessary to assume that the form of the receptors with which adrenaline combines differs in different tissues" (CLARK, 1937).

The acceptance of the receptor concept was a gradual one. This is well illustrated by a discussion held in 1943, on "Modes of Drug Action" (see DALE, 1943). The present Volume shows that the ideas put forward by AHLQUIST (1948) five years later still dominate our ideas on adrenergic receptors although there are indications that the concept may have to be modified.

The discovery of the irreversible α-blocking agents (NICKERSON and GOODMAN, 1947) raised hopes that these compounds might be useful in elucidating the chemistry of the α-receptors. NICKERSON (1957), in discussing this problem, refers to the reactivity of dibenamine and dibenzyline with sulphydryl, amino and carboxyl groups; he considered an interaction with sulphydryl groups as the most likely one. BELLEAU (1960) has suggested an interaction with a phosphoryl group in the receptor.

It might be appropriate also to refer to the work of BELLEAU (1958) according to which the α-blocking activity of the haloalkylamines can be accounted for by assuming that they are active in causing displacement of the agonists from the receptors when their molecules are isosteric with the agonists.

The contributions to the present Volume show that the subdivision into α- and β-receptors is still useful, in spite of observations on the metabolic actions of certain catecholamines which seem to limit the usefulness of the concept. There are also recent observations on receptors on neurones in the brain stem which respond to noradrenaline and dopamine with inhibition; these receptors are not blocked by the α- or the β-blockers but they are inhibited by 3,4-dimethoxyphenylethylamine and by bulbocapnine (GONZALEZ-VEGAS and WOLSTENCROFT, 1971a, b).

Another line of approach to the chemical nature of the adrenergic receptors stems from the analysis of the metabolic effects of the catecholamines. The glycogenolytic actions of adrenaline were known already at the time of PAUL TRENDELENBURG's (1924) review (see also CORI, 1931). It was the subsequent work from Carl and Gerty Cori's laboratory (see for instance HEGNAUER and CORI, 1934; SUTHERLAND and CORI, 1951) which established the activating effect of the catecholamines on the enzyme phosphorylase. In the further analysis of this effect it was found that the activation of phosphorylase depended on the action of cyclic 3′, 5′-AMP, and that the catecholamines exerted an activating effect upon the enzyme responsible for the formation of this nucleotide, adenyl cyclase (SUTHERLAND and RALL, 1960a, b). It is generally accepted that the β-effects of the catecholamines are brought about by this activation of adenyl cyclase, through an increase in the intracellular concentration of cyclic AMP, but this is considered probable also for the α-effects of the amines (ROBISON, BUTCHER and SUTHERLAND, 1967).

What is less certain is whether the catecholamines exert a direct action on the enzyme molecule itself, by an allosteric effect upon the enzyme protein. ROBISON et al. (1967) consider the cyclase as part of the receptor complex.

However, other observers consider it unlikely that the adenyl cyclase molecule itself is the receptor (MAYER, 1970). In this connection it seems of interest that the activation of adenyl cyclase of avian red corpuscles, present in large membrane fragments, is lost when these fragments are further broken down (ØYE and SUTHERLAND, 1966). These and similar observations leave the possibility open that between the catecholamines and adenyl cyclase another molecule is interposed. This is similar to ideas discussed some time ago (BLASCHKO, 1960). Such a concept would account for the differences between different types of receptor.

The position of adenyl cyclase as a regulator of intracellular metabolic events is one of the most far-reaching recent contributions that the biochemists have made to our understanding of the mode of action of the catecholamines. The central position of adenyl cyclase in these events can at present be more readily understood if we assume that the receptors are distinct from the cyclase enzyme, which responds with activation to a great variety of other stimuli. The cyclase can be considered as the central point upon which the various stimuli converge. There is no doubt that this point must be very close to the receptors.

We consider the metabolic actions of the catecholamines not as simply additional to their other effects; a metabolic response, mediated by one of the systems that is activated by cyclic AMP, is the basis of many, if not all, the effects that the pharmacologists have studied. Activation of phosphorylase is only one of these responses. Not only is glycogen breakdown activated; glycogen formation is suppressed. And in view of our increasing knowledge of the role of fatty acids as fuel in muscle tissue, the effects of the cyclic nucleotide on the mobilization of fatty acids is particularly important. There are also the effects on protein kinases; these may be of particular interest in relation to the classical pharmacological actions of the catecholamines. These effects are fully discussed by Mrs. HIMMS-HAGEN in this Volume.

In view of the writer's own research interests, it is perhaps not surprising that the biochemical advances have been stressed in this introduction. Biochemical methods have helped in the understanding of catecholamine formation and catabolism, and also in that of their actions on the effector tissues. Biochemical studies have also added to our understanding of the functional unity of the adrenergic system. A new field of study is that of macromolecules involved in the functioning of the adrenergic system. The effects of the nerve growth factor have demonstrated the chemical specificity of a macromolecule, seeking out and acting selectively upon the adrenergic neurones (see LEVI-MONTALCINI and ANGELETTI, 1968). And more recently there has been the study of another specific macromolecule, chromogranin A, which has no known catalytic function. It seems tempting to assume that further research will uncover a physiological role for this substance which is set free when adrenergic structures are stimulated. However, here we have reached the limits of our present knowledge. It is good to know that there still is scope for new discoveries.

The writer is indebted to his co-editor, E. MUSCHOLL, who has taken a major share in this work. He fortunately has made good the writer's shortcomings in pharmacology. We have shared satisfactions and also some disappointments. Of the latter, the main shortcoming is in the fact that the prospective contributor of a chapter on fluorescence-microscopic methods found himself unable to meet our deadline. It is fortunate that this topic has often been comprehensively reviewed in recent years. To our great satisfaction, however, all other manuscripts were delivered, edited and revised within one year, and the literature of the first half of 1970 could be considered by most contributors to this volume.

References

AHLQUIST, R.P.: A study of the adrenotropic receptors. Amer. J. Physiol. **153**, 586—600 (1948).

ARMSTRONG, M.D., MCMILLAN, A., SHAW, K.F.: 3-Methoxy-4-hydroxy-D-mandelic acid, a urinary metabolite of norepinephrine. Biochim. biophys. Acta (Amst.) **25**, 422—423 (1957).

AXELROD, J.: O-Methylation of epinephrine and other catechols *in vitro* and *in vivo*. Science **126**, 400—401 (1957).

— Purification and properties of phenylethanolamine-N-methyl transferase. J. biol. Chem. **237**, 1657—1660 (1962).

— Enzymic oxidation of epinephrine to adrenochrome by the salivary gland. Biochim. biophys. Acta (Amst.) **85**, 247—254 (1964).

— Methylation reactions in the formation and metabolism of catecholamines and other biogenic amines. Pharmacol. Rev. **18**, 95—113 (1966).

— TOMCHIK, R.: Enzymatic O-methylation of epinephrine and other catechols. J. biol. Chem. **233**, 702—705 (1958).

BACQ, Z.M.: La pharmacologie du système nerveux autonome, et particulièrement du sympathique d'après la théorie neurohumorale. Ann. Physiol. Physiochim. biol. **10**, 467—528 (1934).

— La transmission chimique des influx dans le système nerveux autonome. Ergebn. Physiol. **37**, 82—185 (1935).

— The metabolism of adrenaline. Pharmacol. Rev. **1**, 1—27 (1949).

BANKS, P., HELLE, K.: The release of protein from the stimulated adrenal medulla. Biochem. J. **97**, 40C—41C (1965).
BEIN, H.J.: The pharmacology of Rauwolfia. Pharmacol. Rev. **8**, 435—483 (1956).
BELLEAU, B.: The mechanism of drug action at receptor surfaces. Part I. Introduction. A general interpretation of the adrenergic blocking activity of β-haloalkylamines. Canad. J. Biochem. **36**, 731—753 (1958).
— Relationships between agonists, antagonists and receptor sites. In: Ciba Foundation Symposium on Adrenergic Mechanisms, pp. 223—245. Ed. by J.R. VANE, G.E.W. WOLSTENHOLME and MAEVE O'CONNOR. London: Churchill 1960.
— BURBA, J., PINDELL, M., REIFFENSTEIN, J.: Effect of deuterium substitution in sympathomimetic amines on adrenergic responses. Science **133**, 102—104 (1961).
— FANG, M., BURBA, J., MORAN, J.: The absolute optical specificity of monoamine oxidase. J. Amer. chem. Soc. **82**, 5752—5754 (1960).
BERGERET, B., BLASCHKO, H., HAWES, R.: Occurrence of an amine oxidase in horse serum. Nature (Lond.) **180**, 1127—1128 (1957).
BERTLER, Å., ROSENGREN, E.: Occurrence and distribution of dopamine in brain and other tissues. Experientia (Basel) **15**, 10—11 (1959).
BIRKMAYER, W., HORNYKIEWICZ, O.: Der L-3,4-Dioxyphenylalanin (=DOPA)-Effekt bei der Parkinson-Akinese. Wien. klin. Wschr. **73**, 787—788 (1961).
BLASCHKO, H.: The specific action of l-dopa decarboxylase. J. Physiol. (Lond.) **96**, 50P—51P (1939).
— The activity of l(—)-dopa decarboxylase. J. Physiol. (Lond.) **101**, 337—349 (1942).
— Substrate specificity of amino-acid decarboxylases. Biochim. biophys. Acta (Amst.) **4**, 130—137 (1950).
— Amine oxidase and amine metabolism. Pharmacol. Rev. **4**, 415—458 (1952).
— Metabolism of epinephrine and norepinephrine. Pharmacol. Rev. **6**, 23—28 (1954).
— Metabolism and storage of biogenic amines. Experientia (Basel) **13**, 9—12 (1957a).
— Formation of catecholamines in the animal body. Brit. med. Bull. **13**, 162—165 (1957b).
— The development of current concepts of catecholamine formation. Pharmacol. Rev. **11**, 307—316 (1959).
— Chairman's Opening Remarks. In: Ciba Foundation Symposium on Adrenergic Mechanisms, pp. 473—480. Ed. by J.R. VANE, G.E.W. WOLSTENHOLME and MAEVE O'CONNOR. London: Churchill 1960.
— The amine oxidases of mammalian blood plasma. Advanc. comp. Physiol. Biochem. **1**, 67—116 (1962).
— BUFFONI, F.: Pyridoxal phosphate as a constituent of the histaminase (benzylamine oxidase) of pig plasma. Proc. roy. Soc. B. **163**, 45—60 (1965).
— — WEISSMAN, N., CARNES, W.H., COULSON, W.F.: The amine oxidase of pig plasma in copper deficiency. Biochem. J. **96**, 4C—5C (1965).
— CHRUŚCIEL, T.L.: The decarboxylation of amino acids related to tyrosine and their awakening action in reserpine-treated mice. J. Physiol. (Lond.) **151**, 272—284 (1960).
— COMLINE, R.S., SCHNEIDER, F.H., SILVER, M., SMITH, A.D.: Secretion of a chromaffin granule protein, chromogranin, from the adrenal gland after splanchnic stimulation. Nature (Lond.) **215**, 58—59 (1967).
— HAGEN, J.M., HAGEN, P.: Mitochondrial enzymes and chromaffin granules. J. Physiol. (Lond.) **139**, 316—322 (1957).
— LEVINE, W.G.: Observations on phenolases. Neuro-Psychopharmacology, **2**, 435—439. Ed. by E. ROTHLIN. Amsterdam: Elsevier 1961.
— RICHTER, D., SCHLOSSMANN, H.: The inactivation of adrenaline. J. Physiol. (Lond.) **90**, 1—19 (1937a).
— — — The oxidation of adrenaline and other amines. Biochem. J. **31**, 2187—2196 (1937b).
— SMITH, A.D.: Editors, Subcellular and macromolecular aspects of synaptic transmission. Phil. Trans. roy. Soc. B. **261**, 273—437 (1971).
— WELCH, A.D.: Localization of adrenaline in cytoplasmic particles of the bovine adrenal medulla. Naunyn-Schmiedeberg's Arch. exp. Path. Pharmak. **219**, 17—22 (1953).
BLOOM, F.E., IVERSEN, L.L., SCHMITT, F.O.: Editors, Macromolecules in synaptic function. Neurosciences Res. Prog. Bull. Vol. **8**, No. 4, 325—455 (1970).
BUFFONI, F., BLASCHKO, H.: Benzylamine oxidase and histaminase: purification and crystallization of an enzyme from pig plasma. Proc. roy. Soc. B. **161**, 153—167 (1964).
BÜLBRING, E.: The methylation of noradrenaline by minced suprarenal tissue. Brit. J. Pharmacol. **4**, 234—244 (1949).
BURN, J.H., RAND, M.J.: The action of sympathomimetic amines in animals treated with reserpine. J. Physiol. (Lond.) **144**, 314—366 (1958).
— — Sympathetic postganglionic mechanism. Nature (Lond.) **164**, 163—165 (1959).

CANNON, W.B.: Die Notfallsfunktion des sympathico-adrenalen Systems. Ergebn. Physiol. **27**, 380—406 (1928).
— ROSENBLUETH, A.: Autonomic neuro-effector systems. New York: Macmillan 1937.
— URIDIL, J.E.: Some effects on the denervated heart of stimulating the nerves of the liver. Amer. J. Physiol. **58**, 353—364 (1921).
CARLSSON, A., LINDQVIST, M., MAGNUSSON, T.: 3,4-Dihydroxyphenylalanine and 5-hydroxytryptophan as reserpine antagonists. Nature (Lond.) **180**, 1200 (1957).
— ROSENGREN, E., BERTLER, A., NILSSON, J.: Effect of reserpine on the metabolism of catecholamines. In: Psychotropic Drugs, pp. 363—372. Ed. by S. GARATTINI and V. GHETTI. Amsterdam: Elsevier 1957.
CARNES, W.H.: Copper and connective tissue metabolism. Int. Rev. Connective Tissue Res. **4**, 197—232 (1968).
CLARK, A.J.: General pharmacology. In: Handbuch der experimentellen Pharmakologie. Ed. by W. HEUBNER and J. SCHÜLLER. Ergänzungswerk, 4ter Band. Berlin: Julius Springer 1937.
COLLINS, C.G.S., YOUDIM, M.B.H.: Multiple forms of human brain monoamine oxidase. Biochem. J. **117**, 43P (1970).
CORI, C.F.: Mammalian carbohydrate metabolism. Physiol. Rev. **11**, 143—275 (1931).
COTZIAS, G.C., VAN WOERT, M.H., SCHIFFER, I.M.: Aromatic amino acids and modification of Parkinsonism. New Engl. J. Med. **276**, 374—379 (1967).
DALE, H.H.: Nomenclature of fibres in the autonomic system and their effects. J. Physiol. (Lond.) **80**, 10P—11P (1933).
— General introductory address. In: Modes of drug action. A general discussion. Trans. Faraday Soc. **39**, 319—322 (1943).
— Adventures in physiology. The Wellcome Trust: London 1965.
DELLA CORTE, L., PERRINO, I.: Il ruolo delle aminossidasi plasmatiche nel metabolismo della dopamina. Farmaco, Ed. sci. **23**, 204—209 (1968).
DEMIS, D.J., BLASCHKO, H., WELCH, A.D.: The conversion of dihydroxyphenylalanine-2-C^{14} (dopa) to norepinephrine by bovine adrenal medullary homogenates. J. Pharmacol. exp. Ther. **113**, 14—15 (1955).
— — — The conversion of dihydroxyphenylalanine-2-C^{14} (dopa) to norepinephrine by bovine adrenal medullary homogenate. J. Pharmacol. exp. Ther. **117**, 208—212 (1956).
DOUGLAS, W.W.: Stimulus-secretion coupling: the concept and clues from chromaffin and other cells. Brit. J. Pharmacol. **34**, 451—474 (1968).
EHRINGER, R.H., HORNYKIEWICZ, O.: Verteilung von Noradrenalin und Dopamin (3-Hydroxytyramin) im Gehirn des Menschen und ihr Verhalten bei Erkrankungen des extrapyramidalen Systems. Klin. Wschr. **15**, 1236—1239 (1960).
ELLIOTT, T.R.: On the action of adrenalin. J. Physiol. (Lond.) **31**, XX—XXI (1904).
ERÄNKÖ, O.: Distribution of fluorescing islets, adrenaline and noradrenaline in the adrenal medulla of the hamster. Acta endocr. (Kbh.) **18**, 174—179 (1955).
ERWIN, V.G., HELLERMAN, L.: Mitochondrial monoamine oxidase. I. Purification and characterization of the bovine kidney enzyme. J. biol. Chem. **242**, 4230—4238 (1967).
VON EULER, U.S., HILLARP, N.-Å.: Evidence for the presence of noradrenaline in submicroscopic structures of adrenergic axons. Nature (Lond.) **177**, 44—45 (1956).
FALCK, B., HILLARP, N.-Å., THIEME, G., TORP, A.: Fluorescence of catecholamines and related compounds condensed with formaldehyde. J. Histochem. Cytochem. **10**, 348—354 (1962).
GADDUM, J.H., SCHILD, H.: A sensitive physical test for adrenaline. J. Physiol. (Lond.) **80**, 9P—10P (1934).
GONZALEZ-VEGAS, J.A., WOLSTENCROFT, J.H.: Actions of 3,4-dimethoxyphenylethylamine in relation to the effects of catecholamines on brainstem neurones. Brit. J. Pharmacol. **41**, 406P—407P (1971a).
— — Antagonism of noradrenaline and dopamine inhibition of brain-stem neurones by bulbocapnine. J. Physiol. (Lond.) **214**, 16P (1971b).
GOODALL, McC.: Studies of adrenaline and noradrenaline in mammalian heart and suprarenals. Acta physiol. scand. **24**, Suppl. **85**, 7—51 (1951).
— KIRSHNER, N.: Biosynthesis of adrenaline and noradrenaline *in vitro*. J. biol. Chem. **226**, 213—221 (1957).
— — Biosynthesis of epinephrine and norepinephrine by sympathetic nerves and ganglia. Circulation **17**, 366—371 (1958).
GRAEFE, K.H., TRENDELENBURG, U.: The influence of intraneuronal inactivating mechanisms on the membrane-amine pump. Naunyn-Schmiedeberg's Arch. exp. Path. Pharmak. **266**, 336—337 (1970).
GREEN, D.E., RICHTER, D.: Adrenaline and adrenochrome. Biochem. J. **31**, 596—616 (1937).

Greer, C.M., Pinkston, J.O., Baxter, J.H., Jr., Brannon, E.S.: Norepinephrine [β-(3,4-dihydroxyphenyl)-β-hydroxyethylamine] as a possible mediator in the sympathetic division of the autonomic nervous system. J. Pharmacol. exp. Ther. **62**, 189—227 (1938).
Hagen, P.: Biosynthesis of norepinephrine from 3,4-dihydroxyphenylethylamine (dopamine). J. Pharmacol. exp. Ther. **116**, 26 (1956).
— Welch, A.D.: The adrenal medulla and the biosynthesis of pressor amines. Recent Progr. Hormone Res. **12**, 27—44 (1956).
Hare, M.L.C.: Tyramine oxidase. I. A new enzyme system in liver. Biochem. J. **22**, 968—979 (1928).
Hegnauer, A., Cori, G.T.: The influence of epinephrine on chemical changes in isolated frog muscle, J. biol. Chem. **105**, 691—703 (1934).
Hillarp, N.-Å., Lagerstedt, S., Nilson, B.: The isolation of a granular fraction from the suprarenal medulla containing the sympathomimetic catecholamines. Acta physiol. scand. **28**, 251—263 (1953).
Hirsch, J.G.: Spermine oxidase: an amine oxidase with specificity for spermine and spermidine. J. exp. Med. **97**, 345—355 (1953).
Holtz, P., Heise, R., Lüdtke, K.: Fermentativer Abbau von l-Dioxyphenylalanin (dopa) durch Niere. Naunyn-Schmiedeberg's Arch. exp. Path. Pharmak. **191**, 87—118 (1938).
— Palm, D.: Brenzkatechinamine und andere sympathicomimetische Amine. Biosynthese und Inaktivierung, Freisetzung und Wirkung. Ergebn. Physiol. **58**, 1—580 (1966).
Holzbauer, M., Vogt, M.: Depression by reserpine of the noradrenaline concentration in the hypothalamus of the cat. J. Neurochem. **1**, 8—11 (1956).
Johnston, J.P.: Some observations upon a new inhibitor of monoamine oxidase. Biochem. Pharmacol. **17**, 1285—1297 (1968).
Kapeller-Adler, R.: Amine oxidases and methods for their study. New York, London, Sydney, Toronto: John Wiley & Sons 1970.
Kim, H.C., D'Iorio, A.: Possible isoenzymes of monoamine oxidase in rat tissues. Canad. J. Biochem. **46**, 295—297 (1968).
Kopin, I.J.: The influence of false adrenergic transmitters on adrenergic neurotransmission. In: Adrenergic Neurotransmission, pp. 95—104. Ciba Foundation Study Group No. **33**. Ed. by G.E.W. Wolstenholme and Maeve O'Connor. London: Churchill 1968.
Langemann, H.: Enzymes and their substrates in the adrenal gland of the ox. Brit. J. Pharmacol. **6**, 318—324 (1951).
Levi-Montalcini, R., Angeletti, P.V.: Nerve growth factor. Physiol. Rev. **48**, 534—569 (1968).
Loewi, O.: Über humorale Übertragbarkeit der Herznervenwirkung. I. Mitteilung. Pflügers Arch. ges. Physiol. **189**, 239—242 (1921).
— Über humorale Übertragbarkeit der Herznervenwirkung. Naturwissenschaften **10**, 52—55 (1922).
— Quantitative und qualitative Untersuchung über den Sympathicusstoff. Pflügers Arch. ges. Physiol. **237**, 504—514 (1936).
Mayer, S.E.: Adenyl cyclase as a component of the adrenergic receptor. In: Ciba Foundation Symposium on Molecular Properties of Drug Receptors, pp. 43—58. Ed. by Ruth Porter and Maeve O'Connor. London: Churchill 1970.
McEwen, C.M.: Human plasma monoamine oxidase. I. Purification and identification. J. biol. Chem. **240**, 2003—2010 (1965).
Melville, K.I.: The antisympathomimetic action of dioxane compounds (F883 and F933), with specific reference to the vascular responses to dihydroxyphenylethanolamine (Arterenol) and nerve stimulation. J. Pharmacol. exp. Ther. **59**, 317—327 (1937).
Montagu, K.R.: Catechol compounds in rat tissues and in brains of different animals. Nature (Lond.) **180**, 244—245 (1957).
Nagatsu, T., Levitt, M., Udenfriend, S.: Tyrosine hydroxylase. The initial step in norepinephrine biosynthesis. J. biol. Chem. **239**, 2910—2917 (1964).
Nickerson, M.: Nonequilibrium drug antagonism. Pharmacol. Rev. **9**, 246—259 (1957).
— Goodman, L.S.: Pharmacological properties of a new adrenergic blocking agent: N,N-dibenzyl-β-chloroethylamine (Dibenamine). J. Pharmacol. exp. Ther. **89**, 167—185 (1947).
Øye, I., Sutherland, E.W.: The effect of epinephrine and other agents on adenyl cyclase in the cell membrane of avian erythrocytes. Biochim. biophys. Acta (Amst.) **127**, 347—354 (1966).
Partridge, S.M.: Biosynthesis and nature of elastin structures. Fed. Proc. **25**, 1023—1029 (1966).
Peart, W.S.: The nature of splenic sympathin. J. Physiol. (Lond.) **108**, 491—501 (1949).
Pichler, H., Suko, J., Hertting, G.: Action of drugs upon the formation of tritiated water from dl-7-H^3-noradrenaline in the rat. Biochem. Pharmacol. **17**, 1329—1337 (1968).

PLETSCHER, A., SHORE, P.A., BRODIE, B.: Serotonin release as a possible mechanism of reserpine action. Science **122**, 374—375 (1955).

QUASTEL, J.H.: Amine Oxidases. In: Handbook of Neurochemistry. Ed. by A. LAJTHA. Vol. IV, pp. 285—312. New York-London: Plenum Press 1970.

RACKER, E., PROCTOR, H.: Reconstitution of the outer mitochondrial membrane with monoamine oxidase. Biochem. biophys. Res. Commun. **39**, 1120—1125 (1970).

ROBISON, G.A., BUTCHER, R.W., SUTHERLAND, E.W.: Adenyl cyclase as an adrenergic receptor. Ann. N.Y. Acad. Sci. **139**, 703—723 (1967).

SCHNAITMAN, C., ERWIN, V.G., GREENAWALT, J.W.: The submitochondrial localization of monoamine oxidase. J. Cell Biol. **32**, 719—735 (1967).

SCHÜMANN, H.J.: Nachweis von Oxytyramin (Dopamin) in sympathischen Nerven und Ganglien. Naunyn-Schmiedeberg's Arch. exp. Path. Pharmak. **227**, 566—573 (1956).

SJOERDSMA, A.: Catecholamine-drug interaction in man. Pharmacol. Rev. **18**, 673—683 (1966).

SOURKES, T., HENEAGUE, P., TRANO, Y.: Enzymatic decarboxylation of isomers and derivatives of dihydroxyphenylalanine. Arch. Biochem. Biophys. **40**, 185—193 (1952).

STEHLE, R.L., ELLSWORTH, H.C.: Dihydroxyphenylethanolamine (Arterenol) as a possible sympathetic hormone. J. Pharmacol. exp. Ther. **59**, 114—121 (1937).

SUKO, J., LINET, O., HERTTING, G.: Tritiumwasser in Speicheldrüsen, im Speichel und Plasma der Katze nach Injektion von DL-7-H^3-Noradrenalin. Naunyn-Schmiedeberg's Arch. Pharmak. exp. Path. **256**, 439—449 (1967).

SUTHERLAND E. W., CORI C. F.,: Effect of hyperglycemic factor and epinephrine on liver phosphorylase. J. biol. Chem. **188**, 531—543 (1951).

— RALL, T.W.: The relation of adenosine-3',5'-phosphate and phosphorylase to the actions of catecholamines and other hormones. Pharmacol. Rev. **12**, 265—299 (1960a).

— — The relation of adenosine-3',5'-phosphate to the action of catecholamines. In: Ciba Foundation Symposium on Adrenergic Mechanisms, pp. 295—304. Ed. by J.R. VANE, G.E.W. WOLSTENHOLME and MAEVE O'CONNOR. London: Churchill 1960b.

TIPTON, K.F.: The presence of flavine-adenine dinucleotide in preparations of pig-brain mitochondria. Biochem. J. **104**, 36P—37P (1967).

— The prosthetic groups of pig brain mitochondrial monoamine oxidase. Biochim. biophys. Acta (Amst.) **159**, 451—459 (1968).

TRENDELENBURG, P.: Adrenalin und adrenalinverwandte Substanzen. In: Handbuch der experimentellen Pharmakologie, pp. 1130—1293. Ed. by A. HEFFTER. Berlin: Julius Springer 1924.

— Die Hormone. Ihre Physiologie und Pharmakologie. Erster Band. Berlin: Julius Springer 1929.

UDENFRIEND, S., WYNGAARDEN, J.B.: Precursors of adrenal epinephrine and norepinephrine *in vivo*. Biochim. biophys. Acta (Amst.) **20**, 48—52 (1956).

VOGT, M.: The concentration of sympathin in different parts of the central nervous system under normal conditions and after the administration of drugs. J. Physiol. (Lond.) **123**, 451—481 (1954).

WEIL-MALHERBE, H., BONE, A.D.: Intracellular distribution of catecholamines in the brain. Nature (Lond.) **180**, 1050—1051 (1957).

YAMADA, H., YASUNOBU, K.T.: Monoamine oxidase. I. Purification, crystallization and properties of plasma monoamine oxidase. J. biol. Chem. **237**, 1511—1516 (1962).

YOUDIM, M.B.H., SANDLER, M.: Isoenzymes of soluble monoamine oxidase from human placental and rat-liver mitochondria. Biochem. J. **105**, 43P (1967).

ZELLER, E.A., BARSKY, J., BERMAN, E.R., FOUTS, J.R.: Action of isonicotinic acid hydrazide and related compounds on enzymes of brain and other tissues. J. Lab. clin. Med. **40**, 965—966 (1952).

Note added in proof: Recent work on amine oxidases is reviewed in:

COSTA, E., SANDLER, M.: Editors, Monoamine oxidases: new vistas. New York: Raven Press (in press).

Chapter 2

The Chromaffin System

R. E. Coupland

With 11 Figures

I. Introduction

Staining characteristics have frequently been used for the identification and classification of cells or tissues, and elements referred to as chromaffin cells, basophils, eosinophils and chromophobes immediately spring to mind. The term "chromaffin" was introduced by Kohn (1900, 1902, 1903,) in respect of the reaction of cells of the adrenal medulla and elements topographically and developmentally associated with sympathetic neurons — particularly in the pre- and paravertebral chains and plexuses of the abdomen.

The term "chromaffin" implies an affinity for chrome salts, and in the normal chromaffin reaction as well as its more recent improvements, which have been achieved by the use of mixtures having a pH *c* 6, the amine is oxidized and chromium is bound to phenolic and indolic complexes (Coupland, 1954, 1965a); subsequent staining reactions often reflect the presence of chrome complexes.

A single staining characteristic is rarely sufficiently specific to allow one to make a worthwhile biological classification of cells or tissues. In consequence other factors such as developmental origin, structure and biochemistry must be taken into account in defining and classifying these elements. In the present work the criteria previously detailed (Coupland, 1965a) have been applied in identifying elements as chromaffin cells. Thus a normal chromaffin cell is one which develops from neuroectoderm, is innervated by pre-ganglionic sympathetic nerve fibres, is capable of synthesizing and secreting catecholamines and of storing them in sufficient concentration to give a positive chromaffin reaction.

This definition excludes from the designation as chromaffin cells mast cells of various forms which give a positive chromaffin reaction as a result of their dopamine or 5-hydroxytryptamine (5HT) content as well as the 5HT-containing enterochromaffin cells. Furthermore, the adrenergic sympathetic neurons and phaeochromoblasts which meet all criteria except that of a positive chromaffin reaction following fixation in potassium dichromate are also excluded. The latter are, however, justifiably designated as chromaffin cell precursors.

Since the chromaffin reaction develops as a result of the catecholamine content of the cell and its intensity is proportional to the concentration of the amine, the reaction varies under physiological and experimental conditions. There is, however, no evidence that under normal physiological conditions the amine content of a chromaffin cell can be so depleted as to result in its failure to give a positive chromaffin reaction, though in experimental circumstances, and in particular after insulin hypoglycaemia or reserpine administration (Coupland, 1958, 1959) severe depletion of some or all chromaffin cells occurs so that a negative staining reaction results.

The sensitivity of the chromaffin reaction for localizing biogenic amines in tissues is relatively low even though it is improved by buffering the fixative to pH 5.6—6 (COUPLAND, 1965a). More sensitive techniques are the use of biochemical assay of tissue extracts combined with electron microscopy following glutaraldehyde fixation followed by silver impregnation (TRAMEZZANI et al., 1964), glutaraldehyde-osmium tetroxide (COUPLAND et al., 1964; COUPLAND and HOPWOOD, 1966), or glutaraldehyde-potassium dichromate fixation (WOOD and BARRNETT, 1964), or the application of the formaldehyde-fluorescent reaction for biogenic amines of FALCK et al. (1962) which can be made qualitative and quantitative by use of microspectrophotometry in conjunction with light microscopy (CASPERSSON et al., 1966). These techniques are of more value than the routine chromaffin reaction for identifying catecholamines in normal nervous tissue and in neural tumours, but for positive identification of amines should not be divorced from amine assay. All electron histochemical techniques involving initial fixation in glutaraldehyde depend for the identification of adrenaline and noradrenaline storing granules on the formation *in situ* of an insoluble polymer with noradrenaline and the loss of adrenaline (COUPLAND and HOPWOOD, 1966). Subsequent treatment allows the binding of an electron dense substance to the polymer and in the writer's experience osmium tetroxide is the most useful in the case of the adrenal gland. Dichromate followed by osmium tetroxide would appear to be more useful in the case of amine-storage vesicles in nerve fibres (BLOOM and BARRNETT, 1966).

II. Distribution of Chromaffin Cells in Vertebrates

The comparative anatomy of chromaffin tissue has been reviewed by the writer (COUPLAND, 1965a), and only recent contributions will be considered below. During the past five years workers have concerned themselves more with the identification and localization of cells storing adrenaline and/or noradrenaline than with the overall distribution of chromaffin tissue.

1. Invertebrates

Since ROAF and NIERENSTEIN (1907) and ROAF (1911) reported that the purple gland of *Nucella lapillus* contained "chromaffin cells" and that extracts had a pressor effect on intravenous injection in the rabbit, little or no work has been carried out on the structure or biochemistry of this organ. In consequence it is not possible to adequately classify the constituent elements.

The reports of EULER (1953) and ÖSTLUND (1954) on the presence of pressor substances in invertebrates including octopus, whelk, mussel and snail have been extended and supplemented by DAHL et al. (1962) who applied fluorescent microscopy and chemical assay to cerebral and visceral ganglia of the bivalve *Anodonta piscanalis* and the snail *Helix pomatia*. Groups of nerve cells which contain either 5-hydroxytryptamine or a catecholamine (probably dopamine) were demonstrated. Other neurons were apparently free from monoamines.

2. Vertebrates

Cyclostomata: The chemical nature of chromaffin cells described by GIACOMINI (1902) in the walls of the posterior cardinal veins of *Petromyzon marinus* and *Lampetra planeri* does not appear to have been determined. Further observations have however been made on the hearts of cyclostomes following reports of chromaffin cells in the heart wall (JOHNELS and PALMGREN, 1960), and the presence of large quantities of catecholamines in extracts of these organs (Östlund, 1954; Euler and Fänge, 1961). Bloom et al. (1961, 1962, 1963) described dendritic cells containing catecholamines in the hearts of both *Lampetra* and *Myxine*. Amine-containing cells lying on the surface of muscle bundles in the atrium and sinus venosus, and less frequently in the other chambers of the hearts of lampreys are separated from the lumina by only a thin endothelium. The cells vary in shape but are often multipolar and elongated; they contain adrenaline, noradrenaline or both amines.

Elasmobranchii: The distribution of chromaffin tissue in dogfish and rays was described in detail (Coupland, 1965a). Subsequent work by the writer on male and female forms of the dogfish *Scylliorhinus canicula* using the chemical and fluorimetric assay techniques of Euler and Hamberg (1949) and Udenfriend (1962), has demonstrated the presence of adrenaline and noradrenaline in the suprarenal bodies of the species with noradrenaline forming 70—80% of the total amine. No difference was noted in the amine content of the anterior, middle and posterior bodies. These findings are in keeping with the observations of Shepherd and West (1952) on the amine content of the suprarenal bodies of *Squalus acanthias*. Amine assays of suprarenal bodies have been correlated with electron microscopic examination after fixation by the glutaraldehyde-osmium tetroxide sequence and subsequent staining with uranyl acetate and lead citrate. Adrenaline- and noradrenaline-storing cells have been identified in adult forms of both sexes, with noradrenaline-storing elements predominating.

Cells containing mixtures of amines have not been identified (Coupland, 1971).

In the male dogfish *(S. canicula)* some of the peripheral cells of the caudal suprarenal bodies give a weak or negative chromaffin reaction and a negative iodate reaction; in some cases these non-reactive cells form a relatively distinct peripheral zone. A few scattered cells having similar staining properties may also be identified in the periphery of the caudal bodies of the female dogfish, but are less numerous, and do not form such a distinct zone. Because of the negative iodate reaction these peripheral cells were thought by Olivereau (1959) to be adrenaline-storing elements. Sacarrão (1966) denied the presence of any sexual difference. Recent work of the writer (Coupland, 1971) has, however, demonstrated that these peripheral cells contain sparsely scattered highly electron dense membrane-bound noradrenaline granules 20—250 nm diameter, indicative of the presence of primary amine (Fig. 1). Indeed, the size of these granules approximate to amine-storage granules which may be identified in the soma of sympathetic neurons of the same species, and though there is no evidence from either cell form, or internal structure to suggest that these peripheral elements are true neurons, one is reminded of Vincent's (1898) suggestion that transitional cells, intermediate in type between chromaffin cells and sympathetic neurons, may exist in *S. canicula*.

Amphibia: The presence of specific adrenaline- and noradrenaline-storing cells in the frog *(Rana temporaria)* adrenal glands has been demonstrated by the writer (Coupland, 1971) after glutaraldehyde-osmium tetroxide fixation combined with fluorimetric assay of extracts. Cells containing mixtures of the two amines were not observed. Adrenaline- and noradrenaline-storing cells have also been identified in the toad, *Bufo arenarum*, Hensel (Piezzi, 1965). Typical cholinergic-type nerve endings have been observed by the writer on both types of chromaffin cells.

The occurrence of two types of synapse on the chromaffin cells of the toad's adrenal gland was reported by Piezzi (1966). One was described as containing small (300—500 Å) electron lucent synaptic vesicles and was clearly a typical cholinergic-type ending. The other so-called ending contained vesicles which showed electron dense cores and a diameter of 700—1,300 Å. This latter type of granule is in all respects similar to the larger vesicles, with electron dense centres described by the writer in the pre-terminal region of adrenal medullary nerve

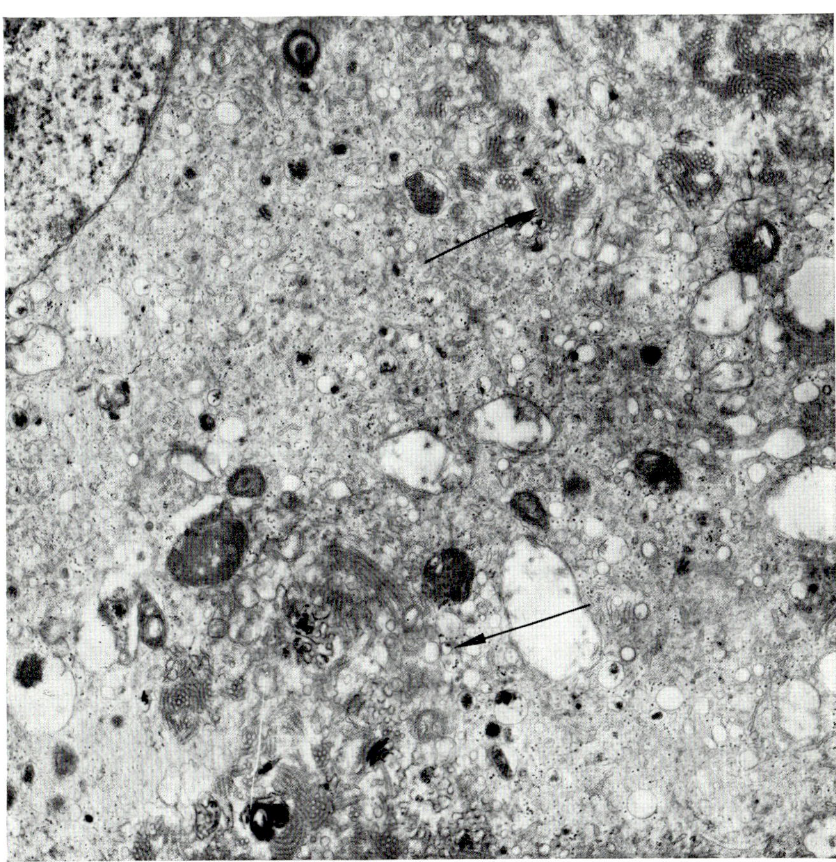

Fig. 1. Electron micrograph showing a peripheral cell of a posterior suprarenal body of male dogfish containing small electron dense inclusions typical of primary amine, lysosomes and aggregates of cytoplasmic tubules (arrowed). Fixed in glutaraldehyde/osmium tetroxide × 14,500

fibres in the rat (Coupland, 1965c), and from the illustrations of Piezzi (1966) together with his description which includes a statement that the so-called type II ending contains microtubules as well as granulated vesicles and mitochondria, the writer believes that the so-called type II ending is the pre-terminal region of a cholinergic nerve and not a true synaptic ending. Nerve endings containing both types of vesicles have been observed by the writer on chromaffin cells of the frog on a number of occasions (Fig. 2).

Extracts of the carotid labyrinths of the frog *(R. temporaria)* have been shown by Banister et al. (1967) to contain substantial amounts of adrenaline and only traces of noradrenaline and dopamine. The amine-containing cells were identified with the formaldehyde-fluorescence technique, but the concentration of amine was insufficient to result in a positive chromaffin reaction.

Reptiles: The work of HOUSSAY et al. (1962) and WASSERMANN and TRAMEZZANI (1963) has demonstrated that the pattern of a peripheral distribution of noradrenaline-storing cells and a more central arrangement of adrenaline-storing elements, described by WRIGHT and JONES (1955) in the adrenal of the green

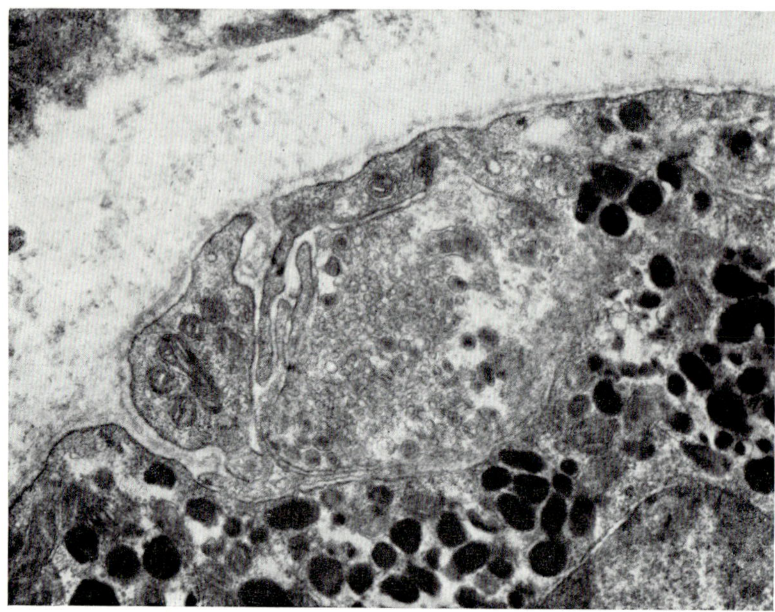

Fig. 2. Electron micrograph showing a nerve ending on a noradrenaline-storing chromaffin cell of frog adrenal. Note the presence of both electron dense and electron lucent synaptic vesicles. Fixed in glutaraldehyde/osmium tetroxide × 24,000

lizard *(Lacerta viridis)* also occurs in the snake *(Xenodon merremii)*, lizard *(Teius teyou)* and yacare *(Caiman latirostris)*. In the tortoise *(Phrynops hilarii)* the distribution of the two types of cell is more random.

Birds: Chromaffin cells are rather uniformly and diffusely distributed in small groups throughout the avian adrenal. Light and electron microscopy after appropriate fixation and staining demonstrate the presence of both adrenaline- and noradrenaline-storing cells in cellular islands or cords and apparently without obvious relationship to their proximity to cortical elements (COUPLAND, 1965a, 1971). No evidence of a zonal distribution of adrenaline and noradrenaline secreting cells was obtained.

The presence of specific adrenaline- and noradrenaline-storing cells has been demonstrated electron microscopically (COUPLAND, 1971), and no evidence of the presence of mixtures of the two types of granules within a single chromaffin cell has been obtained. In some cells chromaffin granules were observed within what appear to be autophagic vacuoles (Fig. 3); this association has not been observed in normal mammal adrenal glands.

Mammals: The distribution of chromaffin cells in mammals was reviewed by COUPLAND (1965a). In postnatal specimens the largest individual collections of chromaffin cells form the adrenal medullas. Scattered cells or small groups are commonly associated with the pre-vertebral sympathetic plexuses, and the paravertebral sympathetic chains and their visceral branches in the neck, thorax, abdomen and pelvis. The largest extra-adrenal collections of chromaffin cells normally lie adjacent to the abdominal aorta in the pre- and para-aortic positions. Small groups of cells are associated with the sympathetic plexuses of the heart

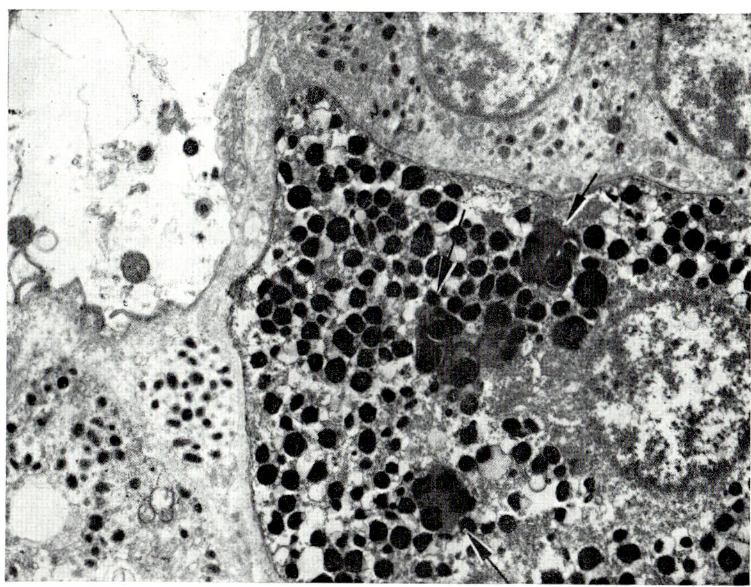

Fig. 3. Electron micrograph showing adrenaline- and noradrenaline-storing cells of domestic fowl adrenal gland. Note chromaffin granules within dark bodies (autophagic vacuoles; arrowed) of noradrenaline-storing cell. Glutaraldehyde/osmium tetroxide × 3,000

and great vessels, with the ganglia or interganglionic fibres and splanchnic branches of the sympathetic chains in the abdomen and pelvis, and with individual ganglia or interganglionic nerve fibres.

By the use of chemical assay in conjunction with both light and electron histochemistry the adrenal medullas of most adult mammals except rabbits and guinea-pigs have been shown to be composed normally of both adrenaline- and noradrenaline-storing cells. In adult forms the two amines are stored in specific cells and mixed storage elements do not normally exist. During foetal and the first few days of postnatal life individual cells containing mixtures of adrenaline and noradrenaline granules are occasionally observed (COUPLAND and WEAKLEY, 1968, 1970; ELFVIN, 1967a). The primary amine is the first to appear during morphogenesis and noradrenaline-storing cells and granules predominate during early foetal life. Later adrenaline-storing granules and cells appear, and in animals like the rabbit which have a predominantly adrenaline-secreting adrenal medulla they are the predominant cell type during the last third of foetal life (COUPLAND and WEAKLEY, 1968).

Adrenaline becomes the predominant amine in both foetal rabbit and rat adrenal glands after the twentieth day of gestation (BRUNDIN, 1965; ROFFI, 1964, 1968), but since the gestation period is longer in the rabbit this implies a relatively earlier onset of methylation in this form. In man adrenaline appears early in foetal life in the human adrenal medulla (COUPLAND, 1953; GREENBERG and LIND, 1961) comprising *c* 50% of total catecholamine during the second half of gestation.

Unlike the adrenal medulla extra-adrenal chromaffin tissue shows little or no change in amine content during foetal life. In both man and rabbit (Coupland, 1953; Coupland and MacDougall, 1966; Greenberg and Lind, 1961) noradrenaline forms the predominant amine (>90%) throughout foetal life. In post-natal rabbits *c* 90% of the catecholamine is still noradrenaline at the age of three months. Although it is difficult or impossible to localize discrete collections of extra-adrenal chromaffin cells in man after the age of three years (Coupland, 1954, 1965a) the finding that noradrenaline is the sole or predominant amine in extra-adrenal phaeochromocytomas, while adrenaline is commonly in excess in adrenal medullary tumors (Euler et al., 1955; Euler and Ström, 1957; Hunter et al., 1963), coupled with the excess of the primary amine during late foetal and early post-natal life (Coupland, 1953; West et al., 1953; Greenberg and Lind, 1961) makes it likely that noradrenaline continues to be the predominant amine of human extra-adrenal chromaffin tissue after birth.

Specific adrenaline- and noradrenaline-storage cells and granules have been identified in the adrenal glands of adult man, cat, mouse, bovine and rat. In man, cat, mouse and rat groups of noradrenaline-storing chromaffin cells form islands which are scattered throughout the adrenal medulla and may have some specific relation to blood vessels (Coupland, 1965a). In bovines, sheep and pigs (Coupland, 1965a) adrenaline-storing cells lie mainly in the periphery of the adrenal medulla and are closely associated with venous sinuses draining from the adjacent cortex. In the hamster noradrenaline-storing cells are peripherally distributed (Eränkö, 1955).

Evidence for the presence of amine-storing cells in the superior cervical ganglion of the adult albino rat has been presented by Siegrist et al. (1966), Grillo (1966), Williams (1967a and b), Elfvin (1968), and Matthews and Raisman (1969). Elfin (1968) has observed a similar cell in the inferior mesenteric ganglion of the rabbit.

The fate and function of extra-adrenal chromaffin cells are still subjects of debates. Electron microscopic evidence of degeneration of extra-adrenal chromaffin bodies in the newborn mouse has been presented by Virágh and Korényi Both (1967). These changes are in keeping with previous findings (Coupland, 1960, 1965a) in work using the light microscope. In all mammals so far examined there appears to be a reduction in number of extra-adrenal chromaffin cells during the post-natal phase, though substantial collections persist up to adult life in the guinea-pig, and rabbit, and until late childhood in man. In the rat the early and near complete disappearance of the main abdominal para-aortic chromaffin body, which normally occurs during the first week after birth, may be prevented by the daily administration of adreno-cortical hormone (Lempinen, 1964).

3. The Carotid Body

The chromaffinity of the carotid body was reported by Stilling (1892). Although commonly classified as a para-ganglion, no agreement has been reached regarding the chromaffin nature of the cells comprising this structure. This subject has been reviewed by Adams (1958) and Coupland (1965a). The chief or glomus type I cells are polygonal, arranged in cords or lobules and may be either non-chromaffin or chromaffin in staining reaction. Other cells are more irregular in form and considered to be supporting (sustentacular or glomus type II) cells. Sympathetic and parasympathetic nerve fibres innervate this organ. Silver staining allows the chief cells to be designated argyrophil and non-argyrophil.

Histochemical reactions for catecholamines, including the iodate reaction (Hillarp and Hökfelt, 1953) and the fluorescent reaction of Falck et al. (1962) have been applied by Muratori and Battaglia (1960a and b), Muratori (1962a), Muratori et al. (1965), and Muratori et al. (1966) to cervico-thoracic paraganglia, including carotid and aortic bodies of cat, chick, rabbit, cow and pig. The authors claimed to have demonstrated the presence of noradrenaline in individual glomus cells, but unfortunately amine assays were not performed. Electron microscopic evidence for the presence of primary aromatic amines (interpreted as being noradrenaline) in cells of the carotid body of the rat and newborn cat was presented by Battaglia (1966), and Muratori et al. (1965).

Other workers have shown that the histochemically reactive amines of the carotid body are not always noradrenaline. Thus, Chiocchio et al. (1966) histochemically identified the presence of primary aromatic amine in the carotid body of the cat, and showed by assay that *c* 60% of this was dopamine with some 35% noradrenaline. The presence of 5-hydroxytryptamine in the human carotid body has been demonstrated by Hamberger et al. (1966) using fluorescent microspectrophotometry. According to Dearnaley et al. (1968) assay reveals that dopamine is present in the carotid body of the rabbit, but in the calf only noradrenaline was identified by Muscholl et al. (1960).

The fine structure and organisation of the carotid bodies of cat and rabbit (Garner and Duncan, 1958), rat (Hoffman and Birrell, 1958; Lever et al., 1959; Biscoe and Stehbens, 1967), horse and dog (Höglund, 1967) and dog (Kobayashi, 1968) have been determined. From these works it would appear that under normal conditions the chief cells contain variable numbers of membrane-bound inclusion granules which are either highly or moderately electron dense, and that the less well granulated cells may also contain membrane-bound cytoplasmic vacuoles. Kobayashi (1968) noted that chromaffin cells were similar to non-chromaffin elements so far as nuclear appearance was concerned, but that they differed from each other in relative concentration of granules and electron density of granules; chromaffin cells had granules of high electron density and homogeneous appearance up to 0.3 μ diameter, while non-chromaffin cells contained fewer granules 0.1—0.2 μ diameter which were only moderately electron dense. It is possible, therefore that the two types of chief cells may synthesize and store different amines. Electron microscopic evidence of what appears to be exocytosis with discharge of granule contents from glomus cells has been presented by Kobayashi (1968).

Chromaffin and non-chromaffin glomus type I cells are separated from blood by capillary endothelium, pericytes, pericapillary space with connective tissue fibres and cell processes and sustentacular cells, and the latter elements largely exclude them from contact with connective tissue spaces. From the illustrations of Biscoe and Stehbens (1967) the supporting (sustentacular, glomus type II) cells bear at least a superficial resemblance to the Schwann cells of the adrenal medulla (Coupland, 1965b and c), and abdominal para-aortic bodies (Coupland and Weakley, 1970), which embrace chromaffin cells with slender processes.

Synaptic nerve endings have been observed on both chromaffin and non-chromaffin chief cells (Kobayashi, 1968) and some resemble the cholinergic endings on the cells of the adrenal medulla illustrated by Coupland (1965c). The similarity in form of endings on chromaffin cells in the two situations suggests the possibility of a similar, i.e. efferent, function, and this conclusion is supported by morphological and electrophysiological findings of Biscoe et al. (1970) following nerve sections which provided evidence of efferent ending on type I cells. The place of origin or ending of afferent nerve fibres (see Biscoe et al., 1967, Biscoe and SAMPSON, 1967) is still unknown. No definite changes have been observed in the glomus cells following section of either the glosso-pharyngeal or sympathetic nerve fibres to the body, though evidence of degeneration of nerve fibres was obtained. According to HOFFMAN and BIRELL (1958) the osmophilic granules of glomus type I cells are reduced in number in conditions of anoxia. According to WOODS (1967) glomus type I cells of the rabbit have higher cytochrome oxidase and carbonic anhydrase than the type II (sustentacular) cells, while the latter contain more monoamine oxidase. The carotid body receives a sympathetic innervation; some of these nerve fibres are destined for blood vessels (BISCOE and PURVES, 1967a, b), but some are of importance in the response of the chemoreceptors to general stimuli such as limb movement. Efferent nerve fibres of intra-cranial origin pass through the sinus nerve (BISCOE et al., 1970), and modify the afferent discharge during hypoxia (NEIL and O'REGAN, 1969; SAMPSON and BISCOE, 1970), and so complete a feedback system.

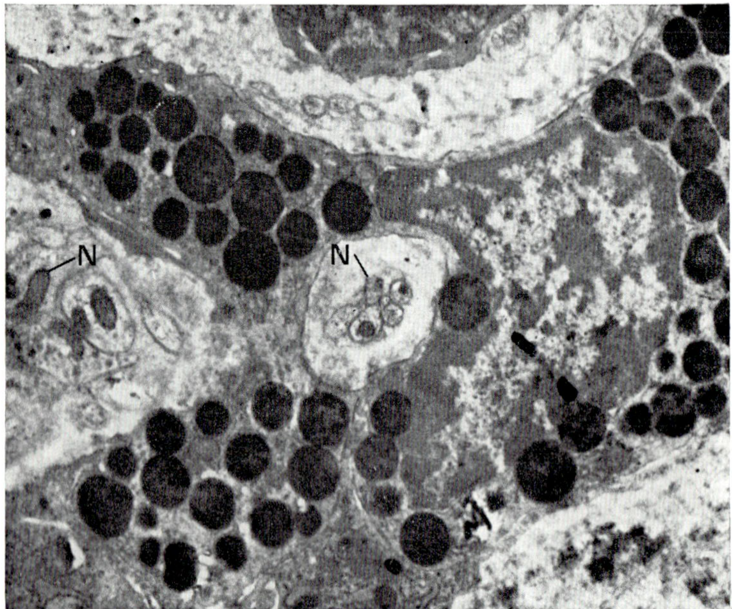

Fig. 4. Electron micrograph showing mast cell in submucosa of rat duodenum closely associated with nerve fibres (N). Fixed in glutaraldehyde/osmium tetroxide × 10,500

Collections of epithelioid cells which are structurally similar to those of the carotid body occur in the cervico-thoracic region adjacent to the main branches of aorta (PALKAMA and HOPSU, 1965), the pulmonary arteries, atria of the heart, and along cranial nerve, especially the glossopharyngeal. The subject has been reviewed by DE KOCH (1959), BOYD (1961), and MURATORI (1959, 1962b).

4. Peripheral Chromaffin Cells

No specific evidence has been adduced to support the claims of ADAMS-RAY and NORDENSTAM (1956) and BURCH and PHILLIPS (1958) for the existence of chromaffin cells in the periphery, i.e. adjacent to blood vessels in the limbs, including the dermis. All cells so described possess characteristics more typical of melanophores (ALLEGRA and MARCHESELLI, 1960) or mast cells than chromaffin cells (COUPLAND and HEATH, 1961a; COUPLAND, 1963; MATZ and SKINNER, 1962) and the fact that nerve fibres may lie close to such elements (NORDENSTAM and WESTER, 1964) in no way proves that they are chromaffin elements, since in the submucosa of the gut nerve fibres have been observed by the writer lying adjacent to or even passing through mast cells (Fig. 4). According to MÖLLER (1964) catecholamines disappear from the skin following reserpine treatment and sympathetic denervation, indicating a close connection of cutaneous noradrenaline with the sympathetic innervation of the skin.

There is no evidence to suggest that mast cells make a substantial contribution to peripheral synthesis or storage of noradrenaline, even though mouse and hamster mast cells are capable of taking up and storing a variety of exogenous amines (ERÄNKÖ and KAUKO, 1965), or taking up dopa and metabolising it as far as dopamine (DAY and GREEN, 1962; ADAMS-RAY et al., 1965). The occurrence of dopamine-containing mast cells in the gut and other viscera of ungulates (COUPLAND and HEATH, 1961b) is undisputed, however, but in view of the developmental origin, structure and lack of innervation, these elements are better considered to be mast cells which give a positive chromaffin reaction than chromaffin cells if the latter term is to have any real functional significance.

III. The Functional Anatomy of the Chromaffin Cell

Accounts of the fine structure of adrenal chromaffin cells include those of COUPLAND (1965a, b and c), and COUPLAND and WEAKLEY (1968, 1970) on rat and rabbit, YATES (1963, 1964) on hamster, ELFVIN (1967a and b) on rat, and FLETCHER (1964) on guinea-pig. The structure of the chromaffin cells of the human adrenal medulla has been considered by BENEDECZKY and LAPIS (1968) and YOKOYAMA and TAKAYASU (1969) in papers which also relate to phaeochromocytomas. A comparative survey of the ultra-structure of chromaffin cells of the suprarenal bodies of dogfish, and adrenal glands of frog, domestic fowl, mouse, cat, bovine and man has been published by the writer (COUPLAND, 1971). The following generalisations can now be made:

The typical feature of a chromaffin cells in all species is the presence of membrane-bound electron dense vesicles which, since the work of BLASCHKO and WELCH (1953), are known to store the majority of the cell complement of catecholamines. The use of assay techniques in association with fixation in glutaraldehyde followed by osmium tetroxide (COUPLAND and HOPWOOD, 1966; COUPLAND, 1971) allows one to classify chromaffin cells of adult forms of all species into types viz. adrenaline-storing and noradrenaline-storing cells. Under normal circumstances adult adrenal or suprarenal chromaffin cells may store either adrenaline or noradrenaline granules, but not mixtures of the two types. However, under experimental conditions (COUPLAND and MACDOUGALL, 1966) during foetal life and shortly after birth both adrenaline and noradrenaline granules may be observed within the same adrenal chromaffin cell (COUPLAND and WEAKLEY, 1968, 1970; ELFVIN, 1967a). In extra-adrenal chromaffin cells of the rabbit a few granules having the morphological characteristics of adrenaline-storing granules have been observed alongside many noradrenaline-storing granules in specific cells (COUPLAND and WEAKLEY, 1970), but the majority of chromaffin cells contain only noradrenaline-storing granules.

Adrenaline- and noradrenaline-storing chromaffin granules show species differences in relative sizes (Table I) and size alone is of little value in determining the amine-storage-type of a particular cell. Identification must therefore depend upon the use of appropriate electron histochemical techniques in conjunction with amine assay.

Table 1. *Average diameter of chromaffin granules (nm) in adrenaline (A) and noradrenaline (N) cells*

Dogfish		Frog		Domestic fowl		Rat		Cat		Man	
A	N	A	N	A	N	A	N	A	N	A	N
219	227	179	141	168	224	153	135	185	181	175	135

1. Structure of Chromaffin Granules

HILLARP (1959) showed that water comprises some 68.5% of the wet weight of bovine chromaffin granules, and that the dried form was made up of 35% protein, 22% lipid, 20% catecholamine and 15% ATP. The granule proteins have been categorized by the elegant work of the Blaschko group at the University of Oxford and their associates, and may be considered (see SMITH, 1968) to be comprised of two classes: first a group of enzymes (ATPase, cytochrome b-559 and dopamine-β-hydroxylase), and second, proteins without known enzymic activity. A large part of the protein complement (*c* 77%) is water soluble (HILLARP, 1958). The remainder may be structural protein. According to BLASCHKO et al. (1966) the main component of soluble protein (chromogranin A) has a molecular weight of about 75,000. A study of the amino acid composition of chromogranin A (SMITH and WINKLER, 1967) has revealed the presence of a number of polar amino acids with some 26% w/w being comprised of glutamic acid. Hence this soluble protein carries a high negative change, as does ATP and may be directly concerned in the binding of catecholamine.

Soluble protein including chromogranin A has been demonstrated in chromaffin granules in tissue sections using an immunohistochemical technique (HOPWOOD, 1968a). In cells fixed in glutaraldehyde the protein is denaturated and retained within the granule and is partly responsible for the image seen with the electron microscope. In the noradrenaline-storing granule catecholamine is also retained following precipitation (COUPLAND and HOPWOOD, 1966) and accounts for the high electron density and homogenous appearance of these structures, Adrenaline is, however, lost from adrenaline-storing granules and in its absence the precipitated binding substance appears finely granular and moderately electron dense. The loss of adrenaline and *in situ* precipitation of noradrenaline following glutaraldehyde fixation forms the basis of the differential fixation/staining reaction for the two types of granules (COUPLAND et al., 1964; TRAMEZZANI et al., 1964). The moderately electron dense finely granular image of the adrenaline-storing granule is probably produced mainly by denaturated protein, though since lipids have also been demonstrated biochemically (BLASCHKO et al., 1967; SMITH and WINKLER, 1967) and histochemically (HOPWOOD, 1968b) these may also be partly responsible. A characteristic feature of the granule lipid is its high molar ratio of cholesterol to lipid phosphorus, and the presence of substantial amounts of lysolecithin in the phospholipid fraction (WINKLER et al., 1967).

The basophilia of adrenaline-storing cells and eosinophilia of noradrenaline-storing cells (COUPLAND, 1965a) observed after fixation in buffered (pH 5.8—7) formaldehyde can now be explained in light of work on the chemical composition of chromaffin granules and the knowledge that aldehyde fixation results in precipitation or denaturation of protein, and (over the range pH 5.8—7.4) of primary catecholamine (Coupland and Hopwood, 1966; Hopwood, 1967a), while amine loss rather than precipitation occurs with ethanol. Thus in aldehyde fixed tissues basophilic dyes get ready access to the carboxyl groups of protein (Hopwood, 1967b) on the adrenaline-storing granules, but are at least partly prevented from binding to the protein of noradrenaline-storing granules by primary catecholamine precipitated *in situ*.

The contents of the amine depleted (due to fixation, dehydration, etc) adrenaline-storage granule usually fails to show evidence of a specific internal pattern. However, evidence of subunits and a three-dimensional pattern has been obtained on a number of occasions with partially depleted or disorganised noradrenaline-storing granules and very occasionally with adrenaline-storing granules in both sections of intact adrenal medullas and of isolated granule preparations (Coupland, 1971).

2. Cell Organelles

In addition to catecholamine-storing chromaffin granules, chromaffin cells contain a full spectrum of cytoplasmic organelles (Figs. 5, 6) including slightly elongated mitochondria with typical cristae, lysosomes, multivesicular bodies, Golgi membranes, centrioles, small amounts of rough endoplasmic reticulum and free ribosomes; microtubules and/or microfibrils also occur.

Adrenaline- and noradrenaline-storing cells differ from each other with respect to the pattern of distribution of cytoplasmic organelles and inclusions. Cytoplasmic organelles and inclusions are relatively uniformly scattered in adrenaline-storing cells while in noradrenaline-storing cells the centrosphere is larger and freer from organelles or inclusions other than the Golgi elements and centrioles (Figs. 5 and 6). Granular material may be identified in some Golgi cisternae and vesicles in both types of cell; some give a positive acid phosphatase reaction and reactive lysosomes are normally seen around the periphery of the Golgi region. Hence the Golgi complex is probably concerned with lysosome formation (Coupland et al., 1968, 1971). However, some of the Golgi zone granular material does not react for acid phosphatase. Instead in noradrenaline-storing cells it appears homogeneously highly electron dense after glutaraldehyde/osmium tetroxide fixation indicating the presence of primary amine (dopamine or noradrenaline). Thus some of the small granular aggregates are chromaffin granules. The primary amine has not been identified in the Golgi zone in adult adrenaline-storing cells, and hence in the absence of an acid phosphatase reaction it is difficult to decide which granular contents are lysosomal and which are chromaffin granules.

The close functional relationship between chromaffin granules and lysosomes similar to those observed by Smith and Farquhar (1966) in the mammotrophs of the anterior pituitary has not been observed in the mammalian adrenal medulla. However, elements with an appearance identical with typical chromaffin granules have been observed by the writer in the lysosome-like dark bodies of the domestic fowl (Fig. 3) and cytolysomes have been seen by Virágh and Korényi Both (1967) in the extra-adrenal chromaffin bodies of the mouse. These findings would suggest that in some species lysosomal activity and autophagic vacuole formation may be involved in the intracellular destruction of chromaffin granules.

In the developing chromaffin cell free ribosomes are very numerous and are often arranged in groups which may have a helical form or form rosettes (Coupland and Weakley, 1968, 1970). Concentric arrays of rough endoplasmic reticulum have been observed in the cells of newborn animals (Coupland and Weakley, 1970), but in older forms endoplasmic reticulum is usually either thinly and diffusely distributed throughout the cell or forms small stacks. Changes in endoplasmic reticulum and other organelles during cell secretion or synthesis have not been assessed quantitatively. Yates (1964), however, reported an increase in the amount of endoplasmic reticulum and of ribosomes after a single injection of reserpine in the hamster.

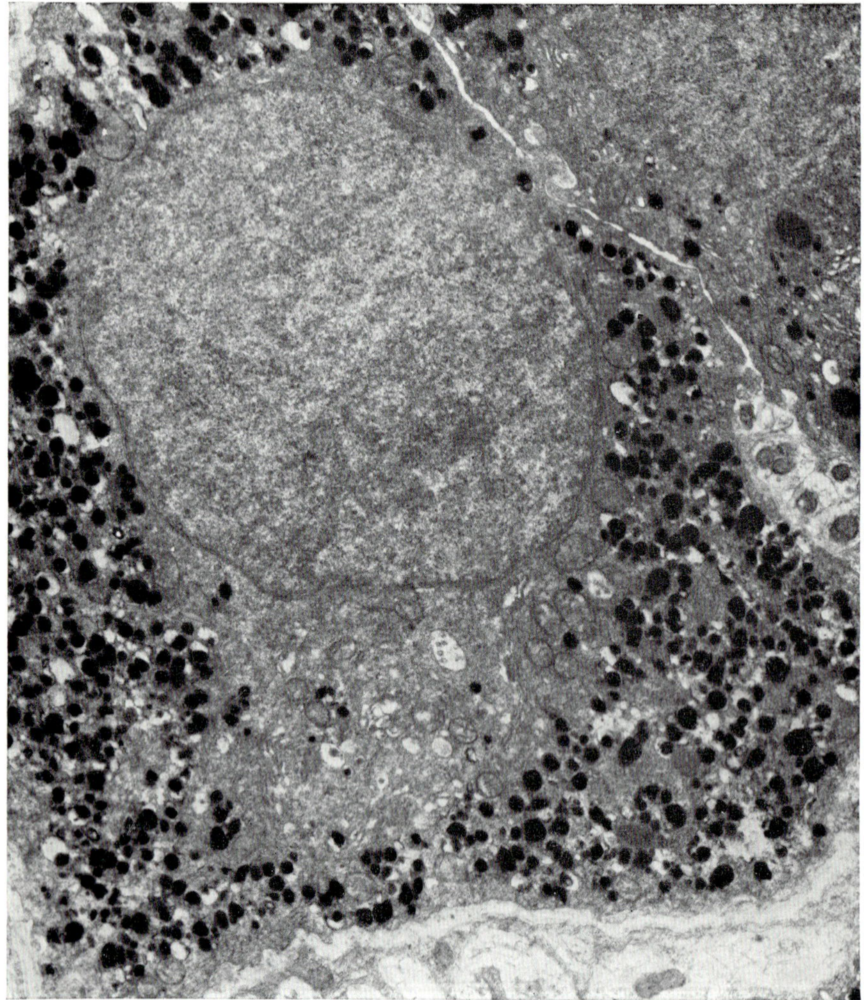

Fig. 5. Electron micrograph of noradrenaline-storing cell of rat adrenal medulla showing clearly defined Golgi zone and adjacent cytoplasm containing relatively few chromaffin granules. Glutaraldehyde/osmium tetroxide × 9,450

The plasma membrane of chromaffin cells typically show a unit membrane structure, with a width or 75—80 Å. Cells may be close packed with spaces of *c* 150—200 Å between plasma membranes, but larger intercellular spaces or canaliculi free from connective tissue elements, and sometimes containing cilia or bare nerve fibres, are often observed in regions where more than two cells lie in association with each other. These spaces are separated from the connective tissue elements and their associated tissue fluid by a distinct basement membrane which bridges the open end of the intercellular space (Fig. 8). Hence substances passing between the canaliculi and general connective tissue spaces must cross the bridging basement membrane. The plasma membranes of opposed chromaffin cells often show simple desmosomes characterised by a localised thickening and increase in density

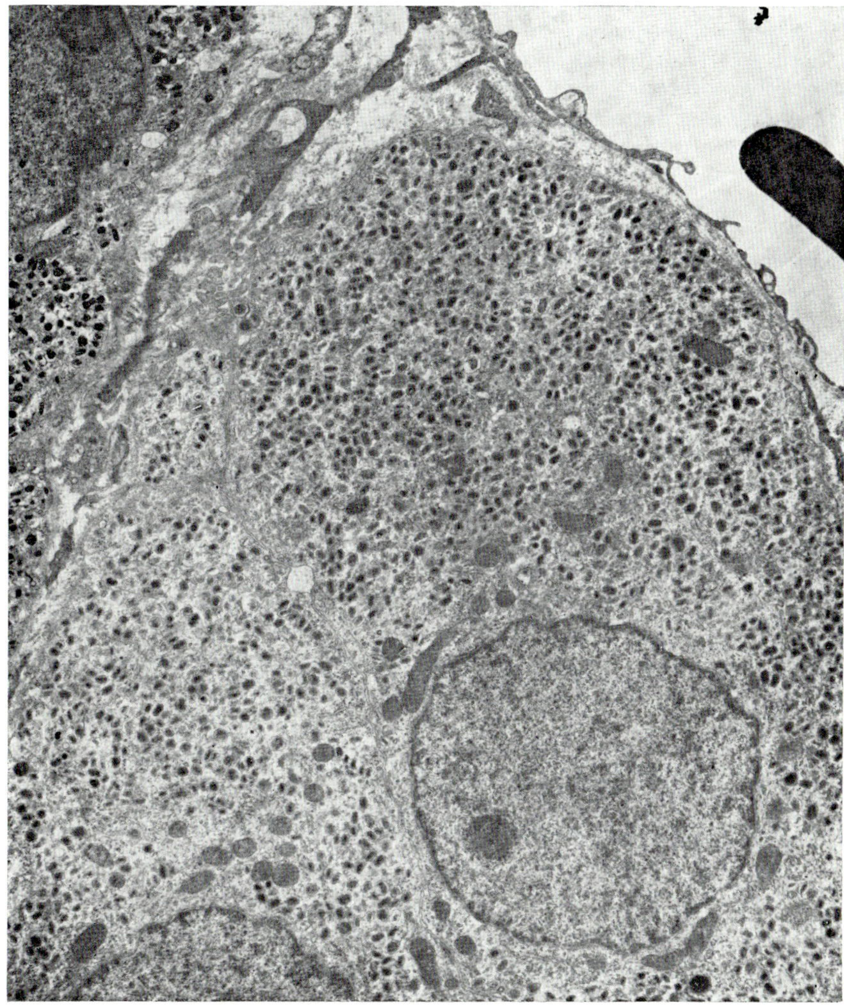

Fig. 6. Electron micrograph of adrenaline-storing cell of rat adrenal medulla showing relatively even distribution of cytoplasmic organelles and inclusions. Glutaraldehyde/osmium tetroxide × 4,050

of the layers of the plasma membranes. Tight junctions and typical maculae densa with cytoplasmic fibrils have not been observed in the rat (Coupland, 1965a), rabbit or human adrenal medulla. In the guinea-pig attachment of intracellular filaments to desmosome-like regions has been observed by Gorgas (1968).

Cilia are commonly observed arising from chromaffin cells and extend into intracellular canaliculi or tunnels formed by finger-like invaginations of plasma membrane, or into canalicular intercellular spaces. They often show an irregular arrangement of fibrils, and patterns varying between 6+2 to 9+2 have been observed, though the more central pair is often eccentric, and an 8+2 pattern has most often been noted (Coupland, 1965a; Coupland and Weakley, 1968, 1970). As yet it has not been possible to ascribe a definite function to these structures, and it is possible that the 8+2 pattern represents the displacement of a peripheral fibril of a sensory cilium, or that they are rather atavistic motor cilia. This latter possibility must be seriously considered in view of the fact that 9+2 cilia have also been observed (Coupland and Weakley, 1970).

The nucleus of the mature chromaffin cell is relatively vesicular showing a moderate diffuse fine granularity and one to three nucleoli. In some cells granular nuclear material forms aggregates adjacent to the inner nuclear membrane with discontinuities in aggregates opposite nuclear pores. Mitotic figures are not uncommonly seen in developing chromaffin cells during foetal life (Jackson, 1919; Mitchell, 1948; Coupland and Weakley, 1968), and have been observed in neo-natal tissue *in vitro* (Coupland and MacDougall, 1966). They have been observed in well granulated cells as well as in ones in which granules are sparsely distributed. They are, however, rare in specimens from normal adult animals. Evidence of mitotic activity in chromaffin cells of year-old Italian and Wistar rats has been provided by Malvadi et al. (1968) following colchicine injection. The number in a whole adrenal medulla dropped from between 12 and 16 at 60—80 days to 6 or 7 in a 350-day old animal. Highest mitotic activity was observed at noon. Degenerative changes are rarely observed within the cells of the normal adrenal medulla, but these changes are not uncommon in extra-adrenal chromaffin cells of 5—10-day old mice (Virágh and Korényi Both, 1967) at a time when the main pre-aortic chromaffin body (Coupland, 1960) is breaking up. Degenerating cells have not been observed within the equivalent body in the rabbit (Coupland and Weakley, 1970), but the latter persists until old age. The degenerative changes observed in the extra-adrenal chromaffin cells of the mouse, coupled with the presence of autophagic vacuoles containing secretion granules in otherwise intact cells, reflect cessation of secretory activity followed, in some cases, by cell death.

3. Formation of Chromaffin Granules

Electron microscopic evidence for the presence of small chromaffin granules within the Golgi membranes has been presented by Yates (1963), Coupland (1965a), Elfvin (1967a) and Coupland and Weakley (1968, 1970). In noradrenaline-storing cells, after glutaraldehyde-osmium tetroxide fixation, small collections of highly electron dense granular material, indicative of the presence of primary amine, have been observed within Golgi zone vesicles in both foetal and post-natal specimens (Coupland, 1965a; Coupland and Weakley, 1968, 1970). In adrenaline-storing cells similar granular material fails to give electron histochemical reactions for noradrenaline. These findings suggest that in the normal rabbit, where excessive depletion of the amine content of the chromaffin cells has not been induced by drugs or other methods, the synthetic phases of catecholamine production are rapidly completed, and that virtually all amine stored in association with binding proteins is in the final form, i.e. noradrenaline or adrenaline according to the cell type. This situation does not apply to glands which have been intensely stimulated, e.g. in the case of the cat adrenal following depletion by acetylcholine (Butterworth and Mann, 1957), and rat following reserpine induced depletion (Callingham and Mann, 1958; Coupland, 1959). In these cases following near total depletion of the glands noradrenaline reaches a normal or higher than normal concentration more rapidly than adrenaline, and the normal proportion of two amines was not realised until some 3 weeks after the initial depletion. Small chromaffin granules are not restricted to the Golgi membranes, however, and so it is possible that, as suggested by RATZENHOFER and MÜLLER (1967) a ubiquitous formation of chromaffin granules from endoplasmic reticulum occurs.

Chromaffin granules of different sizes appear to be randomly arranged throughout the cell and no evidence of zonation with respect to size (and hence presumably maturity) has been obtained (COUPLAND, 1971). Hence, there is no evidence to suggest that once granules leave the Golgi zone, or the endoplasmic reticulum if the Golgi region is bypassed, they move towards the cell surface and reach an optimum size prior to discharge of contents. One assumes that in a population of granules size and age are directly related. Histograms showing size distribution of granules show a deviation to the left of mean (COUPLAND, 1970) indicating that relatively few granules reach old age. Hence, the majority must be discharged or otherwise disappear after a relatively short life span.

4. Adrenaline-Noradrenaline Storage

Although both adrenaline and noradrenaline may be stored in separate granules within the same chromaffin cell during foetal and early post-natal life (COUPLAND and WEAKLEY, 1968, 1970; ELFVIN, 1967a) mixtures of adrenaline- and noradrenaline-storing granules are not normally seen in adult specimens of dogfish suprarenal bodies or in the adrenal chromaffin cells of frog, domestic fowl, rat, rabbit, cat, bovine or man (COUPLAND, 1971). Some of the predominantly noradrenaline-storing cells of the extra-adrenal chromaffin tissue of the adult rabbit do, however, appear to contain mixtures of the two amines (COUPLAND and WEAKLEY, 1970).

Injections of tritiated dihydroxyphenylalanine (dopa; ELFVIN et al., 1966) result after only 30 min in a general labelling of chromaffin cells in regions rich in chromaffin granules. No selective labelling of the Golgi region occurred. This result is not unexpected, since tyrosine hydroxylation (LADURON and BELPAIRE, 1968) and dopamine production normally takes place in the cytosol (BLASCHKO et al., 1955), after which dopamine is taken up and β-hydroxylated within the large granule fraction by the dopamine β-hydroxylase (KIRSHNER, 1959). It would seem probable therefore that some of the small collections of granular material observed within the Golgi vesicles represents recently synthesized binding substance (in particular the proteins chromogranin) and dopamine β-hydroxylase, and that under normal circumstances, in common with the binding substance present in chromaffin granules elsewhere in the cell, chromogranins take up catecholamine from the adjacent cytosol. Following injections of the tritiated dopa to normal mice and hamsters a more rapid turnover rate was observed by ELFVIN et al. (1966) in adrenaline-storing cells, though radioactivity persisted in both types of chromaffin cells for at least 1 week after injection.

5. Adrenaline versus Noradrenaline Storage

It is now known that the conversion of noradrenaline to adrenaline is controlled by the activity of a methylating enzyme, phenylethanolamine-N-methyl transferase (PNMT) which is located within the cytosol (KIRSHNER and GOODALL, 1957). Work carried out independently and simultaneously in a number of centres has demonstrated the importance of local concentrations of corticosteroids in the control of methylation. Thus COUPLAND and MACDOUGALL (1966) demonstrated by both assay and electron histochemistry that the presence of high physiological concentrations of corticosterone induced adrenaline storage in organ cultures of extra-adrenal chromaffin cells which normally store only or predominantly noradrenaline. 11-deoxycorticosterone is without this effect (Coupland, 1968) hence the 11-oxy group is important in the inductive process. Lempinen (1964) showed that injections of cortisone or hydrocortisone to rats prevented the normal post-natal involution of extra-adrenal chromaffin tissue, and indeed caused it to increase in volume. 11-deoxycorticosterone was without effect, however, while ACTH prevented the disappearance of the cells but did not stimulate increase in volume. Subsequently, Lempinen (1966) and Eränkö et al. (1966) demonstrated by fluorescence microscopy and chromatography that injections of hydrocortisone into young rats, not only prevents involution, but results in the appearance of adrenaline in the extra-adrenal cells. Injection of hydrocortisone into neonatal rats increases both the adrenaline content of extra-adrenal chromaffin tissue and activity of PNMT (Roffi and Margolis, 1966). Injections of hydrocortisone and ACTH have similar effects on the amine content, and PNMT activity of adrenal glands of hypophysectomized foetal rabbits and rats (Roffi, 1968).

Administration of dexamethasone and ACTH was found by Wurtman and Axelrod (1966) to prevent the fall in adrenal PNMT activity following hypophysectomy: ACTH acting indirectly via the adrenal cortex. The effect was prevented by simultaneous treatment with actinomycin D or puromycin, indicating that the increase in enzyme activity consequent upon steroid administration involved protein synthesis, and that the steroid probably acts through its effect on RNA transcription. Aldosterone, testosterone propprionate and oestradiol valerate were without effect on PNMT activity as were gonadotrophins (Wurtman, 1966). Later Wurtman (1968) reported differences in the distribution, activity, physical properties and response to hypophysectomy of PNMT of frog and rat. Enzyme activity in the frog did not fall after hypophysection. Further support for the role of corticosteroids in PNMT induction and activity has been provided by Pohorecky and Rust (1968) using hypophysectomized rats, and Leach and Lipscomb (1969) working with intact animals. PNMT activity has been found to change within a few minutes or hours of hypophysectomy or the injection of steroids or ACTH, while adrenaline concentration changes over a period of days or weeks.

This recent work supports and extends previous morphological and biochemical observations (Coupland, 1953) which suggested that the presence of locally high concentrations of adrenocortical steroids in mammalian adrenal medullary vascular sinuses was responsible for the appearance of the secondary amine. The influence of steroids on methylation in lower forms has still to be determined though recent work carried out in this laboratory (Barber and Coupland, unpublished) suggests that PNMT activity does respond to changes in concentrations of corticosteroids providing physiological rather than pharmacological doses are used.

6. Discharge of Contents of Chromaffin Granules

In well fixed tissue chromaffin granules are only observed within the cytoplasm of chromaffin cells, and the majority show a peripheral membrane which is complete and has a typical unit membrane structure. A few granules do show a broken outer peripheral membrane which is considered by the writer to be an artefact of preparation since, following intense neurogenic stimulation of chromaffin cells by insulin hypoglycaemia or amine discharge induced by reserpine. The swollen chromaffin granules commonly exhibit various degrees of swelling, but still retain intact limiting membranes.

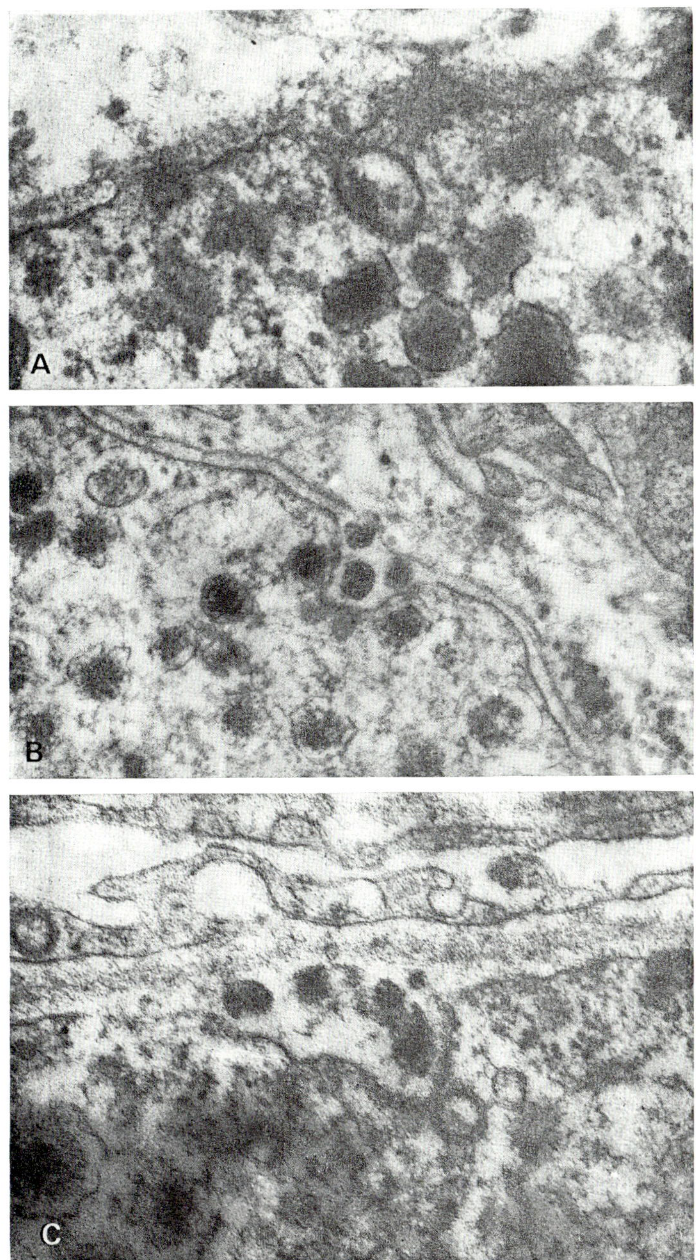

Fig. 7A—C. Electron micrographs of rat adrenal chromaffin cells fixed in osmium tetroxide showing possible sequence of events (A—C) during exocytosis of chromaffin granules. Note thinning of basement membrane over site of discharge and disintegration of contents as they escape. A and C × 72,000; B × 36,000

The mechanism of discharge has been debated for some years. Morphological observations (Coupland, 1965a and b; Diner, 1967) have demonstrated what appears to be the fusion of granule membranes with plasma membrane, and discharge of the contents of the granule into the surrounding tissue spaces or intercellular spaces (Fig. 7). These findings are in accord with biochemical evidence that during secretion induced by nerve stimulation, or by the application of a parasympathomimetic drug, granule amine, ATP and soluble protein are released in molar proportions similar to those existing in the intact granule, but that there is no loss of soluble components of the cytosol or of granule membranes during the discharge process (Banks and Helle, 1965; Schneider et al., 1967; Sage et al., 1967; Viveros et al., 1969).

It is, however, possible that some drugs capable of producing catecholamine depletion do so by other means, e.g. reserpine in low doses (Yates, 1963, 1964; Viveros et al., 1969) may affect the cells in a different way and without causing intracytoplasmic rupture of the membranes of chromaffin granules, may allow amine to diffuse across the cytoplasm and to pass through binding and transfer sites on the plasma membrane. In keeping with this suggestion Elfvin (1967b) noted a reduction in the density of the contents of chromaffin granules and the occurrence of small patches of electron dense material on the plasma membrane of adrenal medullary chromaffin cells following reserpinization of rats. Appearances suggestive of fusion of granule *contents* with plasma membranes have also been observed on occasions by the writer in normal rat adrenal glands. These observations, together with the report of Lever (1971) that the appearance of discontinuous limiting membranes on chromaffin granules may reflect secretory changes rather than preparation artefacts, justify caution in generalizing about the mechanism of amine secretion. Hence, it would seem reasonable to conclude that though exocytosis is almost certainly operative in the discharge process in some or many instances, other mechanisms, probably involving selective transport of the soluble contents of granules across the plasma membrane, may operate in certain circumstances.

IV. Innervation of Chromaffin Cells

1. Adrenal Medulla

The chromaffin cells are innervated by preganglionic sympathetic nerve fibres derived from neurons whose cell bodies lie between T3 and L3 (Tournade et al., 1925; Young, 1939; Maycock and Heslop, 1939; Kiss, 1951; Robinson and Monro, 1958; Coupland, 1965a). The preganglionic fibres pass mainly through the greater thoracic splanchnic nerves, but a few may run in the lower thoracic and upper two lumbar splanchnic nerves to reach the adrenal glands. Innervation in the cat is predominantly ipsilateral (Marley and Prout, 1968), and this state of affairs probably holds true for other forms.

Morphological evidence for the cholinergic nature of the nerve fibres and endings was initially based upon light microscopic evidence using the cholinesterase technique (Koelle, 1950; Coupland and Holmes, 1958), and structural evidence based upon the presence of non-granulated synaptic vesicles in nerve endings (Coupland, 1965b and c). More recently the cholinergic nature of the endings has been demonstrated by electron histochemistry (Lewis and Shute, 1969; Mastrolia and Coupland, unpublished).

In adult mammals nerve fibres form synaptic endings on chromaffin cells. At the zone of contiguity the opposed plasma membranes show regions of increased electron density, and the synaptic region may lie on the same plane as the remainder of the surface of the cell, or may lie in a depression or tunnel produced by invagination of the cell surface (Fig. 8). One or more endings may be observed on a single chromaffin cell, and a single nerve fibre has been observed making synaptic

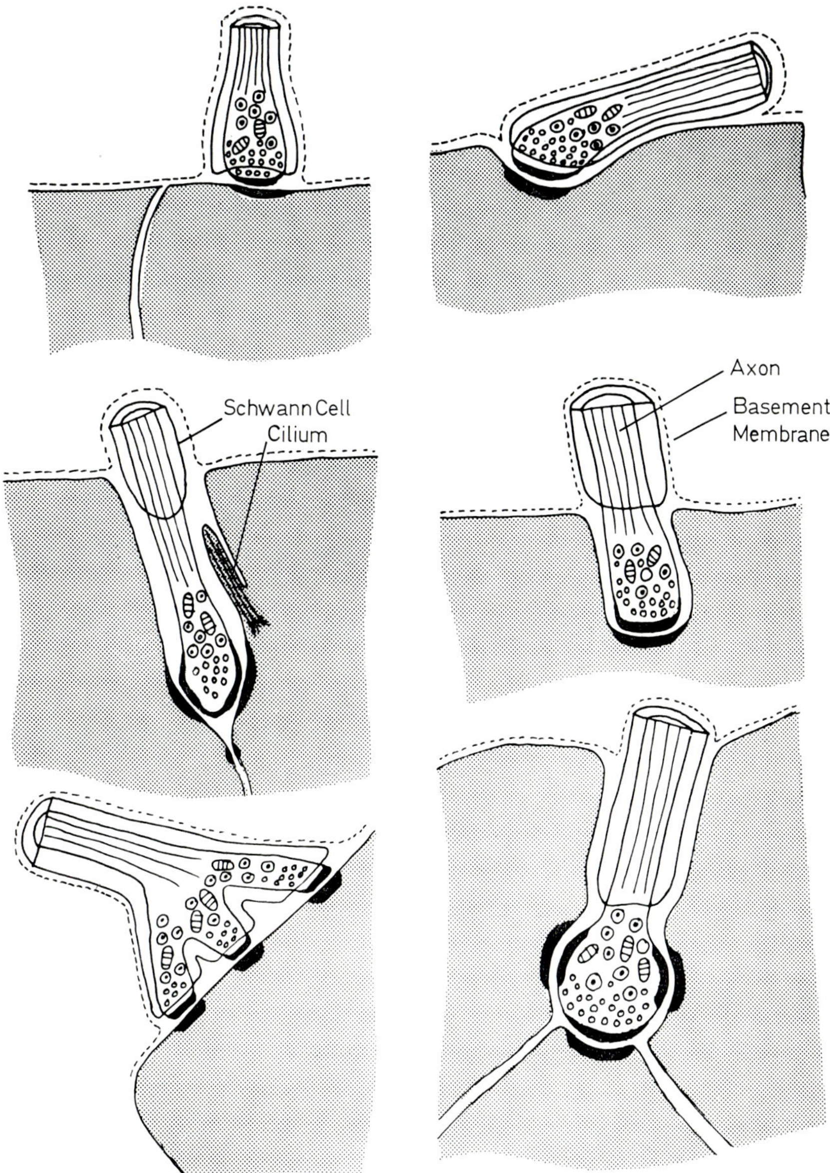

Fig. 8. Diagram illustrating the different forms of nerve endings observed by the writer in association with adrenal chromaffin cells

contact with up to three chromaffin cells (Coupland, 1965c). Some nerve fibres enter intercellular canaliculi before ending, and as they do so, the basement membrane of the Schwann cell associated with the nerve fibre fuses with that of the chromaffin cell or its satellite Schwann cell, and the Schwann cell covering of the axon terminates at, or shortly after, that point. Where nerve fibres are in close proximity to connective tissue elements and adjacent spaces they are always covered on the connective tissue aspect or aspects by Schwann cell cytoplasm and associated basement membrane.

Although nerve axons containing synaptic vesicles have been observed in contiguity with chromaffin cells during foetal life (COUPLAND and WEAKLEY,

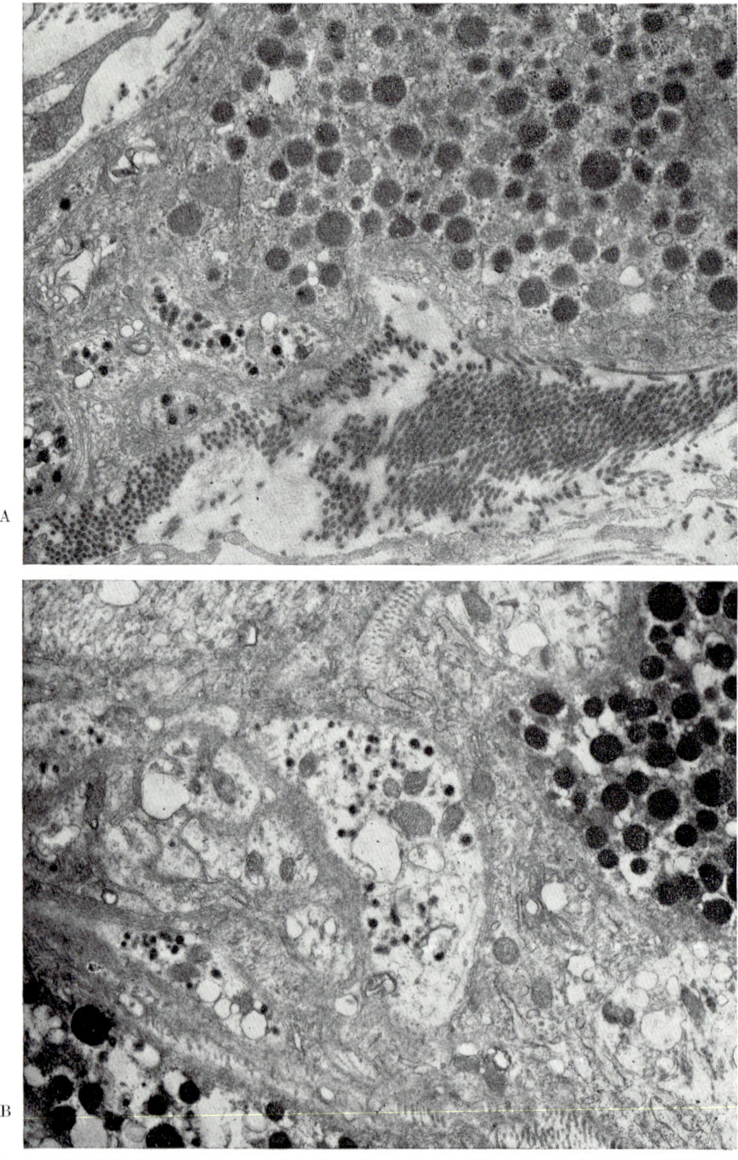

Fig. 9A and B. Electron micrographs showing nerve fibres containing vesicles with highly electron dense contents (primary amine) in close proximity to an adrenaline-storing cell (A) and a noradrenaline-storing cell (B) of dogfish suprarenal body. Glutaraldehyde/osmium tetroxide × 10,800

1968) typical thickenings of pre- and post-synaptic membranes are not usually observed before birth, though the typical complement of synaptic vesicles is observed in the endings during both foetal and post-natal life. Two types of synaptic vesicles may be recognised in cholinergic nerve endings associated with chromaffin cells (COUPLAND, 1965a and c; COUPLAND and WEAKLEY, 1968, 1970). The first type is found predominantly in the region of the synapse and after fixation in osmium tetroxide or glutaraldehyde takes the form of small rounded or slightly elongated vesicles *c* 40 nm in mean diameter and having electronlucent centres. After similar fixation the second type of vesicle is larger, average diameter 80—100 nm, and after the above fixatives possesses a core which exhibits a

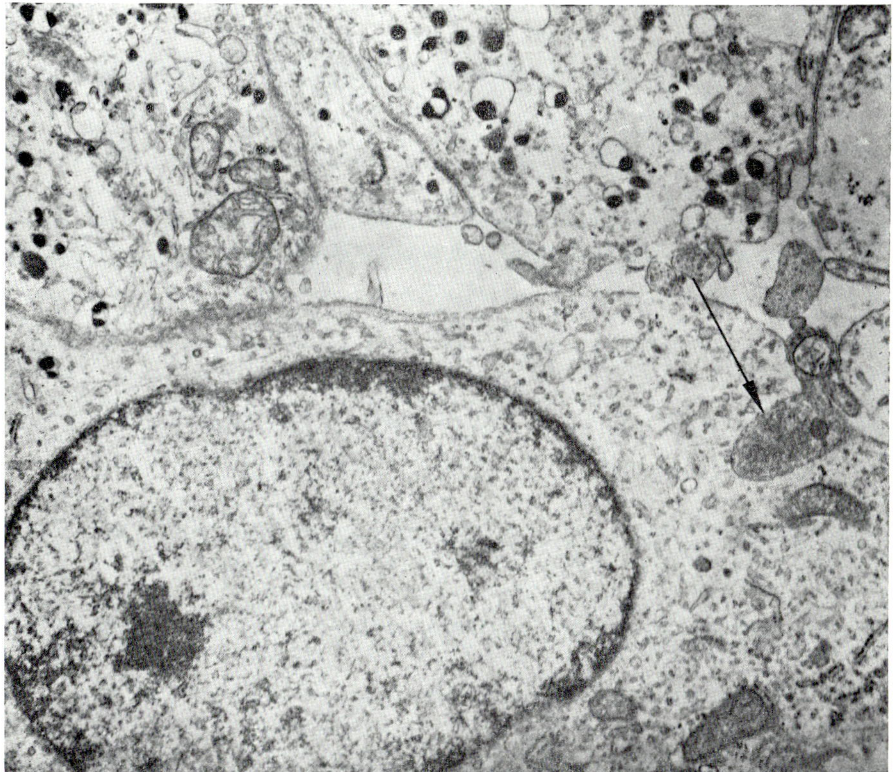

Fig. 10. Electron micrograph showing nerve ending (arrow) on an extra-adrenal chromaffin cell of a human foetus (three-months old). × Glutaraldehyde/osmium tetroxide × 15,000

fine moderately electron dense granularity. These larger granulated vesicles are most numerous in the pre-terminal part of the axon where they may outnumber the small vesicles. Only occasional granulated vesicles are observed in the synaptic region where the small vesicles preponderate. The functional significance of the large granulated vesicle is at present unknown, but there is no evidence to suggest that it represents a site of catecholamine storage. Similar large granulated vesicles in nerve endings in the brain do not respond to injections of reserpine in a fashion characteristic of amine storage granules (FUXE et al., 1965). The small electronlucent vesicles correspond to the elements isolated by DE ROBERTIS et al. (1963) and WHITTAKER et al. (1964) and considered to represent sites of storage of acetylcholine.

While noradrenaline-storing cells appear to be innervated in a relatively haphazardous fashion, adrenaline-storing cells often show distinct polarity with the venous pole of cells being free from nerve fibres and endings. According to LEWIS and SHUTE (1969) noradrenaline-storing cells are more richly innervated than adrenaline-storing cells, but this difference has not been observed by the writer.

The same pattern of innervation of chromaffin cells to that described above has been observed by the writer in the adrenal bodies of birds (domestic fowl), and amphibia (Fig. 2). Cholinergic nerve endings have not, however, been observed on chromaffin cells of suprarenal bodies of dogfish, though nerve fibres containing noradrenergic-type vesicles have been seen in close proximity to chromaffin cells (Fig. 9).

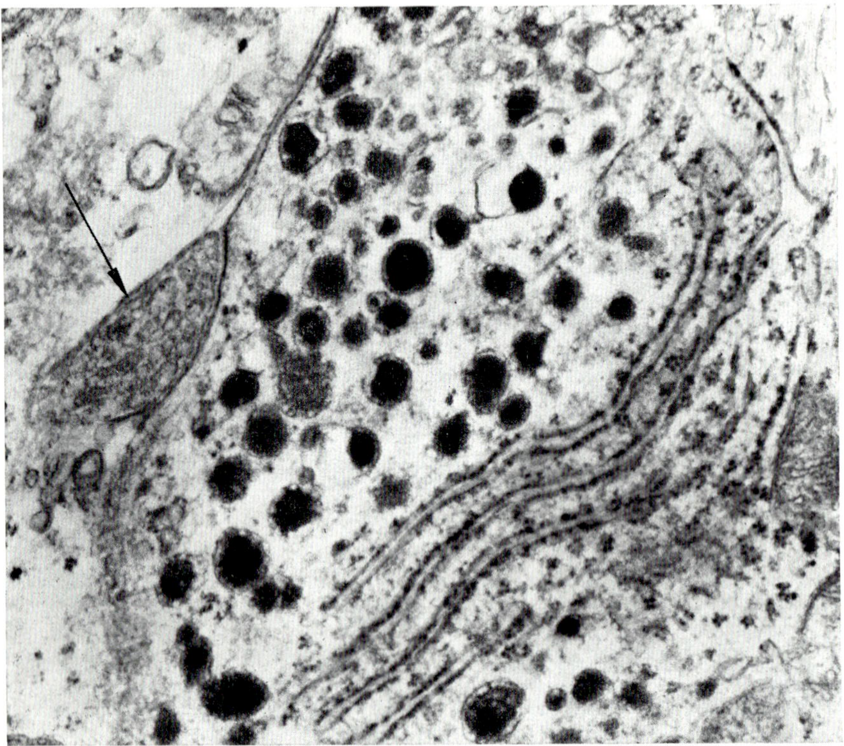

Fig. 11. Electron micrograph showing a nerve ending (arrow) on an extra-adrenal chromaffin cell of a three-month-old human foetus. Glutaraldehyde/osmium tetroxide × 40,000

2. Extra-Adrenal Chromaffin Cells

In spite of a careful search in many specimens few nerve fibres have been observed in intimate association with extra-adrenal chromaffin cells of the pre-aortic region, i.e. of the para-aortic bodies including organs of Zuckerkandl. The majority of nerve fibres associated with these structures are of large calibre and clearly in transit to other areas. Occasional small synaptic-type endings containing small electronlucent vesicles have been observed in human foetuses (Figs. 10 and 11). Only a few atypical endings were observed on chromaffin cells of the rabbit pre-aortic body (COUPLAND and WEAKLEY, 1968, 1970). Synaptic endings were not described by VIRÁGH and KORÉNYI BOTH (1967) on chromaffin cells of the mouse pre-aortic bodies. More recent work (COUPLAND and MASTROLIA, 1970, unpublished) using an electron histochemical technique for cholinesterase has revealed the presence of sparsely distributed cholinergic endings of fine nerve fibres on these cells in early post-natal rabbit specimens.

Typical cholinergic-type synapses have been observed, however, by SIEGRIST et al. (1966) on granulated cells of the superior cervical ganglion of the rat. More recently WILLIAMS (1967a, b) and MATTHEWS and RAISMAN (1969) observed both afferent cholinergic type endings, and what appeared to be efferent synapses on a different face of the granulated cells of the superior cervical ganglion of cat and rat. Hence, at least some of these granulated cells would appear to occupy the position of and possibly act as interneurons. However, the possibility that they may also secrete externally into the tissue spaces has not been excluded.

No evidence has been obtained which would suggest that the extra-adrenal chromaffin cells of the mammalian abdomen have the form or function of interneurons, and from their general morphological features a typical endocrine role would seem to be far more probable. It is, therefore, possible that some of the granulated cells observed in the superior cervical ganglion may be typical extra-adrenal chromaffin cells similar to those described previously in man and lower forms (COUPLAND, 1965a), while others, characterized by having smaller inclusions granules, and probably an insufficient concentration of amine to give a positive chromaffin reaction (though they would fluoresce after formaldehyde treatment) may be interneurons.

Current morphological (COUPLAND and WEAKLEY, 1968, 1970) and physiological/pharmacological (MUSCHOLL and VOGT, 1964) evidence suggests that the majority of these extra-adrenal chromaffin cells are only sparsely innervated and their function in homeostasis is currently unclear.

References

ADAMS, W. E.: The Comparative Morphology of the Carotid Body and Carotid Sinus. Springfield, Ill.: Charles C. Thomas 1958.

ADAMS-RAY, J., DAHLSTRÖM, A., FUXE, K., HÄGGENDAL, J.: Formation and storage of dopamine in hamster mast cells following administration of dopa. J. Pharm. Pharmacol. **17**, 252—253 (1965).

— NORDENSTAM, H.: Un système des cellules chromaffines dans la peau humaine. Lyon chir. **52**, 125—129 (1956).

ALLEGRA, F., MARCHESELLI, W.: Sulla presunta esistenza di un sistema di cellule chromaffini nelle cute umana. Minerva derm. **30**, 373—376 (1960).

BANISTER, R.J., PORTIG, P.J., VOGT, M.: The content and localization of catecholamines in the carotid labyrinths and aortic arches of *Rana temporaria*. J. Physiol. (Lond.) **192**, 529—535 (1967).

BANKS, P., HELLE, K.: The release of protein from the stimulated adrenal medulla. Biochem. J. **97**, 40—41 C (1965).

BATTAGLIA, G.: Osservazioni ultrastrutturali sul glomo carotideo del ratto. Boll. Soc. ital. Biol. sper. **152**, 1581—1584 (1966).

BENEDECZKY, I., LAPIS, K.: Vergleichende elektronen-mikroskopische Untersuchungen am Nebennierenmark und Phäochromocytom des Menschen. Beitr. path. Anat. **137**, 403—438 (1968).

BISCOE, T.J., LALL, A., SAMPSON, S.R.: Electron microscopic and electrophysiological studies on the carotid body following intracranial section of the glossopharyngeal nerve. J. Physiol. (Lond.) **208**, 133—152 (1970).

— PURVES, M.J.: Observations on carotid body chemoreceptor activity cervical sympathetic discharge in the cat. J. Physiol. (Lond.) **190**, 413—424 (1967a).

— — Factors affecting the cat carotid chemoreceptor and cervical sympathetic activity with special reference to passive hind-limb movements. J. Physiol. (Lond.) **190**, 425—441 (1967b).

BISCOE, T.J., SAMPSON, S.R.: Spontaneous activity recorded from the cut central end of the carotid sinus nerve of the cat. Nature (Lond.) **216**, 294 (1967).
— — PURVES, M.J.: Stimulus response curves of single carotid body chemoreceptor afferent fibres. Nature (Lond.) **215**, 654—655 (1967).
— STEHBENS, W.E.: Ultrastructure of the denervated carotid body. Quart. J. exp. Physiol. **52**, 31—36 (1967).
BLASCHKO, H., FIREMARK, H., SMITH, A.D., WINKLER, H.: Lipids of the adrenal medulla. Lysolecithin, a characteristic constituent of chromaffin granules. Biochem. J. **104**, 545 to 549 (1967).
— HAGEN, P., WELCH, A.D.: Observations on the intracellular granules of the adrenal medulla J. Physiol. (Lond.) **129**, 27—49 (1955).
— SMITH, A.D., WINKLER, H.: Untersuchungen an Eiweißfraktionen der chromaffinen Granula. Naunyn-Schmiedeberg's Arch. exp. Path. Pharmak. **253**, 23 (1966).
— WELCH, A.D.: Localization of adrenaline in cytoplasmic particles of the bovine adrenal medulla. Naunyn-Schmiedeberg's Arch. exp. Path. Pharmak. **219**, 17—22 (1953).
BLOOM, F.E., BARRNETT, R.J.: Fine structural localization of noradrenaline in vesicles of autonomic nerve endings. Nature (Lond.) **210**, 599—601 (1966).
BLOOM, G., ÖSTLUND, E., EULER, U.S. v.: A specific granular secretory cell in the heart of cyclostomes. Mem. Soc. Endocr. **12**, 255—263 (1962).
— — — LISHAJKO, F., RITZÉN, M., ADAMS-RAY, J.: Studies on catecholamine-containing granules of specific cells in cyclostome hearts. Acta physiol. scand. **53**, Suppl. 185 (1961).
— — FÄNGE, R.: Functional aspects of cyclostome hearts in relation to recent structural findings: The Biology of Myxine. Eds. A. Brodal and R. Fänge, pp. 340—351. Oslo: Universitetsforlaget 1963.
BOYD, J.D.: The inferior aortico-pulmonary glomus. Brit. med. Bull. **17**, 127—131 (1961).
BRUNDIN, T.: Catecholamines in adrenals from fetal rabbits. Acta physiol. scand. **63**, 509 to 510 (1965).
BURCH, G.E., PHILLIPS, J.H.: Chromaffin reacting cells in human digital skin. Circulat. Res. **6**, 416—423 (1958).
BUTTERWORTH, K.R., MANN, M.: The adrenaline and noradrenaline content of the adrenal gland of the cat following depletion by acetylcholine. Brit. J. Pharmacol. **12**, 415—421 (1957).
CALLINGHAM, B.A., MANN, M.: Adrenaline and noradrenaline content of the adrenal gland of the rat following depletion with reserpine. Nature (Lond.) **181**, 423—424 (1958).
CASPERSSON, T., HILLARP, N.-Å., RITZÉN, M.: Fluorescence microspectrophotometry of cellular catecholamines and 5-hydroxytryptamine. Exp. Cell Res. **42**, 415—428 (1966).
CHIOCCHIO, S.R., BISCARDI, A.M., TRAMEZZANI, J.H.: Catecholamines in the carotid body of the cat. Nature (Lond.) **212**, 834—835 (1966).
COUPLAND, R.E.: On the morphology and adrenaline-noradrenaline content of chromaffin tissue. J. Endocr. **9**, 194—203 (1953).
— Observations on the chromaffin reaction. J. Anat. (Lond.) **88**, 142—151 (1954).
— The effects of insulin, reserpine and choline 2:6-xylylether bromide on the adrenal medulla and on medullary autografts in the rat. J. Endocr. **17**, 191—196 (1958).
— The catecholamine content of the adrenal medulla of the rat following reserpine-induced depletion. J. Endocr. **18**, 154—161 (1959).
— Post-natal distribution of the abdominal chromaffin tissue in the guinea-pig, mouse and white rat. J. Anat. (Lond.) **94**, 244—256 (1960).
— Mast cells and chromaffin cells. Ann. N.Y. Acad. Sci. **103**, 139—150 (1963).
— The Natural History of the Chromaffin Cell. London: Longmans 1965a.
— Electron microscopic observations on the structure of the rat adrenal medulla. I. The Ultrastructure and organization of chromaffin cells in the normal rat adrenal medulla. J. Anat. (Lond.) **99**, 231—254 (1965b).
— Electron microscopic observations on the structure of the rat adrenal medulla. II. Normal innervation. J. Anat. (Lond.) **99**, 255—272 (1965c).
— Corticosterone and methylation of noradrenaline by extra-adrenal chromaffin tissue. J. Endocr. **41**, 487—490 (1968).
— Observations on the form and size distribution of chromaffin granules and on the identity of adrenaline- and noradrenaline-storing chromaffin cells in vertebrates and man. Mem. Soc. Endocr. **19**, 611—635 (1971).
— HEATH, I.D.: Chromaffin cells, mast cells and melanin. I. The granular cells of the skin. J. Endocr. **22**, 59—69 (1961a).
— — Chromaffin cells, mast cells and melanin. II. The chromaffin cells of the liver capsule and gut in ingulates. J. Endocr. **22**, 71—76 (1961b).
— HOLMES, R.L.: The distribution of cholinesterase in the adrenal glands of the rat, cat and rabbit. J. Physiol. (Lond.) **141**, 97—106 (1958).

Coupland, R. E., Hopwood, D.: The mechanism of the differential staining reaction for adrenaline- and noradrenaline-storage granules in tissues fixed in glutaraldehyde. J. Anat. (Lond.) **100**, 227—243 (1966).

— Macdougall, J. D.: Adrenaline formation in noradrenaline-storing chromaffin cells *in vitro* induced by corticosterone. J. Endocr. **36**, 317—324 (1966).

— Mastrolia, L., Weakley, B. S.: Different localization of lysosomal enzymes in adrenaline- and noradrenaline-storing cells of rat adrenal medulla. J. Anat. (Lond.)**103**, 582 (1968).

— — — Localization of acid phosphatase in the adrenal medulla of the albino rat. In: Histochemistry of Nervous Transmission, ed. O. Eränkö. Amsterdam: Elsevier 1971 (in press).

— Pyper, A. S., Hopwood, D.: A method of differentiating between noradrenaline- and adrenaline-storing cells in the light and electron microscope. Nature (Lond.) **201**, 1240 to 1242 (1964).

— Weakley, B. S.: Developing chromaffin tissue in the rabbit: an electron microscopic study. J. Anat. (Lond.) **102**, 425—455 (1968).

— — Electron microscopic observations on the adrenal medulla and extra-adrenal chromaffin tissue of the postnatal rabbit. J. Anat. (Lond.) **106**, 213—231 (1970).

Dahl, E., Falck, B., Lindqvist, M., Mecklenburg, C. v.: Monoamines in mollusc neurons. Kungl. Fysiog. Säll. Lund. **32**, 89—91 (1962).

Day, M., Green, J. P.: The uptake of amino acids and the synthesis of amines by neoplastic mast cells in culture. J. Physiol. (Lond.) **164**, 210—226 (1962).

Dearnaley, D. P., Fillenz, M., Woods, R. I.: The identification of dopamine in the carotid body of the rabbit. In: Arterial chemoreceptors, ed. R. W. Torrance, pp. 189—192. Oxford-Edinburgh: Blackwell 1968.

DeKoch, L. L.: The carotid body system of the higher vertebrates. Acta anat. (Basel) **37**, 265—279 (1959).

DeRobertis, E., De Lores Arnaiz, R. G., Salganicoff, L., De Iraldi, P. A., Zieher, L. M.: Isolation of synaptic vesicles and structural organization of the acetylcholine system within brain nerve endings. J. Neurochem. **10**, 225—235 (1963).

Diner, O.: L'expulsion des granules de la médullo-surrénale chez le hamster. C. R. Acad. Sci. (Paris) **265**, 616—619 (1967).

Elfvin, L.-G.: The development of the secretory granules in the rat adrenal medulla. J. Ultrastruct. Res. **17**, 45—62 (1967a).

— Effects of reserpine on the surface structure of chromaffin cells in the rat adrenal medulla. J. Ultrastruct. Res. **21**, 459—473 (1967b).

— A new granule containing nerve cell in the inferior mesenteric ganglion of the rabbit. J. Ultrastruct. Res. **22**, 37—44 (1968).

— Appelgren, L. E., Ullberg, S.: High resolution autoradiography of the adrenal medulla after injection of tritiated dihydroxyphenylalanine (dopa). J. Ultrastruct. Res. **14**, 277 to 293 (1966).

Eränkö, O.: Distribution of fluorescing islets, adrenaline and noradrenaline in the adrenal medulla of the hamster. Acta endocr. (Kbh.) **18**, 174—179 (1955).

— Kauko, L.: Uptake of monoamines by mesenteric mast cells of the mouse. Acta physiol. scand. **64**, 283—284 (1965).

— Lempinen, M., Räisänen, L.: Adrenaline and noradrenaline in the organ of Zuckerkandl and adrenals of newborn rats treated with hydrocortisone. Acta physiol. scand. **66**, 253 to 254 (1966).

Euler, U. S. v.: Presence of catecholamines in visceral organs of fish and invertebrates. Acta physiol. scand. **28**, 297—305 (1953).

— Fänge, R.: Catecholamines in nerves and organs of *Myxine glutinosa*, *Squalus acanthias* and *Gadus callarias*. Gen. comp. Endocr. **1**, 191—194 (1961).

— Gemzell, C. A., Ström, G., Westman, A.: Report of a case of phaeochromocytoma with special regard to preoperative diagnostic problems. Acta med. scand. **153**, 127—136 (1955).

— Hamberg, U.: Colorimetric determination of noradrenaline in the presence of adrenaline. Science **110**, 561 (1949).

— Ström, G.: Phaeochromocytoma. Present status of diagnosis and treatment of phaeochromocytoma. Circulation **15**, 5—13 (1957).

Falck, B., Hillarp, N.-Å., Thieme, G., Torp, A.: Fluorescence of catecholamines and related compounds condensed with formaldehyde. J. Histochem. Cytochem. **10**, 348—354 (1962).

Fletcher, J. R.: Light and electron microscopic studies of the effect of reserpine on the adrenal medulla of the guinea pig. Exp. Cell Res. **36**, 579—591 (1964).

Fuxe, E., Hökfelt, B., Nilsson, O.: A fluorescence and electron microscopic study on certain brain regions rich in monoamine terminals. Amer. J. Anat. **117**, 33—46 (1965).

Garner, C. M., Duncan, D.: Observations on the fine structure of the carotid body. Anat. Rec. **130**, 691—700 (1958).

Giacomini, E.: Contributo alla conoscenza delle capsule surrenali nei Ciclostomi. Sulle capsule surrenali dei Petromizonti. Monit. zool. ital. **13**, 143—162 (1902).

Gorgas, K.: Über Fibrillärstrukturen im Nebennierenmark von Haus- und Wildmeerschweinchen (Cavia aperea f. porcellus L. und Cavia aperea tschudii Fitzinger). Z. Zellforsch. **87**, 377—388 (1968).

Greenberg, R. E., Lind, J.: Catecholamines in tissues of the human fetus. Pediatrics **27**, 904—911 (1961).

Grillo, M. A.: Electron microscopy of sympathetic tissues. Pharmacol. Rev. **18**, 387—399 (1966).

Hamberger, B., Ritzén, M., Wersäll, J.: Demonstration of catecholamines and 5-hydroxytryptamine in the human carotid body. J. Pharmacol. Therap. **152**, 197—201 (1966).

Hillarp, N.-Å.: Isolation and some biochemical properties of the catecholaminegranules in the cow adrenal medulla. Acta physiol. scand. **43**, 82—96 (1958).

— Further observations on the state of the catecholamines stored in adrenal medullary granules. Acta physiol. scand. **47**, 271—279 (1959).

— Hökfelt, B.: Evidence of adrenaline and noradrenaline in separate adrenal medullary cells. Acta physiol. scand. **30**, 55—68 (1953).

Hoffman, H., Birrell, J. H. W.: The carotid body in normal and anoxic states: an electron microscopic study. Acta anat. (Basel) **32**, 297—311 (1958).

Höglund, R.: An ultrastructural study of the carotid body of horse and dog. Z. Zellforsch. **76**, 568 (1967).

Hopwood, D.: The effect of formaldehyde fixation and dehydration on ox adrenal medulla with respect to the chromaffin reaction and post-chroming. Histochemie **10**, 98—106 (1967a).

— Adrenal medullary basophilia in ox, pig and sheep. A histochemical, immunohistochemical and cell fractionation study. Histochemie **11**, 268—279 (1967b).

— An immunohistochemical study of the adrenal medulla of the ox. Histochemie **13**, 323 to 330 (1968a).

— A histochemical analysis of adrenal lipids in ox and sheep. Histochemie **14**, 270—281 (1968b).

Houssay, B., Wassermann, G. F., Tramezzani, J. H.: Formation et sécrétion differentielles d'adrénaline et de noradrénaline surrénales. Arch. int. Pharmacodyn. **140**, 84—91 (1962).

Hunter, R. B., Marshall, P. B., Oram, F. J.: Catechol amine excretion in normal persons and in cases of pheochromocytoma. Quart. J. exp. Med. **32**, 225—242 (1963).

Jackson, C. M.: The postnatal development of the suprarenal gland. Amer. J. Anat. **25**, 221—289 (1919).

Johnels, A. G., Palmgren, A.: "Chromaffin" cells in the heart of *Myxine glutinosa*. Acta zool. (Stockh.) **41**, 313—314 (1960).

Kirshner, N.: Biosynthesis of adrenaline and noradrenaline. Pharmacol. Rev. **11**, 350—357 (1959).

— Goodall, McC.: Formation of adrenaline from noradrenaline. Biochem. biophys. Acta (Amst.) **24**, 658—659 (1957).

Kiss, T.: Experimentell-morphologische Analyse der Nebenniereninnervation. Acta anat. (Basel) **13**, 81—89 (1951).

Kobayashi, S.: Fine structure of the carotid body of the dog. Arch. histol. jap. **30**, 95—120 (1968).

Kohn, A.: Über den Bau und die Entwicklung der sog. Carotisdrüse. Arch. mikr. Anat. **56**, 81—184 (1900).

— Das chromaffine Gewebe. Z. ges. Anat. 3, Ergebn. Anat. Entwickl.-Gesch. **12**, 253—348 (1902).

— Die Paraganglien. Arch. mikr. Anat. **62**, 263—365 (1903).

Koelle, G.: The histochemical differentiation of types of cholinesterase and their localization in tissues of the cat. J. Pharmacol. Therap. **100**, 158—179 (1950).

Laduron, P., Belpaire, F.: Tissue fractionation and catecholamines. II. Intracellular distribution patterns of tyrosine hydroxylase, dopa decarboxylase, dopamine-beta-hydroxylase, phenylethanolamine n-methyltransferase and monoamine oxidase in adrenal medulla Biochem. Pharmacol. **17**, 1127—1140 (1968).

Leach, C. S., Lipscomb, H. S.: Adrenal cortical control of adrenal medullary function. Proc. Soc. exp. Biol. (N.Y.) **130**, 448—451 (1969).

Lempinen, M.: Extra-adrenal chromaffin tissue of the rat and the effect of cortical hormones on it. Acta physiol. scand. **62**, Suppl. 231, 1—91 (1964).

— Effect of hydrocortisone on histochemically demonstrable catecholamines of the para-aortic body of the rat. Acta physiol. scand. **66**, 251—252 (1966).

LEVER, J.D.: In: Subcellular Organization and Function in Endocrine Tissues ed. H. Heller. Mem. Soc. Endocr. (in press).

— LEWIS, P.R., BOYD, J.D.: Observations on the fine structure and histochemistry of the carotid body in the cat and rabbit. J. Anat. (Lond.) **93**, 478—490 (1959).

LEWIS, P.R., SHUTE, C.C.D.: An electron microscopic study of cholinesterase distribution in the rat adrenal medulla. J. Microscopy **89**, 181—194 (1969).

MALVALDI, G., MENCACCI, P., VIOLA-MAGNI, M.P.: Mitoses in the adrenal medullary cells. Experientia (Basel) **24**, 475—476 (1968).

MARLEY, E., PROUT, G.I.: Innervation of the cat's adrenal medulla. J. Anat. (Lond.) **102**, 257—274 (1968).

MATZ, L.R., SKINNER, S.L.: Evidence against presence of chromaffin cells in human skin. Circulat. Res. **11**, 418—422 (1962).

MATTHEWS, M.R., RAISMAN, G.: The ultrastructure and somatic efferent synapses of small granule-containing cells in the superior cervical ganglion. J. Anat. (Lond.) **103**, 255—282 (1969).

MAYCOCK, W.D'A., HESLOP, T.S.: An experimental investigation of the nerve supply of the adrenal medulla of the cat. J. Anat. (Lond.) **73**, 551—558 (1939).

MITCHELL, R.M.: Histological changes and mitotic activity in rat adrenal during postnatal development. Anat. Rec. **101**, 161—185 (1948).

MÖLLER, H.: On catecholamines of the skin. Acta derm.-venereol. (Stockh.) **44**, Suppl. 55, 1—16 (1964).

MURATORI, G.: Istofisiologia comparata delle zone aortico-arteriose pressorecettive e degli annessi dispositive chemorecettori (paraganglio carotico, paraganglio succlario, paraganglio aortico-polmonare). Monit. zool. ital. **68**, Suppl. 17—84 (1959).

— Numero e topografia dei paragangli aortico-polmonari nel gatto e nel coniglio neonati. Boll. Soc. ital. Biol. sper. **38**, 50—53 (1962a).

— Histological observations on the cervico-thoracic paraganglia of amniotes. Arch. int. Pharmacodyn. **140**, 217—226 (1962b).

— BATTAGLIA, G.: Osservazioni sulla reazione iodaffine nel paraganglio carotico. Boll. Soc. ital. Biol. sper. **36**, 402—405 (1960a).

— — Sulla reazione iodaffine nei paraganglia aortico-abdominali e nei paragangli cervio-toracici del gatto. Boll. Soc. ital. Biol. sper. **36**, 1405—1408 (1960b).

— — MODONESI, G.: Dimonstrazione istochimica della noradrenalina nel cromaffine cervico-toracico e aortico-abdominale degli amnioti. II. Osservazioni al microscopio elettronico. Boll. Soc. ital. Biol. sper. **41**, 1185—1186 (1965).

— CHIARINI, C., BATTAGLIA, G.: Dimonstrazione delle catecolamine nel cromaffine cervico-toracico dei mammiferi mediante la microscopia a fluorescenza. Riv. istochim. **12**, 1—10 (1966).

MUSCHOLL, E., RAHN, K.-H., WATZKA, M.: Nachweis von Noradrenalin im Glomus caroticum. Naturwissenschaften **47**, 324 (1960).

— VOGT, M.: Secretory response of extramedullary chromaffin tissues. Brit. J. Pharmacol. **22**, 193—203 (1964).

NEIL, E., O'REGAN, R.G.: Effect of sinus and aortic nerve efferents on arterial chemoreceptor function. J. Physiol. (Lond.) **200**, 69P—70P (1969).

NORDENSTAM, H., WESTER, P.O.: Chromaffin granules in certain arteries. Acta med. scand. **176**, 633—637 (1964).

OLIVEREAU, M.: Mise en évidence d'adrénaline et de noradrénaline dans le tissu chromaffine d'un poisson sélacien la roussette. Ann. Endocr. (Paris) **20**, 645—653 (1959).

ÖSTLUND, E.: The distribution of catecholamines in lower animals and their effect on the heart. Acta physiol. scand. **31**, Suppl. 112, 1—67 (1954).

PALKAMA, A., HOPSU, V.K.: The presence of a carotid body like structure between the right subclavian and common carotid arteries. Ann. Med. exp. Fenn. **43**, 169—173 (1965).

PIEZZI, R.S.: Two types of chromaffin cells in the adrenal gland of the "Bufo arenarum" Hensel. Acta physiol. lat. -amer. **15**, 96—100 (1965).

— Two types of synapses in the chromaffin tissue of the toad's adrenal. Acta physiol. lat.-amer. **16**, 282—285 (1966).

POHORECKY, L., RUST, J.H.: Studies on the cortical control of the adrenal medulla in the rat. J. Pharmacol. Therap. **162**, 227—238 (1968).

RATZENHOFER, M., MÜLLER, O.: Ultrastructure of adrenal medulla of the prenatal rat. J. Embryol. exp. Morph. **18**, 13—25 (1967).

ROAF, H.E.: The situation in the mantle of *Purpura lapillus* of the cells which yield a pressor substance. Quart. J. exp. Physiol. **4**, 89—92 (1911).

— NIERENSTEIN, M.: The physiological action of the extract of the hypobranchial gland of *Purpura lapillus*. J. Physiol. (Lond.) **36**, V—VIIIP (1907).

Robinson, R., Monro, A. F.: Adrenal activity in subjects with complete transverse lesions of the spinal cord. Nature (Lond.) **182**, 805 (1958).

Roffi, J.: Dosage de l'adrénaline et de la noradrénaline dans les surrénales du foetus de lapin au cours de la gestation. J. Physiol. (Paris) **56**, 434—435 (1964).

— Influence des corticosurrénales sur la synthèse d'adrénaline chez le foetus et le nouveau-né de rat et de lapin. J. Physiol. (Paris) **60**, 455—494 (1968).

— Margolis, F.: Synthèse d'adrénaline dans le tissu chromaffine extra-surrénalien, chez le Rat nouveau-né, sous l'effet de l'hydrocortisone ou de la corticostimuline. C. R. Acad. Sci. (Paris) **263**, 1496—1499 (1966).

Sacarrão, G. F.: Quelques remarques sur les corps suprarénaux des sélaciens. Arq. Museu Bocage (2a serié) **1**, 1—9 (1966).

Sage, H. J., Smith, W. J., Kirshner, N.: Mechanism of secretion from the adrenal medulla. I. A microquantitative immunologic assay for bovine adrenal catecholamine storage vesicle protein and its application to studies of the secretory process. Molec. Pharmacol. **3**, 81—89 (1967).

Sampson, S. R., Biscoe, T. J.: Efferent control of the carotid body chemoreceptor. Experientia (Basel) **26**, 261—262 (1970).

Schneider, F. H., Smith, A. D., Winkler, H.: Secretion from the adrenal medulla: biochemical evidence for exocytosis. Brit. J. Pharmacol. **31**, 94—104 (1967).

Shepherd, D. M., West, G. B.: Differentiation of chromaffin cells. J. Pharm. Pharmacol. **5**, 216 (1952).

Siegrist, G., Ribaupierre, F. de, Dolivo, M., Rouiller, C.: Les cellules chromaffines des ganglions cervicaux supérieurs du rat. J. Microscopie **5**, 791—794 (1966).

Smith, A. D.: Biochemistry of adrenal chromaffin granules. In: The Interaction of Drugs and Subcellular Components on Animal Cells, pp. 239—292. Ed. by P. N. Campbell. London: Churchill 1968.

— Winkler, H.: Purification and properties of an acidic protein from chromaffin granules of bovine adrenal medulla. Biochem. J. **103**, 483—492 (1967).

Smith, R. E., Farquhar, M. G.: Lysosome function in the regulation of the secretory process in cells of the anterior pituitary gland. J. Cell Biol. **31**, 319—347 (1966).

Stilling, H.: Du ganglion intercarotidien. Inaug. Diss., Lausanne. Trav. Fac. Univ. Lausanne 321—331 (1892).

Tournade, A., Chabrol, M., Wagner, P.-E.: Le système nerveux adrénaline-sécréteur. C. R. Soc. Biol. (Paris) **93**, 933 (1925).

Tramezzani, J. H., Chiocchio, S., Wassermann, C. F.: A technique for light and electron microscopic identification of adrenaline- and noradrenaline-storing cells. J. Histochem. Cytochem. **12**, 890—899 (1964).

Udenfriend, S.: Aminoacids, amines and other metabolites. In: Fluorescence Assay in Biology and Medicine, pp. 144—151. London: Academic Press 1962.

Vincent, S.: The comparative histology of the suprarenal capsules. Int. Mschr. Anat. Physiol. **15**, 282—326 (1898).

Virágh, S., Korényi Both, A.: The fine structure of abdominal paraganglia in the newborn mouse. Acta Biol. Hung. **18**, 161—179 (1967).

Viveros, O. H., Arqueros, L., Kirshner, N.: Mechanism of secretion from the adrenal medulla. V. Retention of storage vesicle membranes following release of adrenaline. Molec. Pharmacol. **5**, 342—349 (1969).

Wassermann, G. F., Tramezzani, J. H.: Separate distribution of adrenaline- and noradrenaline-secreting cells in the adrenal of snakes. Gen. comp. Endocr. **3**, 480—489 (1963).

West, G. B., Shepherd, D. M., Hunter, R. B., Macgregor, A.: The function of the organs of Zuckerkandl. Clin. Sci. **12**, 317—325 (1953).

Whittaker, V. P., Michaelson, I. A., Kirkland, R. J. A.: The separation of synaptic vesicles from nerve-ending particles (synaptosomes). Biochem. J. **90**, 293—303 (1964).

Williams, T. D.: Electron microscopic evidence for an autonomic interneuron. Nature (Lond.) **214**, 309—310 (1967a).

— The question of the intraganglionic (connector) neuron of the autonomic nervous system. J. Anat. (Lond.) **101**, 603—604 (1967b).

Winkler, H., Strieder, N., Ziegler, E.: Über Lipide, insbesondere Lysolecithin, in den chromaffinen Granula verschiedener Species. Naunyn-Schmiedebergs Arch. Pharmak. exp. Path. Pharmak. **256**, 407—415 (1967).

Wood, J. G., Barrnett, R. J.: Histochemical demonstration of norepinephrine at a fine structural level. J. Histochem. Cytochem. **12**, 197—209 (1964).

Woods, R. I.: Distribution of cytochrome oxidase, monoamine oxidase and carbonic anhydrase in the carotid body of the rabbit. Nature (Lond.) **213**, 1240 (1967).

Wright, A., Jones, I. C.: Chromaffin tissue in the lizard adrenal gland. Nature (Lond.) **175**, 1001—1002 (1955).

WURTMAN, R.J.: Control of epinephrine synthesis in the adrenal medulla by the adrenal cortex: hormonal specificity and dose-response characteristics. J. Endocrinology **79**, 608—614 (1966).

— Species differences in inducibility of phenyl ethanolamine N-methyl transferase. Endocrinology **82**, 584—590 (1968).

— AXELROD, J.: Control of enzymatic synthesis of adrenaline in the adrenal medulla by adrenal cortical steroids. J. biol. Chem. **241**, 2301—2305 (1966).

YATES, R.D.: An electron microscopic study of the effects of reserpine on adreno-medullary cells of the Syrian hamster. Anat. Rec. **146**, 29—45 (1963).

— A light and electron microscopic study correlating the chromaffin reaction and granule ultrastructure in the adrenal medulla of the Syrian hamster. Anat. Rec. **149**, 237—249 (1964).

YOKOYAMA, M., TAKAYASU, H.: An electron microscopic study of the human adrenal medulla and phaeochromocytoma. Urol. int. (Basel) **24**, 79—95 (1969).

YOUNG, J.Z.: Partial degeneration of the nerve supply of the adrenal. A study in autonomic innervation. J. Anat. (Lond.) **73**, 540—550 (1939).

Chapter 3

Electron Microscopy of Catecholamine-Containing Structures

FLOYD E. BLOOM

With 17 Figures

I. Introduction

Interest in the fine structure of catecholamine containing cells has centered mainly upon the identification of the cellular organelles which store the catecholamines. This is a natural prerequisite since, with rare exceptions, there is no way to ascertain that the cells being examined do actually contain catecholamines without a documented specific cytochemical method. As a result, most reviews of the subject have quite properly emphasized approaches to the identification of cytochemically reactive tissue catecholamines (see BLOOM and GIARMAN, 1968; HÖKFELT, 1968a, b; TRANZER et al., 1969; BLOOM, 1970; JAIM-ETCHEVERRY and ZIEHER, 1970), with considerably less emphasis given to a description of the fine structural characteristics of these cells (GRILLO, 1966; HÖKFELT, 1969). Therefore, the present chapter will not only attempt to cover critical analysis of the currently available cytochemical methods for catecholamines, but also to highlight current concepts of the fine structure as well.

II. Identifying Catecholamine-Containing Cellular Organelles

Certain cells, such as the chromaffin cells of the adrenal medulla and the sympathetic ganglioneurons, must obviously contain catecholamines. If it were possible to study these cells as model systems for identifying the catecholamines, the methods could then be applied to those cells in the rest of the sympathetic and central nervous system in which catecholamine storage is much less certain. The first task, therefore, is to consider the approaches by which it is possible to make such identifications in tissue examined with the electron microscope.

1. Identification Criteria

The following criteria are useful considerations against which to evaluate the reliability of the cytochemical identification of noradrenaline, adrenaline or dopamine.

1. The electron stain selectively reacts with the desired substance *in vitro*.
2. The distribution of the reactive tissue sites agrees with light microscopic histochemical and cellular biochemical analyses. Thus, almost all quantitative ultrastructural evaluations of staining methods for monoamines are predicated upon the fluorescence histochemistry (see VAN ORDEN et al., 1966; FUXE et al., 1965, 1966; BLOOM and AGHAJANIAN, 1968a; HÖKFELT, 1968a, b; LEVER et al., 1968), and synaptic vesicle fraction analyses of nerve ending particles (see WHITTAKER, 1966).

3. The reactive sites should fluctuate in proportion to the amount of amine in the tissue when pharmacological depletion studies, loading studies, or catabolic inhibition cause fluctuations in the biochemically measurable levels.

4. The tissue elements reacting to the staining method should be confirmed by autoradiographic studies in which radioactive amine is physiologically introduced into the tissue pool of monoamine, and then serves as a separate marker for the sites binding the substance. This criterion has several subrequirements of its own, which must also be examined critically (see BLOOM, 1970).

5. Destruction of the nerve pathways which give rise to the monoamine-containing fibers should remove all the axons which gave a positive staining reaction. This criterion can be satisfied relatively easily for the peripheral nervous system, where the classical neuroanatomy is well established, although, in actual practice, it has not been regularly applied. In the central nervous system this criterion is difficult to apply since nerve tracts can not be selectively lesioned by surgical techniques; in this respect, the use of 6-hydroxydopamine (THOENEN and TRANZER, 1968) is quite relevant (BLOOM et al. 1969; HÖKFELT and UNGERSTEDT, 1969).

6. The staining sites should be confirmed by auxiliary cytochemical methods such as the demonstration of relevant synthetic or catabolic enzymes. Only monoamine oxidase (BOADLE and BLOOM, 1969) appears to be approachable from this standpoint.

2. Chemical Basis for the Selective Staining of Catecholamines

While there were numerous light microscopic reactions described for identifying the monoamines histochemically in adrenal medullary chromaffin cells (see PEARSE, 1961), these reactions depended upon the development of specific colored end-products and were not directly applicable to the electron microscope. Before 1965, the only available electron microscopic cytochemical reactions on catecholamines were based upon the use of OsO_4 as a combined fixative and electron stain (DE ROBERTIS and PELLEGRINO DE IRALDI, 1961a, b; GRILLO and PALAY, 1962; RICHARDSON, 1958, 1962, 1963, 1964). The "osmiophilic" subcellular precipitate was taken as an indicator of catecholamine content because such amines were "known to be potent reducing substances" (DE ROBERTIS and PELLEGRINO DE IRALDI, 1961a, b). This latter statement was, in turn, based upon *in vitro* tests.

Similar reasoning lies behind the use of $KMnO_4$ as a fixative producing more reliable reactions on catecholamine containing tissues (RICHARDSON, 1966; HÖKFELT, 1967a—d, 1968a, b, 1969; HÖKFELT and JONSSON, 1968).

If tissue monoamine stores could be approximated by an aqueous solution of the amine, then test tube reactions might help explain the reactivity of these substances with the commonly used electron microscopic fixatives (Table 1). These tests indicate that a very large spectrum of natural and synthetic catecholamines will "reduce" OsO_4 and $KMnO_4$, forming gross precipitates. However, from the reported data, it is uncertain whether such precipitates indicate insoluble polymers of the oxidized amines, or of the reduced metallic oxidants, or of some coordination complex between the two. However it is only the electron-opacity of the precipitate which is most crucial to an identification of reactive cellular sites.

Two questions immediately derived are the retention of the monoamine in its tissue site during the fixation process with OsO_4 or $KMnO_4$ and the subsequent oxidation-reduction reaction indicated by the test tube experiments. Because of their slow penetration into tissue, OsO_4 and $KMnO_4$ are commonly used in immersion fixation at 3—5° C, by which it is hoped to slow autolysis of cellular

Table I. *Reaction of Monoamines with Staining Fixatives*

Test for Reaction:	OsO_4 [a]	Formaldehyde [b]	Glutaraldehyde [c]	$KMnO_4$ [d]	Glutal. + $K_2Cr_2O_7$ [e]	Glutal. + Ag [f]	Glutal. OsO_4 [h]
Amine							
Noradrenaline	+	0	+	++	++	++	+
Adrenaline	+	0		++		+	
Dopamine	+	0	+	++	++	+	
Serotonin	+	0	+	++	++	+	+
5-OH dopamine [i]	+			++			+
6-OH dopamine	0			++			
Alpha-methyl noradrenaline				++			
Metaraminol	0			++			

References: [a] Van Orden et al. (1966); [b] Hopsu and Makinnen (1966); [c] Wood and Barrnett (1964), Coupland et al. (1964); Solcia et al. (1969); [d] Hökfelt and Jonsson (1968); [e] Wood and Barrnett (1964); Jaim-Etcheverry and Zieher (1969); [f] Tramezzani et al. (1964); Cannata et al. (1968); [g] Solcia et al. (1969); [h] Coupland et al. (1964); Machado (1967); Tranzer and Thoenen (1967a); Tranzer et al. (1969); [i] Tranzer and Thoenen (1967a).

organelles. However, the cooler temperature is also likely to influence the reactivity of the fixative and of the available reactive groups in the tissue, as well as the relative extraction of reactive tissue components.

The reactions undergone by OsO_4 and $KMnO_4$ as they react with tissue have been reviewed in detail (Bloom, 1970). Despite the large number of investigations into the nature of these reactions (see Adams et al., 1967; Hökfelt and Jonsson, 1968), it is still not certain which of the many reactions contribute to the electronopacity of the tissue and which to the reduction of the oxidants.

Furthermore, the tissue groups reacting with these substances are not well characterized aside from being "reducing substances" (see Hake, 1965; Pearse, 1961) although tissue proteins are thought to be particularly decomposed by MnO_4 (Lenard and Singer, 1968). The reduced form of $KMnO_4$, MnO_2, occurs in nature as a grey-black precipitate which would be expected to be somewhat electron-opaque.

These metallic oxidants do not provide much well fixed tissue for examination because they are most commonly employed as immersion fixatives: small pieces of the tissue are dissected and immersed in the cooled solutions. In this fashion, only the outer surfaces are exposed to the fixative, and in each case there has been considerable previous manipulation of the tissues. On the other hand, the advent of aldehyde fixatives (Sabatini et al., 1963) made it feasible to fix organs for electron microscopy by intravascular perfusion. Thus the tissues could be fixed more rapidly, with less functional compromise, and with considerably better preservation of a greater proportion of the fine structure, not to mention lower cost. In such cases it was necessary to react the glutaraldehyde fixed tissues with OsO_4 in order to develop the electron opacity of the membranes and organelles, although it is obvious that this only complicates interpretation of the cytochemistry of the reactions. When solutions of glutaraldehyde are mixed with monoamines in the test tube, obvious yellowish precipitates can be seen to form with noradrenaline, but not with adrenaline which is a secondary amine (Table 1). This reaction is believed to be an addition of the aldehydes to the terminal side chain amines (see BLOOM, 1970).

As a dialdehyde, polymer formation might also proceed by this reaction (see COUPLAND and HOPWOOD, 1966) and could account for the majority of the yellow precipitate mentioned above. However, each noradrenaline molecule has only 1 reactive site, and each glutaraldehyde only 2; therefore, if the observed 1:1 ratio in the final precipitate is valid (COUPLAND and HOPWOOD, 1966), the exact structure of such a polymer is difficult to visualize. The reaction of the monoamines

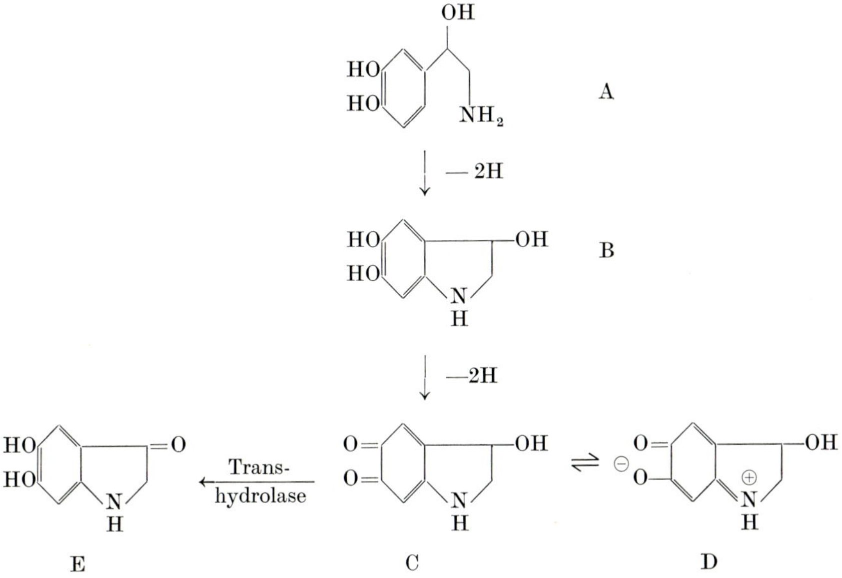

Fig. 1. Diagrammatic reaction scheme for the oxidation of catecholamines by oxidants, as might be expected to occur during the fixation of tissue with fixatives such as OsO_4 or $KMnO_4$. Each of the intermediates might contribute to the eventual production of an electron-opaque deposit within storage organelles of catecholamine containing cells. The final transhydrolation step might result in the removal of the label from carbon atom 7, the site of most H^3-noradrenaline radioactivity

with glutaraldehyde does not alter the reducing power of these substances, hence, we would expect that the monoamine-glutaraldehyde polymer should also be capable of reacting with the oxidants. Clearly the complex of aldehyde and monoamine can reduce alkaline silver salts to the metal (TRAMEZZANI et al., 1964; CANNATA et al., 1968).

Rather precise organic chemical observations have been made on the formation of pigments from catecholamines, since this is the main route for the formation of melanins (see PEARSE, 1961) and aminochromes (see HEACOCK, 1965). In the case of the naturally occurring catecholamines, the reaction is believed to be: (Fig. 1). The aminochromes represent the natural form of catechol-polymers such as melanin, which are known to be electron-opaque in electron microscopic investigations of melanophores (RILEY and FORTNER, 1963). This indicates that equivalently electron-opaque products might be expected to occur from monoamines if the proper cytochemical production method were available.

Regardless of the success of tests carred out *in vitro*, only application to tissues can evaluate the relative sensitivity of the method. Thus, the first attempts at specific localizations of catecholamines by electron microscopy tested the adrenal medullary cell, in which there were high concentrations of catecholamines. WOOD and BARRNETT (1964) showed that adrenal medulla fixed in glutaraldehyde and exposed to acidic solutions of $K_2Cr_2O_7$ (the chromaffin reaction) resulted in selective opacification of the chromaffin granules of noradrenaline-containing cells, but not adrenaline-containing cells. The latter remained unstained until the pH of the $K_2Cr_2O_7$ approached neutrality. Subsequently COUPLAND et al. (1964); COUPLAND and HOPWOOD (1966) showed the same cytochemical separation between noradrenaline cells and adrenaline cells occurred if neutral OsO_4 (Fig. 2) were substituted for $K_2Cr_2O_7$. The latter reaction appears superficially to be less selective since the OsO_4 also makes multiple organelles and membranes electron-opaque whereas the former method results in much greater opacification of chromaffin granules than other cytoplasmic structures.

In both cases the reaction seems to be based upon the selective retention in the tissue of the primary amine, while adrenaline is lost either in the acidic rinses or during the exposure to osmium. In the reaction scheme proposed by COUPLAND, it should be noted that the "negative" reaction given by the adrenaline-containing granules is not completely negative, but that the adrenaline granules exhibit a fibrillar, moderately electron-opaque central matrix, which may be due to granule proteins (see BLOOM and AGHAJANIAN, 1968b).

The condensation of glutaraldehyde with noradrenaline in the chromaffin granule matrix also appears to account for the positive staining of the slightly opaque chromaffin granules exposed to ammoniacal silver after glutaraldehyde fixation (TRAMEZZANI et al., 1964; CANNATA et al., 1968). On the other hand, adrenal medullary tissue fixed in $KMnO_4$ shows no electron opacity within the chromaffin granules of the adrenaline cell type (DUNCAN and YATES, 1967), and small opaque precipitates in the noradrenaline type (HÖKFELT, personal communication).

By virtue of the biochemical data on subcellular binding of noradrenaline (GLOWINSKI et al., 1965; DE ROBERTIS, 1966; WHITTAKER, 1966; PELLEGRINO DE IRALDI and DE ROBERTIS, 1964) cytochemists now have a great deal of background information with which to analyze the problem of fine structural localization. As described elsewhere in this volume, the subcellular distribution of tissue adrenaline was first studied on homogenates of the adrenal medulla (BLASCHKO and WELCH, 1953) and splenic nerve (VON EULER and HILLARP, 1956). In these tissues and in several sympathetically innervated organs analyzed later (see STJARNE, 1966; POTTER, 1967; IVERSEN, 1967; ROTH et al., 1968), the monoamine content was richest in the microsomal fragments containing particulate

Fig. 2a and b. Adrenal medulla of hamster (a) and rat (b) fixed with glutaraldehyde before further processing to differentiate the contents of the chromaffin vesicles histochemically. In both illustrations, the noradrenaline-containing cells are at upper left (N) and the adrenaline-containing cells at lower right (A). 2a was prepared by the dichromate method of WOOD and BARRNETT (1964); 2b was prepared by the routine OsO_4 procedure of COUPLAND et al., 1964. Several peripheral autonomic axons (PA) can be seen coursing between the cells in 2b, and making a specialized contact with the noradrenaline cell. Note that the electron opacity of the noradrenaline-containing cells is greatly increased relative to the adrenaline cells. (Magnification × 35,000; sources for a, unpublished micrograph of WOOD and BARRNETT, for b, unpublished micrograph of BLOOM)

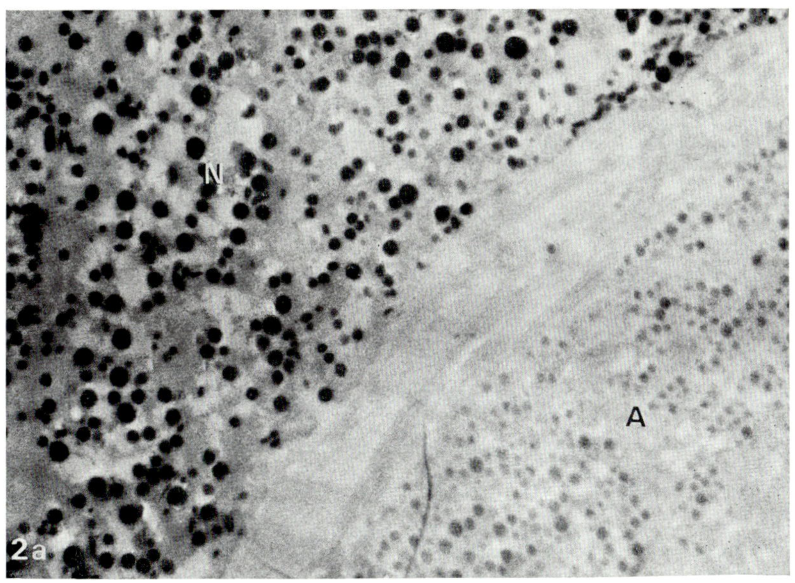

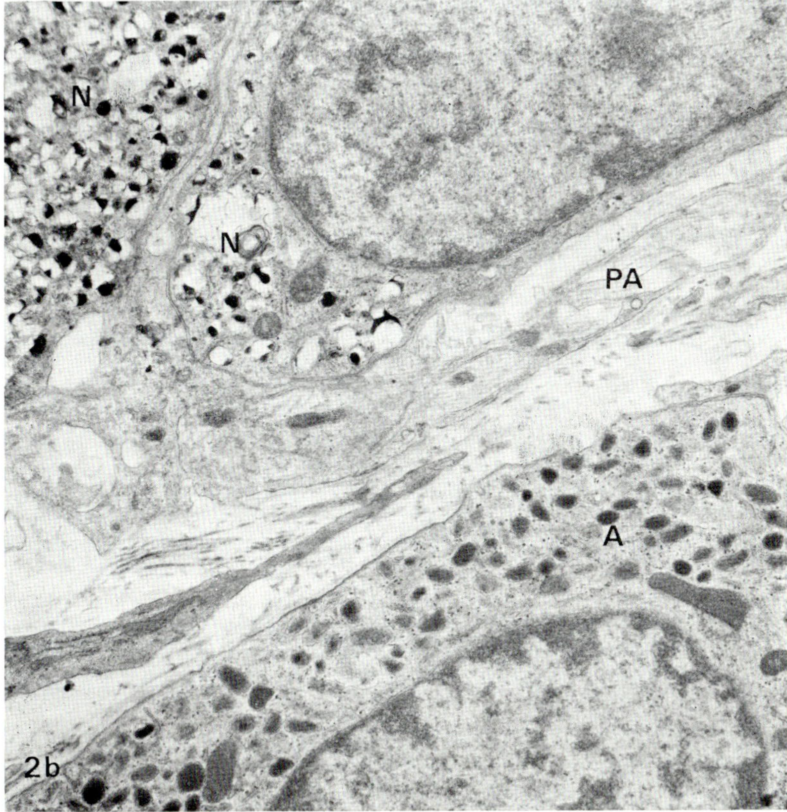

Fig. 2

Table II. *Studies on Fine Structure of Peripheral Catecholamine-Containing Tissues*

Tissue	Fine Structure	Pharmacology	Autoradiography (A) Denervation (D)
1. Adrenal Medulla	Coupland (1965)		Elfvin et al. (1966) (A)
	Elfvin (1965, 1967)		
	Tramezzani et al. (1964)		
	Wood and Barrnett (1964)		
2. Brown Fat	Ochi et al. (1969)		
3. Carotid Body	Grimley and Glenner (1968)	Duncan and Yates (1967)	Chen and Yates (1969) (A)
		Chen et al. (1969)	
		Zapata et al. (1969)	
4. Ciliary Body		Nishida et al. (1969)	
5. Ganglia	Elfvin (1963a, b, 1968)	Clementi et al. (1965)	Grillo (1966) (D)
	Taxi (1961, 1969)	Hökfelt (1969)	
	Siegrist et al. (1968)	Van Orden et al. (1969)	
	Williams (1967)		
6. Heart	Thaemert (1966)		Wolfe and Potter (1963) (A)
			Potter (1967) (D)
7. Intestine	Richardson (1958)	Taxi and Droz (1970)	Taxi and Droz (1966b, 1970) (A)
	Grillo and Palay (1962)		
	Gabella (1967)		
	Pick et al. (1967)		
8. Iris	Richardson (1964, 1966)	Hökfelt (1967a, 1969)	Roth and Richardson (1969) (D)
	Hökfelt (1966a)		
9. Juxta Glomerular Apparatus	Barajas and Latta (1968)		
10. Lacrimal Gland	Ruskell (1967)		
11. Lung	Fillenz (1969)		
12. Nictitating Membrane . .		Van Orden et al. (1967b)	Van Orden et al. (1967b) (D)
13. Pancreas (endocrine) . . .	Legg (1967)		Esterhuizen et al. (1968a, b) (A)
	Shorr and Bloom (1970)		
14. Pineal	Anderson (1965)	de Robertis and Pellegrino de Iraldi (1961a, b)	Wolfe et al. (1962) (A)
	Arstila and Hopsu (1964)	Pellegrino de Iraldi and de Robertis (1961, 1963, 1964)	Budd and Salpeter (1969) (A)
	Wolfe (1965)	Bondareff (1966)	Taxi and Droz (1966a) (A)
	Wartenberg and Baumgarten (1969)	Bondareff and Gordon (1966)	Pellegrino de Iraldi et al. (1965) (D)
	Bondareff (1965)	Bloom and Giarman (1967, 1970)	

Table II (continued)

Tissue	Fine Structure	Pharmacology	Autoradiography (A) Denervation (D)
	Pellegrino de Iraldi and de Robertis (1964) Machado (1967)	Pellegrino de Iraldi and Guedet (1969)	
15. Spleen	Fillenz (1970)	Tranzer and Thoenen (1967a)	
16. Sympathetic Axons . . .	Elfvin (1968) Roth et al. (1968)	Banks et al. (1969)	Stjärne et al. (1970) (A) Kapeller and Mayor (1969) (D)
17. Vas Deferens	Richardson (1962) Merrillees (1968)	Richardson (1963) Bloom and Barrnett (1966) Hökfelt (1966b) Tranzer and Thoenen (1967b) 1968a, b) Farrell (1968) Van Orden et al. (1966, 1967a)	Taxi and Droz (1966b) (A) Tranzer and Thoenen (1968a) (D)
18. Vasculature	Siggins and Bloom (1969, 1970) Devine (1967) Devine and Simpson (1967)	Siggins and Bloom (1969, 1970) Devine and Simpson (1968) Graham et al. (1969)	Siggins and Bloom (1969, 1970) (A) Devine and Simpson (1968) (A) Graham et al. (1968) (A) Lever et al. (1968) (A) Siggins and Bloom (1969, 1970) (D) Devine (1969) (D)

structures on the order of 30—200 mμ in size by electron microscopy. This binding of monoamines to these particulate elements in homogenates has thereafter been referred to trivially as the "storage granule" or granular amine fraction, in an implied reference to the chromaffin granules.

When subcellular fractionation studies were extended to the central nervous system (see de Robertis, 1966; Whittaker, 1966) the catecholamines could be found in those fractions of the homogenate which contained pinched off nerve endings and in which synaptic vesicles could be seen. Because the greatest enhancement in specific concentration of acetylcholine occurred when rather pure collections of the synaptic vesicles were obtained from acetylcholine-rich nerve ending fractions, it is widely considered that the major portion of the particulate monoamine is also contained within synaptic vesicles. Nevertheless. highly purified vesicle fractions containing monoamines have not been prepared due in part to lack of methods to retain the amines within the particles during the separation procedures (see Whittaker, 1966; Michaelson, 1967).

III. Localization of Catecholamines in Nervous Tissues

1. Peripheral Sympathetic Nerve Terminals

The possibility that sympathetic nerve terminals could be morphologically distinguished from other types of nerve terminals arose when multiple types of synaptic vesicles were observed in the nerves to the pineal (de Robertis and Pellegrino de Iraldi, 1961 a, b) and to the intestine (Grillo and Palay, 1962). The newly described vesicles were distinguished by the electron-opacity of their contents after fixation with OsO_4 and on the basis of their size.

a) Small Granular Vesicles

These vesicles measure 40—60 mμ and have variable degrees of internal electron-opacity, dependent upon the type of fixation and the tissue. The small granular vesicles appear to be most easily demonstrated in the nerves to the pineal but have now been observed in a wide variety of sympathetically innervated tissues (Table 2). Studies upon lower vertebrates and invertebrates had not successfully demonstrated the existence of small granular vesicles (Taxi, 1969; Best and Noel, 1969; Robinson and Burnstock, unpublished; Siggins and Bloom, unpublished), until the recent work of Mancini and Frontali (1970) on the cockroach brain. Even within the various regions of the sympathetic nervous system of the same species of animal, there are considerable differences in the ease with which the small granular vesicles can be demonstrated. These tissue differences can only be partially explained in terms of relative extent of inner-

Fig. 3a and b. Nerve terminals of sympathetic nerves to pineal of untreated rat, fixed by perfusion with glutaraldehyde and routine exposure to OsO_4, showing the variation in the number and extent to which the large granular vesicles (arrows) and small granular vesicles have become electron opaque. Electron lucent (agranular) vesicles have the same relative electron opacity of the mitochondria (M). Some of the relatively agranular vesicles in b appear to be ellipsoidal in shape, while the fully granular vesicles are more spherical. (Magnification × 35,000; source, Bloom, unpublished material)

Fig. 4. Nerve terminals of sympathetic axons to pineal of untreated rat prepared by the $KMnO_4$ immersion protocol of Hökfelt (1967a—d). Many of the small granular vesicles appear to be full of electron-opaque material (*), while others are only partially opaque. The axon at upper left exhibits a large granular vesicle, in which the electron opaque material takes the form of a fibrillar amorphous deposit on the inner surface of the vesicle membrane. (Magnification × 100,000; source, Crayton and Bloom, unpublished material)

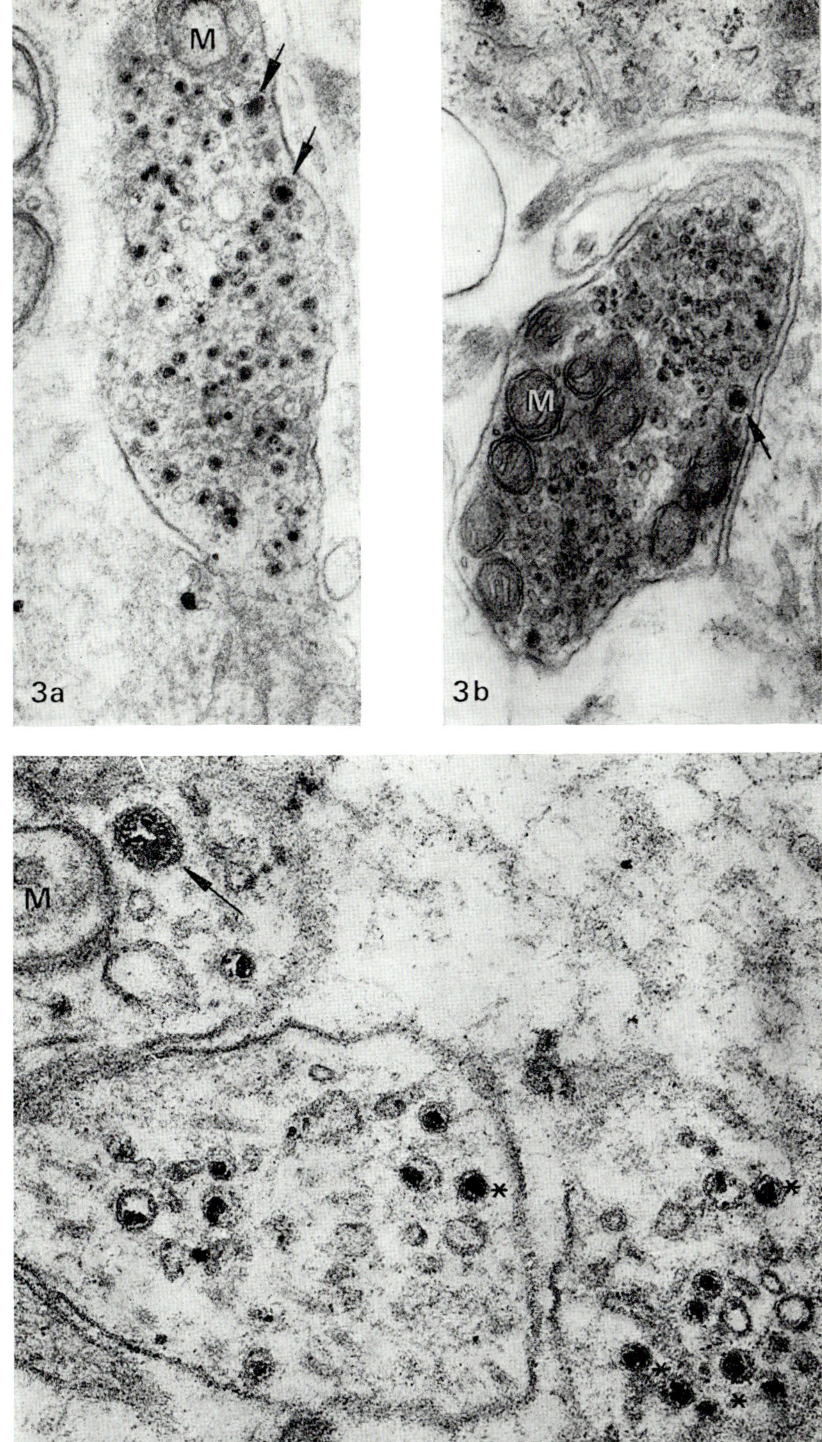
M
3a
M
3b
M
4

vation, the relative content or turnover rates of noradrenaline or the neural activity prior to and during fixation, although these factors must obviously be of importance. The main difference appears to be in the methods used for fixation. In the same tissues, the ease of demonstrating the granular deposits in the synaptic vesicles of peripheral sympathetic nerves occurs in the following decreasing order: 3% $KMnO_4$ (Richardson, 1966; Hökfelt, 1967a, 1968a, b; Van Orden et al., 1969; Bloom and Giarman, 1970, Fig. 4) > glutaraldehyde-dichromate-OsO_4 (Tranzer and Snipes, 1968; Tranzer et al., 1969) > glutaraldehyde/OsO_4 (Bloom and Barrnett, 1966; Van Orden et al., 1966, 1967a, b; Machado, 1967; Bloom and Giarman, 1970; Pellegrino de Iraldi and Gueudet, 1969) > formaldehyde OsO_4 (Bondareff, 1965) > OsO_4 (de Robertis and Pellegrino de Iraldi, 1961a, b; Grillo and Palay, 1962; Grillo, 1966). However, these differences between the fixatives can not be explained on the extent to which the fixative retains the tissue monoamine (Hökfelt and Jonsson, 1968; Bloom and Giarman, 1970; Taxi, 1968; Taxi and Droz, 1970; Devine and Laverty, 1968) or on the relative preservation of tissue fine structure.

Does the presence of small granular vesicles (Figs. 3, 4, 5, 6) serve to indicate monoamines directly? Several lines of evidence strongly suggest that it does. With the "proper" fixation, such nerves can be seen in all sympathetically innervated tissues (Richardson, 1966; also see reviews by Bloom and Giarman, 1968; Jaim-Etcheverry and Zieher, 1970; Tranzer et al., 1969; Bloom, 1970). Nerves with small granular vesicles disappear when the sympathetic axons are surgically severed (Pellegrino de Iraldi et al., 1965; Van Orden et al., 1967b), and are not seen after immunosympathectomy (Richardson et al., cited by Sjöqvist et al., 1965) or when degeneration is due to 6-hydroxydopamine (Devine and Laverty, 1968; Tranzer and Thoenen, 1968a; Devine, 1969; Siggins and Bloom, 1970; Fig. 7). Such nerves can be localized independently of fixation by electron microscopic autoradiography after labelling with H^3-Noradrenaline (Wolfe et al., 1962, Fig. 5; Wolfe and Potter, 1963; Devine and Simpson, 1968; Taxi and Droz, 1966a, b, 1970; Esterhuizen et al., 1968a, b; Graham et al., 1968; Lever et al., 1968; Budd and Salpeter, 1969) or H^3-dihydroxyphenylalanine (Taxi and Droz, 1966a, b). Finally, the small granular vesicles seen after OsO_4 or $KMnO_4$ fixation can be depleted with sympathetic nerve stimulation (Richardson, 1963; Hökfelt, 1968a, b), as well as by drugs (see Table II).

The next question which arises is whether the deposit which makes these vesicles morphologically unique from other synaptic vesicles of the same size range (such as those seen in neuro-muscular junction and other non-adrenergic peripheral junctions) is in itself indicative of the relative monoamine content. Considerable data favor equating the granular deposit with catecholamine storage. The relative numbers of small granular vesicles per nerve terminal tend to decrease with amine depletion by reserpine (Pellegrino de Iraldi and de Robertis,

Fig. 5. Electron microscopic autoradiograph localizing radioactive norepinephrine over nerve terminals of the rat pineal. Tissue fixed with intravascular osmium tetroxide 30 min following the injection of 12.5 μg of radioactive noradrenaline. The silver grains are concentrated over the nerve terminals in which small granular vesicles can be clearly seen. (Magnification × 42,000; source, David E. Wolfe)

Fig. 6. Nerves to pineal of rat pretreated with one dose of 5-hydroxydopamine (10 mg/Kg, IV, 30 min) and fixed as tissue in Fig. 4. Vesicles are now somewhat enlarged and almost all vesicles contain heavily opaque, but irregular precipitates. (Magnification × 100,000; source, Bloom, unpublished material)

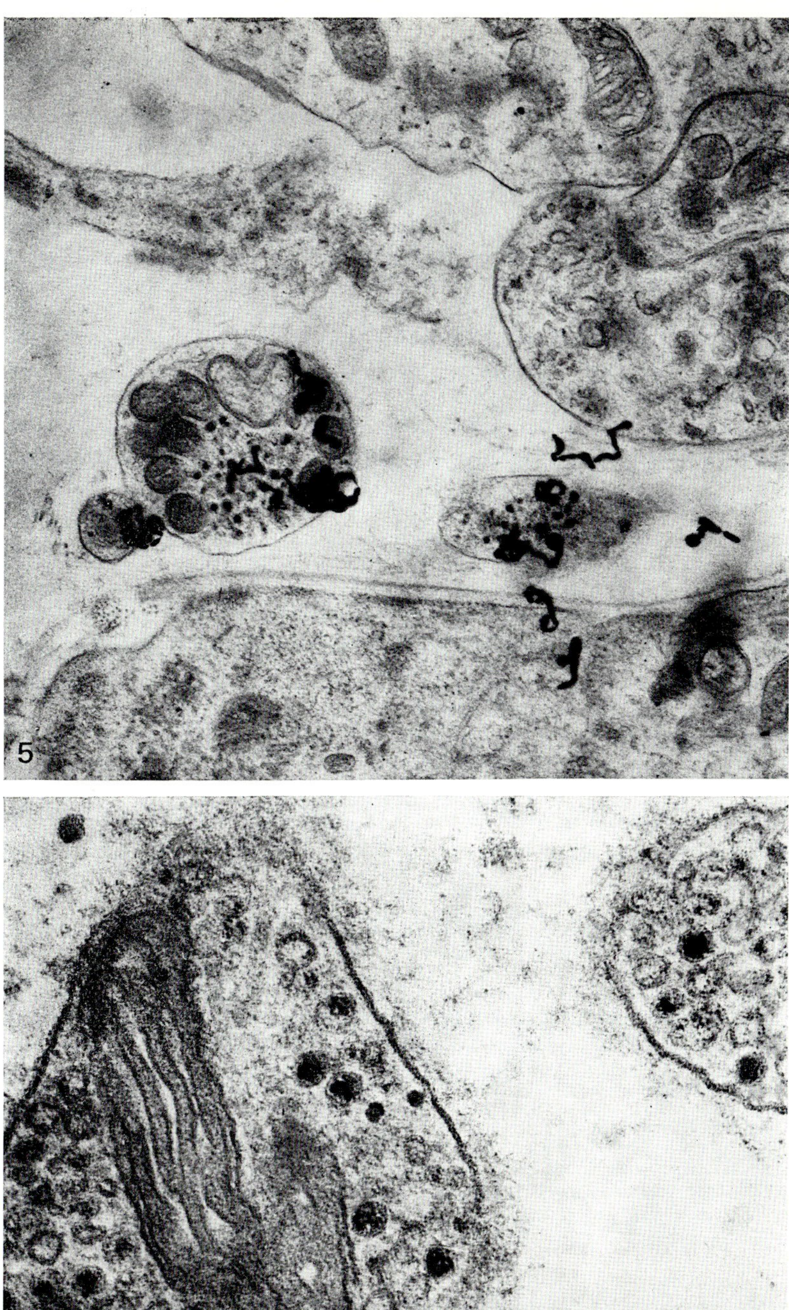
5
6

1961, 1963; Richardson, 1963; Clementi, 1965; Clementi et al., 1965; Hökfelt, 1966b; Van Orden et al., 1966) metaraminol (Bondareff and Gordon, 1966) or α-methylmetatyrosine (Bloom and Barrnett, 1966; Van Orden et al., 1966) and can be enhanced or restored by monoamine oxidase inhibitors (Pellegrino de Iraldi and de Robertis, 1963; Van Orden et al., 1967a) with or without dihydroxyphenylalanine (Pellegrino de Iraldi and de Robertis, 1964; Clementi, et al., 1965) or by loading with noradrenaline (Van Orden et al., 1966), with α-methylnoradrenaline (Bondareff, 1966; Hökfelt, 1967a, c, 1968a, b) or with 5-hydroxydopamine (Tranzer and Thoenen, 1967a, 1968b, Fig. 6).

There are also data which tend to refute that the granular deposits are actually catecholamine. Success or failure in the demonstration of the vesicle granularity with a particular fixative chemical is not proportional to the amount of radioactive catecholamine retained in the tissue (Devine and Simpson, 1968; Hökfelt and Jonsson, 1968; Taxi, 1968, 1969; Bloom and Giarman, 1970) or in homogenate fractions (Whittaker, 1966; Michaelson et al., 1968; Michaelson, 1967; Potter, 1967). By autoradiography, heavy deposits of silver grains can frequently be seen over axons in which the granular vesicles exhibit only minimal granularities (Lever et al., 1968; Devine and Simpson, 1968; Esterhuizen et al., 1968a, b; Budd and Salpeter, 1969; Taxi, 1969) indicating, at the least, that catecholamines can occur within the vicinity of the vesicles without the vesicles being granular. These arguments could be explained away most simply by proposing that fixation was adequate to bind the catecholamine to the tissue, but incorrect for producing the electron opaque deposits. However, the small granular vesicles seen after $KMnO_4$ fixation exhibit fewer autoradiographic grains than do other portions from identical tissue prepared with glutaraldehyde/OsO_4, where there are multiple autoradiographic grains but fewer small granular vesicles (Bloom and Giarman, 1970; Taxi, 1969) Were it not for these observations, there would be no reason to doubt the conclusion that the presence of the intravesicular granularity is indicative of the catecholamine. However, these as yet unexplained observations indicate the need for caution before reaching such a conclusion, particularly when considered in the light of observations on noradrenaline in the central nervous system and in neuronal cell bodies (see below).

An additional feature complicating the quantitative interpretation of the small granular vesicle precipitate arises from observations that certain "adrenergic" nerves may also store 5-hydroxytryptamine (Bloom and Giarman, 1967, 1968; Jaim-Etcheverry and Zieher, 1970; Pellegrino de Iraldi and Gueduet, 1969). On the basis of biochemical experiments, it can be estimated that more than half of the monoamine contained in the nerves to the rat pineal may be 5-hydroxytryptamine rather than noradrenaline (Neff et al., 1969). This may be one explanation for the ease with which the small granular vesicles in the pineal nerves are demonstrated with various fixatives (see above). It is, therefore, of considerable interest that depletion of the 5-hydroxytryptamine following syn

Fig. 7. Vascular nerves in frog retrolingual membrane after exposure to topical 6-hydroxydopamine and fixation 5 days later with glutaraldehyde and OsO_4. The nerves with electron opaque axoplasm (arrows) disappear as the noradrenaline fluorescent axons and sympathetic nerve activity are lost. Axon in center shows loss of synaptic vesicles (*). Note that axon at far left appears normal and may be assumed to be cholinergic. (Magnification × 40,000; from Siggins and Bloom, 1969, 1970)

Fig. 8. Autoradiographic localization of H^3-noradrenaline applied topically to normal frog retrolingual membrane 2 hours before fixation with glutaraldehyde and OsO_4. Grains are located over terminals which are filled mainly with large electron-opaque granular vesicles. (Magnification × 25,000; from Siggins and Bloom, 1969, 1970)

thesis inhibition with p-chlorophenylalanine produces loss of the small granular vesicles with glutaraldehyde/OsO_4 fixation but not with primary fixation by

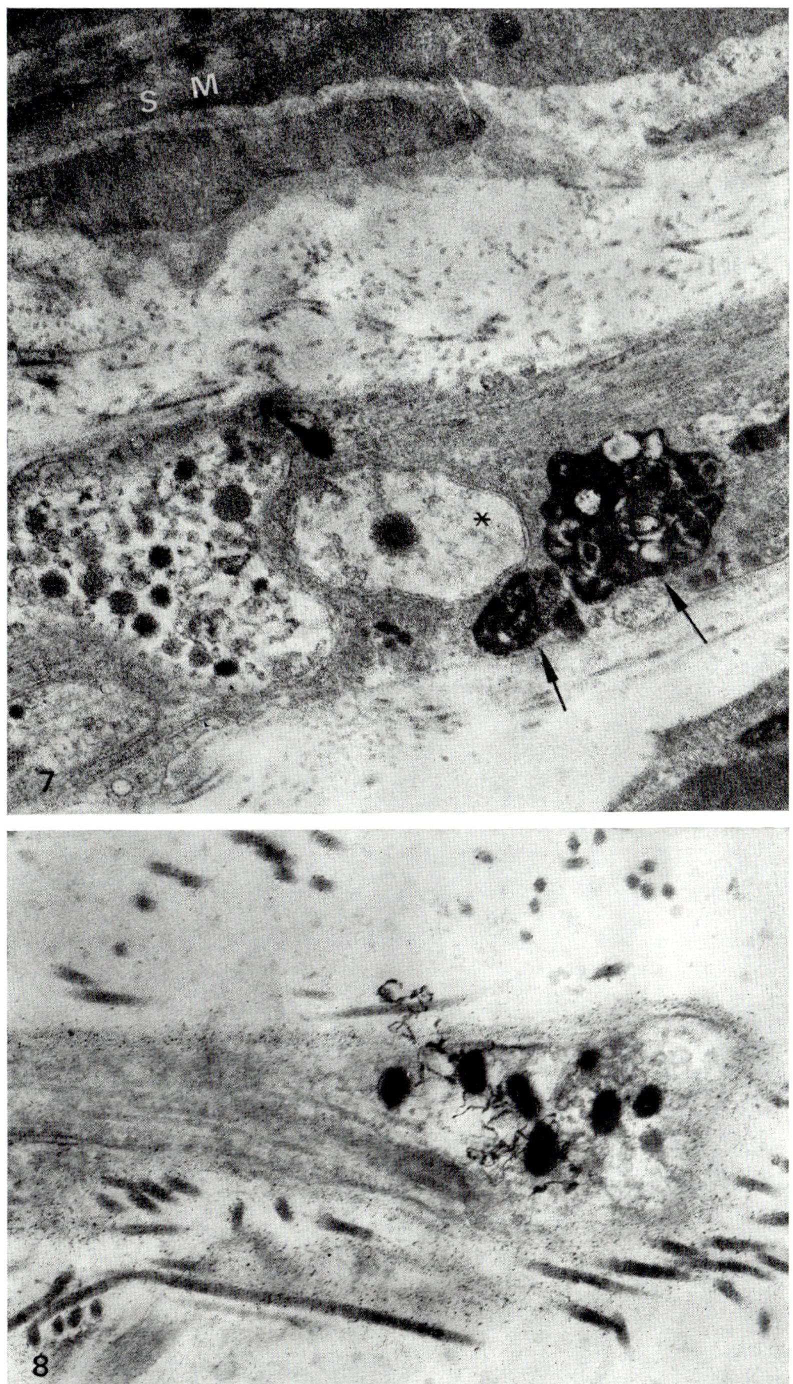

either OsO_4 (Pellegrino de Iraldi and Gueudet, 1969) or $KMnO_4$ (Bloom and Giarman, 1967, 1970). Such observations thus provide the possibility of untold complicating factors in the cytochemical production of small granular vesicle precipitates.

b) Large Granular Vesicles

In addition to the small granular vesicles, peripheral sympathetic nerves also contain larger vesicles 80—120 mμ in size (Grillo and Palay, 1962). These large granular vesicles exhibit a more fibrillar electron-opaque deposit, but with less electron opacity than the small granular vesicles. The large granular vesicles constitute about 1—5% of the vesicles in various peripheral adrenergic nerve terminals (Bondareff, 1965; Van Orden et al., 1966, 1967a, b) but are also seen in nerve terminals classically considered to be cholinergic, such as the pre-ganglionic axons to a variety of sympathetic ganglia (Taxi, 1961, 1965; Grillo and Palay, 1962; Grillo, 1966; Clementi et al., 1965). The same type of large granular vesicle appears to be the main form of granular synaptic vesicle seen in the retina (Pellegrino de Iraldi and Jaim-Etcheverry, 1967b) and in the nervous systems of lower vertebrates and invertebrates (Best and Noel, 1969; Siggins and Bloom, 1970, Fig. 8; Van Orden et al., 1969). The relative electron-opacity of these larger granular vesicles appears to be unrelated to the amount of monoamine in the tissue (Bondareff, 1965; Bloom and Barrnett, 1966). Statistical interpretation of autoradiographs of pineal nerves indicates no relative increase in the number of grains over these vesicles with respect to the small granular vesicle (Budd and Salpeter, 1969). Nevertheless, despite these negative correlations, some evidence suggests that the large granular vesicles participate in the monoamine storage process of peripheral nerves. Loading tissue with 5-hydroxydopamine and examining it after glutaraldehyde/OsO_4 fixation reveals increased electron-opacity over the large granular vesicles in adrenergic nerve terminals, but not the large granular vesicles in pre-ganglionic cholinergic axons (Tranzer and Thoenen, 1967a, 1968b). Similar selective increases in the electron-opacity of the large granular vesicles of adrenergic nerves have been seen after noradrenaline loading and $KMnO_4$ fixation (Hökfelt, 1968a, b, 1969). These observations may reflect biochemical differences not only among the large granular vesicles, but in the uptake specificities of the axonal membrane (Tranzer and Thoenen, 1967a, 1968b) as well. In addition, when ligature constrictions of peripheral nerve trunks cause accumulation of biochemically and histochemically demonstrable noradrenaline (Dahlström, 1967), it is mainly the large granular vesicles which are found in increased numbers above the constriction on electron microscopic observation (Kapeller and Mayor, 1969). Recent quantitative studies on the vesicular components of the splenic innervation show that only the large granular vesicles are found in the splenic nerve trunk, while large and small vesicles are found in the nerve terminals within the spleen (Geffen and Ostberg, 1969; Fillenz, 1970). A similar increase in large granular vesicles has also been observed in peripheral sympathetic nerves in which colchicine has been used to impair axoplasmic flow (Dahlström and Hökfelt, personal communication). The large granular vesicles which accumulate after physical constriction of axons seem to be more labile to drug treatments than normal large granular vesicles (Kapeller and Mayor, 1969; Banks et al., 1969).

2. Central Nerve Terminals

Prior to 1967 small granular vesicles could not be demonstrated in the central nervous system, and all attention was devoted to the central large granular vesicles (Fig. 9). These vesicles can be presumed to indicate central monoamines because some large granular vesicles react positively with the WOOD-BARRNETT procedure (WOOD, 1966). The large granular vesicles also appear in fractions of brain homogenates rich in nerve terminals obtained from noradrenaline-rich

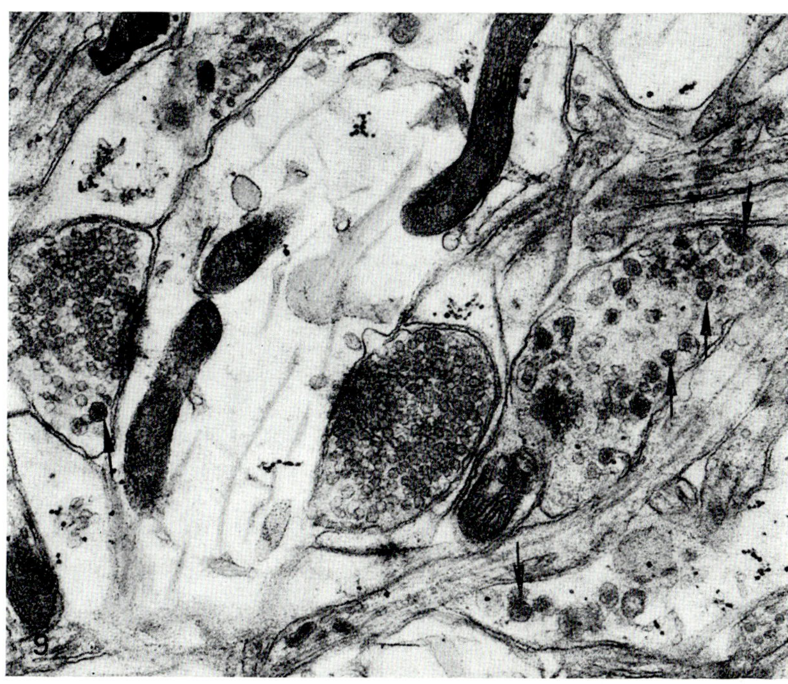

Fig. 9. Periventricular nucleus of the rat hypothalamus fixed by perfusion with glutaraldehyde and routine exposure to OsO_4, illustrating the occurrence of numerous large granular vesicles (arrows) in synaptic terminals and axons. All the small synaptic vesicles associated with the large granular vesicles are agranular. (Manification × 35,000; BLOOM and BARRNETT, unpublished material)

areas of the hypothalamus (DE ROBERTIS et al., 1965). The large granular vesicles were present in the majority of nerve terminals identified by autoradiography as containing H^3-noradrenaline (AGHAJANIAN and BLOOM, 1966, 1967a, b; LENN, 1967; DESCARRIES and DROZ, 1968a, b, 1970; Fig. 10). Furthermore, large granular vesicles are seen in the nerve terminals which degenerate after lesions of monoamine pathways (RAISMAN, 1969). The distribution of central nerve terminals containing several large granular vesicles varies throughout the rat central nervous system in relatively good correlation with the total reported regional content of noradrenaline but not of the dopamine (BLOOM and AGHAJANIAN, 1968a).

According to some authors, large granular vesicles are less frequent after depletion of central noradrenaline stores (PELLEGRINO DE IRALDI et al., 1963; BAK, 1965, 1967; ISHII et al., 1965; MATSUOKA et al., 1965; SHIMIZU and ISHII, 1965; HALARIS et al., 1967; ISHII, 1967) and increase in frequency after treatment with monoamine oxidase inhibitors and monoamine precursors (PELLEGRINO DE IRALDI et al., 1963; HASHIMOTO et al., 1965; ISHII, 1967; PELLEGRINO DE IRALDI and JAIM-ETCHEVERRY, 1967a; PFEIFFER et al., 1968; ZAMBRANO, 1968). Others disagree (FUXE et al., 1965; BLOOM and AGHAJANIAN, 1968a; HÖKFELT, 1968a, b).

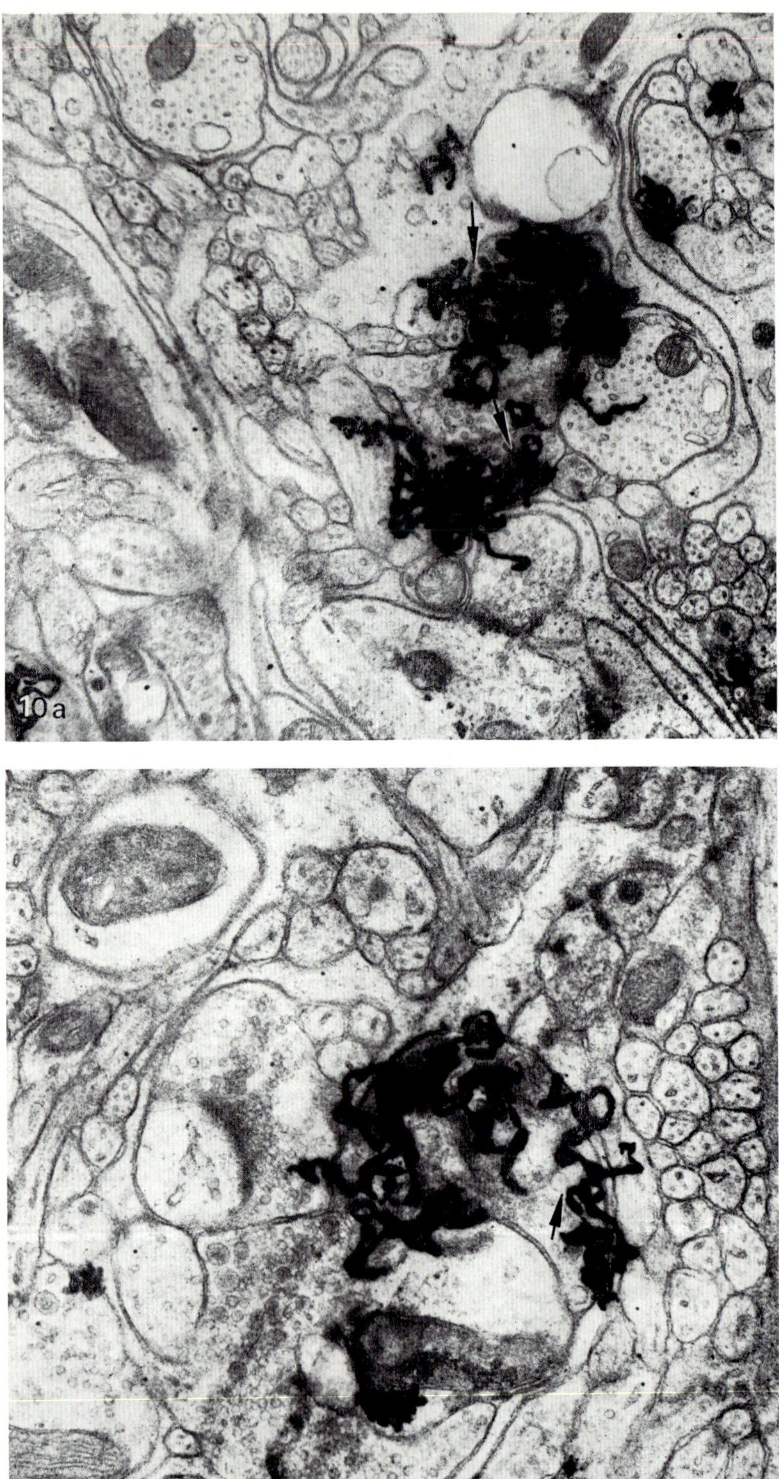
10 a
10 b

Fig. 10a and b. Autoradiographic localization of d,l-7-H^3-noradrenaline in periventricular nucleus of rat hypothalamus; tissue fixed by perfusion with glutaraldehyde two hours after the intracisternal injection of 50 μC (1 μg) of amine. Autoradiographic protocol followed that of Aghajanian and Bloom (1967a); Ilford L-4 emulsion developed after 6 weeks exposure. In a, two preterminal axons are completely covered with autoradiographic grains, although occasional large granular vesicles can be seen (arrows). In b, a nerve terminal making specialized contact with a small dendritic process is also covered with a large cluster of grains; only one large vesicle can be seen clearly (arrow) and its electron-opacity is not marked. Grain clusters such as these have not been seen over any other structures except nerve terminals or preterminal axons. (Magnifications, a, × 25,000; b, × 40,000; from Bloom, unpublished material)

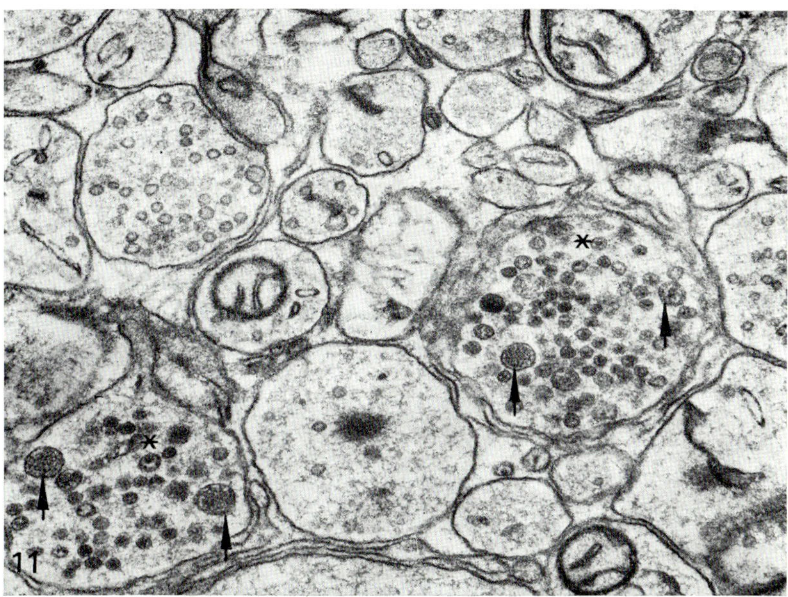

Fig. 11. Periventricular zone of hypothalamus of untreated rat, incubated as a slice in α-methylnoradrenaline (1 μg/ml) and fixed in $KMnO_4$. Two nerve terminals contain several large granular vesicles (arrows) which are surrounded by numerous small granular vesicles (*). Compare with Figs. 9 and 10. (Magnification × 40,000; modified from Hökfelt, 1968a, with permission of the author)

By using an electron-opaque stain for protein which does not depend on an oxidation-reduction reaction (Bloom and Aghajanian, 1968b) the authors concluded that most of the large granular vesicle electron opacity after glutaraldehyde/OsO_4 was due to a proteinaceous component in their internal matrix (Bloom and Aghajanian, 1968a). This latter conclusion was also directly applicable to the peripheral large granular vesicles and chromaffin granules (see also Jaim-Etcheverry and Zieher, 1969).

However, with the successful application of MnO_4 fixation to the central nervous system (Hökfelt, 1967a, c, 1968a, b; Hökfelt and Jonsson, 1968) large granular vesicles could no longer be considered to be the only potential storage organelle for central monoamines. By fixing thin slices of brain tissue with $KMnO_4$, Hökfelt (1968a, b) was able to observe small granular vesicles in nerve terminals in hypothalamus, locus coeruleus, and median eminence of untreated rats (Fig. 11). After incubation of the slices in α-methylnoradrenaline (1—10 μg/ml), small granular vesicles could be seen frequently in terminals from caudate nucleus, locus coeruleus, and supra-chiasmatic nucleus; their appearance could be blocked if the animals or the incubating media offered exposure to drugs capable of blocking the uptake or storage processes. Furthermore, nerves capable of binding α-methylnoradrenaline disappear from the caudate after lesions of the substantia nigra (HÖKFELT and UNGERSTEDT, 1969). By fixing slices of cockroach brain with $KMnO_4$ after incubation in 10 μg/ml of α-methylnoradrenaline, small granular vesicles can be found, but not with any other preparative technique (MANCINI and FRONTALI, 1970).

These observations clarify the relative importance of large granular vesicles in the identification of the noradrenaline-containing central and peripheral nerve terminals, and suggest that they be interpreted cautiously in this respect. However, certain cautions must also be placed upon the interpretation of the small granular vesicles. As in the peripheral nervous system, there is an unexplained discrepancy in the retention of brain noradrenaline and the appearance of the small granular vesicles. In the brain, there is the additional problem that 2 other types of small granular vesicles appear not to be correlated with monoamine content; such vesicles can be seen in the rabbit brain, despite reserpine treatment (TRANZER et al., 1969) and can be produced in glutaraldehyde-fixed brain by exposure to OsO_4 at elevated temperatures (BLOOM and AGHAJANIAN, 1968c and Fig. 12), although this latter procedure appears to "leech" out the radioactive noradrenaline, Furthermore, the "hot osmium" small granular vesicles persist after administration of reserpine, and do not increase in frequency after inhibition of monoamine oxidase. The success of the "hot osmium" technique may depend upon the fact that osmium vapors are more effective sources of electron opaque "osmium black" precipitates (see BLOOM, 1970), but their persistence despite depletion of amines suggests they react with some vesicle component distinct from the monoamine. Furthermore, by injecting 6-hydroxydopamine (THOENEN and TRANZER, 1968; TRANZER and THOENEN, 1967b, 1968b) intracerebrally, central catecholamine degeneration can now also be followed by both fine structure and biochemistry (Figs. 13, 14, 15, BLOOM et al., 1969; URETSKY and IVERSEN, 1969). Thus both types of granular vesicles should be subjected to tests for the satisfaction of the criteria proposed above. As in the peripheral nervous system, the large granular vesicles in the brain do not appear to be the exclusive organelles of noradrenaline-containing neurons. Terminals fixed with $KMnO_4$ and showing small granular vesicles (HÖKFELT, 1968a) constitute less than $^1/_2$ the number of terminals showing large granular vesicles with glutaraldehyde/OsO_4 (BLOOM and AGHAJANIAN, 1968a) when the same brain regions are quantitated. The relative number of nerve terminals showing small granular vesicles after intraventricular injection of 5-hydroxydopamine (TRANZER and THOENEN, 1967a, b; TRANZER et al., 1969;

Fig. 12. Normal rat hypothalamus fixed by perfusion with glutaraldehyde and exposed to OsO_4 in solution at 60° C. In contrast to results with standard glutaraldehyde/OsO_4 sequence on brain (see Fig. 9), numerous irregular electron-opaque deposits are seen in both the small and large synaptic vesicles in terminal at right; at left, terminal is filled with typical agranular vesicles. (Magnification × 50,000; unpublished micrograph from BLOOM and AGHAJANIAN, 1968c)

Fig. 13. Periventricular nucleus from rat hypothalamus prepared by standard glutaraldehyde perfusion and exposure to OsO_4. However, in this case, the animal was perfused, two hours after an intracisternal injection of 5-hydroxydopamine (200 μg), resulting in the visualization of numerous electron opaque deposits within the small synaptic vesicles of the preterminal axon in the center (arrows). Note that the synaptic vesicles surrounding the large granular vesicles (*arrows) in the two axons at bottom have remained agranular. (Magnification × 100,000; from BLOOM, unpublished material)

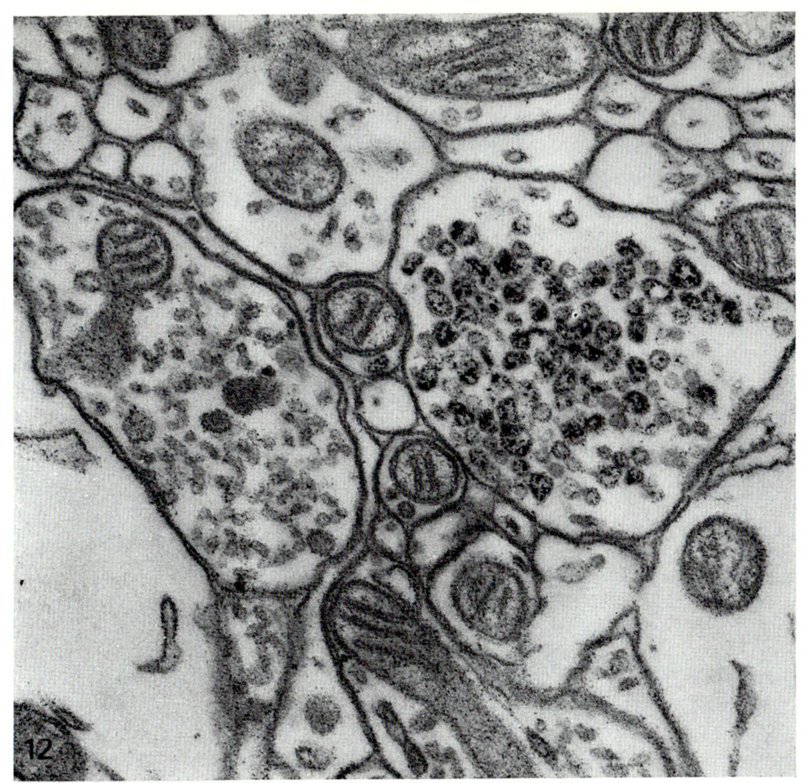
12

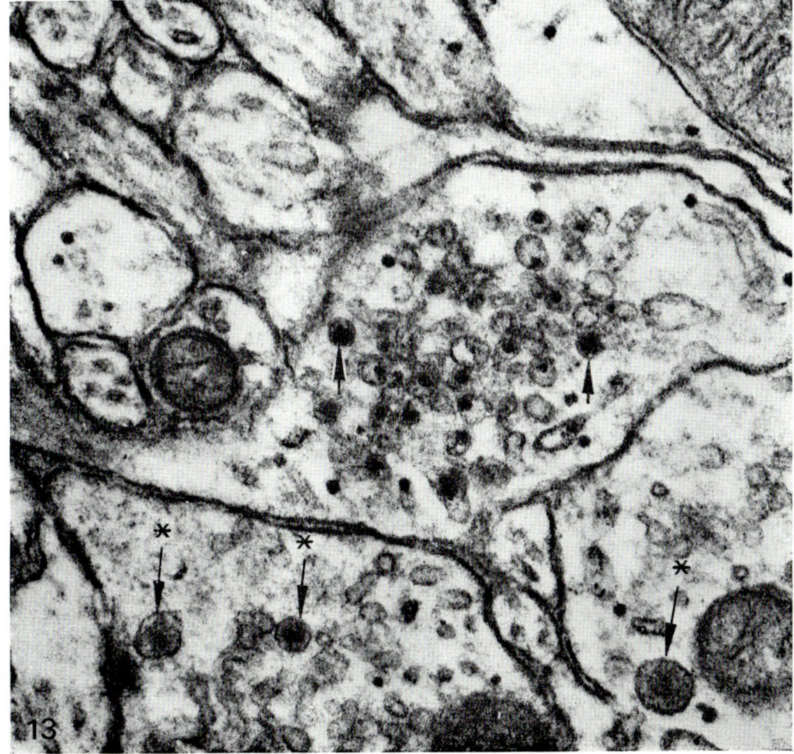
13

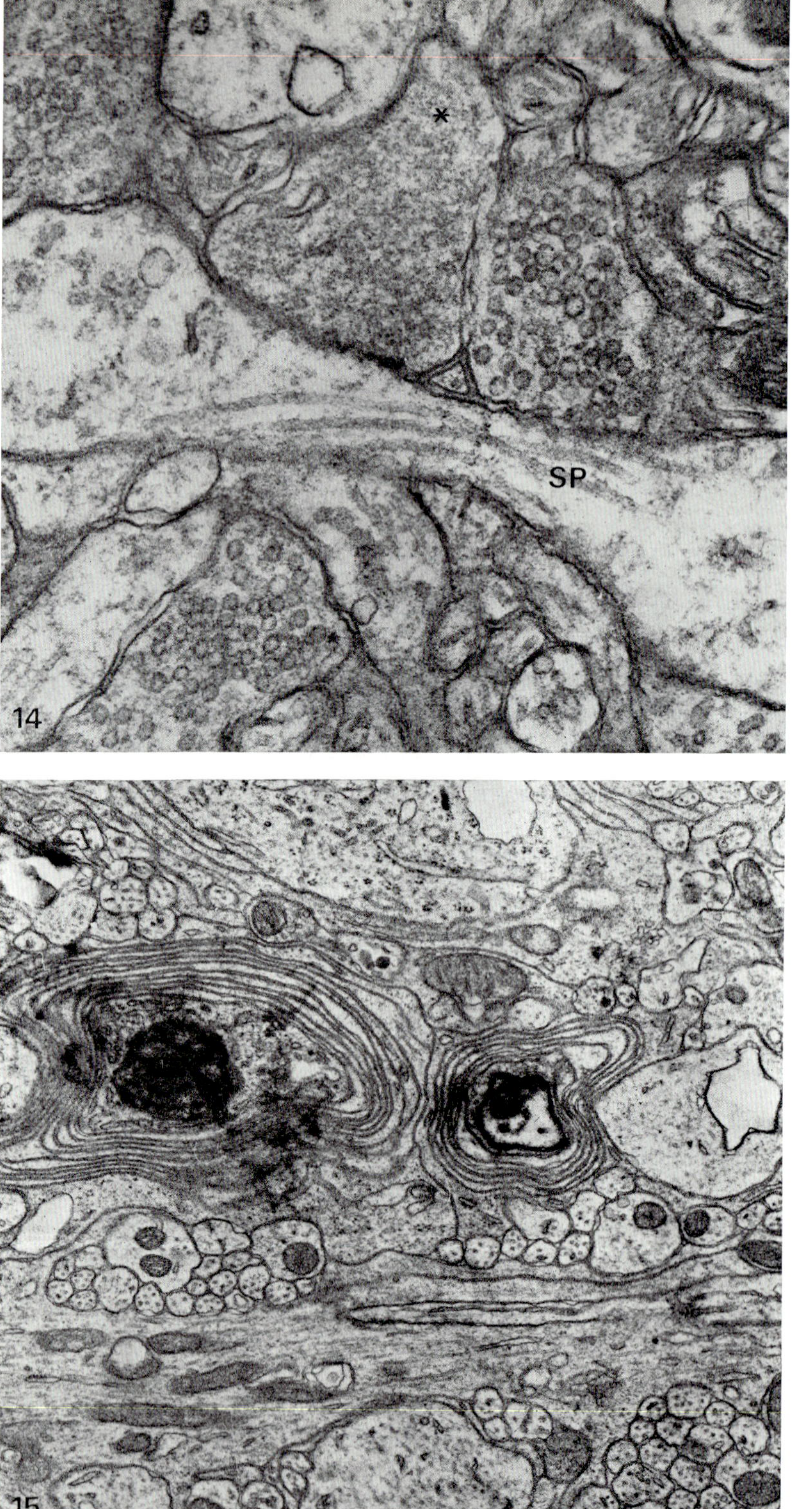
*
SP
14
15

RICHARDS and TRANZER, 1970; BLOOM and CRAYTON, 1970) is even smaller (Fig. 13).

A final note of caution regarding the interpretation of large granular vesicles in the brain relates to their frequent confusion with neurosecretory granules (KOBAYASHI et al., 1965; RINNE, 1966; MONROE, 1967).

3. Localizing Catecholamines in Neuronal Cell Bodies and Non-terminal Axons

Since the association between small granular vesicles and noradrenaline stores holds reasonably well for the nerve terminals, one might expect similar vesicles would be found to store the amine present in the cell body and along the axons. From fluorescence histochemical observations (DAHLSTRÖM and FUXE, 1964), the cell bodies normally fluoresce after gaseous formaldehyde, and this fluorescence is greatly augmented by pretreating the animals with monoamine oxidase inhibitors. This experiment has been performed by two separate groups using electron microscopy to search for a cellular organelle which increases in number following such treatment; in both cases no such organelle could be found (LENN, 1965; FUXE et al., 1966).

When sympathetic ganglia are subjected to subcellular fractionation, little or no particulate storage form of noradrenaline is found in the rat (FISCHER and SNYDER, 1965), although substantially more noradrenaline is associated with the particulate fractions of the bovine stellate ganglia (SCHÜMANN et al., 1966). Furthermore, no matter which fixative procedure is successful in revealing the small granular vesicles of the terminals, it has rarely been possible to see such vesicles within the cytoplasm of the cell body unless MnO_4 salts are used (GRILLO, 1966; HÖKFELT, 1968a, b; TRANZER et al., 1969; VAN ORDEN et al., 1969). On the other hand, the cell bodies of both central and peripheral noradrenaline-containing neurons do exhibit autoradiographic labeling with H^3-noradrenaline (DESCARRIES and DROZ, 1968a, b, 1970; TAXI, 1969) particularly when monoamine oxidase has been inhibited. However, in the latter cases, the labeling appears to be somewhat random with respect to perikaryal organelles, although the activity within the cells is clearly greater than the surrounding tissues. DESCARRIES has suggested (personal communication) that some type of macromolecular material may be present within such cells to bind the noradrenaline once it has entered the cell; such a macromolecule could represent an "extra vesicular" type of binding. Similar suggestions were also put forward to account for the autoradiographic localization of H^3-noradrenaline over bovine splenic nerve axons in which no vesicles (neither large granular vesicles or small granular vesicles) could

Fig. 14. Caudate of rat perfused as material in Figs. 9, 10 and 13; this animal was pretreated with a monoamine oxidase inhibitor (pargyline 50 mg/Kg IV) 30 min prior to receiving a single intracisternal injection of 6-hydroxydopamine, and perfused 8 hours after this latter treatment. In this field, three nerve terminals are seen in contact with a long dendritic spine (SP). Note that the synaptic vesicles of the terminal in the center (*) appear very indistinct and that the axoplasm has become relatively increased in electron-opacity; such changes are the earliest detectable alterations in fine structure observed reproducibly. (Magnification × × 60,000; from BLOOM, KUPRYS and BATTENBERG, unpublished)

Fig. 15. Periventricular hypothalamus of rat treated with 3 injection sequences of intracisternal 6-hydroxydopamine (BLOOM et al., 1969) and perfused with glutaraldehyde 7 days after last treatment. Note the extremely dense residua of two degenerated axons are wrapped in multiple lamellae of glia membranes. (Magnification × 25,000; from BLOOM, KUPRYS and BATTENBERG, unpublished)

be seen (Stjärne et al., 1970). Loading of cell body organelles with 5-hydroxydopa or 5-hydroxydopamine has been seen in the hypothalamus of the lizard (Baumgarten et al., 1969; Wartenberg and Baumgarten, 1969) but not in mammalian brain (Tranzer, personal communication). Thus, for the present, we must conclude that the monoamine cell bodies are even more difficult sites in which to localize these substances. Both small granular vesicles and large granular vesicles occur in and around the Golgi zones of the cell bodies, as well as in isolated areas of both the perikaryon and dendrites (Hökfelt, 1967a—c, 1969) but, it is not known whether they are present in sufficient numbers to account for the amine content measurable by biochemical or fluorescence histochemical approaches.

IV. Cytology of Catecholamine-Containing Cells

Having gone to considerable lengths to be able to specify that a given cell does contain catecholamines on the basis of certain cytochemical reactions with its synaptic or secretory vesicles, we can belatedly proceed to examine the cytology of these cells.

1. The Chromaffin Cells

The secretory cells of the adrenal medulla have been investigated with the electron microscope multiple times (see Coupland, 1965; Elfvin, 1965, 1967; Elfvin et al., 1966; Diner, 1967). The chromaffin cells have a generally uniform appearance and are organized in epithelial sheets grouped around capillary sinusoids. At the junctions between adjacent chromaffin cells, the surface of the two cells exhibits a specialized zonula adherens form of intracellular contact. The membrane bounded chromaffin granules constitute the major cytoplasmic organelle; their size varies between 50 and 350 mμ and the electron opacity of the central matrix is fixation dependent (see above and Duncan and Yates, 1967). The chromaffin granules appear to be packaged in the membranes of the Golgi zones. In comparison to the amount of protein (2—5 μg/ml plasma per minute in the calf; Blaschko et al., 1967) liberated (Banks and Helle, 1965; Blaschko et al., 1965; Kirshner et al., 1965) from the cells with the catecholamines, there is surprisingly little rough endoplasmic reticulum. A small number of lysosomes (Bradbury et al., 1966; Holtzman and Dominitz, 1968) and multivesicular bodies, as well as numerous mitochondria can also be observed. Under certain conditions, some chromaffin granules also exhibit staining for acid phosphatase (Holtzman and Dominitz, 1968). The cell surface has received much attention in the search for clues into cytophysiologic observations on the mode of the catecholamine secretion. Although random pictures compatible with a rather gross form of exocytosis have been published (Coupland, 1965; Elfvin, 1965) no reliable statistical tests on intact tissue have been reported. In most mammalian species

Fig. 16. Superior cervical ganglion of rat fixed by perfusion with glutaraldehyde and routine exposure to OsO_4, 30 min after intravenous injection of 5-hydroxydopamine (10 mg/Kg). The perikaryonal cytoplasm is filled with multiple large vesicles filled with electron-opaque material (arrow); such vesicles can also be seen near Golgi membranes (G) and near a specialized synaptic contact with a small dendritic spine of an adjacent neuron (arrow s). This cell has many of the characteristics of the intraganglionic chromaffin neuron. A more typical preganglionic axo-dendritic synaptic contact is seen at upper right (arrow a). (Magnification × 20,000; from Bloom, unpublished)

Fig. 17. A noradrenaline containing cell from the carotid body of an untreated cat, fixed with glutaraldehyde and reacted with the Ag^+ method of Tramezzani et al. (1964). A granular silver precipitate can be seen on or over the majority of the cytoplasmic granules in this chief cell. (Magnification × 21,000; donated by Chiocchio and Tramezzani)

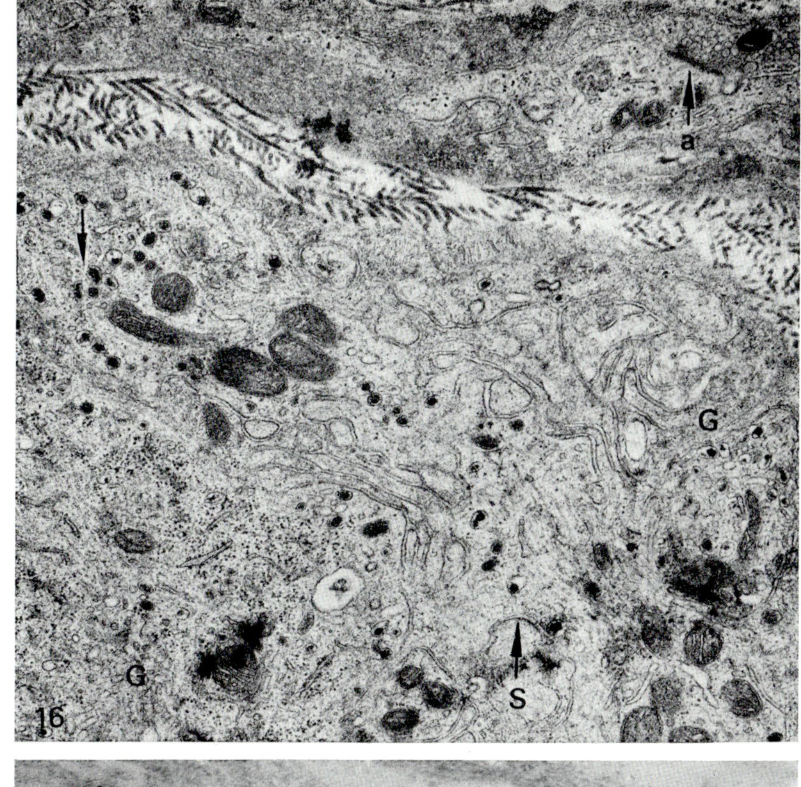
a
G
G
S
16

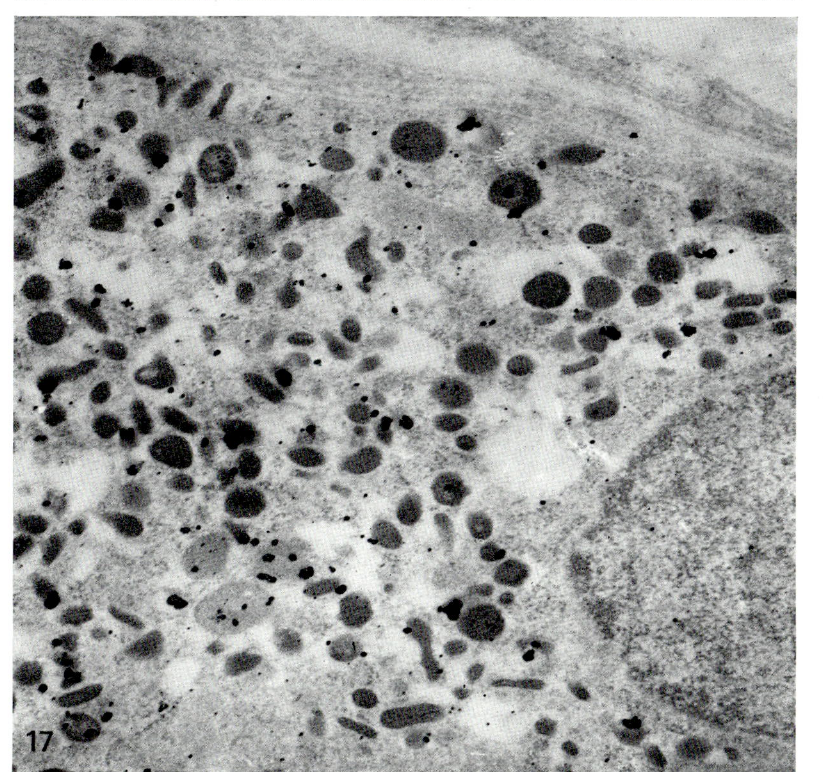
17

the adrenal chromaffin cells receive synaptic connections from preganglionic nerve fibers, and ganglionic neurons have also been noted within the medulla itself.

2. Chromaffin Neurons

In her review of 1966, Grillo mentioned that detailed analysis of cervical sympathetic ganglia had revealed a cell type which had the cytological characteristics of both neurons and chromaffin cells. Their cytoplasm was filled with somewhat smaller, but otherwise typical chromaffin-like granules (see Fig. 16), but in addition to receiving preganglionic synapses these cells also appeared to be prejunctional in specialized intercellular contacts with both ganglion neurons and with other chromaffin cells. Williams (1967) found similar details and proposed that these cells could function as interneurons within the ganglia. These cells form only a small proportion of the neuronal cell population within the ganglia, but have now been described by several different groups examining varied sympathetic ganglia (Siegrist et al., 1968; Elfvin, 1968; Van Orden et al., 1969; Matthews and Raisman, 1969; Shorr and Bloom, 1970). They are most frequently found in groups of 3—5, clustered around ganglionic capillaries (Fig. 16). It is not clear whether these cells function as interneurons or represent reserve ectopic chromaffin tissue, but they do seem to represent an intermediate state between the purely secretory medullary cell and the non-endocrine sympathetic neurons. It will be quite important to study such cells by electrophysiologic approaches.

3. Carotid Body Chemoreceptors

While it has been well known that the carotid bodies of several mammalian species contain relatively large amounts of all three natural catecholamines (see Dearnaly et al., 1968; Zapata et al., 1969) their form of catecholamine storage and the functional purpose of the monoamines were not known. Recently these cells have been studied by several different groups (Duncan and Yates, 1967; Grimley and Glenner, 1968; Zapata et al., 1969; Chen and Yates, 1969; Chen et al., 1969). The primary cells are called chief cells (or glomus Type I cells) and contain osmiophilic cytoplasmic granules of the size range observed in medullary chromaffin cells (Fig. 17). The electron opacity of the cytoplasmic granules disappears upon fixation with $KMnO_4$ (as does that of the medullary chromaffin cells, see Duncan and Yates, 1967), but when fixed with glutaraldehyde and OsO_4 the granules do not change in appearance even after severe depletion of catecholamines with reserpine. The chief cells also resemble medullary cells in that they receive multiple synaptic contacts. They resemble ganglion neurons in that they are completely surrounded by glia-like "sustentacular" cells. However, their physiologic role remains unclear, in that there is no observable morphological correlate to electrical or chemical hyperactivity (Zapata et al., 1969). Duncan and Yates have suggested that the chief cells are directly responsive to chemical stimulation, and respond by releasing catecholamines which in some way activate the contacting nerve fibers. More correlative work is needed on this second interesting intermediate catecholamine tissue.

4. Sympathetic Neurons

Ganglion cells have been described for a variety of sympathetic ganglia. Grillo (1966) described that specialized forms of intercellular contact may occur between adjacent cell bodies, although no known electrophysiologic correlate of this has been described. The cells are only moderate in size in the mammal (less than 25 μ on the average) considering the extremely widespread ramifications of their terminal axonal arborization. The majority of synaptic contacts in the mammal are axodendritic (Fig. 16, ELFVIN, 1963a, b) but in the frog synapses occur exclusively on the soma (TAXI, 1961, 1965). Numerous large granular vesicles can be seen near the Golgi zone, while the smaller granular vesicles can be seen accumulated in groups throughout the cytoplasm of the soma and dendrites (GRILLO, 1966; HÖKFELT, 1969). The surface of the ganglion cell is completely surrounded by Schwann cells (also termed satellite cells) which wrap around the synaptic contacts of the soma and dendritic tree. Some of the Schwann cells may bear ciliated processes (GRILLO and PALAY, 1963).

5. Sympathetic Axons and Terminals

Beyond the fact that the sympathetic axons are unmyelinated, yet enclosed within the cytoplasm of Schwann cells, there are few other structural details of note. These axons contain all the routinely described cellular organelles including microtubules, mitochondria, and large granular vesicles (see ROTH et al., 1968). In an extensive series of investigations, KAPELLER and MAYOR (1969) have investigated the morphologic changes ensuing upon the placement of a ligature constriction around these axons. The terminals, particularly with regard to the vesicular contents, have already been described. The point to be remembered about the terminations of the sympathetic axons is that each axon has multiple dilated regions at which synaptic vesicles are accumulated; but at no point — including the ultimate termination of the axon — does the axon come into any form of specialized contact with the glands or smooth muscle cell it innervates (RICHARDSON, 1963, 1964; THAEMERT, 1966; FARRELL, 1968; MERRILLEES, 1968).

6. Central Neurons and Terminals

The few existing papers on the cytology of central catecholamine neurons were written in days prior to the development of reproducible fixation techniques and should be repeated before presence or absence of structural peculiarites can be decided. Many such cells exhibit multiple forms of granular organelles (LENN, 1965; FUXE et al., 1965) but the relation to the catecholamines is dubious. After $KMnO_4$ fixations, HÖKFELT (1967d) has reported the observation of small granular vesicles in the cytoplasm of neurons in the locus coeruleus. There is little more to be said regarding the cytology of the terminals, except that they seem to form mainly axodendritic synapses, and can vary substantially in size (see HÖKFELT, 1968a, b; HÖKFELT and UNGERSTEDT, 1969; DESCARRIES and DROZ, 1970; BLOOM and AGHAJANIAN, 1968a).

V. Conclusions

The use of electron microscopy to explore the cytophysiology of catecholamine containing cells has concentrated upon techniques for demonstrating the nature of the catecholamine storing cellular organelles. Now that several useful techniques exist for such localizations, it may be expected that greater detailed descriptions of the intercellular relations of these cells, particularly in the central nervous system, will soon be forthcoming. Of particular interest, will be studies aimed at clarifying the differences in the composition of the synaptic vesicles of the central and peripheral neurons which synthesize and release catecholamines, and the cellular role played by the vesicles in these processes.

References

Adams, C. W. M., Abdulla, Y. H., Bayliss, O. B.: Osmium tetroxide as a histochemical and histological reagent. Histochemie **9**, 68—77 (1967).

Aghajanian, G. K., Bloom, F. E.: Electron microscopic autoradiography of rat hypothalamus after intraventricular H^3-norepinephrine. Science (N.Y.) **153**, 308—310 (1966).

— — Localization of tritiated serotonin in rat brain by electron microscopic autoradiography. J. Pharmacol. exp. Ther. **156**, 23—30 (1967a).

— — Electron microscopic localization of tritiated norepinephrine in rat brain: Effects of drugs. J. Pharmacol. exp. Ther. **156**, 407—416 (1967b).

Anderson, E.: The anatomy of bovine and ovine pineals. J. Ultrastruct. Res. Suppl. **8**, 1—80 (1965).

Arstila, A. W., Hopsu, V. K.: Studies on the rat pineal gland. I. Ultrastructure. Ann. Acad. Scient. Fennicae S. B. 113 (1964).

Bak, I. J.: Electron microscopic observations in the substantia nigra of mouse during reserpine administration. Experientia (Basel) **21**, 568—570 (1965).

— The ultrastructure of the substantia nigra and caudate nucleus of the mouse and the cellular localization of catecholamines. Exp. Brain Res. **3**, 40—57 (1967).

Banks, P., Helle, K.: The release of protein from the stimulated adrenal medulla. Biochem. J. **97**, 40C—41C (1965).

— Kapeller, K., Mayor, D.: The effects of iproniazid and reserpine on the accumulation of granular vesicles and noradrenaline in constricted adrenergic nerves. Brit. J. Pharmacol. **37**, 10—18 (1969).

Barajas, L., Latta, H.: Structure of the juxtaglomerular apparatus. Circulation Research **21**, Suppl. 2, 15—28 (1968).

Baumgarten, H. G., Braak, H., Wartenberg, H.: Demonstration of dense core vesicles by means of pyrogallol derivatives in noradrenaline containing neurons from the organon vasculosum hypothalami of *Lacerta*. Z. Zellforsch. **95**, 396—404 (1969).

Best, J. B., Noel, J.: Complex synaptic configutations in planarian brain. Science **164**, 1070—1071 (1969).

Blaschko, H., Welch, A. D.: Localization of adrenaline in cytoplasmic particles of the bovine adrenal medulla. Naunyn-Schmiedeberg's Arch. exp. Path. Pharmak. **219**, 17—22 (1953).

Blaschko, H. K. F., Comline, R. S., Schneider, F. A., Silver, M., Smith, A. D.: Secretion of a chromaffin granule protein, chromogranin, from the adrenal gland after splanchnic stimulation. Nature (Lond.) **215**, 58—59 (1967).

Bloom, F. E.: The fine structural localization of biogenic monoamines in nervous tissue. Int. Rev. Neurobiol. **13**, 45—70 (1970).

— Aghajanian, G. K.: An electron microscopic analysis of large granular synaptic vesicles of the brain in relation to monoamine content. J. Pharmacol. Exp. Therap. **159**, 261—273 (1968a).

— — Fine structural and cytochemical analysis of the staining of synaptic junctions with phosphotungstic acid. J. Ultrastruct. Res. **22**, 361—375 (1968b).

— — An osmiophilic substance in brain synaptic vesicles not related to catecholamine content. Experientia (Basel) **24**, 1225—1227 (1968c).

— Algeri, S., Groppetti, A., Revuelta, A., Costa, E.: Lesions of central norepinephrine terminals with 6-OH-dopamine: Biochemistry and fine structure. Science **166**, 1284—1286 (1969).

— Barrnett, R. J.: Fine structural localization of norepinephrine in vesicles of autonomic nerve endings. Nature (London) **210**, 599—601 (1966).

— Crayton, J. W.: Electron microscopic localization of biogenic amines. In: Methods in Investigative and Diagnostic Endocrinology (S. Berson, R. Yalow, R. Dorfman, E. Rall and I. Kopin, eds.). North-Holland Publishing Co. in press.

— Giarman, N. J.: Fine structure of granular vesicles in pineal autonomic nerve endings after serotonin depletion. Anat. Rec. **157**, 351 (1967).

— — Physiologic and pharmacologic considerations of biogenic amines in the nervous system. Ann. Rev. Pharmacol. **8**, 229—258 (1968).

— — The effects of p-Cl-phenylalanine on the content and cellular distribution of 5-HT in the rat pineal gland: combined biochemical and fine structural observations. Biochem. Pharmacol. (1970).

Boadle, M. C., Bloom, F. E.: A method for the fine structural localization of monoamine oxidase activity. J. Histochem. Cytochem. **17**, 331—340 (1969).

Bondareff, W.: Submicroscopic morphology of granular vesicles in sympathetic nerves of rat pineal body. Z. Zellforsch. **67**, 211—218 (1965).

— Localization of alpha-methyl norepinephrine in sympathetic nerve fibers of the pineal body. Exp. Neurol. **16**, 131—135 (1966).

Bondareff, W., Gordon, B.: Submicroscopic localization of norepinephrine in sympathetic nerves of rat pineal. J. Pharmacol. exp. Ther. **153**, 42—47 (1966).

Bradbury, S., Smith, A.D., Winkler, H.: The demonstration of lysosomes in the bovine adrenal medulla. Experientia (Basel) **22**, 142—144 (1966).

Budd, G.C., Salpeter, M.M.: The distribution of labeled norepinephrine within sympathetic nerve terminals studied with electron microscope radioautography. J. Cell Biol. **41**, 21—32 (1969).

Cannata, M.A., Chiocchio, S.R., Tramezzani, J.H.: Specificity of the glutaraldehyde silver technique for catecholamines and related compounds. Histochemie **12**, 253—264 (1968).

Chen, I.-L., Yates, R.D.: Electron microscopic radioautographic studies of the carotid body following injections of labeled biogenic amine precursors. J. Cell Biol. **42**, 794—803 (1969).

— — Duncan, D.D.: The effects of reserpine and hypoxia on the amine-storing granules of the hamster carotid body. J. Cell Biol. **42**, 817—826 (1969).

Clementi, F.: Modifications ultrastructurelles provoquées par quelques médicaments sur les terminaisons nerveuses adrénergiques et sur la médullaire/ surrénale. Experientia (Basel) **21**, 171—172 (1965).

— Mantegazza, P., Botturi, M.: A pharmacologic and morphologic study on the nature of the dense-core granules present in the pre-synaptic endings of sympathetic ganglia. Int. J. Neuropharmacol. **5**, 281—285 (1965).

Coupland, R.E.: Electron microscopic observations on the structure of the rat adrenal medulla. I. The ultrastructure and organization of chromaffin cells in the normal adrenal medulla. J. Anat. **99**, 231—254 (1965).

— Hopwood, D.: Mechanism of a histochemical reaction differentiating between adrenaline — and noradrenaline — storing cells in the microscope. Nature **209**, 590—591 (1966).

— Pyper, A.S., Hopwood, D.: A method for differentiating between noradrenaline — and adrenaline — storing cells in the light and electron microscope. Nature **201**, 1240—1242 (1964).

Dahlström, A.: The intraneuronal distribution of noradrenaline and the transport and life-span of amine storage granules in the sympathetic adrenergic neuron. Arch. Pharmakol. exp. Path. **257**, 93—114 (1967).

— Fuxe, K.: Evidence for the existence of monoamine-containing neurons in the central nervous system. I. Demonstration of monoamines in the cell bodies of brain stem neurons. Acta physiol. scand. **62**, Suppl. 232, 1—55 (1964).

Dearnaley, D.P., Fillenz, M., Woods, R.I.: The identification of dopamine in the rabbit's carotid body. Proc. roy. Soc. B **170**, 195—203 (1968).

De Robertis, E.: Adrenergic endings and vesicles isolated from brain. Pharmacol. Rev. **18**, 413—424 (1966).

— Pellegrino de Iraldi, A.: A plurivesicular component in adrenergic nerve endings. Anat. Record **139**, 299 (1961a).

— — Plurivesicular secretory processes and nerve endings in the pineal gland of the rat. J. biophys. biochem. Cytol. **10**, 361—372 (1961b).

— — Rodriguez de Lores Arnaiz, G., Zieher, L.M.: Synaptic vesicles from the rat hypothalamus. Isolation and norepinephrine content. Life Sci. **4**, 193—201 (1965).

Descarries, L., Droz, B.: Electron microscope radioautographic detection of norepinephrine-H^3 in the central nervous system of the rat. Fourth European Regional Conference on Electron Microscopy, p. 527—528 (1968a).

— — Neurobiologie — Incorporation de noradrénaline — ^3H (NA-^3H) dans le systéme nerveux central du rat adulte. Etude radio-autographique en microscopie électronique. C.R. Acad. Sci. Paris **266**, 2480—2482 (1968b).

— — Intraneural distribution of exogenous norepinephrine in the central nervous system of the rat. J. Cell Biol. **44**, 385—399 (1970).

Devine, C.E.: Electron microscope autoradiography of rat arteriolar axons after noradrenaline infusion. Proc. of the Univ. of Otago Med. Sch. **45**, 7—8 (1967).

— The fine structure of vascular axons after treatment with 6-hydroxydopamine. Proc. of the Univ. of Otago Med. Sch. **47**, 4—6 (1969).

— Laverty, R.: Fixation for electron microscopy and the retention of ^3H-noradrenaline by tissues. Experientia (Basel) **24**, 1156—1157 (1968).

— Simpson, F.O.: The fine structure of vascular sympathetic neuromuscular contacts in the rat. Amer. J. Anat. **121**, 153—174 (1967).

— — Localization of tritiated norepinephrine in vascular sympathetic axons of the rat intestine and mesentery by electron microscope radioautography. J. Cell Biol. **38**, 184—192 (1968).

Diner, O.: L'expulsion des granules de la médullosurrénale chez le Hamster. C.R. Acad. Sci. Paris **265**, 616—619 (1967).

Duncan, D., Yates, R.: Ultrastructure of the carotid body of the cat as revealed by various fixatives and the use of reserpine. Anat. Record **157**, 667—682 (1967).
Elfvin, L.-G.: The ultrastructure of the superior cervical ganglion of the cat. J. Ultrastruct. Res. **8**, 403—440 (1963a).
— Electron microscopic studies on the splenic nerve, the superior cervical ganglion, and the sympathetic trunk of the cat. Doctoral Thesis, Karolinska Institutet (1963b).
— The fine structure of the cell surface of chromaffin cells in the rat adrenal medulla. J. Ultrastruct. Res. **12**, 263—286 (1965).
— The development of the secretory granules of the rat adrenal medulla. J. Ultrastruct. Res. **17**, 45—62 (1967).
— A new granule-containing nerve cell in the inferior mesenteric ganglion of the rabbit. J. Ultrastruct. Res. **22**, 37—44 (1968).
— Appelgren, L. E., Ullberg, S.: High resolution autoradiography of the adrenal medulla after injection of tritiated dihydroxyphenylalanine (DOPA). J. Ultrastruct. Res. **14**, 277—293 (1966).
Esterhuizen, A.C., Graham, J.D.P., Lever, J.D., Spriggs, T.L.B.: Catecholamines and acetylcholinesterase distribution in relation to noradrenaline release. An enzyme histochemical and autoradiographic study on the innervation of the cat nictitating muscle. Brit. J. Pharmacol. **32**, 46—56 (1968b).
— Spriggs, T.L.B., Lever, J.D.: Nature of islet-cell innervation in the cat pancreas. Diabetes **17**, 33—36 (1968a).
Euler, U.S. von, Hillarp, N.-Å.: Evidence for the presence of noradrenaline in submicroscopic structures of adrenergic axons. Nature (Lond.) **177**, 44 (1956).
Farrell, K. E.: Fine structure of nerve fibers in smooth muscle of the vas deferens in normal and reserpinized rats. Nature **217**, 279—281 (1968).
Fillenz, M.: Innervation of pulmonary capillaries. Experientia (Basel) **25**, 842 (1969).
— The innervation of the cat spleen. Proc. roy. Soc. B **174**, 459—468 (1970).
Fischer, J.E., Snyder, S.: Disposition of norepinephrine-H^3 in sympathetic ganglia. J. Pharmacol. **150**, 190—195 (1965).
Fuxe, K.: Evidence for the existence of monoamine neurons in the central nervous system. III. The monoamine nerve terminal. Z. Zellforsch. **65**, 573—596 (1965).
— Hökfelt, T., Nilsson, O.: A fluorescence and electronmicroscopic study on certain brain regions rich in monoamine terminals. Amer. J. Anat. **117**, 33—46 (1965).
— — — Reinius, S.: A fluorescence and electron microscopic study on central monoamine nerve cells. Anat. Record **155**, 33—40 (1966).
Gabella, G.: Dense-core vesicles in nerve fibres of intestinal circular muscle layer. J. Microscopie **6**, 863—866 (1967).
Geffen, L.B., Livett, B.G., Rush, R.A.: Immunohistochemical localization of protein components of catecholamine storage vesicles. J. Physiol. **204**, 593—605 (1969).
— Ostberg, A.: Distribution of granular vesicles in normal and constricted sympathetic neurones. J. Physiol. **204**, 583—592 (1969).
Glowinski, J., Kopin, I.J., Axelrod, J.: Metabolism of [^{3}H] norepinephrine in the rat brain. J. Neurochem. **12**, 25—30 (1965).
Graham, J. D. P., Lever, J.D., Spriggs, T. L. B.: An examination of adrenergic axons around pancreatic arterioles of the cat for the presence of acetylcholinesterase by high resolution autoradiographic and histochemical methods. Brit. J. Pharmacol. **33**, 15—20 (1968).
— — — The effect of morphine dependence on the vesicular content of adrenergic nerves in relation to arteriolar smooth muscle in the pancreas of the rat. Brit. J. Pharmacol. **37**, 19—23 (1969).
Grillo, M.A.: Electron microscopy of sympathetic tissues. Pharmacol. Rev. **18**, 387—399 (1966).
— Palay, S.L.: Granule-containing vesicles in the nervous system. In: Electron Microscopy, S.S. Breese, Jr. edit., Vol. 2, U-1. New York: Academic Press 1962.
— — Ciliated Schwann cells in the autonomic nervous system of the adult rat. J. Cell Biol. **16**, 430—436 (1963).
Grimley, P.M., Glenner, G.G.: Ultrastructure of the human carotid body — a perspective on the mode of chemoreception. Circulation **37**, 648—664 (1968).
Hake, T.: Studies on the reactions of OsO_4 and $KMnO_4$ with amino acids, peptides and proteins. Lab. Invest. **14**, 1208—1212 (1965).
Halaris, A., Ruther, E., Matussek, N.: Effect of a benzoquinolizine (RO 4—1284) on granulated vesicles of the rat brain. Z. Zellforsch. **76**, 100—107 (1967).
Hashimoto, Y., Ishii, S., Ohi, Y., Imaizumi, R.: The effects of DOPA on the norepinephrine and dopamine contents and on the granulated vesicles of the hypothalamus of reserpinized rats. Jap. J. Pharmacol. **15**, 395—400 (1965).
Heacock, R.A.: The aminochromes. Advan. Heterocyclic Chem. **5**, 205—257 (1965).

HÖKFELT, T.: Electron microscopic observations on nerve terminals in the intrinsic muscles of the albino rat iris. Acta physiol. scand. **67**, 255—256 (1966a).
— The effect of reserpine on the intraneuronal vesicles of the rat vas deferens. Experientia (Basel) **22**, 56 (1966b).
— Electron microscopic studies on brain slices from regions rich in catecholamine nerve terminals. Acta physiol. scand. **69**, 119—120 (1967a).
— The possible ultrastructural identification of tubero-infundibular dopamine-containing nerve endings in the median eminence of the rat. Brain Res. **5**, 121—123 (1967b).
— Ultrastructural studies on adrenergic nerve terminals in the albino rat iris after pharmacological and experimental treatment. Acta physiol. scand. **69**, 125—126 (1967c).
— On the ultrastructural localization of noradrenaline in the central nervous system of the rat. Z. Zellforsch. **79**, 110—117 (1967d).
— Electron microscopic studies on peripheral and central monoamine neurons, Tryckerielaget Ivar Haeggstrom A.B. Stockholm: Doctoral Thesis 1968a.
— In vitro studies on central and peripheral monoamine neurons at the ultrastructural level. Z. Zellforsch. **91**, 1—74 (1968b).
— Distribution of noradrenaline storing particles in peripheral adrenergic neurons as revealed by electron microscopy. Acta physiol. scand. **76**, 427—440 (1969).
— JONSSON, G.: Studies on reaction and binding of monoamines after fixation and processing for electron microscopy with special reference to fixation with potassium permanganate. Histochemie **16**, 45—67 (1968).
— UNGERSTEDT, U.: Electron and fluorescence microscopical studies on the nucleus caudatus putamen of the rat after unilateral lesions of ascending nigro-neostriatal dopamine neurons. Acta physiol. scand. **76**, 415—426 (1969).
HOLTZMAN, E., DOMINITZ, R.: Cytochemical studies of lysosomes, Golgi apparatus and endoplasmic reticulum in secretion and protein uptake by adrenal medulla cells of the rat. J. Histochem. Cytochem. **16**, 320—336 (1968).
HOPSU, V.K., MAKINNEN, E.O.: Two methods for demonstration of noradrenaline-containing adrenal medullary cells. J. Histochem. Cytochem. **14**, 434—435 (1966).
ISHII, S.: Morphological studies on the distribution and properties of the granulated vesicles in the brain. Arch. Histol. Jap. **28**, 355—376 (1967).
— SHIMIZU, N., MATSUOKA, M., IMAIZUMI, R.: Correlation between catecholamine content and numbers of granulated vesicles in rabbit hypothalamus. Biochem. Pharmacol. **14**, 183—184 (1965).
IVERSEN, L.L.: The uptake and storage of noradrenaline in sympathetic nerves. Cambridge: Univ. Press 1967.
JAIM-ETCHEVERRY, G., ZIEHER, L.M.: Selective demonstration of a type of synaptic vesicle by phosphotungstic acid staining. J. Cell Biol. **42**, 855—860 (1969).
— — Ultrastructural aspects of neurotransmitter storage in adrenergic nerves. Proc. 1st Intl. Symp. on Cell Biol. and Cytopharmacol. (in press).
KAPELLER, K., MAYOR, D.: An electron microscopic study of the early changes proximal to a constriction in sympathetic nerves. Proc. Roy. Soc. B. **172**, 39—51 (1969).
KIRSHNER, N., SAGE, H.J., SMITH, W.J.: Mechanism of secretion from the adrenal medulla. II. Release of catecholamines and storage vesicle protein in response to chemical stimulation. Mol. Pharmacol. **3**, 254—265 (1965).
KOBAYASHI, H., HIRANO, T., OOTA, Y.: Electron microscopic and pharmacological studies on the median eminence and pars nervosa. Archives d'Anatomie Microscopique **54**, 277—294 (1965).
LEGG, P.G.: The fine structure and innervation of the beta and delta cells in the islet of Langerhans of the cat. Z. Zellforsch. **80**, 307—321 (1967).
LENARD, J., SINGER, S.J.: Alteration of the conformation of proteins in red blood cell membranes and in solution by fixatives used in electron microscopy. J. Cell Biol. **37**, 117—121 (1968).
LENN, N.J.: Electron microscopic observations on monoamine-containing brain stem neurons in normal and drug treated rats. Anat. Record **153**, 399—406 (1965).
— Localization of uptake of tritiated norepinephrine by rat brain in vivo and in vitro using electron microscopy. Amer. J. Anat. **120**, 377—389 (1967).
LEVER, J.D., SPRIGGS, T.L.B., GRAHAM, J.D.P.: A formol-fluorescence, fine-structural and autoradiographic study of the adrenergic innervation of the vascular tree in the intact and sympathectomized pancreas of the cat. J. Anat. **101**, 15—33 (1968).
MACHADO, A.B.M.: Straight OsO_4 versus glutaraldehyde-OsO_4 in sequence as fixatives for the granular vesicles in sympathetic axons of the rat pineal body. Stain Technol. **42**, 293—300 (1967).
MANCINI, G., FRONTALI, N.: On the ultrastructural localization of catecholamines in the beta lobes (Corpora Pedunculata) of *Periplaneta americana*. Z. Zellforsch. **103**, 341—350 (1970).

Matsuoka, M., Ishii, S., Shimizu, N., Imaizumi, R.: Effect of WIN 18501—2 on the content of catecholamine containing granules in the rabbit hypothalamus. Experientia (Basel) **21**, 1—5 (1965).
Matthews, M.R., Raisman, G.: The ultrastructure and somatic efferent synapses of small granule-containing cells in the superior cervical ganglion. J. Anat. **105**, 255—282 (1969).
Merrillees, N.C.R.: The nervous environment of individual smooth muscle cells in the guinea pig vas deferens. J. Cell Biol. **37**, 794—818 (1968).
Michaelson, I.A.: The subcellular distribution of acetylcholine, choline acetyltransferase, and acetyl cholinesterase in nerve tissue. Ann. N.Y. Acad. Sci. **144**, 387—410 (1967).
— Taylor, P.W., Richardson, K.C., Titus, E.: Uptake and metabolism of d,l,norepinephrine by subcellular particles of rat heart. J. Pharmacol. exp. Ther. **160**, 277—291 (1968).
Monroe, B.G.: A comparative study of the ultrastructure of the median eminence, infundibular stem, and neural lobe of the hypophysis of the rat. Z. Zellforsch. **76**, 405—432 (1967).
Neff, N.H., Barrett, R.E., Costa, E.: Kinetic and fluorescent histochemical analysis of the serotonin compartments in rat pineal gland. Europ. J. Pharmacol. **5**, 348—356 (1969).
Nishida, S., Trotter, J., Sears, M.L.: Innervation of the chamber angle of the guinea pig eye. Exp. Eye Res. **8**, 143—146 (1969).
Ochi, J., Konishi, M., Yoshikawa, H.: Morphologischer Nachweis der sympathischen Innervation des braunen Fettgewebes bei der Ratte. Z. Anat. Entwickl.-Gesch. **129**, 259—267 (1969).
Pearse, A.G.E.: Histochemistry, theoretical and applied, 2nd ed. Boston, Mass: Little Brown and Co. 1961.
Pellegrino de Iraldi, Duggan, F., de Robertis, E.: Adrenergic synaptic vesicles in the anterior hypothalamus of the rat. Anat. Record. **145**, 521—531 (1963).
— Gueudet, R.: Catecholamines and serotonin in granulated vesicles of nerve endings in the pineal gland of the rat. Int. J. Neuropharmacol. **8**, 9 (1969).
— Jaim-Etcheverry, G.: Ultrastructural changes in the nerve endings of the median eminence after nialamide-DOPA administration. Brain Res. **6**, 614—618 (1967a).
— — Granulated vesicles in retinal synapses and neurons. Z. Zellforsch. **81**, 283—296 (1967b).
Pellegrino de Iraldi, A., de Robertis, E.: Action of reserpine on the submicroscopic morphology of the pineal gland. Experientia (Basel) **17**, 122—123 (1961).
— — Action of reserpine, iproniazid and pyrogallol on nerve endings of the pineal gland. Int. J. Neuropharmacol. **2**, 231—239 (1963).
— — Ultrastructure and function of catecholamine containing systems. Proc. 2nd Int. Congr. Endocrinology **83**, 355—363 (1964).
— Zieher, L.M., de Robertis, E.: Ultrastructure and pharmacological studies of nerve endings in the pineal organ. Prog. Brain Res. **10**, 389—421 (1965).
Pfeiffer, A.K., Szato, S., Polkouits, M., Okros, I.: Correlation between noradrenaline content of the brain and the number of granular vesicles in rat hypothalamus during nialamid administration. Exp. Brain Res. **5**, 79—86 (1968).
Pick, J., de Lemos, C., Cranella, A.: Fine structure of nerve terminals in the human gut. Anat. Record. **159**, 131—146 (1967).
Potter, L.T.: Role of intraneuronal vesicles in the synthesis, storage and release of noradrenaline. Circulation Res. Suppl. III, 13—24 (1967).
Raisman, G.: Neuronal plasticity in the septal nuclei of the adult cat. Brain Res. **14**, 25—48 (1969).
Richards, J.G., Tranzer, J.P.: The ultrastructural localization of amine storage sites in the central nervous system with the aid of a specific marker, 5-hydroxydopamine. Brain Res. **17**, 463—470 (1970).
Richardson, K.C.: Electromicroscopic observations on Auerbach's plexus in the rabbit with special reference to the problem of smooth muscle innervation. Amer. J. Anat. **103**, 99—136 (1958).
— The fine structure of autonomic nerve endings of the rat vas deferens. J. Anat. **96**, 427—442 (1962).
— The fine structure of tissues following isolation in oxygenated saline for prolonged periods. Anat. Rec. **145**, 275 (1963).
— The fine structure of the albino rabbit iris with special reference to the identification of adrenergic and cholinergic nerves and nerve endings in its intrinsic muscles. Amer. J. Anat. **114**, 173—206 (1964).
— Electron microscopic identification of autonomic nerve endings. Nature (Lond.) **210**, 756 (1966).
Riley, V., Fortner, J.G.: The pigment cell: Molecular, biological and clinical aspects. Ann. N.Y. Acad. Sci. **100**, 1—13 (1963).
Rinne, U.K.: Ultrastructure of the median eminence of the rat. Z. Zellforsch. **74**, 98—122 (1966).

ROTH, C.D., RICHARDSON, K.C.: Electron microscopical studies on axonal degeneration in the rat iris following ganglionectomy. Am. J. Anat. **124**, 341—360 (1969).

ROTH, R.H., STJÄRNE, L., BLOOM, F.E., GIARMAN, N.J.: Light and heavy norepinephrine storage particles in the rat heart and in bovine splenic nerve. J. Pharmacol. exp. Ther. **162**, 203—212 (1968).

RUSKELL, G.L.: Vasomotor axons of the lacrimal glands of monkeys and the ultrastructural identification of sympathetic terminals. Z. Zellforsch. **83**, 321—333 (1967).

SABATINI, D.D., BENSCH, K.G., BARRNETT, R.J.: Cytochemistry and electron microscopy. The preservation of cellular ultrastructure and enzymatic activity. J. Cell Biol. **17**, 19—58 (1963).

SALPETER, M.M., BACHMANN, L., SALPETER, E.E.: Resolution in electron microscope radioautography. J. Cell Biol. **41**, 1—20 (1969).

SCHÜMANN, H.J., SCHMIDT, K., PHILIPPU, A.: Storage of norepinephrine in sympathetic ganglia. Life Sci. **5**, 1809—1815 (1966).

SHIMIZU, U., ISHII, S.: Electron microscopic observation of catecholamine-containing granules in the hypothalamus and area postrema and their changes following reserpine injection. Arch. Histol. Jap. **24**, 489—497 (1965).

SHORR, S.S., BLOOM, F.E.: Fine structure of islet-cell innervation in the pancreas of normal and alloxan-treated rats. Z. Zellforsch. **103**, 12—25 (1970).

SIEGRIST, G., DOLIVO, M., DUNANT, Y., FOROGLOV-KERAMEUS, C., DE RIBAUPIERRE, F., ROULLIER, C.: Ultrastructure and function of the chromaffin cells in the superior cervical ganglion of the rat. J. Ultrastruct. Res. **25**, 381—407 (1968).

SIGGINS, G.R., BLOOM, F.E.: Structure-function relationship of neurovascular control after 6-hydroxydopamine. Pharmacologist **11**, 263 (1969).

— — Cytochemical and physiological effects of 6-hydroxydopamine on peri-arteriolar nerves. Circulation Res. (1970).

SJÖQVIST, F., TITUS, E., MICHAELSON, I.A., TAYLOR, P., RICHARDSON, K.C.: Uptake and metabolism of d,l norepinephrine-7-H^3 in tissues of immunosympathectomized mice and rats. Life Sci. **4**, 1125—1133 (1965).

SOLCIA, E., SAMPIETRO, R., CAPELLA, C.: Differential staining of catecholamines, 5-hydroxytryptamine and related compounds in aldehyde-fixed tissues. Histochemie **17**, 273—283 (1969).

STJÄRNE, L.: Storage particles in noradrenergic tissues. Pharmacol. Rev. **18**. 425—432 (1966).

— ROTH, R.H., BLOOM, F.E., GIARMAN, N.J.: Norepinephrine concentrating mechanisms in sympathetic nerve trunks. J. Pharmacol. exp. Ther. **171**, 70—79 (1970).

TAXI, J.: Etude au microscope électronique de ganglions sympathétiques de grenouille. Bull. Ass. Anat. (Nancy) **47**, 794—798 (1961).

— Contribution a l'étude des connexions des neurones moteurs du système nerveux autonome. Annal. Sci. Natur. (Zool.) 12e gérie **7**. 413—674 (1965).

— Sur la fixation et la signification du contenu dense des vesicules des fibres adrénergiques étudiées au microscope électronique. Comp. Rend. Acad. Bulgare Sci. **21**, 1229—1231 (1968).

— Morphological and cytochemical studies on the synapses in the autonomic nervous system. Progr. Brain Res. **31**, 5—20 (1969).

— DROZ, B.: Étude de l'incorporation de noradrénaline-^{3}H (NA-^{3}H) et de 5-hydroxytryptophane-^{3}H (5-HTP-^{3}H) dans l'epiphyse et le ganglion cervical supérieur. C.R. Acad. Sci. (Paris) **263**, 1326—1329 (1966a).

— — Étude de l'incorporation de noradrénaline-^{3}H (NA-^{3}H) et de 5-hydroxytryptophane (5-HTP-^{3}H) dans les fibres nerveuses du canal déférent et de l'intestin. C.R. Acad. Sci. (Paris) **263**, 1237—1240 (1966b).

— — Radioautographic studies of the accumulation of some biogenic amines in the autonomic nervous system. In: Dynamics of the Neuron, S. BARONDES, ed. New York: Academic Press (in press).

THAEMERT, J.C.: Ultrastructural interrelationships of nerve processes and smooth muscle cells in three dimensions. J. Cell Biol. **28**, 37—49 (1966).

THOENEN, H., TRANZER, J.P.: Chemical sympathectomy by selective destruction of adrenergic nerve endings with 6-hydroxydopamine. Naunyn-Schmiedeberg's Arch. Pharmak. exp. Path. **261**, 271—288 (1968).

TRAMEZZANI, H.H., CHIOCCHIO, S.R., WASSERMAN, J.H.: A technique for light and electron microscopic identification of adrenalin and noradrenalin storing cells. J. Histochem. Cytochem. **12**, 890—899 (1964).

TRANZER, J.P., SNIPES, R.L.: Fine structural localization of noradrenaline in sympathetic nerve terminals: a critical study of the influence of fixation. In: Fourth European Regional Conference on Electron Microscopy, Rome 519 (1968).

Tranzer, J.P., Thoenen, H.: Electron microscopic localization of 5-hydroxydopamine (3,4,5-trihydroxyphenyl-ethylamine), a new "false" sympathetic transmitter. Experientia (Basel) **23**, 743—745 (1967a).

— — Ultramorphologische Veränderungen der sympathischen Nervenendigungen der Katze nach Vorbehandlung mit 5- und 6-Hydroxy-Dopamin. Naunyn-Schmiedeberg's Arch. Pharmak. exp. Path. **257**, 343—344, (1967b).

— — An electron microscopic study of selective acute degeneration of sympathetic nerve terminals after administration of 6-hydroxydopamine. Experientia (Basel) **24**, 155—156 (1968a).

— — Various types of amine-storing vesicles in peripheral adrenergic nerve terminals. Experientia (Basel) **24**, 484—485 (1968b).

— — Snipes, R.L., Richards, J.G.: Recent developments on the ultrastructural aspects of adrenergic nerve endings in various experimental conditions. Progr. Brain Res. **31**, 33—46 (1969).

Uretsky, N.J., Iversen, L.L.: Effects of 6-hydroxydopamine on noradrenaline-containing neurones in the rat brain. Nature (Lond.) **221**, 557 (1969).

Van Orden, L.S., Bensch, K.G., Giarman, N.J.: Histochemical and functional relationships of catecholamines in adrenergic nerve endings. II. Extravesicular norepinephrine. J. Pharmacol. exp. Ther. **155**, 428—439 (1967a).

— — Langer, S.Z., Trendelenburg, U.: Histochemical and fine structural aspects of the onset of denervation supersensitivity in the nictitating membrane of the spinal cat. J. Pharmacol. exp. Ther. **157**, 274—283 (1967b).

— Bloom, F.E., Barrnett, R.J., Giarman, N.J.: Histochemical and functional relationships of catecholamines in adrenergic nerve endings. I. Participation of granular vesicles. J. Pharmacol. exp. Ther. **154**, 185—199 (1966).

— Schaefer, J.M., Burke, J.P.: Identification of two norepinephrine storage compartments in nerve terminals by histochemistry and electron microscopy. Pharmacologist **11**, 178 (1969).

Wartenberg, H., Baumgarten, H.G.: Über die elektronenmikroskopische Identifizierung von noradrenergen Nervenfasern durch 5-Hydroxydopamin und 5-Hydroxydopa im Pinealorgan der Eidechse *(Lacerta muralis)*. Z. Zellforsch. **94**, 252—260 (1969).

Whittaker, V.P.: Catecholamine storage particles in the central nervous system. Pharmacol. Rev. **18**, 401—412 (1966).

Williams, T.H.: Electron microscopic evidence for an autonomic interneuron. Nature (Lond.) **214**, 309—310 (1967).

Wolfe, D.E.: The epiphyseal cell: An electron microscopic study of its intercellular relationships and intracellular morphology in the pineal body of the albino rat. Progr. Brain Res. **10**, 332—376 (1965).

— Potter, L.T., Richardson, K.C., Axelrod, J.: Localizing tritiated norepinephrine in sympathetic axons by electron microscope autoradiography. Science **138**, 440—442 (1962).

— — Localization of norepinephrine in the atrial myocardium. Anat. Rec. **145**, 301 (1963).

Wood, J.G.: Electron microscopic localization of amines in central nervous tissue. Nature (Lond.) **209**, 1131—1133 (1966).

— Barrnett, R.J.: Histochemical demonstration of norepinephrine at a fine structural level. J. Histochem. Cytochem. **12**, 197—209 (1964).

Zambrano, D.: The effect of nialamide and L-DOPA on the synaptic endings of the neurosecretory neurons of the supraoptic nucleus of the rat. Neuroendocrinology **3**, 99—106 (1968).

Zapata, P., Hess, A., Bliss, E.L., Eyzaguirre, C.: Chemical, electron microscopic and physiological observations on the role of catecholamines in the carotid body. Brain Res. **14**, 473—496 (1969).

Chapter 4

Catecholamines in the Invertebrates

JOHN H. WELSH

With 10 Figures

I. Introduction

There are a number of reasons for the rapidly growing interest in the distribution of catecholamines in the invertebrates. Most important among these is the availability of new methods for the isolation, identification, and assay of the individual amines, and for their cellular localization. In applying these newer methods, most workers have been attempting to answer one or more of the following questions: 1. How general is the occurrence of catecholamines throughout the animal kingdom? 2. How are they distributed in different organs, tissues and cells? 3. How do their relative amounts compare in different animal phyla? 4. How does the distribution of the catecholamines compare with that of 5-hydroxytryptamine (5-HT)? 5. What are the functional roles of the catecholamines in the invertebrates? 6. Will a study of their modes of action in the invertebrates aid in an understanding of their modes of action in the vertebrates?

This chapter will review the available literature that deals with the identification and estimation of levels of individual catecholamines in various whole animals, in nervous systems of representative species of the major invertebrate phyla, and in a few non-nervous tissues or their products. Dopamine will be shown to be the dominant catecholamine in the invertebrates, with noradrenaline usually present in smaller amounts and adrenaline generally absent or, if demonstrable, present only in trace amounts. A second aim will be to review the studies on the cellular localization of catecholamines as revealed by the fluorescence histochemical method of FALCK and HILLARP. This highly useful method has shown that catecholamines of the invertebrates are found principally in their nervous systems and in neurones that often may be identified as sensory, internuncial, motor, or „modulator" (i. e., having a neurohormonal role).

Our knowledge of the formation, storage, release, and destruction or removal of catecholamines in the invertebrates is less complete than is our knowledge of these events in the vertebrates, or at least in the mammals, hence these aspects will receive less attention. Likewise, the functional roles of the catecholamines in the invertebrates are still poorly understood. However, there is growing evidence that dopamine may act as a neurotransmitter. Some of this evidence will be set forth.

Rather than deal in turn with each of these several topics (i. e., quantitative levels, cellular distribution, metabolism, and function) and discuss all of the invertebrate phyla under each topic, it appears desirable to organize the material by individual phyla. This has certain advantages. It recognizes the great diversity of the invertebrates and the probable relationships between the phyla. Assuming that these relationships are somewhat as indicated in Fig. 1, any striking differences seen between phyla might reflect their phylogenetic history and level of organization. For example, the arthropods are certainly more highly evolved and specialized than are the coelenterates or flatworms, while the annelids and molluscs are rather closely related phyla. However, there are so many "missing links" among present-day invertebrates that it is impossible to determine whether a given biochemical system, such as the catecholamine system has been "handed on" from phylum to phylum, or has evolved *de novo* a number of times in different phyla. Regardless of the problem of relationships among the invertebrates, we shall see that one or more of the catecholamines has been found in representatives of most of the major phyla. The minor invertebrate phyla (not shown in Fig. 1) have yet to be examined for the possible presence of catecholamines.

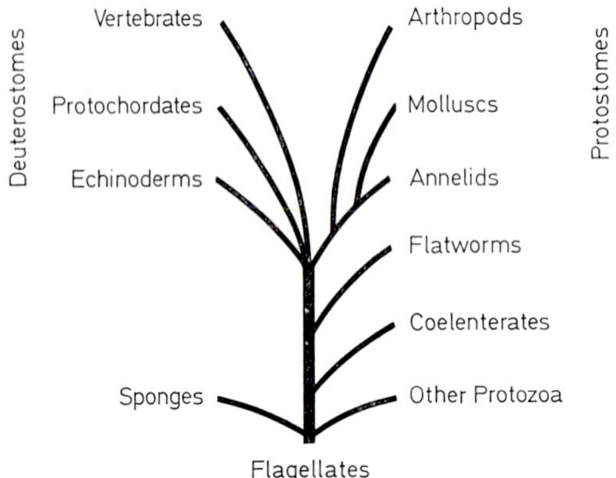

Fig. 1. A schema showing the probable relationships of the major groups of invertebrates discussed in this review

At the time this chapter was written, some 50 species of invertebrates belonging to 10 of the major phyla had been examined for their content of catecholamines, either of whole animals or of various parts, especially nervous tissues. The data are summarized in Table 1. The more reliable identifications of the individual catecholamines are those obtained by the more recently developed methods for extracting and concentrating the amines that include adsorption on alumina, followed by elution and chromatography. The more recent estimates of levels of the catecholamines have been made by spectrofluorometry or, when restricted by the small amount of available tissue, by quantitative thin layer chromatography.

The fluorescence-histochemical method of FALCK and HILLARP (see FALCK, 1962; FALCK and OWMAN, 1965; CORRODI and JONSSON, 1967) for visualizing cells that contain catecholamines or 5-HT has been used with much success in studies on a variety of fresh water and terrestial invertebrates. Tissues of marine animals are less suited for this method if freezedried before exposure to formaldehyde vapors, infiltration and sectioning. This is presumably due to the high salt content of the dried tissue. However, satisfactory results have been obtained with tissues that can be dried, treated, and examined as whole mounts (e. g., COOKE and GOLDSTONE, 1970), or frozen and sectioned before drying and subsequent exposure to formaldehyde vapors (e.g., COTTRELL and PENTREATH, 1970).

A rather good correlation is generally seen between the levels of monoamines obtained for a given invertebrate tissue and the numbers of nerve cells and fibres showing a fluorescence characteristic for catecholamines (green) or 5-HT (yellow). Examples of this will be cited.

Table 1. *The quantitative distribution of catecholamines in some representative invertebrates*

Phylum and Species	Tissue	Dopamine	Noradrenaline	Adrenaline	Method of Assay	Reference
			μg/g wet tissue*			
PROTOZOA						
Crithidia fasiculata	whole animals	n.d.**	0.1—0.2	n.d.	Fluorometry	Janakidevi et al. (1966)
Tetrahymena pyriformis . .	whole animals	n.d.	0.25—0.35	0.13—0.15	Fluorometry	Janakidevi et al. (1966)
Spirostomum sp.	whole animals	—	n.d.	—	S.F.***	Applewhite et al. (1969)
COELENTERATA						
Actinia equina	whole animals	14.1 ± 5.5 ng/g	4.7 ± 0.6 ng/g	< 0.2 ng/g	S.F.	Carlyle (1969a)
PLATYHELMINTHES						
Dugesia tigrina	whole animals	1.3	0.9	n.d.	chromatrogaphy	Welsh and King (1970)
Procotyla fluviatilis	whole animals	1.5	n.d.	n.d.	chromatography	Welsh and King (1970)
Procotyla fluviatilis	whole animals	0.6; 1.7	n.d.; 0.2	n.d.	S.F.	Sweeney (pers. comm.)
ANNELIDA						
Lumbricus terrestris	nerve cord	—	0.32	1.4	bioassay	Östlund (1954)
Lumbricus terrestris	nerve cord	3.0	1.5	n.d.	chromatography	Rude (1969a)
Lumbricus terrestris	nerve cord	3.0; 3.8	—	—	S.F.	Stephens and Welsh (unpublished)
Lumbricus terrestris	nerve cord	"trace"	NA+A < 1.0		?	Myhrberg (1967)
Lumbricus terrestris	"brain"	—	NA+A 2.0		?	Myhrberg (1967)
Hirudo medicinalis	nerve cord	1.9	1.0	—	S.F.	Stephens and Welsh (unpublished)
Hirudo medicinalis	nerve cord	n.d.	n.d.	—	S.F.	Marsden and Kerkut (1969)
Golfingia (= Phascolosoma) sp.	brain and nerve cord	4.5	—	—	S.F.	Stephens and Welsh (unpublished)

* Unless otherwise indicated.
** n.d. = none detected.
*** S.F. = spectrofluorometry.

Table 1 (continued)

Phylum and Species	Tissue	Dopamine	Noradrenaline	Adrenaline	Method of Assay	Reference
MOLLUSCA						
Class Gastropoda						
Helix pomatia	cerebral ganglia	7.25	n.d.	n.d.	S.F.	DAHL et al. (1962, 1966)
Helix pomatia	nerve ring	2—4	—	—	—	CARDOT (1963)
Helix pomatia	"brain"	5.5	n.d.	n.d.	S.F.	SEDDEN et al. (1968)
Helix pomatia	"brain"	6	0.08	—	chromatography and bioassay	OSBORNE and COTTRELL (1970)
Helix pomatia	heart	0.5	0.75—1	—	chromatography and bioassay	OSBORNE and COTTRELL (1970)
Helix aspersa	"brain"	5.5	n.d.	n.d.	S.F.	SEDDEN et al. (1968)
Planorbis corneus	"brain"	9.53	n.d.	—	S.F.	MARSDEN and KERKUT (1970)
Melongena corona	ganglion ring	63	n.d.	n.d.	S.F.	SWEENEY (1963)
Lunatia heros	ganglion ring	27	n.d.	n.d.	S.F.	SWEENEY (1963)
Busycon canaliculatum	ganglion ring	14	n.d.	n.d.	S.F.	SWEENEY (1963)
Buccinum undatum	cerebral gang.	17.3	n.d.	n.d.	S.F.	DAHL et al. (1966)
Buccinum undatum	optic tentacles	"trace"	—	—	S.F.	DAHL et al. (1966)
Class Pelecypoda						
Mercenaria mercenaria	pooled ganglia	261	n.d.	n.d.	S.F.	SWEENEY (1963)
Mercenaria mercenaria	pooled ganglia	22	n.d.	n.d.	S.F.	KERKUT et al. (1966)
Spisula solida	pooled ganglia	40—50	5—6	n.d.	chromatography and S.F.	COTTRELL (1967)
Spisula solida	visceral ganglia	80	—	—	chromatography and S.F.	COTTRELL (1968)

Table 1 (continued)

Phylum and Species	Tissue	Dopamine	Noradrenaline	Adrenaline	Method of Assay	Reference
Spisula solida	cerebral ganglia	80	—	—	chromatography and S.F.	COTTRELL (1968)
Spisula solida	pedal ganglia	195	—	—	chromatography and S.F.	COTTRELL (1968)
Spisula solidissima	pooled ganglia	26	n.d.	n.d.	S.F.	SWEENEY (1963)
Mytilus edulis	pooled ganglia	35	n.d.	n.d.	S.F.	SWEENEY (1963)
Modiolus modiolus	pooled ganglia	85	n.d.	n.d.	S.F.	SWEENEY (1963)
Ensis directus	pooled ganglia	37	n.d.	n.d.	S.F.	SWEENEY (1963)
Mya arenaria	pooled ganglia	96	n.d.	n.d.	S.F.	SWEENEY (1963)
Aequipecten irradians	pooled ganglia	74	n.d.	n.d.	S.F.	SWEENEY (1963)
Anodonta piscinalis	cerebral ganglia	11.6	—	—	S.F.	DAHL et al. (1966)
Anodonta piscinalis	visceral ganglia	19.2	—	—	S.F.	DAHL et al. (1966)
Anadonta piscinalis	pedal ganglia	47.2	—	—	S.F.	DAHL et al. (1966)
Sphaerium sulcatum	whole animals	5.2 ± 1.6 ng/animal	3.5 ± 1.2 ng/animal	n.d.	S.F.	SWEENEY (1968)
Class Cephalopoda						
Eledone cirrhosa	"brain"	8—13	2—5	n.d.	chromatography and S.F.	COTTRELL (1967)
Octopus vulgaris	salivary glands	n.d.	1—3	n.d.	chromatography and bioassay	v. EULER (1953)
ARTHROPODA						
Class Crustacea						
Carcinus maenas	ganglia	0.5—1.0	< 0.5	n.d.	chromatography and S.F.	COTTRELL (1967)
Hyas araneus	ganglia	< 0.5	< 0.5	n.d.	chromatography and S.F.	COTTRELL (1967)

Table 1 (continued)

Phylum and Species	Tissue	Dopamine	Noradrenaline	Adrenaline	Method of Assay	References
Class Insecta						
Tenebrio molitor (larvae)	whole	10—15	1.3; 2.2	0.01; 0.061	bioassay	Östlund (1954)
Tenebrio molitor (adults)	whole	2—4	1.1	0.15	bioassay	Östlund (1954)
Tenebrio molitor (larvae)	ant. portion	1—4	0.011; 0.05	0.15; 0.18	bioassay	Östlund (1954)
Tenebrio molitor (adults)	post. portion	10—15	0.93; 0.94	0.093; 0.094	bioassay	Östlund (1954)
Apis mellifica (worker)	whole adults	5—10	0.75	0.05	bioassay	Östlund (1954)
Apis mellifica (worker)	whole larvae	2—4	0.3	< 0.01	bioassay	Östlund (1954)
Pieris brassicae	whole larvae	—	0.33	< 0.005	Fluorometry	v. Euler (1961)
Periplaneta americana	head ganglia	2.5 ± 0.6	0.37 ± 0.04	—	S.F.	Frontali and Häggendal (1969)
Acheta domesticus	developing eggs at 156 hrs.	93.5	—	—	S.F.	Furneaux and McFarlane (1965a)
ECHINODERMATA						
Asterias rubens	radial nerves	3—8	0.5—2	n.d.	chromatography and S.F.	Cottrell (1967)
Echinus esculentus	radial nerves	2.5—7	1.5—3.5	n.d.	chromatography and S.F.	Cottrell (1967)
UROCHORDATA						
Ciona intestinalis	whole animals	—	< 0.005	< 0.003	Fluorometry	v. Euler (1961)
CEPHALOCHORDATA						
Branchiostoma lanceolatum	whole animals	—	0.16	< 0.005	Fluorometry	v. Euler (1961)

Some of the early literature on the occurrence of adrenaline or an adrenaline-like substance in the invertebrates was reviewed by HANSTRÖM (1939). More recent reviews of invertebrate pharmacology (CRESCITELLI and GEISSMAN, 1962; COTTRELL and LAVERACK, 1968) contain sections on the catecholamines. The first extensive study of catecholamines in invertebrates and lower vertebrates was by ÖSTLUND (1954), but in this study most extracts were made from entire animals.

Note added in proof: For the isolation of arterenone from the sclerotized cuticle of the desert locust and other insects see:

ANDERSEN, S. O.: Isolation of arterenone (2-amino-3′,4′-hydroxyacetophenone) from hydrolysates of sclerotized insect cuticle. J. Insect Physiol. **16**, 1951—1959 (1970).

— BARRETT, F. M.: The isolation of ketocatechols from insect cuticle and their possible role in sclerotization. J. Insect Physiol. **17**, 69—83 (1971).

II. Catecholamines in the Major Invertebrate Phyla

1. Protozoa

Only a few species of protozoans have been examined for the possible presence of catecholamines. BAYER and WENSE (1936) claimed that extracts from *Paramecium* contained a sympathomimetic substance that, in biological tests, and from certain of its chemical properties, appeared to be adrenaline. An extract of the marine flagellate, *Noctiluca miliaris*, when assayed on the fowl's rectal caecum appeared to contain an adrenaline-like substance (ÖSTLUND, 1954). Using a fluorometric assay, JANAKIDEVI et al. (1966) found noradrenaline and adrenaline in extracts of the ciliate, *Tetrahymena pyriformis*, but only noradrenaline in *Crithidia fasciculata*, a ciliate protozoan (Table 1). DOPA and dopamine were not found. These authors found that labelled phenylalanine, tyrosine and dihydroxyphenylalanine were incorporated into the catecholamines of *Tetrahymena* but only the latter two into the noradrenaline of *Crithidia*.

BLUM (1967) has shown that certain drugs known to act on the catecholamine system affect growth and glycogen metabolism in *Tetrahymena*. The effect of reserpine on growth and catecholamine content of *Tetrahymena* has also been studied (BLUM et al., 1966).

APPLEWHITE et al. (1969) could detect no noradrenaline in *Spirostomum*.

The occurrence of catecholamines in protozoans is of considerable interest in view of the primitive nature of this group and the relationships of certain of its members (the chlorophyll-containing flagellates) with the algae. Catecholamines are known to be present in several plants and fruits (e.g., UDENFRIEND et al., 1959) and it is conceivable that the protozoans "inherited" the catecholamine system from plant-like ancestors from which they arose. Additional protozoans should be examined for the possible presence of catecholamines.

2. Porifera (Sponges)

An indication of the possible presence of catecholamines in sponges is given by the histochemical study by LENTZ (1966) of *Sycon (Scypha) ciliatum*. Certain mesenchymal cells were found to react in a manner suggesting the presence of adrenaline; others appeared to contain noradrenaline; and some cells were found that reacted in a manner characteristic for monoamine oxidase.

Further study of the sponges, using more specific methods for identifying the catecholamines, will be required to make more certain their presence in members of this phylum.

3. Coelenterata

This phylum includes the radially symmetrical animals such as hydra, sea anemones, and jelly fish. It is characterized by the presence of nematocysts (stinging organelles) that inject a paralyzing venom into the prey and by the presence of the most primitive of present-day nervous systems. Numerous sensory cells are present, especially in tentacles, and a "nerve net" with mostly nonpolarized synapses is a characteristic feature of the coelenterate nervous system.

Further anatomical and functional details concerning coelenterate and other invertebrate nervous systems may be found in the monumental treatise — *Structure and Function in the Nervous Systems of Invertebrates* by BULLOCK and HORRIDGE (1965).

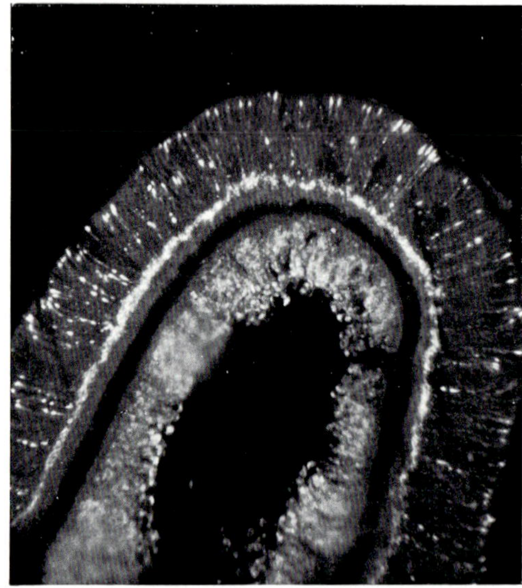

Fig. 2. Longitudinal section through the distal part of a tentacle of *Metridium senile*, showing the green-fluorescing sensory neurones as revealed by the method of FALCK and HILLARP for catecholamines. [From Fig. 1C, DAHL, E. et al., Quart. J. micr. Sci. **104**, 531 (1963a)]

One of the earliest applications of the histochemical fluorescence method of FALCK and HILLARP in a study of invertebrates was that by DAHL et al. (1963a and b) on certain coelenterates. They found in the tentacles of two sea anemones, *Metridium senile* and *Tealia felina*, numerous sensory cells (or possibly sensory-motor neurones) that exhibited a green fluorescence after freeze-drying and treatment with formaldehyde gas (Fig. 2). The conditions of the reaction suggested the presence of primary catecholamines rather than adrenaline. In the hydrozoan, *Hydractinia echinata*, no fluorescent neurones were found.

Using histochemical methods other than that of FALCK and HILLARP, catecholamine-containing neurones have been reported by WOOD and LENTZ (1964) to be present in *Hydra littoralis* and *Metridium senile*. Reference to a paper by PLOTNIKOVA and GOVYRIN (1966) on catecholamine-containing nervous elements in coelenterates and certain other invertebrates is cited by KLEMM (1968a).

Identifiable catecholamines were not detected on chromatograms of extracts of three species of coelenterates, including *Metridium*, by ÖSTLUND (1954). However, CARLYLE (1969a) has identified DOPA, dopamine and noradrenaline in extracts of the sea anemone, *Actinia equina*. The levels in whole body extracts were found to be low (Table 1). This would be expected if these substances are present mainly in sensory cells of the tentacles.

Pharmacological studies of muscle preparations of the anemones, *Calliactis parasitica* and *Metridium senile*, by Ross (1960a and b) failed to show any clear evidence for an adrenergic innervation of these muscles. CARLYLE (1969b), likewise, failed to obtain any direct evidence for the involvement of catecholamines in the responses of an isolated muscle preparation from *Actinia equina*. However, CARLYLE did observe changes in excitability of whole *Actinia* after treatment with reserpine and reports that these changes, in many experiments, could be reversed by noradrenaline and dopamine. These pharmacological findings of Ross and of CARLYLE might be explained by a restricted localization of catecholamines to sensory cells in sea anemones.

4. Platyhelminthes (Flatworms)

This phylum includes the free-living flatworms (Turbellaria), the parasitic flukes (Trematoda), and the tapeworms (Cestoda). It is the most primitive group of bilaterally symmetrical animals and the first to show centralization and cephalization of the nervous system. The triclad turbellarians (planarians) are among the more widely studied invertebrates. Their nervous system is more advanced than that of the coelenterates and many basic neuronal features of the higher invertebrates and the vertebrates are seen in their diverse types of neurones (see BULLOCK and HORRIDGE, 1965).

DAHL et al. (1963a and b) made brief mention of finding adrenergic sensory neurones in turbellarians by means of the histochemical method of FALCK and HILLARP. This led WELSH and WILLIAMS (1970) to examine certain species of planarians by the same method. A small white planarian, *Phagocata oregonensis*, especially favorable for study as whole mounts, was most thoroughly examined but two other species, *Procotyla fluviatilis* and *Dugesia tigrina* were included in the study. Nerve cells reacting in a manner that indicated the presence of primary catecholamines and others containing 5-HT were found distributed throughout the nervous systems of these planarians. Figure 3 is a schematic representation of the nervous system of *Phagocata* showing the approximate locations, but not the exact numbers, of neurones in which monoamines could be demonstrated by their characteristic fluorescence. The nervous systems of *Procotyla* and *Dugesia* were found to differ only slightly from that of *Phagocata*.

WELSH and KING (1970) have confirmed the presence of catecholamines in planarians by means of extraction and thin-layer chromatography. Extracts of *Dugesia tigrina* yielded dopamine (av. 1.3 μg/g whole animals) and noradrenaline (av. 0.9 μg/g). Single lots of *Phagocata* and *Procotyla* gave chromatographic evidence of only dopamine (approximately 1.5 μg/g whole animals). In an independent study of *Procotyla*, SWEENEY (personal communication) found 1.7 μg/g dopamine and 0.2 μg/g noradrenaline in one lot and 0.6 μg/g of dopamine and no detectable noradrenaline in a second lot.

5-HT (1.5—3.4 μg/g whole animals) has been found in two species of *Dugesia* (WELSH and MOORHEAD, 1960) and in *Procotyla* (3.7 and 6.6 μg/g) by SWEENEY (personal communications).

From the histochemical studies, it appears that certain sensory, internuncial, and motor neurones of these planarians contain primary catecholamines. The amounts of catecholamines in these cells must be very high since their total volume constitutes a small fraction (less than 1 %) of the volume of an individual animal.

In addition to monoaminergic neurones, planarians are also known to have cholinergic and neurosecretory neurones (see Lentz, 1968a and b). It is remarkable that four of the well-known chemical types of neurones of higher animals are present in the nervous systems of representatives of the most primitive existing animals having a centralized nervous system.

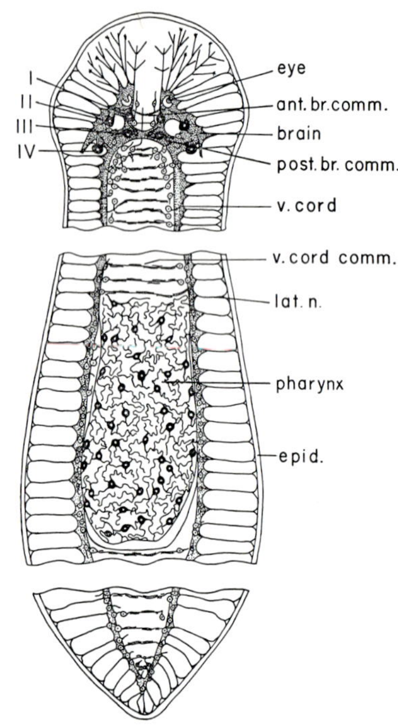

Fig. 3. Diagram of nervous system of *Phagocata oregonensis* as seen by induced fluorescence. Stippled areas of brain and ventral cords indicate green-fluorescing fibre tracts and neuropiles. The four pairs of large catecholamine cells of the brain (I, II, III, IV) and the fluorescing nerve net of the pharynx are shown in black. Yellow-fluorescing (5-HT-containing) nerve cells are shown in white. Ventral cord commissures and lateral nerves contain both green and yellow-fluorescing nerve fibers. The extensive branching of lateral nerves and the peripheral plexus of both types of fluorescing neurons have been omitted from this schema. ant. br. comm. = anterior brain commissure. post. br. comm. = posterior brain commissure. v. cord = ventral cord. v. cord. comm. = ventral cord commissure. lat. n. = lateral nerve. epid. = epidermis. [From Fig. 1, Welsh, J.H. and L.D. Williams, J. comp. Neurol. **138**, 103 (1970)]

The summary of a study of the distribution of monoamine-containing neurones in the planarian, *Dendrocoelum lacteum*, by Plotnikova and Kuzmina (1968) has recently come to the writer's attention. Using the histochemical fluorescence method of Falck and Hillarp they have found fluorescing neurones in the central and peripheral portions of the nervous system, including that of the pharynx. They also note that certain sensory cells show a bright green fluorescence.

5. Nemertinea (Ribbon Worms)

This phylum consists of a relatively small group of unsegmented worms that are mostly larger and more advanced than the flatworms. Reutter (1969a) has examined a common European species, *Lineus sanguineus*, for the presence of monoamines, using the method of Falck and Hillarp. Specific fluorescence was seen only in the nervous system and only green-fluorescing (catecholamine-containing) elements were found. Only a few green-fluorescing cells were noted in the brain. Green-fluorescing plexuses were seen in frontal organs, the proboscis, and the mouth-foregut region. Reutter concludes that the catecholamine-containing neurones of the frontal organ are probably sensory, while those of the other plexuses may be motor. The reaction time indicated the presence of dopamine or noradrenaline or a mixture of these primary amines.

In a later study (Reutter, 1969 b), histochemical observations on *Lineus* were made during regeneration of the foregut.

6. Annelida (Segmented Worms)

The major classes of annelids are the Polychaeta (mostly marine), the Oligochaeta (fresh water or terrestial), and the Hirudinea or leeches (mostly aquatic).

Historically, the common earthworm, *Lumbricus terrestris*, and the medicinal leech, *Hirudo medicinalis*, occupy unique positions among the invertebrates as regards the discovery of monoaminergic neurones. In 1903, Poll and Sommer described chromaffin cells in certain leeches, including *Hirudo*. Later, Biedl (1910) showed that extracts of leech ganglia contained an adrenaline-like substance. Gaskell (1914) confirmed these observations and also described chromaffin cells in the ventral ganglia of the polychaetes, *Eunice gigantea* and *Aphrodite aculeata*, and in the oligochaete, *Lumbricus herculeus (L. terrestris)*.

In each of the ventral ganglia of *Hirudo*, Gaskell found six chromaffin cells: one pair of very large cells — the "colossal" cells, described earlier by Retzius (1891) — and two pairs of smaller cells. Having observed that adrenaline caused acceleration in the rate of pulsation of the lateral blood sinuses of *Hirudo*, as did stimulation of lateral nerves from the ganglia, Gaskell (1914, 1919) concluded that the chromaffin cells innervated the lateral sinuses and released adrenaline as a regulator of the sinus beat. Gaskell suggested that in *Lumbricus* and other annelids, the chromaffin cells had a similar role in the regulation of blood flow. For many years the "adrenergic" nature of the chromaffin cells of annelids was accepted and further histochemical studies (e.g., Vialli, 1934; Lancaster, 1939; Ziller-Perez, 1942; Bianchi, 1962) tended to support this view. The finding of 5-HT in the nervous systems of *Hirudo* and *Lumbricus*, as well as in nervous systems of many other invertebrates (Welsh and Moorhead, 1960), and the availability of a histochemical method that distinguished between catecholamine- and 5-HT-containing neurones led to further examination of *Hirudo* and *Lumbricus*.

Several studies of the nervous system of *Hirudo*, using the Falck and Hillarp method have now shown that the chromaffin cells of Gaskell and others fluoresce in a manner characteristic for 5-HT rather than for the catecholamines (Kerkut et al., 1967 a; Ehinger, et al., 1968; Rude, 1969 b; Marsden and Kerkut, 1969). The presence of 5-HT in the large chromaffin cells of *Hirudo* (the colossal cells of Retzius) has been confirmed by means of microspectrofluorometry (Ehinger et al., 1968; Rude et al., 1969) and by chromatography and spectrofluorometry of extracts of dissected and pooled colossal cell bodies (Rude et al., 1969).

Green-fluorescing cell bodies have been found in the fused head and anal ganglia of *Hirudo* (Rude, 1969 b; Marsden and Kerkut, 1969) but none have been regularly seen in the ventral ganglia. However, located in each of the paired antero-lateral nerves of the ventral ganglia, there is a green (catecholamine) cell, whose axon enters the ganglion and divides to send one process anteriorly and the other in a posterior direction (Ehinger et al., 1968; Rude, 1969 b; Marsden and

KERKUT, 1969). The neuropiles of the fused head ganglia and those of the ventral ganglia fluoresce in a manner that indicates a majority of catecholamine-containing fibers generally mixed with fewer 5-HT-containing fibers (RUDE, 1969b; MARSDEN and KERKUT, 1969).

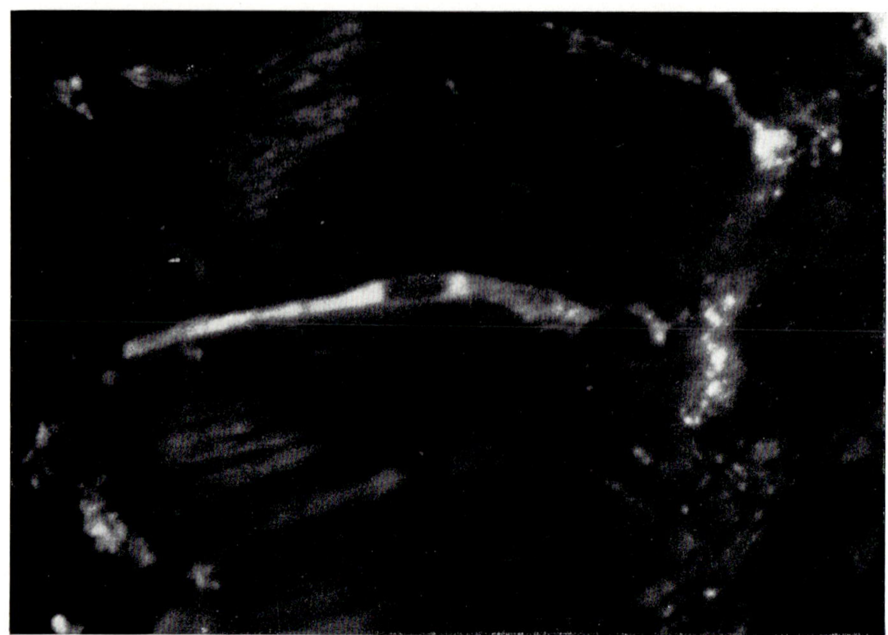

Fig. 4. A green-fluorescing sensory cell in the integument of the earthworm, *Lumbricus terrestris*. [From Fig. 9a, MYHRBERG, H.E., Z. Zellforsch. **81**, 311 (1967)]

Fluorescence studies of the nervous system of *Lumbricus* (RUDE, 1966; MYHRBERG, 1967) have shown the presence of many more yellow (5-HT) cells in each ganglion than are present in *Hirudo* ganglia. Each ventral ganglion, however, has only one pair (MYHRBERG, 1967), or possibly two pairs (RUDE, 1966), of green cells. A pair of green-fluorescing fiber tracts run the entire length of the ventral nerve cord. Numerous green fibers in the lateral nerves of each ganglion enter these tracts (RUDE, 1966). Many green-fluorescing sensory cells are present in certain epidermal regions of *Lumbricus*, especially the clitellum (Fig. 4) and prostomium (MYHRBERG, 1967; RUDE, 1966).

In the polychaete, *Nephtys caeca*, CLARK (1966) found three pairs of green-fluorescing cells and 15 to 18 pairs of yellow cells in each segment of the ventral nerve cord. About 30 pairs of green cells and seven pairs of yellow cells were found in the brain. Numerous green and yellow fibers run longitudinally in the cord. Many green sensory cells were seen in the epidermis but no fluorescing cells were found in association with the antennae or the eyes.

These histochemical studies of *Hirudo*, *Lumbricus* and *Nephtys* show that yellow-fluorescing cells are more numerous than the green-fluorescing cells in their central nervous systems. However, there are many green fibers in the neuropiles which are probably very largely the central axons of peripheral sensory cells. Spectrofluorometric assays of extracts of nerve cords of five species of annelids gave levels of 5-HT ranging from 3.1—10.4 μg/g wet tissue (WELSH and MOORHEAD, 1960).

Catecholamines are not as easily isolated, identified and assayed as is 5-HT, especially when levels are low and amounts of tissue are limited. This accounts, in part, for the variability in the results from the few studies on annelids (Table 1). RUDE (1969a) used thin layer chromatography in her study of the nerve cord of *Lumbricus*. Dopamine (3 μg/g) and noradrenaline (1.5 μg/g) were found but no adrenaline could be detected. DOPA was occasionally seen. MARSDEN and KERKUT (1969) could detect neither dopamine nor noradrenaline by means of spectrofluorometry in extracts of *Hirudo* nerve cords, but in one determination only, STEPHENS and WELSH (unpublished) obtained a value of 1.9 μg dopamine/g and of 1.0 μg noradrenaline/g.

Dopamine would appear to be the dominant catecholamine in *Lumbricus* and *Hirudo* nervous systems while adrenaline would appear to be absent.

Little is known concerning the physiological roles of the catecholamines in annelids. Some of the early pharmacological studies (e.g., GASKELL, 1914, 1919; WELLS, 1937; WU, 1939) suggest dual innervation of certain muscles, especially visceral, with acetylcholine and adrenaline often showing opposing actions. Since there are numerous catecholamine-containing epidermal sensory cells in annelids (RUDE, 1966; CLARK, 1966; MYHRBERG, 1967) that apparently send axons into the nerve cords to form neuropiles and fiber tracts, one might predict that the neurotransmitter of these neurones will be shown to be a catecholamine.

The setal muscles of the clitellar segment of *Lumbricus* are innervated by green-fluorescing fibers (MYHRBERG, 1967). This might be a suitable place for a study of catecholamine transmitter action.

7. Mollusca

Quantitative distribution. More species of molluscs have been examined for the presence of catecholamines than in any other phylum of invertebrates. However, representatives of only three of the six classes have thus far been studied. These are Gastropoda, Pelecypoda (or Bivalvia) and the Cephalopoda. The majority of the quantitative estimates have been made on nervous tissues. Dopamine has been found in very large amounts ranging from 5 μg/g to over 200 μg/g of wet central nervous tissue (Table 1). No other group of animals is known to contain such high levels of dopamine in their nervous system.

Noradrenaline has been detected and levels estimated in the ganglia of only four species of molluscs and the levels found are lower than those for dopamine. It is conceivable that the extra-ordinary high levels of dopamine have permitted its estimation in such small amounts of tissue that low levels of noradrenaline have sometimes been undetected. The difficulties that can be encountered in the spectrofluorometric assay of derivatives of the catecholamines before they are chromatographically separated are well-known. It may be significant that COTTRELL (1967) identified and estimated dopamine and noradrenaline in *Spisula solida* and *Eledone cirrhosa* ganglia by means of chromatography followed by elution and spectrofluorometric assay (Table 1).

There is no evidence for the occurrence of adrenaline in the nervous systems of molluscs.

Most of the determinations of dopamine levels in molluscs have been made on pooled ganglia of different types, but in two studies the cerebral, visceral and pedal ganglia of bivalve molluscs have been separately examined. DAHL et al. (1966) found much more dopamine in pedal ganglia of *Anodonta piscinalis* than in the other ganglia and the same was found in *Spisula solida* by COTTRELL (1967). DAHL et al. (1966) observed a denser neuropile of green-fluorescing fibers in the pedal ganglia of *Anodonta* than in other ganglia. A similar situation has been reported in *Sphaerium sulcatum* by Sweeney (1968). These fibers originate from numerous sensory cells in the foot (Dahl et al., 1963b; Sweeney, 1968), and their abundance, relative to other ganglia, might account for the high levels of dopamine observed in pedal ganglia.

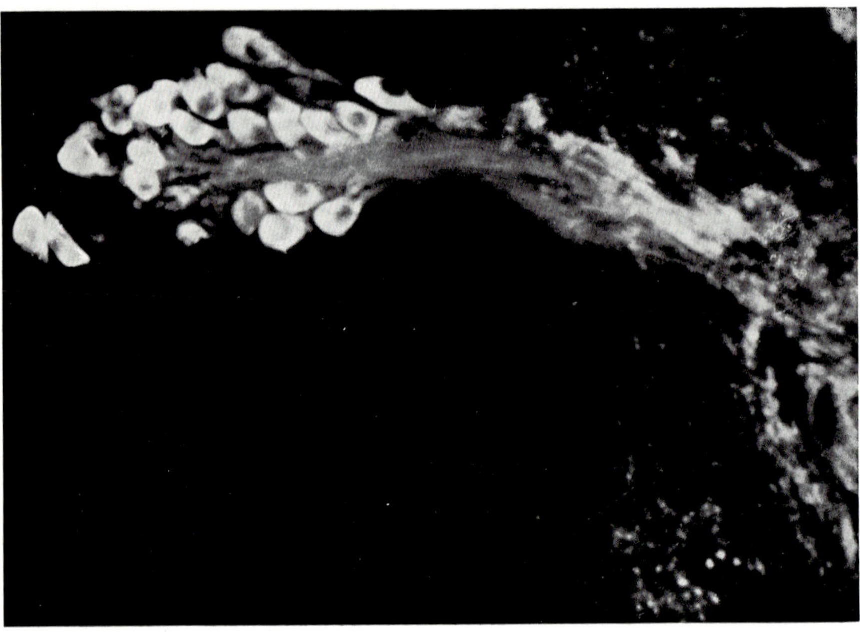

Fig. 5. A group of small dopamine-containing neurones from the cerebral ganglion of *Helix pomatia*. [From Fig. 2, Dahl, E. et al., Z. Zellforsch. **71**, 489 (1966)]

A variety of amines have been isolated from the venom-producing posterior salivary glands of several species of cephalopods (for references see Hartman et al., 1960; Ghiretti, 1960). These include acetylcholine, histamine, tyramine, octopamine and 5-HT. Noradrenaline was found in extracts of posterior salivary glands of *Octopus vulgaris* by von Euler (1953). Bioassay yielded a noradrenaline equivalent of 1—3 μg/g fresh tissue. Chromatography gave a spot corresponding with noradrenaline. Dopamine and adrenaline appeared not to be present. Hartmann et al. (1960) reported the presence of dopamine in the posterior salivary glands of *Octopus appollyon* and *Octopus bimaculatus* but noradrenaline and adrenaline were not definitely identified.

Distribution of catecholamine-containing neurones: The high levels of dopamine in the nervous systems of gastropod and pelecypod molluscs and its probable role as a neurotransmitter in molluscs (see below) lend particular interest to the identification and distribution of their catecholamine-containing nerve cells. Several histochemical fluorescence studies have been made and the findings will be briefly summarized.

Gastropoda: The nervous systems of such gastropod molluscs as snails (e.g. *Helix*), sea hares (e.g. *Aplysia*) and nudibranchs (e.g. *Anisodoris*) contain unusually large nerve cells that are readily identified in living material. These are under intensive study in several laboratories and it is desirable that their individual chemical types (e.g. cholinergic, adrenergic, serotonergic, neurosecretory) be determined; also, where possible, that the type of innervation of a given cell be histochemically demonstrated, thereby indicating the probable neurotransmitter acting on that cell.

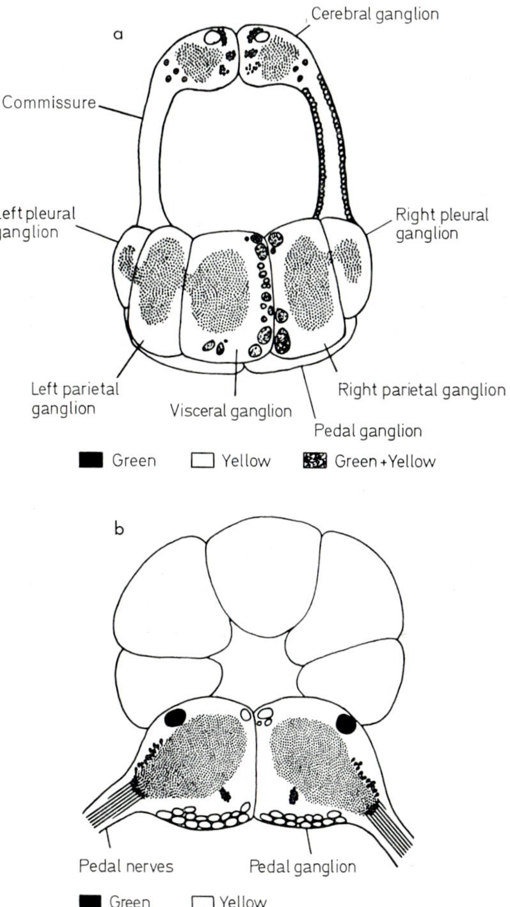

Fig. 6a. Diagram of the central ganglia of *Helix aspersa* showing the locations of the fluorescing cell bodies and neuropiles (stippled areas). b. Diagram showing the positions of fluorescing cells in the pedal ganglia of *Helix aspersa*. The black areas near the upper edge of each ganglion represent the otocysts. [Fig. 6a from Fig. 8, and 6b from Fig. 9, of Sedden, C.B. et al., Symp. Zool. Soc. (Lond.) No. 22, 19 (1968)]

One of the first invertebrates to be studied by the method of Falck and Hillarp was the pulmonate snail, *Helix pomatia* (Dahl et al., 1962). In this and a later report (Dahl et al., 1966), the distribution of fluorescing cells and fibers in the ganglionic ring was described. In the cerebral ganglia clusters of small green cells were seen and many intensely green fibers in the neuropile (Fig. 5). A green or yellow fluorescence was seen in some of the larger cells. Most of the ganglion cells did not develop a specific fluorescence but green varicose fibers appeared to make synaptic contact with them. This was especially noted in the suboesophageal ganglia.

The distribution of catecholamine- and 5-HT-containing cells in *Helix aspersa* has also been reported (Kerkut et al., 1967b; Sedden et al., 1968). Figures 6a and b from the latter paper summarize their findings. Of particular interest is their observation that certain neurones of the visceral and right parietal ganglia appear to contain both dopamine and 5-HT. When snails are injected with DOPA these cells show a distinct increase of green fluorescence; when injected with 5-hydroxytryptophan the yellow fluorescence is increased.

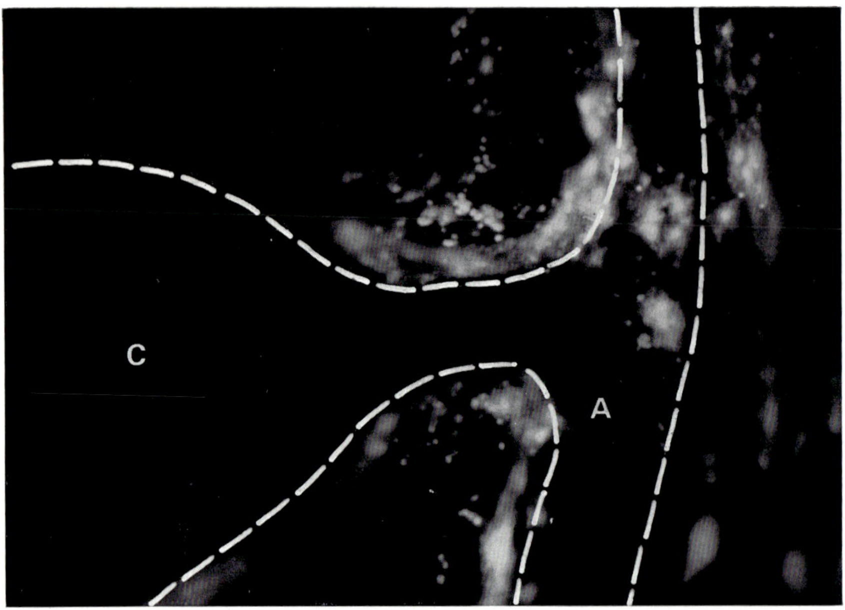

Fig. 7. Part of a large (500 μ), non-fluorescing cell (C) from a ganglion of *Strophocheilus oblongus* showing green-fluorescing nerve endings in the region of the axon hillock and proximal segment of the axon (A). The spherical, fluorescing dots are auto-fluorescent pigment granules. [Photo supplied by C.P. Jaeger]

An histochemical study of a Brazilian land snail, *Strophocheilus oblongus*, carried out in the author's laboratory, resulted in findings that correspond in many respects with those on *Helix* (Jaeger et al., 1971) Neuropiles contain green-fluorescing fibers, many of which appear to come from peripheral sensory cells. Green fibers seem to make synaptic contact at the region of the axon hillock and the proximal segment of the axon of certain very large non-fluorescing cells (Fig. 7). Some large cells show evidence of containing both a primary catecholamine and 5-HT. When first examined in UV-light they have a mixed yellow-green fluorescence. After a few minutes of irradiation the yellow fades, leaving a uniformly green colour in the cytoplasm.

In other studies on gastropods, catecholamine-containing sensory cells have been found in *Buccinum undatum* (Dahl et al., 1966); monoamine-containing axons have been seen in the cardiac nerves of *Mercenaria mercenaria* (Loveland, 1963), of *Strophocheilus* (Jaeger et al., 1971), and of *Helix pomatia* (Cottrell and Osborne, 1969; Cardot, 1969a); fluorescing cells have been mapped in ganglia of *Planorbis corneus* (Marsden and *Kerkut*, 1970); and the localization of monoamines in the cerebral ganglia of *Lymnaea stagnalis* has been described by SAKHAROV and ZS.-NAGY, 1968).

Pelecypoda: In histochemical studies of bivalve molluscs, an abundance of peripheral, monoamine-containing sensory cells has been noted (DAHL et al., 1963b; SWEENEY, 1965, 1968). Many of the green-fluorescing fibers of the ganglionic neuropiles apparently are the central processes of these sensory cells. In *Anodonta piscinalis,* the extent and intensity of the green-fluorescing fibers of the neuropiles increases from cerebral to visceral to pedal ganglia (DAHL et al., 1966). Since the levels of dopamine in these ganglia show a corresponding increase in the same order (Table 1), it is probable that much of the dopamine resides in these neuropiles.

In support of the evidence that the green-fluorescing fibers of the neuropiles of *Anodonta piscinalis* may come largely from peripheral sensory cells is the observation of ZS.-NAGY (1967) that there are relatively few green-fluorescing cell bodies in the ganglia of *Anodonta cygnea,* while yellow-fluorescing cells are numerous. However, from depletion and recovery studies, ZS.-NAGY suggests "that the yellow cells are transformed periodically into green cells and conversely".

The fresh-water bivalve mollusc, *Sphaerium sulcatum,* was selected by SWEENEY (1968) for a study of the distribution of monoamine-containing neurones since small individuals (less than 5 mm in length) could be serially sectioned. This permitted an unusually complete mapping of the anatomical distribution of the monoamines. Dopamine and noradrenaline were found present in extracts of whole *Sphaerium* in approximately equal amounts (Table 1). 5-HT was also found.

There are very few large nerve cell bodies in bivalve molluscs, hence they are less well suited for physiological and pharmacological studies on individual cells than are the gastropods.

Nerve fibers showing a yellow-green fluorescence, believed to be due to dopamine, have been found in the intestine of the bivalve mollusc, *Tapes watlingi* (DOUGAN and MCLEAN, 1970). It is postulated that they innervate intestinal smooth muscle.

Metabolism: An increase in the catecholamines of optic ganglia of *Eledone moschata,* after the injection of DOPA into the circulation, was observed by BERTACCINI (1961). CARDOT (1963) incubated ganglia and hearts of *Helix pomatia* with added DOPA and pyridoxal phosphate and observed an active synthesis of dopamine. KERKUT et al. (1966) injected DOPA into *Helix aspersa* and measured the levels of both DOPA and dopamine in the ganglia over a period of 6 hours. SWEENEY (1968) injected tritiated DOPA into the bivalve, *Mercenaria mercenaria.* Dopamine-H^3 appeared in the ganglia within 1 hour after injection. Isolated ganglia also converted DOPA-H^3 to dopamine-H^3. These results indicate an active DOPA decarboxylase in molluscan nervous systems. The low levels of noradrenaline, or its apparent absence in some species of molluscs, suggest that dopamine β-hydroxylase activity is low or this enzyme is absent from some species.

Little is known concerning the nature of catecholamine stores in molluscan nervous systems. Using the method of WOOD (1966) for localizing amines by electron microscopy, COTTRELL (1968) has observed electron dense vesicles about 300—1000 Å in diameter in the neuropile of ganglia of *Spisula solida.* However, 5-HT and catecholamines are both present in the ganglia and the WOOD reaction does not distinguish between these two types of monoamines.

Other electron microscopic studies have been made on molluscan neuropiles and certain tissues believed to contain dopaminergic fibers. GERSCHENFELD (1963) observed clear synaptic vesicles, slightly larger dense-cored synaptic vesicles, and neurosecretory vesicles in the neuropiles of the slug, *Vaginula solea,* and the snails,

Cryptomphallus aspersa and *Helix pomatia*. He concluded that the dense-cored vesicles could contain either 5-HT or a catecholamine. Dense-cored vesicles (av. diameter of 1000 Å), and believed to contain dopamine, have been seen in the neuropiles of *Anodonta cygnea* by Zs.-Nagy (1968). Certain nerve fibers in the heart of *Helix pomatia* contain dense-cored vesicles that are stained by the Wood reaction for amines. Other fibers contain typical neurosecretory vesicles (Cottrell and Osborne, 1969).

Until a study has been made of an identifiable neurone known to contain a catecholamine, such as that of Rude et al. (1969), on the giant Retzius cells of *Hirudo*, or that of Cottrell and Osborne (1970) on the large yellow-fluorescing cells of the cerebral ganglia of *Limax* the certain identification of catecholamine-containing vesicles in molluscan neurones will not have been realized. The single, large, green-fluorescing cell found in the right pedal ganglion of *Planorbis* by Marsden and Kerkut (1970) would appear to be ideal for such a study.

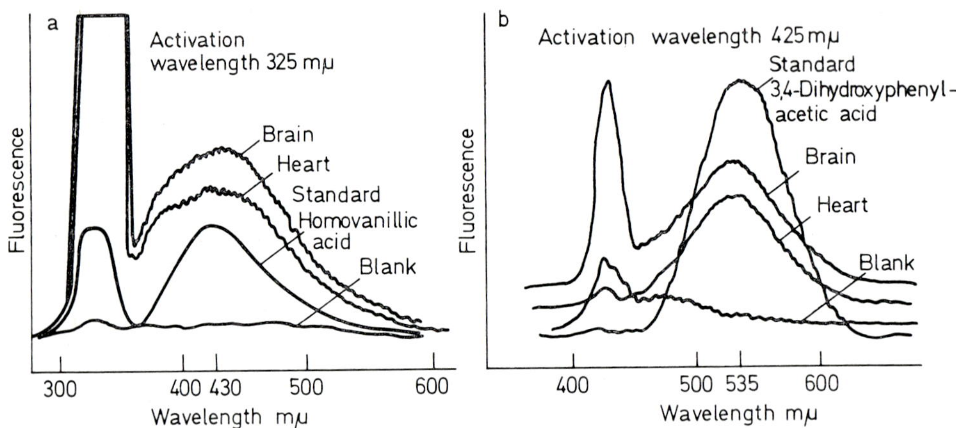

Fig. 8a and b. Fluorescence spectra of heart and brain extracts of *Helix aspersa* showing the presence of (a) homovanillic acid and (b) 3,4-dihydroxyphenylacetic acid. [From Fig. 2, Osborne, N.N. and G.A. Cottrell, Comp. Gen. Pharmacol. **1**, 43 (1970)]

It is well-established that reserpine reduces the levels of monoamines in molluscan nerve tissue (Piccinelli, 1958; Bertaccini, 1961; Mirolli, 1964; Mirolli and Welsh, 1964; Dahl et al., 1966; Kerkut et al., 1966; Cottrell, 1968). Dopamine was found to be reduced from a control level of 5.5 μg/g of ganglionic tissue to 0.5 μg/g, 48 hours after the injection of a high dose of reserpine into *Helix aspersa* (Kerkut et al., 1966). Cottrell (1968) obtained about 50% decrease in dopamine levels of *Spisula* ganglia after animals had been maintained for 5—7 days in sea water containing reserpine.

That dopamine acts as a neurotransmitter in molluscs appears highly probable but the manner in which it is inactivated is not yet fully established. Blaschko and collaborators (e.g., Blaschko and Hope, 1957) failed to detect amine oxidase activity in various tissues of some species of molluscs and, where demonstrable, the activity was very low. Studies on *Helix* nervous systems led Cardot (1963), Dahl et al. (1966) and Kerkut et al. (1969) to conclude that monoamine oxidase was probably absent. Sweeney (1969a and b) could obtain no evidence for the presence of this enzyme in ganglia of *Mercenaria*, although weak activity was noted in *Mercenaria* digestive gland and gill tissue. However, Osborne and Cot-

TRELL (1970) have been able to demonstrate dopamine and noradrenaline metabolites in extracts of ganglia and hearts of *Helix aspersa*. Using spectrofluorometric and chromatographic methods for detecting phenolic acids, OSBORNE and COTTRELL (1970) have shown that the dopamine metabolites, 3,4-dihydroxyphenylacetic acid and homovanillic acid, and the corresponding metabolities of noradrenaline, 3,4-dihydroxymandelic acid and vanillinmandelic acid, are present in both ganglionic and heart extracts of *Helix*. Figure 8, reproduced from their paper, shows the spectrofluorometric evidence for the presence of dopamine metabolites in extracts of heart and "brain". These results appear to indicate that monoamine oxidase is present in the central nervous system and the heart of *Helix aspersa* although the level of activity may be low.

Evidence for the oxidation of dopamine in homogenates of heart and ganglia of *Helix pomatia* by cytochrome oxidase has been presented by CARDOT (1969b).

That released dopamine in molluscan nervous systems may be actively returned to dopamine stores is suggested by results obtained by SWEENEY (personal communication). He has found that tritiated dopamine injected into intact *Mercenaria* is accumulated above circulating levels only in the ganglia. Isolated pedal ganglia also concentrate dopamine H^3. For example, after a 10 min incubation in 0.1 μ M of dopamine-H^3, the tissue to medium ratio is 4.5. After bathing ganglia in isotope-free sea water for one hour the tritium label chromatographs as dopamine.

Dopamine as a Neurotransmitter:

In addition to the chemical and histochemical evidence for dopaminergic neurones in molluscs there is growing pharmacological evidence that dopamine plays a role as a neurotransmitter in this group. This evidence comes, in part, from studies on identifiable neurones in ganglia of *Helix* and *Aplysia*.

KERKUT and WALKER (1961, 1962), using intracellular recordings of individual cells, found a number of spontaneously active cells in *Helix aspersa* ganglia that were hyperpolarized by dopamine (threshold 10^{-9} to 10^{-11} g/ml applied to surface of cell), accompanied by a decrease in the frequency of the action potentials or complete inhibition. Certain other cells were found to be depolarized and excited by dopamine. Subsequently, the pharmacological properties of these cells were studied in greater detail (WALKER et al., 1968; WOODRUFF et al., 1970). On cells that were inhibited by dopamine, ergometrine was found to be the most effective antagonist (Fig. 9).

A study of the structure-activity relationships of dopamine and a series of related compounds has been made on the spontaneously active cells of *Helix aspersa* that are inhibited by dopamine (WOODRUFF and WALKER, 1969). N-methyldopamine was found to be equiactive with dopamine; (—)-noradrenaline was, on the average, 25 times less potent than dopamine, and (—)-adrenaline 92 times less potent. Evidence indicates that dopamine receptors different from vertebrate α- or β-receptors are present in these neurones.

One of the large cells of the right parietal ganglion of *Helix aspersa* exhibits the interesting phenomenon of synaptic inhibition of long duration (KERKUT et al., 1969). Stimulation of the left pallial nerve results in long-lasting inhibition for a duration of 3 sec to several minutes following a single stimulus. Dopamine hyperpolarizes this cell by increasing its permeability to potassium and stops spontaneous activity. Ergometrine blocks the inhibition resulting from nerve stimulation as well as that from applied dopamine.

TAUC (1958) was the first to observe the phenomenon of "inhibition of long duration" (ILD) in molluscan neurones. In studies on *Aplysia depilans* and *Helix pomatia* he found certain cells that responded to brief stimulation by a long-lasting hyperpolarization that did not result from a repetitive inhibitory input. In a later study of these cells in *Aplysia*, they were shown to have a non-cholinergic excitatory input and to be hyperpolarized by catecholamines (Gerschenfeld

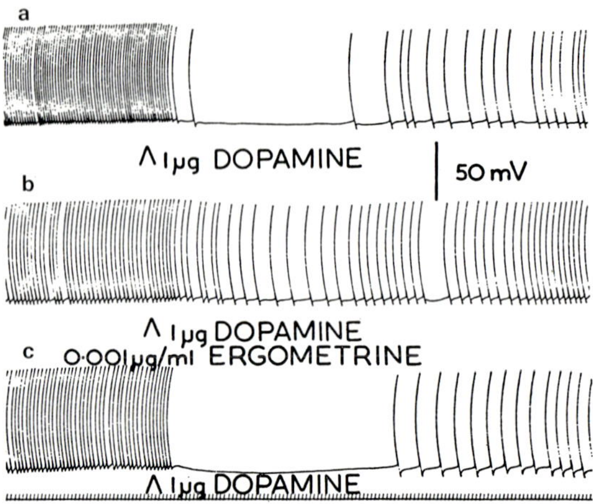

Fig. 9a—c. The effect of ergometrine on the response of an identified cell (Cell 2) of the right parietal ganglion of *Helix aspersa* to dopamine. a. the effect of 1 µg of dopamine applied over the cell on its spontaneous activity. b. the effect of pretreatment with 0.001 µg/ml ergometrine on the response to 1 µg dopamine. c. the effect of 1 µg dopamine after washing the preparation with Ringer. Time interval 1 sec. Portions of the record between a and b and between b and c have been deleted. [From Fig. 6, Walker, R.J. et al., Comp. Biochem. Physiol. **24**, 455 (1968)]

and Tauc, 1964). These and other studies on various types of neurones in *Aplysia* and certain land snails have been reviewed by Tauc (1967). Since then, further studies in Tauc's laboratory have demonstrated a two-component postsynaptic inhibition of certain *Aplysia* neurones, the first phase of which is blocked by d-tubocurarine and the second, later phase, is not blocked by any acetylcholine antagonist that was tested (Kehoe, 1967). One interpretation suggested that the second phase might result from released dopamine, known to produce prolonged hyperpolarization when applied by electrophoretic injection onto the cell body. In a further study of *Aplysia* cells that exhibit synaptic inhibition of long duration, Ascher (1968) has examined the ionic mechanism underlying the inhibition produced by the normal input to the cell or by injecting dopamine onto its surface and finds that it is apparently due to a selective increase in permeability to potassium ions.

Other indications of a neurotransmitter or regulatory role for dopamine in molluscs derive from studies on molluscan hearts. Adrenaline and noradrenaline have long been known to have an excitor action on many molluscan hearts (see review by Krigsman and Divaris, 1955). In studies of the relative activities of the catecholamines, Greenberg (1960) found dopamine to be approximately ten times as active as adrenaline or noradrenaline on the heart of *Mercenaria* (= Venus) *mercenaria*, while Chong and Phillis (1965) report that dopamine is 100 times as active as noradrenaline on the heart of *Tapes watlingi*. In view of the histochemical demonstration of catecholamine-containing neurones in molluscan cardioregulatory nerves, referred to earlier, these pharmacological studies take on added significance.

Dopamine has been shown to relax "catch" in the anterior byssus retractor muscle of *Mytilus edulis* (Northrop, 1964; Twarog, unpublished). By means of intracellular recordings, Hidaka (1969) has shown that these muscle fibres are hyperpolarized by dopamine (threshold below 10^{-8}M).

8. Arthropoda

In contrast with the annelids and molluscs the few arthropods that have been examined have low levels of catecholamines in their nervous systems (Table 1). In two species of crabs, Cottrell (1967) found a measurable amount of dopamine (0.5—1.0 μg/g) in the ventral ganglia of *Carcinus maenas*, but less than 0.5 μg/g in ganglia of *Hyas araneus*. However, in pericardial (neurohemal) organs of crabs, Cooke and coworkers (unpublished) have found appreciable amounts of dopamine. These organs also contain more 5-HT than any other nervous structures in crabs (Maynard and Welsh, 1959; Welsh and Moorhead, 1960).

The only quantitative estimate of catecholamines in insect nervous tissue by spectrofluorometry appears to be that of Frontali and Häggendal (1969) on head ganglia of *Periplaneta* (Table 1). Östlund (1954), using chromatography and bioassays, found relatively large amounts of dopamine in larvae of *Tenebrio molitor* (mealworms) and in whole adult honeybees *(Apis mellifica)*. As the result of more recent work (Karlson et al., 1962; Sekeris and Karlson, 1966) it has been established that dopamine in *Tenebrio* is a precursor of N-acetyldopamine which is involved in the tanning of insect cuticle.

From the eggs of the house cricket, *Acheta domesticus*, Furneaux and McFarlane (1965a) isolated and identified DOPA, dopamine and N-acetyldopamine. Dopamine is present in larger amounts than either of the others. Its maximum concentration (about 93 μg/g live eggs) occurs 156 hours after the beginning of development. They conclude that the N-acetyldopamine is probably involved in tanning of the cuticle. In a later study, Furneaux and McFarlane (1965b) found DOPA, dopamine and N-acetyldopamine in eggs of three other species of crickets but not in eggs of *Musca domestica* or in whole ootheca of *Blatella germanica*. Based on these observations they suggested a possible relationship between catecholamines and water absorption in insect eggs.

Some of the dopamine found in extracts of whole adult honey bees by Östlund (1954) must have come from the venom and venom glands since Micheal Owen (personal communication) has found high levels of dopamine and lesser amounts of noradrenaline in the venom of the honey bee and in that of the wasp, *Vespula maculata*. This makes an interesting addition to the complex mixtures of biogenic amines and kinins that have been isolated from hymenopteran venoms (e.g., Bhoola et al., 1961; Habermann, 1968).

The localization of monoamine-containing neurones in crustaceans has been studied by means of the method of Falck and Hillarp in a crayfish, *Astacus astacus*, by Elofsson et al. (1966) and in crabs, by Goldstone and Cooke (1971). In the crayfish the majority of fluorescing cells exhibit a green fluorescence that is mainly due to dopamine. In the brain these cells and fibres occur principally in the protocerebrum. Green-fluorescing cells and fibers are also present in three of the "optic ganglia", that is, the medulla externa, medulla interna, and medulla terminalis of the eyestalk, but not in the lamina terminalis which receives primary sensory neurones from the retina. Green-fluorescing cells and fibers are also present in the suboesophageal and first thoracic ganglia. Other ganglia of the ventral nerve cord were not examined. The only yellow-fluorescing cells seen in *Astacus* were a pair of large cells in the region of the brain proper adjacent to the olfactory lobes; one yellow cell in each eyestalk; and at least one yellow cell in the suboesophageal ganglion. Elofsson et al. (1968) report the presence of green-fluorescing fibers in the nerve plexus of the hindgut of *Astacus*.

Goldstone and Cooke (1971) have made a similar study of the distribution of fluorescing structures in the nervous system of the green crab, *Carcinus maenas*. In the brain of *Carcinus*, fluorescing cell bodies are located in three regions: anterior, posterior and superior-lateral cell groups. In the anterior group, 5 to 10 pairs of small (30 μ) green- and yellow-fluorescing cells send axons into the optic peduncles. Clusters of smaller (10 μ) green- and yellow-fluorescing cells contribute axons to neuropiles, from which fibers also enter the optic peduncles. Two or three pairs of fluorescing cells are present in the superior-lateral cell groups. Two pairs of large (50 μ) green-fluorescing cells are located in the posterior region of the brain. Other smaller fluorescing cells are in this region. Near the exit of each oesophageal connective there is a single large (75 μ) green-fluorescing cell. Each connective (commissural) ganglion has a green cell (90 μ) whose axon runs anteriorly into the brain and then reverses its direction, proceeds back through the connective to the ventral ganglion, and exits to contribute endings in neurohemal organs that will be discussed later.

In *Carcinus*, and other crabs, the ventral ganglia are fused to form a ring-like mass of cell bodies, fiber tracts and neuropiles. The majority of fluorescing cells in this ganglionic mass are located in anterior and posterior regions. In the anterior region (corresponding to the suboesophageal ganglion of the crayfish) there are 10 to 15 pairs of small, green-fluorescing cells. In that part representing the last thoracic segment there are three pairs of yellow-fluorescing cells. In the most posterior portion, consisting of fused abdominal ganglia, one pair of large (80—90μ) green-fluorescing cells lies in a dorsal midline. The axon of each branches and four large green fibers leave the ganglion to enter the abdomen.

In a separate study, Cooke and Goldstone (1970) have found that the paired pericardial organs and their anterior ramifications (both of which are neurohemal structures) receive green-and yellow-fluorescing axons. The pericardial organs were earlier shown to contain multibranched neurosecretory axons (Alexandrowicz, 1953; Maynard, 1961), that release cardioexcitor materials into the circulation (Cooke, 1964). Cooke and Goldstone have now found that a small number of monoamine-containing axons enter the pericardial organs by way of segmental nerves from the ventral ganglion. On each side, one yellow and one green axon also send branches into the anterior ramification. These fluorescing axons branch and rebranch to produce a dense array of fine varicose fibers and terminal "blebs" at the surfaces of the neurohemal organs that are exposed to the hemolymph (Fig. 10). The largest green-fluorescing axon that enters each pericardial organ has been shown in *Carcinus maenas* to come from the large green cell soma located in the connective ganglia.

Berlind et al. (1970) have failed to find evidence that dopamine and 5-HT function in the release of neuropeptides from crab pericardial organs.

The stomatogastric ganglion of the lobster, *Homarus vulgaris*, has been shown to have some yellow-green fluorescing cells and a fluorescent neuropile (Osborne and Dando, 1970).

The distribution of catecholamine-containing neurones in the brain and suboesophageal ganglion of the cockroach, *Periplaneta americana*, has been examined by Frontali and Norberg (1966) and Frontali (1968). Green-fluorescing cells and neuropiles were found in the three major divisions of the brain (protocerebrum, deutocerebrum and tritocerebrum) as well as in the suboesophageal ganglion. No clear evidence was obtained for the presence of 5-HT-containing neurones.

Klemm (1968a) has described the distribution of green-fluorescing cells and fibers in certain caddis flies (Trichoptera), especially in *Limnephilus politus*. Green cells were always seen in several areas of the brain and in the suboesophageal ganglion. No yellow-fluorescing structures were seen in the central nervous system, but Klemm (1968b) found two pairs of yellow-fluorescing cells in the frontal ganglion of the stomatogastric nervous system of *Limnephilus*. In all other parts of the stomatogastric system no monoamine-containing structures were seen.

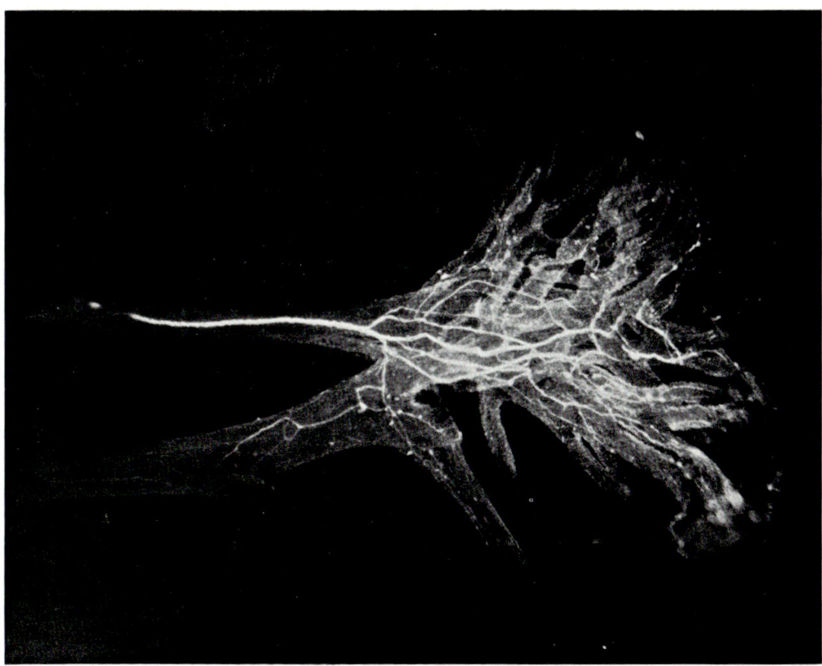

Fig. 10. Photograph of a whole mount of the posterior region of a pericardial (neurohemal) organ of the crab, *Cardisoma guanhumi*, showing the green-fluorescing, multibranched terminals of the axon of a cell located in one of the connective ganglia. [Photo supplied by Cooke I.M. and M.W Goldstone]

In other histochemical fluorescence studies of the sympathetic nervous system of insects, Plotnikova (1968) found three green-fluorescing median areas in the metathoracic ganglion of *Locusta migratoria* which are believed to be part of the vegetative nervous system and Chanussot et al. (1969) find neuropiles rich in catecholamine-containing fibers in the ingluvial (foregut) ganglion of *Schistocerca gregaria* and *Blaberus craniifer*. This latter study includes an investigation of the ultrastructure of these fibers. The ultrastructural localization of catecholamines in the brain of *Periplaneta americana* has been investigated by Mancini and Frontali (1967, 1970).

There is little or no direct evidence for a neurotransmitter role for the catecholamines in arthropods. From histochemical studies it would appear that most of the catecholamine-containing neurones are internuncials with their terminals in the complex neuropiles where neurotransmitter phenomena are not readily studied. Adrenaline has long been known to have an excitor action on many arthropod hearts (for references see Krijgsman, 1952; Treherne, 1966). There is no evidence for an adrenergic innervation of arthropod cardiac muscle or of cardiac ganglion cells, but either might be influenced by circulating catecholamines. In the crabs, at least, possible sources of blood-borne dopamine are the pericardial organs referred to earlier.

9. Echinodermata

Adrenaline is known to oppose the action of acetylcholine on a variety of echinoderm organs and muscle preparations (for references see WELSH, 1966). While large amounts of acetylcholine have been found in extracts of radial nerves of a variety of echinoderms (personal communications from G.A. COTTRELL and from L.S. ROBERTS to WELSH, 1966; PENTREATH and COTTRELL, 1968), until recently there had been no evidence for the presence of catecholamines in this phylum. ÖSTLUND (1954) failed to find conclusive evidence for any adrenaline-like substance in extracts of whole bodies of a sea cucumber, a sea urchin and a brittle star. However, an amine oxidase has been found by BLASCHKO and HOPE (1957) in several species of echinoderms. COTTRELL (1967) has now shown that considerable amounts of dopamine and noradrenaline are present in radial nerves of the sea urchin, *Echinus esculentus*, and the starfish, *Asterias rubens* (Table 1).

The localization of monoamines in the nervous systems of representative echinoderms has been studied by COBB (1969) and COTTRELL and PENTREATH (1970). COBB made his observations on an Australian starfish, *Patiriella calcar*, and a sea urchin, *Heliocidaris erythrogramma*, using the procedure of FALCK and HILLARP. In sections of radial nerve cords of this sea urchin, hundreds of fine (0.2 μ to 1 μ in diameter) yellow-green fluorescing fibers and some small fluorescent bodies, probably unipolar nerve cells, were seen. Large numbers of fluorescent cell bodies were found in the epithelial layer covering the cord. The radial nerve cord of *Patiriella* differs from that of *Heliocidaris* in two respects: fewer fluorescing cell bodies were seen in the epithelium of the cord and the fluorescent fibers were restricted to the ectoneural portion of the cord. In each tubefoot of both the sea urchin and starfish, a group of fluorescent fibers was seen. A fluorescing nerve plexus was found in the oesophagus of the sea urchin. No fluorescing sensory cells were seen. COBB concludes that the fluorescence that he observed suggests the presence of a primary catecholamine.

In a study of formaldehyde-induced fluorescence in tissues of the European starfish, *Asterias rubens*, and brittle star, *Ophiothrix fragilis*, COTTRELL and PENTREATH (1970) overcame some of the difficulties encountered in the freeze-drying and infiltration of tissues of marine animals, especially when hard structures are present, by sectioning frozen tissue and then drying the sections over P_2O_5 before exposure to formaldehyde gas. In general, their findings are in agreement with those of COBB (1969). Catecholamine fluorescence was found only in neurones of the ectoneural portion of the nervous system. In the starfish this is the sensory-associative division, while the hyponeural portion is believed to consist mainly of motor neurones. In contrast with the findings of COBB (1969) on the starfish, *Patiriella*, no amine-containing cell bodies were definitely identified in the radial nerve cords of *Asterias*. Green-fluorescing fiber tracts and networks were observed in the tube feet. These were continuous with the fluorescing fiber system of the radial nerve cords. When *Asterias* were maintained in sea water containing reserpine for three or four days the movements and coordination of "stepping" of the tube feet (podia) were distinctly abnormal.

Both COBB, and COTTRELL and PENTREATH conclude that the fluorescing neurones of the echinoderms that they have studied are mainly internuncial neurones. However, certain of the pharmacological responses of isolated echinoderm preparations (see WELSH, 1966) suggest the possibility of a double innervation of some echinoderm muscles by cholinergic and adrenergic neurones. This, and certain other questions concerning the functional roles of the primary catecholamines in echinoderms, call for further study.

10. Hemichordata, Urochordata and Cephalochordata

These groups of invertebrates have features that show a relationship with the echinoderms as well as with the vertebrates. Hence, in a consideration of the phylogenetic distribution of the biogenic amines, their presence or absence in these groups is of particular interest. Unfortunately, little is known concerning the occurrence of catecholamines in these animals. ÖSTLUND (1954) found no evidence for the presence of catecholamines in whole body extracts of *Ciona intestinalis,* a urochordate, nor did VON EULER (1961). In extracts of whole *Branchiostoma lanceolatum,* a cephalochordate, VON EULER (1961) found an appreciable amount of noradrenaline. If the noradrenaline is restricted to the nervous system, as in most invertebrates that have been examined, its level there must be rather high. The possible presence of dopamine in *Branchiostoma* has not been investigated. Localization studies of catecholamines in these primitive chordates have yet to be made.

In studies of other biogenic amines, acetycholine has been found in very large amounts (20—120 μg/g wet tissue) in cerebral ganglia of *Ciona intestinalis* (FLOREY, 1963) and *Ciona* muscle appears to have a cholinergic innervation (FLOREY, 1967). While 5-HT could not be demonstrated in extracts of cerebral ganglia of *Ciona,* it was found in other tissues, where its major source may be enterochromaffin cells (WELSH and LOVELAND, 1968). Cerebral ganglia of *Ciona* and other primitive chordates should be examined for the possible presence of catecholamines.

III. Summary and Concluding Remarks

By means of the newer methods for isolating, identifying, and estimating amounts, one or more of the catecholamines have been found in representatives of the major invertebrate phyla. In the great majority of invertebrates that have been examined, dopamine is the dominant catecholamine. Noradrenaline, when shown to be present, is at levels lower than those of dopamine. In most invertebrates, adrenaline appears to be absent.

The cellular localization of the primary catecholamines and 5-HT in the invertebrates is now known in a number of representative species. Use of the histochemical fluorescence method of FALCK and HILLARP has shown that the catecholamines are present almost exclusively in nervous systems. From the most primitive type of nervous system — that found in the coelenterates — to the nervous systems of the highly specialized arthropods, nerve cells have been found that, after exposure to formaldehyde gas, fluoresce in a manner specific for catecholamines. These neurones may be any of the three basic types: sensory, internuncial or associative, and motor. Catecholamine-containing neurones of all three types appear to be present in the earliest centralized nervous system, that of the flatworms. Primary sensory neurones containing catecholamines are numerous in certain coelenterates, flatworms, annelids and molluscs. Their presence in arthropods and echinoderms is still uncertain.

Where quantitative estimates of dopamine levels have been made on isolated portions of nervous systems (e.g., pelecypod molluscs), there is a good correlation between the levels of dopamine and the numbers of green-fluorescing cells and extent of the fluorescing neuropiles. Relatively small amounts of dopamine and noradrenaline have been found in the few arthropod nervous systems that have been examined and the numbers of green-fluorescing neurones are small relative to the numbers found in certain molluscs that have high levels of dopamine in their nervous systems.

Dopamine, presumably of non-nervous origin, has been found in the venom glands and venom of the honey bee and wasp, and in the posterior salivary glands of octopus. The dopamine of certain insects that serves as a precursor to N-acetyldopamine, a substance involved in the tanning of the insect cuticle, is also presumably of non-nervous origin although its actual source seems not to have been explored.

In this review, major attention has been given to the distribution of catecholamines among the major invertebrate phyla, and to their cellular localization in nervous systems. Only in dealing with the molluscs has the literature on the metabolism, storage, release, and possible function of the catecholamines, especially dopamine, been given much consideration. In most other groups little is known concerning these matters. To the extent that present knowledge allows, one may conclude that the metabolism, storage, and release of catecholamines are essentially similar in the molluscs and in the higher vertebrates. Certain problems such as the exact identification of the catecholamine storage vesicles have been difficult to resolve in electron microscope studies of molluscan, and other, nervous systems. This is due, in part, to the frequent intermingling of the axons of catecholamine-containing and 5-HT-containing neurones and the possibility that the vesicles are similar in the two types of neurones. In the molluscs, a further complication is the almost certain presence of both a catecholamine and 5-HT in certain neurones. If final proof of this is forthcoming, there will remain the interesting question of the manner in which these two types of amines are stored in, and released from, the same cell.

From studies on identifiable neurones of *Helix* and *Aplysia*, there is growing evidence that dopamine acts as a neurotransmitter. Certain large, nonfluorescing cells in ganglia of *Strophocheilus* have an abundance of green-fluorescing nerve fibers (and presumably nerve endings) in the region of the axon hillock and the proximal segment of the axon. Dopamine mimics the effects of stimulating nerves that innervate certain identifiable *Helix and Aplysia* neurones. Results of pharmacological studies on such cells are consistent with the view that these nerves contain dopaminergic axons.

A second, possible role of dopamine in certain invertebrates is that of a blood-borne neurohumoral agent, or "modulator". The pericardial organs of certain crustaceans are known to be neurohemal structures consisting, in large part, of the multibranched terminals of at least three types of axons: dopamine-containing, 5-HT-containing and neurosecretory. The neurosecretory endings are known to release neuropeptides when their axons are stimulated electrically. These are cardioexcitor substances but may regulate other processes in the animal. Dopamine and 5-HT may also be released in a similar manner and carried in the blood to act on the heart and other target organs.

Certain molluscan hearts have also been shown to be innervated by nerves made up of axons of several types, including catecholamine-containing fibers. Rather than directly innervating cardiac muscle, these several types of axons have swollen endings that appear quite comparable to those of certain known neurohemal structures. As in the pericardial organs, these molluscan heart structures would appear to release substances (including dopamine) into the circulation to act not only upon the heart but on more distant targets.

Although there is an endless supply of invertebrate species yet to be examined for their content, localization, and functional roles of the catecholamines, certain facts are already well established. Among these are the early appearance of catecholamines in the evolving nervous system; their presence in all invertebrate nervous systems that have been adequately examined; and the relatively large amounts of dopamine that have been found.

References

ALEXANDROWICZ, J.S.: Nervous organs in the pericardial cavity of the decapod Crustacea. J. Mar. Biol. Ass. U. K. **31**, 563—580 (1963).

APPLEWHITE, P.B., GARDNER, F.T., LAPAN, E.: Physiology of habituation learning in a protozoan. Trans. N. Y. Acad. Sci. Ser. II **31**, 842—849 (1969).

ASCHER, P.: Electrophoretic injections of dopamine on *Aplysia* neurons. J. Physiol. (Lond.) **198**, 48—49P (1968).

BAYER, G., WENSE, T.: Über den Nachweis von Hormonen in einzelligen Tieren. II. Mitt. Adrenalin (Sympathin) im *Paramecium*. Pflügers Arch. ges. Physiol. **237**, 651—653 (1936).

BERLIND, A., COOKE, I.M., GOLDSTONE, M.W.: Do the monoamines in crab pericardial organs play a role in peptide neurosecretion? J. exp. Biol. **53**, 669—677 (1970).

BERTACCINI, G.: A Discussion in *Regional Neurochemistry*. S.S. Kety and J. Elkes, eds. Oxford: Pergamon Press 1961.

BHOOLA, K.D., CALLE, J.D., SCHACHTER, M.: Identification of acetylcholine, 5-hydroxytryptamine, histamine, and a new kinin in hornet venom (*V. crabro*). J. Physiol. (Lond.) **159**, 167—182 (1961).

BIANCHI, S.: Richerche istochemiche e fluoromicroscopiche su neuroni cromaffini degli Irudinei. Arch. Zool. ital. (Torino) **47**, 339—351 (1962).

BIEDL, A.: Über das Adrenalgewebe bei Wirbellosen. 8th Int. Congress Zool. Graz, 503—505 (1910).

BLASCHKO, H., HOPE, D.B.: Observations on the distribution of amine oxidase in invertebrates. Arch. Biochem. Biophys. **69**, 10—15 (1957).

BLUM, J.J.: An adrenergic control system in *Tetrahymena*. Proc. nat. Acad. Sci. (Wash.) **58**, 81—88 (1967).

— KIRSHNER, N., UTLEY, J.: The effect of reserpine on growth and catecholamine content of *Tetrahymena*. Mol. Pharmacol. **2**, 606 (1966).

BULLOCK, T.H., HORRIDGE, G.A.: *Structure and Function in the Nervous Systems of Invertebrates*. San Francisco: W.H. Freeman 1965.

CARDOT, J.: Sur la présence de dopamine dans le système nerveux et ses relations avec la décarboxylation de la dioxyphénylalanine chez le Mollusque *Helix pomatia*. C. R. Acad. Sci. (Paris) **257**, 1364—1366 (1963).

— Mise en évidence de monoamines dans les fibres nerveuses du coeur des Mollusques *Helix pomatia* Linné et *Archachatina marginata* Swainson par l'histochimie de fluorescence. C. R. Acad. Sci. (Paris) **269**, 345—347 (1969a).

— Recherches sur l'oxydation *in vitro* de la dopamine par le coeur et les ganglions nerveux du Mollusque *Helix pomatia* (L.): la cytochrome oxydase. C. R. Soc. Biol. (Paris) **163**, 873—877 (1969b).

CARLYLE, R.F.: The occurrence of catecholamines in the sea anemone *Actinia equina*. Brit. J. Pharmacol. **36**, 182P (1969a).

— The occurrence of pharmacologically active substances in, and the action of drugs on, preparations of the sea anemone *Actinia equina*. Brit. J. Pharmacol. **37**, 532—533P (1969b).

CHANUSSOT, B., DANDO, J., MOULINS, M., LAVERACK, M.S.: Mise en évidence d'une amine biogène dans le système nerveux stomatogastrique des Insectes. Étude histochimique et ultrastructurale. C.R. Acad. Sci. (Paris) **268**, 2101—2104 (1969).

CHONG, G.C., PHILLIS, J.W.: Pharmacological studies on the heart of *Tapes watlingi*, a mollusc of the family Veneridae. Brit. J. Pharmacol. **25**, 481—496 (1965).

CLARK, M.E.: Histochemical localization of monoamines in the nervous system of the polychaete *Nephtys*. Proc. roy. Soc. B **165**, 308—327 (1966).

COBB, J.L.S.: The distribution of mono-amines in the nervous system of echinoderms. Comp. Biochem. Physiol. **28**, 967—971 (1969).

COOKE, I.M.: Electrical activity and release of neurosecretory material in crab pericardial organs. Comp. Biochem. Physiol. **13**, 353—366 (1964).

— GOLDSTONE, M.W.: Fluorescence localization of monoamines in crab neurosecretory structures. J. exp. Biol. **53**, 651—668 (1970).

CORRODI, H., JONSSON, G.: The formaldehyde fluorescence method for the histochemical demonstration of biogenic monoamines. J. Histochem. Cytochem. **15**, 65—78 (1967).

Cottrell, G. A.: Occurrence of dopamine and noradrenaline in the nervous tissue of some invertebrate species. Brit. J. Pharmacol. **29**, 63—69 (1967).
— Amines in molluscan nervous tissue and their subcellular localization. In: *Invertebrate Neurobiology*, J. Salanki, ed. New York: Plenum 1968.
— Laverack, M. S.: Invertebrate pharmacology. Ann. Rev. Pharmacol. **8**, 273—298 (1968).
— Osborne, N. N.: Localization and mode of action of cardioexcitatory agents in molluscan hearts. In: *Comparative Physiology of the Heart: Current Trends*. Experientia Suppl. 15, F. V. McCann, ed. (1969).
— — Serotonin in a subcellular position. Nature (Lond.) **225**, 470—472 (1970).
— Pentreath, V. W.: Localization of catecholamines in the nervous system of a starfish, *Asterias rubens*, and of a brittlestar, *Ophiothrix fragilis*. Comp. Gen. Pharmacol. **1**, 73—81 (1970).
Crescitelli, F., Geissman, T. A.: Invertebrate pharmacology: selected topics. Ann. Rev. Pharmacol. **2**, 143—192 (1962).
Dahl, E., Falck, B., Lindqvist, M., von Mecklenburg, C.: Monoamines in mollusc neurons. Kgl. Fysiogr. Sällsk. Lund Förh. **32**, 89—92 (1962).
— — von Mecklenburg, C., Myhrberg, H.: An adrenergic nervous system in sea anemones. Quart. J. micr. Sci. **104**, 531—534 (1963a).
— — — — Adrenergic sensory neurons in invertebrates. Gen. comp. Endocr. **3**, (1963b).
— — — — Rosengren, E.: Neuronal localization of dopamine and 5-hydroxytryptamine in some mollusca. Z. Zellforsch. **71**, 489—498 (1966).
Dougan, D. F. H., McLean, J. R.: Evidence for the presence of dopaminergic nerves and receptors in the intestine of a mollusc, *Tapes watlingi*. Comp. Gen. Pharmacol. **1**, 33—46 (1970).
Ehinger, B., Falck, B., Myhrberg, H. E.: Biogenic monoamines in *Hirudo medicinalis*. Histochemie **15**, 140—149 (1968).
Elofsson, R., Kauri, T., Nielsen, S.-O., Strömberg, J.-O.: Localization of monoaminergic neurons in the central nervous system of *Astacus astacus* Linné (Crustacea). Z. Zellforsch. **74**, 464—473 (1966).
— — — — Catecholamine-containing nerve fibers in the hind-gut of the crayfish *Astacus astacus L.* (Crustacea, Decapoda). Experientia (Basel) **24**, 1159 (1968).
Euler, U. S. v.: Presence of catecholamines in visceral organs of fish and some invertebrates. Acta physiol. scand. **28**, 297—305 (1953).
— Occurrence of catecholamines in Acrania and invertebrates. Nature (Lond.) **190**, 170—171 (1961).
Falck, B.: Observations on the possibilities of the cellular localization of monoamines by a fluorescence method. Acta physiol. scand. **56**, Suppl. 197 (1962).
— Owman, C.: A detailed methodological description of the fluorescence method for the cellular demonstration of biogenic monoamines. Acta Univ. Lund, Section 11, No. 7 (1965).
Florey, E.: Acetylcholine and cholinesterase in tunicates. Comp. Biochem. Physiol. **8**, 327—330 (1963).
— Cholinergic neurons in tunicates: an appraisal of the evidence. Comp. Biochem. Physiol. **22**, 617—627 (1967).
Frontali, N.: Histochemical localization of catecholamines in the brain of normal and drug-treated cockroaches. J. Insect Physiol. **14**, 881—886 (1968).
— Häggendal, J.: Noradrenaline and dopamine content in the brain of the cockroach *Periplaneta americana*. Brain Res. **14**, 540—542 (1969).
— Norberg, K.-A.: Catecholamine containing neurons in the cockroach brain. Acta physiol. scand. **66**, 243—244 (1966).
Furneaux, P. J. S., McFarlane, J. E.: Identification, estimation, and localization of catecholamines in eggs of the house cricket, *Acheta domesticus* (L.). J. Insect Physiol. **11**, 591—600 (1965a).
— — A possible relationship between the occurrence of catecholamines and water absorption in insect eggs. J. Insect Physiol. **11**, 631—635 (1965b).
Gaskell, J. F.: The chromaffine system of annelids and the relation of this system to the contractile vascular system in the leech, *Hirudo medicinalis*. Phil. Trans. B **205**, 153—212 (1914).
— Adrenalin in annelids. J. gen. Physiol. **2**, 73—85 (1919).
Gerschenfeld, H. M.: Observations on the ultrastructure of synapses in some pulmonate molluscs. Z. Zellforsch. **60**, 258—275 (1963).
— Tauç, L. Différent aspects de la pharmacologie des synapses dans le système nerveux central des mollusques. J. Physiol. (Paris) **56**, 360—361 (1964).
Ghiretti, F.: Toxicity of octopus saliva against Crustacea. Ann. N.Y. Acad. Sci. **90**, 726—741 (1960).

Goldstone, M.W., Cooke, I.M.: Histochemical localization of monoamines in the crab central nervous system. Z. Zellforsch. **116**, 7—19 (1971).

Greenberg, M.J.: The responses of the *Venus* heart to catechol amines and high concentrations of 5-hydroxytryptamine. Brit. J. Pharmacol. **15**, 365—374 (1960).

Habermann, E.: Biochemie, Pharmakologie und Toxikologie der Inhaltsstoffe von Hymenopterengiften. Ergebn. Physiol. **60**, 220—325 (1968).

Hanström, B.: *Hormones in Invertebrates*. Oxford: Clarendon Press 1939.

Hartman, W.J., Clark, W.G., Cyr, S.D., Jordan, A.L., Leibhold, R.A.: Pharmacologically active amines and their biogenesis in the octopus. Ann. N.Y. Acad. Sci. **90**, 637—666 (1960).

Hidaka, T.: Dopamine hyperpolarizes and relaxes *Mytilus* muscle. Amer. Zool. **9**, 1108 (1969).

Jaeger, C.P., Jaeger, E.C., Welsh, J.H.: Localization of monoamine-containing neurones in the nervous system of *Strophocheilus oblongus* (Gastropoda). Z. Zellforsch. **112**, 54—68 (1971).

Janakidevi, K., Dewey, V.C., Kidder, G.W.: The biosynthesis of catecholamines in two genera of protozoa. J. biol. Chem. **241**, 2576—2578 (1966).

Karlson, P., Sekeris, C.E., Sekeri, K.E.: Zum Tyrosinstoffwechsel der Insekten. VI. Identifizierung von N-Acetyl-3,4-dihydroxy-β-phenyläthylamin (N-Acetyl-dopamin) als Tyrosinmetabolit. Hoppe-Seylers Z. physiol. Chem. **327**, 86—94 (1962).

Kehoe, J.: Pharmacological characteristics and ionic bases of a two component postsynaptic inhibition. Nature (Lond.) **215**, 1503—1505 (1967).

Kerkut, G.A., Horn, N., Walker, R.J.: Long-lasting synaptic inhibition and its transmitter in the snail *Helix aspersa*. Comp. Biochem. Physiol. **30**, 1061—1074 (1969).

— Sedden, C.B., Walker, R.J.: The effect of DOPA, α-methyl DOPA and reserpine on the dopamine content of the brain of the snail, *Helix aspersa*. Comp. Biochem. Physiol. **18**, 921—930 (1966).

— — — Cellular localization of monoamines by fluorescence microscopy in *Hirudo medicinalis* and *Lumbricus terrestris*. Comp. Biochem. Physiol. **21**, 687—690 (1967a).

— — — Uptake of DOPA and 5-hydroxytryptophan by monoamine-forming neurones in the brain of *Helix aspersa*. Comp. Biochem. Physiol. **23**, 159—162 (1967b).

— Walker, R.J.: The effects of drugs on the neurones of the snail *Helix aspersa*. Comp. Biochem. Physiol. **3**, 143—160 (1961).

— — The specific chemical sensitivity of *Helix* nerve cells. Comp. Biochem. Physiol. **7**, 277—288 (1962).

Klemm, N.: Monoaminhaltige Strukturen im Zentralnervensystem der Trichoptera (Insecta). Teil I. Z. Zellforsch. **92**, 487—502 (1968a).

— Monoaminerge Zellelemente im stomatogastrichen Nervensystem der Trichopteren (Insecta). Z. Naturforsch. **23b**, 1279—1280 (1968b).

Krijgsman, B.J.: Contractile and pacemaker mechanisms of the heart of arthropods. Biol. Rev. **27**, 320—346 (1952).

— Divaris, G.A.: Contractile and pacemaker mechanisms of the heart of molluscs. Biol. Rev. **30**, 1—39 (1955).

Lancaster, S.: Nature of the chromaffin nerve cells in certain annulates and arthropods. Trans. Amer. microsc. Soc. **58**, 90—96 (1939).

Lentz, T.L.: Histochemical localization of neurohumors in a sponge. J. exp. Zool. **162**, 171—180 (1966).

— *Primitive Nervous Systems*. New Haven: Yale Univ. Press 1968a.

— Histochemical localization of acetylcholinesterase activity in a planarian. Comp. Biochem. Physiol. **27**, 715—718 (1968b).

Loveland, R.E.: Some aspects of cardio-regulation in *Mercenaria mercenaria*. Ph. D. Thesis. Harvard University 1963.

Mancini, G., Frontali, N.: Fine structure of the mushroom body neuropile of the brain of the cockroach, *Periplaneta americana*. Z. Zellforsch. **83**, 334—343 (1967).

— — On the ultrastructural localization of catecholamines in the beta lobes (corpora pedunculata) of *Periplaneta americana*. Z. Zellforsch. **103**, 341—350 (1970).

Marsden, C.A., Kerkut, G.A.: Fluorescent microscopy of the 5-HT- and catecholamine-containing cells in the central nervous system of the leech *Hirudo medicinalis*. Comp. Biochem. Physiol. **31**, 851—862 (1969).

— — The occurrence of monoamines in *Planorbis corneus:* a fluorescence microscopic and microspectrometric study. Comp. Gen. Pharmacol. **1**, 101—116 (1970).

Maynard, D.M.: Thoracic neurosecretory structures in Brachyura. I. Gross anatomy. Biol. Bull. **121**, 316—329 (1961).

— Welsh, J.H.: Neurohormones of the pericardial organs of brachyuran crustacea. J. Physiol. (Lond.) **149**, 215—227 (1959).

Mirolli, M.: The effects of reserpine on molluscs. Ph. D. Thesis. Cambridge, Mass.: Harvard University 1964.
— Welsh, J.H.: The effects of reserpine and LSD on molluscs. In: *Comparative Neurochemistry*. D. Richter, ed. Oxford: Pergamon Press 1964.
Myhrberg, H.E.: Monoaminergic mechanisms in the nervous system of *Lumbricus terrestris* (L.). Z. Zellforsch. **81**, 311—343 (1967).
Northrop, R.B.: Pharmacological responses of the anterior byssus retractor muscle of *Mytilus* to dopamine, serotonin, and methysergide. Amer. Zool. **4**, 423 (1964).
Osborne, N.N., Cottrell, G.A.: Occurrence of noradrenaline and metabolites of primary catecholamines in the brain and heart of *Helix*. Comp. Gen. Pharmacol. **1**, 1—10 (1970).
— Dando, M.R.: Monoamines in the stomatogastric ganglion of the lobster, *Homarus vulgaris*. Comp. Biochem. Physiol. **32**, 327—331 (1970).
Östlund, E.: The distribution of catechol amines in lower animals and their effect on the heart. Acta physiol. scand. **31**, Suppl. 112 (1954).
Pentreath, V.W., Cottrell, G.A.: Acetylcholine and cholinesterase in the radial nerve of *Asterias rubens*. Comp. Biochem. Physiol. **27**, 775—785 (1968).
Piccinelli, D.: Effect of reserpine on indole-alkylamine and phenylalkylamine levels in tissues of lower vertebrates and molluscs. Arch. int. Pharmacodyn. **117**, 452—459 (1958).
Plotnikova, S.I.: The structure of the sympathetic nervous system of insects. In: *Neurobiology of Invertebrates*. J. Salanki, ed. pp. 59—68. New York: Plenum Press 1968.
— Kuzmina, L.V.: Distribution of monoamine-containing nervous elements in Planaria, *Dendrocoelum lacteum* (Turbellaria). J. evol. Biochem. Physiol. suppl. 1968. Physiology and Biochemistry of Invertebrates, pp. 23—29, Leningrad.
Plotnikova, S.N., Govyrin, W.A.: Die Verteilung katecholaminhaltiger Nervenelemente bei einigen Vertretern der Coelenteraten und Protostomier. Arch. anat. gistol. embriol. **50**, 79—87 (1966).
Poll, H., Sommer, A.: Über phaeochrome Zellen in Centralnervensystem des Blutegels. Verh. physiol. Ges. Berl. **10**, 549 (1903).
Retzius, G.: Zur Kenntnis des centralen Nervensystems der Hirudineen. Biol. Unters. Neue Folge **2**, 13—15 (1891).
Reutter, K.: Biogene Amine in Nervensystem von *Lineus sanguineus Rathke* (Nemertini). Z. Zellforsch. **94**, 391—406 (1969a).
— Das Verhalten des aminergen Nervensystems während der Regeneration des Vorderdarms von *Lineus sanguineus* Rathke (Nemertini). Z. Zellforsch. **102**, 283—292 (1969b).
Ross, D.M.: The effects of ions and drugs on neuromuscular preparations of sea anemones. I. On preparations of the column of *Calliactis* and *Metridium*. J. exp. Biol. **37**, 732—752 (1960a).
— II. On sphincter preparations of *Calliactis* and *Metridium*. J. exp. Biol. **37**, 753—774 (1960b).
Rude, S.: Monoamine-containing neurons in the nerve and body wall of *Lumbricus terrestris*. J. comp. Neurol. **128**, 397—412 (1966).
— Catecholamines in the ventral nerve cord of *Lumbricus terrestris*. Comp. Biochem. Physiol. **28**, 747—752 (1969a).
— Monoamine-containing neurons in the central nervous system and peripheral nerves of the leech, *Hirudo medicinalis*. J. comp. Neurol. **136**, 349—372 (1969b).
— Coggeshall, R.E., van Orden, L.S., 3rd: Chemical and ultrastructural identification of 5-hydroxytryptamine in an identified neuron. J. Cell Biol. **41**, 832—854 (1969).
Sakharov, D.A., Zz.-Nagy, I.: Localization of biogenic monoamines in cerebral ganglia of *Lymnaea stagnalis* L. Acta biol. hung. **19**, 145—157 (1968).
Sedden, C.B., Walker, R.J., Kerkut, G.A.: The localization of dopamine and 5-hydroxytryptamine in neurones of *Helix aspersa*. Symp. Zool. Soc. (Lond.) No. **22**, 19—32 (1968).
Sekeris, C.E., Karlson, P.: Biosynthesis of catecholamines in insects. Pharmacol. Rev. **18**, 89—94 (1966).
Sweeney, D.C.: Dopamine: Its occurrence in molluscan ganglia. Science **139**, 1051 (1963).
— Histochemical and pharmacological indications that dopamine may be a neurohumor in molluscs. Amer. Zool. **5**, 671 (1965).
— The anatomical distribution of monoamines in a fresh-water bivalve mollusc, *Sphaerium sulcatum* (L.). Comp. Biochem. Physiol. **25**, 601—613 (1968).
— Absence of monoamine oxidase activity in several invertebrate nervous systems. Amer. Zool. **9**, 582 (1969a).
— The synthesis of dopamine from DOPA in the ganglia of *Mercenaria mercenaria* (Mollusca, Pelecypoda). Comp. Biochem. Physiol. **30**, 903—907 (1969b).
Tauc, L.: Processus postsynaptiques d'excitation et d'inhibition dans le soma neuronique de l'Aplysie et de l'Escargot. Arch. ital. Biol. **96**, 78—110 (1958).
— Transmission in invertebrate and vertebrate ganglia. Physiol. Rev. **47**, 521—593 (1967).

TREHERNE, J.E.: *The Neurochemistry of Arthropods.* Cambridge: University Press 1966.

UDENFRIEND, S., LOVENBERG, W., SJOERDSMA, A.: Physiologically active amines in common fruits and vegetables. Arch. Biochem. Biophys. **85**, 487—491 (1959).

VIALLI, M.: Le cellule cromaffini dei gangli nervosi negli Irudinei. Atti Soc. Ital. Sci. Nat. **73**, 57—73 (1934).

WALKER, R.J.: Certain aspects of the pharmacology of *Helix* and *Hirudo* neurons. In: *Neurobiology of Invertebrates.* J. Salanki, ed. pp. 227—253. New York: Plenum Press 1968.

— WOODRUFF, G.N., GLAIZNER, B., SEDDEN, C.B., KERKUT, G.A.: The pharmacology of *Helix* depamine receptor of specific neurones in the snail, *Helix aspersa.* Comp. Biochem. Physiol. **24**, 455—469 (1968).

WELLS, G.P.: Studies on the physiology of *Arenicola marina* L. I. The pace-maker role of the oesophagus, and the action of adrenaline and acetylcholine. J. exp. Biol. **14**, 117—157 (1937).

WELSH, J.H.: Neurohumors and neurosecretion. In: *Physiology of Echinodermata.* R.A. Boolootian, ed. New York: Interscience 1966.

— KING, E.C.: Catecholamines in planarians. Comp. Biochem. Physiol. **36**, 683—688 (1970).

— LOVELAND, R.E.: 5-Hydroxytryptamine in the ascidian, *Ciona intestinalis* L. Comp. Biochem. Physiol. **27**, 719—722 (1968).

— MOORHEAD, M.: The quantitative distribution of 5-hydroxytryptamine in the invertebrates, especially in their nervous systems. J. Neurochem. **6**, 146—169 (1960).

— WILLIAMS, L.D.: Monoamine-containing neurons in planaria. J. comp. Neurol. **138**, 103—116 (1970).

WOOD, J.G.: Electron microscopic localization of amines in central nervous tissue. Nature (Lond.) **209**, 1131—1133 (1966).

— LENTZ, T.L.: Histochemical localization of amines in *Hydra* and in the sea anemone. Nature (Lond.) **201**, 88—90 (1964).

WOODRUFF, G.N., WALKER, R.J.: The effect of dopamine and other compounds on the activity of neurones of *Helix aspersa;* structure-activity relationships. Int. J. Neuropharmacol. **8**, 279—289 (1969).

— — KERKUT, G.A.: Actions of ergometrine on catecholamine receptors in the guinea-pig vas deferens and in the snail brain. Comp. Gen. Pharmacol. **1**, 61—66 (1970).

WU, K.S.: On the physiology and pharmacology of the earthworm gut. J. exp. Biol. **16**, 184—197 (1939).

ZILLER-PEREZ, H.V.: On the chromaffin cells of the nerve ganglia of *Hirudo medicinalis* L. J. comp. Neurol. **76**, 367—394 (1942).

ZS.-NAGY, I.: Histochemical demonstration of biogenic monoamines in the central nervous system of the lamellibranch mollusc *Anodonta cygnea* L. Acta biol. hung. **18**, 1—8 (1967).

ZS.-NAGY, L.: Histochemical and electron-microscopic studies on the relation between dopamine and dense-core vesicles in the neurons of *Anodonta cygnea* L. In: *Neurobiology of Invertebrates.* J. Salanki, ed. pp. 69—84. New York: Plenum Press 1968.

Note added in proof: For recent literature on catecholamines in insects see also:

ANDERSEN, S.O.: Isolation of arterenone (2-amino-3′,4′-dihydroxyacetophenone) from hydrolysates of sclerotized insect cuticle. J. Insect Physiol. **16**, 1951—1959 (1970).

BAGNOLI, P., BRUNELLI, M., MAGNI, F., VIOLA, M.: The identification of a flash-inhibiting substance from the male gonads of *Luciola lusitanica* (Charp.). Arch. ital. Biol. (in press).

CARLSON, A.D.: Neural control of firefly luminescence. Advanc. Insect Physiol. **6**, 51—96 (1969).

SMALLEY, K.N.: Adrenergic transmission in the light organ of the firefly, *Photinus pyralis.* Comp. Biochem. Physiol. **16**, 467—477 (1965).

Chapter 5

The Distribution of Catecholamines in Vertebrates

MARGARETHE HOLZBAUER and D. F. SHARMAN

I. Introduction

Three catecholamines have been definitely identified as being present in many vertebrate tissues. These are (—)-adrenaline ((—)-2-[3,4-dihydroxyphenyl] methylethan-2-olamine), (—)-noradrenaline ((—)-2-[3,4-dihydroxyphenyl] ethan-2-olamine) and dopamine (2-[3,4-dihydroxyphenyl] ethylamine). In addition there are several reports which demonstrate the presence of the precursor amino acid L-DOPA ((—)-2-[3,4-dihydroxyphenyl] alanine) but many of these are based on a minimum of experimental evidence and some are conflicting in their observations. N-methyl adrenaline (AXELROD, 1960) and N-methyldopamine (epinine) (MÄRKI et al., 1962) have also been extracted from vertebrate tissues or body fluids. There may be other catecholamines present which have yet to be isolated.

The first hormone to be chemically identified was a catecholamine. Although adrenaline was extracted from the adrenal gland, isolated (ABEL and CRAWFORD, 1897; TAKAMINE, 1901; ALDRICH, 1901) and synthesized (STOLZ, 1904; DAKIN, 1905), ABEL and TAVEAU (1905) were still able to bring forward objections to the identity of the isolated material with the synthetic product. The fluorimetric methods of analysis which are applied to the estimation of catecholamines, on their own, yield much less chemical information than was available to these earlier workers yet the presence of a fluorescent material in a solution after a few simple procedures is often accepted as sufficient proof for the presence of a catecholamine in the material which has been extracted. Although for most purposes the current fluorimetric analytical methods are suited to the detection of changes in the concentration of tissue catecholamines, near the lower limit of their range of sensitivity they tend to become unreliable and the distinction between estimation and identification must be rigidly observed. There are many reports on the presence or concentration of catecholamines in tissues which are not confirmed on more detailed investigation. In addition the concentration of a catecholamine in a tissue is subject to biological variation. Thus it is frequently very difficult to decide which of the many reported concentrations of catecholamines in vertebrate tissues is the one to cite in a review such as this. We have decided to give, where possible, the results obtained by different authors using different methods of analysis and also results in which the same procedure has been applied to many different tissues. In this way we hope that a clearer picture will emerge. The values given are usually mean values but some single observations have been included. It is felt that to include a standard error of the mean does not have any value unless the number of observations is also given. In many cases this information is not available and if included here for every example would complicate the presentation which is intended to show where the catecholamines have been found and to indicate the amounts present.

The development of fluorescence histochemical methods for the localisation and identification of monoamines in tissues has proved to be most valuable in extending the knowledge of the distribution of catecholamines. Observations made with these methods will be included here as providing further evidence for the presence of catecholamines in tissues but the methods themselves will not be discussed in detail.

II. Methods Used for the Estimation and Identification of Catecholamines in Tissues and Body Fluids

Many of the earlier methods for the estimation of catecholamines were based on pharmacological responses to these substances. As early as 1912, ELLIOTT showed that the response of the blood pressure to adrenaline in the spinal cat could be used to measure the adrenaline in the adrenal gland. Among other tissues which have been used as test preparations for the estimation of catecholamines are the rat uterus (DE JALON et al., 1945), the blood vessels of the rabbit ear (PAGE and GREEN, 1948; DE LA LANDE and HARVEY, 1965), the rectal caecum of the hen (BARSOUM and GADDUM, 1935; VON EULER, 1948a) and the blood pressure of the rat (SHIPLEY and TILDEN, 1947; CRAWFORD and OUTSCHOORN, 1951). The use of biological preparations for the assay of catecholamines has been reviewed by GADDUM (1959) and VANE (1966). Bioassay if carried out with proper controls and with carefully purified tissue extracts is very sensitive and can be very specific, but it is time consuming and not very accurate. An improvement in accuracy was sought in chemical methods of assay.

Of several colorimetric methods, that of VON EULER and HAMBERG (1949a) was probably the most successful. It was based on the formation of a red colour when adrenaline and noradrenaline are oxidised with iodine and was used in the demonstration of noradrenaline in the adrenal gland (VON EULER and HAMBERG, 1949b) and a similar method was used by EHRINGER and HORNYKIEWICZ (1960) to estimate the concentration of dopamine in the human brain. Colorimetric methods were not sensitive or specific enough to measure the small amounts of catecholamines found in most tissues. Analytical methods based on the formation of fluorescent derivatives of catecholamines have proved sensitive enough to enable a more detailed examination of vertebrate tissues for the presence of catecholamines to be carried out. Only two types of chemical reaction have formed the basis of all of these assays. The first of these, usually termed the trihydroxyindole procedure (THI) from the chemical structure of the products formed from adrenaline and noradrenaline, is the more specific procedure. The catecholamine is oxidised and the molecular structure of the product is rearranged in concentrated alkali in the presence of a stabilising agent. The fluorescence of this solution can be measured directly or the pH can be adjusted before the measurement is made, a procedure which is necessary for the estimation of dopamine. The fluorescence is usually measured at wavelengths of activation and fluorescence which give the best specificity to the procedure. More than one catecholamine can be measured in the same solution by varying the conditions of oxidation or by making use of the differences in the characteristics of the fluorescence of the products from the different catecholamines. The history and chemistry of this reaction has been reviewed by VON EULER (1959) and VENDSALU (1960). Some detailed reports of its application have been given by LUND (1949), VON EULER and FLODING (1955), VON EULER and LISHAJKO (1961), SOURKES and MURPHY

(1961), Anton and Sayre (1962), Häggendal (1963a) and Laverty and Taylor (1968).

The second procedure by which a fluorescent derivative of the catecholamines can be made is based on the condensation of catechol compounds with 1,2-diaminoethane. First described for the estimation of adrenaline by Natelson et al. (1949), the procedure has been criticised for its lack of specificity (Valk and Price, 1956). However, the procedure is very sensitive and when combined with careful extraction and purification procedures can be used in the estimation and identification of catecholamines and related compounds (Montagu, 1957; von Euler and Lishajko, 1957; Laverty and Sharman, 1965).

The specificity of any method of estimating catecholamines also depends upon the procedures used to prepare extracts for testing. The earliest biological estimations were carried out on simple extracts of tissues usually made with protein precipitants such as acid ethanol or trichloroacetic acid and the specificity of the method resided in the test preparation. In 1938 Shaw described how adrenaline was adsorbed onto aluminium hydroxide at pH 8—8.5 but not at pH 4. Lund (1949) replaced aluminium hydroxide with aluminium oxide and this method has been used to extract catechol compounds from tissue extracts by many workers. The catechols can be eluted from the alumina with dilute acid. Unfortunately this extraction procedure seems to be regarded by some as having an absolute specificity for catechol compounds. This is not so since, for example, Wieland (1942) and Fromageot et al. (1948) have clearly shown that aluminium oxide can also act as an ion exchange material and will take up amino acids at a neutral or slightly alkaline pH.

Ion exchange resins have also often been employed to extract catecholamines. The procedure most often used is based on that of Bertler et al. (1958) who used the strong cation exchange resin, Dowex-50. The catecholamines can be separated by elution chromatography (Bertler et al., 1958; Häggendal, 1962).

Shore and Olin (1958) described a simple solvent (n-butanol) extraction method which extracts basic substances from tissues or tissue extracts and gives a solution to which the trihydroxyindole procedure can be applied. It is simple and rapid but not very specific and was improved by Chang (1964) who combined it with the aluminium oxide extraction procedure.

Paper chromatography has also been used to purify tissue extracts. Vogt (1954) employed the method described by James (1948) and by Crawford and Outschoorn (1951) in mapping the distribution of adrenaline and noradrenaline in the dog brain. A separation of the acetyl derivatives of catecholamines by paper chromatography (Hagopian et al., 1961) has formed the basis of the methods used for the estimation of catecholamines by Goldstein et al. (1959), Laverty and Sharman (1965) and Crawford and Yates (1970).

Recently methods based on the formation of radioactive derivatives of catecholamines have been reported and that described by Saelens et al. (1967) appears to be specific for the measurement of noradrenaline but the method developed by Nikodijevic et al. (1969) may have a wider application. In the former method noradrenaline is converted to radioactive adrenaline by the enzymic transfer of a radioactive methyl group to the amino nitrogen using the enzyme phenylethanolamine-N-methyl transferase. The radioactive product is purified by paper chromatography and measured by liquid scintillation counting. The latter method employs the enzyme catechol-O-methyl transferase to introduce a radioactive methyl group at the 3-position on the phenyl ring of noradrenaline and may have a more general application to the estimation of other catechol compounds.

Gas chromatography has found little application, as yet, to the estimation of catecholamines, but urinary dopamine has been estimated using this technique by CLARKE et al. (1967).

Mass spectrometry will no doubt provide very good evidence for the identification of small amounts of catecholamines in tissues. Dopamine has been identified by KNOCHE et al. (1969) by mass spectrometry of its 1-dimethylaminonaphthalene-5-sulphonyl (dansyl) derivative as being present in the carotid body of the horse.

Some of the concentrations of catecholamines given in this review may be higher than the true concentrations but it is less likely that they are too low since the methods employed, *if used correctly*, will always measure the catecholamines present in an extract but they may not exclude all other substances.

III. Distribution of Catecholamines in Tissues and Body Fluids

1. Catecholamines in Cyclostomata (Hagfishes and Lampreys)

The concentrations of adrenaline and noradrenaline, which have been estimated to be present in tissues of some cyclostomata, are listed in Table 1. The heart contains large amounts of both catecholamines, compared with mammalian species. Adrenaline is the major catecholamine in the heart of *Lampetra fluviatilis*. Its concentration is higher in the auricle than in the ventricle and most of the amine is probably contained in the chromaffin cells found in this organ (BLOOM et al., 1961; STABROVSKII, 1967). The latter author also found an increase in the adrenaline content of the heart of *Lampetra fluviatilis* after muscular exercise.

In the heart of *Myxine glutinosa*, adrenaline is the main catecholamine present in the ventricle, whereas there is more noradrenaline than adrenaline in the auricle and the portal heart.

In both species the heart is normally insensitive to catecholamines (ÖSTLUND, 1954). However, after treatment with reserpine, which decreases the natural catecholamine content, adrenaline and noradrenaline had a positive inotropic and chronotropic effect (BLOOM et al., 1961). There is no evidence for the existence of cardioregulatory nerve fibres (VON EULER and FÄNGE, 1961).

2. Catecholamines in Euselachii

Noradrenaline is present in higher concentrations than adrenaline in most tissues analysed from members of this sub-class (Tables 2 and 3). A regional analysis of the catecholamines in the brain of *Squalus acanthias* was carried out by VON EULER (1961). The uneven distribution of noradrenaline shows a similarity to that in the mammalian brain.

VON EULER (1953) found that the sympathetic ganglia along the central dorsal blood vessels contained both adrenaline (2.8 μg/mg) and noradrenaline (6.8 μg/mg) and observed that the tissue contained many chromaffin cells.

3. Catecholamines in Teleostii (Bony fishes)

Many organs from different species of this class of animals have been analysed for their catecholamine content. Tables 4 and 5 show some of the reported values for the concentrations of adrenaline and noradrenaline present in different organs. There is little experimental evidence to demonstrate the function of catecholamines in the tissues of bony fishes. Denervation of the swim bladder of *Gadus callarius* (cod) did not result in a decrease in the catecholamine content of this organ (VON EULER and FÄNGE, 1961). Changes in the concentration of catecholamines in the blood and tissues of bony fishes have been observed. STABROVSKII (1969) reported that the tissues of some fishes which were migrating over long distances contained more catecholamines than the same tissues of fishes which were leading a more stationary existence (Table 5). A rise in the concentration of adrenaline in the liver and the heart and a 10—100 fold increase in the plasma concentrations of adrenaline and noradrenaline were observed when *Salmo gairdneri* was grasped or chased (NAKANO and TOMLINSON, 1967). Similarly, a threefold increase in the blood catecholamine concentration was seen after disturbing *Cyprinus carpio* (MAZEAUD, 1964). BOEHLKE et al. (1967) reported diurnal variation in the concentration of noradrenaline in the plasma of *Ictalurus punctatus* (channel catfish). The concentration was lowest in the morning (3 μg/l.) and highest in the afternoon (46 μg/l.).

The cellular localisation of catecholamines has been studied in several organs of fishes using fluorescence histochemistry. In *Salmo irideus*, after treatment of the tissue with formaldehyde, fine fluorescing fibres were seen in the hypothalamus and there was a layer of green fluorescing cells with protrusions into the ventricular lumen beneath the ependymal border (BERTLER et al., 1963). Using the same methods BAUMGARTEN and BRAAK (1967) found catecholamine-containing cell groups in the hypothalamus of *Carassius auratus* and BAUMGARTEN (1967) reported fluorescing fibres in the gut, the splanchnic nerve and in nerve cells of a ganglion on the oesophagus of *Tinca vulgaris*. From histochemical tests the author concluded that dopamine might be present in these tissues. LUPPA et al. (1968) found fluorescence which was attributable to monoamines in the neuro-secretory neurons in the urophysis of *Cyprinus carpio*. JUORIO (personal communication) has found that dopamine is present in the brain of *Carassius auratus* in addition to adrenaline and noradrenaline.

4. Catecholamines in Amphibia

Amphibian tissues were used in the earliest studies on catecholamines. A pressor active substance from the adrenal glands of frogs was described by SZYMONOWICZ (1896). Adrenaline was isolated and crystallised from the parotid gland of *Bufo agua* (the tropical toad) by ABEL and MACHT (1912). They found that the crude venom contained up to 6.7% of adrenaline. CALDEYRO and PATETTA (1946) and BACQ and LECOMTE (1947) studied the secretion of sympathomimetic substances from the parotid gland of *Bufo arenarum Hensel* and observed that denervation of the gland caused a decrease in the secretion of adrenaline. Earlier observations on the presence of adrenaline in the secretion from the skin and the parotid glands of toads have been reviewed by GESSNER (1938). LOEWI (1936) identified the adrenaline in the heart of the frog by biological and fluorescence methods and concluded that in the frog the "Sympathicus Stoff" was identical with adrenaline.

The concentrations of catecholamines in different organs of amphibia are listed in Tables 6—10. Adrenaline is the dominant catecholamine in most organs. Exceptions are found in the peripheral organs of some newts and salamanders (see Table 6). In the adrenal glands, the concentrations of adrenaline and noradrenaline are usually similar. The sympathetic chain in *Rana catesbeiana* contains more noradrenaline (10.1 μg/g) than adrenaline (2.9 μg/g) (AZUMA et al., 1965).

FALCK et al. (1963) demonstrated the presence of adrenergic nerve fibres in the heart of *Rana temporaria* by fluorescence microscopy but could not find any fluorescing chromaffin cells. Environmental temperature changes did not affect the catecholamine content of the heart of *Rana catesbeiana* (AZUMA et al., 1965). Six weeks after denervation of the heart the catecholamine content was not decreased if the frogs were kept at low temperatures. They died if they were kept at 18—22° C.

Seasonal variations occur in the catecholamine concentration of amphibian tissues. DONOSO and SEGURA (1965) found that, in *Bufo arenarum*, there was a lower plasma adrenaline concentration in summer and that the concentration of noradrenaline decreased in the autumn. The average concentrations of adrenaline and noradrenaline in the plasma were 0.6 μg/100 ml and 0.7 μg/100 ml respectively. SEGURA et al. (1967) found that there was a lower adrenaline concentration in the brain of *Bufo arenarum Hensel* during hibernation which coincided with a slow EEG-pattern. Seasonal variations in the catecholamine content of the adrenal gland of *Bufo arenarum Hensel* have been observed by RAPELA and GORDON (1956). The adrenaline concentration was low in summer and high in winter. The changes in the noradrenaline content were not so pronounced. Some observations on the catecholamine concentrations in the eye of the frog and the toad are listed in Table 10.

Small amounts of dopamine have been found in amphibian tissues. ANGELAKOS et al. (1965) estimated the concentration of dopamine in the heart of *Rana pipiens*. The highest concentrations were in the sinus venosus which contains the pacemaker (see Table 8). There was little, if any, dopamine present in the heart of *Rana temporaria* (FALCK et al., 1963). GROBECKER et al. (1966) were unable to find DOPA or dopamine in the heart, adrenals or skin of *Rana temporaria*. Dopamine has also been found during the embryonic development of *Rana pipiens*. CASTON (1962) observed that dopamine was the first catecholamine to be detected (27 ng/embryo at stage 15) (stages according to SHUMWAY, 1940). Noradrenaline appeared at stage 16 (19 ng/embryo) and adrenaline at stage 17 (13.3 ng/embryo). At stage 18 the embryos contained 40 ng dopamine, 71 ng noradrenaline and 50 ng adrenaline.

In the carotid labyrinth of *Rana temporaria* BANISTER et al. (1967) found 0.4—1.0 μg dopamine per g tissue. They also determined adrenaline and noradrenaline (2—7 μg/g) in the carotid labyrinth and the aortic arch of this species, using bioassay methods after paper chromatography and also by fluorescence methods. The concentrations of catecholamines in the brain of *Rana temporaria* have been determined by JUORIO (personal communication) using the method of LAVERTY and SHARMAN (1965) and obtained the following values. Ventral regions of the cerebral hemispheres: adrenaline 0.50 μg/g, noradrenaline 0.17 μg/g, dopamine 0.23 μg/g; Thalamus + hypothalamus + optic lobes: adrenaline 0.50 μg/g, noradrenaline 0.14 μg/g, dopamine 0.23 μg/g; Hypothalamus: adrenaline 2.93 μg/g, noradrenaline 0.52 μg/g, dopamine 1.06 μg/g.

MÄRKI et al. (1962) extracted the venom of the parotid gland of *Bufo marinus*, and with the aid of column chromatography on aluminium oxide columns, two-dimensional paper chromatography and fluorescence characteristics they identified adrenaline, noradrenaline and dopamine in a ratio of approximately 4:1:2. N-methyl-dopamine was present in the same concentration as noradrenaline.

The fluorescence histology of amphibian tissue was studied by McLEAN and BURNSTOCK (1966, 1967a). Fluorescing fibres in the smooth muscle bands and accompanying blood vessels were observed in the lung of toads. In the wall of the lung and the vago-sympathetic trunk there were also catecholamine containing ganglion cells which were able to take up ^{3}H-noradrenaline. Adrenergic fibres in the smooth muscles of the bladder of toads and frogs are rare. BURNSTOCK (1969) reported that there was 1.86 μg/g wet weight adrenaline and 0.23 μg/g wet weight noradrenaline in the bladder of *Rana catesbeiana*. BROUWER and VAN DE VEERDONK (1969) studied the fluorescence microscopy of the skin of *Xenopus laevis* and found a green fluorescing strip below the epidermis. Only dopamine could be identified in extracts of the skin.

ITURRIZA (1967) concluded from fluorescence histology of the pineal gland of *Bufo arenarum* that this organ does not possess an active adrenergic nerve system. Adrenergic fibres in the pars intermedia of the pituitary gland of *Bufo arenarum* which were in close relation to the cells containing colloid vesicles were reported by ENEMAR et al. (1967).

5. Catecholamines in Reptilia

Noradrenaline and adrenaline have been estimated in organs of some reptiles. Noradrenaline was present in higher concentrations than adrenaline in all of the organs examined with the exception of the adrenal gland (Table 11). A very high concentration of noradrenaline (16.4 μg/g) was found in the vas deferens of the Greek tortoise *(Testudo graeca)* by SJÖSTRAND (1965a). ANTON and SAYRE (1964) found dopamine in the heart, brain, kidney and liver of the turtle. There was an especially high concentration of dopamine in the spleen of this animal. The identity of the compound measured in the spleen was verified by paper chromatography. JUORIO (1969) studied the distribution of dopamine in the brain of a turtle *(Geochelone chilensis)* (Table 12) and found high concentrations in the area of the nucleus basalis, a part of the brain which has functions similar to those of the basal ganglia of the mammalian brain where large amounts of dopamine are also found. As in the mammal treatment with reserpine reduces the concentration of the cerebral dopamine in this turtle. However, no effects of reserpine on the behaviour of this animal were observed. The large noradrenaline concentrations present in the kidneys of some Testudines are probably associated with chromaffin tissue.

In reptiles the chromaffin tissue exists both in association with the interrenal elements and with sympathetic neurones. In the adrenal of the lizard *Lacerta viridis*, one group of chromaffin cells embraces the cortex and is thickened in the dorsal region of the gland. There is histochemical evidence that these cells contain mainly noradrenaline (WRIGHT and CHESTER-JONES, 1955). Another group of chromaffin cells forms tongues and islets between the adrenal cortical cells. These cells contain adrenaline. In the snake adrenal gland, the peripheral chromaffin tissue is placed like a ribbon longitudinally over the surface of the gland and the central chromaffin tissue intermingles with cortical tissue (WASSERMANN and TRAMEZZANI, 1963). The chromaffin tissue in the centre of the gland contains phenylethanolamine-N-methyl transferase (WURTMAN et al., 1967b).

Fluorescence microscopic studies of the lung (MCLEAN and BURNSTOCK, 1967a), the urinary bladder (MCLEAN and BURNSTOCK, 1967b) and the large intestine (READ and BURNSTOCK, 1968) of *Trachysaurus rugosus* (the sleepy lizard) have demonstrated the presence of adrenergic nerves.

ZARAFONETIS and KALAS (1960) found catecholamines in the freeze dried venom of the snakes *Agkistrodon piscivorus*, *Crotalus atrox* and *Crotalus adamanteus* ANTON and GENNARO (1965) were unable to confirm this observation. No catecholamines were found in the venom of *Heloderma horridum* (ZARAFONETIS and KALAS, 1960).

6. Catecholamines in Birds

Studies on the distribution of catecholamines in birds are few. Naturally, most observations have been made on the chicken *(Gallus domesticus)* and some have been made on the pigeon *(Columba livia)*. Investigations on other species have been sporadic.

From the figures given in Tables 13 and 14 it would seem that, in general, there is a higher relative concentration of adrenaline in avian tissues than there is in the corresponding mammalian tissues. This does not apply to the adrenal glands of birds where, as in mammals, there are cell groups which contain either adrenaline or noradrenaline (ERÄNKÖ, 1957) and GHOSH (1962), on the basis of histological observations, has shown that the percentage of adrenaline in this tissue in a series of birds ranged from 0 in *Phalacrocorax niger* (cormorant) to 95% in *Corvus splendens* (Indian house crow).

The subcellular distribution of adrenaline and noradrenaline in the adrenal gland of the chicken has been studied by SCHÜMANN (1957). As had been previously observed with the bovine adrenal gland (EADE, 1956) granules containing mainly adrenaline could be separated from granules containing very high percentages of noradrenaline.

The formation of catecholamines in the embryo of the chicken has been studied (BOUCEK and BOCKLAGE-BOURNE, 1962; LEIBSON and STABROVSKII, 1962; IGNARRO and SHIDEMAN, 1968a and b; and MANUKHIN et al., 1969). Dopamine has been detected in the embryo after 2 days incubation and noradrenaline and adrenaline appear after 3 days. The formation of the catecholamines is preceded by the appearance of the precursor amino acid DOPA. In view of the few but widely varying estimates of this amino acid in chicken tissues using apparently reliable and reasonably specific methods further investigations must be made before the figures given here for the concentrations of DOPA can be accepted as the true values.

The distribution of catecholamines in the brain of the pigeon and the chicken has been determined in greater detail than in the other avian organs. There is, however, disagreement on the relative concentration of adrenaline in the brain of the pigeon and the chicken. The differences appear to be partly methodological in origin and partly due to the differences in the concentration of adrenaline in different strains of chicken and partly due to the increase of the relative concentration of adrenaline in the brain which occurs with age (JUORIO and VOGT, 1970; CALLINGHAM and SHARMAN, 1970).

Fluorescence histochemistry has been used to study the innervation of some avian tissues. AKESTER and MANN (1969) have suggested that the fluorescing nerve fibres in the renal portal valve in the chicken contain adrenaline whereas DOLEŽEL and ZLÁBEK (1969) have found that noradrenaline is present. BELL (1969) has examined the innervation of the anterior mesenteric artery of the chicken and concluded that the fluorescing nerve fibres contain noradrenaline. EVERETT and MANN (1967) have reported that fluorescence histochemistry of the intestine of the chick indicates the presence of adrenaline.

STURKIE and LIN (1968) have found that there is a higher concentration of noradrenaline in the blood plasma of female chickens than in that of males. There was no difference in the adrenaline concentration.

7. Catecholamines in Mammals

a) Nervous System

Brain

The presence of noradrenaline and adrenaline in the mammalian central nervous system was detected by VON EULER (1946) and HOLTZ (1950) using bioassay methods. At first the amines were thought to be associated with vasomotor nerves. The regional distribution of these two amines in the brain was described by VOGT (1954) who also used bioassay but employed paper chromatographic separation of the amines to ensure the specificity of the results. In addition it was shown (VOGT, 1954) that cervical sympathectomy did not affect the concentration of adrenaline and noradrenaline in the hypothalamus of the cat. This result was confirmed and extended to dopamine in rat brain tissues by BERTLER and ROSENGREN (1959a) using fluorimetric assay procedures. The concentration of the amines indicated that there were more catecholamine containing nerves in the hypothalamus than would be expected for vasomotor control alone. MONTAGU (1956a, 1957) examined extracts of brain tissue for catechol compounds using paper chromatography, paper electrophoresis and separation on ion exchange resins. The results showed that substances behaving like adrenaline and noradrenaline on paper chromatography were present in brain tissue. In addition, a third substance which the author concluded was probably dopamine was also present. Human brain, taken 30 hours after death, was shown to contain DOPA (3,4-dihydroxyphenylalanine) (MONTAGU, 1957). No clear evidence for the presence of DOPA in the brains of species other than man has been reported. SANO et al. (1959) have described the distribution of this amino acid in the human brain and MATSUOKA et al. (1964) have given estimates for its concentration and distribution in the rabbit. However, ANTON and SAYRE (1964) were unable to detect DOPA in the brains of several species. Improved methods for the analysis of this amino acid are required.

In 1958 BERTLER et al. described a method for the estimation of adrenaline and noradrenaline in tissues involving adsorption of the amines onto a small column of ion exchange resin and showed that eluates from the column, when derived from brain tissue extracts, contained substances which behaved like noradrenaline and dopamine on paper chromatography. LAVERTY and SHARMAN (1965) acetylated the amines present in extracts of brain tissue and found that substances which showed the properties of the acetyl derivatives of adrenaline, noradrenaline and dopamine could then be isolated.

The concentrations of adrenaline, noradrenaline and dopamine in different parts of the brains of different mammalian species are given in Tables 15—22.

Tables 15—22 show that, in general, the distribution of catecholamines is similar in the brains of different mammalian species. Some discrepancies between the results obtained by different methods are present. These can arise from differences in dissection. GLOWINSKI and IVERSEN (1966), POPOV et al. (1967) and VALZELLI and GARATTINI (1968) have given details of their dissection procedure for the rat brain and REIS et al. (1968) illustrated their dissection of the cat brain. Sometimes the differences are due to the lack of absolute specificity in the methods used. The estimation of noradrenaline in striatal tissues seems to present such a problem. When analysed by the more specific procedures, the caudate nucleus is found to contain very little noradrenaline, but several of the fluorimetric analyses indicate the presence of a higher concentration of this amine. It remains to be determined whether this difference is due to errors inherent in the methods used or the presence of another substance in this tissue.

Some of the differences in the estimates of the concentrations of catecholamines in the brain tissue might have their origin in the natural variations that can occur. The concentrations of catecholamines increases with age from birth to the adult state (BEAUVALLET et al., 1961; KARKI et al., 1962; PSCHEIDT and HIMWICH, 1966; AGRAWAL et al., 1968) and can vary with the season of the year (MONTAGU, 1956b, 1959; BEAUVALLET et al., 1962) and strains or genera (SCUDDER et al., 1966).

Various forms of stress are known to change the concentration of noradrenaline in the brain (VOGT, 1954; BARCHAS and FREEDMAN, 1963; MAYNERT and LEVI, 1964; MOORE and LARIVIERE, 1964). Circadian and ultradian rhythms in the concentrations of catecholamines have been observed in the brain of the rat (SCHEVING et al., 1968; FRIEDMAN and WALKER, 1968; MANSHARDT and WURTMAN, 1968) in which the concentration of an amine can vary by 15—20% around the 24 hours mean value. A detailed analysis of the concentrations of noradrenaline in regions of the cat brain has been made by REIS et al. (1968). These authors found that circadian rhythms in the concentration of noradrenaline were only observed in some parts of the brain, but the variation in concentration in those parts was up to threefold. Changes in the cerebral concentrations of catecholamines may also occur during hibernation. UUSPÄÄ (1963a) found a reduction in the concentration of noradrenaline in the brain of the hedgehog *(Erinaceus europaeus)* from 0.62 μg/g when awake to 0.43 μg/g when hibernating. There was little change in the concentration of adrenaline or dopamine. However, DRASKÓCZY and LYMAN (1967) observed no differences in the concentrations of noradrenaline and adrenaline in the brain of the ground squirrel *(Citellus tridecemlineatus)* in the awake and hibernating states. In *Citellus lateralis*, TWENTE et al. (1970) have also observed little change in brain catecholamines during the hibernating cycle except for a fall in noradrenaline in the medulla-pons region when the animals were active.

Another problem which has aroused discussion is the significance of the presence of adrenaline in cerebral tissue. The early observations on the presence of this amine in the brain were made with biological tests. In 1962 GUNNE examined brain tissue from the hen, pig, rat, ox and guinea-pig by means of ion exchange resin chromatography and compared the extracts so obtained in bioassay and fluorimetric tests. He showed that adrenaline was present in the brain of the hen, pig and rat but was unable to confirm the presence of this amine in the brain of the ox or the guinea-pig. The formation and metabolism of adrenaline in the brain and the possibility that it might have a separate function in the central nervous system has been discussed by BARCHAS et al. (1969).

Spinal Cord

Sympathomimetic activity was detected in extracts of the spinal cord by VON EULER (1946) who suggested that it was due to the presence of noradrenaline. The concentration of noradrenaline in different parts of the grey matter of the spinal cord of the dog was estimated by VOGT (1954) to be between 0.11 and 0.24 μg/g. The lowest concentration was found in the posterior horns. The observations of these two authors were based on biological assays.

In 1962 MCGEER and MCGEER analysed the spinal cords from six species for their contents of catecholamines using aluminium oxide in the extraction procedure and converted the catecholamines to hydroxyindole derivatives for fluorimetric estimation. The values found for noradrenaline plus adrenaline were similar to those obtained by bioassay. These authors also estimated the concentrations of dopamine and DOPA in the spinal cord to be higher than the concentration of noradrenaline. However, other authors (MAGNUSSON and ROSENGREN, 1963; ANTON and SAYRE, 1964; ANDÉN, 1965 and LAVERTY and SHARMAN, 1965) have been unable to confirm the results of MCGEER and MCGEER (1962) in respect of the concentration of DOPA or dopamine. Table 23 shows the concentrations of catecholamines estimated to be in the spinal cord. The distribution of catecholamines in different parts of the spinal cord has been studied by MCGEER and MCGEER (1962), ANDÉN (1965) and ANDERSON and HOLGERSON (1966). These authors have all shown that the grey matter contains more noradrenaline than the white matter, a result which corresponds with fluorescence histochemical observations. The concentration of noradrenaline is highest at the sacral end of the spinal cord.

Pineal Gland

The presence of catecholamines in the bovine pineal gland was detected by GIARMAN and DAY (1958). PELLEGRINO DE IRALDI and ZIEHER (1966) estimated both noradrenaline (7.59 μg/g gland) and dopamine (34.3 μg/g gland) in the pineal gland of the rat. They also demonstrated that the noradrenaline was associated with the sympathetic innervation since decentralisation or extirpation of the superior cervical ganglia resulted in a reduction of the concentration of noradrenaline in the pineal gland. The tissue content of dopamine was unaltered by these procedures.

A circadian rhythm in the content of noradrenaline in the pineal gland has been demonstrated in the rat (WURTMAN and AXELROD, 1966; WURTMAN et al., 1967a), and it is correlated with the daily light changes since it no longer occurred when animals were blinded or kept under constant light or dark conditions. A similar rhythm in the noradrenaline concentration of the pineal gland has been reported for the cat (REIS et al., 1968).

Cerebrospinal Fluid

The noradrenaline in the cerebrospinal fluid of the dog was estimated by VOGT (1954), using bioassay, to be 5 μg/litre. With a fluorimetric method based on condensation with 1,2-diaminoethane, WEIL-MALHERBE and LIDDELL (1954) found 0.9 μg/litre adrenaline and 2.46 μg/litre noradrenaline in the cerebrospinal fluid of neurological patients. MANGER et al. (1959) using a similar method obtained values of about 1 μg/litre for the total "epinephrine-like substance" in human cerebrospinal fluid. DENCKER et al. (1967) have applied the THI procedure to the problem of estimating the catecholamines in cerebrospinal fluid. They obtained a mean noradrenaline concentration of 0.5 ± 0.03 μg/litre from 68 patients with mental disease. In a few other cases the concentration was high, up to 16.4 μg/litre. In one case only was adrenaline detected. Dopamine was not found. As in blood plasma some of the noradrenaline in the cerebrospinal fluid was in an acid hydrolysable form.

Peripheral Nerves and Ganglia

Evidence for the identity of the sympathomimetic substance in adrenergic nerves with (—)-noradrenaline was obtained by VON EULER (1948a) using bioassay and a colorimetric method of analysis. This author showed that adrenaline was also present in cattle nerves (VON EULER, 1948b, 1949). Adrenaline was estimated in peripheral nervous tissues by VOGT (1954) using the response of the rat uterus stimulated by carbachol after separation of the catecholamines by paper chromatography. The presence of dopamine in cattle nerves and ganglia was clearly demonstrated by SCHÜMANN (1956) who examined extracts of these tissues by means of paper chromatography and used colour, fluorescence and biological tests for the identification of dopamine. This author confirmed the presence of noradrenaline but could not detect adrenaline by chemical means. LAVERTY and SHARMAN (1965 and unpublished) were also unable to detect adrenaline in the sympathetic nerves and ganglia of the dog by a fluorimetric method. Adrenaline does not seem to comprise more than a very small proportion of the catecholamines in peripheral nerve. Some estimations of the concentrations of the catecholamines in peripheral nervous tissues are given in Table 24. The large and variable concentrations of adrenaline and noradrenaline seen in the mesenteric ganglia and hypogastric nerve of the dog is due to the presence of chromaffin tissue (VOGT, 1963).

b) Eye

Examples of catecholamine concentrations in parts of the eye in some mammalian species are given in Table 25.

A rich network of fluorescing nerve fibres in the iris of several species was demonstrated by FALCK (1962), MALMFORS (1965) and ERÄNKÖ and RÄISÄNEN (1966). By combining the results obtained with fluorescence microscopy and chemical estimation, DAHLSTRÖM et al. (1966) were able to calculate the noradrenaline content of one varicosity of an adrenergic nerve in the iris to be 4.2×10^{-3} pg.

A detailed study of the autonomic innervation of the eye in monkey, cat and rabbit (LATIES and JACOBOWITZ, 1966) showed large species differences. No adrenergic nerves were found in the cornea of the monkey, whereas the same tissue of cat and rabbit contained an abundance of adrenergic nerves. The iris sphincter muscle and the ciliary muscle showed variable densities of adrenergic fibres, but the choroid was always innervated with very many fibres. HÄGGENDAL and MALMFORS (1965) demonstrated dopamine containing cell bodies and nerve fibres in the inner part of the inner nuclear layer of the retina. In the choroid a rich plexus of adrenergic neurones was seen to wrap around the vessels. They also found that the main catecholamine in the retina was dopamine. The noradrenaline in the choroid disappeared after cervical sympathectomy whereas the dopamine was unaffected.

BERNHEIMER (1964) demonstrated the presence of DOPA in the iris and the choroid including the pigment epithelium of the retina and also in the tapetum fibrosum of the eye of the calf. As all these tissues contain pigments he suggested that the DOPA serves as the precursor of melanin. DRUJAN et al. (1965) observed a decrease in the dopamine concentration in the retina of the rabbit after exposure to light for four hours. NICHOLS et al. (1967) exposed rats, rabbits and guinea-pigs to light for one hour and found an increase in the concentration of dopamine in the retina of the rat and in the posterior half of the eyeball of the rabbit and guinea-pig. These latter authors confirmed their observations with fluorescence microscopy.

c) Adrenal Gland

Adrenal Medulla

Numerous estimates of the adrenaline and noradrenaline content of the mammalian adrenal gland have been published. The total amount of catecholamines and also the relative amount of adrenaline in the gland varies from species to species. Tables are available in GOODALL (1951), WEST (1955), VON EULER (1956) and VON EULER (1963b). In Table 26 representative figures for a number of species are listed in order of the relative amount of adrenaline. The concentration must depend on the ratio between cortical and medullary tissue in individual animals. Some of the observed species differences are due to the ways in which the animals were killed. LUND (1951), for example, observed that adrenals from anaesthetised dogs contained only one half of the amount of adrenaline found in non-anaesthetised dogs. Fear or other forms of stress are known to deplete the adrenal medulla. In the cottontail rabbit *Sylvilagus floridanus* the total amount of catecholamines contained in the adrenal gland is about 40% higher in animals kept isolated than in animals kept in groups (McKinney et al., 1970). The high percentage of noradrenaline in the adrenal of the whale (Burn et al., 1951; Rastgeldi, 1951) and the low percentage in the rabbit (Hökfelt and McLean, 1950) seem to be representative for these species. Goodall (1951) concluded that aggressive, hunting animals have relatively more noradrenaline in their adrenals.

Young animals have more noradrenaline in their glands. With increasing age adrenaline becomes the dominant amine. This was observed by Holton (1951) in cattle, by Shepherd and West (1951) in man, cat, rabbit, guinea-pig and dog and confirmed by Cession-Fossion and Vandermeulen (1963) for the rabbit. In the rat, however, the ratio of adrenaline to noradrenaline in the adrenal remained essentially constant between birth and 200 days of age (Eränkö and Räisänen, 1956). Roffi (1968) found more adrenaline than noradrenaline in the adrenal of the rat and rabbit embryo.

There are also seasonal variations in the concentrations of adrenal catecholamines. Suomalainen and Uuspää (1958) and Uuspää (1963b) have reported that the adrenaline concentration in the adrenal glands of the hibernating hedgehog is higher than when the animal is awake.

Butterworth and Mann (1960, 1962) observed that the relative amount of adrenaline present in the adrenal gland is the same in the left and right adrenal glands of cats and also in the adrenal glands of litter-mates. This is independent of the litter size and the appearance of the kittens and is similar to the adrenaline percentage in the mother. In cats from different litters the relative amount of adrenaline varies between 20% and 80%.

The presence of 2 different cell types in the adrenal medulla, one of them containing adrenaline and the other noradrenaline, was demonstrated histochemically, using oxidation with potassium iodate, by Hillarp and Hökfelt (1953). This procedure causes rapid pigment formation with noradrenaline but not with adrenaline. Adrenal glands of rat, guinea-pig, rabbit, cat, dog, sheep, cow, horse and domestic fowl were treated in this way and it was found that the pigments formed were mainly localized within certain cells whose number varied more or less directly with the content of noradrenaline. Eränkö (1951) observed that after fixation of adrenal glands with formalin some medullary cells exhibit a strong fluorescence in ultraviolet light. When the catecholamines were extracted from parts of the same tissue slices of the adrenals of the hamster (Eränkö, 1955a) and the cat (Eränkö, 1955b) as were used for the histology and the amines separated by paper chromatography and estimated biologically, it was found that the noradrenaline content of the cells which fluoresced strongly after formalin fixation was much higher than that of the remaining medullary cells which were found to contain more adrenaline.

Podgornaya (1967) studied the distribution of noradrenaline and adrenaline cells in the adrenal medulla using histochemical methods in 20 different mammalian species, including the tiger, northern deer and mink.

Dopamine in the Adrenal Gland

There are small amounts of dopamine in the adrenal gland. The presence of dopamine in the sheep adrenal gland was reported by Goodall (1951). Shepherd and West (1953) investigated the adrenal glands of some other species using bioassay methods after paper chromatography to determine adrenaline and noradrenaline and a colour reaction on the chromatogram to estimate dopamine. Some estimates of the concentration of dopamine in the adrenal gland are summarized in Table 27. Dengler (1957) analyzed extracts of sheep adrenal glands for dopamine using paper chromatography and colorimetry and found that 2%

of the catecholamines in this tissue consists of dopamine. Dopamine was also found in the adrenal gland of the goat by VANDERMEULEN and CESSION-FOSSION (1968) and in the rabbit (BERTLER et al., 1960). SHARMAN (unpublished observations) could not detect dopamine in the adrenal gland of rats ($<$ 10 ng/adrenal). The same glands contained 45 μg noradrenaline/adrenal and 180 μg adrenaline/adrenal. SHEPHERD and WEST (1953) were unable to detect dopamine in extracts from pig, dog, cat, rabbit or adult human adrenal glands. Both dopamine and its precursor DOPA have been reported to be present in the adrenal gland of the sloth (PHILLIPOT et al., 1965).

HEMPEL and MÄNNL (1967) found radioactive dopamine in adrenal venous blood of cats which had been injected with tritiated tyrosine. They calculated that the cat normally secretes 0.01 μg of dopamine/min/adrenal (HEMPEL and MÄNNL, 1969). Studies on the subcellular distribution of dopamine in the adrenal glands of the ox and cow (EADE, 1958) and the sheep (LISHAJKO, 1968) showed that it is present in a "large-granule" fraction.

MATLINA and RACHMANOVA (1967) measured catecholamines in the adrenal gland of the rat using a fluorescence method. They found an apparently high concentration of dopamine but concluded that there might be another substance present which gave rise to a fluorescence under the conditions used to estimate dopamine. The values they obtained for adrenaline and noradrenaline are similar to those reported by other authors.

N-methyladrenaline

The presence of N-methyladrenaline in the adrenal medulla of monkey, rat, rabbit and guinea-pig was demonstrated by AXELROD (1960) using column chromatography on aluminium oxide, two dimensional paper chromatography, a colour reaction with potassium ferricyanide, and the formation of the O-methyl derivative, N-methylmetanephrine. This latter substance has been extracted from human urine (ITOH et al., 1962).

d) Extramedullary Chromaffin Tissue

Islands of chromaffin tissue, termed paraganglia, are found behind the peritoneum round the large blood vessels. The largest accumulation of these cells was described by ZUCKERKANDL (1901) and is known as the organ of ZUCKERKANDL. The paraganglia are large during embryonic life and early childhood and then atrophy. BIEDL and WIESEL (1902) and FULK and MACLEOD (1916) observed "adrenaline-like" biological activity in extracts of these organs. In the newborn child the organs of ZUCKERKANDL were found to contain more "adrenaline-like" activity than the two adrenal glands together (ELLIOTT, 1913). A detailed analysis of the catecholamine content of human ZUCKERKANDL organs was carried out by WEST et al. (1953) using paper chromatography and bioassay methods. The total amount of noradrenaline present in the organ increased from 4 μg at 15 weeks of gestation to its highest value, 14—28 μg, on the day of birth. In 1—2 year old children the content of noradrenaline in the organ was 2 μg whereas in older children noradrenaline was no longer detected. Adrenaline was found in the organ of ZUCKERKANDL only after birth. The amounts were 2—5 μg in children up to 5 years old. At birth the amount of noradrenaline contained in the paraganglia was more than double the amount contained in one adrenal gland at this time.

SHEPHERD and WEST (1952) also studied the catecholamines contained in the paraganglia of several species of laboratory animals. On the day of birth the noradrenaline content of the paraganglia of the guinea-pig was about 10 μg, that of the rabbit 5—12 μg, of the dog 15 μg and of the cat 10—25 μg. With the exception of the cat there was more noradrenaline in the organ of Zuckerkandl than in the adrenal gland. In these species no adrenaline, dopamine or DOPA was detected in the paraganglia at any age.

Brundin (1966) used column chromatography and fluorimetric methods in a study of the catecholamines in the paraganglia of the foetal and newborn rabbit. At 29 days of gestation 4.5 μg noradrenaline was found in the paraganglia of the rabbit foetus and only 0.5 μg in its adrenal glands. The noradrenaline content was 6.5—7.4 μg during the first week and fell to 2.4—5.2 μg at 4 weeks of age. These quantities are in agreement with the figures obtained by Shepherd and West (1952). Neither adrenaline nor dopamine was found to be present in this tissue. The adrenaline contents in the paraganglia which were reported earlier (Brundin et al., 1966) were probably due to technical difficulties.

Vogt (1963) found large chromaffin bodies inside the inferior mesenteric ganglion and the hypogastric nerve in young dogs. In adult dogs and puppies the noradrenaline concentrations in the hypogastric nerve ranged from 0.14—16.2 μg/g and the adrenaline concentrations from 0.03—13.5 μg/g. The concentrations were dependent on the amount of chromaffin tissue present. These catecholamines frequently prove resistant to the depleting action of reserpine, in contrast to catecholamines in other nerves (Vanov and Vogt, 1963).

The question of an innervation of extramedullary chromaffin tissue is still debated. Perfusates of the inferior mesenteric ganglion of dogs and its chromaffin cell islets contained noradrenaline (0.7—40 ng/min) and adrenaline (0.7—25 ng/min). There was little change after stimulation of the inferior splanchnic nerve or the ascending mesenteric nerves. Infusions of acetylcholine or nicotine, however, caused increases in the released catecholamines of up to 900% (Muscholl and Vogt, 1964).

The small amounts of adrenaline in most extra-adrenal chromaffin tissue and the absence of adrenaline from the chromaffin tissue in lower vertebrates in which the adrenal medulla and cortex are completely separated (Coupland, 1953) gave rise to the suggestion that the adrenal cortex is required for the methylation of noradrenaline. Shepherd and West (1951) correlated the ratio between adrenal medullary and cortical tissue with the relative amount of adrenaline present in the glands. Wurtman and Axelrod (1965) studied the activity of the enzyme phenylethanolamine-N-methyl transferase in the adrenal of rats and found it significantly decreased after hypophysectomy and increased when dexamethasone was given for 6 days. A small fall in the concentration of adrenaline in the adrenal gland occurred after hypophysectomy. In the adrenal gland of the snake *Xenodon merremii*, the enzyme activity was much higher in those parts of the glands where cortical tissue intermingles with chromaffin tissue than in those parts which contain only chromaffin tissue (Wurtman et al., 1967b). Rubin et al. (1968) removed as much medullary tissue as possible from the bisected glands taken from anaesthetised cats and estimated the catecholamines contained in the "medulla" and in the "cortex" to which several layers of medullary cells were attached. Sixty-nine percent of the catecholamines in the "medulla" was adrenaline whereas ninety-five percent of the catecholamines in the "cortex" consisted of adrenaline. In contrast Eränkö (1955a) found that, in the adrenal medulla of the hamster, the adrenaline-containing cells were located in the centre of the medulla and the noradrenaline-containing cells in the periphery, adjoining the adrenal cortex.

There are also chromaffin cells present in the tissues of ruminants. These contain dopamine and also stain as mast cells. Their contribution to the catecholamine content of ruminant tissues is discussed in the sections concerned with individual mammalian organs.

e) Heart

Table 28 contains some estimates of the concentrations of catecholamines found in the mammalian heart. The major catecholamine is noradrenaline. There is a regional distribution of this amine in the heart which is similar in all the species studied. The highest concentration is found in the right atrium and the concentrations in the atria are higher than in the ventricles. Those regions which have the highest amine concentrations also show the greatest number of adrenergic neurones and nerve terminals when studied by fluorescence microscopy (ANGELAKOS et al., 1963). In the cat, removal of the right stellate ganglion caused a fall of the noradrenaline concentrations in all parts of the heart, whereas removal of the left stellate ganglion caused a fall of the noradrenaline concentrations only in the left auricle and the left ventricle (HERTTING and SCHIEFTHALER, 1964). Homologous heart grafts in puppies lose their catecholamines within 72 hours (WEGMANN et al., 1962). LEDUC et al. (1955) related the catecholamine content of the rat heart to its nitrogen content and found it to be 3.03 ng of adrenaline and 15.7 ng of noradrenaline per mg nitrogen. A small percentage of the catecholamines in the heart of rat, mouse, guinea-pig and cat is located in chromaffin cells within the atrial parasympathetic ganglia of the heart. These chromaffin cells are innervated by postganglionic parasympathetic fibres from the same ganglion and send short neurons mainly to blood vessels (JACOBOWITZ, 1967).

Dopamine was first found in the heart of the sheep by GOODALL (1951). The high concentrations of dopamine in the heart of ruminantes can probably be referred to the dopamine which is contained in the mast cells of this species (CARLSSON, 1959). A high dopamine concentration was also found in the sino atrial node of the rabbit and histochemical studies of this region showed a high density of fluorescent fibres and fibre bundles (ANGELAKOS et al., 1963). MIYAHARA (1962) has reported the presence of DOPA (0.4—1.0 μg/g) in different regions of the dog heart.

f) Lung

The catechol compounds contained in the lungs of cattle and sheep were investigated by VON EULER and LISHAJKO (1957) and by SCHÜMANN (1958). The former authors employed a chromatographic separation on a starch column followed by condensation with 1,2-diaminoethane to demonstrate the presence of both noradrenaline and dopamine in extracts of ruminant lung tissue. SCHÜMANN (1958) used adsorption onto aluminium hydroxide and paper chromatographic separation and colorimetry, fluorimetry and bioassay to identify dopamine in sheep and cattle lung.

A wider distribution of dopamine in tissues other than the lung was demonstrated by BERTLER et al. (1959) in the cow, sheep and goat. It was shown also (BERTLER et al., 1959; FALCK et al., 1959) that the dopamine was associated with a granular chromaffin cell which was not found in the tissues of the pig, cat, rabbit, guinea-pig or rat. Although BERTLER et al. (1959) observed that the concentration of dopamine did not always parallel the density of the mast cells in ruminant tissues, further experiments using fluorescence histochemical methods has led to the conclusion that in ruminants the mast cells store dopamine (FALCK et al., 1964b). The possibility of a relation between the dopamine-containing cells and the adrenergic innervation of the ruminant lung has been considered by HEBB et al. (1968) who concluded that the proximity of some cells to nerve fibres was not of special significance. The concentrations of catecholamines in the lungs of some different species estimated by different analytical procedures is given in Table 29.

g) Kidney

Some estimates of the concentrations of catecholamines in the kidney are given in Table 30. The regional distribution of catecholamines in the kidney of the dog was studied by McKenna and Angelakos (1968). Adrenergic fibres were seen to run with the interlobar and arcuate arteries and along the afferent arterioles There were also nerve terminals on the vasa recta of the outer medulla. Nerve fibres were never seen on the glomeruli, the efferent arterioles or the tubuli. There was good agreement between the density of fluorescing fibres and the noradrenaline content of the different regions of the kidney.

The adrenergic nerves of the kidney have their origin in the aortico-renal ganglion (Doležel, 1967). After denervation of the kidney the noradrenaline content of the organ decreases (von Euler and Purkhold, 1951 (sheep); Nagatsu et al., 1969 (dog)) whereas in the cat, decentralisation by cutting the left splanchnic nerve causes a slight increase in the noradrenaline content (Rehn, 1958).

h) Thyroid Gland

Estimates of the concentrations of catecholamines in the thyroid gland are given in Table 31.

The dopamine in the thyroid of the sheep is located in mast cells, the number of which can vary in different animals (Jaim-Etcheverry and Zieher, 1968). This might explain the difference in the dopamine concentrations found by Falck et al. (1964a) and the former authors.

i) Reproductive Organs

Male Sex Organs

The main catecholamine present in the male sex organs is noradrenaline (Table 32). It is present in adrenergic neurones and nerve terminals. Adrenaline was sometimes found but only in small amounts. However, Sjöstrand (1965b) reported much larger concentrations of adrenaline in the caudal prostate of *Macaca irus*. This tissue was found to contain a large number of fluorescing cells after treatment with formaldehyde. The male genital organs are innervated by nerves which originate in the inferior mesenteric ganglion, the lumbo-sacral region of the spinal cord and in ganglion cells within the tissue walls. The short adrenergic neurones of these latter ganglion cells innervate the smooth muscle of the different accessory sex organs and contain over 90% of the noradrenaline found in these organs. They do not degenerate after sectioning the hypogastric nerves and the noradrenaline content of the organs does not as a rule fall after denervation. Denervation, however, causes a loss of the fluorescent fibres normally seen in the walls of the blood vessels (Sjöstrand, 1965b).

As can be seen in Table 32 the vasa deferentia in all of the species given contain especially high concentrations of noradrenaline. This tissue was used by Dahlström et al. (1966) to calculate the amount of noradrenaline present in a single fluorescing nerve varicosity as 5.9×10^{-3} pg. Specific granules were isolated from the vas deferens and the vesicular gland of the bull (von Euler and Lishajko, 1966) from which noradrenaline was released at $^1/_3$ of the rate at which it was released from granules obtained from the splenic nerve. Castration and testosterone had but little effect on the noradrenaline concentrations in the vasa deferentia and seminal vesicles of the guinea-pig (Ryd and Sjöstrand, 1967).

A detailed analysis of the catecholamines contained in human male sex organs obtained at operations was carried out by Baumgarten et al. (1968). No dopamine or adrenaline was detected. Fluorescence histology showed that adrenergic nerves in the testes were only present in the blood vessels. In the other organs they were also present in the smooth muscle. Table 33 gives estimates of the concentrations of catecholamines in the penis and associated tissues.

Female Sex Organs

As in the male sex organs, the main catecholamine found in the female genital tract is noradrenaline. It is contained in the adrenergic nerve terminals and neurones originating, as in the male, from the inferior mesenteric ganglion and the lumbo sacral ganglia of the sympathetic chain (long, vasomotor nerves) and from peripheral sympathetic ganglia which are especially abundant in the uterine wall near the utero-vaginal junction in several species (short neurones, ending in non vascular smooth muscle fibres) (Sjöberg, 1967). Some nerves which did not supply blood vessels were observed in the parenchyma of the ovary (Owman and Sjöberg, 1966; Owman et al., 1967).

Examples of catecholamine concentrations in the uterus of several species are given in Table 34. Variations in the catecholamine concentrations were observed during the oestrous cycle. In the rat, the largest amount of adrenaline was found in the uterus on the day of oestrous and the uptake of ^{3}H-adrenaline but not of ^{3}H-noradrenaline was increased (Wurtman et al., 1963). On the day of oestrous the concentration of adrenaline in the blood of the aorta was also increased (Green and Miller, 1966) and it is possible that at this phase the uterus is able to accumulate some of this circulating adrenaline. Variations in the catecholamine contents of several tissues of the female reproductive tract were also observed during pregnancy. In the rabbit the noradrenaline content of the uterus and vagina more than doubled during the first 12 days and fell again toward the end of pregnancy. It also increased in the oviduct and remained high. No change in the concentration of noradrenaline occurred in the ovary (Rosengren and Sjöberg, 1968). Cha et al. (1965) found an increase in the noradrenaline content of the uterus on days 18—20 of pregnancy and a fall towards the end of pregnancy in the rat. Rudzik and Miller (1962) and Spratto and Miller (1968a) observed an increase in the uterine adrenaline content and in uterine weight after the administration of oestrogens to rats. These changes were independent of the presence of the adrenal medulla (Spratto and Miller, 1968b). Wurtman et al. (1964) studied the subcellular distribution of ^{3}H-adrenaline in the uterus of the rat after an injection of this radioactive amine. In immature rats, after treatment with an oestrogen, they found an increase in the total amount of ^{3}H-adrenaline but no increase in ^{3}H-adrenaline in the fraction containing the granulated vesicles. Sjöberg (1968a) reported an increased noradrenaline content in the neurones of the muscle coat of the vagina and uterus after administration of 17β-oestradiol to rabbits.

j) Gastro-intestinal Tract

Table 35 shows examples of the concentrations of catecholamines in different parts of the gastro-intestinal tract of several mammalian species. The concentrations of adrenaline were very low in all species examined and the noradrenaline concentrations were also low. Dopamine was just detectable in non-ruminants. High concentrations of dopamine were found in the gastro-intestinal tract of ruminants, especially in the sheep. The bulk of the amine was found in the mucosa. This tissue contains abundant chromaffin cells (Falck et al., 1959) which are of the same type as those present in the liver and lung of ruminants, but show a stronger chromaffin reaction. In the goat they are present in the lamina propria around the bottom of the crypts and in the sheep they are mainly in submucosal connective tissue (BERTLER et al., 1959). Fluorescence microscopy of the intestine of the guinea-pig showed fluorescing fibres in the Auerbach plexus and in the Meissner plexus and a pericellular network around non-fluorescing ganglion cells (READ and BURNSTOCK, 1968).

Catecholamines were also found in the gastric juice of the dog (KAZAROVA and ESAYAN, 1966) in concentrations of 1—10 ng/ml. In man dopamine (0.02—0.1 μg/ml) and noradrenaline (0.015 μg/ml in 1 out of 4 experiments) was detected only after an injection of histamine or insulin (HÄGGENDAL, 1967).

k) Liver

Noradrenaline, adrenaline and dopamine can be extracted from the liver. Except in the ruminants, noradrenaline is the major catecholamine present. The noradrenaline in the liver disappears after the organ is denervated (VON EULER and PURKHOLD, 1951). In the ruminants, dopamine is stored in mast cells (FALCK et al., 1964b). These authors found that mast cells, which showed a strong fluorescence after treatment of the tissue with formaldehyde, were located in the liver capsule, in the connective tissue adjacent to the capsule and in the connective tissue septa within the liver. They were not present in the parenchyma. The dopamine content of a single mast cell was estimated to be $0.4—0.5 \times 10^{-5}$ μg.

The fluorescence histology of the liver tissue of the dog, cat, guinea-pig, rat and mouse was investigated by UNGVÁRY and DONATH (1969). In these species the adrenergic fibres were confined to the blood vessels where they formed a network between the adventitia and the media. The nerve supply to the hepatic arteries is most abundant in cats and dogs. There is also a rich adrenergic innervation of the hepatic veins and the branches of the hepatic portal veins. The large hepatic veins of the dog have a particularly dense adrenergic innervation before the entry into the vena cava. This may be concerned with the blood storage function of the liver in this species. There are few adrenergic fibres to be found in the bile ducts. No convincing evidence for an adrenergic innervation of the parenchyma or the Kupffer cells of the liver was obtained. The fine fibres which were found in the peripheral parts of the lobuli were thought to innervate the arterial sinusoids.

Values for the concentrations of catecholamines in the liver of some mammalian species are listed in Table 36.

l) Spleen

As shown in Table 37, the noradrenaline concentration in the mammalian spleen is usually more than 10 times higher than the concentration of adrenaline or dopamine. An exception was the observation by VAN DEN BRUEL et al. (1967) who found more adrenaline than noradrenaline in the spleen of the European muskrat (see Table 37). The concentration of catecholamines in the spleen when the organ is relaxed and filled with blood will be different from when it is contracted. Some authors have therefore expressed the catecholamine concentration in the spleen as the amount present per mole of DNA-phosphorus. BROWN et al. (1966) reported a value for the cat spleen of 1.53 moles noradrenaline/mole DNA-phosphorus ($\times 10^{-3}$) (sic). STREET and ROBERTS (1969) found 14.68 ng adrenaline/μ mole DNA-P and 50.2 ng noradrenaline/μ mole DNA-P in the cat spleen. STREET and ROBERTS (1969) also identified and estimated dopamine in the cat's spleen. In one group of 22 cats they found 4.82 (S.E. $\pm$ 1.16) ng/μ mole DNA-P, in another group of 9 cats 33.8 (S.E. $\pm$ 8.6). The authors did not know of any apparent difference in these two groups of cats. Decentralization of the spleen by cutting the left splanchnic nerve caused a slight increase in the noradrenaline content of the spleen (REHN, 1958; BROWN et al., 1966). Three months after postganglionic denervation the noradrenaline content of the spleen was decreased by more than 90% (VON EULER and PURKHOLD, 1951).

GILLESPIE and KIRPEKAR (1966) studied the catecholamine fluorescence developed in the spleen after formaldehyde treatment and found that it was confined to nerve fibres in the smooth muscles of the capsule, the arteries and veins.

m) Salivary Glands

Catecholamines have been estimated in the salivary glands of a few species. Some of the observations are listed in Table 38.

Sympathetic denervation causes a loss of noradrenaline, but not of adrenaline from the submaxillary gland of the rat (VON EULER and RYD, 1963). Ligation of the secretory duct does not cause a decrease in the noradrenaline content of the salivary gland (ANDÉN et al., 1966b) or in the number of adrenergic nerve terminals which can be seen by fluorescence microscopy. However, the monoamine oxidase activity in the tissue disappears and the uptake of noradrenaline is very much reduced. Fluorescence microscopy of the normal submaxillary gland, parotid gland and sublingual gland of the dog (FUJIWARA et al., 1966) and of the submaxillary gland of the rat (ANDÉN et al., 1966b) showed a network of fibres round the acini and some in the walls of the blood vessels. The ducts are devoid of adrenergic innervation. NORBERG and OLSON (1965) found fibres round the acini only in the serous glands but not in the mainly mucous sublingual gland.

n) Pancreas

Detailed investigations into the occurrence of biogenic amines in the mammalian endocrine pancreas were summarised by CEGRELL (1968). Noradrenaline and dopamine were found in the pancreas of several species (Table 39) and there is evidence that dopamine is present in higher concentrations in the younger animal than in the adult. Adrenaline could not be detected.

In cattle and sheep, dopamine is the predominant catecholamine in the pancreas (SCHÜMANN, 1959).

FALCK and HELLMANN (1963) studied monoamine fluorescence in the pancreas of the duck and 5 different mammalian species. They found a few adrenergic nerve fibres which mainly supplied blood vessels in the exocrine parenchyma. In the cat and the dog there was a fine network of fibres around small bundles of islet cells in the islets of Langerhans. Monoamine fluorescence was seen in some islet cells in cat, horse, dog and duck, but not in rat and mouse. In the guinea-pig no adrenergic innervation of the islet cells was found (FALCK and HELLMANN, 1964). CEGRELL et al. (1964) observed a catecholamine fluorescence in the A cells of the duck and pigeon pancreas and in the B cells of the guinea-pig pancreas, but not in the A cells of guinea-pig, rat or mouse pancreas.

o) Catecholamines in the Walls of Blood Vessels

The first detailed investigation into the occurrence of biologically active substances in the walls of blood vessels was carried out by SCHMITERLÖW (1948). He found sympathomimetic vasoactive substances in the aorta of horse, cattle, dog and pig and in a number of smaller vessels in the horse. The greatest activities were extracted from the renal artery, the superior vena cava, the portal vein and the coronary arteries. VON EULER and LISHAJKO (1958) identified 3,4-dihydroxyphenylacetic acid, 3,4-dihydroxymandelic acid and dopamine in addition to adrenaline and noradrenaline in pooled extracts of bovine splenic vessels.

FAREDIN et al. (1961) estimated the catecholamines in the vessels of normal dogs and dogs with Goldblatt clamps on their renal arteries. Three to eight months later the adrenaline content of the blood vessels of the latter dogs was higher than in the control animals, whereas the noradrenaline content was lower. This was independent of the development of hypertension in the operated dogs.

Especially high concentrations of noradrenaline were reported for arteries and veins of the mesenteric vascular tree by GENEST et al. (1969) when compared with that in the small vessels of the hind leg. The authors discuss the possible connections between the high noradrenaline concentrations and the acute response of the mesenteric vessels in maintaining the blood pressure.

MAXWELL et al. (1968) found that 75% of the noradrenaline in the thoracic aorta of the rabbit is located in the adventitia, the remainder is found in the media-intimal layers.

Table 40 gives estimates of the concentrations of catecholamines in the walls of blood vessels in several species.

p) Carotid Body

The possibility that catecholamines may play a role in the chemoreceptor function of the carotid body has encouraged the investigation of this tissue. The histological tests described by HILLARP and HÖKFELT (1953) for the demonstration of adrenaline and noradrenaline were applied to this tissue by PRIĬMAK (1959). It was found that chromaffin cells were present in the carotid body of the rabbit and the cat but not in mice, rats, guinea-pigs or sables. In the cat and the rabbit, the noradrenaline test was positive for specific cells. The concentrations of catecholamines which have been estimated to be present in the carotid body in four species are given in Table 41. DEARNALEY et al. (1968) carefully analysed the catecholamines in the carotid body of the rabbit and identified noradrenaline and dopamine by means of chromatography and fluorescence reactions. Fluorescence analysis indicated that the proportion of adrenaline was not more than 10% of the total noradrenaline and adrenaline present. The dopamine appeared to be present in cells which gave rise to an intense fluorescence after formaldehyde treatment. Dopamine has also been identified in extracts of the carotid body of the horse by means of mass spectrometry (KNOCHE et al., 1969).

q) Adipose Tissue

As can be seen from Table 41, the main catecholamine in mammalian adipose tissue is noradrenaline. Its concentration is highest in the interscapular (brown fat) fat tissue, where it is located in adrenergic neurones and nerve terminals.

Fluorescence microscopy of interscapular and mediostinal brown fat of the rat showed fluorescing fibres on blood vessel walls and fine networks round individual fat cells (WIRSÉN, 1965; WIRSÉN and HAMBERGER, 1967; DERRY et al., 1969). The latter fibres have their origin in ganglion cells within the fat. Their fluorescence remains after reserpine treatment and immunosympathectomy. The fluorescence of the long adrenergic nerve fibres in the blood vessel walls disappears under these circumstances (DERRY et al., 1969).

Denervation of the interscapular fat bodies of the rat and the mouse causes the noradrenaline to disappear within 24 hours. Noradrenaline can still be found in the fat tissue 3—6 hours after denervation but exposure of the animals to cold no longer causes lipid mobilisation (SIDMAN et al., 1962; WEINER et al., 1962).

r) Skeletal Muscle

Small amounts of dopamine, adrenaline and noradrenaline have been found in the skeletal muscle. Fluorescing nerve fibres were seen in the walls of the blood vessels and within the muscle tissue itself (FUXE and SEDVALL, 1965) after treatment of skeletal muscle with formaldehyde. Examples of catecholamine concentrations in mammalian skeletal muscles are listed in Table 42. GOVYRIN (1965) estimated the adrenaline and noradrenaline content of the triceps brachii of the cat before and after sympathetic denervation. Seven days after denervation the noradrenaline had disappeared, and even 3 years later no noradrenaline could be detected in the muscle. However the adrenaline content remained unchanged. The author concluded from this observation that the adrenaline must be contained in structures other than sympathetic nerves. A large number of chromaffin cells was found in the abdominal muscles of the sheep and goat (BERTLER et al., 1959). The dopamine in these muscles is probably contained in the chromaffin mast cells.

s) Skin

The concentration of noradrenaline and adrenaline in human skin was estimated by ADAMS-RAY (1956) using bioassay. The concentrations of noradrenaline ranged from 0.025—0.96 μg/g and those of adrenaline from 0.005—0.08 μg/g (these values assume a misprint of mg/g in the published work). The presence of DOPA in skin was indicated by the experiments of FOSTER and BROWN (1957). CEGRELL et al. (1967) have extracted catechol derivatives from the skin of young pigmented mice and found that dopamine and DOPA are present in approximately equal amounts (0.2—0.8 μg/g). The concentration of DOPA in the pigmented skin of rabbits, dogs and guinea-pigs has been estimated by CEGRELL et al. 1970). Most of the DOPA was found in the hair. It is concluded, that when present in skin, dopamine is stored in mast cells and that most of the DOPA is associated with the hair matrix. The noradrenaline in the skin reflects the presence of a sympathetic innervation.

t) Catecholamines in Blood

The history of the estimation of catecholamines in blood is almost the history of the measurement of adrenaline and noradrenaline. The concentrations of these substances in blood is an index of the balance between their formation, release, metabolism and excretion. The concentrations of catecholamines in plasma are very low and their estimation has required that methods be used at the limit of their sensitivity. However, methods are now available which can give reliable estimates of the concentration of adrenaline and noradrenaline in blood. CALLINGHAM (1968) in his review on this subject concludes that in human plasma the normal resting value for noradrenaline is 0.2—0.4 ng/ml and for adrenaline 0.0—0.2 ng/ml in venous plasma and 0.1—0.3 ng/ml in arterial plasma. Such results are obtained when the methods described by COHEN and GOLDENBERG (1957a, b) [A.F.], VENDSALU (1960) [R.F.], ANTON and SAYRE (1962) [A.F.], HÄGGENDAL (1963a) [R.F.] and KLENSCH (1966) [R.F.] are used correctly. That different methods now give similar results is good evidence that the substances measured are indeed adrenaline and noradrenaline. However, HOLZBAUER and VOGT (1954) were unable to detect (< 1 ng/ml) noradrenaline in human or dog peripheral plasma using a biological assay method. HÄGGENDAL (1963b) has found that adrenaline and noradrenaline can be present in human plasma in the form of acid hydrolysable conjugates and some of the catecholamine may be bound to a specific protein (MIRKIN et al., 1966). An association of catecholamines with blood platelets has been demonstrated by WEIL-MALHERBE and BONE (1958) in the human and by BORN et al. (1958) in the pig. The latter authors showed that the platelets could take up adrenaline and noradrenaline against a concentration gradient. However VENDSALU (1960) has concluded that although the concentration of catecholamines in the platelets is higher than in plasma, the contribution of platelet bound amines to the total in platelet rich plasma is insignificant.

There is little information on the occurrence of dopamine in blood plasma. STREET and ROBERTS (1969) have reported the presence of dopamine in the plasma of the cat under chloralose anaesthesia, and it is also present in the blood of the sheep anaesthetised with halothane and the conscious goat (KELLY et al., 1970). It remains to be seen whether the dopamine in the blood of ruminants is derived from the mast cells in these species.

u) Catecholamines in Urine

HOLTZ and CREDNER (1942) examined the properties of a pressor substance present in urine and concluded that it was dopamine which they showed could be formed in the tissues by the decarboxylation of DOPA. It was later shown (HOLTZ et al., 1947) that the biological properties of the substance which was now called "urosympathin" could be ascribed to a mixture of dopamine, noradrenaline and a small amount of adrenaline. HOLTZ et al. (1950) and SCHÜMANN (1950) found that most of the biological activity of urosympathin could be accounted for by noradrenaline.

It was demonstrated by VON EULER and HELLNER (1951) by means of paper chromatography, bioassay and colorimetry, that urine contains the three catecholamines adrenaline, noradrenaline and dopamine.

The concentration of these amines in the urine varies under normal physiological conditions and the vast number of observations which have been made are beyond the scope of this review. An indication of the variation in the amounts found in human and rat urine is given in Table 44. Catecholamines have been estimated in the urine of other species. Among these are the pig (CUNNINGHAM, 1967; BALDWIN et al., 1969), cow (VON EULER and HELLNER, 1951), dog (MILLAR and BENFEY, 1958; DE SCHAEPDRYVER et al., 1959), mouse (LE BLANC et al., 1967) sloth (PHILLIPOT et al., 1965) and monkey (HARRISON and SEATON, 1966). Part of the catecholamine content of the urine is present in a conjugated form which can be hydrolysed by boiling with dilute acid. In man the conjugated form appears to be a sulphate ester (RICHTER, 1940; WEIL-MALHERBE, 1964) whereas in the rabbit, conjugation with glucuronic acid takes place (CLARK and DRELL, 1954).

v) Cells which can Form Catecholamines

In a number of mammalian tissues there are cells which normally contain very little or no adrenaline, noradrenaline or dopamine and which after the administration of L-DOPA are found to develop an intense green fluorescence when the tissues are treated with formaldehyde for fluorescence histology. The fluorescence can be developed within 30 min of the administration of L-DOPA and may be obtained for longer than 20 hours afterwards. If the animals are pretreated with an inhibitor of the enzyme DOPA-decarboxylase then the formation of fluorescence in these cells after L-DOPA is inhibited. In some cases a fluorescence can be developed after D-DOPA but it is thought that this amino acid is first racemised to the L-form before being taken up by the cells. It is concluded that the development of the fluorescence is due to the presence, in these cells, of dopamine formed by decarboxylation of the administered amino acid.

There are cells, which respond in this way, in the skin of the mouse, rabbit and hamster but they are not present in the skin of the adult guinea-pig. These cells also stain as mast cells (ADAMS-RAY et al., 1964; CEGRELL et al., 1967). ADAMS-RAY et al. (1964) suggest that the cells normally store another catecholamine which cannot condense with formaldehyde to give a fluorescent product, and have suggested that a substance like N-methyl-adrenaline might be considered. ERSPAMER and VIALLI (1952) and ERSPAMER (1959) have extracted leptodactyline (m-hydroxyphenylethyltrimethylammonium) from the skin of amphibia of the genus *Leptodactylus* and ERSPAMER and GLÄSSER (1960) have shown that this substance is pharmacologically active with nicotinic and neuromuscular blocking properties. The possibility of naturally-occurring quaternary catecholamines might also be considered. Other cells which can be made to develop fluorescence after L-DOPA administration include parafollicular cells in the thyroid gland of the mouse (LARSON et al., 1966), and islet cells in the pancreas of the mouse and guinea-pig (CEGRELL, 1967, 1968).

There are also "enterochromaffin-like" cells in the stomach of the rat (HÅKANSON and OWMAN, 1966; HÅKANSON et al., 1967) and in the gastro-intestinal tract of the human foetus (FALCK et al., 1967). HÅKANSON et al. (1969) have described three different systems of monoamine storing cells in the gastrointestinal tract of foetal and neonatal rats. These are the "enterochromaffin-type" cells which contain the non-mast cell store of gastric histamine and which will form dopamine if L-DOPA is administered, two types of mast cells one of which will take up L-DOPA and the enterochromaffin cells which do not appear to take up this amino acid. Some of these cells show the ability to take up and decarboxylate L-DOPA only in the foetus or neonatal state. It would seem that many cells which can synthesise and store amines in the body pass through a stage in their development where they can form and store dopamine from L-DOPA. Some retain this ability although they are not normally exposed to L-DOPA.

The endothelial cells of the blood capillaries in the brain are also able to take up and decarboxylate L-DOPA but not D-DOPA or dopamine. The endothelial lining of non-capillary intracerebral blood vessels does not contain such cells (BERTLER et al., 1966). No fluorescence could be developed in the endothelium of peripheral capillaries. In the retina and the optic nerve, parts of the eye which originate from the neural crest, the capillaries also contained cells in which a fluorescence could be developed after L-DOPA. These cells were absent from capillaries in the area postrema, the median eminence and the choroid plexus of the pig and also were not found in parts of the median surface of the olfactory bulb in the mouse, regions of the brain where there is no blood-brain barrier.

Explanation of Symbols Used in Tables

A = adrenaline		DOPA = dihydroxyphenylalanine		PC. = paper chromatography	
A. = alumina		E_1 = enzyme assay; SAELENS et al. (1967)		R. = resin	
AC. = acetylation		E_2 = enzyme assay; NIKODIJEVIC et al. (1969)		S = solvent extraction	
B. = bioassay		F. = fluorescence		— = not tested	
C. = colorimetry		N = noradrenaline		O = not detected	
CC. = column chromatography				μg/g = μg/g tissue	
D = dopamine					

Table 1. *Catecholamines in the Lamprey and the Hagfish* (Class: Marsipobranchii, Sub-Class: Cyclostomata)

Order and species		Concentrations in μg/g tissue: Heart A	Heart N	Brain A	Brain N	Vagus nerve A	Vagus nerve N	Kidney A	Kidney N	Pronephros A	Pronephros N	Skeletal muscle A	Skeletal muscle N	Liver A	Liver N	Method	Reference
HYPERORATII:																	
Lampetra fluviatilis	Whole heart	19.1	5.0													PC.B.	AUGUSTINSSON et al. 1956
	Auricle	41.2	19.0	—	—	—	—	—	—	—	—	—	—	—	—		
	Ventricle	12.5	0.8														
	Auricle	130.0	6.3	—	—	—	—	—	—	—	—	—	—	—	—	A.F.	ÖSTLUND et al., 1960
	Ventricle	28.0	—														
	Whole heart*	99.6	12.1	—	0.34	—	—	0.1	0.49	—	—	0.01	0.21	0.03	0.13	R.F.	STABROVSKII, 1967
	Auricle	127.1	16.0														
	Ventricle	81.0	11.6														
	Large vessels	1.2	5.0														
	Auricle*	130.0	—	—	—	—	—	—	—							A.F.	BLOOM et al., 1961
	Ventricle	30.0	—							—	—	—	—	—	—		
HYPEROTRETI:																	
Myxine glutinosa	Whole heart	5.0	0.83	—	—	—	—	—	—	—	—	—	—	—	—	PC.B.	ÖSTLUND, 1954
	Auricle	13.0	47.0	—	—	—	—	—	—	—	—	—	—	—	—	A.F.	ÖSTLUND et al., 1960
	Ventricle	45.0	6.0														
	Portal heart	2.6	51.0														
	Auricle*	12.5	45.0	—	—	—	—	—	—	—	—	—	—	—	—	A.F.	BLOOM et al., 1961
	Ventricle	45.0	5.0														
	Portal heart	5.0	55.0														
		—	—	< 0.02	< 0.02	—	—	—	—	—	—	—	—	—	—	A.F.	v. EULER, 1961
	Auricle	8.1	18.0	—	—	0.84	2.4	< 0.02	16.0	< 0.02	6.3	< 0.01	0.06	—	—	A.F.	v. EULER and FÄNGE, 1961
	Ventricle	59.0	6.5														
	Portal heart	3.1	58.0														

* Chromaffin cells demonstrated in the heart.

Table 2. *Catecholamines in Cartilaginous Fishes* (Class: Selachii, Sub-Class: Euselachii)

Order and species	Heart			Brain			Kidney		Skeletal muscle		Liver		Spleen		Intestine		Interrenal tissue		Method	Ref.
	Concentrations in $\mu g/g$ tissue																			
		A	N		A	N	A	N	A	N	A	N	A	N	A	N	A	N		
PLEUROTREMATA:																				
Squalus acanthias		—	—		—	—	30.0	50.0*	—	—	<0.04	0.04	—	—	—	—	—	—	B.	1
		—	—	Whole brain	0.03	0.04	0.13	0.93**	—	—	—	—	0.022	0.08	—	—	8.0	52.0	PC.B.	2
		—	—	Whole brain	0.11	0.37	—	—	—	—	—	—	—	—	—	—	—	—	A.F.	3
				Telencephalon	0.12	0.49														
				Optic lobes	0.20	0.31														
				Diencephalon	0.31	0.55														
				Hypothalamus	0.33	0.44														
				Pituitary gland	0.41	1.5														
				Cerebellum	0.011	0.056														
				Medulla oblongata	0.13	0.25														
	Auricle	<0.02	0.78		—	—	1.9	19.0	—	—	—	—	0.025	0.096	0.03	0.33	—	—	A.F.	4
	Ventricle	<0.02	0.09																	
	Whole heart	0.03	0.10																	
	Whole heart	0.02	0.07	Whole brain	0.08	0.05	5.8	9.5	0.01	0.04	0.01	0.01	0.03	0.02	—	—	—	—	A.F.	5
HYPOTREMATA:																				
Raja batis	Whole heart	0.025	0.87		—	—	0.027	0.29	—	—	—	—	—	—	—	—	95.0	100.0	PC.B.	6
Dasyatis pastinaca	Whole heart	0.17	0.29	Whole brain	0.11	0.08	0.19	0.76	0.02	0.08	0.02	0.02	0.03	0.27	—	—	—	—	A.F.	7

* includes abdominal blood vessels; ** includes some interrenal tissue.

References: 1. v. EULER, 1953; 2. ÖSTLUND, 1954; 3. v. EULER, 1961; 4. v. EULER and FÄNGE, 1961; 5. STABROVSKII, 1969; 6. ÖSTLUND, 1954; 7. STABROVSKII, 1969.

Table 4. *Catecholamines in Bony Fishes* (Class: Pisces, Sub-Class: Neopterygii)

Concentrations in μg/g tissue

Species	Heart		Brain		Anterior kidney		Skeletal muscle		Liver		Spleen		Intestine		Stomach		Blood μg/l		Method	Ref.
	A	N	A	N	A	N	A	N	A	N	A	N	A	N	A	N	A	N		
ORDER: ISOPONDYLI																				
Salmo salar	0.04	0.03	—	—	—	—	—	—	0.02	0.02	0.042	0.03	—	—	—	—	—	—	A.B.	1
	0.18	0.40	—	—	—	—	—	—	—	—	—	—	—	—	—	—	—	—	F.	2
	—	—	—	—	—	—	—	—	—	—	—	—	0.04	0.06	0.08	0.06	—	—	F.	3
Salmo Gairdneri	0.02	0.02	—	—	4.7	4.5	0.003	0.022	0.02	0.03	—	—	—	—	—	—	4.0 (Plasma)	3.3	A.F.	4
Salmo irideus	—	—	A + N 6.3		—	—	—	—	—	—	—	—	—	—	—	—	—	—	R.F.	5
ORDER: HAPLOMI																				
Esox lucius	0.04	0.06	—	—	—	—	—	—	0.04	0.03	0.04	0.03	—	—	—	—	—	—	A.B.	6
ORDER: OSTARIOPHYSI																				
Cyprinus carpio	—	—	—	—	—	—	—	—	—	—	—	—	—	—	—	—	1.5 (Whole blood)	16.0	A.F.	7
	0.05	0.46	0.02	0.19	0.05	0.84	0.02	0.10	0.05	0.13	0.04	0.22	—	—	—	—	—	—	R.F.	8
				Kidney body	0.12	0.60														
Carassius auratus	♀0.23 ∅ ♂0.20 ∅	0.28 ∅ 0.27 ∅	♀0.45 ∅ ♂0.41 ∅	0.12 ∅ 0.11 ∅	—	—	—	—	—	—	—	—	—	—	—	—	—	—	R.F.	9
	—	—	*	0.49	—	—	—	—	—	—	—	—	0.64	*	0.35	*	—	—	S.F.	10
Ictalurus punctatus	—	—	—	—	—	—	—	—	—	—	—	—	—	—	—	—	4.0 (Plasma)	3.0—46.0	A.F.	11

Species	Heart		Brain		Vagus		Sympathetic chain		Anterior kidney		Kidney body		Liver		Spleen		Swim bladder		Method	Ref.
	A	N	A	N	A	N	A	N	A	N	A	N	A	N	A	N	A	N		
ORDER: ANACANTHINI																				
Gadus callarius	—	—	—	—	—	—	—	—	—	—	—	—	—	—	0.12	0.04	—	—	PC.B.	12
	—	—	0.03	0.27	—	—	—	—	—	—	—	—	—	—	—	—	—	—	A.F.	13
	0.17	<0.02	0.03	0.27	0.41	0.17	1.8	<0.02	45.0	<0.02	0.39**	<0.02	—	—	0.16	0.06	0.11	1.1	A.F.	14
ORDER: PERCOMORPHI																				
Lucioperca lucioperca	0.02	0.12	—	—	—	—	6.4	38.0	—	—	2.7	9.2	0.01	0.02	0.02	0.03	—	—	B.	15

* It is assumed that this catecholamine could not be detected.
** Included some chromaffin cell groups from dorsal sympathetic chain.
∅ No units given in original paper. We assume μg/g tissue.

References: 1. v. EULER, 1953; 2. GANNON and BURNSTOCK, 1969; 3. NORTH, 1965; 4. NAKANO and TOMLINSON, 1967; 5. BERTLER et al., 1963; 6. v. EULER, 1953; 7. MAZEAUD, 1964; 8. STABROVSKII, 1968; 9. JOFRE and IZQUIERDO, 1967; 10. BRODIE et al., 1964; 11. BOEHLKE et al., 1967; 12. ÖSTLUND, 1954; 13. v. EULER, 1961; 14. v. EULER and FÄNGE, 1961 15. v. EULER, 1953.

Table 3. *Catecholamines in the Chromaffin Tissue of Some Cartilaginous Fishes*

Species	Adrenaline mg/g	Nor-adrenaline mg/g	Method	Reference
Squalus acanthias . . .	3.10	6.70	A.F.	v. EULER and FÄNGE, 1961
Squalus acanthias. . . .	0.90	2.40	PC.B.	SHEPHERD et al. 1953
Scylliorhinus canicula .	1.15	2.20		
Scylliorhinus stellaris . .	0.85	1.90		
Mustelis canis	1.00	2.20		
Torpedo marmorata . . .	0.15	0.60		

Table 6. *Catecholamines in Salamanders and Newts*
(Class: Amphibia, Order: Caudata)

Genus and species	Concentrations in μg/g tissue						
	Heart		Brain	Stom-ach	Small intes-tine	Me-thod	Reference
	A	N	A	N	N		
Sub-order: AMBYSTOMATOIDEA							
Axolotl tigrinum	—	0.36	0.75	0.67	0.38	S.F.	BRODIE et al. 1964*
Sub-order: SALAMANDROIDEA							
Desmognathus	—	0.94	1.24	1,1	3.0		
Sub-order: PROTEIDA							
Necturus maculosus	—	<0.17	0.39	1.3	0.22		
Newt (unspecified)	0.01	0.57	—	—	—	A.F.	ANGELAKOS et al., 1965

* No figures were given for noradrenaline in brain tissue and for adrenaline in the heart, stomach and small intestine. It is assumed that in these tissues these amines could not be detected.

Table 5. *Mean Catecholamine Concentrations in Different Organs of Bony Fishes Found in the Black Sea* (STABROVSKII, 1969)

Species	Concentrations in μg/g tissue											
	Kidney		Liver		Heart		Brain		Skeletal muscle		Spleen	
	A	N	A	N	A	N	A	N	A	N	A	N
Trachurus mediterraneus pontus	11.0	12.6	0.12	0.01	0.41	0.03	0.15	0.02	0.04	0.02	0.31	0.06
Pamatomus saltatrix	12.2	15.1	0.03	0	0.12	0	0.16	0.16	0.04	0.07	0.18	0.18
Mugil auratus	6.0	7.2	0.08	0.08	0.10	0	0.10	0.05	0.04	0.01	0.11	0.15
Mullus barbatus ponticus	18.4	21.8	0.09	0	0.33	0	0.14	0	0.07	0.04	0.36	0
Spicara smaris	26.8	9.1	0.05	0.02	0.20	0	0.14	0	0.02	0.01	0.21	0.09
Diplodus annularis	5.1	2.9	0.02	0	0.30	0	0.07	0	0.02	0	0.02	0.65
Sciaena umbra	4.4	2.8	0.04	0	0.11	0	0.08	0.02	0.03	0	0.13	0.06
Scorpaena porcus	0.80	0.47	0.02	0	0.10	0	0.12	0	0.01	0	0.18	0.02
Trachinus draco	0.52	2.5	0.02	0	0.12	0.01	0.12	0	0.02	0	0.17	0
Uranoscopus scaber	0.70	0.6	0.02	0	0.09	0	0.19	0	0.02	0	0.14	0

0 = None detected.

The fishes are arranged in order of their activity. The first groups of fishes are migrating and cover long distances. They contain higher concentrations of adrenaline in their adrenals; at least 5 observations were made to obtain these mean values.

Table 7. *Catecholamines in the Toad* (Class: Amphibia, Order: Salientia, Sub-Order: Procoela)

Species		Heart			Concentrations in µg/g tissue Brain		Stomach		Small intestine		Bladder		Lung		Method	Reference
		A	N		A	N	A	N	A	N	A	N	A	N		
Bufo americanus	Whole heart	1.8	*	Whole brain	0.83	*	0.5	0.64	*	0.95	—	—	—	—	S.F.	BRODIE et al., 1964
Bufo marinus	Whole heart	7.6	*	Whole brain	2.40	*	1.2	1.1	3.4	*	—	—	—	—		
		—	—		—	—	—	—	—	—	1.4	0.17	0.72	0.12	F.	BURNSTOCK, 1969
		—	—		—	—	0.34	0.04	0.83	0.36	—	—	—	—	F.	NORTH, 1965
	Sinus venosus	4.92	0.06		—	—	—	—	—	—	—	—	—	—	A.F.	ANGELAKOS et al., 1965
	Atria	3.89	0.08													
	Ventricle	5.58	<0.01													
	Whole heart	5.43	0.03													
Bufo terrestris	Sinus venosus	3.58	0.13		—	—	—	—	—	—	—	—	—	—		
	Atria	2.14	0.04													
	Ventricle	2.08	<0.01													
	Whole heart	2.09	0.01													
Bufo arenarum Hensel		—	—	Olfactory bulb	0.9	0.2		—	—	—	—	—	—	—	A.F.	SEGURA and BISCARDI, 1967
				Brain vesicles	1.0	0.2										
				Mesencephalon	1.2	0.3										
				Rhombencephalon	1.0	0.2										
				Hypothalamus	2.9	1.3										
Hyla aura		—	—		—	—	0.38	0,13	—	—	—	—	—	—	F.	NORTH, 1965

* It is assumed that this catecholamine could not be detected.

Table 8. *Catecholamines in the Frog* (Class: Amphibia, Order: Salientia, Sub-Order: Diplasiocoela)

Species		Concentrations in μg/g tissue Heart A	Heart N	Heart D	Brain A	Brain N	Liver A	Liver N	Spleen A	Spleen N	Skeletal muscle A	Skeletal muscle N	Stomach A	Stomach N	Small intestine A	Small intestine N	Skin A	Skin N	Method	Reference
Rana cinerea	Whole heart	0.96	*	—	0.8	*	—	—	—	—	—	—	—	—	0.44	*	—	—	S.F.	Brodie et al., 1964
Rana pipiens	Whole heart	1.2	*	—	2.1	*	—	—	—	—	—	—	0.46	0.44	0.61	>0.06	—	—		
	Sinus venosus**	2.96	0.08	1.51	—	—	—	—	—	—	—	—	—	—	—	—	—	—	A.F.	Angelakos et al., 1965
	Atria**	1.61	<0.05	0.17	—	—	—	—	—	—	—	—	—	—	—	—	—	—	R.F.	
	Ventricle**	2.77	<0.01	0.2	—	—	—	—	—	—	—	—	—	—	—	—	—	—		
Rana catesbeiana	Sinus venosus	0.41	0.01	—	—	—	—	—	—	—	—	—	—	—	—	—	—	—		
	Atria	0.14	0.01	—	—	—	—	—	—	—	—	—	—	—	—	—	—	—		
	Ventricle	0.12	<0.01	—	—	—	—	—	—	—	—	—	—	—	—	—	—	—		
	Whole heart	0.12	<0.01	—	—	—	—	—	—	—	—	—	—	—	—	—	—	—		
	Whole heart	1.52	<0.01	—	1.0	0.46	0.17	—	0.16	—	0.03	—	—	—	—	—	—	—	A.F.	Azuma et al., 1965
Rana temporaria	Whole heart	0.9	0.19	—	—	—	0.04	0.03	0.29	0.63	—	—	—	—	—	—	—	—	A.B.	Östlund, 1954
	Whole heart	1.48	<0.02	***	—	—	—	—	—	—	—	—	—	—	—	—	0.07	***	PC. F.	Grobecker et al., 1966
	Atria	0.94	—	—	—	—	—	—	—	—	—	—	—	—	—	—	—	—		
	Ventricle	1.76	—	—	—	—	—	—	—	—	—	—	—	—	—	—	—	—		
	Atria	1.50	0.01	<0.01	—	—	—	—	—	—	—	—	—	—	—	—	—	—	R.F.	Falck et al., 1963
	Ventricle	1.90	0.01	<0.01	—	—	—	—	—	—	—	—	—	—	—	—	—	—		
Rana (unspecified)	Whole heart	1.86	0.11	—	0.52	0.25	0.1	0.02	0.63	<0.005	—	—	—	—	—	—	—	—	A.F.	Anton and Sayre, 1962

* It is assumed that noradrenaline could not be detected. ** Pooled tissues. *** DOPA, dopamine or noradrenaline could not be detected.

Table 9. *Adrenaline and Noradrenaline in the Adrenal of the Toad and the Frog*

Genus	Adrenaline	Noradrenaline	Units	Method	Reference
Bufo arenarum Hensel	4.3—5.4	1.2—2.4	mg/g adrenal	PC. B.	Houssay et al., 1950
Bufo vulgaris japonica	0.25	0.15	mg/kg body wt.	C.	Inoue and Akimoto, 1959
Bufo (unspecified)	0.13	0.11	mg/kg body wt.	C.	Kamo, 1962
Rana (unspecified)	3	4	μg/frog	B.	West, 1951
Rana (unspecified)	137	167	μg/g adrenal	A.F.	Anton and Sayre, 1962
Rana temporaria	96	156	μg/kg body wt.*	PC. B.	Grobecker et al., 1966
Rana catesbeiana	1100	1830	μg/g adrenal	A.F.	Azuma et al., 1965

* Dopamine could not be detected.

Table 10. *Catecholamine Content of the Retina (Including the Pigment Epithelium) of Toad and Frog*

Genus	Condition	Adrenaline μg/g	Noradrenaline μg/g	Dopamine μg/g	Method	Reference
Bufo **(unspecified)**	4 hr, daylight	0.13	Traces	0.17	A.F.	DRUJAN et al., 1965
	dark	0.21	Traces	0.31		
Bufo marinus	5 min, strong electric light	0.49	—	—	A.F.	DRUJAN and DIAZ BORGES, 1968
	dark	0.60	—	—		
Rana **(unspecified)**	4 hr, daylight	0.81	Traces	0.86	A.F.	DRUJAN et al., 1965
	dark	0.98	Traces	1.37		

Table 12. *Dopamine in Different Regions of the Brain of a Tortoise (Geochelone chilensis* (Gray))
JUORIO, 1969, METHOD: R.F.

Brain region	Dopamine μg/g
Nucleus basalis + cortex olfactorius + septum . .	2.53
Nucleus basalis + cortex olfactorius	3.66
Septum	0.46
Epistriatum + area lateralis + area dorsalis + area medialis	0.47
Olfactory lobe	0.08
Cerebral hemisphere	0.80
Thalamus + hypothalamus + midbrain + medulla + cerebellum	0.24
Cervical spinal cord.	<0.05

Table 11. *Catecholamines in Reptiles* (Class: Reptilia, Order: Testudines)

Species		Adrenal A	Adrenal N	Spleen A	Spleen N	Heart	Heart A	Heart N	Brain A	Brain N	Kidney A	Kidney N	Liver A	Liver N	Ovary A	Ovary N	Pancreas A	Pancreas N	Method	Reference
						Concentrations in $\mu g/g$ tissue														
Chrysemis d'orbignyi	♂	3370	700	—	—		—	—	—	—	—	—	—	—	—	—	—	—	A.F.	MARQUES and SERRANO, 1960
	♀	3030	900	—	—		—	—	—	—	—	—	—	—	—	—	—	—		
Chrysemis picta		—	—	—	—	Whole heart	A+N	0.48	—	—	A+N	91.16	A+N	0.12	—	—	—	—	A.F.	MUSACCHIA et al., 1962
Chelydra serpentina		—	—	<0.01	0.32	Atrium	0.035	0.37	—	—	—	—	—	—	—	—	<0.01	0.25	A.F.	AZUMA et al., 1965
						Ventricle	0.02	0.42	—	—	—	—	—	—	—	—	—	—		
Turtle (unspecified)		2500	3750	—	—	—	—	—	—	—	—	—	—	—	—	—	—	—	PC.B.	WEST, 1955
Turtle (unspecified)		—	—	—	—	Atrium	0.17	1.08	—	—	—	—	—	—	—	—	—	—	S.F.	FRIEDMAN and BHAGAT, 1962
						Ventricle	0.07	0.44	—	—	—	—	—	—	—	—	—	—		
Turtle (unspecified)		895	509	0.11	0.42	Whole heart	0.09	0.43	0.28	0.93	5.23	46.0	0.06	0.04	0.17	0.04	—	—	A.F.	ANTON and SAYRE, 1962
Turtle (unspecified)		—	—	0.06	0.42	Whole heart	0.09	0.43	0.12	0.44	1.5	34.9	0.06	0.04	—	—	—	—	A.F.	ANTON and SAYRE, 1964
				Dopamine	44.7	Dopamine	0.11		Dopamine	0.57	Dopamine	0.59	Dopamine	0.60	—	—	—	—		

(Order: Crocodylia)

Species	Adrenal A	Adrenal N	Spleen A	Spleen N	Heart A	Heart N	Brain A	Brain N	Kidney A	Kidney N	Liver A	Liver N	Lung A	Lung N	Method	Reference
Alligator (unspecified)	373	322	0.3	2.0	0.16	1.2	0.10	0.28	1.6	11.0	0.03	0.08	0.05	0.33	A.F.	ANTON and SAYRE, 1962

(Order: Squamata, Sub-Order: Sauria)

Species	Brain N	Heart A	Heart N	Stomach N	Small intestine N	Bladder A	Bladder N	Lung A	Lung N	Method	Reference
Sauria cyanogenis	1.6	—	6.4	0.76	0.85	—	—	—	—	S.F.	BRODIE et al., 1964
Tiliqua rugosa	—	0.34	2.54	—	—	—	—	—	—	A.F., B.	COOPER et al., 1966
Trachysaurus rugosus	—	—	—	—	—	0.11	0.4	—	—	F.	MCLEAN and BURNSTOCK, 1967b
Trachysaurus rugosus	—	—	—	—	—	—	—	0.04	0.45	F.	MCLEAN and BURNSTOCK, 1967c

(Order: Squamata, Sub-Order: Serpentes)

Species	Spleen A	Spleen N	Heart A	Heart N	Kidney A	Kidney N	Liver N	Lung A	Lung N	Poison gland A	Poison gland N	Venom A+N		Adrenal A	Adrenal N	Method	Reference
Agkistrodon piscivorus	—	—	—	—	—	—	—	—	—	—	—	1.41		—	—	S.F.	ZARAFONETIS and KALAS, 1960
	0.10	0.43	0.07	0.64	0.46	0.98	—	0.07	0.10	0.05	0.72	—		—	—	A.F.	ANTON and SAYRE, 1962
	—	—	—	—	—	—	0.10	—	—	—	—	<0.01		—	—	A.F.	ANTON and GENNARO, 1965
Xenodon merremii	—	—	—	—	—	—	—	—	—	—	—	—	Central:	940	220	A.F.	WASSERMANN and TRAMEZZANI, 1963
													Peripheral:	10	630		
	—	—	—	—	—	—	—	—	—	—	—	—	Whole gland	2130	1360		HOUSSAY et al., 1962
Bothrops jararaca	—	—	—	—	—	—	—	—	—	—	—	—	Whole gland	500—2500 "Adrenin"		B.	VALLE and PORTO, 1945
Crotalus atrox	—	—	—	—	—	—	—	—	—	—	—	0.55		—	—	S.F.	ZARAFONETIS and KALAS, 1960
Crotalus adamanteus	—	—	—	—	—	—	—	—	—	—	—	0.47		—	—	S.F.	ZARAFONETIS and KALAS, 1960
	—	—	—	0.82	—	0.82	0.24	—	0.20	—	0.23	<0.01		—	—	A.F.	ANTON and GENNARO, 1965

Table 13. *The Concentration of Catecholamines in Peripheral Tissues of Birds* (Class: Aves)

Order and species	Age and strain	Tissue	Adrenaline µg/g	Noradrenal. µg/g	Dopamine µg/g	DOPA µg/g	Method	Reference
ORDER: GALLI-FORMES *Gallus domesticus* (chicken)	Domestic fowl	Heart	—	0.24	—	—	A.F.	v. EULER, 1963a
	Chicks aged 1—56 days	Heart	0.73—1.20	0.20—0.54	—	—	S.F.	CALLINGHAM and CASS 1966
	Chicks aged 28 days	Heart	0.20	0.14	3.92	5.09	R.PC.F.	MANUKHIN et al., 1969
	White Leghorn chicks aged 28 days	Heart	6.7 ng/mg protein	2.0 ng/mg protein	0.073 ng/mg protein	0.045 ng/mg protein	A.F.	IGNARRO and SHIDEMAN, 1968a
	White Leghorn adult kept at 25°C for 20 weeks	Heart: Right atrium	2.351	0.735	—	—	A.F.	LIN and STURKIE, 1968
		Left atrium	0.589	0.393	—	—		
		Ventricle	0.134	0.090	—	—		
	Domestic fowl	Liver	—	0.095	—	—	A.F.	v. EULER, 1963a
		Spleen	—	0.56	—	—		
	Chicks aged 28 days	Spleen	0.76	0.39	5.30	10.12	R.PC.F.	MANUKHIN et al., 1969
	Domestic fowl	Stomach muscle	—	0.063	—	—	A.F.	v. EULER, 1963a
		Small intestine	—	0.19	—	—		
	Chicks aged 28 days	Intestine	0.11	0.19	2.74	0.51	R.PC.F.	MANUKHIN et al., 1969
	Domestic fowl	Vas deferens	1.4	9.1	—	—	A.F.	SJÖSTRAND, 1965a
	Chicks aged 1—56 days	Adrenal gland	2500—3500	2500—3500	—	—	S.F.	CALLINGHAM and CASS, 1966
	White Leghorn adult kept at 25°C for 20 weeks	Adrenal gland	3610	1390	—	—	A.F.	LIN and STURKIE, 1968
		Venous blood plasma	6.076 µg/l	1.564 µg/l	—	—		
	Domestic fowl	Adrenal gland	8000	2000	—	—	B.	SHEPHERD and WEST, 1951
	White Leghorn 3rd day of incubat.	Egg yolk	204 ng/g protein	23.5 ng/g protein	—	—	A.F.	IGNARRO and SHIDEMAN, 1968b
ORDER: PASSERI-FORMES SUB-ORDER: PASSERES *Pica pica* (magpie)	Unspecified	Heart	—	0.6—1.1	—	—	A.F.	v. EULER, 1963a
		Liver	—	0.1—0.29	—	—		
		Spleen	—	2.2	—	—		

Table 13. (continued)

Order and species	Age and strain	Tissue	Adrenaline µg/g	Noradrenaline µg/g	Dopamine µg/g	DOPA µg/g	Method	Reference
ORDER: COLUMBIFORMES *Columba livia* (pigeon)	Unspecified	Heart	0.03	0.74	0.09	None detected <0.05	A.F.	ANTON and SAYRE, 1964
		Heart	—	0.952	—	—	A.F.	LINÉT et al., 1967
		Liver	0.02	0.24	0.13	None detected <0.05	A.F.	ANTON and SAYRE, 1964
		Liver	—	1.14 (NA + A)	0.28	—	R.F.	APRISON and TAKAHASHI, 1965
		Adrenal gland	1.35	1.65	—	—	B.	WEST, 1955
ORDER: ANSERIFORMES	Unspecified							
Cygnus olor (Mute swan)		Testis and epididymis	None detected	5.16; 5.50	None detected	—	R.F.	BAUMGARTEN and HOLSTEIN, 1968
Branta canadiensis (Canada goose)		Blood plasma	1.3 µg/l	3.1 µg/l	—	—	A.F.	DONOSO, 1962
Anas platyrynchas L. (Mallard)		Blood plasma	2.7 µg/l	8.3 µg/l	—	—		
Anas boschas L. (Domesticated duck)		Blood plasma	3.0 µg/l	6.6 µg/l	—	—		
Egyptian goose		Blood plasma	7.7 µg/l	5.9 µg/l	—	—		
ORDER: CHARADRIIFORMES *Larus argentatus P.* (Herring gull)	Unspecified	Blood plasma	2.1 µg/l	15.0 µg/l	—	—		

Table 14. *Concentration (μg/g) of Catecholamines in Avian Brain*
(Class: Aves)

Order and species	Age and/or strain	Tissue	Adrenaline	Noradrenaline	Dopamine	Method	Ref.
ORDER: GALLIFORMES *Gallus domesticus* (Chicken)	Adult	Brain	—	0.60	—	S.F.	1
	Chick	Brain	0.037; 0.030	0.066; 0.051	0.13; 0.19	A.R.F.	2
	1—56 days	Brain	0.08—0.10	0.18—0.22	—	S.F.	3
	Adult White Leghorn	Pallium	—	0.49	0.81	S.F.	4
		Striatum	—	0.40	1.13		
		Diencephalon and mesencephalon	—	0.98	0.19		
		Pons and medulla	—	0.85	0.24		
		Cerebellum	—	0.47	0.09		
		Cervical spinal cord	—	0.14	0.07		
		Thoracic spinal cord	—	0.18	0.05		
		Lumbar spinal cord	—	0.15	0.06		
	Adult Rhode Island Red and Plymouth Rock	Nucleus basalis anterior part	—	0.37	2.80	Adrenaline and corres-	5
		Nucleus basalis posterior part	—	0.39	0.40	ponding noradrenaline	
		Epibasalis complex	—	0.23	0.07; 0.02	PC.B.	
		Thalamus	0.64	0.88	—	Dopamine and	
		Hypothalamus	1.01	1.42	—	some nor-	
		Medulla	0.35	0.45; 0.42	—	adrenaline	
		Optic lobes	0.07	0.23; 0.23	<0.04	R.F.	
		Cerebellum	<0.02	0.21; 0.12	<0.04		
		Thalamus, hypothalamus, midbrain and medulla	—	—	0.19		
	Adult Rhode Island Red	Hypothalamus	0.65	1.45	—	PC.B.	6
	Adult Plymouth Rock	Hypothalamus	0.66	1.61	—	PC.B.	
	Adult White Leghorn	Diencephalon	0.21	0.99	—	Ac.PC.F.	
	Unspecified strain 4—8 weeks old	Ventral diencephalon (hypothalamus)	0.11	0.70	0.08	R.F.	7
		Dorsal diencephalon (thalamus)	0.19	1.0	0.11		

Table 14. (continued)

Order and species	Age and/or strain	Tissue	Adrenaline	Noradrenaline	Dopamine	Method	Ref.
ORDER: GALLIFORMES *Gallus domesticus* (Chicken)	"Ross 1" cocks 6 months	Cerebral hemispheres	0.03; 0.01	0.27; 0.29	0.47; 0.42	Ac.PC.F.	8
		Optic lobes	0.04; 0.02	0.40; 0.31	0.01; <0.01		
		Diencephalon and mesencephalon	0.40; 0.40; 0.18	1.36; 1.01; 0.67	0.12; 0.09		
		Cerebellum	<0.01; <0.01	0.27; 0.20	<0.01; 0.01		
		Medulla	0.14; 0.07	0.47; 0.28	0.02; 0.02		
	"Ross 1" cocks 7 day	Hypothalamus	0.15; 0.16	0.83; 0.89	0.28; 0.31		
ORDER: ANSERIFORMES *Cairina moschata* (Muscovy duck)		Nucleus basalis anterior part	—	—	3.61	R.F.	9
		Nucleus basalis posterior part	—	—	0.55		
		Epibasalis complex	—	—	0.04		
		Thalamus, hypothalamus, midbrain and medulla	—	—	<0.01		
		Optic lobes	—	—	<0.01		
		Cerebellum	—	—	<0.01		
ORDER: PASSERIFORMES SUB-ORDER: PASSERES *Lonchura punctulata* (Spice finch)		Nucleus basalis anteriorpart	—	—	7.5	R.F.	10
		Nucleus basalis posterior part	—	—	1.45; 1.44		
		Epibasalis complex	—	—	0.07		
		Thalamus, hypothalamus, midbrain and medulla	—	—	0.16		
		Optic lobes	—	—	<0.03		
		Cerebellum	—	—	<0.03		
		Hypothalamus	0.5	2.0	—	PC.B.	
ORDER: COLUMBIFORMES *Columba livia*	Unspecified	Whole brain	—	0.38	—	S.F.	11
		Whole brain	0.02	0.25	0.29	A.F.	12
		Whole brain	—	0.353	0.403	A.F.	13
		Telencephalon except palaeostriatum and neostriatum	—	0.27	0.35	R.F.	14
		Palaeostriatum and neostiratum	—	0.52	1.5		
		Diencephalon	—	0.88	0.05		
		Mesencephalon	—	0.89	0.05		
		Area of mesencephalic [illegible]		5.2	0.67		

Order and species	Age and/or strain	Tissue	Adrenaline	Noradrenaline	Dopamine	Method	Ref.
ORDER: COLUMBIFORMES		Cerebellum	—	0.16	0.01		
		Medulla	—	0.50	0.03		
Columba livia (Pigeon)	White Carneaux cocks	Telencephalon	None detected	0.52	1.00	Noradrenaline S.F. Dopamine R.F.	15
		Diencephalon and optic lobes		0.86	0.23		
		Cerebellum		0.25	0.13		
		Pons-medulla		0.96	0.26		
	Unspecified	Cerebral hemispheres, thalamus, hypothalamus, midbrain and medulla	—	0.27	0.52	Noradrenaline and adrenaline PC.B.	16
		Cerebral hemispheres	—	0.22	0.61	Noradrenaline and dopamine R.F.	
		Epibasalis complex	0.04	0.16	0.04		
		Nucleus basalis	—	0.36	2.00		
		Nucleus basalis anterior part	0.11	0.40	3.00		
		Nucleus basalis posterior part	0.05	0.17	0.60		
		Thalamus, hypothalamus, midbrain and medulla	—	0.34; 0.79	0.09		
		Thalamus	0.24	0.75	—		
		Hypothalamus	0.38	1.50	0.15		
		Optic lobes	0.06	0.34	<0.01		
		Medulla and part of midbrain	0.06	0.42	—		
		Cerebellum	<0.03	0.14	<0.02		
		Spinal cord	<0.02	0.06	<0.03		
		Diencephalon	0.1	0.93	—	Ac.PC.F.	17
		Hypothalamus	0.1	0.71	—	PC.B.	
		Diencephalon	None detected	0.60; 0.90	0.08; 0.08	R.F.	18

Reference: 1. BRODIE et al., 1964; 2. MONTAGU, 1957; 3. CALLINGHAM and CASS, 1966; 4. PSCHEIDT and HABER, 1965; 5. JUORIO and VOGT, 1967; 6. JUORIO and VOGT, 1970; 7. FALCK et al., 1969; 8. CALLINGHAM and SHARMAN, 1970; 9. JUORIO and VOGT, 1967; 10. JUORIO and VOGT, 1967; 11. BRODIE et al., 1964; 12. ANTON and SAYRE, 1964; 13. LINÉT et al., 1967; 14. BERTLER et al., 1964; 15. APRISON and TAKAHASHI. 1965; 16. JUORIO and VOGT, 1967; 17. JUORIO and VOGT, 1970; 18. FALCK et al., 1969.

Table 15. *Catecholamines in the Brain of the Rabbit*

Species	Tissue	Noradrenal. μg/g	Dopam. μg/g	Method	Reference
ORDER: LAGOMORPHA FAMILY: LEPORIDAE *Oryctolagus cuniculus*	Whole brain	0.29	0.32	R.F.	Bertler and Rosengren, 1959b
	Hypothalamus	1.07	—	PC.B.	Sanan and Vogt, 1962
	Cortex	0.08	0.27	R.F.	Matsuoka et al., 1964
	Pons	0.08	0.32		
	Cerebellum	0.06	0.34		
	Medulla oblongata	0.05	0.18		
	Corpora quadrigemina	0.05	0.51		
	Thalamus	0.22	0.27		
	Hypothalamus	0.81	0.47		
	Caudate nucleus	0.85	4.28		
	Lentiform nucleus	0.20	1.87		
	Hypothalamus	1.52	0.20	AC.PC.F.	Laverty and Sharman, 1965
	Midbrain	0.59	0.18		
	Massa intermedia of thalamus	0.36	0.10		
	Caudate nucleus	0.025; 0.017	—	PC.B.	Sharman and Vogt, 1965
		0.33; 0.18	—	R.F.	
		0.045; 0.027	—	AC.PC.F.	
	Caudate nucleus	—	5.25	R.F.	Lisch et al., 1968
	Caudate nucleus	—	8.8	R.F.	O'Keeffe et al., 1970
	Hypothalamus	1.27; 0.94	0.19		

Table 16. *Catecholamines in the Brain of Rodents*
(Order: Rodentia)

Species	Tissue	Noradrenal. μg/g	Dopamine μg/g	Method	Ref.
SUB-ORDER: MYOMORPHA FAMILY: MURIDAE SUB-FAMILY: MURINAE *Rattus norvegicus* (rat)	Whole brain	0.49	0.60	R.F.	1
		0.32 (Adrenaline 0.04)	0.68	A.F.	2
		0.28	0.49	S.F.	3
	Caudate nucleus	0.27	6.39	AC.PC.F.	4
	Hypothalamus	1.29	0.14		
	Midbrain	0.55	0.13		
	Cerebral cortex	0.18	<0.01		
	Cortex (telencephalon without striatum)	0.24	} 7.5 6.7* Combined 1.2* (bracketed: Cortex to Hippocampus)	A.F.	5
	Caudate nucleus, putamen and globus pallidus	0.25		*R.F.	*6
	Midbrain, thalamus and subthalamus	0.37			
	Hypothalamus	1.79			
	Hippocampus	0.20			
	Cerebellum	0.17			
	Medulla oblongata and pons	0.72	0.06*		
	Mesencephalon	—	0.23*		
	Tuberculum olfactorium + nucleus accumbens + septum + nucleus interstitialis striae terminalis	—	1.3*		
	Olfactory bulb and tract	0.53	1.4	A.F.	7
	Frontal and parietal neo-pallium with approx. 20% of hippocampus	0.27	0.27		
	Main part of hippocampus amygdaloid body, palaeopallium and a small part of neopallium	0.52	0 63		

Table 16. (continued)

Species	Tissue	Noradrenal. µg/g	Dopamine µg/g	Method	Ref.
Rattus norvegicus (rat)	Main mass of the head of the caudate nucleus, putamen, globus pallidus, main part of corpus callosum and fornix	0.57	2.4		
	Main part of thalamus and epithalamus, fornix, tail of the caudate nucleus and cerebral peduncle	0.65	0.91		
	Hypothalamus	1.5	1.3		
	Inferior and superior colliculi	0.51	1.7		
	Tegmentum, part of cerebral peduncle and sometimes a small part of pons	0.64	1.2		
	Entire cerebellum	0.28	0.36		
	Pons, corpus trapezoideum and part of medulla oblongata	0.70	0.84		
	Medulla oblongata and some medulla spinalis	0.52	1.05		
	Cerebral hemispheres	0.17	0.50	S.F.	8
	Hypothalamus	0.73	0.52		
	Thalamus	0.35	0.22		
	Corpora quadrigemina	0.28	0.15		
	Medulla oblongata	0.32	0.09		
	Corpus striatum	0.71	5.25		
	Cerebellum	0.10	none detected		
	Olfactory bulbs	0.26	0.19		
	Mesencephalic area	0.31	0.26		
	Pons	0.35	0.10		
	Crux cerebri	0.40	0.54		
	Floor of 4th ventricle	0.60	0.53		
	Frontal cortex	0.19	0.06		
	Occipital cortex	0.15	0.09		
	Limbic area	0.16	0.03		
Mus musculus (mouse)	Whole brain	0.4	1.2	R.F.	9
		0.497	0.824	A.F.	10
		0.48	0.70	S.F.	11
		0.621	—	E_2	12
		µg/g protein			
	Cerebellum	3.49	—	E_1	13
	Lower brainstem	7.39	—		
	Upper brainstem with pons and tegmentum	6.26	—		
	Hypothalamus	13.20	—		
	Olfactory bulb	11.20	—		
		µg/g			
SUB-ORDER: HYSTRICOMORPHA FAMILY: CAVIDAE *Cavia porcellus* (guinea-pig)	Whole brain	0.38	0.34	R.F.	14
		0.32	0.70	A.F.	15
		0.31	0.68	A.F.	16

References: 1. Bertler and Rosengren, 1959b; 2. Anton and Sayre, 1964; 3. Valzelli and Garattini, 1968; 4. Laverty and Sharman, 1965; 5. Glowinski and Iversen, 1966; 6. Anden et al., 1966a; 7. Popov et al. 1967; Valzelli and Garattini, 1968; 9. Carlsson and Lindqvist, 1962; 10. Smith, 1963; 11. Fleming et al., 1965; 12. Nikodijevic et al., 1969; 13. Saelens et al., 1967; 14. Bertler and Rosengren, 1959b; 15. Paulsen and Hess, 1963; 16. Anton and Sayre, 1964.

Table 17. *Catecholamines in the Brain of the Cat*
(Order: Carnivora, Sub-Order: Fissipeda, Family: Felidae)

Species	Tissue	Nor-adrenaline µg/g	Dop-amine µg/g	Method	Reference
Felis catus (cat)	Whole brain	0.22	0.28	R.F.	BERTLER and ROSENGREN, 1959b
	Cerebral hemispheres (not corpus striatum and hippocampus)				
	rostral part	0.22	0.08		
	caudal part	0.23	0.10		
	Caudate nucleus	0.22	8.00		
	Lentiform nucleus	0.20	1.90		
	Hippocampus	0.14	0.08		
	Hypothalamus	2.01	0.75		
	Diencephalon (excluding hypothalamus)	0.34	0.16		
	Mesencephalon	0.43	0.19		
	Pons	0.52	0.11		
	Medulla oblongata	0.39	0.08		
	Cerebellum	0.13	0.02		
	Anterior hypothalamus	3.6	—	S.F.	KUNTZMAN et al., 1961
	Posterior hypothalamus	2.0	—		
	Septum	1.5	—		
	Midbrain reticular formation	1.4	—		
	Central grey matter	1.2	—		
	Olfactory tubercle	0.95	—		
	Pontile reticular formation	0.97	—		
	Medial geniculate	0.50	—		
	Neocortex	0.49	—		
	Hypnogenic zone of Hess	0.45	—		
	Amygdala	0.30	—		
	Caudate nucleus	0.36	—		
	Pyriform cortex	0.35	—		
	Auditory cortex	0.35	—		
	Cochlear nucleus	0.32	—		
	Inferior colliculus	0.26	—		
	Thalamus (whole)	0.17	—		
	Pons	0.25	—		
	Intralaminar and midline nuclei	0.40	—		
	Basal thalamic area	1.00	—		
	Cingulate cortex	0.35	—		
	Association cortex	0.21	0.30	A.F.	MCGEER et al., 1963
	Sensory cortex	0.11	0.13		
	Orbital cortex	0.28	0.30		
	Septal region	0.70	1.62		
	Caudate nucleus	0.41	3.12		
	Midbrain	0.50	0.53		
	Hypothalamus	2.22	0.70		
	Thalamus	0.22	0.50		
	Amygdala, fornix + hippocampus	0.17	0.21		
	Cingulate gyrus	0.27	0.58		
	Quadrigeminal plate	0.40	1.59		
	Pons	0.20	0.32		
	Medulla	0.36	0.32		
	Neocerebellum	0.12	0.20		
	Archicerebellum	0.17	0.14		
	Cervical cord	0.34	0.45		

Table 17a. *Diurnal Variations in the Noradrenaline Content of the Brain of the Cat*

Species	Tissue	Time	Noradrenaline µg/g	Method	Reference
Felis catus (cat)	Cervical spinal cord	0700	0.103	A.F.	Reis et al., 1968
		1300	0.161		
		1900	0.343		
		0100	0.150		
	Pons	0700	0.275		
		1300	0.416		
		1900	0.283		
		0100	0.308		
	Superior colliculus	0700	0.141		
		1300	0.568		
		1900	0.166		
		0100	0.385		
	Substantia nigra and lateral tegmentum	0700	0.250		
		1300	0.544		
		1900	0.241		
		0100	0.431		
	Lateral thalamus	0700	0.203		
		1300	0.451		
		1900	0.278		
		0100	0.368		
	Hypothalamus: region of tuber cinereum	0700	2.420		
		1300	2.317		
		1900	3.737		
		0100	2.534		
	Hypothalamus: anterior hypothalamus region	0700	1.931		
		1300	2.975		
		1900	3.978		
		0100	3.571		
	Medulla	24 hr mean	0.313		
	Cerebellum	24 hr mean	0.375		
	Inferior colliculus	24 hr mean	0.230		
	Periaquaeductal grey matter and interpeduncular nucleus	24 hr mean	0.775		
	Red nucleus-medial tegmentum	24 hr mean	0.695		
	Habenula	24 hr mean	1.380		
	Medial thalamus	24 hr mean	0.494		
	Mamillary bodies	24 hr mean	0.377		
	Tuber cinereum	24 hr mean	2.801		
	Lateral division of hypothalamus	24 hr mean	0.801		
	Nucleus of diagonal band	24 hr mean	1.289		
	Amygdala-entorhinal cortex	24 hr mean	0.325		
	Olfactory bulb	24 hr mean	0.252		
	Olfactory tubercle	24 hr mean	0.537		
	Hippocampus	24 hr mean	0.195		
	Caudate nucleus	24 hr mean	0.102		
	Globus pallidus	24 hr mean	0.263		
	Septum	24 hr mean	0.599		
	Sensorimotor cortex	24 hr mean	0.333		

Table 18. *Catecholamines in the Brain of the Dog*
(Order: Carnivora, Sub-Order: Fissipeda, Family: Canidae)

	Tissue	Noradrenaline µg/g	Adrenaline µg/g	Method	Reference
Canis familiaris (dog)	*Diencephalon*			PC. B.	VOGT, 1954
	Corpora mammillaria	0.41	0.17 (Corpora mammillaria to Medial thalamic nuclei)		
	Regio preoptica	0.28			
	Remainder of hypothalamus	1.03			
	Medial thalamic nuclei	0.24			
	Mesencephalon				
	Stratum griseum centrale	0.42	—		
	"Midbrain" (excluding colliculi, basis pedunculi and brachium colliculi inferioris)	0.37	—		
	Red nucleus and fossa interpeduncularis	0.26	—		
	Medulla oblongata				
	Region of nuclei X and XII	0.31	—		
	Formatio reticularis				
	posterior part	0.34	—		
	anterior part	0.36	—		
	Area acustica	0.39	—		
	Central part of floor of fourth ventricle	0.27	—		
	Area postrema	1.04			
	Pons, ventromedial; superior colliculi; inferior colliculi; cortex (average); medial geniculate body; nucleus (and funiculus) gracilis and cuneatus	0.1—0.2			
	Grey matter				
	Lateral thalamic nuclei; lateral geniculate body; cerebellar cortex; amygdaloid nuclei; caudate nuclei; some cortical areae; tuber olfactorium; cornu ammonis (grey matter)	<0.1			
	White matter				
	Brachium conjunctivum; corpus callosum; pyramid; cerebellar fibres; cornu ammonis (white matter); optic nerve; album centrale	<0.1			
	Whole brain	0.16	0.19	R.F.	BERTLER and ROSENGREN, 1959b
	Cerebral hemispheres (not corpus striatum and hippocampus)				
	rostral part	0.13	0.07		
	caudal part	0.12	0.08		
	Caudate nucleus	0.10	5.90		
	Lentiform nucleus	0.08	1.63		
	Hippocampus	0.14	0.13		
	Hypothalamus	0.76	0.26		
	Diencephalon (excluding hypothalamus)	0.17	0.09		
	Mesencephalon	0.33	0.20		
	Pons	0.41	0.10		
	Medulla oblongata	0.37	0.13		
	Cerebellum	0.06	0.03		
	Caudate nucleus	0.09	9.9	R.AC.PC.F.	LAVERTY and SHARMAN, 1965
	Hypothalamus	1.35	0.25		
	Massa intermedia of thalamus	0.17	0.05		
	Midbrain	0.43	0.33		
	Cerebral cortex	0.16	0.01		
	Palaeocerebellum	0.05	0.003		

Table 19. *Catecholamines in the Brain of Ruminants*
(Order: Artiodactyla, Sub-Order: Ruminantia, Family: Bovidae)

Species	Tissue	Nor-adrenaline µg/g	Dopamine µg/g	Method	Reference
Ovis aries (sheep)	Whole brain	0.21	0.29	R.F.	BERTLER and ROSENGREN, 1959b
	Cerebral hemispheres (cxeluding striatum and hippocampus)				
	rostral part	0.16	0.12		
	caudal part	0.13	0.02		
	Caudate nucleus	0.13	6.68; 11.78*	AC.PC. F.*	*LAVERTY and SHARMAN, 1965
	Lentiform nucleus	0.10	4.78		
	Hippocampus	0.15	0.06		
	Hypothalamus	1.15	0.19		
	Diencephalon (excluding hypothalamus)	0.28	0.16		
	Mesencephalon	0.47	0.24		
	Pons	0.58	0.04		
	Medulla oblongata	0.46	0.17		
	Cerebellum	0.06	0.03		
	Superior hypothalamus	3.01	0.27	AC.PC. F.	LAVERTY and SHARMAN, 1965
	Inferior hypothalamus	1.44	0.21		
	Massa intermedia of thalamus	0.70	0.34		
	Pituitary stalk and median eminence	0.32	5.05		
Capra hircus (goat)	Caudate nucleus	—	10.9	AC.PC. F.	LAVERTY and SHARMAN, 1965
	Superior hypothalamus	1.48	0.15		
	Medial hypothalamus	1.81	0.10		
	Inferior hypothalamus	2.16	0.11		
	Massa intermedia of thalamus — medial	0.34	0.31		
	Massa intermedia of thalamus — lateral	0.12	0.46		
	Anterior midbrain	0.29	0.41		
	Medial anterior midbrain	0.45	0.27		
	Medial posterior midbrain	0.55	0.14		
	Posterior midbrain	0.34	0.04		
	Pituitary stalk and media eminence	0.16	2.0		

Table 20. *Catecholamines in the Brain of the Pig*
(Order: Artiodactyla, Sub-Order: Suiformes, Family: Suidae)

Species	Tissue	Noradrenaline µg/g	Dopamine µg/g	Method	Reference
Sus scrofa domesticus (pig)	Whole brain	0.14	0.22	R.F.	BERTLER and ROSENGREN, 1959b
	Cerebral hemispheres (excluding corpus striatum and hippocampus)				
	rostral part	0.09	0.08		
	caudal part	0.09	0.05		
	Caudate nucleus	0.21	6.1		
	Lentiform nucleus	0.03	3.6		
	Hippocampus	0.09	0.04		
	Hypothalamus	0.83	0.88		
	Diencephalon (not hypothalamus)	0.18	0.11		
	Mesencephalon	0.31	0.14		
	Pons	0.25	0.06		
	Medulla oblongata	0.22	0.05		
	Cerebellum	0.10	0.01		
	Median eminence and infundibular stem region	0.78	0.85	A.F.	RINNE and SONNINEN, 1968
	Mediobasal hypothalamus	1.97	0.14		
	Remainder of hypothalamus	0.61	0.13		
	Pituitary gland				
	Pars distalis	0.01	0.01	R.F.	BJÖRKLUND et al., 1967
	Pars intermedia				
	proximal portion	0.01	0.18		
	distal portion	0.03	0.62		
	Neural lobe	0.04	0.32		

Table 21. *Catecholamines in the Brain of the Monkey*
(Order: Primates, Sub-Order: Anthropoidea, Family: Cercopithecidae)

Species	Tissue	Nor-adrenaline µg/g	Dop-amine µg/g	Method	Reference
Macaca mulatta (monkey)	Pons and medulla	0.49		S.F.	PSCHEIDT and HIMWICH, 1963
	Midbrain and hypothalamus	0.77			
	Caudate nucleus	0.36			
	Thalamus	0.56			
	Hippocampus + amygdala	0.29			
	"Lenticular thalamic mass" (lateral thalamic nuclei, internal capsule, putamen and globus pallidus)	0.29; 0.35			
	Temperal pole	0.20; 0.24			
	Various cortical structures	0.17			
	Amygdala-hippocampus-fornix	0.11	0.18	A.F.	WADA and MCGEER, 1966
	Thalamus	0.27	0.11		
	Basal ganglia	0.37	1.59		
	Cingulate gyrus	0.18	0.18		
	Pons	0.30	0.27		
	Midbrain	0.38	0.39		
	Caudate nucleus	0.32	3.50		
	Medulla	0.37	0.25		
	Septal region	0.49	0.28		
	Quadrigeminal plate	1.02	0.76		
	Hypothalamus	7.10	1.69		
	Archicerebellum	0.06	0.08		
	Neocerebellum	0.14	0.08		
	Striatum	0.26	7.5	A.F.	Calculated from POIRIER et al., 1966
	Caudate nucleus	—	10.3	R.F.	O'KEEFFE et al., 1970
	Putamen	—	12.4		
	Substantia nigra	—	0.8		

Table 23. *Catecholamines in the Spinal Cord*

Species	Tissue	Nor-adrenaline µg/g	Dopamine µg/g	DOPA µg/g	Method	Reference
Oryctolagus cuniculus (rabbit)	Spinal cord	0.16	0.84	0.33	A.F.	MCGEER and MCGEER, 1962
		0.03	0.02	<0.05	A.F.	ANTON and SAYRE, 1964
		0.15	0.01 or less	—	R.F.	MAGNUSSON and ROSENGREN,
Rattus norvegicus (rat)	Spinal cord	0.15	1.00	0.67	A.F.	MCGEER and MCGEER, 1962
		0.11	0.02	<0.05	A.F.	ANTON and SAYRE, 1964
Cavia porcellus (guinea-pig)	Spinal cord	0.17	0.06	<0.05	A.F.	ANTON and SAYRE, 1964
Felis catus (cat)	Spinal cord	0.19	0.45	0.40	A.F.	MCGEER and MCGEER, 1962
		0.05	0.05	<0.05	A.F.	ANTON and SAYRE, 1964
	Thoracic and lumbar cord	0.08; 0.16	0.010; 0.007	—	R.AC.PC.F.	LAVERTY and SHARMAN, 1965
(kitten, 10 days old)	Spinal cord	0.36	—	—	S.F.	ANDERSON and HOLGERSON, 1966
Canis familiaris (dog)	Spinal cord	0.06	0.02	<0.05	A.F.	ANTON and SAYRE, 1964
	Thoracic and lumbar cord	0.10	0.008	—	R.AC.PC.F.	LAVERTY and SHARMAN, 1965
Bos taurus (cattle)	Spinal cord	0.10	0.20	0.18	A.F.	MCGEER and MCGEER, 1962
Homo sapiens (man)	Spinal cord	0.13	0.32	0.35		

Table 22. *Catecholamines in Human Brain*

	Tissue	Noradrenaline μg/g 1	2	3	Dopamine μg/g 1	2	3	Method	Reference
Homo sapiens (man) adult	*Telencephalon*							1. Noradrenaline R.F. Dopamine R.C.	EHRINGER and HORNYKIEWICZ, 1960
	Cortex (various areas)		0	0		0.02	0	2. A.R.F.	SANO et al., 1959
			0.06	0.03		0.17	0.06	3. R.F.	BERTLER, 1961
	Caudate nucleus	0.09	0.04	0.04	3.5	5.74	3.12		
	Putamen	0.12	0.07	0.02	3.7	8.25	5.27		
	Globus pallidus	0.15	0.02	0.05	0.5	1.01	0.32		
	Nucleus amygdalae	0.21	0.06		0.6	0.13			
	Septal region	0.31			0.3				
	Septum and fornix		0.17			0.07			
	Diencephalon								
	Thalamus (whole)	0.13			0.3				
	Thalamus (medial)	0.22	0.09	0.09	0.4	0.46	0.03		
	Thalamus (rostral)		0	0.02		0.11	0.07		
	Thalamus (lateral)		0.04	0.04		0.30	0.01		
	Hypothalamus	1.25	1.11		0.8	1.12			
	Anterior part			0.96			0.18		
	Intermediate part			1.19			0.14		
	Posterior part			0.31			0.22		
	Mesencephalon								
	Nucleus ruber	0.30	0.23	0.22	0.70	1.17	0.19		
	Substantia nigra	0.21	0.07	0.04	0.9	0.38	0.40		
	Corpora quadrigemina	0.12	0.15		0.4	0.07			
	Superior colliculus			0.12			0.13		
	Inferior colliculus			0.15			0.10		
	Rhombencephalon								
	Grey matter in floor of fourth ventricle	0.35			0.6				
	Dorsal part of medulla including floor of fourth ventricle			0.13			—0.01 (sic)		
	Medulla oblongata		0.14			0.17			
	Pons	0.13		0.04	0.2		0		
	Dorsal part		0.15			0.08			
	Central part		0.02			0.07			
	Cerebellum								
	Cerebellum		0.01			0			
	Cerebellar cortex			0.02			0.02		
	Nucleus dentatus	<0.06	0.01	0.01	<0.5	0.03	0.08		

Table 24. *Catecholamines in Peripheral Nervous Tissue*

Species	Tissue	Adrenaline µg/g	Nor-adrenaline µg/g	Dop-amine µg/g	Method	Ref.
Mus musculus (mouse)	Stellate and superior cervical ganglia	approx. 3	14	—	S.F.	1
Rattus norvegicus (rat)	Superior cervical ganglion	0.26	19.8	—	S.F.	2
	Stellate ganglion	0.12	27.1	—		
	Superior cervical ganglion	7.3	—	—	PC.B.	3
Oryctolagus cuniculus (rabbit)	Superior cervical ganglion	0.34	4.5	—	PC.B.	4
	Solar ganglion	1.5	6.7	—		
	Superior cervical ganglion	—	3.5	0.85	AC.PC.F.	5
	Stellate ganglion	—	13.0	4.64		
Felis catus (cat)	Superior cervical ganglion	0.14	3.5	—	PC.B.	6
	Stellate ganglion	0.09	2.9	—		
	Inferior mesenteric ganglion	0.4—15.6	9.6—46.2	—		
	Splenic nerve	0.23	2.5	—		
	Thoracic chain	0.02	0.7	—		
	Abdominal chain	0.10	1.6	—		
	Superior cervical ganglion	—	5.26	0.82	AC.PC.F.	7
	Stellate ganglion	—	2.82	1.32		
	Superior cervical ganglion	0.19	6.86	—	R.F.	8
Canis familiaris (dog)	Hypogastric nerve	0.09—1.23	1.7—3.6	—	PC.B.	9
	Mesenteric ganglia	39.0 ⌀	40.2 ⌀	—		
	Inferior mesenteric ganglion	31.0 ⌀	76.6 ⌀	—	PC.B.	10
	Splenic nerve	—	12.2	0.45	R.AC.PC.F.	11
	Cardiac nerve	—	7.8	0.78		
	Sympathetic chain	—	2.2	0.17		
	Superior cervical ganglion	—	26.5	2.00		
	Inferior cervical ganglion	—	5.5	0.80		
	Stellate ganglion	—	15.9	1.53		
Ovis aries (sheep)	Splenic nerve	—	5—8	—	B	12
	Mesenteric nerve	—	1—3.5	—		
	Thoracic and lumbar sympathetic chain	—	1—4	—		
	Sciatic nerve	—	0.2	—		
	Stellate ganglion	—	4.07	1.48	AC.PC.F.	13
Capra hircus (goat)	Stellate ganglion	—	1.95	0.85	AC.PC.F.	14
	Sympathetic trunk	—	1.2	0.6	R.F.	15
	Sciatic nerve	—	0.1	0.4		
Bos taurus (cattle)	Splenic nerve	0.2—0.5*	8.5—18.5	—	B.	16
	Mesenteric nerve	—	1.5—3.0	—		*17
	Splanchnic nerve	—	4.0	—		
	Sympathetic trunk (neck)	—	0.6	—		
	Thoracic and lumbar sympathetic chain	—	2.5—4.9	—		
	Saphenous nerve	—	0.2—1.0	—		
	Phrenic nerve	—	0.15—0.25	—		
	Short ciliary nerve	—	0.4	—		
	Vagus	—	0.1	—		
	Superior cervical ganglion	—	1.0	—		
	Splenic nerve	—	8.6	2.5	A.F.	18

References: 1. CRAIN and WIEGAND, 1961; 2. Calculated from KLINGMAN, 1965; 3. VOGT, unpublished; 4. MUSCHOLL and VOGT, 1958; 5. LAVERTY and SHARMAN, 1965; 6. MUSCHOLL and VOGT, 1958; 7. LAVERTY and SHARMAN, 1965; 8. KIRPEKAR et al., 1962; 9. MUSCHOLL and VOGT, 1958; 10. VANOV and VOGT, 1963; 11. LAVERTY and SHARMAN, 1965; 12. V. EULER, 1956; 13. LAVERTY and SHARMAN, 1965; 14. LAVERTY and SHARMAN, 1965; 15. CARLSSON, 1959; 16. V. EULER, 1956; *V. EULER, 1948b; 18. V. EULER and LISHAJKO, 1957.

⌀ contains chromaffin tissue.

Table 25. *Catecholamines in the Eye*

Species	Tissue	Adrenaline	Nor-adrenaline	Dop-amine	Me-thod	Ref.
Rattus			ng/iris:			
norvegicus	Iris	—	4.6	—	R.F.	1
(rat)			ng/retina:			
	Retina	Dark: —	—	3.3	S.F.	2
		Light: —	—	5.2		
	Iris + ciliary body		µg/g tissue:			
		—	3.7	—	E_1	3
Oryctolagus			ng/eye:			
cuniculus	Retina	—	0.15	9.2	R.F.	4
(rabbit)	Choroid	—	10.00	0		
			µg/g tissue:			
	Retina	—	<0.01	0.09	R.F.	5
	Choroid	—	0.26	0.06		
			µg/g tissue:			
	Retina	Dark: Traces	Traces	2.20	A.F.	6
		Light: Traces	Traces	1.27		
			ng/eye:			
	Posterior segment of	Dark: —	16.5	8.8	S.F.	7
	eyeball	Light: —	22.7	13.7		
Cavia			ng/eye:			
porcellus	Posterior segment of	Dark: —	16.2	3.5	S.F.	8
(guinea-	eyeball	Light: —	19.3	4.8		
pig, albinic)						
Felis catus			µg/g tissue:			
(cat)	Iris	—	5.0	—	R.F.	9
	Nictitating membrane	—	2.4	—	R.F.	10
	(smooth muscle)	—	4.3	—	A.F.	11
Bos taurus			µg/g tissue:			
(cattle)	Retina	0.005	0.05	—	A.B.	12
	Lens + vitreous body	—	0.0005	—		
	Iris + ciliary body	0.02	0.39	—		
	Aqueous humour*	0—0.75	0—1.3 µg/ 100 ml			
			µg/g tissue:			
				DOPA**		
	Lens	—	<0.02	—	A.PC.F.	13
	Vitreous body	—	<0.01	—		
	Retina***	—	<0.01	—		
	Tapetum fibrosum	—	0.04	0.5—1.0		
	Choroid + pigment epithelium of retina	—	0.10	1.90		
	Iris	—	0.38	2.40		

* from cow and horse combined
** identified, probably values underestimated
*** without pigment epithelium

References: 1. Dahlström et al., 1966; 2. Nichols et al., 1967; 3. Iversen and Jarrott, 1970; 4. Häggendal and Malmfors, 1963; 5. Häggendal and Malmfors, 1965; 6. Drujan et al., 1965; 7. Nichols et al., 1967; 8. Nichols et al., 1967; 9. Andén and Henning, 1966; 10. Kirpekar et al., 1962; 11. Smith et al., 1966; 12. Dunér et al., 1954; 13. Bernheimer, 1964.

Table 26. *Catecholamines in the Adrenal Glands of Different Mammals (Method: B.)*

	Adrenaline + noradrenaline µg/g	% Adrenaline	Reference
Whale	2070	17	BURN et al., 1951
Lion	530	45	GOODALL, 1951
Squirrel	200	50	v. EULER (unpublished)
Pig	2150	51	WEST, 1955
Wildebeest	1430	58	GOODALL, 1951
Cat	970	59	WEST, 1955
Gazelle	920	61	GOODALL, 1951
Goat	2230	63	WEST, 1955
Dik-Dik	120	64	
Sheep	750	67	
Cow	1750	71	
Dog	1500	73	
Ox	1620	74	
Mouse	1000	75	
Horse	840	80	
Macacus	330	81	
Sloth	713	83	PHILLIPOT et al., 1965
Zebra	1930	83	GOODALL, 1951
Man	600	83	
Hare	350	88	
Rat	1230	91	
Hamster	400	92	WEST, 1955
Rabbit	480	98	
Guinea-pig	150	98	
Baboon	830	100	

Table 27. *Catecholamines in the Adrenal gland*

Species	Adrenaline µg/g	Noradrenaline µg/g	Dopamine µg/g	Method	Reference
Adrenal medullary tissue					
Ovis aries	2000	1600	350	PC.B.	SHEPHERD and WEST, 1953
Bos taurus:					
Ox	4000	1500	35		
Cow	4000	1250	17		
Homo sapiens	1260	314	0		
Sus scrofa	4000	4000	0		
Whole gland					
Capra hircus	515	1041	7.8	A.F.	VANDERMEULEN and CESSION-FOSSION, 1968

Table 28. *Catecholamines in the Mammalian Heart*

Species	Heart tissue	Adrenaline µg/g	Nor-adrenaline µg/g	Dop-amine µg/g	Method	Reference
Erinaceus europaeus (hedgehog)	Whole heart: active	0.045	0.59	0.01	R.F.	UUSPÄÄ, 1963a
	Whole heart: hibernating	0.054	0.65	0.025		
Oryctolagus cuniculus (rabbit)	Right atrium	0.05	3.03	—	PC.B.	MUSCHOLL, 1959
	Left atrium	0.02	1.51	—		
	Atrial septum	0.06	1.62	—		
	Right ventricle	0.03	1.98	—		
	Left ventricle	0.02	1.52	—		
	Ventricular septum	—	1.59	—		
	Apex	0.03	1.82	—		
	Sino-atrial node (SAN)	<0.01	2.63	3.42	A.F.	ANGELAKOS et al., 1963
	Right atrium without SAN	0.07 ∅	3.48	0.29		
	Left atrium	<0.01	1.70	0.07°		
	Right ventricle	0.13	3.14	0.08		
	Left ventricle	0.07	1.85	0.03		
	Whole heart	0.15	1.20	0.04	A.F.	ANTON and SAYRE, 1964
Citellus tridecem-lineatus (Ground squirrel)	Whole heart: active:	0.12	1.29	—	R.A.F.	DRASKÓCZY and LYMAN, 1967
	Whole heart: hibernating	0.05	1.00	—		
Ondatra zibethica (European muskrat)	Whole heart (acclimatized animal)	0.21	0.12	—	A.F.	VAN DEN BRUEL et al., 1967
Rattus norvegicus (rat)	Whole heart	0.04	0.72	0	PC.C.B.	GOODALL, 1951
	Whole heart	0.02	0.65	—	A.C.B.	HÖKFELT, 1951
	Whole heart	0.16	0.53	—	A.F.B.	MONTAGU, 1956a
	Right atrium	—	1.49	—	PC.B.	MUSCHOLL, 1959
	Left atrium	—	1.14	—		
	Right ventricle	—	0.70	—		
	Left ventricle	—	0.40	—		
	Whole heart	0.05	0.27	0.03	A.F.	ANTON and SAYRE, 1964
	Auricle	—	3.65	—	S.A.F.	CHANG and SU, 1967
	Ventricle	—	1.66	—		
	Whole heart	—	0.67	—	A.F.	DE SCHRYVER et al., 1969
	Whole heart	—	0.86	—	E_2	NIKODIJEVIC et al., 1969
	Atria + right ventricle	—	1.1—1.8***	—	R.F.	BORCHARD and VOGT, 1970
Mus musculus (mouse)	Whole heart	—	0.55	—	R.F.	SHARMAN et al., 1962
	Whole heart	0.03*	0.4; 0.8**	0.01*	R.F.	LAVERTY et al., 1965
	Whole heart	—	0.9	—	E_2	NIKODIJEVIC et al., 1969
Cavia porcellus (guinea-pig)	Right atrium	0.23	4.11	—	PC.B.	MUSCHOLL, 1959
	Left atrium	0.14	2.73	—		
	Right ventricle	0.09	1.57	—		
	Left ventricle	0.06	1.30	—		
	Right atrium	0.99	4.63	1.39	A.F.	ANGELAKOS et al., 1963
	Left atrium	<0.01	3.11	0.68		
	Right ventricle	0.31	2.21	0.08		
	Left ventricle	0.25	1.96	0.06		
	Whole heart	0.20	1.80	0.06	A.F.	ANTON and SAYRE, 1964
	Right ventricle	—	2.15	—	A.F.	SPANN et al., 1964
	Left ventricle	—	1.82	—		
	Whole heart	—	2.14	—	E_2	NIKODIJEVIC et al., 1969
Canis familiaris (dog)	Right atrium + right auricle	—	2.70	—	S.F.	SHORE et al., 1958
	Right ventricle + apex + papillary muscle	—	1.40	—		
	Atrio-ventricular node	—	1.40	—		
	Left ventricle + papillary muscle	—	1.70	—		
	Tricuspidal valve	—	0.1	—		
	Semilunar valve	—	not detected	—		
	Mitral valve	—	not detected	—		

Table 28. (continued)

Species	Heart tissue	adrenaline µg/g	Nor-adrenaline µg/g	Dop-amine µg/g	Method	Reference
	Right atrium	<0.04	1.51	0.78	R.F.	MIYAHARA, 1962
	Left atrium	<0.04	1.05	0.68		
	Right ventricle	<0.04	1.01	0.44		
	Left ventricle	<0.04	0.86	0.43		
	Atria	0.24	2.98	—	S.F.	FRIEDMAN and BHAGAT, 1962
	Ventricles	0.14	1.09	—		
	Right atrium	—	1.96	—	A.F.	KLOUDA, 1963
	Left atrium	—	1.13	—		
	Right ventricle	—	0.80	—		
	Left ventricle	—	0.62	—		
	Ventricular septum	—	0.67	—		
	Whole heart	—	—	<0.06	A.F.	WEGMANN, 1963
	Whole heart	0.11	1.01	0.05	A.F.	ANTON and SAYRE, 1964
	Sino-arterial node (SAN)	0.09	1.94	—	A.F.	SHINDLER et al., 1968
	Right atrium without SAN	0.08	1.38	—		
	Sino-atrial node	—	1.80	2.0	A.F.	ANGELAKOS et al., 1969
Felis catus (cat)	Right atrium	0.048	1.24	—	PC.B.	MUSCHOLL, 1959
	Left atrium	0.031	0.61	—		
	Atrial septum	—	0.81	—		
	Right ventricle	0.035	1.15	—		
	Left ventricle	0.029	0.88	—		
	Ventricular septum	—	0.76	—		
	Apex	—	0.57	—		
	Papillary muscle from left ventricle	—	0.60	—		
	Right atrium	—	1.50	—	A.F.	HERTTING and SCHIEFTHALER, 1964
	Left atrium	—	1.20	—		
	Atrial septum	—	1.45	—		
	Right ventricle	—	1.55	—		
	Left ventricle	—	1.60	—		
	Ventricular septum	—	1.40	—		
	Whole heart	0.06	0.44	0.07	A.F.	ANTON and SAYRE, 1964
	Whole heart	—	2.08	—	R.F.	THOENEN et al., 1967
Ovis aries (sheep)	Whole heart	0.15	0.79	identified	PC. B.	GOODALL, 1951
	Whole heart	—	1.00	0.3	R.F.	CARLSSON, 1959
	Whole heart	—	1.00	0.3	R.F.	BERTLER et al. 1959
	Whole heart	0.17	1.05	—	A.F.	ANTON and SAYRE, 1962
Capra hircus (goat)	Whole heart	—	1.4	0.5	R.F.	CARLSSON, 1959
	Whole heart	—	1.4; 1.4	0.5; 0.7	R.F.	BERTLER et al., 1959
Bos taurus (cattle)	Auricle	0.028	0.29	—	PC. B.	GOODALL, 1951
	Ventricle	0.059	0.22	—		
	Whole heart	—	1.0	1.5	R.F.	CARLSSON, 1959
	Whole heart	—	1.0	1.5	R.F.	BERTLER et al., 1959
	Pericardium (visceral)	—	0.1	0.7		
Saimiri sciureus (squirrel monkey)	Right atrium	—	1.4	—	S.F.	ORDY et al., 1966
	Left atrium	—	0.6	—		
	Right ventricle	—	1.3	—		
	Left ventricle	—	0.9	—		
Homo sapiens (man)	Whole heart	0.18	1.04	—	A.F.	ANTON and SAYRE, 1962

* of this order; ** 2 different strains; *** noradrenaline concentration increases with age; ∅ in 1 out of 3; ° in 1 out of 2.

Table 29. *Catecholamines in the Lung*

Species	Noradrenaline µg/g	Dopamine µg/g
Oryctolagus cuniculus, Rabbit	0.0[3]; 0.08[5]; 0.18[6]	0.2[3]; 0.30[6]
Rattus norvegicus, Rat	0.1[3]; 0.18[6]	0.0[3]; 0.18[6]
Mus musculus, Mouse	0.11[6]	0.15[6]
Cavia porcellus, Guinea-pig	0.2[3]; 0.16[6]	0.22[6]
Canis familiaris, Dog	0.1[3]; 0.01, 0.028[2]; 0.35[6]	0.0[3]; 0.2, 0.4[2]; 0.24[6]
Felis catus, Cat	0.3[3]; 0.47[6]	0.0[3]; 0.44[6]
Sus scrofa, Pig	0.1[3]	0.0[3]
Capra hircus, Goat	0.1[3]; 0.39[6]	5.3[3]; 6.45[6]
Ovis aries, Sheep	0.1[3]; 0.0—0.1[4]; 0.09[2]	6.9[3]; 3.6—9.8[4]; 24.2[3]
Bos taurus, Cattle	0.1[3]; 0.0—0.1[4] 0.01—0.04[1]; 0.014[2]	9.5[3]; 3.5—15[4]; 1.0[1]; 1.1[2]
Homo sapiens, Man	0.14[6]	0.59[6]

Reference	Method
[1] VON EULER and LISHAJKO, 1957	A.CC.F.B.
[2] SCHÜMANN, 1958	A.C.F.
[3] CARLSSON, 1959	R.F.
[4] BERTLER et al., 1959	R.F.
[5] SHORE, 1959	S.F.
[6] AVIADO and SADAVONGVIVAD 1970	S.F.

Table 30. *Catecholamines in the Mammalian Kidney*

Species	Tissue	Adrenaline µg/g	Nor-adrenaline µg/g	Dop-amine µg/g	Method	Reference
Oryctolagus cuniculus (rabbit)	Whole kidney	—	0.17	—	S.F.	SHORE, 1959
	Whole kidney	0.02	0.16	0.02	A.F.	ANTON and SAYRE, 1964
Rattus norvegicus (rat)	Whole kidney	—	0.25	—	R.PC.F.	DE SCHAEPDRYVER et al., 1963
	Whole kidney	0.03	0.10	0.03	A.F.	ANTON and SAYRE, 1964
Cavia porcellus (guinea-pig)	Whole kidney	0.11	0.44	0.04	A.F.	ANTON and SAYRE, 1964
Canis familiaris (dog)	Whole kidney	—	—	0.11	A.F.	WEGMANN, 1963
	Whole kidney	0.05	0.32	0.03	A.F.	ANTON and SAYRE, 1964
	Subcapsular cortex	—	0.17	—	A.F.	MCKENNA and ANGELAKOS, 1968
	mid cortex	—	0.25	—		
	Juxta medullary cortex	—	0.42	—		
	outer medulla	—	0.39	—		
	inner medulla	—	0.04	—		
	Renal cortex	—	0.50	—	A.F.	NAGATSU et al., 1969
	Renal medulla	—	0.20	—		
Felis catus (cat)	Whole kidney	0.04	0.27	—	A.B.	REHN, 1958
	Whole kidney	0.03	0.29	0.07	A.F.	ANTON and SAYRE, 1964
Ovis aries (sheep)	Whole kidney	0.06	0.50	—	A.B.	v. EULER and PURKHOLD, 1951

Table 31. *Catecholamines in the Thyroid Gland*

	Adrenaline µg/g	Nor-adrenaline µg/g	Dop-amine µg/g	Method	Reference
Cavia porcellus (guinea-pig)	0.26	0.27	—	A.F.	ANTON and SAYRE, 1962
Ovis aries (sheep)	—	—	0.13	R.F.	FALCK et al., 1964a
	—	0.37	4.51	R.F.	JAIM-ETCHEVERRY and ZIEHER, 1968
Homo sapiens (man)	0.04	0.27	—	A.F.	ANTON and SAYRE, 1962

Table 32. *Catecholamines in Male Sex Organs* (Concentrations in μg/g tissue)

Species	Prostate			Vas deferens		Seminal vesicle			Epididymis			Testis		Method	Ref.
	Part	A	N	A	N	Part	A	N	Part	A	N	A	N		
Erinaceus europaeus (hedgehog)	Whole gland	0.13*	0.79	0	8.7		—	—		—	—	—	—	A.F.	1
Oryctolagus cuniculus (rabit)	Whole gland	0	2.2	0	6.7	+ coagulating gland	—	3.2		—	—	—	—	A.F.	2
		—	—	0.22	6.9		—	—	Caput	<0.05	0.23	<0.05	0.04	A.F.	3
									Cauda	0.17	3.41				
Rattus norvegicus (rat)	+ ampullary gland	0	1.57	0	7.9	+ coagulating gland	0	1.26		—	—	—	—	A.F.	4
	+ ampullary gland	0	1.60	0	15.4	+ coagulating gland	0	1.80		—	—	—	—	A.F.	5
		—	—	0.05	9.7		—	—	Caput	<0.05	0.08	<0.05	0.03	A.F.	6
									Cauda	0.07	0.54				
		—	—	—	8.9		—	—		—	—	—	—	E_1	7
Mus musculus (mouse)		—	—	0	5.4		—	0.99		—	—	—	—	A.F.	8
Cavia porcellus (guinea-pig)	+ coagulating gland	0	0.40	0	10.0		0	4.3		—	—	—	—	A.F.	9
		—	—	—	10.0		—	3.7		—	—	—	—	A.F.	10
		—	—	0.3	12.8		—	—	Caput	0.38	0.25	<0.05	0.02	A.F.	11
									Cauda	0.37	3.07				
		—	—	0	10.7		—	—		—	—	—	—	S.A.F.	12
		—	—	—	9.1		—	—		—	—	—	—	E_1	13
Canis familiaris (dog)	+ coagulating gland	0.31**	0.05 to 4.0	—	1.16		—	—		—	—	—	—	A.F.	14

Table 32. (continued)

Species	Prostate			Vas deferens		Seminale vesicle			Epididymis			Testis		Method	Ref.
	Part	A	N	A	N	Part	A	N	Part	A	N	A	N		
Alopex lagopus (arctic fox)	Whole gland	0	1.46	—	1.15		—	—		—	—	—	—	A.F.	15
Felis catus (cat)	+ coagulating gland	0	4.2	0	4.4		—	—		—	—	—	—	A.F.	16
		—	—	0.12	6.7		—	—	Caput	<0.05	1.14	<0.05	0.21	A.F.	17
									Cauda	0.07	1.15				
Sus scrofa (boar)	body	0	0.84	0	6.7		0	1.06		—	—	—	—	A.F.	18
Bos taurus (bull)	body	0	8.8	0	9.3		0	10.70		—	—	—	—	A.F.	19
Ovis aries (ram)	Whole gland	0	0.56	0	10.3		0	8.9		—	—	—	—	A.F.	20
Macaca irus (monkey)	Cranial	2.7—7.3	4.7	0.9—21.9	16.6		1.5	3.8							
	Caudal	29.9—212	35.5							—	—	—	—	A.F.	21
Homo sapiens (man)		—	—	—	—		—	—		—	—	0.12	0.54	A.F.	22
		—	—	0	1.18		—	—		—	—	—	—	A.F.	23
	(Hyperplastic)	0	0.15	0	1.43		—	—	Caput + Corpus	—	0.84	—	0.07	R.F.	24
									Cauda	—	1.04				

* present in 1 out of 3 samples
** present in 1 out of 6 samples

Reference: 1. SJÖSTRAND, 1965b; 2. SJÖSTRAND, 1965b; 3. ELIASSON and RISLEY, 1968; 4. SJÖSTRAND, 1965b; 5. SJÖSTRAND and SWEDIN, 1967; 6. ELIASSON and RISLEY, 1968; 7. IVERSEN and JARROTT, 1970; 8. SJÖSTRAND, 1965b; 9. SJÖSTRAND, 1965b; 10. RYD and SJÖSTRAND, 1967; 11. ELIASSON and RISLEY, 1968; 12. PALAIC and PANISSET, 1969; 13. IVERSEN and JARROTT, 1970; 14. SJÖSTRAND, 1965b; 15. SJÖSTRAND, 1965b; 16. SJÖSTRAND, 1965b; 17. ELIASSON and RISLEY, 1968; 18. SJÖSTRAND, 1965b; 19. SJÖSTRAND, 1965b; 20. SJÖSTRAND, 1965b; 21. SJÖSTRAND, 1965b; 22. ANTON and SAYRE, 1962; 23. SJÖSTRAND, 1965b; 24. BAUMGARTEN et al., 1968.

Table 33. *Catecholamines in the Penis*

Species	Tissue	Adrenaline μg/g	Noradrenaline μg/g	Dopamine μg/g	Method	Reference
Oryctolagus cuniculus (rabbit)	Corpus cavernosum penis	0.04	0.28	—	R.F.	PENTTILA, 1966
	Corpus cavernosum urethrae	0.17	1.15	—		
Bos taurus (bull)	Corpus cavernosum penis:					
	Middle part	0.01	0.01	0.36		
	Proximal part	0.03	0.01	0.50		
	Corpus cavernosum urethrae:					
	Glans penis	0.02	0.01	0.44		
	Pars spongiosa	0.03	0.03	0.32		
	Musculus retractor penis:					
	Proximal portion	0.02	3.80	0.37	R.F.PC.	KLINGE, 1970
	Middle portion	0.02	3.70	0.34		
	Distal portion	0.01	1.90	0.20		

Table 34. *Catecholamines in the Female Reproductive Tract*

Species	Organ	Catecholamine μg/g Adrenaline	Catecholamine μg/g Noradrenal.	Catecholamine (μg/pair) Adrenaline	Catecholamine (μg/pair) Noradrenal.	Method	Ref.
Oryctolagus cuniculus (rabbit)	Uterus	0.13**	0.23**	—	—	S.F.	1
	Uterus	<0.01	1.08	—	—	A.F.	2
	Uterus	—	—	—	0.75	R.F.	3
	Ovary	—	—	—	0.04		
	Oviduct	—	—	—	0.3		
	Vagina	—	—	—	0.5		
Rattus norvegicus (rat)	Uterus	—	—	<0.01*, 0.2**	0.11*, 0.11**	R.S.	4
	Uterus	—	—	0.04*, 0.09**	—	S.F.	5
	Uterus	0.04*, 0.1**	0.33*, 0.66**	—	—	S.F.	6
	Uterus	<0.01	0.25	—	—	A.F.	7
	Uterus (ovariectomised)	0.13	0.23	—	—	S.F.	8
	Ovary	0.05	0.20	—	—	A.F.	9
Cavia porcellus (guinea-pig)	Uterus	<0.01	0.65	—	—	A.F.	10
	Uterus	—	0.75	—	0.52	R.F.	11
	Ovary	0.15	0.74	—	—	A.F.	12
Felis catus (cat)	Uterus	<0.01	1.71	—	—	A.F.	13
Homo sapiens (woman)	Uterus	0.13	0.08	—	—	S.F.	14
	Uterus:						
	fundus	—	0.12	—	—	R.F.	15
	corpus	—	0.16	—	—		
	cervix	—	0.45	—	—		
	Ovary	—	0.86	—	—		
	Oviduct:						
	ampulla	—	0.34	—	—		
	isthmus	—	0.49	—	—		
	intramural	—	0.33	—	—		

* dioestrus; ** oestrus.

References: 1. CHA et al., 1965; 2. GUTMAN and WEIL-MALHERBE, 1967; 3. ROSENGREN and SJÖBERG, 1968; 4. OSKARSSON, 1960; 5. WURTMAN et al., 1963; 6. CHA et al., 1965; 7. GUTMAN and WEIL-MALHERBE, 1967; 8. GILES and MILLER, 1967; 9. ANTON and SAYRE, 1962; 10. GUTMAN and WEIL-Malherbe, 1967; 11. SJÖBERG, 1968b; 12. ANTON and SAYRE, 1962; 13. GUTMAN and WEIL-Malherbe, 1967; 14. CHA et al., 1965; 15. OWMAN et al., 1967.

Table 35. *Catecholamines in the Gastro-Intestinal Tract*

Species	Organ	Adrenaline µg/g	Noradrenaline µg/g	Dopamine µg/g	Method	Reference
Oryctolagus cuniculus (rabbit)	Gastric mucosa	—	0.19	—	S.F.	SHORE, 1959
	Small intestine	—	0.30	—		
	Ileum	—	0.41	0.12	S.F., R.F.	COLLINS and WEST, 1968
Rattus norvegicus (rat)	Stomach	—	0.36	—	S.F.	BOGDANSKI et al., 1963
	Stomach	—	—	0—0.1	R.F.	HÅKANSON et al., 1967
	Small intestine	—	0.35	—	S.F.	BOGDANSKI et al., 1963
	Duodenum + upper jejunum	—	0.22	—	PC. B.	GÖRÖG and SZPORNY, 1961
	Ileum	—	0.37	0.09	S.F., R.F.	COLLINS and WEST, 1968
	Caecum	<0.1	0.98	<0.1	R.F.	STRANDBERG et al., 1966
	Pyloric antrum	—	0.42	—	S.F.	KLINGMAN et al., 1964
	Duodenum and proximal jejunum	—	0.61	—		
	Jejunum	—	0.47	—		
	Distal jejunum and most proximal ileum	—	0.37	—		
	Distal ileum	—	0.28	—		
	Caecum	—	0.40	—		
Canis familiaris (dog)	Jejunum: total	—	0.003	0.16	A.PC.F.	SCHÜMANN, 1959
	Jejunum mucosa	—	0.003	0.20		
	Jejunum muscularis	—	—	<0.05		
	Colon: total	—	0.02	0.30		
	Stomach:				R.F.	KAZAROVA and ESAYAN, 1966
	Lesser curvature:					
	muscularis	0.029	0.053	—		
	mucose membrane	0.037	0.213	—		
	Greater curvature:					
	muscularis	0.020	0.097	—		
	mucose membrane	0.021	0.281	—		
Bos taurus (cattle)	Jejunum: total	—	0.04	16.0	A.PC.F.	SCHÜMANN, 1959
	Jejunum mucosa	—	0.05	27.9		
	Jejunum muscularis	—	0.06	6.0		
	Colon: total	—	—	18.3		
	Duodenum: total	—	0.1	4.4	R.F.	BERTLER et al., 1959
Ovis aries (sheep)	Jejunum: total	—	0.01	1.85	A.PC.F.	SCHÜMANN, 1959
	Jejunum mucosa	—	0.007	2.76		
	Jejunum muscularis	—	0.003	1.12		
	Colon: total	—	0.004	4.30		
	Duodenum: total	—	—	4.2	R.F.	BERTLER et al., 1959
Capra hircus (goat)	Third stomach	—	0.1	0.2	R.F.	BERTLER et al., 1959
	Duodenum: total	—	0.2, 0.4	6.3, 2.1		
	Jejunum: total	—	0.2, 0.2	4.0, 2.0		
	Colon: total	—	0.2, 0.2	2.5, 1.9		

Table 36. *Catecholamines in the Liver*

Species	Tissue	Adrenaline µg/g	Noradrenaline µg/g	Dopamine µg/g	Method	Reference
Oryctolagus cuniculus (rabbit)	Whole liver	—	0.11	—	S.F.	SHORE, 1959
	Whole liver	0.01	0.08	0.02	A.F.	ANTON and SAYRE, 1964
Rattus norvegicus (rat)	Whole liver	0.002	0.06	—	A.F., B.	HÖKFELT, 1951
	Whole liver	0.02	0.08	—	A.F.,PC.,B.	MONTAGU, 1956a
	Whole liver	0.004	0.04	—	A.F.	LEDUC, 1961
	Whole liver	—	0.10	—	A., PC., F.,	DE SCHAEPDRYVER et al., 1963
	Whole liver	0.01	0.02	0.03	A.F.	ANTON and SAYRE, 1964
Canis familiaris (dog)	Whole liver	—	—	<0.06	A.F.	WEGMAN, 1963
	Whole liver	0.07	0.25	0.02	A.F.	ANTON and SAYRE, 1964
Felis catus (cat)	Whole liver	0.02	0.27	0.07	A.F.	ANTON and SAYRE, 1964
Bos taurus (cattle)	Whole liver	—	0.1, 0.0	2.5, 2.5*	R.F.	BERTLER et al., 1959
	Capsule	—	0.2, 0.1, 0.5	17.0, 7.0, 7.8*		
	Parenchyma	—	0.3, 0.1	1.75, 0.55*		
	Whole liver	—	—	1.5*	A.PC., F.	SCHÜMANN, 1959
Ovis aries (sheep)	Whole liver	0.08	0.33	—	A.B.	v. EULER and PURKHOLD, 1951
	Whole liver	—	—	0.4*	A.PC., F.	SCHÜMANN, 1959
	Whole liver	—	0.2	0.3*	R.F.	BERTLER et al., 1959
	Capsule	—	0.4	1.4*		
	Parenchyma	—	0.2	0.1*		
Capra hircus (goat)	Capsule	—	0.2, 0.5	1.6, 7.3*	R.F.	BERTLER et al., 1959
	Parenchyma	—	0.1, 0.1	1.6, 1.6*		

* MAST CELLS PRESENT

Table 38. *Catecholamines in Salivary Glands*

Species	Gland	Adrenaline µg/g	Nor-adrenaline µg/g	Dop-amine µg/g	Method	Reference
Rattus norvegicus (rat)	Submaxillary	—	1.33	—	A.F.	BENMILOUD, 1963
		0.05	0.95	—	A., B.	v. EULER and RYD, 1963
		—	1.60	—	R.F.	ANDÉN et al., 1966b
		—	0.22	—	R.F.	JONASON, 1969
		—	2.1	—	E_1	IVERSEN and JARROTT, 1970
Canis familiaris (dog)	Submaxillary	—	1.21	—	R.F.	FUJIWARA et al., 1966
	Parotid	—	0.85	—		
	Sublingual	—	0.20	—		
Felis catus (cat)	Salivary glands (unspecified)	—	1.40	—	A.B.	v. EULER, 1956
	Submaxillary	0.01	0.73	—	R.F.	STRÖMBLAD, 1960
Bos taurus (cattle)	Salivary glands (unspecified)	—	0.4—2.2	—	A.B.	v. EULER, 1956
	Parotid	—	—	0.41	A.PC.F.C.	SCHÜMANN, 1959
Ovis aries (sheep)	Submaxillary	0.1—0.3	0.4—1.2	—	A.B.	v. EULER and PURKHOLD, 1951
	Parotid	0.03—0.19	0.48—2.2	—		

Table 37. *Catecholamines in the Spleen*

Species		Adrenaline µg/g	Noradrenaline µg/g	Dopamine µg/g	Method	Reference
Oryctolagus cuniculus (rabbit)		—	0.69	—	S.F.	Shore, 1959
		0.04	1.01	0.04	A.F.	Anton and Sayre, 1964
Rattus norvegicus (rat)		0.009	0.43	—	A.B.	Hökfelt, 1951
		0.032	0.51	—	A.F.	Leduc, 1961
		—	1.1	—	S.F.	Levi-Montalcini and Angeletti, 1962
		—	0.73	—	A.F.	Benmiloud, 1963
		0.070	0.47	0.02	A.F.	Anton and Sayre, 1964
		0	0.40	—	A.F.	Iwata et al., 1968
Ondatra zibethica (European muskrat)		0.72	0.53	—	A.F.	van den Bruel et al., 1967
Mus musculus (mouse)		—	0.50	—	S.F.	Levi-Montalcini and Angeletti, 1962
		0.04	0.23	—	A.F.	Anton and Sayre, 1962
Cavia porcellus (guinea-pig)		0.06	0.86	0.05	A.F.	Anton and Sayre, 1964
		—	0.4	—	B.	Bacq and Fischer, 1947
Canis familiaris (dog)		—	—	0.24	A.F.	Wegmann, 1963
		0.05	1.31	0.03	A.F.	Anton and Sayre, 1964
		—	2.10	—	A.F.	Nagatsu et al., 1969
Felis catus (cat)		0.04	0.83	—	A.B.	Rehn, 1958
		0.27	2.10	0.12	A.F.	Anton and Sayre, 1964
		—	4.32	—	R.F.	Thoenen et al., 1967
Bos taurus (cattle)	Whole spleen	—	1.0	0.8	R.F.	Bertler et al., 1959
	Spleen capsule	—	0.7, 0.2	0.4, 0.6		
Capra hircus (goat)		—	4.6, 6.8	1.0, 1.0	R.F.	Bertler et al., 1959
Ovis aries (sheep)		0.01	3.5	—	A.B.	v. Euler and Purkhold, 1951
		—	—	0.4*	A.PC.F.	Schümann, 1959
		—	1.9	0.9	R.F.	Bertler et al., 1959
Homo sapiens (man)		0.02	0.08	—	A.F.	Anton and Sayre, 1962

* Dopamine was 35% of the total catecholamines.

Table 39. *Catecholamines in the Pancreas*

Species		Noradrenaline µg/g	Dopamine µg/g	Method	Reference
Cavia porcellus (guinea-pig)					
Newborn:	albino	0.39	0.11	R.F.	CEGRELL and FALCK, 1968
	pigmented	0.41	1.74		
1 week old:	pigmented	0.36	0.41		
1 month old:	pigmented	0.22	0.01		
adult:	pigmented	0.43	0.03		
Sus scrofa (pig)					
8—10 weeks		0.18	0.27	R.F.	CEGRELL et al., 1968
5 months		0.31	0.47		
Bos taurus (cattle)		—	0.20	A.PC.F.	SCHÜMANN, 1959
Ovis aries (sheep)		—	0.62		
Homo sapiens (human fetus, 21—23 weeks gestation)		0.42	<0.01	R.F.	CEGRELL, 1968

Table 40. *Catecholamines in Blood Vessel Walls*

Species	Vessel	Adrenaline µg/g	Noradrenaline µg/g	Method	Ref.
Oryctolagus cuniculus (rabbit)	Aorta	—	0.24	B.	1
	Central artery of the ear	0.08	0.90	A.F.	2
	Aorta:			R.F.	3
	Media + intima	—	0.25		
	Adventitia	—	0.79		
	Total	—	0.53		
Cavia porcellus (guinea-pig)	Aorta	0.32	—	F.	4
Canis familiaris (dog)	Lung vessels:			A.B.PC.	5
	Arteries	0.02	0.63		
	Veins	0.02	0.44		
	Thoracic aorta	—	0.43		
	Femoral artery	—	0.55		
	Mesenteric artery	—	0.51		
	Portal vein	—	0.45		—
	Mesenteric vein	—	0.42		
	Aortic arch	—	1.3	S.F.	6
	Pulmonary artery	—	1.1		
	Superior vena vaca	—	not detected		
	Femoral artery	0.04	0.47	A.F.	7
	Carotid artery	0.06	1.11		
	Renal artery	0.07	1.45		
	Coeliac artery	0.08	1.44		
	Abdominal aorta	0.09	1.37		
	Superior mesenteric vascular tree:			A.F.	8
	Small arteries	—	5.1		
	Small veins	—	4.7		
	Superior mesenteric artery: trunk	—	2.0		
	Superior mesenteric vein: trunk	—	2.0		

Table 40 (continued)

Species	Vessel	Adrenaline µg/g	Noradrenaline µg/g	Method	Ref.
Canis familiaris (dog)	Aorta	—	1.6		
	Renal artery	—	1.8		
	Carotid artery	—	1.6		
	Femoral artery	—	0.9		
	Pulmonary artery	—	1.0		
	Saphenous artery:				
	Fibular branch	—	2.0		
	Plantar branch	—	2.5		
	Artery in rectus abdominus	—	not detected		
Bos taurus (cattle)	Splenic arteries	0.04	0.36	A.B.PC.	9
	Splenic veins	0.01	0.36		
	Lung vessels (∅ >2 mm)				
	Arteries	0.02	0.35		
	Veins	0.02	0.27		

References: 1. MACMILLAN and RAND, 1962; 2. DE LA LANDE and HEAD, 1967; 3. MAXWELL et al., 1968; 4. POLIKARPOVA, 1961; 5. V. EULER and LISHAJKO, 1958; 6. SHORE et al., 1958; 7. FAREDIN et al., 1961; 8. GENEST et al., 1969; 9. V. EULER and LISHAJKO, 1958.

Table 41. *Catecholamines in the Carotid Body*

Species	Adrenaline µg/g	Noradrenaline µg/g	Dopamine µg/g	Method	Reference
Oryctolagus cuniculus (rabbit)	—	1.51	20—40	R.F.	DEARNALEY et al., 1968
Felis catus (cat)	0.008—0.020 µg/body	0.08—0.10 µg/body	0.06—0.20 µg/body	R.F.	CHIOCCHIO et al., 1966
Sus scrofa (pig)	—	0.07—0.81	—	PC. B.	RAHN, 1961
Bos taurus (calf)	<0.002	1—5.1	—	PC. B.	MUSCHOLL et al., 1960
	—	0.86—5.1	—	PC. B.	RAHN, 1961

Table 42. *Noradrenaline Concentrations in Mammalian Adipose Tissue (µg/g)*

Species	Inter-scapular (brown)	Epididymal	Perirenal	Retro-peritoneal	Sub-cutaneous	Omen-tal	Method	Ref.
Citellus tridecemlineatus (ground squirrel)								
active	0.98	—	—	—	—	—	R.A.F.	1
hibernating	0.42	—	—	—	—	—		
Oryctolagus cuniculus (rabbit)	0.19	0.15	—	—	—	—	S.F.	2
	0.19	—	—	—	—	—	S.F.	3
	0.04	0.02	—	—	—	—	A.F.	4
	0.09	—	0.08	0.12	0.01	—	A.F.	5
Rattus norvegicus (rat)								
(Sprague Dawley) .	0.15	0.12	—	—	—	—	S.F.	6
(unspecified). . . .	—	0.12∅	—	—	—	—	S.F.	7
(Sprague-Dawley) .	0.48	—	—	—	—	—	A.F.	8
(Wistar)	1.40	0.042	—	—	—	—	A.F.	9
(Wistar)	—	0.002†	—	—	—	—	S.F.	10
(Sprague-Dawley) .	0.17	0.03	0.03	0.03	—	—	A.F.	11
(Wistar)	0.57	0.05	0.09	—	—	—		
(unspecified). . . .	1.02	—	—	—	—	—	A.F.	12
Mus musculus (mouse)	0.5*	0.06**	—	—	—	—	A.F.	13
	0.77	—	—	—	—	—	A.F.	14

* adrenaline: 0.05 µg/g; ** adrenaline: 0.006 µg/g; ∅: dopamine not detected; † adrenaline: 0.001 µg/g.

Table 42 (continued)

Species	Inter-scapular (brown)	Epididymal	Perirenal	Retro-peritoneal	Sub-cutaneous	Omen-tal	Method	Ref.
Cavia porcellus (guinea-pig)	0.31	0.11	0.56	0.30	—	—	A.F.	15
	0.25	—	—	—	—	—	A.F.	16
Canis familiaris (dog)	—	—	—	—	—	0.12	S.F.	17
Felis catus (cat)	0.18	—	0.7	0.12	0.11	0.11	A.F.	18
Homo sapiens (man)								
♂	—	—	—	—	0.15	—	A.F.	19
♀	—	—	—	—	0.01	—	A.F.	

References: 1. DRASKÓCZY and LYMAN, 1967; 2. PAOLETTI et al., 1961; 3. SMITH et al., 1962; 4. STOCK and WESTERMANN, 1963; 5. SPANO et al., 1967; 6. PAOLETTI et al., 1961; 7. SMITH et al., 1962; 8. WEINER et al., 1962; 9. STOCK and WESTERMANN, 1963; 10. HRŮZA et al., 1966; 11. SPANO et al., 1967; 12. BIECK et al., 1967; 13. SIDMAN et al., 1962; 14. STOCK and WESTERMANN, 1963; 15. STOCK and WESTERMANN, 1963; 16. SPANO et al., 1967; 17. SMITH et al., 1962; 18. SPANO et al., 1967; 19. SPANO et al., 1967.

Table 43. *Catecholamines in Skeletal Muscle*

Species	Muscle	Adrenaline μg/g	Nor-adrenaline μg/g	Dop-amine μg/g	Method	Reference
Rattus norvegicus (rat)	Triceps brachii	0.25*	0.27*	—	A.F.	GOVYRIN, 1965
	Gluteal muscle	—	0.058	—	A.F.	SCHRYVER et al., 1969
Canis familiaris (dog)	Thigh muscle	0.021	0.039	—	B.	RAAB and GIGEE, 1955
	Unspecified	0.006	0.005	—	A.F.	BOYARSKY et al., 1966
Felis catus (cat)	Unspecified	—	0.03	—	A.B.	v. EULER, 1956
	Triceps brachii	0.4*	0.5*	—	A.F.	GOVYRIN, 1965
Bos taurus (cattle)	Unspecified	—	0.04	—	A.B.	v. EULER, 1956
Ovis aries (sheep)	Unspecified	—	0.03—0.07	—	A.B.	v. EULER, 1956
	Abdominal	—	0	0.2, 0.15	R.F.	BERTLER et al., 1959
Capra hircus (goat)	Abdominal	—	0.0, 0.1	0.4, 1.0	R.F.	BERTLER et al., 1959

* These values are μg/g dry wt.

Table 44. *Catecholamines in Urine*

Species		Adrenaline μg/24 hr	Noradrenal. μg/24 hr	Dopamine μg/24 hr	Method	Reference
Rattus norvegicus (rat)	Unhydrolysed urine	0.00—0.66	2.5—4.8	28—62	A.F.	Ranges of means obtained with rats of different weights LEDUC, 1961
	Hydrolysed urine	0.4—0.72	1.12—1.95	—	R.F.	CRAWFORD and LAW, 1958
	Unhydrolysed urine	0.18—0.44	0.73—1.3	—		
Homo sapiens (man)	Hydrolysed urine	2.7—22.4	11.5—63	100—200	A.C.B. A.B.	v. EULER et al., 1951 v. EULER and HELLNER, 1951
	Unhydrolysed urine	0.6—12.6	7.0—58	—	A.B.	KÄRKI, 1956
	Unhydrolysed urine	3.2—31.0	25.4—130.4	26—595	A.F.	DRUJAN et al., 1959
	Unhydrolysed urine	5.2—20.5	3.9—33.9	—	R.F.	SHARMAN, 1960
	Hydrolysed urine Psychiatric patients	7—23	26—112	343—735	AC.PC.F.	Calculated from GOLDSTEIN et al., 1959, assuming a daily excretion of 1.4 g creatinine.

References

Abel, J.J., Crawford, A.C.: On the blood pressure raising constituent of the suprarenal capsule. Bull. Johns Hopk. Hosp. 8, 151—157 (1897).

— DeM. Taveau, R.: On the decomposition products of epinephrin hydrate. J. biol. Chem. **1,** 1—32 (1905).

— Macht, D.I.: Two crystalline pharmacological agents obtained from the tropical toad *Bufo agua*. J. Pharmacol. exp. Ther. **3**, 319—377 (1912).

Adams-Ray, J.: L'hypertonie des veinules de la peau dans les cas d'etat pathologique et chez les individus bien portants. Acta neuroveg. (Wien) **14**, 283—287 (1956).

— Dahlström, A., Fuxe, K., Hillarp, N.-Å.: Mast cells and monoamines. Experientia (Basel) **20**, 80—82 (1964).

Agrawal, H.C., Glisson, S.N., Himwich, W.A.: Developmental changes in monoamines of mouse brain. Int. J. Neuropharmacol. **7**, 97—101 (1968).

Akester, A.R., Mann, S.P.: Adrenergic and cholinergic innervation of the renal portal valve in the domestic fowl. J. Anat. (Lond.) **104**, 241—252 (1969).

Aldrich, T.B.: A preliminary report on the active principle of the suprarenal gland. Amer. J. Physiol. **5**, 457—461 (1901).

Andén, N.-E.: Distribution of monoamines and dihydroxyphenylalanine decarboxylase activity in the spinal cord. Acta physiol. scand. **64**, 197—203 (1965).

— Fuxe, K., Hamberger, B., Hökfelt, T.: A quantitative study on the nigro-neostriatal dopamine neuron system in the rat. Acta physiol. scand. **67**, 306—312 (1966a).

— Henning, M.: Adrenergic nerve function, noradrenaline level and noradrenaline uptake in cat nictitating membrane after reserpine treatment. Acta physiol. scand. **67**, 498—504 (1966).

— Norberg, K.A., Olson, L.: The adrenergic nerves of rat salivary glands after excretory duct ligation. Acta physiol. scand. **66**, 501—506 (1966b).

Anderson, E.G., Holgerson, L.O.: The distribution of 5-hydroxytryptamine and norepinephrine in cat spinal cord. J. Neurochem. **13**, 479—485 (1966).

Angelakos, E.T., Fuxe, K., Torchiana, M.L.: Chemical and histochemical evaluation of the distribution of catecholamines in the rabbit and guinea pig hearts. Acta physiol. scand. **59,** 184—192 (1963).

— Glassman, P.M., Millard, R.W., King, M.: Regional distribution and subcellular localization of catecholamines in the frog heart. Comp. Biochem. Physiol. **15**, 313—324 (1965).

— King, M., Millard, R.W.: Regional distribution of catecholamines in the hearts of various species. Ann. N.Y. Acad. Sci. **156**, 219—240 (1969).

Anton, A.H., Gennaro, J.F.: Norepinephrine and serotonin in the tissues and venoms of two pit vipers. Nature (Lond.) **208**, 1174—1175 (1965).

— Sayre, D.F.: A study of the factors affecting the aluminium oxide — trihydroxyindole procedure for the analysis of catecholamines. J. Pharmacol. exp. Ther. **138**, 360—375 (1962).

— — The distribution of dopamine and dopa in various animals and a method for their determination in diverse biological material. J. Pharmacol. exp. Ther. **145**, 326—336 (1964).

Aprison, M.H., Takahashi, R.: Biochemistry of the avian central nervous system II. 5-hydroxytryptamine, acetylcholine, 3,4-dihydroxyphenylethylamine and norepinephrine in discrete areas of the pigeon brain. J. Neurochem. **12**, 221—230 (1965).

Augustinsson, K.B., Fänge, R., Johnels, A., Östlund, E.: Histological, physiological and biochemical studies on the heart of two cyclostomes, hagfish *(Myxine)* and lamprey *(Lampetra)*. J. Physiol. (Lond.) **131**, 257—276 (1956).

Aviado, D.M., Sadavongvivad, C.: Pharmacological significance of biogenic amines in the lungs: noradrenaline and dopamine. Brit. J. Pharmacol. **38**, 374—385 (1970).

Axelrod, J.: N-Methyladrenaline, a new catecholamine in the adrenal gland. Biochim. biophys. Acta (Amst.) **45**, 614—615 (1960).

Azuma, T., Binia, A., Vischer, M.B.: Adrenergic mechanisms in the bull frog and turtle. Amer. J. Physiol. **209**, 1287—1294 (1965).

Bacq, Z.M., Fischer, P.: Nature de la substance sympâthicomimétique extraite des nerfs ou des tissus des mammifères. Arch. int. Physiol. **55**, 73—91 (1947).

— Lecomte, J.: Composition de la sécrétion des glandes paratoïdes de Bufo arenarum H. après énervation. C. R. Soc. Biol. (Paris) **141**, 861—862 (1947).

Baldwin, B.A., Ingram, D.L., LeBlanc, J.: The effects of environmental temperature and hypothalamic temperature on the excretion of catecholamines in the urine of the pig. Brain Res. **16**, 511—515 (1969).

Banister, R.J., Portig, P.J., Vogt, M.: The content and localization of catecholamines in the carotid labyrinths and aortic arches of *Rana temporaria*. J. Physiol. (Lond.) **192,** 529—535 (1967).

Barchas, J.D., Ciaranello, R.D., Steinman, A.M.: Epinephrine formation in mammalian brain. Biol. Psychiat. **1**, 31—48 (1969).

— Freedman, D.: Response to physiological stress. Biochem. Pharmacol. **12**, 1232—1235 (1963).

Barsoum, G.S., Gaddum, J.H.: The pharmacological estimation of adenosine and histamine in blood. J. Physiol. (Lond.) **85**, 1—14 (1935).

Baumgarten, H.G.: Vorkommen und Verteilung adrenerger Nervenfasern im Darm der Schleie *(Tinca vulgaris cuv.)* Z. Zellforsch. **76**, 248—259 (1967).

— Braak, H.: Catecholamine im Hypothalamus vom Goldfisch *(Carassius auratus)*. Z. Zellforsch. **80**, 246—263 (1967).

— Falck, B., Holstein, A.-F., Owman, Ch., Owman, T.: Adrenergic innervation of the human testis, epididymis, ductus deferens and prostate: A fluorescence microscopic and fluorimetric study. Z. Zellforsch. **90**, 81—95 (1968).

— Holstein, A.-F.: Adrenerge Innervation im Hoden und Nebenhoden vom Schwan *(Cygnus olor)*. Z. Zellforsch. **91**, 402—410 (1968).

Beauvallet, M., Fugazza, J., Solier, M.: Sur les variations du taux de la noradrénaline dans le tissue cérébral du rat en fonction de l'age et du sexe. J. Physiol. (Paris) **53**, 267—268 (1961).

— — — Nouvelles recherches sur les variations saisonnières de la noradrénaline cérébrale. J. Physiol. (Paris) **54**, 289—290 (1962).

Bell, C.: Indirect cholinergic vasomotor control of intestinal blood flow in the domestic chicken. J. Physiol. (Lond.) **205**, 317—327 (1969).

Benmiloud, M.: The bretylium-like effect of guanethidine. Life Sci. **1**, 9—15 (1963).

Bernheimer, H.: Über das Vorkommen von Katecholaminen und von 3,4-dihydroxyphenylalanin *(DOPA)* im Auge. Naunyn-Schmiedeberg's Arch. exp. Path. Pharmak. **247**, 202 to 213 (1964).

Bertler, Å.: Occurrence and localization of catecholamines in the human brain. Acta physiol. scand. **51**, 97—107 (1961).

— Carlsson, A., Rosengren, E.: A method for the fluorimetric determination of adrenaline and noradrenaline in tissues. Acta physiol. scand. **44**, 273—292 (1958).

— Falck, B., Gottfries, C.G., Ljunggren, L., Rosengren, E.: Some observations on adrenergic connections between mesencephalon and cerebral hemispheres. Acta pharmacol. (Kbh.) **21**, 283—289 (1964).

— — Hillarp, N.-Å., Rosengren, E., Torp, A.: Dopamine and chromaffin cells. Acta physiol. scand. **47**, 251—258 (1959).

— — von Mecklenburg, C.: Mono-aminergic mechanisms in special ependymal areas in the rainbow trout, *Salmo irideus*. Gen. comp. Endocr. **3**, 685—686 (1963).

— — Owman, Ch., Rosengren, E.: The localization of monoaminergic blood-brain barrier mechanisms. Pharmacol. Rev. **18**, 369—385 (1966).

— Hillarp, N.-Å., Rosengren, E.: Some observations on the synthesis and storage of catecholamines in the adrenaline cells of the suprarenal medulla. Acta physiol. scand. **50**, 124—131 (1960).

— Rosengren, E.: Brain catecholamine content after sectioning the adrenergic nerves to the brain vessels. Acta physiol. scand. **47**, 362—364 (1959a).

— — Occurrence and distribution of catecholamines in brain. Acta physiol. scand. **47**, 350—361 (1959b).

Bieck, P., Stock, K., Westermann, E.: Über die Bedeutung des Serotonins im Fettgewebe. Naunyn-Schmiedeberg's Arch. exp. Path. Pharmak. **256**, 218—236 (1967).

Biedl, A., Wiesel, J.: Über die funktionelle Bedeutung der Nebenorgane des Sympathicus (Zuckerkandl) und der chromaffinen Zellgruppen. Pflügers Arch. ges. Physiol. **91**, 434—461 (1902).

Björklund, A., Falck, B., Rosengren, E.: Monoamines in the pituitary gland of the pig. Life Sci. **6**, 2103—2110 (1967).

Bloom, G., Östlund, E., von Euler, U.S., Lishajko, F., Ritzén, M., Adams-Ray, J.: Studies on catecholamine containing granules of specific cells in cyclostome hearts. Acta physiol. scand. Suppl. 185 (1961).

Boehlke, K.W., Tiemeier, O.W., Eleftheriou, B.E.: Diurnalrhythm in plasma epinephrine and norepinephrine in the channel catfish *(Ictalurus punctatus)*. Gen. comp. Endocr. **8**, 189—192 (1967).

Bogdanski, D.F., Bonomi, L., Brodie, B.B.: Occurrence of serotonin and catecholamines in brain and peripheral organs of various vertebrate classes. Life Sci. **2**, 80—84 (1963).

Borchard, F., Vogt, M.: Noradrenaline content of the heart of the adrenal demedullated rat. Brit. J. Pharmacol. **38**, 50—55 (1970).

Born, G.V.R., Hornykiewicz, O., Stafford, A.: The uptake of adrenaline and noradrenaline by blood platelets of the pig. Brit. J. Pharmacol. **13**, 411—414 (1958).

BOUCEK, R.J., BOCKLAGE BOURNE, B.: Catecholamines of the allantoic fluid in the developing chick embryo. Nature (Lond.) **193**, 1181—1182 (1962).
BOYARSKY, S., KIRSHNER, N., LABAY, P.: Catecholamine content of the normal dog ureter. Invest. Urol. **4**, 97—102 (1966).
BRODIE, B.B., BOGDANSKI, D.F., BONOMI, L.: Formation, storage and metabolism of serotonin (5-hydroxytryptamine) and catecholamines in lower vertebrates. In: Comparative Neurochemistry, pp. 367—377. Ed. by D. Richter. Oxford: Pergamon Press 1964.
BROUWER, E., VAN DE VEERDONK, F.C.G.: Identification of a catecholamine in the skin of the toad *Xenopus laevis* and the relation to the physiological melanophore reaction. Experientia (Basel) **25**, 391—392 (1969).
BROWN, G.L., DEARNALEY, D.P., GEFFEN, L.B.: Noradrenaline content of the decentralised spleen. J. Physiol. (Lond.) **187**, 32—34P (1966).
BRUEL, VAN DEN, W., CESSION-FOSSION, A., VANDERMEULEN, R., LECOMTE, J.: Teneur en catecholamine de quelques organes *d'Ondatra zibethica*. C.R. Soc. Biol. (Paris) **161**, 1474—1476 (1967).
BRUNDIN, T.: Studies on the preaortal paraganglia of newborn rabbits. Acta physiol. scand. **70**, Suppl. 290 (1966).
— HAMBERGER, B., NORBERG, K.-A.: Postnatal changes in the preaortal paraganglia of rabbits. Acta physiol. scand. **66**, 255—256 (1966).
BURN, J.H., LANGEMANN, H., PARKER, R.H.O.: Noradrenaline in whale suprarenal medulla. J. Physiol. (Lond.) **113**, 123—128 (1951).
BURNSTOCK, G.: Evolution of the autonomic innervation of visceral and cardiovascular systems in vertebrates. Pharmacol. Rev. **21**, 247—324 (1969).
BUTTERWORTH, K.R., MANN, M.: Proportion of noradrenaline to adrenaline in the adrenal glands of litter mate cats. Nature (Lond.) **187**, 785 (1960).
— — A quantitative comparison of the sympathomimetic amine content of the left and right adrenal gland of the cat. J. Physiol. (Lond.) **162**, 473—484 (1962).
CALDEYRO, R., PATETTA, M.A.: Diminished adrenaline concentration in the parotid secretion of Bufo arenarum H. after sympathetic enervation. Arch. Soc. Biol. Montevideo **13**, 1—6 (1946). Cited from Chem. Abstr. **41**, 2495 (1947).
CALLINGHAM, B.A.: The catecholamines. Adrenaline; Noradrenaline. Hormones in Blood. 2nd Ed. Vol. **2**. London, New York: Academic Press 1968.
— CASS, R.: Catecholamines in the chick. Physiology of the domestic fowl, pp. 279—285. Ed. by C. Horton-Smith and E.C. Amoroso. Edinburgh: Oliver and Boyd Ltd. 1966.
— SHARMAN, D.F.: The concentration of catecholamines in the brain of the domestic fowl *(Gallus domesticus)*. Brit. J. Pharmacol. **40**, 1—5 (1970).
CARLSSON, A.: The occurrence, distribution and physiological role of catecholamines in the nervous system. Pharmacol. Rev. **11**, 490—493 (1959).
— LINDQVIST, M.: *In vivo* decarboxylation of a-methyl DOPA and a-methylmetatyrosine. Acta physiol. scand. **54**, 87—94 (1962).
CASTON, J.D.: Appearance of catecholamines during development of *Rana pipiens*. Develop. Biol. **5**, 468—482 (1962).
CEGRELL, L.: The occurrence of biogenic monoamines in the mammalian endocrine pancreas. Acta physiol. scand. Suppl. 314, 1—7 (1968).
— FALCK, B.: The development of monoamine containing cells in guinea-pig pancreas. Acta physiol. scand. Suppl. 314, 24—34 (1968).
— — HELLMAN, B.: Monoaminergic mechanisms in the endocrine pancreas. The structure and metabolism of the pancreatic islets. Proc. 3rd intern. symp. Uppsala, Stockholm, 1964, pp. 429—435. Ed. by S.E. Brodin et al.
— — ROSENGREN, A.M.: Catechol derivatives in the skin of young mice. Acta Univ. Lund. Sect. II. No. 30, 1—5 (1967).
— — — Extraction of DOPA from the integument of pigmented animals. Acta physiol. scand. **78**, 65—69 (1970).
— — ROSENGREN, E.: Monoamines in the pig pancreas with special reference to the endocrine part. Acta physiol. scand. Suppl. 314, 8—13 (1968).
CESSION-FOSSION, A., VANDERMEULEN, R.: Teneur de catecholamines de la medullosurrenale du lapereau. C.R. Soc. Biol. (Paris) **157**, 1845—1846 (1963).
CHA, K.-S., LEE, W.-C., RUDZIK, A., MILLER, J.W.: A comparison of catecholamine concentrations of uteri from several species and the alterations which occur during pregnancy. J. Pharmacol. exp. Ther. **148**, 9—13 (1965).
CHANG, C.-C.: A sensitive method for spectrophotofluorometric assay of catecholamines. Int. J. Neuropharmacol. **3**, 643—649 (1964).
— SU, C.Y.: Effect of cold stress on the subcellular distribution of noradrenaline in the rat heart. J. Pharm. Pharmacol. **19**, 73—77 (1967).

Chiocchio, S.R., Biscardi, A.M., Tramezzani, J.H.: Catecholamines in the carotid body of the cat. Nature (Lond.) **212**, 834—835 (1966).

Clark, W.G., Drell, W.: Isolation of epinephrine monoglucuronide. Fed. Proc. **13**, 343 (1954).

Clarke, D.D., Wilk, S., Gitlow, S.E., Franklin, M.J.: Gas chromatographic determination of dopamine at the nanogram level. J. Gas Chromatogr. **5**, 307—310 (1967).

Cohen, G., Goldenberg, M.: The simultaneous fluorimetric determination of adrenaline and noradrenaline in plasma — I. J. Neurochem. **2**, 58—70 (1957a).

— — The simultaneous fluorimetric determination of adrenaline and noradrenaline in plasma — II. J. Neurochem. **2**, 71—80 (1957b).

Collins, G.G.S., West, G.W.: Some pharmacological actions of diethyldithiocarbamate on rabbit and rat ileum. Brit. J. Pharmacol. **32**, 402—409 (1968).

Cooper, C.J., de la Lande, I.S., Tyler, M.J.: The catecholamines in lizard heart. Aust. J. exp. Biol. med. Sci. **44**, 205—210 (1966).

Coupland, R.E.: On the morphology and adrenaline-noradrenaline content of chromaffin tissue. J. Endocr. **9**, 194—203 (1953).

Crain, S.M., Wiegand, R.G.: Catecholamine levels of mouse sympathetic ganglia following hypertrophy produced by salivary nerve growth factor. Proc. Soc. exp. Biol. (N.Y.) **107**, 663—665 (1961).

Crawford, T.B.B., Law, W.: The urinary excretion of adrenaline and noradrenaline by rats under various experimental conditions. Brit. J. Pharmacol. **13**, 35—43 (1958).

— Outschoorn, A.S.: The quantitative separation of adrenaline and noradrenaline in biological fluids and tissue extracts. Brit. J. Pharmacol. **6**, 8—19 (1951).

— Yates, C.M.: A method for the estimation of the catecholamines and their metabolites in brain tissue. Brit. J. Pharmacol. **38**, 56—71 (1970).

Cunningham, H.M.: Anabolic response and catecholamine excretion following isocarboxazide administration to pigs. J. Animal. Sci. **26**, 345—351 (1967).

Dahlström, A., Häggendal, J., Hökfelt, T.: The noradrenaline content of varicosities of sympathetic adrenergic nerve terminals in the rat. Acta physiol. scand. **67**, 289—294 (1966).

Dakin, H.D.: The synthesis of a substance allied to adrenalin. Proc. roy. Soc. B. **76**, 491—497 (1905).

Dearnaley, D.P., Fillenz, M., Woods, R.I.: The identification of dopamine in the rabbits carotid body. Proc. roy. Soc. B. **170**, 195—203 (1968).

Dencker, S.J., Häggendal, J., Ilves-Häggendal, M.: Presence of free and conjugated noradrenaline in human cerebrospinal fluid. Acta physiol. scand. **69**, 140—146 (1967).

Dengler, H.: Occurrence of hydroxytyramine in the adrenal. Naunyn-Schmiedeberg's Arch. exp. Path. Pharmak. **231**, 373—377 (1957).

Derry, D.M., Schoenbaum, E., Steiner, G.: Two sympathetic nerve supplies to brown adipose tissue of the rat. Canad. J. Physiol. Pharmacol. **47**, 57—63 (1969).

Doležel, S.: Monoaminergic innervation of the kidney. Aorticorenal ganglion — a sympathetic monoaminergic ganglion supplying the renal vessels. Experientia (Basel) **23**, 109—111 (1967).

— Zlábek, K.: Über einen monoaminergen Mechanismus im Nierenpfortadersystem der Vögel. Z. Zellforsch. **100**, 521—535 (1969).

Donoso, A.O.: Concentration de l'adrénaline et de la noradrénaline dans le plasma de quelques espèces d'oiseaux. Action de divers facteurs. C.R. Soc. Biol. (Paris) **156**, 790—795 (1962).

— Segura, E.T.: Seasonal variations of plasma adrenaline and noradrenaline in toads. Gen. comp. Endocr. **5**, 440—443 (1965).

Draskoćzy, P.R., Lyman, C.P.: The turnover of catecholamines in active and hibernating ground squirrels. J. Pharmacol. exp. Ther. **155**, 101—111 (1967).

Drujan, B.D., Diaz Borges, J.M.: Adrenaline depletion induced by light in the dark adapted retina. Experientia (Basel) **24**, 676—677 (1968).

— — Alvarez, N.: Relationship between the contents of adrenaline, noradrenaline and dopamine in the retina and its adaptational state. Life Sci. **4**, 473—477 (1965).

— Sourkes, T.L., Layne, D.S., Murphy, G.F.: The differential determination of catecholamines in urine. Canad. J. Biochem. **37**, 1153—1159 (1959).

Dunér, H., von Euler, U.S., Pernow, B.: Catecholamines and substance P in the mammalian eye. Acta physiol. scand. **31**, 113—118 (1954).

Eade, N.R.: Differential sedimentation of noradrenaline in homogenates of adrenal medullary granules. J. Physiol. (Lond.) **132**, 53P—54P (1956).

— The distribution of the catecholamines in homogenates of the bovine adrenal medulla. J. Physiol. (Lond.) **141**, 183—192 (1958).

Ehringer, H., Hornykiewicz, O.: Verteilung von Noradrenalin und Dopamin (3-Hydroxytyramin) im Gehirn des Menschen und ihr Verhalten bei Erkrankungen des extrapyramidalen Systems. Klin. Wschr. **38**, 1236—1239 (1960).

ELIASSON, R., RISLEY, P. L.: Adrenergic innervation of the male reproductive organs of some mammals. III. Distributions of noradrenaline and adrenaline. Acta physiol. scand. **73**, 311—319 (1968).

ELLIOTT, T. R.: The control of the suprarenal glands by the splanchnic nerves. J. Physiol. (Lond.) **44**, 374—409 (1912).

— Note on the quantitative estimation of adrenalin. J. Physiol. (Lond.) **46**, 15—17P (1913).

ENEMAR, A., FALCK, B., ITURRIZA, F. C.: Adrenergic nerves in the *pars intermedia* of the pituitary in the toad, *Bufo arenarum*. Z. Zellforsch. **77**, 325—330 (1967).

ERÄNKÖ, O.: On the histochemistry of the rat adrenal medulla. Acta physiol. scand. **25**, Suppl. 89, 22—23 (1951).

— Distribution of fluorescing islets, adrenaline and noradrenaline in the adrenal medulla of the hamster. Acta endocr. (Kbh.) **18**, 174—179 (1955a).

— Distribution of fluorescing islets, adrenaline and noradrenaline in the adrenal medulla of the cat. Acta endocr. (Kbh.) **18**, 180—188 (1955b).

— Distribution of adrenaline and noradrenaline in the hen adrenal gland. Nature (Lond.) **179**, 417—418 (1957).

— RÄISÄNEN, L.: Adrenaline and noradrenaline in the adrenal medulla during postnatal development of the rat. Endocrinology **60**, 753—760 (1956).

ERSPAMER, V.: Isolation of Leptodactyline (m-hydroxyphenylethyltrimethylammonium) from extracts of leptodactylus skin. Arch. Biochem. Biophys. **82**, 431—438 (1959).

— GLÄSSER, A.: The pharmacological actions of (m-hydroxyphenethyl) trimethylammonium (Leptodactyline). Brit. J. Pharmacol. **15**, 14—22 (1960).

— VIALLI, M.: Ricerce preliminari sulle indolalchilamine e sulle fenilalchilamine degli estratti di pelle di anfibio. Ric. Sci. **22**, 1420—1425 (1952).

EULER, U. S., VON: A specific sympathomimetic ergone in adrenergic nerve fibres (sympathin) and its relations to adrenaline and noradrenaline. Acta physiol. scand. **12**, 73—97 (1946).

— Identification of the sympathomimetic ergone in adrenergic nerves of cattle (Sympathin N) with laevo-noradrenaline. Acta physiol. scand. **16**, 63—74 (1948a).

— Assay of noradrenaline and adrenalin in extracts of nerves and tissues. Nature (Lond.) **162**, 570—571 (1948b).

— The distribution of sympathin N and sympathin A in spleen and splenic nerves of cattle. Acta physiol. scand. **19**, 207—214 (1949).

— Presence of catecholamines in visceral organs of fish and invertebrates. Acta physiol. scand. **28**, 297—305 (1953).

— Noradrenaline. Springfield, Ill.: Charles C. Thomas 1956.

— The development and applications of the trihydroxyindole method for catecholamines. Pharmacol. Rev. **11**, 262—268 (1959).

— Occurrence and distribution of catecholamines in fish brain. Acta physiol. scand. **52**, 62—64 (1961).

— In: Comparative Endocrinology. Ed. by VON EULER and HELLER. Vol. 1, Adrenergic Neurohormones, pp. 209—238. New York and London: Academic Press 1963a.

— In: Comparative Endocrinology. Ed. by VON EULER and HELLER. Vol. 2. Chromaffin cell Hormones, pp. 258—290. New York and London: Academic Press 1963b.

— FÄNGE, R.: Catecholamines in nerves and organs of *Myxine glutinosa*, *Squalus acanthias* and *Gadus callarias*. Gen. comp. Endocr. **1**, 191—194 (1961).

— FLODING, I.: A fluorimetric micromethod for differential estimation of adrenaline and noradrenaline. Acta physiol. scand. **33**, Suppl. 118, 45—62 (1955).

— HAMBERG, U.: Colorimetric determination of noradrenaline and adrenaline. Acta physiol. scand. **19**, 74—84 (1949a).

— — L-Noradrenaline in the suprarenal medulla. Nature (Lond.) **163**, 642—643 (1949b).

— — HELLNER, S.: β-(3,4-dihydroxyphenyl) ethylamine (hydroxytyramine) in normal human urine. Biochem. J. **49**, 655—658 (1951).

— HELLNER, S.: Excretion of noradrenaline, adrenaline and hydroxytyramine in urine. Acta physiol. scand. **22**, 161—167 (1951).

— LISHAJKO, F.: Dopamine in mammalian lung and spleen. Acta physiol. pharmacol. neerl. **6**, 295—303 (1957).

— — Catecholamines in the vascular wall. Acta physiol. scand. **42**, 333—341 (1958).

— — Improved technique for the fluorimetric estimation of catecholamines. Acta physiol. scand. **51**, 348—356 (1961).

— — A specific kind of noradrenaline granules in the vesicular gland and the vas deferens of the bull. Life Sci. **5**, 687—691 (1966).

— PURKHOLD, A.: Effect of sympathetic denervation on the noradrenaline and adrenaline content of the spleen, kidney, and salivary glands in the sheep. Acta physiol. scand. **24**, 212—217 (1951).

— RYD, G.: Effect of sympathetic denervation and adrenalectomy on the catecholamine content of the rat submaxillary gland. Acta physiol. scand. **59**, 62—66 (1963).

Everett, S.D., Mann, S.P.: Catecholamine release by histamine from isolated intestine of the chick. Europ. J. Pharmacol. **1**, 310—320 (1967).
Falck, B.: Observations on the possibilities of the cellular localization of monoamines by a fluorescence method. Acta physiol. scand. **56**, Suppl. 197 (1962).
— Häggendal, J., Owman, C.: The localisation of adrenaline in adrenergic nerves in the frog. Quart. J. exp. Physiol. **48**, 253—257 (1963).
— Håkanson, R., Owman, C., Sjöberg, N.-O.: Monoamine storing cells of enterochromaffin type in gastrointestinal tract of human fetus. Acta physiol. scand. **71**, 403—404 (1967).
— Hellman, B.: Evidence for the presence of biogenic amines in pancreatic islets. Experientia (Basel) **19**, 139—140 (1963).
— — A fluorescent reaction for monoamines in the insulin producing cells of the guinea pig. Acta endocr. (Kbh.) **45**, 133—138 (1964).
— Hillarp, N.-Å., Torp, A.: Some observations on the histology and histochemistry of the chromaffin cells probably storing dopamine. J. Histochem. Cytochem. **7**, 323—328 (1959).
— Larson, B., von Mecklenburg, C., Rosengren, E., Svenaeus, K.: On the presence of a second specific cell system in mammalian thyroid gland. Acta physiol. scand. **62**, 491—492 (1964a).
— Ljunggren, L., Nordgren, L.: Diencephalic catecholamines in chick and pigeon. Life Sci. **8**, 889—893 (1969).
— Nystedt, T., Rosengren, E., Stenflo, J.: Dopamine and mast cells in ruminants. Acta pharmacol. (Kbh.) **21**, 51—58 (1964b).
Faredin, I., Benko, A., Winter, M., Botos, A.: Catecholamine content of the arterial walls in experimental hypertension. Experientia (Basel) **17**, 225 (1961).
Fleming, R.M., Clark, W.G., Fenster, E.D., Towne, J.C.: A single extraction method for the simultaneous fluorometric determination of serotonin, dopamine and norepinephrine in brain. Analyt. Chem. **37**, 692—696 (1965).
Foster, M., Brown, S.R.: The production of DOPA by normal pigmented mammalian skin. J. biol. Chem. **225**, 247—252 (1957).
Friedman, A.H., Bhagat, B.: The concentration of catecholamines in the turtle heart and vagal escape. J. Pharm. Pharmacol. **14**, 764 (1962).
— Walker, C.A.: Circadian rhythms in rat mid-brain and caudate nucleus biogenic amine levels. J. Physiol. (Lond.) **197**, 77—85 (1968).
Fromageot, C., Jutisz, M., Lederer, E.: Séparations chromatographiques d'acides aminés et de peptides. IV. Séparation en quatre groupes. Biochim. biophys. Acta (Amst.) **2**, 487—498 (1948).
Fujiwara, M., Tanaka, T., Hiroshi, H., Okegawa, T.: Cytological localization of noradrenaline, monoamine oxidase and acetylcholinesterase in salivary glands of dog. J. Histochem. Cytochem. **14**, 483—494 (1966).
Fulk, M.E., Macleod, J.J.R.: Evidence that the active principle of the retroperitoneal chromophil tissue has the same physiological actions as the active principle of the suprarenal glands. Amer. J. Physiol. **40**, 21—29 (1916).
Fuxe, K., Sedvall, G.: The distribution of adrenergic nerve fibres to the blood vessels in skeletal muscle. Acta physiol. scand. **64**, 75—85 (1965).
Gaddum, J.H.: Bioassay Procedures. Pharmacol. Rev. **11**, 241—249 (1959).
Gannon, B., Burnstock, G.: Excitatory adrenergic innervation of the fish heart. Comp. Biochem. Physiol. **29**, 765—773 (1969).
Genest, J., Simard, S., Rosenthal, J., Boucher, R.: Norepinephrine and renin content in arterial tissue from different vascular beds. Canad. J. Physiol. Pharmacol. **47**, 87—91 (1969).
Gessner, O.: Tierische Gifte. Handb. exp. Pharmak. Erg. **6**, 1—83, Berlin: Springer 1938.
Ghosh, A.: A comparative study of the histochemistry of the avian adrenals. Gen. comp. Endocr. Suppl. **1**, 75—80 (1962).
Giarman, N.J., Day, N.: Presence of biogenic amines in the bovine pineal body. Biochem. Pharmacol. **1**, 235 (1958).
Giles, R.E., Miller, J.W.: The catechol-O-methyl transferase activity and endogenous catecholamine content of various tissues in the rat and the effect of administration of U-0521 (3′,4′-dihydroxy-2-methylpropiophenone). J. Pharmacol. exp. Ther. **158**, 189—194 (1967).
Gillespie, J.S., Kirpekar, S.M.: The histological localization of noradrenaline in the cat spleen. J. Physiol. (Lond.) **187**, 69—79 (1966).
Glowinski, J., Iversen, L.L.: Regional studies of catecholamines in the rat brain — I. The disposition of [^{3}H] norepinephrine, [^{3}H] dopamine and [^{3}H] DOPA in various regions of the brain. J. Neurochem. **13**, 655—669 (1966).
GöröG, P., Szporny, L.: Effect of Vincamin on the noradrenaline content of rat tissue. Biochem. Pharmacol. **8**, 259—262 (1961).

GOLDSTEIN, M., FRIEDHOFF, A.J., SIMMONS, C.: A method for the separation and estimation of catecholamines in urine. Experientia (Basel) **15**, 80—81 (1959).

GOODALL, McC.: Studies of adrenaline and noradrenaline in mammalian heart and suprarenals. Acta physiol. scand. **24**, Suppl. 85 (1951).

GOVYRIN, V.A.: Epinephrine and norepinephrine in skeletal muscle. Fed. Proc. **24**, T 865—867 (1965).

GREEN, R.D., MILLER, J.W.: Catecholamine concentrations: Changes in plasma of rats during estrous cycle and pregnancy. Science **151**, 825—826 (1966).

GROBECKER, H., HOLTZ, P., MÜLLER, H.K.: Die Wirkung von α-Methyldopa und Dopa auf den Brenzcatechinamingehalt des Herzens, der Nebennieren und der Haut des Frosches sowie auf die Melanophoren der Froschhaut. Naunyn-Schmiedeberg's Arch. Pharmak. exp. Path. **255**, 474—490 (1966).

GUNNE, L.-M.: Relative adrenaline content in brain tissue. Acta physiol. scand. **56**, 324—333 (1962).

GUTMAN, Y., WEIL-MALHERBE, H.: Subcellular distribution of norepinephrine in uteri of some species. Nature (Lond.) **214**, 108—109 (1967).

HÄGGENDAL, J.: On the use of strong exchange resins for determinations of small amounts of catecholamines. Scand. J. clin. Lab. Invest. **14**, 537—544 (1962).

— An improved method for fluorimetric determination of small amounts of adrenaline and noradrenaline in plasma and tissues. Acta physiol. scand. **59**, 242—254 (1963a).

— The presence of conjugated adrenaline and noradrenaline in human blood plasma. Acta physiol. scand. **59**, 255—260 (1963b).

— The presence of dopamine in human gastric juice. Acta physiol. scand. **71**, 127—128 (1967).

— MALMFORS, T.: Evidence of dopamine-containing neurons in the retina of rabbits. Acta physiol. scand. **59**, 295—296 (1963).

— — Identification and cellular localisation of the catecholamines in the retina and the choroid of the rabbit. Acta physiol. scand. **64**, 58—66 (1965).

HAGOPIAN, M., DORFMAN, R.I., GUT, M.: A method for the isolation and separation of catecholamines and their transformation products from biological media. Analyt. Biochem. **2**, 387—390 (1961).

HÅKANSON, R., LILYA, B., OWMAN, C.: Properties of a new system of amine storing cells in the gastric mucosa of the rat. Europ. J. Pharmacol. **1**, 188—199 (1967).

— OWMAN, C.: Distribution and properties of amino acid decarboxylase in gastric mucosa. Biochem. Pharmacol. **15**, 489—499 (1966).

— — SJÖBERG, N.-O.: Three different systems of monoamine storing cells in the gastrointestinal tract of fetal and neonatal rats. Acta physiol. scand. **75**, 213—220 (1969).

HARRISON, T.S., SEATON, J.F.: Tissue content of epinephrine and norepinephrine following adrenal medullectomy. Amer. J. Physiol. **210**, 599—600 (1966).

HEBB, C., KASA, P., MANN, S.: The relation between nerve fibres and dopamine cells in the ruminant lung. Histochem. J. **1**, 166—175 (1968).

HEMPEL, K., MÄNNL, H.F.K.: Resting secretion of dopamine from the adrenal glands of the cat *in vivo*. Experientia (Basel) 919—920 (1967).

— — Dopamin, ein neuer Bestandteil des Nebennieren-Inkrets. Naunyn-Schmiedeberg's Arch. exp. Path. Pharmak. **263**, 222 (1969).

HERTTING, G., SCHIEFTHALER, T.: The effect of stellate ganglion excision on the catecholamine content and the uptake of ^{3}H-norepinephrine in the heart of the cat. Int. J. Neuropharmacol. **3**, 65—69 (1964).

HILLARP, N.-Å., HÖKFELT, B.: Evidence of adrenaline and noradrenaline in separate adrenal medullary cells. Acta physiol. scand. **30**, 55—67 (1953).

HÖKFELT, B.: Noradrenaline and adrenaline in mammalian tissues. Acta physiol. scand. **25**, Suppl. 92 (1951).

— McLEAN, J.: The adrenaline and noradrenaline content of the suprarenal glands of the rabbit under normal conditions and after various forms of stimulation. Acta physiol. scand. **21**, 258—270 (1950).

HOLTON, P.: High concentration of nor-adrenaline in calves' suprarenals. Nature (Lond.) **167**, 858—859 (1951).

HOLTZ, P.: Über die sympathicomimetische Wirksamkeit von Gehirnextrakten. Acta physiol. scand. **20**, 354—362 (1950).

— CREDNER, K.: Die enzymatische Entstehung von Oxytyramin im Organismus und die physiologische Bedeutung von Dopadecarboxylase. Naunyn-Schmiedeberg's Arch. exp. Path. Pharmak. **200**, 356—388 (1942).

— — KRONEBERG, G.: Über das sympathomimetische pressorische Prinzip des Harns — („Urosympathin"). Naunyn-Schmiedeberg's Arch. exp. Path. Pharmak. **204**, 228—243 (1947).

— KRONEBERG, G., SCHÜMANN, H.-J.: Über das „Urosympathin" des Tierharns. Naunyn-Schmiedeberg's Arch. exp. Path. Pharmak. **209**, 364—374 (1950).

Holzbauer, M., Vogt, M.: The concentration of adrenaline in the peripheral blood during insulin hypoglycaemia. Brit. J. Pharmacol. **9**, 249—252 (1954).
Houssay, B.A., Gerschman, R., Rapela, C.E.: Adrénaline et Noradrénaline de la surrénale du crapaud normal ou hypophysoprive. C.R. Soc. Biol. (Paris) **144**, 1227—1228 (1950).
— Wassermann, G.F., Tramezzani, J.H.: Formation et sécrétion differentielles d'adrénaline et de noradrénaline surrénales. Arch. int. Pharmacodyn. **140**, 84—91 (1962).
Hrůza, Z., Albrecht, I., Jelinková, M., Erdösova, R.: Adrenaline and its effect in adaptation to trauma. Physiol. bohemoslov. **15**, 434—438 (1966).
Ignarro, L.J., Shideman, F.E.: Appearance and concentrations of catecholamines and their biosynthesis in the embryonic and developing chick. J. Pharmacol. exp. Ther. **159**, 38—48 (1968a).
— — Norepinephrine and epinephrine in the embryo and embryonic heart of the chick: Uptake and subcellular distribution. J. Pharmacol. exp. Ther. **159**, 49—58 (1968b).
Inoue, M., Akimoto, H.: Seasonal variations in the noradrenaline and adrenaline contents of the toad's adrenal. Kumamoto med. J. **12**, 7—11 (1959).
Itoh, C., Yoshinaga, K., Sato, T., Ishida, N., Wada, Y.: Presence of N-methylmetadrenaline in human urine and tumour tissue of phaeochromocytoma. Nature (Lond.) **193**, 477—478 (1962).
Iturriza, F.C.: Histochemical demonstration of biogenic monoamines in the pineal gland of the toad, *Bufo arenarum*. J. Histochem. Cytochem. **15**, 301—303 (1967).
Iversen, L.L., Jarrott, B.: Modification of an enzyme radiochemical assay procedure for noradrenaline. Biochem. Pharmacol. **19**, 1841—1843 (1970).
Iwata, H., Fujimoto, S., Nishikawa, T., Hano, K.: Pharmakologische Untersuchungen bei Thiamin-Mangel. I. Änderungen des Katecholamingehalts im Gewebe. Experientia (Basel) **24**, 378—380 (1968).
Jacobowitz, D.: Histochemical studies of the relationship of chromaffin cells and adrenergic nerve fibers to the cardiac ganglia of several species. J. Pharmacol. exp. Ther. **158**, 227 to 240 (1967).
Jaim-Etcheverry, G., Zieher, L.M.: Cytochemical localization of monoamine stores in sheep thyroid gland at the electron microscope level. Experientia (Basel) **24**, 593—595 (1968).
Jalon, P.G. De, Bayo, J.B., Jalon, M.G. De: Sensible y nuevo metodo de valoracion de adrenalina en utero aislado de rata. Farmacoter. act. **2**, 313—318 (1945).
James, W.O.: Demonstration and separation of noradrenaline, adrenaline and methyladrenaline. Nature (Lond.) **161**, 851—852 (1948).
Jofre, I.J., Izquierdo, J.A.: The concentration of adrenaline and noradrenaline in the brain and the heart of the goldfish *Carassius auratus*. J. Pharm. Pharmacol. **19**, 340—341 (1967).
Jonason, J.: Effects of Reserpine on the noradrenaline content of atrophied rat salivary glands. Acta physiol. scand. **75**, 73—77 (1969).
Juorio, A.V.: Distribution of dopamine in the brain of a tortoise *Geochelone chilensis* (Gray). J. Physiol. (Lond.) **204**, 503—509 (1969).
— Vogt, M.: Monoamines and their metabolites in avian brain. J. Physiol. (Lond.) **189**, 489—518 (1967).
— — Adrenaline in bird brain. J. Physiol. (Lond.) **209**, 757—763 (1970).
Kärki, N.T.: The urinary excretion of noradrenaline and adrenaline in different age groups, its diurnal variation and the effect of muscular work on it. Acta physiol. scand. **39**, Suppl. 132 (1956).
Karki, N., Kuntzman, R., Brodie, B.B.: Storage, synthesis and metabolism of monoamines in the developing brain. J. Neurochem. **9**, 53—58 (1962).
Kamo, M.: Effect of reserpine on the noradrenaline and adrenaline content of the adrenal gland in the toad. Acta med. Nagasaki. **6**, 71—73 (1962).
Kazarova, E.K., Esayan, N.A.: Noradrenaline and adrenaline of dog stomach wall and gastric juice. Biol. Zh. Arm. **19**, 58—64 (1966) (Armenian).
Kelly, M., Sharman, D.F., Tegerdine, P.: Dopamine in the blood of the ruminant. J. Physiol. (Lond.) **210**, 130P (1970).
Kirpekar, S.M., Cervoni, P., Furchgott, R.F.: Catecholamine content of the cat nictitating membrane following procedures sensitizing it to norepinephrine. J. Pharmacol. exp. Ther. **135**, 180—190 (1962).
Klensch, H.: Der basale Noradrenalinspiegel im peripheren venösen Blut des Menschen. Pflügers Arch. ges. Physiol. **290**, 218—224 (1966).
Klinge, E.: The catecholamine content of the bull retractor penis muscle. Acta physiol. scand. **78**, 103—109 (1970).
Klingman, G.I.: Catecholamine levels and DOPA decarboxylase activity in peripheral organs and adrenergic tissues in the rat after immunosympathectomy. J. Pharmacol. exp. Ther. **148**, 14—21 (1965).

KLINGMAN, G.I., KARDAMAN, S., HABER, J.: Amine levels, monoamine oxidase and DOPA-decarboxylase activities in the gastrointestinal tract of the rat. Life Sci. **3**, 1355—1360 (1964).
KLOUDA, M.A.: Distribution of catecholamine in the dog heart. Proc. Soc. exp. Biol. (N.Y.) **112**, 728—729 (1963).
KNOCHE, H., ALFES, H., MOELLMAN, H.: Biogenic amines in the carotid body: identification of dopamine by mass spectrometry. Experientia (Basel) **25**, 515—516 (1969).
KUNTZMAN, R., SHORE, P.A., BOGDANSKI, D., BRODIE, B.B.: Micro analytical procedures for fluorometric assay of brain DOPA-5HTP decarboxylase, norepinephrine and serotonin and a detailed mapping of decarboxylase activity in brain. J. Neurochem. **6**, 226—232 (1961).
DE LA LANDE, I.S., HARVEY, J.A.: A new and sensitive bioassay for catecholamines. J. Pharm. Pharmacol. **17**, 589—593 (1965).
— HEAD, R.J.: The catecholamines in the central artery of the rabbit ear. Aust. J. exp. Biol. med. Sci. **45**, 707—710 (1967).
LARSON, B., OWMAN, C., SUNDLER, F.: Monoaminergic mechanisms in parafollicular cells of the mouse thyroid gland. Endocrinology **78**, 1109—1114 (1966).
LATIES, A.M., JACOBOWITZ, D.: A comparative study of the autonomic innervation of the eye in monkey, cat and rabbit. Anat. Rec. **156**, 383—396 (1966).
LAVERTY, R., SHARMAN, D.F.: The estimation of small quantities of 3,4-dihydroxyphenylethylamine in tissues. Brit. J. Pharmacol. **24**, 538—548 (1965).
— — VOGT, M.: Action of 2,4,5-trihydroxyphenylethylamine on the storage and release of noradrenaline. Brit. J. Pharmacol. **24**, 549—560 (1965).
— TAYLOR, K.M.: The fluorometric assay of catecholamines and related compounds. Improvements and extensions to the hydroxyindole technique. Analyt. Biochem. **22**, 269—279 (1968).
LEBLANC, J., ROBINSON, D., SHARMAN, D.F., TOUSIGNANT, P.: Catecholamines and short term adaptation to cold in mice. Amer. J. Physiol. **213**, 1419—1422 (1967).
LEDUC, J.: Catecholamine production and release in exposure and acclimation to cold. Acta physiol. scand. **53**, Suppl. 183 (1961).
— DUBREUIL, R., D'IORIO, A.: Distribution of adrenaline and noradrenaline in the normal and hyperthyroid rat following adrenaline administration. Canad. J. Biochem. **33**, 283 to 288 (1955).
LEIBSON, L.G., STABROVSKII, E.M.: Adrenaline and noradrenaline content of the adrenal glands of the chick embryo. Fiziol. Zh. (Mosk.) **48**, 857—863 (1962) (Russian).
LEVI-MONTALCINI, R., ANGELETTI, P.U.: Noradrenaline and monoamine oxidase content in immunosympathectomized animals. Int. J. Neuropharmacol. **1**, 161—164 (1962).
LIN, Y.-C., STURKIE, P.D.: Effect of environmental temperature on the catecholamines of chickens. Amer. J. Physiol. **214**, 237—240 (1968).
LINÉT, O., WIDHALM, S., HERTTING, G.: The influence of experimental thiamine avitaminosis on catecholamine levels in hearts and brains of pigeons. Int. J. Neuropharmacol. **6**, 337 to 339 (1967).
LISCH, H.-J., AIGNER, A., HORNYKIEWICZ, O.: Dopamin-Stoffwechsel im Nucleus caudatus des Kaninchens nach partieller Hemmung der Gehirn-Monoaminoxydase mittels Nialamid. Naunyn-Schmiedeberg's Arch. exp. Path. Pharmak. **261**, 289—298 (1968).
LISHAJKO, F.: Occurrence and some properties of dopamine — containing granules in the sheep adrenal. Acta physiol. scand. **72**, 255—256 (1968).
LOEWI, O.: Quantitative und qualitative Untersuchungen über den Sympathicusstoff. Pflügers Arch. ges. Physiol. **237**, 504—514 (1936).
LUND, A.: Fluorimetric determination of adrenaline in blood. III. A new sensitive and specific method. Acta pharmacol. (Kbh.) **5**, 231—247 (1949).
— Release of adrenaline and noradrenaline from the spurarenal gland. Acta pharmacol. (Kbh.) **7**, 309—320 (1951).
LUPPA, H., WEISS, J., FEUSTEL, G.: Histochemische Untersuchungen zur Lokalisation von Acetylcholinesterase, Monoaminoxydase und Monoaminen im kaudalen neurosekretorischen System von *Cyprinus carpio*. Z. Zellforsch. **89**, 499—508 (1968).
MACMILLAN, W.H., RAND, M.J.: The effects in rabbits of thyroidectomy and treatment with triiodothyronin on the sensitivity to noradrenaline and the content of noradrenaline in aorta and spleen. J. Pharm. Pharmacol. **14**, 257—267 (1962).
MÄRKI, F., AXELROD, J.J., WITKOP, B.: Catecholamines and methyltransferases in the South American toad. Biochim. biophys. Acta (Amst.) **58**, 367—369 (1962).
MAGNUSSON, J., ROSENGREN, E.: Catecholamines of the spinal cord normally and after transection. Experientia (Basel) **19**, 229 (1963).
MALMFORS, T.: Studies on adrenergic nerves. Acta physiol. scand. **64**, Suppl. 248 (1965).
MATLINA, E.SCH., RACHMANOVA, T.B.: Adrenaline, noradrenaline, dopamine and DOPA in the blood and tissues of white rats in craniocerebral trauma. Bull. exp. Biol. Med. **63**, 55—57 (1967) (Russian).

Manger, W.M., Wakim, K.G., Bollman, J.L.: Chemical quantitation of epinephrine and norepinephrine in plasma. Springfield, Ill.: Charles C. Thomas 1959.
Manshardt, J., Wurtman, R.J.: Daily rhythm in the noradrenaline content of rat hypothalamus. Nature (Lond.) **217**, 574—575 (1968).
Manukhin, B.N., Pustovoitova, Z.E., Vyaz'mina, N.M.: The content of catecholamines and DOPA in tissues of chick embryo and chicken. Zh. Evol. Biol. Fiziol. V, 42—48 (1969).
Marques, M., Serrano, L.: Adrenaline and noradrenaline in the adrenals of normal and hypophysectomised turtles. Rev. bras. Biol. **20**, 251—256 (1960).
Matsuoka, M., Yoshida, H., Imaizumi, R.: Distribution of catecholamines and their metabolites in rabbit brain. Biochim. biophys. Acta (Amst.) **82**, 439—441 (1964).
Maxwell, R.A., Eckhardt, S.B., Wastila, W.B.: Distribution of endogenous norepinephrine in adventitial and media-intimal layers of rabbit aorta and the capacity of these layers to bind tritiated norepinephrine. J. Pharmacol. exp. Ther. **161**, 34—39 (1968).
Maynert, E.W., Levi, R.: Stress induced release of brain norepinephrine and its inhibition by drugs. J. Pharmacol. exp. Ther. **143**, 90—95 (1964).
Mazeaud, M.: Influence de divers facteurs sur l'adrénalinémie et la noradrénalinémie de la carpe. C.R. Soc. Biol. (Paris) **158**, 2018—2021 (1964).
McGeer, E.G., McGeer, P.L.: Catecholamine content of spinal cord. Canad. J. Biochem. **40**, 1141—1151 (1962).
McGeer, P.L., McGeer, E.G., Wada, J.A.: Central Aromatic amine levels and behavior. II. Serotonin and catecholamine levels in various cat brain areas following administration of psychoactive drugs or amine procursors. Arch. Neurol. (Chic.) **9**, 81—89 (1963).
McKenna, O.C., Angelakos, E.T.: Adrenergic innervation of the canine kidney. Circulat. Res. **22**, 345—354 (1968).
McKinney, T.D., Baldwin, D.M., Giles, R.H., Jr.: Effects of differential grouping on adrenal catecholamines in the cottontail rabbit. Physiol. Zool. **43**, 55—59 (1970).
McLean, J.R., Burnstock, G.: Histochemical localization of catecholamines in the urinary bladder of the toad *(Bufo marinus)*. J. Histochem. Cytochem. **14**, 538—548 (1966).
— — Innervation of the lungs of the toad *(Bufo marinus)*. II. Fluorescent histochemistry of catecholamines. Comp. Biochem. Physiol. **22**, 767—773 (1967a).
— — Innervation of the urinary bladder of the sleepy lizard *(Trachysaurus rugosus)*. I. Fluorescent histochemical localization of catecholamines. Comp. Biochem. Physiol. **20**, 667—673 (1967b).
— — Innervation of the lungs of the sleepy lizard *(Trachysaurus rugosus)*. I. Fluorescent histochemistry of catecholamines. Comp. Biochem. Physiol. **22**, 809—813 (1967c).
Millar, R.A., Benfey, B.G.: The fluorimetric estimation of adrenaline and noradrenaline during haemorrhagic hypotension. Brit. J. Anaesth. **30**, 158—165 (1958).
Mirkin, B.L., Brown, D.M., Ulstrom, R.A.: Catecholamine binding Protein: Binding of tritium to a specific protein fraction of human plasma following *in vitro* incubation with tritiated noradrenaline. Nature (Lond.) **212**, 1270—1271 (1966).
Miyahara, M.: Catecholamine metabolism in heart muscle. Jap. Circulat. J. (Ni.) **26**, 1—7 (1962).
Montagu, K.A.: Adrenaline and noradrenaline concentrations in rat tissues. Biochem. J. **63**, 559—565 (1956a).
— Seasonal variations of noradrenaline and adrenaline concentrations in rat tissue. Nature (Lond.) **178**, 417—418 (1956b).
— Catechol compounds in rat tissues and in brains of different animals. Nature (Lond.) **180**, 244—245 (1957).
— Seasonal changes of the catechol compounds present in rat tissues. Biochem. J. **71**, 91—99 (1959).
Moore, K.E., Lariviere, E.W.: Effects of stress and d-amphetamine on rat brain catecholamines. Biochem. Pharmacol. **13**, 1098—1100 (1964).
Musacchia, X.J., Jellinek, M., Cooper, T.: Effect of hibernation and cold torpor on tissue catecholamine content. Proc. Soc. exp. Biol. (N.Y.) **110**, 856—857 (1962).
Muscholl, E.: Die Konzentration von Noradrenalin und Adrenalin in den einzelnen Abschnitten des Herzens. Naunyn-Schmiedeberg's Arch. exp. Path. Pharmak. **237**, 350—364 (1959).
— Rahn, K.H., Watzka, M.: Nachweis von Noradrenalin im Glomus caroticum. Naturwissenschaften **47**, 325 (1960).
— Vogt, M.: The action of reserpine on the peripheral sympathetic system. J. Physiol. (Lond.) **141**, 132—155 (1958).
— — Secretory responses of extramedullary chromaffin tissue. Brit. J. Pharmacol. **22**, 193—203 (1964).
Nagatsu, T., Rust, L.A., DeQuattro, V.: The activity of tyrosine hydroxylase and related enzymes of catecholamine biosynthesis and metabolism in dog kidney — Effects of denervation. Biochem. Pharmacol. **18**, 1441—1446 (1969).

NAKANO, T., TOMLINSON, N.: Catecholamine and carbohydrate concentrations in Rainbow trout *(Salmo Gairdnerii)* in relation to physical disturbance. J. Fish. Res. Bd. Can. **24**, 1701—1715 (1967).

NATELSON, S., LUGOVOY, J.K., PINCUS, J.B.: A new fluorometric method for the determination of epinephrine. Arch. Biochem. **23**, 157—158 (1949).

NICHOLS, C.W., JACOBOWITZ, D., HOTTENSTEIN, M.: The influence of light and dark on the catecholamine content of the retina and choroid. Invest. Ophthal. **6**, 642—646 (1967).

NIKODIJEVIC, B., DALY, J., CREVELING, C.R.: Catechol-O-methyl transferase. I. An enzymatic assay for cardiac norepinephrine. Biochem. Pharmacol. **18**, 1577—1584 (1969).

NORBERG, K.-A., OLSON, L.: Adrenergic innervation of the salivary glands in the rat. Z. Zellforsch. **68**, 183—189 (1965).

NORTH, W.G.: Estimations of catecholamines in vertebrate tissues. Fourth Year Honours Thesis, University of Melbourne 1965, cited from Burnstock, 1969.

ÖSTLUND, E.: The distribution of catecholamines in lower animals and their effect on the heart. Acta physiol. scand. **31**, Suppl. 112 (1954).

— BLOOM, G., ADAMS-RAY, J., RITZÉN, M., SIEGMAN, M., NORDENSTAM, H., LISHAJKO, F., VON EULER, U.S.: Storage and release of catecholamines, and the occurrence of a specific submicroscopic granulation in hearts of cyclostomes. Nature (Lond.) **188**, 324—325 (1960).

O'KEEFFE, R., SHARMAN, D.F., VOGT, M.: Effect of drugs used in psychoses on cerebral dopamine metabolism. Brit. J. Pharmacol. **38**, 287—304 (1970).

ORDY, J.M., SAMOVAJSKI, T., SCHROEDER, D.: Concurrent changes in hypothalamic and cardiac catecholamine levels after anesthetics, tranquilizers and stress in a subhuman primate. J. Pharmacol. exp. Ther. **152**, 445—457 (1966).

OSKARSSON, V.: Influence of ovarian hormones and denervation on the catecholamines of the rat uterus. Acta Endocr. **34**, 38—44 (1960).

OWMAN, C., ROSENGREN, E., SJÖBERG, N.-O.: Adrenergic innervation of the human female reproductive organs: a histochemical and chemical investigation. Obstet. and Gynec. **30**, 763—773 (1967).

— SJÖBERG, N.-O.: Adrenergic nerves in the female genital tract of the rabbit. With remarks on cholinesterase-containing structures. Z. Zellforsch. **74**, 182—197 (1966).

PAGE, I.H., GREEN, A.A.: Perfusion of rabbit's ear for study of vasoconstrictor substances. Methods in Medical Research. Ed. V.R. POTTER. The Year Book Publishers Inc. Chicago, Vol. 1, 123—129 (1948).

PALAÍC, D., PANISSET, J.-C.: The effect of nerve stimulation and angiotensin on the accumulation of ^{3}H-norepinephrine and the endogenous norepinephrine level in guinea pig vas deferens. Biochem. Pharmacol. **18**, 2693—2700 (1969).

PAOLETTI, R., SMITH, R.L., MAICKEL, R.R., BRODIE, B.B.: Identification and physiological role of noradrenaline in adipose tissue. Biochem. biophys. Res. Commun. **5**, 424—429 (1961).

PAULSEN, E.C., HESS, S.M.: The rate of synthesis of catecholamines following depletion in guinea pig brain and heart. J. Neurochem. **10**, 453—459 (1963).

PELLEGRINO DE IRALDI, A., ZIEHER, L.M.: Noradrenaline and dopamine content of normal, decentralised and denervated pineal gland of the rat. Life Sci. **5**, 149—154 (1966).

PENTTILA, O.: Acetylcholine, biogenic amines and enzymes involved in their metabolism in penile erectile tissue. Ann. Med. exp. Fenn. Suppl. 44 (1966).

PHILLIPOT, E., GOFFART, M., DRESSE, A.: Le système surrénalo-sympathique chez le paresseux *(Choloepus hoffmanni* Peters). Arch. int. Physiol. Biochim. **73**, 476—504 (1965).

PODGORNAYA, G.: Morphological and histochemical studies of the medulla of the adrenal in mammals. Arkh. Anat. Gistol. Embriol. **52**, 22—30 (1967) (Russian).

POIRIER, L.J., SOURKES, T.L., BOUVIER, G., BOUCHER, R., CARABIN, S.: Striatal amines, experimental tremor and the effect of harmaline in the monkey. Brain **89**, 37—52 (1966).

POLIKARPOVA, L.I.: Content of adrenaline and its oxidation products in blood vessel walls of guinea pigs exposed to ionizing radiation. Radibiologiya (Buc.) **1**, 899—902 (1961).

POPOV, N., POHLE, W., ROSLER, V., MATTHIES, H.: Regionale Verteilung von γ-Aminobuttersäure, Glutaminsäure, Asparaginsäure, Dopamin, Noradrenalin und Serotonin im Rattenhirn. Acta biol. med. germ. **18**, 695—702 (1967).

PRIIMAK, E.K.: Distribution of adrenaline and noradrenaline in cells of the carotid body. Dokl. Akad. Nauk SSSR, Otd. Biol. **128**, 618—621 (1959).

PSCHEIDT, G.R., HABER, B.: Regional distribution of dihydroxyphenylalanine and 5-hydroxytryptophan decarboxylase and of biogenic amines in the chicken central nervous system. J. Neurochem. **12**, 613—618 (1965).

— HIMWICH, H.E.: Reserpine, monoamine oxidase inhibitors and distribution of biogenic amines in monkey brain. Biochem. Pharmacol. **12**, 65—71 (1963).

— — Biogenic amines in various brain regions of growing cats. Brain Res. **1**, 363—368 (1966).

RAAB, W., GIGEE, W.: Specific avidity of the heart muscle to absorb and store epinephrine and norepinephrine. Circulat. Res. **3**, 553—558 (1955).

Rahn, K.H.: Morphologische Untersuchungen am Paraganglion caroticum mit histochemischem und pharmakologischem Nachweis von Noradrenalin. Anat. Anz. **110**, 140—159 (1961).

Rapela, C.E., Gordon, M.F.: Seasonal variations in the adrenaline and noradrenaline contents of the adrenals of the toad *Bufo arenarum*. C.R. Soc. Biol. (Paris) **150**, 1290—1291 (1956).

Rastgeldi, S.: Adrenaline and noradrenaline in the whale suprarenal gland. Acta physiol. scand. **23**, 44—46 (1951).

Read, J.B., Burnstock, G.: Comparative histochemical studies of adrenergic nerves in the enteric plexuses of vertebrate large intestine. Comp. Biochem. Physiol. **27**, 505—517 (1968).

Rehn, O.N.: Effect of decentralisation on the content of catecholamines in the spleen and kidney of the cat. Acta physiol. scand. **42**, 309—312 (1958).

Reis, D.J., Weinbren, M., Corvelli, A.: A circadian rhythm of norepinephrine regionally in cat brain: Its relationship to environmental lighting and to regional diurnal variations in brain serotonin. J. Pharmacol. exp. Ther. **164**, 135—145 (1968).

Richter, D.: The inactivation of adrenaline *in vivo* in man. J. Physiol. (Lond.) **98**, 361—374 (1940).

Rinne, U.K., Sonninen, V.: The occurrence of dopamine and noradrenaline in the tubero-hypophysial system. Experientia (Basel) **24**, 177—178 (1968).

Roffi, J.: Évolution des quantités d'adrénaline et de noradrénaline dans les surrénales des foetus et des nouveau-nés de rat et de lapin. Ann. Endocr. (Paris) **29**, 277—300 (1968).

Rosengren, E., Sjöberg, N.-O.: Changes in the amount of adrenergic transmitter in the female genital tract of rabbit during pregnancy. Acta physiol. scand. **72**, 412—424 (1968).

Rubin, R.P., Cohen, M.S., Harman, S.M., Roer, E.M.: The localization of adrenaline-rich medullary chromaffin cells adjacent to the adrenal cortex. J. Endocr. **41**, 541—545 (1968).

Rudzik, A.D., Miller, J.W.: The effect of altering the catecholamine content of the uterus on the rate of contractions and the sensitivity of the myometrium to relaxin. J. Pharmacol. exp. Ther. **138**, 88—95 (1962).

Ryd, G., Sjöstrand, N.O.: Effect of castration and testosterone administration on the noradrenaline content of the vas deferens and the seminal vesicle of the guinea pig. Experientia (Basel) **23**, 816—817 (1967).

Saelens, J.K., Schoen, M.S., Kovacsics, G.B.: An enzyme assay for norepinephrine in brain tissue. Biochem. Pharmacol. **16**, 1043—1049 (1967).

Sanan, S., Vogt, M.: Effect of drugs on the noradrenaline content of brain and peripheral tissue and its significance. Brit. J. Pharmacol. **18**, 109—127 (1962).

Sano, I., Gamo, T., Kakimoto, Y., Taniguchi, K., Takesada, M., Nishinumani, K.: Distribution of catechol compounds in human brain. Biochim. biophys. Acta (Amst.) **32**, 586 to 587 (1959).

De Schaepdryver, A.F., Preziosi, P., Van der Stricht, J.: Urinary adrenaline and noradrenaline output after medullo-adrenalectomy in dogs. Arch. int. Pharmacodyn. **121**, 468—477 (1959).

— Taquini, A.C., Jr., Bernard, P., Heymans, C.: Tissue catecholamines in chronic renal hypertension. Arch. int. Pharmacodyn. **142**, 260—266 (1963).

Scheving, L.E., Harrison, W.H., Gordon, P., Pauly, J.E.: Daily fluctuation (circadian and ultradian) in biogenic amines of the rat brain. Amer. J. Physiol. **214**, 166—173 (1968).

Schmiterlöw, C.G.: The nature and occurrence of pressor and depressor substances in extracts from blood vessels. Acta physiol. scand. **16**, Suppl. 56 (1948).

De Schryver, C., Mertens-Strythagen, J., Becsei, I., Lammerant, J.: Effect of training on heart and skeletal muscle catecholamine concentration in rats. Amer. J. Physiol. **217**, 1589—1592 (1969).

Schümann, H.-J.: Zur Pharmakologie des Arterenols und Adrenalins. Naunyn-Schmiedeberg's Arch. exp. Path. Pharmak. **209**, 340—349 (1950).

— Nachweis von Oxytyramin (Dopamin) in sympathischen Nerven und Ganglien. Naunyn-Schmiedeberg's Arch. exp. Path. Pharmak. **227**, 566—573 (1956).

— The distribution of adrenaline and noradrenaline in chromaffin granules from the chicken. J. Physiol. (Lond.) **137**, 318—326 (1957).

— Über den Hydroxytyramin- und Noradrenalingehalt der Lunge. Naunyn-Schmiedeberg's Arch. exp. Path. Pharmak. **234**, 282—290 (1958).

— Über den Hydroxytyramingehalt der Organe. Naunyn-Schmiedeberg's Arch. exp. Path. Pharmak. **236**, 474—482 (1959).

Scudder, C.L., Karczmar, A.G., Everett, G.M., Gibson, J.E., Rifkin, M.: Brain catecholamines and serotonin levels in various strains and genera of mice and a possible interpretation for the correlations of amine levels with electroshock latency and behaviour. Int. J. Neuropharmacol. **5**, 343—351 (1966).

SEGURA, E.T., BISCARDI, A.M.: Changes in brain epinephrine and norepinephrine induced by afferent electrical stimulation in the isolated toad head. Life Sci. **6**, 1599—1603 (1967).
— — APELBAUM, J.: Seasonal variations of brain epinephrine, norepinephrine and 5-HT associated with changes in the EEG of the toad, *Bufo arenarum* Hensel. Comp. Biochem. Physiol. **22**, 843—850 (1967).
SHARMAN, D.F.: The significance of pharmacologically active amines in animal tissues and body fluids. Ph. D. Thesis, University of Edinburgh (1960).
— VANOV, S., VOGT, M.: Noradrenaline content in the heart and spleen of the mouse under normal conditions and after administration of some drugs. Brit. J. Pharmacol. **19**, 527—533 (1962).
— VOGT, M.: The noradrenaline content of the caudate nucleus of the rabbit. J. Neurochem. **12**, 62 (1965).
SHAW, F.H.: The estimation of adrenaline. Biochem. J. **32**, 19—25 (1938).
SHEPHERD, D.M., WEST, G.B.: Noradrenaline and the suprarenal medulla. Brit. J. Pharmacol. **6**, 665—674 (1951).
— — Noradrenaline in accessory chromaffin tissue. Nature (Lond.) **170**, 42—43 (1952).
— — Hydroxytyramine and the adrenal medulla. J. Physiol. (Lond.) **120**, 15—19 (1953).
— — ERSPAMER, V.: Chromaffin bodies of various species of dogfish. Nature (Lond.) **172**, 509 (1953).
SHINDLER, R., HARAKAL, C., SEVY, R.W.: Catecholamine content of the sinoatrial node and common right atrial tissue. Proc. Soc. exp. Biol. (N.Y.) **128**, 798—800 (1968).
SHIPLEY, R.E., TILDEN, J.H.: A pithed rat preparation suitable for assaying pressor substances. Proc. Soc. exp. Biol. (N.Y.) **64**, 453—455 (1947).
SHORE, P.A.: A simple technique involving solvent extraction for the estimation of norepinephrine and epinephrine in tissues. Pharmacol. Rev. **11**, 276—277 (1959).
— COHN, V.H., JR., HIGHMAN, B., MALING, H.M.: Distribution of norepinephrine in the heart. Nature (Lond.) **181**, 848—849 (1958).
— OLIN, J.S.: Identification and chemical assay of norepinephrine in brain and other tissues. J. Pharmacol. exp. Ther. **122**, 295—300 (1958).
SHUMWAY, W.: Stages in the normal development of *Rana pipiens*. I. External form. Anat. Rec. **78**, 139—147 (1940).
SIDMAN, R.L., PERKINS, M., WEINER, N.: Noradrenaline and adrenaline content of adipose tissues. Nature (Lond.) **193**, 36—37 (1962).
SJÖBERG, N.-O.: The adrenergic transmitter of the female reproductive tract: Distribution and functional changes. Acta physiol. scand. Suppl. 305 (1967).
— Increase in transmitter content of adrenergic nerves in the reproductive tract of female rabbits after estrogen treatment. Acta endocr. (Kbh.) **57**, 405—413 (1968a).
— Considerations on the cause of disappearance of the adrenergic transmitter in uterine nerves during pregnancy. Acta physiol. scand. **72**, 510—517 (1968b).
SJÖSTRAND, N.-O.: High noradrenaline content in the vas deferens of the cock and the tortoise. Experientia (Basel) **21**, 96 (1965a).
— The adrenergic innervation of the vas deferens and the accessory male genital glands. Acta physiol. scand. **65**, Suppl. 257 (1965b).
— SWEDIN, G.: Effect of chronic hypogastric denervation on the noradrenaline content of the vas deferens and the accessory male reproductive glands of the rat. Experientia (Basel) **23**, 817—818 (1967).
SMITH, C.B.: Enhancement by reserpine and α-methyl DOPA of the effects of d-amphetamine upon the locomotor activity of mice. J. Pharmacol. exp. Ther. **142**, 343—350 (1963).
— TRENDELENBURG, U., LANGER, S.Z., TSAI, T.H.: The relation of retention of norepinephrine — H^3 to the norepinephrine content of the nictitating membrane of the spinal cat during development of denervation supersensitivity. J. Pharmacol. exp. Ther. **151**, 87—94 (1966).
SMITH, R.L., PAOLETTI, R., BRODIE, B.B.: Identification and assay of noradrenaline in adipose tissue. Biochem. J. **82**, 19P (1962).
SOURKES, T.L., MURPHY, G.F.: Determination of catecholamines and catecholamine acids by differential spectrophotofluorimetry. Methods in Medical Research. Ed. J.H. QUASTEL. Year Book Medical Publishers Inc., Chicago **9**, 147—152 (1961).
SPANN, J.F., JR., CHIDSEY, C.A., BRAUNWALD, E.: Reduction of cardiac stores of norepinephrine in experimental heart failure. Science **145**, 1439—1441 (1964).
SPANO, P.F., VARGUI, L., CRABAI, F., CONGIU, S., GESSA, R., GESSA, G.L.: Contenuto di noradrenalina nel tessuto adiposo di varie specie animali. Boll. Soc. ital. Biol. sper. **43**, 640—643 (1967).
SPRATTO, G.R., MILLER, J.W.: The effect of various oestrogens on the weight, catecholamine content and rate of contractions of rat uteri. J. Pharmacol. exp. Ther. **161**, 1—6 (1968a).
— — An investigation of the mechanism by which estradiol-17β elevates the epinephrine content of the rat uterus. J. Pharmacol. exp. Ther. **161**, 7—13 (1968b).

STABROVSKII, E.M.: The distribution of adrenaline and noradrenaline in the organs of the baltic lamprey *Lampetra fluviatilis* at rest and under various functional stresses. J. evol. Biochem. Physiol. **3**, 216—221 (1967) (Russian).

— Adrenaline and noradrenaline in the organs of the carp *Cyprinus carpio* at rest and under functional stresses. J. evol. Biochem. Physiol. **4**, 337—341 (1968) (Russian).

— Adrenaline and noradrenaline in the organs of elasmobranch and teleost fishes from the black sea. J. evol. Biochem. Physiol. **5**, 38—41 (1969) (Russian).

STOCK, K., WESTERMANN, E.O.: Concentration of norepinephrine, serotonin, and histamine and of amine-metabolizing enzymes in mammalian adipose tissue. J. Lipid. Res. **4**, 297 to 304 (1963).

STOLZ, F.: Über Adrenalin und Alkylaminoacetobrenzcatechin. Ber. dtsch. chem. Ges. **37**, 4149—4154 (1904).

STRANDBERG, K., SEDVALL, G., MIDTVEDT, T., GUSTAFSSON, B.: Effect of some biologically active amines on the cecum wall of germ free rats. Proc. Soc. exp. Biol. (N.Y.) **121**, 699 to 702 (1966).

STREET, D.M., ROBERTS, D. J.: The presence of dopamine in cat spleen and blood. J. Pharm. Pharmacol. **21**, 199—201 (1969).

STRÖMBLAD, B.C.R.: Adrenaline-Noradrenaline content of the submaxillary gland of the cat. Experientia (Basel) **16**, 417—418 (1960).

STURKIE, P.D., LIN, Y.-C.: Sex difference in blood norepinephrine of chickens. Comp. Biochem. Physiol. **24**, 1073—1075 (1968).

SUOMALAINEN, P., UUSPÄÄ, J.: Adrenaline-noradrenaline ratio in the adrenal glands of the hedgehog during summer activity and hibernation. Nature (Lond.) **182**, 1500—1501 (1958).

SZYMONOWICZ, L.: Die Funktion der Nebennieren. Pflügers Arch. ges. Physiol. **64**, 97—164 (1896).

TAKAMINE, J.: The isolation of the active principal of the suprarenal gland. J. Physiol. (Lond.) **27**, 29P—30P (1901).

THOENEN, H., HAEFELY, W., GEY, K.F., HÜRLIMANN, A.: Diminished effect of sympathetic nerve stimulation in cats pretreated with 5-hydroxydopa: formation and liberation of fake adrenergic transmitters. Naunyn-Schmiedeberg's Arch. Pharmak. exp. Path. **259**, 17—23 (1967).

TWENTE, J.W., CLINE, W.H., TWENTE, J.A.: Distribution of epinephrine and norepinephrine in the brain of *Citellus lateralis* during the hibernating cycle. Comp. Gen. Pharmacol. **1**, 47—53 (1970).

UNGVÁRY, G.Y., DONÁTH, T.: On the monoaminergic innervation of the liver. Acta anat. (Basel) **72**, 446—459 (1969).

UUSPÄÄ, V.J.: The catecholamine content of the brain and heart of the hedgehog *(Erinaceus europaeus)* during hibernation and in an active state. Ann. Med. exp. Fenn. **41**, 340—348 (1963a).

— Effects of hibernation on the noradrenaline and adrenaline contents of the adrenal glands in the hedgehog. Ann. Med. exp. Fenn. **41**, 349—354 (1963b).

VALK, A. DET., JR., PRICE, H.L.: The chemical estimation of epinephrine and norepinephrine in human and canine plasma. I. A critique of the ethylene diamine condensation method. J. clin. Invest. **35**, 837—841 (1956).

DOVALLE, J.R., PORTO, A.: A note on the adrenin content of the adrenals of snakes. Mem. Inst. Butantan **18**, 247—250 (1945).

VALZELLI, L., GARATTINI, S.: Biogenic amines in discrete brain areas after treatment with monoamine oxidase inhibitors. J. Neurochem. **15**, 259—261 (1968).

VANDERMEULEN, R., CESSION-FOSSION, A.: Présence de dopamine dans les surrénales de la chèvre *(Capra hircus)*. Arch. int. Physiol. Biochim. **76**, 916—919 (1968).

VANE, J.R.: The estimation of catecholamines by biological assay. Pharmacol. Rev. **18**, 317—324 (1966).

VANOV, S., VOGT, M.: Catecholamine-containing structures in the hypogastric nerve of the dog. J. Physiol. (Lond.) **168**, 939—944 (1963).

VENDSALU, A.: Studies on adrenaline and noradrenaline in human plasma. Acta physiol. scand. **49**, Suppl. 173 (1960).

VOGT, M.: The concentration of sympathin in different parts of the central nervous system under normal conditions and after administration of drugs. J. Physiol. (Lond.) **123**, 451 to 481 (1954).

— Hypogastric nerve of the dog. Nature (Lond.) **197**, 804—805 (1963).

WADA, J.A., MCGEER, E.G.: Central aromatic amines and behaviour. III. Correlative analysis of conditioned approach behaviour on brain levels of serotonin and catecholamines in monkey. Arch. Neurol. (Chic.) **14**, 129—142 (1966).

WASSERMANN, G., TRAMEZZANI, J.H.: Separate distribution of adrenaline and noradrenaline secreting cells in the adrenal of snakes *(Xenodon merremii)*. Gen. comp. Endocr. **3**, 480 to 489 (1963).

WEGMANN, A.: Determination of 3-hydroxytyramine and DOPA in various organs of dog after DOPA infusion. Naunyn-Schmiedeberg's Arch. exp. Path. Pharmak. **246**, 184—190 (1963).
— CHIBA, C., CHRYSOHOU, A., BING, R.J.: Catecholamines in homologous heart grafts. Proc. Soc. exp. Biol. (N.Y.) **109**, 543—545 (1962).
WEIL-MALHERBE, H.: The simultaneous estimation of catecholamines and their metabolites. Z. klin. Chem. **6**, 161—167 (1964).
— BONE, A.D.: The association of adrenaline and noradrenaline with blood platelets. Biochem. J. **70**, 14—22 (1958).
— LIDDELL, D.W.: Adrenaline and noradrenaline in cerebrospinal fluid. J.Neurol. Neurosurg. Psychiat. **17**, 247—249 (1954).
WEINER, N., PERKINS, M., SIDMAN, R.L.: Effect of reserpine on the noradrenaline content of innervated and denervated brown adipose tissue of the rat. Nature (Lond.) **193**, 137—138 (1962).
WEST, G.B.: The nature of avian and amphibian sympathin. J. Pharm. Pharmacol. **3**, 400 to 408 (1951).
— The comparative pharmacology of the suprarenal medulla. Quart. Rev. Biol. **30**, 116—137 (1955).
— SHEPHERD, D.M., HUNTER, R.B., MACGREGOR, A.R.: The functions of the organs of Zuckerkandl. Clin. Sci. **12**, 317—324 (1953).
WIELAND, T.: Quantitative Trennung von Aminosäuren durch Austauschadsorption an Aluminiumoxyd. Hoppe-Seylers Z. physiol. Chem. **273**, 24—30 (1942).
WIRSÉN, C.: Studies in lipid mobilization. Acta physiol. scand. **65**, Suppl. 252 (1965).
— HAMBERGER, B.: Catecholamines in brown fat. Nature (Lond.) **214**, 625—626 (1967).
WRIGHT, A., CHESTER-JONES, J.: Chromaffin tissue in the lizard adrenal gland. Nature (Lond.) **175**, 1001—1002 (1955).
WURTMAN, R.J., AXELROD, J.: Adrenaline synthesis: Control by the pituitary gland and adrenal glucocorticoids. Science **150**, 1464 (1965).
— — A 24 hour rhythm in the content of norepinephrine in the pineal and salivary glands of the rat. Life Sci. **5**, 665—669 (1966).
— — POTTER, L.T.: The disposition of catecholamines in the rat uterus and the effect of drugs and hormones. J. Pharmacol. exp. Ther. **144**, 150—155 (1964).
— — SEDVALL, G., MOORE, R.Y.: Photic and neural control of the 24 hour norepinephrine rhythm in the rat pineal gland. J. Pharmacol. exp. Ther. **157**, 487—492 (1967a).
— — TRAMEZZANI, J.: Distribution of the adrenaline-forming enzyme in the adrenal gland of a snake — *Xenodon merremii*. Nature (Lond.) **215**, 879—880 (1967b).
— CHU, E.W., AXELROD, J.: Relation between the oestrous cycle and the binding of catecholamines in the rat uterus. Nature (Lond.) **198**, 547—548 (1963).
ZARAFONETIS, C.J.D., KALAS, J.P.: Serotonin, catecholamines and amine oxidase activity in the venoms of certain reptiles. Amer. J. med. Sci. **240**, 764—768 (1960).
ZUCKERKANDL, E.: Über Nebenorgane des Sympathicus im Retroperitonealraum des Menschen. Anat. Anz. **19**, Erg. H., 95—107 (1901).

Chapter 6

Synthesis, Uptake and Storage of Catecholamines in Adrenergic Nerves, The Effect of Drugs

U.S. v. Euler

With 9 Figures

A. Introduction

The finding that the sympathomimetic agents in chromaffin cells and in adrenergic nerves are stored in apparently similar subcellular particles has sometimes led to the belief that the mechanisms for uptake, storage and release of the active compounds are identical or at least very similar. Detailed studies, mainly on isolated particles, have shown, however, that although similarities occur, important differences between the properties of the chromaffin cell particles and those in the adrenergic nerves exist. Thus nerve particles after partial depletion readily take up amines from a suspension medium to the original content or even higher in the presence of ATP-Mg^{++}, whereas chromaffin cell particles containing either adrenaline or noradrenaline lack this property. Some drugs like phenoxybenzamine inhibit the release of noradrenaline from nerve particles but enhance the release from adrenal medullary granules. Striking differences in osmotic behaviour between chromaffin cell particles and nerve particles have also been described.

Moreover, there is increasing evidence that not all adrenergic nerve particles are of the same kind. Those appearing in the short adrenergic neurons in the male accessory reproductive organs show a different behaviour from those present in the ordinary adrenergic neurons, e.g. in the spleen. It is possible that the adrenergic nerve particles in the CNS have special properties, although little is known in this respect.

The important question of the mechanism of amine release from the chromaffin cells and adrenergic nerve terminals is still under debate and will not be discussed in this Chapter; it is only mentioned here since certain data indicate that the release mechanisms may differ, not only as regards the spontaneous release rate *in vitro*, but also more fundamentally, with respect to the nature of the releasing process *in vivo*.

B. Adrenergic Nerves

I. Synthesis

1. Main Synthetic Pathway

Synthesis of adrenaline occurs *in vivo* from phenylalanine and tyrosine (Gurin and Delluva, 1947; Udenfriend et al., 1953) and from dopa and dopamine (Udenfriend and Wyngaarden, 1956). The formation of noradrenaline as a step in the synthetic pathway was originally suggested by Blaschko (1939) and by

Holtz (1939) following the discovery of dopa decarboxylase by Holtz et al. (1938). This was confirmed *in vitro* by Goodall and Kirshner (1957) who showed that tyrosine is converted in a sequence to dopa, dopamine, noradrenaline and adrenaline by enzymes in the adrenal medulla. This pathway could later be confirmed also for adrenergic nerves (Goodall and Kirshner, 1958) and for organs containing adrenergic nerves (Spector et al., 1963a).

In the first step tyrosine serves as substrate for the enzyme tyrosine hydroxylase which is present in the axoplasm (Nagatsu et al., 1964). The DOPA formed is transformed to dopamine by L-DOPA decarboxylase which also occurs in the axoplasm. Dopamine is subsequently oxidized to noradrenaline with the aid of the enzyme dopamine-β-hydroxylase which is present in the storage particles (Fig. 1).

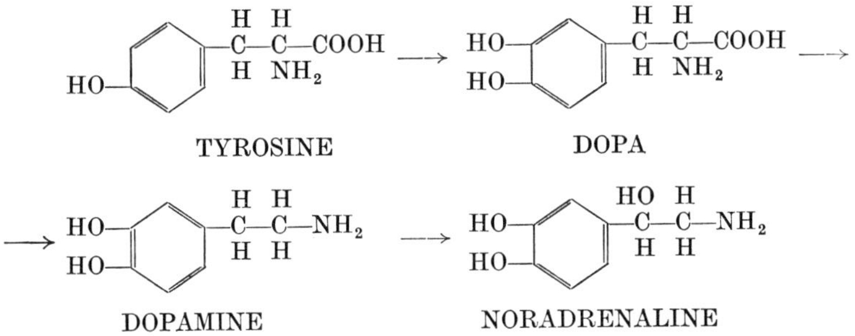

TYROSINE → DOPA → DOPAMINE → NORADRENALINE

Fig. 1. Biosynthetic pathway for noradrenaline

a) Tyrosine Hydroxylase

Since the formation of tyrosine from phenylalanine occurs in a variety of tissues outside the adrenergic neuron it seems appropriate to regard the formation of DOPA from tyrosine as the first synthetic step in this context. Tyrosine, which is generally available in the body fluids, can enter the adrenergic axon, where tyrosine hydroxylase is present. Whether or not special "pump" or "carrier" mechanisms are required for the entrance of tyrosine into the axon is not known, but it has been assumed that this process is facilitated by a "permease".

While tyrosine generally is a poor substrate for amino acid decarboxylases it is transformed into an efficient substrate by hydroxylation in the 3-position of the ring. The active enzyme was isolated and characterized by Nagatsu et al. (1964) (cf. Udenfriend, 1966). It is present in tissues which normally contain noradrenaline or adrenaline. The enzyme requires tetrahydropyridines, e.g. tetrahydrofolic acid, and is activated by divalent iron (Ikeda et al., 1965). Tyrosine hydroxylase catalyzes the oxidation of phenylalanine to tyrosine as well as the following step from tyrosine to DOPA.

The hydroxylation of tyrosine to DOPA is slower than the subsequent decarboxylation and β-hydroxylation and therefore rate limiting (Spector et al., 1963a; Levitt et al., 1965). The activity of the enzyme is inhibited by phenylalanine as well as by DOPA and noradrenaline, which may well constitute a feedback control mechanism, regulating the synthesis rate (Nagatsu et al., 1964).

b) DOPA-Decarboxylase

The second step in the biosynthesis of the adrenergic neurotransmitter, the formation of dopamine from L-DOPA, is catalyzed by an efficient enzyme, L-DOPA decarboxylase, discovered in the mammalian kidney by Holtz et al.

(1938) (cf. BLASCHKO, 1959; HOLTZ, 1959; SOURKES, 1966). The enzyme, which requires pyridoxal-5'-phosphate as co-factor (cf. HOLTZ and PALM, 1964), is cyanide-sensitive; it seems to occur in all tissues containing adrenergic neurons (HOLTZ et al., 1942) or chromaffin cells (LANGEMANN, 1951).

Incubation of noradrenaline or dopamine (but not adrenaline) with the enzymic co-factor causes inactivation of the enzyme and of the amine through formation of Schiff's bases and transformation to tetrahydro isoquinoline derivatives (SCHOTT and CLARK, 1952; HOLTZ and WESTERMANN, 1957).

Since DOPA but not dopamine passes the blood brain barrier, the amino acid has been used in patients with Parkinsonism in order to supply substrate for dopamine formation which is deficient in these cases (BIRKMAYER and HORNYKIEWICZ, 1962).

DOPA-decarboxylase is not highly substrate specific, even if L-DOPA appears to be the best substrate. Ortho and metatyrosine also serve as substrates (BLASCHKO et al., 1949; BLASCHKO, 1950; SOURKES, 1955; BLASCHKO and CHRUSCIEL, 1960), whereas tyrosine is not decarboxylated by the enzyme prepared from the kidney or liver of some animals (HOLTZ et al., 1939; AWAPARA et al., 1964). The finding that N-methyl DOPA is not attacked by mammalian decarboxylase actually formed the basis for the concept of adrenaline formation via a primary amine like dopamine or noradrenaline (BLASCHKO, 1939). On the other hand 5-HTP is a good substrate for the enzyme (HOLTZ and WESTERMANN, 1957; cf. also HAGEN and COHEN, 1966), and also 3,4-dihydroxyphenylserine (DOPS) which is directly decarboxylated to noradrenaline (BLASCHKO et al., 1950; SCHMITERLÖW, 1951).

Decarboxylation of *erythro*-dihydroxyphenylserine and *erythro-m*-hydroxyphenylserine to noradrenaline has been demonstrated with hog kidney extract, and of *erythro*- or *threo*-dihydroxyphenylserine with rat liver homogenate. After injection of *threo*-dihydroxyphenylserine in rats, the (—) isomer of noradrenaline was recovered in urine (HARTMAN et al., 1955b).

The decarboxylation product, dopamine, was first detected in the mammalian heart and the suprarenal medulla (GOODALL, 1950, 1951) and occurs as a natural product in urine (EULER et al., 1951) and in a variety of organs and tissues. In studies of the dopamine content of organs it must be kept in mind, however, that it is not only a precursor for noradrenaline but also occurs as a specific product in certain cells of the chromaffin type in various organs (FALCK et al., 1959), sympathetic nerves (SCHÜMANN, 1956), lungs (EULER and LISHAJKO, 1957), sinus node (ANGELAKOS et al., 1963) and carotid glomus (CHIOCCHIO et al., 1966; LISHAJKO, 1970). Increased amounts of dopamine are found in the urine of patients with phaeochromocytoma. Dopamine also occurs normally in the brain (MONTAGU, 1957) and appears to serve as neurotransmitter in certain areas such as basal ganglia, where its presence has been studied both by direct analysis and by the histochemical fluorescence technique (BERTLER and ROSENGREN, 1959; HORNYKIEWICZ, 1962; FUXE, 1965; CARLSSON, 1966).

Of considerable theoretical and practical interest is the observation that α-methyl DOPA and α-MMT are readily decarboxylated in the mammalian organism and stored in adrenergic nerves as α-methyldopamine, α-methylnoradrenaline and metaraminol (after β-oxidation) (CARLSSON and LINDQVIST, 1962; MAÎTRE and STAEHELIN, 1963; MUSCHOLL and MAÎTRE, 1963; MUSCHOLL, 1965).

c) Dopamine β-hydroxylase

On incubation of homogenates of sympathetic nerves and ganglia with dopamine, the formation of noradrenaline has been established (GOODALL and

Kirshner, 1958), indicating that a hydroxy group is introduced in β-position in the side chain. The transforming enzyme, dopamine-β-hydroxylase was first prepared from adrenal medullary extracts (Levin et al., 1960) and is a copper proteid. The enzyme, which requires ascorbic acid and fumaric acid as co-factors, has been studied in detail by Goldstein et al. (1965) (cf. Kaufman and Friedman, 1965). Its activity is high and similar to that of DOPA-decarboxylase.

The formation of noradrenaline from dopamine has also been demonstrated in isolated nerve granules (Euler and Lishajko, 1968a; Stjärne et al., 1967a).

2. Other Synthetic Pathways

Even meta-tyrosine can be hydroxylated to DOPA, as shown by its subsequent conversion to dopamine (Sourkes et al., 1961b). By ring hydroxylation, metaraminol can be transformed *in vivo* to α-methylnoradrenaline in the guinea pig (Maître and Staehelin, 1965). Interestingly, the amount of α-methylnoradrenaline in the heart exceeded that of noradrenaline.

As already mentioned, 3,4-dihydroxyphenylserine (DOPS) may serve as a precursor to noradrenaline, although no evidence for its presence in the organism has been given. Phenylethylamine (Asatoor and Dalgliesh, 1959) as well as tyramine (Sjoerdsma et al., 1959) occur normally in urine indicating that these amines are formed by decarboxylation of the corresponding amino acids (cf. Lovenberg et al., 1962). After inhibition of monoamine oxidase their excretion is increased. Most of the tyramine found is present in the central nervous system. Apparently the greater part of the tyramine formed in peripheral nervous tissue is oxidized to octopamine (Musacchio and Goldstein, 1963) which is also a natural excretion product in urine (Pisano et al., 1960; Spector et al., 1963b).

In the heart and kidney octopamine could only be demonstrated after inhibition of MAO (Kakimoto and Armstrong, 1962). Posterior salivary glands from *Octopus vulgaris* contain both octopamine (Erspamer and Boretti, 1951) and noradrenaline (Euler, 1953) but the exact stage at which the ring hydroxylation occurs is not known (cf. Blaschko, 1959).

Tyramine and octopamine are apparently to some extent transformed to noradrenaline (Creveling et al., 1962), since administration of these compounds cause an increased excretion of noradrenaline. Some of this may be due to the noradrenaline-releasing effect of the two amines, however.

Liver microsomes from the rabbit can form catechols from the corresponding phenols (dopamine from tyramine, noradrenaline from octopamine) reactions which require NADH (Axelrod, 1963). Non-enzymatic conversion of tyrosine to DOPA (Udenfriend et al., 1954) or of tyramine to dopamine (Holtz and Credner, 1943) has also been demonstrated.

3. Localization of Synthesis. Effect of Precursors

Noradrenaline synthesis takes place in the adrenergic neurons in immediate relation to the storage granules. Of the different enzymes partaking in the formation of the neurotransmitter, only the dopamine-β-hydroxylase has been found to be directly associated with the granules (Potter and Axelrod, 1963a, b) and these are a prerequisite for the final synthetic step (Stjärne and Lishajko, 1967). The newly synthesized noradrenaline is taken up and retained by the granules. The preceding enzymatic transformations from tyrosine are mediated by enzymes present extragranularly in the axoplasm (Stjärne, 1966). It is generally assumed that the enzymes engaged in the synthesis of noradrenaline are transported to the periphery by the axoplasmic flow (cf. Weiss, 1963) like much other material.

After inhibition of synthesis with the decarboxylase inhibitor decaborane-14 in the rabbit, dopamine but not DOPA, restored the deficient response to adrenergic nerve stimulation (BYGDEMAN and EULER, 1966). Although transmitter synthesis normally is adequate to maintain the stores at a level not far from the storage capacity, a certain deficit appears to exist, as concluded from the finding of increased amounts of transmitter in organs after inhibition of nerve activity by decentralization (REHN, 1958) or a neuronal blocker like bretylium (RYD, 1962). An increase of the order of 25—50% over the "normal" content is frequently found on injection of noradrenaline, its precursors, or by exclusion of nerve stimuli.

Access of precursors may also play a role in the rate of synthesis. Thus BALZER and PALM (1962) observed that pretreatment of mice with the MAO inhibitor iproniazid causes an increased influx of ^{14}C-α-aminobutyric acid in the brain. This may also hold true for amino acids serving as noradrenaline precursors (cf. HESS et al., 1959). Alterations in the permeability of the cell membrane may therefore play a part in the action of some MAO inhibitors (EHRINGER et al., 1961).

4. Synthesis Inhibitors

By inhibition of one or more of the enzymatic synthetic steps it should be theoretically possible to diminish the production of the adrenergic neurotransmitter. Such inhibition has been extensively studied partly with the aim to achieve therapeutic results (cf. MUSCHOLL, 1966a).

a) Tyrosine Hydroxylase Inhibitors

Of the three enzymatic steps, the formation of DOPA by tyrosine hydroxylase is the slowest and therefore rate-limiting. Consequently it would seem that an inhibition of this step should be most useful for the purpose of reducing noradrenaline formation. Several kinds of inhibitors have been described.

A certain degree of tyrosine hydroxylase inhibition has been observed with dopacetamide and some congeners in doses of 300 mg/kg (CARLSSON et al., 1963a).

α-Methyltyrosine, which like tyrosine is not a substrate for DOPA decarboxylase (SPECTOR et al., 1965), inhibits tyrosine hydroxylase in contrast to α-methyl DOPA and α-MMT. When α-methyltyrosine is given in amounts that lead to its accumulation in tissue in concentrations higher than those of the natural analogue (5×10^{-5}M), biosynthesis of DOPA is inhibited and the noradrenaline content of the organs lowered. (Fig. 2). On the other hand α-methyltyrosine does not inhibit the formation of dopamine from DOPA or 5-hydroxytryptamine from 5-HTP (Fig. 2).

The inhibition of tyrosine hydroxylase by α-methyltyrosine may cause severe signs of noradrenaline deficiency (SPECTOR et al., 1965). Notwithstanding its inhibitory effect, α-methyltyrosine is to some extent itself hydroxylated in the ring to α-methyl-DOPA and subsequently decarboxylated and β-oxidized to α-methylnoradrenaline (MAÎTRE, 1965).

Effects similar to those of α-methyltyrosine have been demonstrated for its dimethyl ester (H 44/68) (CORRODI and MALMFORS, 1966) which in a dose of 250 mg/kg lowers the noradrenaline stores in rat tissues. Strong inhibitory action has also been reported for 3-iodo-L-tyrosine (GOLDSTEIN and WEISS, 1965).

The noradrenaline depleting effect of H 44/68 has also been shown for adrenergic nerve fibres in the periphery, using the histochemical fluorescence technique of FALCK and HILLARP (CORRODI and MALMFORS, 1966). Of great functional interest is the observation that noradrenaline as well as dopamine strongly inhibit the tyrosine hydroxylase which may form the basis for a feedback control mechanism (NAGATSU et al., 1964; STJÄRNE, 1966).

Inhibition of tyrosine hydroxylase (and of dopamine-β-hydroxylase) has been observed with the pigment antibiotic chrothiomycin (AYUKAWA et al., 1969).

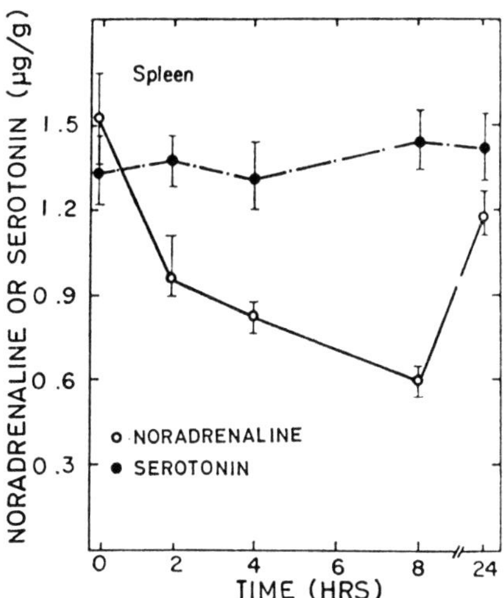

Fig. 2. Levels of noradrenaline and 5-hydroxytryptamine in the spleen of guinea pigs after administration of a single dose of α-methyltyrosine (80 mg/kg i.p.), mean and range (SPECTOR et al., 1965)

b) DOPA Decarboxylase Inhibitors

A number of DOPA decarboxylase inhibitors have been investigated by CLARK and his group (HARTMAN et al., 1955a; CLARK, 1959; CLARK and POGRUND, 1961). Active *in vitro* was e.g. 3-hydroxycinnamic acid although the inhibition *in vivo* was only moderate.

α-Methyl-DOPA and α-MMT exerted a marked inhibitory effect on DOPA decarboxylase as discovered by SOURKES (1954), while α-methylphenylalanine and α-methyltyrosine had only a weak effect. The inhibitory effect could also be shown *in vivo*; thus α-methyl-DOPA diminished the effect of DOPS on the blood pressure which depends on decarboxylation to noradrenaline (SCHMITERLÖW, 1951; DENGLER and REICHEL, 1957). After administration of DOPA to rats *in vivo*, α-methyl-DOPA decreased the excretion of dopamine in urine (MURPHY and SOURKES, 1961).

The fall in noradrenaline-content in various organs observed after α-methyl-DOPA and α-MMT (SOURKES et al., 1961a) does not seem to depend on decarboxylase inhibition since more active hydrazine derivatives lack the effect on the noradrenaline content of the heart and brain. It is therefore assumed that the noradrenaline depleting effect of α-methyl-DOPA and α-MMT is caused by partial substitution of the normal noradrenaline content through the decarboxylated products α-methyldopamine and α-methyl-meta-tyramine which after β-hydroxylation act as false transmitters (WEISSBACH et al., 1960; CARLSSON and LINDQVIST, 1962). This may contribute to the therapeutic effect of α-methyl-DOPA in the treatment of hypertension (OATES et al., 1960), although the β-hydroxylated products are quite efficient as sympathomimetic amines. α-methylnoradrenaline is readily taken up by the normal storage sites in the nerve granules and given off at a similar rate as noradrenaline. This explains the nearly quantitative exchange of noradrenaline for α-methylnoradrenaline (CARLSSON and LINDQVIST, 1962; SCHÜMANN and GROBECKER, 1964). It has been assumed that α-methylnoradrenaline is lost from organs at a slower rate than noradrenaline and also that it causes, by substituting noradrenaline in the CNS, some alteration in the function of the adrenergic system (HOLTZ, 1965; HENNING, 1969).

α) Derivatives of Hydrazine and Hydroxylamine

Strong inhibitory action *in vitro* on the DOPA decarboxylase is exerted by e.g. N-methyl-N (3-hydroxybenzyl)-hydrazine (NSD 1034) (BRODIE et al., 1962; LEVINE and SJOERDSMA, 1964), but this and similar compounds (NSD 1039, 1045) have only little effect on the endogenous amines. These compounds also inhibit the decarboxylation of α-methyl-DOPA and α-MMT (UDENFRIEND and ZALTZMAN-NIRENBERG, 1962), and counteract their blood pressure lowering effect in the hypertensive rat (DAVIS et al., 1963).

β) Decaborane

MERRITT et al. (1965) have shown that the boron hydride decaborane-14 ($B_{10}H_{14}$) lowers the noradrenaline content in the rat brain in doses of 10—20 mg/kg. Decaborane also causes noradrenaline depletion in a variety of tissues, notably the heart, brain and kidney (EULER and LISHAJKO, 1965a). After decaborane treatment the dopamine content in the brain after administration of DOPA is greatly diminished, and in other experiments MERRITT and SCHULTZ (1966) have shown that the decarboxylase activity is greatly lowered. The noradrenaline-depleting effect on the rabbit heart reaches a maximum about 24 hrs after a dose of 4—8 mg/kg intraperitoneally and remains for another 24 hrs whereafter the noradrenaline content gradually returns to normal. In the rabbit decaborane causes a rapid diminution of the response to sympathetic stimulation (BYGDEMAN and EULER, 1966). The effect of decaborane appears to depend on the inactivation of the co-factor pyridoxal-5′-phosphate and can be counteracted by injection of pyridoxine (WYKES and LANDEZ, 1967).

c) Dopamine ß-hydroxylase Inhibitors

Arylalkylamines such as phenylethylamine inhibit the transformation of dopamine to noradrenaline (GOLDSTEIN and CONTRERA, 1961) by competing for the hydroxylating sites of the storage granules.

α) Hydroxybenzyloxyamine

m-Hydroxybenzyloxyamine (NSD 1024) inhibits *in vivo* the formation of noradrenaline from dopamine in the heart (NIKODIJEVIC et al., 1963) and exerts similar inhibitor action on the oxidation of α-methyl-dopamine to α-methylnoradrenaline.

Although N-methyl-N-(3-hydroxybenzyl)-hydrazine (NSD 1034) in low doses is able to prevent the usual rise in noradrenaline in rat brain following a MAO-inhibitor (pargyline) even 200 mg/kg only lowers the normal noradrenaline content by 60% for a few hours (KUNTZMAN et al., 1962).

β) Disulfiram, Tropolone

Disulfiram (antabuse) inhibits aldehyde dehydrogenase and the hydroxylation of dopamine to noradrenaline by dopamine-β-hydroxylase. The active compound is diethyl-dithio-carbamate which is readily formed from disulfiram in the presence of ascorbic acid (ALBERT, 1961; GOLDSTEIN et al., 1964a). It serves as chelator like 8-hydroxy-quinoline, 2,2′-dipyridyl, and EDTA, and inhibits the dopamine-β-hydroxylase which probably is a metal proteid. Also active as inhibitors in this group are 4-methyl- and 4-isopropyltropolone (GOLDSTEIN et al., 1964b)

Disulfiram in a dose of 400 mg/kg lowers the noradrenaline content of the rat heart by about 50% and also prevents the formation and storage of octopamine after administration of tyramine (MUSACCHIO et al., 1964).

The enzyme was found to be relatively insensitive to hormones and reserpine, but was markedly inhibited by thyroxine or benzyloxyamines (NAGATSU et al., 1968).

d) Reserpine

The rapid depletion of noradrenaline stores in organs and adrenergic nerves by reserpine has raised the question as to whether this drug affects synthesis as well as binding to the granules. In experiments with homogenized splenic nerves and with splenic nerve trunk particles the conversion of dopamine to noradrenaline was found to be inhibited by reserpine (STJÄRNE and LISHAJKO, 1966; ROTH and STONE, 1968), suggesting that an altered ability of the granules to take up catecholamines after reserpine treatment prevents the final synthetic step. On the other hand, some observations seem to indicate that reserpine does not seriously impair the noradrenaline synthesis in tissues. Thus GLOWINSKI et al. (1966a) found a considerable degree of noradrenaline synthesis from various precursors in the brain of the reserpinized rat and concluded that synthesis proceeds essentially in a normal fashion, although it may be somewhat hampered by diminished availability of dopamine. Observations on the excretion of free noradrenaline and of 3-methoxy-4-hydroxy mandelic acid in the urine of rats treated with reserpine (WENNMALM, 1968) also support the view that reserpine interferes only to a moderate extent with noradrenaline synthesis (cf. RUTLEDGE and WEINER, 1967).

The fact that noradrenaline synthesis continues even after reserpine depletion of the noradrenaline stores suggests that the ability of the storage particles to take up and bind the product, noradrenaline, is not a prerequisite for its formation. If noradrenaline is not taken up this may be assumed to hold true also for dopamine. Oxidation of dopamine may therefore occur without the amine entering the storage particle.

In the experiments of ROTH and STONE (1968) it was observed that the inhibitory effect of reserpine on noradrenaline synthesis was partly reversed by the MAO inhibitor pargyline in intact nerves, in contrast to isolated nerve particles (STJÄRNE and LISHAJKO, 1966), possibly by increasing the intraaxonal dopamine levels.

The membrane-active drugs prenylamine and phenoxybenzamine also inhibit noradrenaline synthesis at the β-hydroxylation step (STJÄRNE and LISHAJKO, 1966), presumably by preventing access of dopamine to the active sites in the storage particles.

5. Induction and Regulation of Synthesis

Increased adrenergic nerve activity enhances the synthesis of noradrenaline in the nerve terminals as evidenced by the rise in the excretion of noradrenaline in urine (EULER, 1954) and of its metabolites (ARMSTRONG and MCMILLAN, 1959), without lowering of the amounts in the stores.

The effect of nerve stimulation on the synthesis of noradrenaline was first demonstrated for the cat spleen *in vivo*; after 10 min stimulation of its nerves there was no significant reduction of its noradrenaline content in spite of a considerable release of transmitter (EULER and HELLNER-BJÖRKMAN, 1955). Similar results have been obtained on the isolated perfused spleen by DEARNALEY and GEFFEN (1966), who observed a fall of only 7.7% of the original noradrenaline content after nerve stimulation. The outflow of transmitter caused by nerve stimulation (cf. BROWN, 1965) directly indicates that synthesis is increased under these conditions since the transmitter content is practically unchanged. The relative constancy of the noradrenaline content in organs during varying conditions suggests that the regulatory mechanism possesses a high degree of precision. As a likely system it has been proposed that, after noradrenaline release, the lowered concentration at some strategic point in the storage system elicits resynthesis, presumably by removal of an inhibitory action (negative feedback control). This concept has received support by the experimental results of NAGATSU et al. (1964) and UDENFRIEND et al. (1965). Thus the hydroxylation of tyrosine, the rate-limiting step, is significantly inhibited by noradrenaline 2×10^{-4}M in the medium. STJÄRNE (1966) and STJÄRNE et al. (1967b) found that noradrenaline inhibits synthesis to more than 90% even at 2.4×10^{-5}M concentration, and since dopamine formation was less affected, the results suggest inhibition also at the final step (Fig. 3). Binding of noradrenaline to the tyrosine hydroxylase has been reported by IKEDA et al. (1966).

If the concentration of transmitter is increased by a MAO inhibitor, the conversion of labelled tyrosine to noradrenaline is decreased (SPECTOR et al., 1967), which is in harmony with the above concept.

The remarkable and continuous increase in adrenergic transmitter release observed after administration of reserpine in conjunction with a MAO inhibitor (CHESSIN et al., 1957), suggesting increased synthesis, may partly be due to derailment of the regulating system caused by the two drugs in combination. Increased tyrosine hydroxylase activity has been observed in the rat superior cervical ganglia and the rabbit brain stem after reserpine with increased V_{max} for both tyrosine and the pteridine co-factor (MUELLER et al., 1969 a).

The effect of direct and reflex nerve stimulation in increasing noradrenaline synthesis has been observed on various organs (GORDON et al., 1966a, b; ALOUSI and WEINER, 1966; OLIVERIO and STJÄRNE, 1965; AUSTIN et al., 1967; SEDVALL and KOPIN, 1967; WEINER and RABADJIJA, 1968). The effect is not accompanied by an increase in tyrosine hydroxylase activity *in vitro*, which supports the concept of a functional interaction of the product with the synthesizing system.

Noradrenaline synthesis from tyrosine in the isolated guinea pig vas deferens was found to increase 3 times by nerve stimulation (ROTH et al., 1967). The enhancement of synthesis was not dependent on the response of the organ since the same effect was seen when the motor effects of stimulation were inhibited by Hydergine. The effect is not due to increased conversion of dopamine to noradrenaline but is presumably a result of increased tyrosine hydroxylase activity. On the other hand, no increase in synthesis rate occurred on stimulation of the isolated bovine splenic nerve. It is doubtful, however, whether stimulation of the nerve trunk causes release of transmitter as in the isolated organ.

A compensatory increase in adrenal tyrosine hydroxylase activity has been found after chemical sympathectomy produced by 6-hydroxydopamine which destroys the adrenergic nerve endings and depletes the noradrenaline stores (MUELLER et al., 1969b). As shown by DEQUATTRO et al. (1968) sinoaortic denervation of the rabbit caused an increased enzyme activity.

Since the tyrosine hydroxylase activity may also be altered by preganglionic nerve stimulation (THOENEN et al., 1969) it has been suggested that the neural control can be accomplished by two mechanisms 1. rapid changes in end-product inhibition or availability of substrate at the enzyme site, and, 2. gradual alterations in the amount of tyrosine hydroxylase in response to prolonged nerve stimulation (MUELLER et al., 1969a).

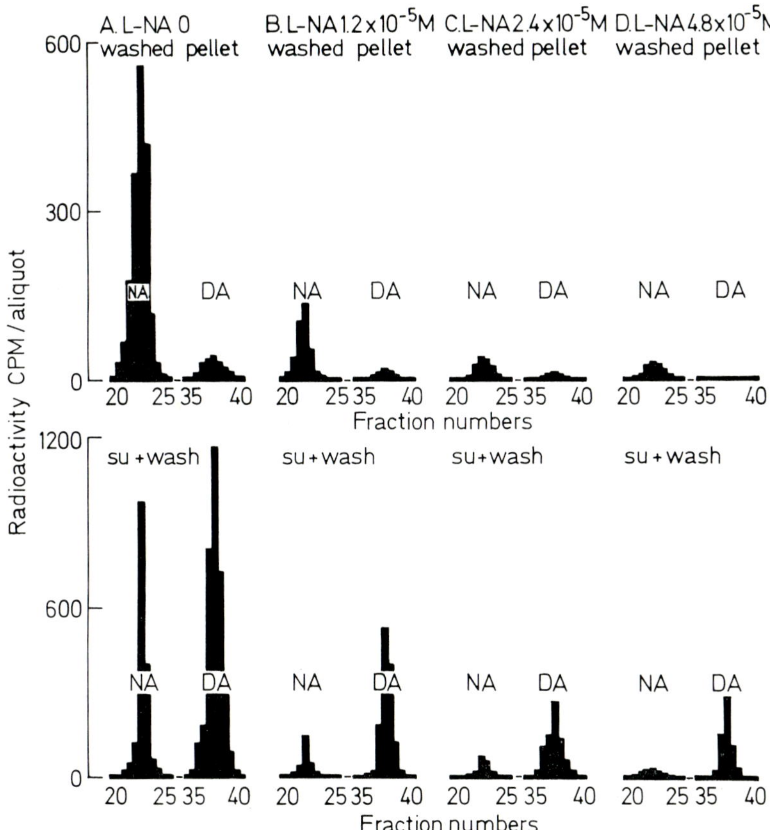

Fig. 3. Inhibition of the noradrenaline and dopamine formation from tyrosine in microsomal fractions of splenic nerve homogenate by addition of noradrenaline to the incubation medium in different concentrations (*A*—*D*). Ion exchange chromatogram fractions. *L-NA*, *NA*, (—)-noradrenaline; *DA*, dopamine; *SU*, supernatant (STJÄRNE et al., 1967b)

Muscular exercise, which strongly increases the noradrenaline output (KÄRKI, 1956), also enhances the activity of tyrosine hydroxylase (AXELROD et al., 1970).

Of drugs which have been reported to stimulate tyrosine hydroxylase, there may be mentioned thyroxine (BAGCHI and MCGEER, 1964) and α-adrenergic blocking agents (DAIRMAN et al., 1968). With the blocking agents no increase in enzyme activity *in vitro* was observed. Since α-adrenergic blockers inhibit noradrenaline uptake in isolated nerve particles as well as release (EULER and LISHAJKO, 1968b) the effect may be the result of either reflexly induced nerve activity or diminished end-product inhibition.

In isolated rat and guinea pig atria and in rat vas deferens angiotensin increases the formation of noradrenaline from tyrosine (BOADLE et al., 1969).

Increased *de novo* synthesis has been seen in the rat heart following hypophysectomy (LANDSBERG et al., 1969). This occurred concomitantly with increased turnover, reflecting thyroid and adrenal deficiency (LANDSBERG and AXELROD, 1968a) and was accompanied by reduced accumulation of ^{3}H-noradrenaline in the rat heart (LANDSBERG and AXELROD, 1968b).

6. Synthesis Rate and Kinetics

The rate of noradrenaline synthesis has been estimated *in vivo* and *in vitro* during different experimental conditions. The rate (measured as μg/g.hr) can be expected to vary widely in different organs as a result of variations in both the rate of release and the size of the stores; the latter may vary from near zero to values of about 10 μg/g depending on the organ.

In order to make results more comparable, data for synthesis rate may be expressed in % of the normal noradrenaline content per g tissue per hr.

PAULSEN and HESS (1963) have reported synthesis rates for noradrenaline of about 0.03 μg/g.hr in the guinea pig heart, depleted after administration of the benzoquinolizine compound, RO 4—1284, or of the methyl ester of methyl reserpate, Su 9064. A similar value for resynthesis was found in the guinea pig brain in which the noradrenaline content was reduced by electroshock.

The amounts of noradrenaline synthesized from tyrosine in the isolated guinea pig heart have been calculated to 0.03—0.05 μg/g.hr (SPECTOR et al., 1963a) but values may be considerably higher at high release rates. Synthesis rate has been calculated on the basis of the disappearance of radioactive noradrenaline incorporated when the organ content was constant (UDENFRIEND and ZALTZMAN-NIRENBERG, 1963; MONTANARI et al., 1963) or by means of the rate of loss of transmitter after synthesis.

Values between 0.03 and 0.10 μg/g.hr have been reported for various organs (CROUT, 1962; POTTER and AXELROD, 1963b; MONTANARI et al., 1963). In the isolated bovine splenic nerve the rate of noradrenaline synthesis from tyrosine was 0.15—0.20 μg/g.hr (ROTH et al., 1967).

At a half-life of 7 hrs for incorporated ^{3}H-noradrenaline, the rate of loss is about 10% per hr and, given a constant total noradrenaline value of 1 μg/g and a regular distribution and release of the label, synthesis proceeds at the rate of 0.1 μg/g.hr. There is some evidence, however, that the release does not affect the stores in a proportionate way but that there is a preference for the release of newly synthesized material. In such case the loss of label is delayed and the rate of synthesis higher than indicated by the half-life (KOPIN et al., 1968).

In perfusion experiments on the isolated guinea pig heart a K_m value for the overall conversion of tyrosine to noradrenaline has been found which is the same as that for tyrosine conversion to DOPA, or 10^{-5}M (SPECTOR et al., 1963a). A more detailed study of the kinetics of bovine adrenal tyrosine hydroxylase has been reported by IKEDA et al. (1966).

The kinetics of the dopamine β-oxidation reaction has been examined in detail by GOLDSTEIN et al. (1968).

The approximate K_m values for the enzymes taking part in catecholamine synthesis are, according to UDENFRIEND (1968)

Tyrosine hydroxylase 1×10^{-5}M
DOPA decarboxylase 4×10^{-4}M
Dopamine-β-hydroxylase 5×10^{-3}M

From these constants UDENFRIEND has concluded that the enzymes must occur in close connection since the intermediates do not accumulate.

II. Uptake

1. Introduction

Normally the adrenergic nerves, like the organs which receive a supply of these nerves, contain a characteristic amount of neurotransmitter, subject to only moderate changes both in loss and gain even under greatly varying activity conditions (EULER, 1951; EULER and HELLNER-BJÖRKMAN, 1955; DEARNALEY and GEFFEN, 1966). This suggests a limited storing capacity, presumably structurally and chemically determined, and normally utilized to an extent allowing only a small or moderate complementary uptake.

Exogenous noradrenaline can be taken up to various extents (RAAB and GIGEE, 1953) but is only temporarily stored. Thus after a limited time the organ content returns to its normal value. The granular stores are capable of taking up and storing also adrenaline; this explains why the uptake in tissues after administration of this amine is more readily detectable: it partly substitutes for noradrenaline in the specific stores (STRÖMBLAD and NICKERSON, 1961; EULER and LISHAJKO, 1963a; ANDÉN, 1964; WESTFALL, 1965).

The availability of radioactively highly labelled noradrenaline has afforded a method of high precision and usefulness, introduced and successfully used in its present form by AXELROD and his co-workers since 1959.

A problem which has not been fully elucidated is whether tracer amounts of highly labelled amines are distributed in a way truly representative of the endogenous distribution in the organism under all conditions.

While uptake studies with the use of semi-tracer amounts of noradrenaline appear at present to give consistent and accurate results, it may under some circumstances be advantageous to study bulk uptake after previous depletion of the stores (cf. p. 202).

For the interpretation and evaluation of uptake experiments distinction has to be made between uptake through the axonal membrane and uptake into the specific stores, particularly since some drugs have different actions on the uptake at these two sites. So far there seems to be no direct method which allows studies to be made of the effect of various drugs and other factors on the uptake through the axonal membrane. However, by comparing the effect of drugs on the total uptake in nerves, for instance by the fluorescence histochemical technique of FALCK and HILLARP, with that in the storage particles, it is sometimes possible to decide whether an uptake inhibition is located at one or the other site. Thus reserpine inhibits noradrenaline uptake in storage particles but not in the axon (MALMFORS, 1965). On the other hand isopropylnoradrenaline is hardly taken up by tissues (ANDÉN et al., 1964; HERTTING, 1964), while it is readily incorporated in isolated particles (EULER and LISHAJKO, 1967b).

Catecholamine uptake in the tissues has become the subject of numerous studies of which only a limited number can be discussed in the present survey. It has been attempted to include those studies in the first place which deal with specific uptake in the normal physiologically relevant stores. An extensive bibliography on uptake is found in the monograph of IVERSEN (1967).

2. Uptake of Catecholamines in Organs and Tissues

Functional uptake of catecholamines was demonstrated as early as 1933 by BURN, who observed a modification of the effect of nerve stimulation after adding adrenaline to the perfusion fluid used for the hindleg of the dog. In most of the studies of amine uptake (e.g. BURN and RAND, 1958) various proportions of the injected amines were in all probability unspecifically located and disappeared relatively rapidly from their deposits. Using highly radioactive catecholamines Axelrod et al. (1959) were able, however, to distinguish for the first time between a specific and a non-specific uptake after injection of 0.1 mg/kg ^{3}H-adrenaline intravenously to mice. They observed that a large proportion of the dose, about 70%, disappeared from the body in some 5 min, whereafter the remaining 30% disappeared more slowly. The experiment thus showed that a certain proportion became bound more firmly and was released at a slow rate. In experiments with highly labelled noradrenaline the results were similar (Whitby et al., 1961), but an interesting difference could be noted, in that a higher proportion of noradrenaline than of adrenaline was specifically bound. As already mentioned, isoprenaline is taken up even less efficiently (Andén et al., 1964). Since all three amines are equally well taken up, and stored by the specific storage particles the differentiation must occur at the axon membrane which therefore appears to constitute a neuronal barrier, allowing preferential uptake of the natural neurotransmitter.

After injection of a large dose of noradrenaline into puppies most of the amine recovered from the heart was located in the soluble fraction of a homogenate after sedimentation, indicating that it was not specifically bound (Wegmann and Kako, 1961). Binding of noradrenaline, administered in large doses, to certain tissues such as smooth muscle cells has been studied by Gillespie (1968) with the aid of the fluorescence technique. For further references see Trendelenburg (1971).

Uptake of catecholamines in brain has recently become the subject of numerous studies after introduction of a technique allowing administration of amines directly into the brain ventricles (Glowinski et al., 1965; Glowinski and Axelrod, 1965). From these and other studies it has become evident that the brain contains specific stores capable of binding catecholamines.

3. Uptake in Adrenergic Nerves

The main specific storage sites for noradrenaline are found in the adrenergic nerves, and it is in agreement with this fact that the distribution of labelled noradrenaline after injection is roughly proportionate to the amount of the transmitter normally present in the different organs (Whitby et al., 1961); this in turn is closely related to the supply of adrenergic nerves. In experiments on the developing rat the accumulation of ^{3}H-noradrenaline occurred parallel to the endogenous noradrenaline content (Iversen et al., 1967). For the distribution of injected label both turnover rate and blood flow in relation to the size of the store are important. If these parameters have low values the conditions for labelling are correspondingly less favourable, as for instance in the adrenal medulla (cf. Wurtman et al., 1964).

Uptake in nerves has been well illustrated by autoradiographic technique. Samorajski et al. (1964) found a deposition of silver over adrenergic nerves in the heart after injection of ^{3}H-noradrenaline in the cat (Fig. 4).

The uptake of radioactive noradrenaline in isolated splenic nerve bundles has been studied by Stjärne et al. (1970a). The concentration of the amine was relatively small, which may be associated with the limited stores.

After degeneration of the adrenergic nerves the transmitter stores are greatly diminished or disappear (Cannon and Lissák, 1939; Goodall, 1951; Euler and Purkhold, 1951). Under these conditions there is a greatly reduced specific uptake of noradrenaline in the organs (Hertting et al., 1961a; Strömblad and Nickerson, 1961). Similarly, after immuno-sympathectomy in rats and mice, the uptake of ^{3}H-noradrenaline is greatly reduced (Zaimis et al., 1965).

A certain uptake nevertheless occurs in the absence of adrenergic nerves but this is presumably of non-specific character (ANDÉN et al., 1963). Nerve free tissue like the placenta lacks endogenous noradrenaline and consequently presents no specific storage sites for uptake of circulating amines under normal conditions (EULER, 1951). It is not known to what extent the placenta takes up catecholamines unspecifically after an injection.

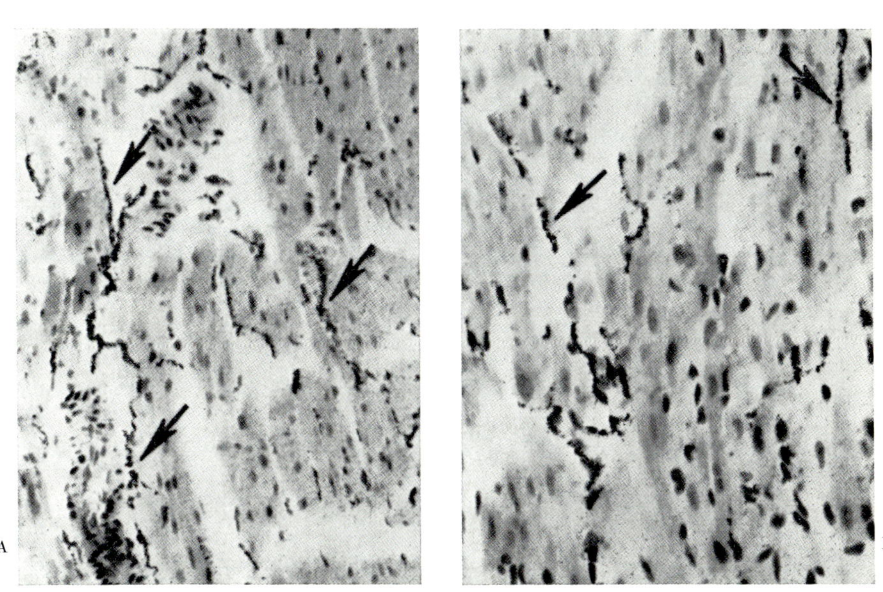

Fig. 4. A Autoradiography of heart muscle 2 min after intravenous injection of ^{3}H-noradrenaline; loci of uptake indicated by arrows. 162×. B Localization of radioactivity in heart muscle 2 hrs after intraperitoneal injection of ^{3}H-noradrenaline. 162× (SAMORAJSKI et al., 1964)

With the histochemical fluorescence technique of FALCK and HILLARP it has been shown that in the rat iris, previously depleted of noradrenaline by reserpine, noradrenaline after injection accumulates in the adrenergic nerve fibres, including the cell bodies and the terminals (HAMBERGER et al., 1964). Combined radioautography and fluorescence technique have also been used, with similar results (GILLESPIE and KIRPEKAR, 1965).

The ease with which noradrenaline is taken up and incorporated in the specific neuronal stores, as evidenced by the rapid uptake in depleted stores (EULER and LISHAJKO, 1965a; BHATTACHARYA, 1968), suggests that some of the released transmitter may be recaptured in the axon, and, depending on the available sites, either bound to specific stores or metabolized.

Precise information as to the proportion of released transmitter recaptured by the axon terminal is for obvious reasons difficult to obtain. Some authors claim that more than 90% of the released transmitter is recaptured (HAEFELY et al., 1964) which would mean that less than 10% of the released transmitter is lost and also that release and uptake are simultaneous processes during continuous adrenergic nerve activity.

As a method of estimating the recapture, use has often been made of drugs which inhibit the passage of the amines through the axonal membrane. Such drugs are cocaine, desipramine, protriptyline and its congeners, and phenoxybenzamine.

It has been reasoned that if re-uptake occurs, a blocking of the membrane should increase the outflow from a perfused organ as a result of nerve stimulation.

While the results obtained with uptake blockers like cocaine (BROWN, 1965) or desipramine (GEFFEN, 1965) at times indicate a weak action on the outflow in the perfused, stimulated cat spleen they generally cause an increase of 2—3 times (cf. STJÄRNE and WENNMALM, 1971). Phenoxybenzamine and other α-blockers, on the other hand, regularly cause a marked increase in the outflow under these conditions.

Although it may be safely assumed that under favourable conditions a certain re-uptake at the axonal level takes place, the importance of this mechanism under normal conditions is difficult to assess. Noradrenaline and its metabolites are continuously present in blood plasma and excreted in urine in amounts which are roughly parallel to the activity of adrenergic nerves. An increased outflow after certain drugs might also depend on releasing action of these drugs per se.

For exogenous circulating amines the temporary uptake in adrenergic axons as well as in extraneuronal tissue probably represents the most important mechanism for the inactivation of the amines (AXELROD, 1965) although the uptake in the specific binding sites may be small.

4. Specific Uptake in Storage Particles

After uptake in adrenergic nerves a certain proportion of released or injected catecholamines is deposited in the storage particles and specifically bound (EULER and LISHAJKO, 1965a; MACKENNA, 1965), as readily observed after previous depletion. This part is not freely diffusible as evidenced by the stability of the particles at low temperature (EULER and LISHAJKO, 1963a), their insensitivity to oxidizing agents (EULER and LISHAJKO, 1967a) and inability to become adsorbed on alumina.

Evidence for the uptake of catecholamines into the specific storage sites has been provided by electron microscope autoradiography, using radioactive noradrenaline which accumulated in sympathetic axons in the rat pineal body (WOLFE et al., 1962). Accumulation of silver grains in the region of the particles in bovine splenic nerves is shown in Fig. 5. The results obtained with the histochemical fluorescence technique are also compatible with this conclusion (CORRODI et al., 1966).

More detailed information on the specific uptake has been obtained by studies on isolated nerve particles. On incubation of a suspension of splenic nerve particles in isotonic sucrose or potassium phosphate there is a continuous release of noradrenaline, increasing in rate with temperature (EULER and LISHAJKO, 1963a, 1967a). The release is partly compensated by re-uptake, depending on the concentration of noradrenaline in the medium as evidenced by the incorporation of labelled noradrenaline in the particles. At a noradrenaline concentration of about 10^{-4}M the reuptake almost wholly compensates for the loss by release at 20°C.

After partial depletion of the noradrenaline content of the particles a net uptake occurs, whereby the uptake of noradrenaline from the incubation medium is greatly facilitated by ATP and other nucleotides in the presence of Mg (EULER and LISHAJKO, 1963b, 1969) (Fig. 6). After re-uptake as well as net uptake the noradrenaline incorporated in particles is released in the same way as the endogenous noradrenaline.

Uptake in particles as well as in organs shows a certain degree of stereoselectivity. Thus the uptake of the (+)-isomers of noradrenaline and adrenaline is considerably smaller than that of the (—)-isomers (ANDÉN, 1964; WESTFALL, 1965;

EULER and LISHAJKO, 1965a) whereas the two isomers are given off at the same rate *in vivo* and from isolated particles.

The amine uptake in nerve particles is not strictly specific since in addition to noradrenaline also adrenaline, isoprenaline, octopamine, α-methylnoradrenaline

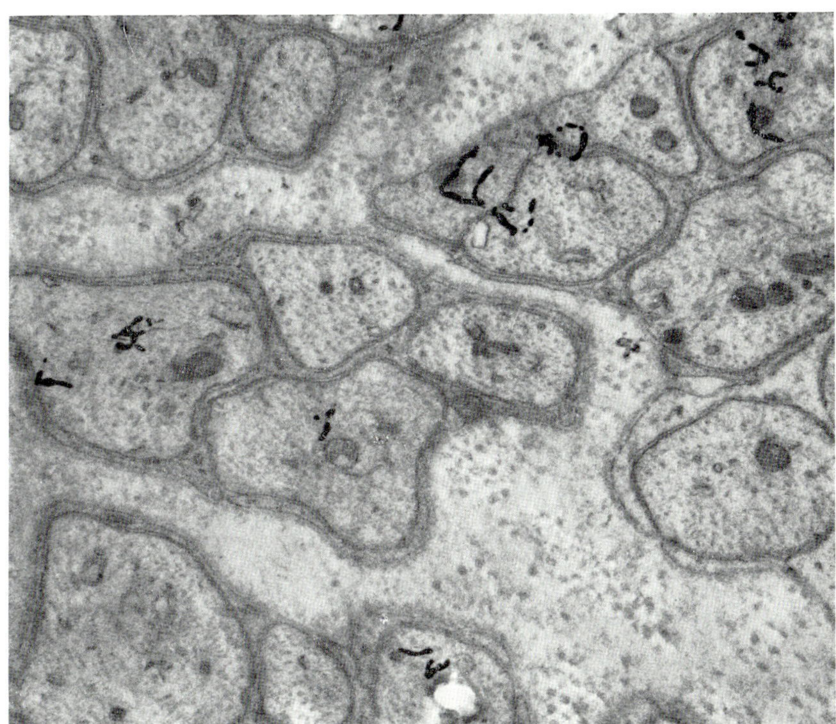

Fig. 5. Autoradiographic electron micrograph of bovine splenic nerve after incubation with ^{3}H-noradrenaline. $\times 25000$ (STJÄRNE et al., 1970a)

and metaraminol can be taken up and stored (EULER and LISHAJKO, 1968a; 1970). A small uptake of dopamine has also been observed after treatment with disulfiram and a MAO-inhibitor (GOLDSTEIN et al., 1964a; MUSACCHIO et al., 1964, 1965a, b). However, even after previous depletion of the noradrenaline stores with decaborane, inhibition of dopamine β-oxidase with disulfiram, and a MAO inhibitor, the uptake of dopamine in the stores is small while noradrenaline is readily taken up (SHAHAB et al., 1971). Infusion of dopamine 1 μg/ml in the isolated rat heart did not cause any substitution of noradrenaline (PESKAR et al., 1968). Some of the dopamine taken up may be stored in dopamine particles present in the heart (ANGELAKOS et al., 1963).

The proportion of uptake of adrenaline in the nerve particles depends on the relative concentrations of adrenaline and noradrenaline (cf. STRÖMBLAD and NICKERSON, 1961; WESTFALL 1965). Whether the specific stores in nerves contain adrenaline in cases of phaeochromocytoma where the plasma concentration may reach values of 3×10^{-7}M adrenaline, is not known, but the proportion of adrenaline would in any event be low.

If uptake of administered catecholamines has taken place at the specific sites it should be possible to demonstrate release of the amine upon nerve stimulation.

This has been shown in the early experiments of BURN (1933) who found that the vasoconstrictor effect of nerve stimulation reappeared in the perfused leg after adding adrenaline to the blood reservoir. Release of labelled amine upon nerve stimulation was shown by HERTTING and AXELROD (1961). After decentralization of the rat salivary gland and the iris the disappearance of labelled noradrenaline was slower than in the normally innervated organs, indicating that the release is enhanced by the normally occurring nerve impulses. Similarly, ganglionic blocking agents slowed the release of ^{3}H-noradrenaline from the heart (HERTTING et al., 1962).

5. Bulk Uptake of Catecholamines after Depletion

While the physiological uptake process is obviously less open to study when the stores are filled to capacity or nearly so, it is possible to study specific uptake after depletion, particularly after giving inhibitors of synthesis which do not seem to interfere with uptake. Thus after decarboxylase inhibition by decaborane-14, which causes a severe depletion of the noradrenaline content of rabbit heart and kidney 24—48 hrs after administration, the injection of noradrenaline in doses of 0.05 mg/kg i.v. or 0.3—0.4 mg/kg intramuscularly rapidly refills the stores to nearly normal values (EULER and LISHAJKO, 1965a). Analysis of subcellular fractions showed that distribution of noradrenaline between particles and supernatant was normal.

The effect of various drugs on the bulk uptake of noradrenaline in the isolated perfused rat heart previously depleted by decaborane has been studied by BHATTACHARYA (1968) (cf. Section B. II. 6).

The histochemical fluorescence technique has also been used for the demonstration of bulk uptake after previous depletion of the endogenous noradrenaline by synthesis inhibitors (CORRODI et al., 1966; MALMFORS and EULER, 1971).

Bulk uptake in the rabbit heart has also been demonstrated after noradrenaline-depletion with prenylamine (MACKENNA, 1965), while the subcellular distribution in different fractions after homogenization was essentially normal.

6. Uptake Estimated by Perfusate Deficit Studies

By measuring the loss of amine in the perfusion fluid after passage through an organ it has been possible to arrive at an estimation of the uptake through the organ. As observed by PAK (1926) and LUND (1951), perfusion of a solution of adrenaline or noradrenaline through the liver leads to an almost complete disappearance of the biological activity of the outflowing solution. BACQ (1937) has found that the kidney also possesses strong inactivating power, and subsequently several organs have been found to remove catecholamines from the perfusion fluid to different extents. An inactivation of this kind is presumably operating continuously under physiological conditions. If no net uptake occurs, removal equals inactivation with the exception of the small percentage excreted unchanged. In man only about 1.5—2% of the infused catecholamines is excreted as such (EULER and LUFT, 1951), indicating that the major part is rapidly metabolized and inactivated.

Of the amount of catecholamines eliminated by the isolated rat heart 90% was retained (LINDMAR and MUSCHOLL, 1964). In the cat spleen 40—70%, depending on the concentration, is lost during the passage, partly by retention, partly by inactivation (GILLESPIE and KIRPEKAR, 1965). In bulk uptake studies after depletion, as much as 40% of the noradrenaline perfused may be taken up and recovered as noradrenaline in the organ when noradrenaline was perfused in a concentration of 10^{-7}M (BHATTACHARYA, 1968). At increasing concentrations of noradrenaline the total amount taken up by the organ as a rule increases (cf. IVERSEN, 1963) and a part of this is temporarily distributed in various kinds of cells (cf. GILLESPIE, 1968). (For discussion of extraneuronal uptake, see TRENDELENBURG, 1971). The ability to remove catecholamines from the perfusing fluid varies considerably in different organs, depending on cell types, vascularization, adrenergic nerve supply and other factors (cf. LUND, 1951).

7. The Uptake Process

It has frequently been stated that the uptake of catecholamines in adrenergic nerves occurs against a concentration gradient. This is true insofar as the concentration of noradrenaline in the plasma after injection of the amine may be considerably lower than the amount of noradrenaline found per unit weight in the tissue, and presumably very much lower than that present at the specific uptake sites. Yet an uptake, e.g. of labelled amines, can be readily demonstrated. Part of this uptake is of exchange character since a steady release and re-uptake appears to take place both at the axonal membrane and at the level of the storage particle. The gradient on the other hand may be largely apparent, since the transmitter amine bound in the storage particles is osmotically inert. Uptake of the transmitter in the stores will then proceed as long as storage sites are available.

As observed by DENGLER et al. (1961) the uptake of ^{3}H-noradrenaline in slices of heart and brain from the cat becomes saturated at a concentration in the medium of 25 ng/ml (1.5×10^{-7}M), when uptake seems to assume the characteristics of diffusion.

The uptake of ^{3}H-noradrenaline in the isolated rat heart has been extensively studied by IVERSEN (1963) using concentrations of 10—1000 ng/ml. The net uptake in the heart increased with time (over a period of 30 min) and with the concentration of ^{3}H-noradrenaline in the medium and reached values of 1.5 μg/g, about three times the normal noradrenaline content. A large part of this noradrenaline is presumably located outside the specific stores, since these amounts cannot be maintained without continuous supply.

From the initial uptake rates the Michaelis-Menten constants have been computed (IVERSEN, 1963). As seen in Table I the K_m for (—)-noradrenaline was estimated at 0.27×10^{-6}M. In later experiments on the iris and ciliary body IVERSEN (1968) found an "affinity constant" of 1.4×10^{-6}M.

Table I. *Kinetic constants for catecholamine uptake in rat heart at perfusion concentrations 10—500 ng/ml* (IVERSEN, 1963)

Compound	K_m $M \times 10^{-6}$	V_{max} μg/min/g heart
(±)-noradrenaline	0.67	0.23
(—)-noradrenaline	0.27	0.20
(+)-noradrenaline	1.39	0.29
(±)-adrenaline	1.40	0.19

In isolated storage particles (EULER and LISHAJKO, 1967a; cf. EULER, 1970) the K_m values for the reuptake of noradrenaline as well as for the ATP-stimulated net uptake were about 1.5×10^{-6}M, which is close to the value reported by IVERSEN for the iris/ciliary body. Similar values were obtained for the uptake of noradrenaline in the perfused lung (HUGHES et al., 1969) and rat iris (JONSSON et al., 1969).

Kinetics of the dopamine-uptake in the isolated rat heart have been studied by PESKAR et al. (1968) who found a value of 0.68×10^{-6}M.

A second uptake process, operating when high concentrations of catecholamines are used in the perfusion medium, has been described by IVERSEN (1965). Binding occurred to some as yet unidentified structures, and at a perfusion concentration of adrenaline of 5 μg/ml the uptake of adrenaline in the rat heart was about 10 μg/g in 5 min or about 15 times the normal content. A large uptake of catecholamines in the spleen has been described by AVAKIAN and GILLESPIE (1968), using analytical and histochemical techniques. Except in adrenergic nerves, uptake was observed in arterial smooth muscle and collagen. For a histochemically visible uptake of this kind, concentrations above 10 μg/ml in the perfusion fluid were required. (For detailed accounts of the uptake studied with high concentrations of catecholamines see IVERSEN [1967] and GILLESPIE [1968]).

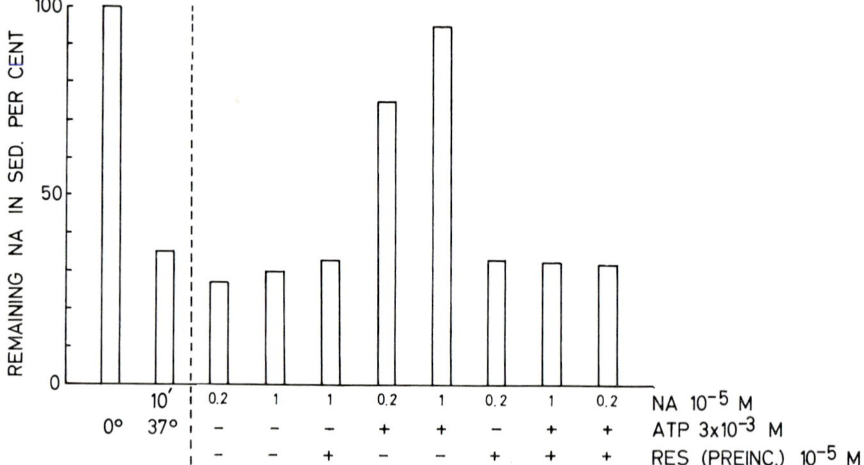

Fig. 6. Isolated splenic nerve particles incubated in phosphate buffer. Per cent noradrenaline of original. After partial depletion (10 min 37°) continued incubation (30 min 20°) with net uptake after addition of ATP. Note no net uptake after reserpine (EULER and LISHAJKO, unpubl.)

The uptake of ^{3}H-noradrenaline in heart slices is also dependent on the presence of Na^{+} in the medium. Substitution of Na^{+} for Li^{+} or K^{+} almost completely blocked the ability of the tissue to concentrate the amine. In isotonic sucrose, however, some uptake occurred (BOGDANSKI and BRODIE, 1966). (For reference see also IVERSEN and KRAVITZ, 1966).

The importance of ATP for catecholamine uptake has been shown for adrenal medullary particles by CARLSSON et al. (1963b) and by KIRSHNER (1962). In isolated adrenergic nerve granules ATP strongly facilitates reuptake as well as net uptake of noradrenaline (EULER and LISHAJKO, 1963b, 1969) (Fig. 6).

Stimulation of noradrenaline uptake in isolated storage particles is also observed with ADP, ITP, CTP and UTP, but not with AMP or cyclic AMP. An interesting difference is noted between nerve particles and adrenal medullary particles, in that the latter show no net uptake of catecholamines after partial depletion (LISHAJKO, 1969). Moreover, uptake in medullary particles is not enhanced by ADP.

It has been assumed that the ATPase present in nerve particles as well as in adrenal medullary particles is in some way involved in the amine uptake process (TAUGNER and HASSELBACH, 1966; PHILIPPU et al., 1967; BURGER et al., 1968). Some observations on the action of metabolic inhibitors are compatible with this concept (EULER and LISHAJKO, 1969).

From the data accumulated it appears that the amine "uptake" is of two principally different kinds, specific uptake in special stores and non-specific accumulation in neurons as well as in other tissue cells. The specific stores seem to be of different kinds and it is generally assumed that the main granular store is supplemented by a more "peripheral" store, perhaps in the axon membrane, from which the immediate release occurs (cf. STJÄRNE, 1964; EULER, 1970).

The final uptake in storage particles is subject to a large number of influences of physical and chemical nature. In addition to temperature, pH, and metabolic factors a variety of drugs act on this process. Reserpine is a potent inhibitor of the ATP-stimulated uptake, but several other drugs have similar though less persistant actions. Most of these cause transmitter depletion *in vivo*.

There are some indications that the uptake process in particles is an active, energy-requiring process. Thus the uptake is greatly facilitated by ATP and apparently dependent on a functioning respiratory chain and oxidative phosphorylation (EULER and LISHAJKO, 1969). The effect of uncouplers suggest that phosphorylation processes are of importance for uptake as well as for retention of the transmitter. Interference with one or several of the mechanisms involved, for instance by drugs, may therefore cause disturbances in uptake and release, and consequently influence the transmitter content of an organ.

The finding that the noradrenaline uptake — both *in vivo* and in isolated particles — is inhibited by α-blockers may be of significance for elucidating the binding mechanism of the transmitter to the receptors in particles as well as in effector cells.

It is worth noticing that many of the findings reported as regards uptake of noradrenaline and other amines in adrenergic neurons and their specific transmitter stores seem to have a certain parallel in the 5-hydroxytryptamine uptake in platelets and their intracellular storage particles (cf. DA PRADA and PLETSCHER, 1968). The platelets in these respects thus appear to behave like "synaptosomes" or free-moving nerve terminals as it were. Blood platelets may therefore in certain ways serve as a model for the more inaccessible adrenergic nerve endings. For amine uptake in "synaptosomes" see the review of WHITTAKER (1966).

8. Uptake of False Transmitters. Multi-Amine Storage

Specific uptake of amines, different from the normal neurotransmitter but capable of binding to the same sites, has been studied both *in vivo*, in perfused organs, and in isolated storage particles. Since these amines may be released in a way similar to that of specifically bound noradrenaline they are often referred to as false transmitters (DAY and RAND, 1963).

Evidence for a stoichiometric exchange of endogenous noradrenaline for metaraminol formed *in vivo* from α-methyl-metatyrosine by decarboxylation and β-oxidation has been provided by CARLSSON and LINDQVIST (1962). MUSCHOLL and MAÎTRE (1963) showed release of α-methylnoradrenaline by nerve stimulation after administration of α-methyl DOPA. Similarly tyramine may be taken up in the nerves and stored and released as octopamine after β-oxidation (KOPIN et al., 1965; cf. MUSCHOLL, 1966a).

False transmitters may be said to have occurred in experiments where adrenaline was injected into an organism in amounts large enough to cause an uptake in adrenergic nerves (RAAB and GIGEE, 1953). Uptake experiments with different catecholamines were made by STRÖMBLAD and NICKERSON (1961), ANDÉN (1964) and ANDÉN et al. (1964), who observed that both (—)- and (+)-adrenaline were taken up by the heart, although in different proportions. When used in sufficiently high doses, (+)-adrenaline or metaraminol could even competitively replace the

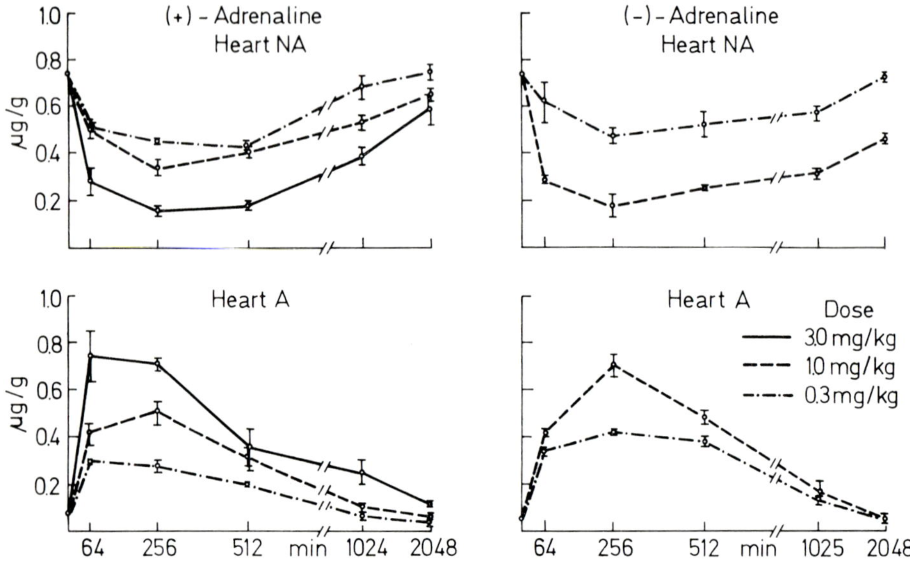

Fig. 7. Noradrenaline and adrenaline in the rat heart after i.m. injection of (—) and (+) adrenaline. Mean and S.E.M. (WESTFALL, 1965)

endogenous noradrenaline to 50—100% in various organs of the rat (ANDÉN and MAGNUSSON, 1963). The substitution process between endogenous noradrenaline and the potential false transmitters (—)- and (+)-adrenaline was studied by WESTFALL (1965) who found an approximately stoichiometric exchange for both isomers in the rat heart. As a sign of the different uptake rates for (—)- and (+)-adrenaline, the adrenaline values after injection of the (—)-isomer were approximately twice as high as for the (+)-isomer (Fig. 7).

The sympathetic nerves of the rat pineal gland contain both noradrenaline and 5-hydroxytryptamine (OWMAN, 1964). As shown by ZWEIG and AXELROD (1969) treatment with the tyrosine hydroxylase inhibitor α-methyltyrosine causes an increase in the pineal 5-hydroxytryptamine, which is synthesized by the parenchymal cells and taken up by the adrenergic nerve terminals. This rise is prevented by dopamine or noradrenaline, suggesting competition for storage sites. On the other hand, tryptophan increases the pineal 5-hydroxytryptamine. These results indicate that adrenergic nerve fibres may also take up and store 5-hydroxytryptamine if this — as in the pineal gland — is normally available in the adjacent cells.

Similar multi-amine storage ability has been described for nerves in a variety of tissue and organs (for references see ZWEIG and AXELROD, 1969) — but in these cases the nerves have been shown to take up foreign amines only after exogenous administration and apparently lack the biosynthetic machinery. An uptake may take place, however, during conditions of increased plasma levels such as may occur in cases of amine-producing tumours.

However, a marked degree of specificity in the ability to take up amines or their precursors has been noted for central neurons (HILLARP et al., 1966). The same is true for organs innervated by peripheral adrenergic nerves (SHAHAB et al., 1971).

9. Effect of Drugs on Catecholamine Uptake in Organs, Nerves and Isolated Particles

Extensive studies on the action of drugs on the uptake of noradrenaline in organs and in isolated nerve particles have been made. Some of these drugs are listed below:

a) Sympathomimetic amines
b) Adrenergic blocking agents
c) Neuronal and ganglionic blockers
d) Psychotropic drugs
e) Enzyme and metabolic inhibitors
f) Various drugs

a) Sympathomimetic Amines

BURGEN and IVERSEN (1965) studied systematically the effect of a large number of sympathomimetic amines on the uptake of ^{14}C-noradrenaline in the isolated perfused rat heart from a solution containing 10 ng/ml (0.6×10^{-7}M). The effects were expressed as ID 50 (drug concentration producing 50% inhibition of noradrenaline uptake). The strongest inhibitory actions on the noradrenaline uptake were exerted by (—)-metaraminol, dopamine, (+)-amphetamine, α-methylnoradrenaline, noradrenaline and tyramine, while isoprenaline had a much weaker effect. This is of interest since isoprenaline is hardly taken up by the axonal membranes. Normetanephrine has also only a moderate inhibitory effect on the uptake.

Amphetamine and tyramine are both noradrenaline releasers and their strong inhibitory effect on noradrenaline uptake may contribute to their relatively strong biological action. The most active inhibitory amines are also readily taken up into tissues.

The following conclusions from the results with the sympathomimetic amines are quoted from BURGEN and IVERSEN (1965) (L stands for (—)):

"(a) β-Hydroxylation produced a decreased affinity for the uptake site. In such compounds the L-enantiomer had a higher affinity than the D-enantiomer.

(b) α-Methylation resulted in a considerable increase in affinity for the uptake site. This effect was also stereochemically specific, in this case the D-enantiomer had considerably more activity than the L-enantiomer.

(c) Phenolic hydroxyl groups enhanced the affinity for the uptake site, para- and meta-substitutions having approximately equal effects. The optimal structure was the 3,4-dihydroxyphenyl group.

(d) N-Substitution decreased the affinity of the drug for the uptake site. This effect was dependent on the size of the N-substituent, bulky substituents having correspondingly greater effects in depressing affinity.

(e) O-Methylation of phenolic hydroxyl groups produced a striking decrease in affinity for the uptake site. Meta-methoxy-compounds had considerably lower affinities than the corresponding para-methoxy compounds.

(f) The phenylethylamine structure could be replaced with saturated five- or six-membered ring structures as in propylhexedrine and cyclopentamine without producing a marked decrease in the affinity for uptake. Even the long chain aliphatic amine tuamine and the indoleamine serotonin had appreciable affinities for the uptake site".

Using the rabbit heart MUSCHOLL and WEBER (1965) tested the effect of various amines on the uptake of α-methyl-noradrenaline with similar results. Amphetamine also inhibits the uptake of ^{3}H-noradrenaline from a depot injected into the lateral ventricles of the brain (GLOWINSKI and AXELROD, 1965).

In a study of the uptake of ^{3}H-noradrenaline in cat tissue slices DENGLER et al. (1961) found that tyramine, ephedrine and (+)-amphetamine in concentrations of 5×10^{-6}M inhibited the uptake 32—57%.

The inhibition of uptake of (—)-metaraminol in rat heart slices by noradrenaline (GIACHETTI and SHORE, 1966) probably signifies that noradrenaline in the concentration used (1.7×10^{-5}M) effectively competes with (—)-metaraminol (5×10^{-7} M) for uptake sites.

On isolated nerve particles EULER and LISHAJKO (1968a) found that indirectly acting amines like tyramine, phenethylamine and amphetamine increase the rate of noradrenaline loss on incubation in potassium phosphate. Most of this effect was due to inhibition of reuptake. Tyramine also inhibits the ATP-facilitated reuptake and net uptake of noradrenaline, partly by competition through the octopamine formed (cf. KOPIN et al., 1965). Uptake of tyramine itself was small. Of other arylamines prenylamine was strongly active as uptake inhibitor.

Incubation of nerve particles with ^{3}H-dopamine caused a considerable uptake of radioactivity which, however, quantitatively corresponded to the extra uptake of noradrenaline. Even when present in a concentration 10 times higher than noradrenaline in the medium, dopamine did not appear bound as such in nerve particles. The inhibitory action of dopamine on the noradrenaline reuptake is presumably a result of a competitive action. When dopamine and noradrenaline both are present in the incubation medium in a concentration of 3×10^{-6}M the reuptake of noradrenaline is inhibited by about 25% (EULER and LISHAJKO, 1968a).

α-Methyl-metatyramine 10^{-4}M inhibits noradrenaline uptake in nerve particles by 65%, while α-methyl-*m*-tyrosine has no effect. The effect of metaraminol, α-methylnoradrenaline and other amines, which are stored in the nerve particles, on the uptake of noradrenaline is dependent on the relative concentrations of noradrenaline and the amine (EULER and LISHAJKO, 1970).

b) Adrenergic Blocking Agents

An inhibitory action of the ^{3}H-noradrenaline uptake in various organs by phenoxybenzamine was observed by HERTTING et al. (1961b). Phentolamine and dichloroisoproterenol in the doses used had no significant action. On testing a number of phenothiazine derivatives ROSELL and AXELROD (1963) found that the inhibitory effect on the noradrenaline uptake in the rat heart was related to their antiadrenergic effect. Chlorpromazine had only a negligible effect on the ^{3}H-noradrenaline uptake in brain (IVERSEN et al., 1966) although it was quite active on the noradrenaline uptake in the heart. Dibenamine had no action on the uptake of noradrenaline in the heart (MUSCHOLL, 1961) or of ^{3}H-noradrenaline in slices of spleen (DENGLER et al., 1961).

BROWN and his co-workers (cf. BROWN, 1965) found that in the perfused cat spleen the α-blockers dibenamine, phenoxybenzamine, phentolamine and Hydergine increased the transmitter outflow at low stimulation frequencies by a factor of 5. This effect was at first interpreted as the result of blockade of the α-receptors in the effector organ but was later attributed to inhibited reuptake (BROWN, 1965). Phenoxybenzamine, as well as Hydergine and phentolamine increased the recovery of infused noradrenaline in the outflow from the perfused spleen from about 30% to about 60—80% (GILLESPIE and KIRPEKAR, 1965).

EISENFELD et al. (1967) found that adrenergic blocking agents, particularly the α-blockers, inhibit also the extraneuronal uptake of noradrenaline in tissues. These agents, in addition, decrease the concentration of the metabolites, which is interpreted as the result of an inhibited extraneuronal transport mechanism.

A number of adrenergic blocking agents have also been tested on the noradrenaline-uptake in isolated nerve particles. All α-blockers tested, including dibenamine, and the majority of β-blockers inhibited reuptake as well as the ATP-stimulated net uptake of noradrenaline to a varying degree (EULER and LISHAJKO, 1968b) suggesting that nerve granules possess an uptake mechanism with certain properties in common with the adrenergic receptors. On the other hand a lack of correlation between receptor and uptake blockade has been reported both with α-adrenergic blockers (THOENEN et al., 1964a) and with β-adrenergic blockers (MUSCHOLL, 1966b). Adrenergic blockers also inhibit the uptake of (—) adrenaline (BORN, 1968) and of ^{3}H-noradrenaline in human blood platelets (BYGDEMAN and JOHNSEN, 1969).

c) Neuronal and Ganglionic Blockers

Of the neuronal blockers, bretylium and TM 10 have little effect on the uptake of ^{3}H-noradrenaline in cat organs, while guanethidine markedly inhibited uptake (HERTTING et al., 1961b; HERTTING, 1965). Bretylium and guanethidine also inhibit noradrenaline uptake in spleen slices (DENGLER et al., 1961).

According to SHORE and GIACHETTI (1966) guanethidine at 5×10^{-6}M blocks an intracellular uptake mechanism and at 10^{-4}M uptake through the axonal membrane. On the other hand guanethidine at 10^{-5}M has no action on release or uptake of noradrenaline in isolated nerve particles and only a weak inhibitory action at 10^{-4}M. This is also seen with β-TM 10 and TM 6 whereas bretylium has no action even at 3×10^{-4}M (EULER and LISHAJKO, 1970).

Hexamethonium seems to have little action on noradrenaline uptake in the heart (LINDMAR and MUSCHOLL 1964), brain (WEIL-MALHERBE et al., 1961) or on isolated particles.

d) Psychotropic Drugs

α) Reserpine

Reserpine strongly inhibits uptake of ^{3}H-noradrenaline in various organs *in vivo* (HERTTING et al., 1961b) and the bulk uptake of noradrenaline after depletion in the perfused rat heart (BHATTACHARYA, 1968). The effect of reserpine is less dramatic in the brain; it blocks the uptake in the pituitary but not in the hypothalamus, cortex or medulla (WEIL-MALHERBE et al., 1961).

An inhibitory action of reserpine on the noradrenaline uptake is also noted on tissue slices (DENGLER et al., 1961).

The initial uptake of catecholamines through axonal or other cell membranes does not seem to be inhibited by reserpine, however (IVERSEN et al., 1965). This is in agreement with histochemical evidence (HAMBERGER et al., 1964) and earlier observations (KOPIN and GORDON, 1962; WEINER and TRENDELENBURG, 1962; LINDMAR and MUSCHOLL, 1964). These results are also in harmony with the findings of ANDÉN et al. (1963) that ^{3}H-noradrenaline can be taken up in tissues of a reserpine-treated animal even after denervation. It is then rapidly metabolized.

GLOWINSKI and AXELROD (1965) observed that whereas amphetamine raises the normetanephrine levels in brain, reserpine augments the O-methylated deaminated metabolites.

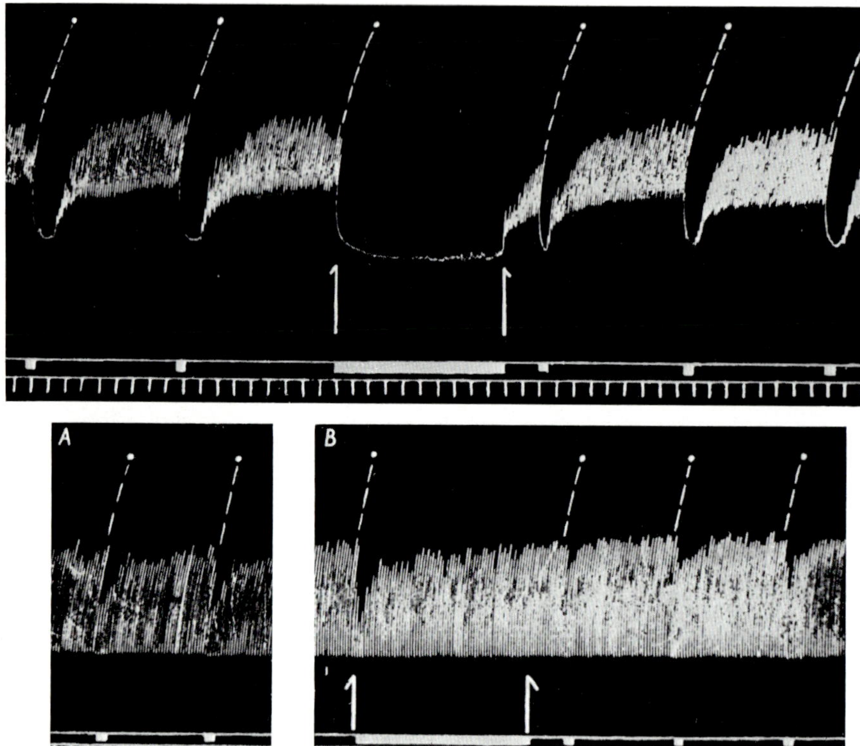

Fig. 8. Upper trace: response of isolated rabbit ileum to pre-arterial nerve stimulation 50/sec for short periods and 5 min. Lower traces: ileum from rabbit pretreated with reserpine. Response to stimulation partially restored by soaking in noradrenaline but readily fatigued (GILLESPIE and MACKENNA, 1961)

Unchanged (LINDMAR and MUSCHOLL, 1964) or even increased removal of noradrenaline from the perfusion fluid passing through organs from reserpine-treated animals (GILLESPIE and KIRPEKAR, 1965) indicates that specific uptake is not essential. Newly synthesized noradrenaline is then partly deaminated by intraneuronal MAO (KOPIN and GORDON, 1962). However, even in reserpine-treated animals a small uptake of noradrenaline can occur at sites which allow temporary restoration of the nerve stimulation effect in an isolated intestinal preparation (GILLESPIE and MACKENNA, 1961) (Fig. 8) or on the circulation of the cat (ROSELL and SEDVALL, 1961; BURN and RAND, 1958). The restored effect is easily fatigued by continuous stimulation of the nerves, suggesting that the uptake in specific stores is very limited, or occurs only in a small pool. The recovery observed after „neuronal rest“ may be explained by refilling of these stores by resynthesis. GILLESPIE and MACKENNA (1961) also observed an acute blocking effect of reserpine added to the organ bath on the effect of adrenergic nerve stimulation, presumably due to delayed refilling of some specific pool even in the presence of nearly normal stores. Effects of a similar kind have been observed by DAY and OWEN (1968) on the rabbit ear and EULER (1969) on guinea pig vas deferens.

Reserpine inhibits the uptake of ^{3}H-noradrenaline in 10 and 18 days old rats but considerably less than in adult animals which may indicate a difference in the specific stores (IVERSEN et al., 1967).

LINDMAR and MUSCHOLL (1965) made the interesting observation that after pretreatment with small doses of reserpine the α-methylnoradrenaline taken up in the rabbit heart after administration of α-methyl-DOPA is not depleted whereas the noradrenaline stores decreased. Whether this difference is due to a less affected uptake or reuptake in particles of α-methylnoradrenaline or depends on firmer binding of this amine has not been established. Similar findings have been made by CARLSSON et al. (1965) on stores in the brain.

The effect of reserpine on isolated nerve particles is to block the net noradrenaline uptake in the presence of ATP (cf. Fig. 6). Whether reuptake is blocked is difficult to ascertain since the normal release is strongly retarded (EULER and LISHAJKO, 1965b).

β) Cocaine

Inhibited tissue uptake as a cause of increased catecholamine action was first suggested by BLASCHKO (1954) who presented this possibility as an explanation of the potentiation of the response to adrenaline by cocaine.

In 1959 MACMILLAN suggested that cocaine, by preventing the uptake of noradrenaline into the tissue stores, increased the amount available for the receptors and thus potentiated its effect. This concept was supported by the finding of TRENDELENBURG (1959) that cocaine delayed the disappearance of noradrenaline from the blood after injection. Direct evidence for the correctness of MACMILLAN's hypothesis was given by MUSCHOLL (1960) and by WHITBY et al. (1960) who observed that cocaine reduced the uptake of circulating noradrenaline in organs and confirmed the increase of its concentration in plasma after injection. This finding has since been amply confirmed in a variety of ways. HUKOVIĆ and MUSCHOLL (1962) showed that cocaine increased the noradrenaline-content of the perfusate from the rabbit heart after sympathetic nerve stimulation by 122%.

Cocaine has been used repeatedly in experiments designed to study recapture of noradrenaline released from organs by nerve stimulation. The results have been variable. Thus TRENDELENBURG (1959), NASMYTH and ANDREWS (1959) and KIRPEKAR and CERVONI (1963) observed only a very modest increase in the outflow of noradrenaline from the stimulated cat spleen after cocaine, certainly not comparable with that seen after phenoxybenzamine. Similar results were obtained by BLAKELEY et al. (1963) who could not detect any action of cocaine on the outflow of noradrenaline after nerve stimulation, while the α-blocker Hydergine caused a large increase like dibenamine and phenoxybenzamine (BROWN and GILLESPIE, 1957). THOENEN et al. (1964b) found an increase of noradrenaline in the outflow of the stimulated spleen after cocaine but still far lower than that observed after phenoxybenzamine. It may be recalled that cocaine increases the effect of adrenaline on the vascular resistance of the perfused human placenta (EULER, 1938). If the effect of cocaine is due to inhibition of reuptake this must occur in non-neuronal tissue in this case.

While cocaine clearly inhibits the uptake of noradrenaline in the tissues, including the adrenergic neurons, this is of a moderate degree, since even large doses of cocaine did not prevent the deposition of radioactive noradrenaline in adrenergic fibres of the heart and vas deferens in mice although the uptake was delayed (SAMORAJSKI et al., 1964) (Fig. 4).

As shown by HERTTING and SCHIEFTHALER (1963) the noradrenaline output of the perfused cat spleen during sympathetic nerve stimulation greatly depends on the flow rate. At low flow rates during vasoconstriction a larger proportion of the released transmitter is re-bound. By blockade of the vasoconstrictor effects or at elevated perfusion pressure the noradrenaline output of the spleen is increased. An enhancement by cocaine of the vasoconstrictor effect of nerve stimulation tends to mask the elevation of overflow of noradrenaline brought about by inhibition of re-uptake at the same time. If the cat spleen is perfused with a constant volume cocaine causes an increase in transmitter output (THOENEN et al., 1964b). The results obtained on the spleen are therefore in accord with those obtained on the heart (HUKOVIĆ and MUSCHOLL, 1962). In this preparation sympathetic stimulation with or without cocaine did not appreciably alter the coronary flow.

Several years ago BLASCHKO (1954) suggested the possibility that potentiation of adrenaline-like action might be brought about by a competitive interference with entry across the cell membrane, causing an amine to be present in an effective concentration for a longer time.

The inhibitory action of cocaine on noradrenaline uptake depends on the concentration ratio of the two compounds (MUSCHOLL, 1961).

Cocaine only moderately inhibited the bulk uptake of noradrenaline in the depleted rat heart (BHATTACHARYA, 1968) particularly when noradrenaline was used in higher concentrations (10^{-6}M). This is in agreement with the conclusion of FURCHGOTT et al. (1963) that cocaine may compete with noradrenaline for common uptake sites.

Cocaine also inhibits the uptake of α-methylnoradrenaline by the isolated rabbit heart (WEBER and MUSCHOLL, 1965). Tetracaine had no effect on the uptake in a concentration with twice the local anesthetic effect. In brain slices no inhibitory action of cocaine is seen on the uptake of ^{3}H-phenylethanolamine, which is an active noradrenaline releaser. The antagonistic action of cocaine on this indirectly acting amine could therefore not be explained by inhibition of amine uptake (ROSS et al., 1968). As observed by BARNETT et al. (1968), cocaine does not inhibit the effect of tyramine on the nictitating membrane in concentrations which potentiate the response to noradrenaline. Similar observations were made by LAGERCRANTZ (1968) on the isolated iris.

γ) Imipramine, Desipramine, Amitriptyline

Imipramine inhibits the uptake of ^{3}H-noradrenaline in heart and spleen (HERTTING et al., 1961b) and after administration in the lateral ventricle the uptake in the brain (GLOWINSKI and AXELROD, 1965). Desipramine (DMI) and amitriptyline acted similarly.

DMI, which is normally a potent inhibitor of noradrenaline uptake (TITUS and SPIEGEL, 1962) and more efficient than cocaine (BARNETT et al., 1968), is ineffective in preventing uptake in the reserpine-pretreated heart (IVERSEN et al., 1965). It is conceivable that reserpine has altered the properties of the cell membrane.

The finding of GEFFEN (1965), previously referred to, that DMI does not increase the outflow of noradrenaline from the isolated perfused spleen on nerve stimulation suggests either that the postulated recapture of transmitter is negligible under the prevailing experimental situation or that desipramine does not reach the release sites.

As reported by IVERSEN et al. (1966) the uptake of noradrenaline in the brain is inhibited by DMI and by amphetamine, but not the uptake of dopamine.

On isolated particles DMI (STJÄRNE et al., 1968), amitriptyline and nortriptyline strongly inhibit release as well as uptake of noradrenaline. DMI also inhibits the noradrenaline releasing effect of tyramine on isolated nerve particles (EULER and LISHAJKO, 1968a).

δ) d-Lysergic Acid Diethylamide

Lysergic acid diethylamide does not affect noradrenaline uptake in organ slices (DENGLER et al., 1961), or in the brain (GLOWINSKI and AXELROD, 1965) but has an increasingly larger inhibitory effect on the noradrenaline uptake in isolated nerve particles when added to the incubation medium to 10^{-6}M or higher.

e) Enzyme and Metabolic Inhibitors

Of the MAO inhibitors, iproniazid inhibits noradrenaline uptake in the hypothalamus but not in the pituitary, whereas pheniprazine was without effect in both cases (WEIL-MALHERBE et al., 1961; HERTTING et al., 1961b). Nialamide and pargyline had no effect on uptake in isolated nerve particles in concentrations up to 10^{-4}M, whereas pheniprazine had a slight releasing effect.

Noradrenaline uptake *in vivo* or in isolated nerve particles was not found to be inhibited by ouabain (WEIL-MALHERBE et al., 1961; HERTTING et al., 1961b; EULER and LISHAJKO, 1965b) whereas inhibition is observed in tissue slices (DENGLER et al., 1961). Recent observations indicate, however, that uptake may be inhibited after a time lag of 10—20 min *in vivo*. (TISSARI et al., 1969; LEITZ and STEFANO, 1970).

Eserine and prostigmine have no action of the outflow of noradrenaline from the perfused spleen on stimulation of its nerves (BLAKELEY et al., 1963) and are also inactive when tested on the release and noradrenaline uptake in isolated nerve particles.

Arsenate and fluoride in high concentrations (10^{-2}—10^{-3}M) do not seem to affect noradrenaline uptake in particles (EULER and LISHAJKO, 1969).

In their study of various metabolic inhibitors on the incorporation of radioactive catecholamines in isolated adrenal medullary granules CARLSSON et al., (1963b) observed that the facilitating effect of ATP plus Mg was inhibited by various compounds. Most active as inhibitors were SH-reagents.

KIRSHNER and SMITH (1966) found that cyanide and iodoacetic acid given together strongly inhibited the catecholamine secretion by acetylcholine from the adrenal gland whereas each substance alone had only little effect. Antimycin or oligomycin also acted as inhibitors only when given in combination.

KIRPEKAR and WAKADE (1968) observed that while iodoacetic acid or dinitrophenol (DNP) 5×10^{-4}M used singly, had a moderate inhibitory effect only, their combined action was marked.

In a study of the action of various metabolic inhibitors on the release and uptake of noradrenaline in nerve particles, EULER and LISHAJKO (1969) found that while cyanide or azide had only little effect on these functions, a number of other agents were active.

Sulphydryl reagents like N-ethylmaleimide (NEM), iodoacetate, iodobenzoate and mercuribenzoate were slightly to moderately active and required high concentrations in order to exert an action. NEM at 3×10^{-4}M inhibited noradrenaline uptake by 40%.

Inhibitors at various sites of the respiratory chain and of oxidative phosphorylation were all active inhibitors of the uptake of noradrenaline in isolated particles, both on reuptake and on the ATP-stimulated net uptake. Thus rotenone, antimycin A, chlorpromazine and oligomycin strongly inhibited uptake. In a concentration of 3×10^{-4}M antimycin completely prevented the ATP-stimulated uptake. Oligomycin was also strongly active.

Uncouplers of oxidative phosphorylation, DNP, carbonyl cyanide *m*-chlorophenylhydrazone (CCP), desaspidin and pentachlorophenol all strongly enhanced spontaneous release and inhibited noradrenaline uptake (EULER and LISHAJKO, 1969).

f) Various Drugs

Nicotine and atropine seem to have no effect on the noradrenaline uptake in tissues or in particles (MUSCHOLL, 1961; EULER and LISHAJKO, 1965b).

A large number of other substances have been studied with regard to their action on the uptake of ^{3}H-noradrenaline in organs *in vivo* or on isolated nerve particles *in vitro*. Of special interest are perhaps the actions of drugs, known to exert actions on the functions of the autonomic nerve system. To this group belong various amines and naturally occurring substances. 5-Hydroxytryptamine, histamine, prostaglandin E_2 (PGE_2) (HEDQVIST, 1970), GABA, angiotensin, vasopressin and oxytocin, insulin and various other peptides were without action on amine uptake.

III. Storage

1. Storage in Subcellular Particles

From analytical data, based on the relative amounts of noradrenaline in splenic nerves and splenic tissue and the probable amount of nerve tissue in the spleen, it was inferred that the amine is accumulated in the nerve terminals (EULER, 1954). Later experiments showed (EULER and HILLARP, 1956) that noradrenaline was bound to a small subcellular particle fraction obtained in the sediment from homogenates of organs and adrenergic nerves by high speed centrifugation. The noradrenaline present in the particles[1] occurred in a bound form as shown by the facts that it was not susceptible to oxidants, nor was it adsorbed on passage through alumina. Moreover, it was not biologically active until released from the granules (EULER, 1958).

Incubation of a suspension of particles in phosphate buffer at 37 °C causes a rapid release of the transmitter with a halftime of about 5 min, whereas it is firmly bound at 0°, no loss being observed in several hours (EULER and LISHAJKO, 1963a).

The cytology of these particles has been studied by electron microscopy. After squeezing of bovine splenic nerves and removal of larger particles a suspension is obtained which contains osmiophilic granules with a diameter of 0.03—0.15 μ (Fig. 9a). (cf. EULER and SWANBECK, 1964). Tissue sections have shown granules of this kind in sympathetic nerve terminals in various organs (DE ROBERTIS and DE IRALDI, 1961; LEVER and ESTERHUIZEN, 1961; RICHARDSON, 1962; HÖKFELT, 1969). The bovine splenic nerve particles have been studied with regard to their physical and chemical properties by LADURON et al. (1966), HÖRTNAGL et al. (1969) and DE POTTER et al. (1969).

While the association of the transmitter with the osmiophilic granules rests beyond doubt, detailed knowledge is still lacking as regards the relative noradrenaline content in granules from the nerve trunk and terminal granules or in granules of different size. After administration of radioactive noradrenaline to animals it has been possible to show that silver grains are located over nerve

1 The subcellular particles storing noradrenaline in adrenergic nerves are often referred to as nerve granules.

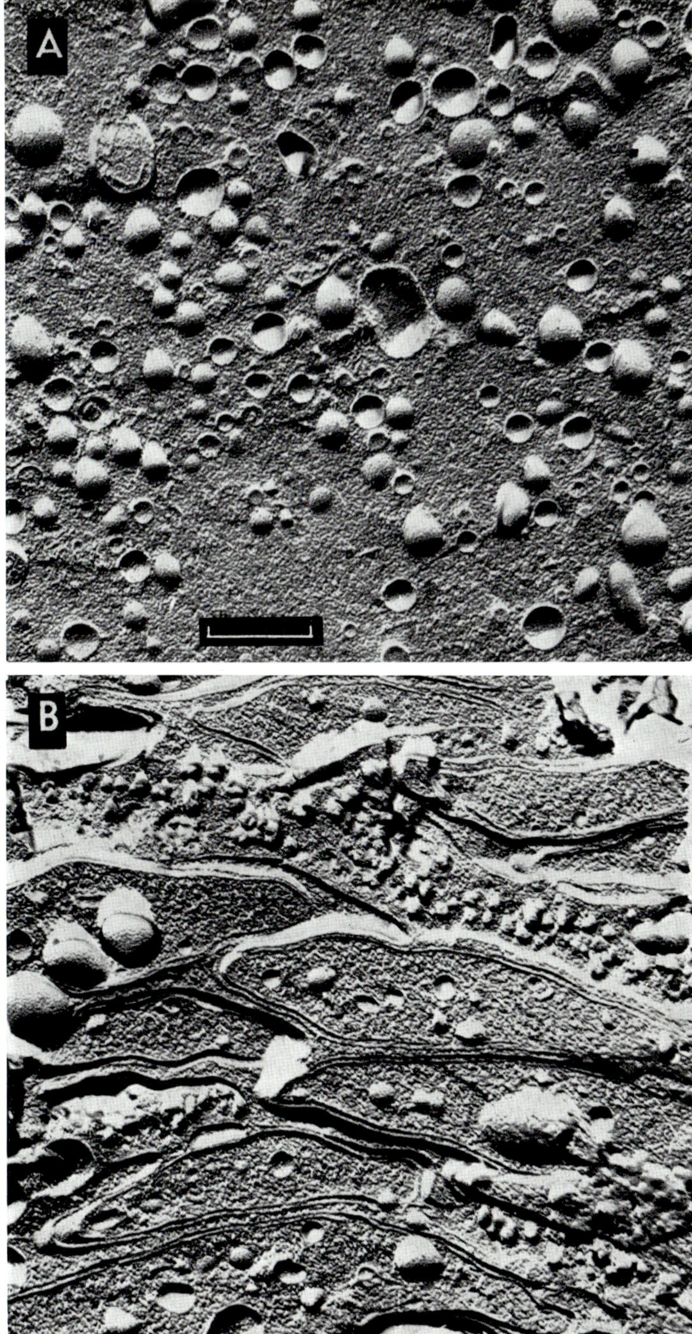

Fig. 9A and B. A: Bovine splenic nerve particles from high speed sediment after homogenization and removal of coarse particles by centrifugation 10 min at 10000× g. B: Bovine splenic nerve axons. Glutaraldehyde fixation. Freezeetching. Marker: 0.2 μ (GEMNE and EULER, unpubl.)

particles in preparations studied by combination of autoradiography and electron microscopy (WOLFE et al., 1962).

Transmitter storage particles appear in the highest number in the terminal swellings of the adrenergic nerves, sometimes tightly packed. In the axon they occur much more sparsely (Fig. 9b); this explains the fact that they have eluded detection for considerable time although their presence in the axoplasm was known. From their relative dispersion and assuming the same relative noradrenaline content in the particles the concentration would be about 100 times higher in the terminal swellings than in the axon. Since the splenic nerve trunk contains about 10 μg/g the concentration in the varicosities would be of the order of 1 mg/g which is similar to that in chromaffin tissue (cf. NORBERG and HAMBERGER, 1964).

Although several possibilities have been suggested for the storage mechanism this is still unknown. Of the various possible modes of storage, binding to nucleotides, proteins, lipoproteins and phospholipids have been suggested (cf. BELLEAU, 1960). For an extensive discussion of this problem the reader is referred to the review by GREEN (1962).

From the results of experiments on uptake *in vivo* and *in vitro* it appears that the catechol group and the β-hydroxyl group in the side chain are essential for the binding in adrenergic storage particles (cf. MUSACCHIO et al., 1965b). As pointed out in section II B 4 the binding characteristics are different in the dopamine particles.

2. Storage Capacity, Noradrenaline Content in Particles

Precise data relating to the noradrenaline storage capacity of the granules at different locations (terminal and extraterminal) and their size in the adrenergic axons cannot be given at present. It has been computed from morphological studies, however, that the average number of granules in a varicosity is of the order of 1000, and from estimations of the number of varicosities and the noradrenaline content of the tissue it is calculated that the average noradrenaline content per granules is 5×10^{-6} pg. or 1.5×10^{4} molecules (DAHLSTRÖM et al., 1966; FOLKOW et al., 1968).

The storage capacity is usually not wholly utilized as judged from the moderate increase of 25—50% observed in the total noradrenaline store in an organ after decentralization, ganglionic blockers or neuronal blockade (cf. Uptake p. 209). Apparently a moderate deficit is upheld during normal impulse traffic.

Whether the lower noradrenaline content in the axon in comparison to that in the terminal swelling simply depends on the greater dispersion of granules in the axon or upon a difference in storage capacity is not known.

3. Stability of Storage Particles

The very high degree of stability of the transmitter storage particles at low temperature is illustrated by the observation that storage of an organ at refrigerator temperature (2—5°C) for 24 hrs does not diminish the yield of noradrenaline extractable from an organ. On storing isolated nerve particles in phosphate buffer for 24 hrs the loss in noradrenaline content is less than 50% of the original content.

At higher temperatures the noradrenaline content of an organ as well as in isolated particles diminishes. Release increases rapidly with temperature. Thus the release constant at 20°C in isotonic phosphate, ph 7.0, is approximately 0.01 or 1% per min, but increases to about 0.15 at 37° (EULER and LISHAJKO, 1967a). The high temperature coefficient (Q_{10} 3—4), has so far not been adequately explained.

4. Free and Particle-bound Noradrenaline in Homogenates of Adrenergic Nerves and in Organs

In the press juice from bovine splenic nerves about 30—40% of the total noradrenaline was recovered in the high speed sediment whereas the remaining part was found in the soluble fraction and in the residue (EULER and LISHAJKO, 1963a). Several authors, using different homogenization procedures have found noradrenaline from various organs, usually the heart, about equally distributed in the coarse particles, the high speed sediment and the soluble fraction (cf. CAMPOS and SHIDEMAN, 1962; BHAGAT, 1963; STITZEL and LUNDBORG, 1967; WESTFALL, 1965; MACKENNA, 1965) and others. These fairly consistent results at first seem to indicate that a certain proportion of the noradrenaline in the adrenergic neurons is either free or loosely bound. In a study of the influence of homogenization on the distribution of noradrenaline between the subcellular fraction, EULER (1966) found, however, that continued treatment of the particle suspension with the homogenizer rapidly lowered the proportion of particle-bound noradrenaline and increased the amount in the soluble portion. Extrapolating back from the rate of continued release from particles, it appeared that the original proportion of soluble noradrenaline only amounted to around 10% or less. The "soluble" fraction may therefore partly be an artifact depending on the mechanical treatment during homogenization. The concept that only a small fraction of the total noradrenaline in the terminal is present in free form is supported by the observation that newly synthetized noradrenaline which cannot be stored, e.g. after reserpine, is either rapidly metabolized or leaves the axon (KOPIN and GORDON, 1962). However, using a standardized technique it seems possible to obtain comparable values which might serve as guidelines for changes caused by various physico-chemical factors or by drugs.

Although most or practically all of the noradrenaline in the terminals may normally occur in a bound form, several observations suggest that there is more than one pool containing the transmitter. TRENDELENBURG (1961) used the term "available noradrenaline" for a certain small fraction which seemed to be released in response to nerve stimulation and various agents, e.g. tyramine. Observations by CROUT et al. (1962) and TRENDELENBURG (1963) are in harmony with the concept that the small available pool can be replenished from a larger pool. It has also been suggested that storage particles near the axonal membrane form a tyramine-releasable pool and take up ^{3}H-noradrenaline preferentially (POTTER and AXELROD, 1963a; CROUT, 1964). Experiments on the isolated guinea pig vas deferens have shown that reserpine in concentrations of 0.25—1 μg/ml rapidly causes neuromuscular inhibition or block (EULER, 1969) which may be due to deficient refilling of a peripheral "available" pool since it is known that reserpine retards the release from the storage granules (EULER and LISHAJKO, 1965b). It has been suggested that the peripheral pool may be associated with or even form a part of the axon membrane (cf. EULER, 1970).

Studies on the specific protein chromogranin A, first demonstrated in adrenal medullary granules, have shown its presence also in the noradrenaline-containing granules of bovine splenic nerve (BANKS et al., 1969). On stimulation of the nerve to the isolated perfused spleen of the calf it was observed (DE POTTER et al., 1969; GEFFEN et al., 1969) that the perfusates contained far more noradrenaline in proportion to chromogranin A and dopamine-β-hydroxylase than the vesicles. These results, like those of STJÄRNE et al. (1970b), which demonstrated that release of transmitter from the stimulated perfused spleen was not accompanied by a release of previously labelled nucleotides, do not speak in favour of exocytosis as a principal mechanism for transmitter release from adrenergic nerves.

5. Effect of Drugs

While the amount of noradrenaline stored in reserpinized tissue is diminished, due to deficient uptake in the particles, there is a striking increase in deaminated metabolites (Kopin and Gordon, 1962; Glowinski and Axelrod, 1965; Glowinski et al., 1966b). After administration of a MAO inhibitor to the reserpinized animal before giving ^{3}H-noradrenaline, it accumulates to almost normal levels. How this noradrenaline is "stored" is not known; it is not even certain that it occurs mainly intraneuronally but it may be present also extraneuronally. In the acutely reserpinized spinal cat preparation the transmitter, protected by a MAO-inhibitor, is constantly leaking out from the terminals and may increase the tissue content of noradrenaline.

The small reserpine-resistent noradrenaline "store", described by Sedvall (1964), Häggendal and Lindqvist (1964), Glowinski et al. (1966b) may be due to retention in particles still able to take up a certain amount of newly synthesized noradrenaline, but releasing it slowly. In this case an additional dose of reserpine might or might not affect this amount, which may represent the balance between a small uptake and slow release. In the reserpine-treated rat heart the small store can be partially released by DMPP (Iversen et al., 1965).

In the reserpine-treated brain DMI or amphetamine hardly affect the accumulation of ^{3}H-noradrenaline, but if the rapid metabolism of the noradrenaline is prevented by a MAO inhibitor like pheniprazine the effects of these drugs again become apparent and the uptake is smaller (Glowinski et al., 1965). Amphetamine in these experiments seems to have a MAO inhibiting effect.

The results of injections of noradrenaline in reserpine pretreated rats have revealed the important fact that the heart of such rats is able to take up and store in a normal manner tracer doses of noradrenaline, but cannot store larger amounts, which are recovered in the supernatant fraction after homogenization (Iversen et al., 1965). Uptake experiments with tracer doses of noradrenaline must therefore be judged with caution.

After administration of amphetamine the normetanephrine level increases in the rat brain whereas after reserpine the O-methylated deaminated metabolites increase. The differences in the metabolic pattern of noradrenaline observed after amphetamine and reserpine moreover suggest the presence of more than one storage form for catecholamines in the brain (Glowinski and Axelrod, 1965).

From studies on the rat brain it has been suggested that reserpine releases noradrenaline mainly from the "supernatant fraction" i.e. from the whole neuron while amphetamine releases from the varicosities (Glowinski et al., 1966b).

Maître and Staehelin (1968) have observed that while cocaine, imipramine and desipramine strongly inhibit the uptake of ^{3}H-noradrenaline in the rat heart, the amount found in the vas deferens was considerably increased, possibly indicating a special storage form in this organ.

The storage in adrenergic nerve particles is influenced by a large number of drugs, as judged by their action on the "spontaneous" release rate (Euler and Lishajko, 1965b). Many of these cause a retardation of the release as observed with reserpine, prenylamine, adrenergic α-blockers, desipramine, nortriptyline, LSD, metabolic inhibitors at the first and second stage of the respiratory chain, oligomycin. Several of these compounds are releasers at higher concentrations.

A releasing action is seen with indirectly acting amines, and uncouplers of oxidative phosphorylation (EULER and LISHAJKO, 1968a, 1969). The releasing effect (also seen with detergents, increased temperature, lysis, and sonication) is apparently in some way associated with the condition of the particle membrane or physico-chemical state of the particle, but may also be induced by metabolic changes.

Several biologically highly active compounds like acetylcholine, histamine, 5-hydroxytryptamine, nicotine, atropine have no effect on the storage and release from particles, whereas cocaine, bretylium and guanethidine have only a weak effect.

Interestingly, there is an exchange between endogenous noradrenaline in the nerve storage particles and exogenous adrenaline in the incubation medium, the rate of which is dependent on the release and the relative concentrations of the amines. This is true also for dopamine (stored as noradrenaline) and tyramine (stored as octopamine).

References

ALBERT, A.: Design of chelating agents for selected biological activity. Fed. Proc. **20**, 137 (1961).

ALOUSI, A., WEINER, N.: The regulation of norepinephrine synthesis in sympathetic nerves: Effect of nerve stimulation, cocaine, and catecholamine-releasing agents. Proc. nat. Acad. Sci. (Wash.) **56**, 1491—1496 (1966).

ANDÉN, N. E.: Uptake and release of dextro- and laevo-adrenaline in noradrenergic stores. Acta pharmacol. (Kbh.) **21**, 59—75 (1964).

— CARLSSON, A., WALDECK, B.: Reserpine-resistant uptake mechanisms of noradrenaline in tissues. Life Sci. **2**, 889—894 (1963).

— CORRODI, H., ETTLES, M., GUSTAFSSON, E., PERSSON, H.: Selective uptake of some catecholamines by the isolated heart and its inhibition by cocaine and phenoxybenzamine. Acta pharmacol. (Kbh.) **21**, 247—259 (1964).

— MAGNUSSON, T.: Functional effect of noradrenaline depletion by α-methyl-m-tyrosine, metaraminol and (+)-adrenaline. Biochem. Pharmacol. **12**, Suppl. p. 66 (1963).

ANGELAKOS, E.T., FUXE, K., TORCHIANA, M.L.: Chemical and histochemical evaluation of the distribution of catecholamines in the rabbit and guinea pig hearts. Acta physiol. scand. **59**, 184—192 (1963).

ARMSTRONG, M.D., MCMILLAN, A.: Studies on the formation of 3-methoxy-4-hydroxy-D-mandelic acid, a urinary metabolite of norepinephrine and epinephrine. Pharmacol. Rev. **11**, 394—401 (1959).

ASATOOR, A.M., DALGLIESH, C.E.: Amines in blood and urine. Biochem. J. **73**, 26P (1959).

AUSTIN, L., LIVETT, B.G., CHUBB, I.W.: In creased synthesis and release of noradrenaline and dopamine during nerve stimulation. Life Sci. **6**, 97—104 (1967).

AVAKIAN, O.V., GILLESPIE, J.S.: Uptake of noradrenaline by adrenergic nerves, smooth muscle and connective tissue in isolated perfused arteries and its correlation with the vasoconstrictor response. Brit. J. Pharmacol. **32**, 168—184 (1968).

AWAPARA, J., PERRY, T.L., HANLY, C., PECK, E.: Substrate specificity of DOPA-decarboxylase. Clin. chim. Acta **10**, 286—289 (1964).

AXELROD, J.: Enzymatic formation of adrenaline and other catechols from monophenols. Science **140**, 499—500 (1963).

— The metabolism, storage and release of catecholamines. Recent Progr. Hormone Res. **21**, 597—619 (1965).

— MUELLER, R.A., THOENEN, H.: Neuronal and hormonal control of lyrosine hydroxylase and phenylethanolamine N-methyltransferase activity. Bayer Symposium II. SCHÜMANN, H.J., KRONEBERG, G., Eds. 1969. Springer Verlag, p. 212—219 (1970).

— WEIL-MALHERBE, H., TOMCHICK, R.: The physiological disposition of H^3-epinephrine and its metabolite metanephrine. J. Pharmacol. exp. Ther. **127**, 251—256 (1959).

AYUKAWA, S., HAMADA, M., KOJIRI, K., TAKEUCHI, T., HARA, T., NAGATSU, T., UMEZAWA, H.: Studies on a new pigment antibiotic, chrothiomycin. J. Antibiot. (Tokyo) **22**, 303—308 (1969).

BACQ, Z.M.: Recherches sur la physiologie et la pharmacologie du système nerveux autonome. XXV. Rôle du foie et des viscères abdominaux dans la déstruction de l'adrénaline. Arch. int. Physiol. **45**, 1—5 (1937).

Bagchi, S.P., McGeer, P.L.: Some properties of tyrosine hydroxylase from the caudate nucleus. Life Sci. **3**, 1195—1200 (1964).

Balzer, H., Palm, D.: Über den Mechanismus der Wirkung des Reserpins auf den Glykogengehalt der Organe. Naunyn-Schmiedeberg's Arch. exp. Path. Pharmak. **243**, 65—84 (1962).

Banks, P., Helle, K.B., Mayor, D.: Evidence for the presence of a chromogranin-like protein in bovine splenic nerve granules. Molec. Pharmacol. **5**, 210—212 (1969).

Barnett, A., Symchowicz, S., Taber, R.I.: The effects of drugs inhibiting catecholamine uptake on tyramine and noradrenaline-induced contractions of the isolated rat vas deferens. Brit. J. Pharmacol. **34**, 484—492 (1968).

Belleau, B.: Relationships between agonists, antagonists and receptor sites. Ciba Foundation Symposium on "Adrenergic Mechanisms", pp. 223—245. London: J. & A. Churchill 1960.

Bertler, Å., Rosengren, E.: Occurrence and distribution of catecholamines in brain. Acta physiol. scand. **47**, 350—361 (1959).

Bhagat, B.: Effect of noradrenaline injection on the catecholamine content of the rat heart. Arch. int. Pharmacodyn. **146**, 47—55 (1963).

Bhattacharya, I.C.: Uptake of noradrenaline in the isolated perfused rat heart after depletion with decaborane. Acta physiol. scand. **73**, 128—138 (1968).

Birkmayer, W., Hornykiewicz, O.: Der L-Dioxyphenylalanin (= L-DOPA)-Effekt beim Parkinson-Syndrom des Menschen: Zur Pathogenese und Behandlung der Parkinson-Akinese. Arch. Psychiat. Nervenkr. **203**, 560—574 (1962).

Blakeley, A.G.H., Brown, G.L., Ferry, C.B.: Pharmacological experiments on the release of the sympathetic transmitter. J. Physiol. (Lond.) **167**, 505—514 (1963).

Blaschko, H.: The specific action of l-dopa decarboxylase. J. Physiol. (Lond.) **96**, 50P—51P (1939).

— Substrate specificity of amino-acid decarboxylases. Biochem. biophys. Acta (Amst.) **4**, 130—137 (1950).

— Metabolism of epinephrine and norepinephrine. Pharmacol. Rev. **6**, 23—28 (1954).

— The development of current concepts of catecholamine formation. Pharmacol. Rev. **11**, 307—316 (1959).

— Burn, J.H., Langemann, H.: The formation of noradrenaline from dihydroxyphenylserine. Brit. J. Pharmacol. **5**, 431—437 (1950).

— Chrusciel, T.L.: The decarboxylation of amino acids related to tyrosine and their awakening action in reserpine-treated mice. J. Physiol. (Lond.) **151**, 272—284 (1960).

— Holton, P., Stanley, G.H.S.: Enzymic formation of pressor amines. J. Physiol. (Lond.) **108**, 427—439 (1949).

Boadle, M.C., Hughes, J., Roth, R.H.: Angiotensin accelerates catecholamine biosynthesis in sympathetically innervated tissues. Nature (Lond.) **222**, 987—988 (1969).

Bogdanski, D.F., Brodie, B.B.: Role of sodium and potassium ions in storage of norepinephrine by sympathetic nerve endings. Life Sci. **5**, 1563—1569 (1966).

Born, G.V.R.: The uptake of adrenaline by human blood platelets. Naunyn-Schmiedeberg's Arch. Pharmak. exp. Path. **259**, 155—156 (1968).

Brodie, B.B., Kuntzman, R., Hirsch, C.W., Costa, E.: Effects of decarboxylase inhibition on the biosynthesis of brain monoamines. Life Sci. **1**, 81—84 (1962).

Brown, G.L.: The release and fate of the transmitter liberated by adrenergic nerves. The Croonian Lecture 1964. Proc. roy. Soc. B. **162**, 1—19 (1965).

— Gillespie, J.S.: The output of sympathetic transmitter from the spleen of the cat. J. Physiol. (Lond.) **138**, 81—102 (1957).

Burgen, A.S.V., Iversen, L.L.: The inhibition of noradrenaline uptake by sympathomimetic amines in the rat isolated heart. Brit. J. Pharmacol. **25**, 34—49 (1965).

Burger, A., Philippu, A., Schümann, J.H.: Untersuchungen zur Bedeutung einer ATPase aus Milznervengranula. Naunyn-Schmiedeberg's Arch. Pharmak. exp. Path. **260**, 101 to 102 (1968).

Burn, J.H.: A pharmacological approach to the cause of asthma. Proc. roy. Soc. Med. **27**, 31—46 (1933).

— Rand, M.J.: The action of sympathomimetic amines in animals treated with reserpine. J. Physiol. (Lond.) **144**, 314—336 (1958).

Bygdeman, S., von Euler, U.S.: Neurotransmitter deficiency and reloading in noradrenaline depleted rabbits. Acta physiol. scand. **68**, 134—140 (1966).

— Johnsen, Ø.: Studies on the effect of adrenergic blocking drugs on catecholamine-induced platelet aggregation and uptake of noradrenaline and 5-hydroxytryptamine. Acta physiol. scand. **75**, 129—138 (1969).

Campos, H.A., Shideman, F.E.: Subcellular distribution of catecholamines in the dog heart. Effects of reserpine and norepinephrine administration. Int. J. Neuropharmacol. **1**, 13—22 (1962).

CANNON, W.B., LISSAK, K.: Evidence for adrenaline in adrenergic neurones. Amer. J. Physiol. **125**, 765—777 (1939).

CARLSSON, A.: Physiological and pharmacological release of monoamines in the central nervous system. Proc. Internat. Wenner-Gren Center Symposium "Mechanisms of release of biogenic amines", held in Stockholm, February 1965, pp. 331—345. U.S. v. EULER, S. ROSELL and B. UVNÄS, Eds. Pergamon Press (1966).

— CORRODI, H., WALDECK, B.: α-Substituierte Dopacetamide als Hemmer der Catechol-O-methyl-transferase und der enzymatischen Hydroxylierung aromatischer Aminosäuren. In den Catecholamin-Metabolismus eingreifende Substanzen. 2. Mitteilung. Helv. chim. Acta **46**, 2271—2285 (1963a).

— DAHLSTRÖM, A., FUXE, K., HILLARP, N.-Å.: Failure of reserpine to deplete noradrenaline neurons of α-methylnoradrenaline formed from α-methyl DOPA. Acta pharmacol. (Kbh) **22**, 270—276 (1965).

— HILLARP, N.-Å., WALDECK, B.: Analysis of the Mg^{++}-ATP dependent storage mechanism in the amine granules of the adrenal medulla. Acta physiol. scand. **59**, Suppl. 215 (1963b).

— LINDQVIST, M.: In-vivo decarboxylation of α-methyl dopa and α-methyl metatyrosine. Acta physiol. scand. **54**, 87—94 (1962).

CHESSIN, M., KRAMER, E.R., SCOTT, C.C.: Modifications of the pharmacology of reserpine and serotonin by iproniazid. J. Pharmacol. exp. Ther. **119**, 453—460 (1957).

CHIOCCHIO, S.R., BISCARDI, A.M., TRAMEZZANI, J.H.: Catecholamines in the carotid body of the cat. Nature (Lond.) **212**, 834—835 (1966).

CLARK, W.G.: Studies on inhibition of l-dopa decarboxylase *in vitro* and *in vivo*. Pharmacol. Rev. **11**, 330—349 (1959).

— POGRUND, R.S.: Inhibition of DOPA decarboxylase *in vitro* and *in vivo*. Circulat. Res. **9**, 721—733 (1961).

CORRODI, H., FUXE, K., HÖKFELT, T.: Refillment of the catecholamine stores with 3, 4-dihydroxyphenylalanine after depletion induced by inhibition of tyrosine-hydroxylase. Life Sci. **5**, 605—611 (1966).

— MALMFORS, T.: The effect of nerve activity on the depletion of the adrenergic transmitter by inhibitors of noradrenaline synthesis. Acta physiol. scand. **67**, 352—357 (1966).

CREVELING, C.R., LEVITT, M., UDENFRIEND, S.: An alternative route for biosynthesis of norepinephrine. Life Sci. **1**, 523—526 (1962).

CROUT, J.R.: Uptake and metabolism of d, l-norepinephrine ($NE\text{-}H^3$) by guinea pig heart *in vivo*. Pharmacologist **4**, 168 (1962).

— The uptake and release of H^3-norepinephrine by the guinea-pig heart *in vivo*. Naunyn-Schmiedeberg's Arch. exp. Path. Pharmak. **248**, 85—98 (1964).

— MUSKUS, A.J., TRENDELENBURG, U.: Effect of tyramine on isolated guinea-pig atria in relation of their noradrenaline stores. Brit. J. Pharmacol. **18**, 600—611 (1962).

DAHLSTRÖM, A., HÄGGENDAL, J., HÖKFELT, T.: The noradrenaline content of the varicosities of sympathetic adrenergic nerve terminals in the rat. Acta physiol. scand. **67**, 289—294 (1966).

DAIRMAN, W., GORDON, R., SPECTOR, S., SJOERDSMA, A., UDENFRIEND, S.: Increased synthesis of catecholamines in the intact rat following administration of α-adrenergic blocking agents. Mol. Pharmacol. **4**, 457—464 (1968).

DA PRADA, M., PLETSCHER, A.: Isolated 5-hydroxytryptamine organelles of rabbit blood platelets: physiological properties and drug-induced changes. Brit. J. Pharmacol. **34**, 591—597 (1968).

DAVIS, R.A., DRAIN, D.J., HORLINGTON, M., LAZARE, R., URBANSKA, A.: The effect of L-α-methyl dopa and N-2-hydroxybenzyl-N-methyl hydrazine (NSD 1039) on the blood pressure of renal hypertensive rats. Life Sci. **2**, 193—197 (1963).

DAY, M.D., OWEN, D.A.A.: The interaction between angiotensin and sympathetic vasoconstriction in the isolated artery of the rabbit ear. Brit. J. Pharmacol. **34**, 499—507 (1968).

— RAND, M.J.: A hypothesis for the mode of action of α-methyldopa in relieving hypertension. J. Pharm. Pharmacol. **15**, 221—224 (1963).

DEARNALEY, D.P., GEFFEN, L.B.: The effect of phenoxy-benzamine on the depletion by nerve stimulation of the noradrenaline of the cat's spleen. J. Physiol. (Lond.) **184**, 75P—76P (1966).

DENGLER, H., REICHEL, G.: Die Beeinflussung der Blutdruckswirkung von Dopa and Dops durch einen Decarboxylase-Inhibitor. Naunyn-Schmiedeberg's Arch. exp. Path. Pharmak. **232**, 324—326 (1957).

DENGLER, H.J., SPIEGEL, H.E., TITUS, E.O.: Uptake of tritium-labeled norepinephrine in brain and other tissues of cat *in vivo*. Science **133**, 1072—1073 (1961).

DE POTTER, W.P., DE SCHAEPDRYVER, A.F., MOERMAN, E.J., SMITH, A.D.: Evidence for the release of vesicle-proteins together with noradrenaline upon stimulation of the splenic nerve J. Physiol. (Lond.) **204**, 102P—104P (1969).

DE QUATTRO, V., MARONDE, R., NAGATSU, T., ALEXANDER, N.: Altered norepinephrine synthesis and storage in the hypertensive buffer denervated rabbit. Fed. Proc. **27**, 240 (1968).

DE ROBERTIS, E., PELLEGRINO DE IRALDI, A.: Plurivesicular secretory processes and nerve endings in the pineal gland of the rat. J. biophys. biochem. Cytol. **10**, 361—372 (1961).

EHRINGER, H., HORNYKIEWICZ, O., LECHNER, K.: Die Wirkung von Methylenblau auf die Monoaminoxydase und den Katecholamin- und 5-Hydroxytryptaminstoffwechsel des Gehirns. Naunyn-Schmiedeberg's Arch. exp. Path. Pharmak. **241**, 568—582 (1961).

EISENFELD, A.J., AXELROD, J., KRAKOFF, L.: Inhibition of the extraneuronal accumulation and metabolism of norepinephrine by adrenergic blocking agents. J. Pharmacol. exp. Ther. **156**, 107—113 (1967).

ERSPAMER, V., BORETTI, G.: Substance of a phenolic and indolic nature present in acetone extracts of the posterior salivary glands of octopoda *(Octopus vulgaris; Octopus macropus* and *Eledone moschata)*. Experientia (Basel) **7**, 271—273 (1951).

EULER, U.S. v.: Action of adrenaline, acetylcholine and other substances on nerve-free vessels (human placenta) J. Physiol. (Lond.) **93**, 129—143 (1938).

— The nature of adrenergic nerve mediators. Pharmacol. Rev. **3**, 247—277 (1951).

— Presence of catechol amines in visceral organs of fish and invertebrates. Acta physiol. scand. **28**, 297—305 (1953).

— Adrenaline and noradrenaline. Distribution and action. Pharmacol. Rev. **6**, 15—22 (1954).

— The presence of the adrenergic neurotransmitter in intraaxonal structures. Acta physiol. scand. **43**, 155—166 (1958).

— Release and uptake of noradrenaline in adrenergic nerve granules. Acta physiol. scand. **67**, 430—440 (1966).

— Acute neuromuscular transmission failure in vas deferens after reserpine. Acta physiol. scand. **76**, 255—256 (1969).

— Effect of some metabolic factors and drugs on uptake and release of catecholamines *in vitro* and *in vivo*. Bayer. Symposium II. KRONEBERG G. and SCHÜMANN, H.J., Eds. 1969. Springer Verlag p. 144—158 (1970).

— HAMBERG, U., HELLNER, S.: β-(3:4-Dihydroxyphenyl) ethylamine (hydroxytyramine) in normal human urine. Biochem. J. **49**, 655—658 (1951).

— HELLNER-BJÖRKMAN, S.: Effect of increased adrenergic nerve activity on the content of noradrenaline and adrenaline in cat organs. Acta physiol. scand. **33**, Suppl. 118, 17—20(1955).

— HILLARP, N.-Å.: Evidence for the presence of noradrenaline in submicroscopic structures of adrenergic axons. Nature (Lond.) **177**, 44—45 (1956).

— LISHAJKO, F.: Dopamine in mammalian lung and spleen. Acta physiol. pharmacol. neerl. **6**, 295—303 (1957).

— — Catecholamine release and uptake in isolated adrenergic nerve granules. Acta physiol. scand. **57**, 468—480 (1963a).

— — Effect of adenine nucleotides on catecholamine release and uptake in isolated adrenergic nerve granules. Acta physiol. scand. **59**, 454—461 (1963b).

— — Stereospecific catecholamine uptake in rabbit hearts depleted by decaborane. Int. J. Neuropharmacol. **4**, 273—280 (1965a).

— — Effect of drugs on the storage granules of adrenergic nerves. In: "Pharmacology of cholinergic and adrenergic transmission". Proc. 2nd Internat. Pharmacol. Meeting, held Prague in August 1963. Czechoslovak Medical Press, Praha, 245—259 (1965b).

— — Reuptake and net uptake of noradrenaline in adrenergic nerve granules with a note on the affinity for l- and d-isomers. Acta physiol. scand. **71**, 151—162 (1967a).

— — The uptake of isoprenaline in nerve granules. Int. J. Neuropharmacol. **6**, 431—434 (1967b).

— — Effect of directly and indirectly acting sympathomimetic amines on adrenergic transmitter granules. Acta physiol. scand. **73**, 78—92 (1968a).

— — Inhibitory action of adrenergic blocking agents on reuptake and net uptake of noradrenaline in nerve granules. Acta physiol. scand. **74**, 501—506 (1968b).

— — Effects of some metabolic co-factors and inhibitors on transmitter release and uptake in isolated adrenergic nerve granules. Acta physiol. scand. **77**, 298—307 (1969).

— LUFT, R.: Noradrenaline output in urine after infusion in man. Brit. J. Pharmacol. **6**, 286—288 (1951).

— PURKHOLD, A.: Effect of sympathetic denervation on the noradrenaline and adrenaline content of the spleen, kidney, and salivary glands in the sheep. Acta physiol. scand. **24**, 212—217 (1951).

— SWANBECK, G.: Some morphological features of catecholamine storing nerve vesicles. Acta physiol. scand. **62**, 487—488 (1964).

FALCK, B., HILLARP, N.-Å., TORP, A.: Some observations on the histology and histochemistry of the chromaffin cells probably storing dopamine. J. Histochem. Cytochem. **7**, 323—328 (1959).

FOLKOW, B., HÄGGENDAL, J., LISANDER, B.: Extent of release and elimination of noradrenaline at peripheral adrenergic nerve terminals. Acta physiol. scand. **72**, Suppl. 307 (1968).
FURCHGOTT, R.F., KIRPEKAR, S.M., RIEKER, M., SCHWAB, A.: Actions and interactions of norepinephrine, tyramine and cocaine on aortic strips of rabbit and left atria of guinea pig and cat. J. Pharmacol. exp. Ther. **142**, 39—58 (1963).
FUXE, K.: The distribution of monoamine nerve terminals in the central nervous system. Acta physiol. scand. **64**, Suppl. 247 (1965).
GEFFEN, L.B.: The effect of desmethylimipramine upon the overflow of sympathetic transmitter from the cat's spleen. J. Physiol. (Lond.) **181**, 69P—70P (1965).
— LIVETT, B.G., RUSH, R.A.: Immunological localization of chromogranins in sheep sympathetic neurones, and their release by nerve impulses. J. Physiol. (Lond.) **204**, 58P—59P (1969).
GIACHETTI, A., SHORE, P.A.: Studies *in vitro* of amine uptake mechanisms in heart. Biochem. Pharmacol. **15**, 607—614 (1966).
GILLESPIE, J.S.: The role of receptors in adrenergic uptake. In Ciba Foundation Study Group No 33 "Adrenergic neurotransmission". pp. 61—72. G.E.W. WOLSTENHOLME and M. O'CONNOR, eds. J. & A. Churchill Ltd. London: 1968.
— KIRPEKAR, S.M.: The inactivation of infused noradrenaline by the cat spleen. J. Physiol. (Lond.) **176**, 205—227 (1965).
— MACKENNA, B.R.: The inhibitory action of the sympathetic nerves on the smooth muscle of the rabbit gut, its reversal by reserpine and restoration by catechol amines and by dopa. J. Physiol. (Lond.) **156**, 17—34 (1961).
GLOWINSKI, J., AXELROD, J.: Effect of drugs on the uptake, release, and metabolism of H^3-norepinephrine in the rat brain. J. Pharmacol. exp. Ther. **149**, 43—49 (1965).
— IVERSEN, L.L., AXELROD, J.: Storage and synthesis of norepinephrine in the reserpine-treated rat brain. J. Pharmacol. exp. Ther. **151**, 385—399 (1966a).
— KOPIN, I.J., AXELROD, J.: Metabolism of 3H norepinephrine in the rat brain. J. Neurochem. **12**, 25—30 (1965).
— SNYDER, S.H., AXELROD, J.: Subcellular localization of H^3-norepinephrine in the rat brain and the effect of drugs. J. Pharmacol. exp. Ther. **152**, 282—292 (1966b).
GOLDSTEIN, M., ANAGNOSTE, B., LAUBER, E., MCKEREGHAN, M.R.: Inhibition of dopamine-β-hydroxylase by disulfiram. Life Sci. **3**, 763—767 (1964a).
— CONTRERA, J.F.: The inhibition of norepinephrine and epinephrine synthesis *in vitro*. Biochem. Pharmacol. **7**, 77—78 (1961).
— JOH, T.H., GARVEY III, T.Q.: Kinetic studies of the enzymatic dopamine β-hydroxylation reaction. Biochemistry **7**, 2724 —2730 (1968).
— LAUBER, E., MCKEREGHAN, M.R.: The inhibition of dopamine-β-hydroxylase by tropolone and other chelating agents. Biochem. Pharmacol. **13**, 1103—1106 (1964b).
— — — Studies on the purification and characterization of 3,4-dihydroxyphenylethylamine β-hydroxylase. J. biol. Chem. **240**, 2066—2072 (1965).
— WEISS, Z.: Inhibition of tyrosine hydroxylase by 3-iodo-l-tyrosine. Life Sci. **4**, 261—264 (1965).
GOODALL, MCC.: Hydroxytyramine in mammalian heart. Nature (Lond.) **166**, 738 (1950).
— Studies of adrenaline and noradrenaline in mammalian heart and suprarenals. Acta physiol. scand. **24**, Suppl. 85 (1951).
— KIRSHNER, N.: Biosynthesis of adrenaline and noradrenaline *in vitro*. J. biol. Chem. **226**, 213—221 (1957).
— — Biosynthesis of epinephrine and norepinephrine by sympathetic nerves and ganglia. Circulation **17**, 366—371 (1958).
GORDON, R., REID, J.V.O., SJOERDSMA, A., UDENFRIEND, S.: Increased synthesis of norepinephrine in the rat heart on electrical stimulation of the stellate ganglia. Mol. Pharmacol. **2**, 610—613 (1966a).
— SPECTOR, S., SJOERDSMA, A., UDENFRIEND, S.: Increased synthesis of norepinephrine and epinephrine in the intact rat during exercise and exposure to cold. J. Pharmacol. exp. Ther. **153**, 440—447 (1966b).
GREEN, J.P.: Binding of some biogenic amines in tissues. In: "Advances in Pharmacology", S. GARATTINI and P.A. SHORE, Eds., Academic Press, **1**, 349—422 (1962).
GURIN, S., DELLUVA, A.M.: The biological synthesis of radioactive adrenaline from phenylalanine. J. biol. Chem. **170**, 545—550 (1947).
HAEFELY, W., HÜRLIMANN, A., THOENEN, H.: A quantitative study of the effect of cocaine on the response of the cat nictitating membrane to nerve stimulation and to injected noradrenaline. Brit. J. Pharmacol. **22**, 5—21 (1964).
HÄGGENDAL, J., LINDQVIST, M.: Disclosure of labile monoamine fractions in brain and their correlation to behaviour. Acta physiol. scand. **60**, 351—357 (1964).

HAGEN, P.B., COHEN, L.H.: Biosynthesis of indolealkylamines. Physiological release and transport of 5-hydroxytryptamine. In: „Handbuch der experimentellen Pharmakologie", Vol. XIX, pp. 182—211. Berlin-Heidelberg-New York: Springer 1966.

HAMBERGER, B., MALMFORS, T., NORBERG, K.-A., SACHS, C.: Uptake and accumulation of catecholamines in peripheral adrenergic neurons of reserpinized animals, studied with a histochemical method. Biochem. Pharmacol. **13**, 841—844 (1964).

HARTMAN, W.J., AKAWIE, R.I., CLARK, W.G.: Competitive inhibition of 3,4-dihydroxyphenylalanine (DOPA) decarboxylase *in vitro*. J. biol. Chem. **216**, 507—529 (1955a).

— POGRUND, R.S., DRELL, W., CLARK, W.G.: Studies on the biosynthesis of arterenol. Enzymatic decarboxylation of diastereoisomers of hydroxyphenylserines. J. Amer. chem. Soc. **77**, 816—817 (1955b).

HEDQVIST, P.: Control by prostaglandin E_2 of sympathetic neurotransmission in the spleen. Life Sci. **9**, Part I, 269—278 (1970).

HENNING, M.: Studies on the mode of action of α-methyldopa. Acta physiol. scand. **76**, Suppl. 322 (1969).

HERTTING, G.: The fate of ^{3}H-iso-proterenol in the rat. Biochem. Pharmacol. **13**, 1119—1128 (1964).

— Effect of drugs and sympathetic denervation on noradrenaline uptake and binding in animal tissues. In: "Pharmacology of cholinergic and adrenergic transmission". Proc. 2nd Internat. Pharmacol. Meeting, Prague held in August 1963. Czechoslovak Medical Press, Praha, 277—288 (1965).

— AXELROD, J.: Fate of tritiated noradrenaline at the sympathetic nerve-endings. Nature (Lond.) **192**, 172—173 (1961).

— — KOPIN, I.J., WHITBY, L.G.: Lack of uptake of catecholamines after chronic denervation of sympathetic nerves. Nature (Lond.) **189**, 66 (1961a).

— — WHITBY, L.G.: Effect of drugs on the uptake and metabolism of H^3-norepinephrine. J. Pharmacol. exp. Ther. **134**, 146—153 (1961b).

— POTTER, L.T., AXELROD, J.: Effect of decentralization and ganglionic blocking agents on the spontaneous release of H^3-norepinephrine. J. Pharmacol. exp. Ther. **136**, 289—292 (1962).

— SCHIEFTHALER, TH.: Beziehung zwischen Durchflußgröße und Noradrenalinfreisetzung bei Nervenreizung der isoliert durchströmten Katzenmilz. Naunyn-Schmiedeberg's Arch. exp. Path. Pharmak. **246**, 13—14 (1963).

HESS, S.M., REDFIELD, B.G., UDENFRIEND, S.: The effect of monoamine oxidase inhibitors and tryptophan on the tryptamine content of animal tissues and urine. J. Pharmacol. exp. Ther. **127**, 178—181 (1959).

HILLARP, N.-Å., FUXE, K., DAHLSTRÖM, A.: Demonstration and mapping of central neurons containing dopamine, noradrenaline, and 5-hydroxytryptamine and their reactions to psychopharmaca. Pharmacol. Rev. **18**, Part I, 727—741 (1966).

HÖKFELT, T.: Distribution of noradrenaline storing particles in peripheral adrenergic neurons as revealed by electron microscopy. Acta physiol. scand. **76**, 427—440 (1969).

HÖRTNAGL, H., HÖRTNAGL, H., WINKLER, H.: Bovine splenic nerve: Characterization of noradrenaline-containing vesicles and other cell organelles by density gradient centrifugation. J. Physiol. (Lond.) **205**, 103—114 (1969).

HOLTZ, P.: Dopadecarboxylase. Naturwissenschaften **27**, 724—725 (1939).

— Role of l-dopa decarboxylase in the biosynthesis of catecholamines in nervous tissue and the adrenal medulla. Pharmacol. Rev. **11**, 317—329 (1959).

— Über den Mechanismus der blutdrucksenkenden Wirkung von α-Methyldopa. In: „Hochdruckforschung. Fortschritte auf dem Gebiet der Inneren Medizin". II. Symposium held in Freiburg 1964. L. HEILMEYER and H.J. HOLTMEIER, Eds. pp. 3—12. Stuttgart: Georg Thieme 1965.

— CREDNER, K.: Oxytyraminbildung aus Tyramin durch Bestrahlung. Naunyn-Schmiedeberg's Arch. exp. Path. Pharmak. **202**, 150—154 (1943).

— — KOEPP, W.: Die enzymatische Entstehung von Oxytyramin im Organismus und die physiologische Bedeutung der Dopadecarboxylase. Naunyn-Schmiedeberg's Arch. exp. Path. Pharmak. **200**, 356—388 (1942).

— — WALTER, H.: Über die Spezifität der Aminosäure-decarboxylasen. Hoppe-Seylers Z. physiol. Chem. **262**, 111—119 (1939).

— HEISE, R., LÜDTKE, K.: Fermentativer Abbau von l-Dioxyphenylalanin (Dopa) durch Niere. Naunyn-Schmiedeberg's Arch. exp. Path. Pharmak. **191**, 87—118 (1938).

— PALM, D.: Pharmacological aspects of vitamin B:. Pharmacol. Rev. **16**, 113—178 (1964).

— WESTERMANN, E.: Hemmung der Glutaminsäuredecarboxylase des Gehirns durch Brenzcatechinderivate. Naunyn-Schmiedeberg's Arch. exp. Path. Pharmak. **231**, 311—332 (1957).

HORNYKIEWICZ, O.: Dopamin (3-Hydroxytyramin) im Zentralnervensystem und seine Beziehung zum Parkinson-Syndrom des Menschen. Dtsch. med. Wschr. **87**, 1807—1810 (1962).

HUGHES, J., GILLES, C.N., BLOOM, F.E.: The uptake and disposition of dl-norepinephrine in perfused rat lung. J. Pharmacol. exp. Ther. **169**, 237—248 (1969).

HUKOVIC, S., MUSCHOLL, E.: Die Noradrenalin-Abgabe aus dem isolierten Kaninchenherzen bei sympathischer Nervenreizung und ihre pharmakologische Beeinflussung. Naunyn-Schmiedeberg's Arch. exp. Path. Pharmak. **244**, 81—96 (1962).

IKEDA, M., FAHIEN, L.A., UDENFRIEND, S.: A kinetic study of bovine adrenal tyrosine hydroxylase. J. biol. Chem. **241**, 4452—4456 (1966).

— LEVITT, M., UDENFRIEND, S.: Hydroxylation of phenylalanine by purified preparations of adrenal and brain tyrosine hydroxylase. Biochem. biophys. Res. Commun. **18**, 482—488 (1965).

IVERSEN, L.L.: The uptake of noradrenaline by the isolated perfused rat heart. Brit. J. Pharmacol. **21**, 523—537 (1963).

— The uptake of catecholamines at high perfusion concentrations in the rat isolated heart: a novel catecholamine uptake process. Brit. J. Pharmacol. **25**, 18—33 (1965).

— The uptake and storage of noradrenaline in sympathetic nerves. Cambridge: The University Press 1967.

— Characteristics of noradrenaline uptake in the iris/ciliary body and other peripheral tissues of the rat. Naunyn-Schmiedeberg's Arch. Pharmak. exp. Path. **259**, 179 (1968).

— AXELROD, J., GLOWINSKI, J.: The effect of antidepressant drugs on the uptake and metabolism of catecholamines in the brain. Proc. Internat. Congress of the Collegium Internat. Neuropsychopharmacologicum, held in Washington, March 1966. Excerpta Medica Internat. Congress Series No 129, 362—366.

— DE CHAMPLAIN, J., GLOWINSKI, J., AXELROD, J.: Uptake, storage and metabolism of norepinephrine in tissues of the developing rat. J. Pharmacol. exp. Ther. **157**, 509—516 (1967).

— GLOWINSKI, J., AXELROD, J.: The uptake and storage of H^3-norepinephrine in the reserpine-pretreated rat heart. J. Pharmacol. exp. Ther. **150**, 173—183 (1965).

— KRAVITZ, E.A.: Sodium dependence of transmitter uptake at adrenergic nerve terminals. Mol. Pharmacol. **2**, 360—362 (1966).

JONSSON, G., HAMBERGER, B., MALMFORS, T., SACHS, C.: Uptake and accumulation of ^3H-noradrenaline in adrenergic nerves of rat iris. Effect of reserpine, monoamine oxidase and tyrosine hydroxylase inhibition. Europ. J. Pharmacol. **8**, 58—72 (1969).

KÄRKI, N.T.: The urinary excretion of noradrenaline and adrenaline in different age groups, its diurnal variation and the effect of muscular work on it. Acta physiol. scand. **39**, Suppl. 132 (1956).

KAKIMOTO, Y., ARMSTRONG, M.D.: On the identification of octopamine in mammals. J. biol. Chem. **237**, 422—427 (1962).

KAUFMAN, S., FRIEDMAN, S.: Dopamine-β-hydroxylase. Pharmacol. Rev. **17**, 71—100 (1965).

KIRPEKAR, S.M., CERVONI, P.: Effect of cocaine, phenoxybenzamine and phentolamine on the catecholamine output from spleen and adrenal medulla. J. Pharmacol. exp. Ther. **142**, 59—70 (1963).

— WAKADE, A.R.: Factors influencing noradrenaline uptake by the perfused spleen of the cat. J. Physiol. (Lond.) **194**, 609—626 (1968).

KIRSHNER, N.: Uptake of catecholamines by a particulate fraction of the adrenal medulla. J. biol. Chem. **237**, 2311—2317 (1962).

— SMITH, W.J.: Metabolic requirements for secretion from the adrenal medulla. Science **154**, 422—423 (1966).

KOPIN, I.J., BREESE, G.R., KRAUSS, K.R., WEISE, V.K.: Selective release of newly synthesized norepinephrine from the cat spleen during sympathetic nerve stimulation. J. Pharmacol. exp. Ther. **161**, 271—278 (1968).

— FISCHER, J.E., MUSACCHIO, J.M., HORST, W.D., WEISE, V.K.: "False neurochemical transmitters" and the mechanism of sympathetic blockade by monoamine oxidase inhibitors. J. Pharmacol. exp. Ther. **147**, 186—193 (1965).

— GORDON, E.K.: Metabolism of norepinephrine-H^3 released by tyramine and reserpine. J. Pharmacol. exp. Ther. **138**, 351—359 (1962).

KUNTZMAN, R., CREVELING, C., HIRSCH, C.W., BRODIE, B.B.: Inhibition of norepinephrine synthesis in mouse brain blockade of dopamine-β-oxidase. Life Sci. **1**, 85—92 (1962).

LADURON, P., DE POTTER, W., DE SCHAEPDRYVER, A.F.: Subcellular distribution of catecholamines in dog spleen. Life Sci. **5**, 457—464 (1966).

LAGERCRANTZ, H.: Potentiation of tyramine effect on the isolated iris muscle by cocaine. Acta physiol. scand. **73**, 58—61 (1968).

LANDSBERG, L., AXELROD, J.: Influence of pituitary, thyroid and adrenal hormones on norepinephrine turnover and metabolism in the rat heart. Circulat. Res. **22**, 559—571 (1968a).
— — Reduced accumulation of ^{3}H-norepinephrine in the rat heart following hypophysectomy. Endocrinology **82**, 175—178 (1968b).
— DE CHAMPLAIN, J., AXELROD, J.: Increased biosynthesis of cardiac norepinephrine after hypophysectomy. J. Pharmacol. exp. Ther. **165**, 102—107 (1969).
LANGEMANN, H.: Enzymes and their substrates in the adrenal gland of the ox. Brit. J. Pharmacol. **6**, 318—324 (1951).
LEITZ, F. H., STEFANO, F. J. E.: Effect of ouabain and desipramine on the uptake and storage of norepinephrine and metaraminol. Europ. J. Pharmacol. **11**, 278—285 (1970).
LEVER, J. D., ESTERHUIZEN, A. C.: Fine structure of the arteriolar nerves in the guinea pig pancreas. Nature (Lond.) **192**, 566—567 (1961).
LEVIN, E. Y., LEVENBERG, B., KAUFMAN, S.: The enzymatic conversion of 3,4-dihydroxyphenylethylamine to norepinephrine. J. biol. Chem. **235**, 2080—2086 (1960).
LEVINE, R. J., SJOERDSMA, A.: Dissociation of the decarboxylase-inhibiting and norepinephrine-depleting effects of α-methyl-dopa, α-ethyl-dopa, 4-bromo-3-hydroxybenzyloxyamine and related substances. J. Pharmacol. exp. Ther. **146**, 42—47 (1964).
LEVITT, M., SPECTOR, S., SJOERDSMA, A., UDENFRIEND, S.: Elucidation of the rate-limiting step in norepinephrine biosynthesis in the perfused guinea-pig heart. J. Pharmacol. exp. Ther. **148**, 1—8 (1965).
LINDMAR, R., MUSCHOLL, E.: Die Wirkung von Pharmaka auf die Elimination von Noradrenalin aus der Perfusionsflüssigkeit und die Noradrenalinaufnahme in das isolierte Herz. Naunyn-Schmiedeberg's Arch. exp. Path. Pharmak. **247**, 469—492 (1964).
— — Die Aufnahme von α-Methylnoradrenalin in das isolierte Kaninchenherz und seine Freisetzung durch Reserpin und Guanethidin *in vivo*. Naunyn-Schmiedeberg's Arch. exp. Path. Pharmak. **249**, 529—548 (1965).
LISHAJKO, F.: Release, reuptake and net uptake of dopamine, noradrenaline and adrenaline in isolated sheep adrenal medullary granules. Acta physiol. scand. **76**, 159—171 (1969).
— Release and uptake of dopamine in isolated granules from a human carotid body tumour. Acta physiol. scand. **79**, 533—536 (1970).
LOVENBERG, W., WEISSBACH, H., UDENFRIEND, S.: Aromatic L-amino acid decarboxylase. J. biol. Chem. **237**, 89—93 (1962).
LUND, A.: Elimination of adrenaline and noradrenaline from the organism. Acta pharmacol. (Kbh.) **7**, 297—308 (1951).
MACKENNA, B. R.: Uptake of catecholamines by the hearts of rabbits treated with Segontin. Acta physiol. scand. **63**, 413—422 (1965).
MACMILLAN, W. H.: A hypothesis concerning the effect of cocaine on the action of sympathomimetic amines. Brit. J. Pharmacol. **14**, 385—391 (1959).
MAÎTRE, L.: Entstehung pressorischer Catecholderivate aus Metaraminol oder α-Methyl-p-Tyrosin (α-MT) im Meerschweinchen. Naunyn-Schmiedeberg's Arch. exp. Path. Pharmak. **251**, 160—161 (1965).
— STAEHELIN, M.: Effect of α-methyl-dopa on myocardial catecholamines. Experientia (Basel) **19**, 573—575 (1963).
— — Presence of α-methyl-noradrenaline ("Corbasil") in the heart of guinea-pigs treated with metaraminol ("Aramine"). Nature (Lond.) **206**, 723—724 (1965).
— — Enhancement of H^3-norepinephrine accumulation in rat vas deferens by cocaine, imipramine, and desmethylimipramine. Experientia (Basel) **24**, 671—672 (1968).
MALMFORS, T.: Studies on adrenergic nerves. The use of rat and mouse iris for direct observations on their physiology and pharmacology at cellular and subcellular levels. Acta physiol. scand. **64**, Suppl. 248 (1965).
— v. EULER, U. S.: Depletion and repletion of noradrenaline in adrenergic nerves of the rat after decaborane treatment. Experientia (Basel) **27**, 417—419 (1971).
MERRITT, J. H., SCHULTZ, E. J.: The effect of decaborane on the biosynthesis and metabolism of norepinephrine in the rat brain. Life Sci. **5**, 27—32 (1966).
— — WYKES, A. A.: Effect of decaborane on norepinephrine content of rat brain. Biochem. Pharmacol. **13**, 1364—1365 (1965).
MONTAGU, K. A.: Catechol compounds in rat tissues and in brains of different animals. Nature (Lond.) **180**, 244—245 (1957).
MONTANARI, R., COSTA, E., BEAVEN, M. A., BRODIE, B. B.: Turnover rates of norepinephrine in hearts of intact mice, rats and guinea pigs using tritiated norepinephrine. Life Sci. **2**, 232—240 (1963).
MUELLER, R. A., THOENEN, H., AXELROD, J.: Increase in tyrosine hydroxylase activity after reserpine administration. J. Pharmacol. exp. Ther. **169**, 74—79 (1969a).
— — — Adrenal tyrosine hydroxylase: Compensatory increase in activity after chemical sympathectomy. Science **163**, 468—469 (1969b).

MURPHY, G.F., SOURKES, T.L.: The action of antidecarboxylases on the conversion of 3,4-dihydroxyphenylalanine to dopamine *in vivo*. Arch. Biochem. **93**, 338—343 (1961).

MUSACCHIO, J.M., GOLDSTEIN, M.: Biosynthesis of norepinephrine and norsynephrine in the perfused rabbit heart. Biochem. Pharmacol. **12**, 1061—1063 (1963).

— KOPIN, I.J., SNYDER, S.: Effects of disulfiram on tissue norepinephrine content and subcellular distribution of dopamine, tyramine and their β-hydroxylated metabolites. Life Sci. **3**, 769—775 (1964).

— — WEISE, V.K.: Subcellular distribution of some sympathomimetic amines and their β-hydroxylated derivatives in the rat heart. J. Pharmacol. exp. Ther. **148**, 22—28 (1965a).

— WEISE, V.K., KOPIN, I.J.: Mechanism of norepinephrine binding. Nature (Lond.) **205**, 606—607 (1965b).

MUSCHOLL, E.: Die Hemmung der Noradrenalin-Aufnahme des Gewebes durch Cocain. Naunyn-Schmiedeberg's Arch. exp. Path. Pharmak. **240**, 8 (1960).

— Effect of cocaine and related drugs on the uptake of noradrenaline by heart and spleen. Brit. J. Pharmacol. **16**, 352—359 (1961).

— Drugs interfering with the storage and release of adrenergic transmitters. In: "Pharmacology of cholinergic and adrenergic transmission". Proc. 2nd Internat. Pharmacol. Meeting, held in Prague, August 1963. Czechoslovak Medical Press, Praha, 291—302 (1965).

— Autonomic nervous system: Newer mechanisms of adrenergic blockade. Ann. Rev. Pharmacol. **6**, 107—128 (1966a).

— Release of catecholamines from the heart. In: "Mechanisms of Release of Biogenic Amines", pp. 247—260. Eds. U.S. v. EULER, S. ROSELL and B. UVNÄS. Oxford: Pergamon Press 1966b.

— MAÎTRE, L.: Release by sympathetic stimulation of α-methylnoradrenaline stored in the heart after administration of α-methyldopa. Experientia (Basel) **19**, 658—659 (1963).

— WEBER, E.: Die Hemmung der Aufnahme von α-Methyl-Noradrenalin in das Herz durch sympathomimetische Amine. Naunyn-Schmiedeberg's Arch. exp. Path. Pharmak. **252**, 134—143 (1965).

NAGATSU, T., LEVITT, M., UDENFRIEND, S.: Conversion of L-tyrosine to 3,4-dihydroxyphenylalanine by cell-free preparations of brain and sympathetically innervated tissues. Biochem. biophys. Res. Commun. **14**, 543—549 (1964).

— VAN DER SCHOOT, J.B., LEVITT, M., UDENFRIEND, S.: Factors influencing dopamine β-hydroxylase activity and epinephrine levels in guinea pig adrenal gland. J. Biochem. **64**, 39—43 (1968).

NASMYTH, P.A., ANDREWS, W.H.H.: The antagonism of cocaine to the action of choline 2,6-xylyl ether bromide at sympathetic nerve endings. Brit. J. Pharmacol. **14**, 477—483 (1959).

NIKODIJEVIC, B., CREVELING, C.R., UDENFRIEND, S.: Inhibition of dopamine β-oxidase *in vivo* by benzyloxyamine and benzylhydrazine analogs. J. Pharmacol. exp. Ther. **140**, 224—228 (1963).

NORBERG, K.-A., HAMBERGER, B.: The sympathetic adrenergic neuron. Acta physiol. scand. **63**, Suppl. 238 (1964).

OATES, J.A., GILLESPIE, L., UDENFRIEND, S., SJOERDSMA, A.: Decarboxylase inhibition and blood pressure reduction by α-methyl-3,4-dihydroxy-dl-phenylalanine. Science **131**, 1890—1891 (1960).

OLIVERIO, A., STJÄRNE, L.: Acceleration of noradrenaline turnover in the mouse heart by cold exposure. Life Sci. **4**, 2339—2343 (1965).

OWMAN, C.: Sympathetic nerves probably storing two types of monoamines in the rat pineal gland. Int. J. Neuropharmacol. **3**, 105—112 (1964).

PAK, C.: Versuche über den Übertritt chemischer Substanzen aus der Gefäßbahn in die Gewebe. Naunyn-Schmiedeberg's Arch. exp. Path. Pharmak. **11**, 42—59 (1926).

PAULSEN, E,C.. HESS, S.M.: The rate of synthesis of catecholamines following depletion in guinea pig brain and heart. J. Neurochem. **10**, 453—459 (1963).

PESKAR, B., HELLMAN, G., HERTTING, G.: Kinetik der Aufnahme und der Transformation von 7-^{3}H-Dopamin im isoliert perfundierten Rattenherzen. Naunyn-Schmiedeberg's Arch. Pharmak. exp. Path. **260**, 186—187 (1968).

PHILIPPU, A., PFEIFFER, R., SCHÜMANN, H.J., LICKFELD, K.: Eigenschaften der Noradrenalin speichernden Granula des sympathischen Ganglion stellatum. Naunyn-Schmiedeberg's Arch. Pharmak. exp. Path. **258**, 251—265 (1967).

PISANO, J.J., CREVELING, C.R., UDENFRIEND, S.: Enzymic conversion of p-tyramine to p-hydroxyphenylethanolamine (Norsynephrin). Biochim. biophys. Acta (Amst.) **43**, 566—568 (1960).

POTTER, L.T., AXELROD, J.: Subcellular localization of catecholamines in tissues of the rat. J. Pharmacol. exp. Ther. **142**, 291—298 (1963a).

— — Studies on the storage of norepinephrine and the effect of drugs. J. Pharmacol. exp. Ther. **140**, 199—206 (1963b).

RAAB, W., GIGEE, W.: Die Katecholamine des Herzens. Naunyn-Schmiedeberg's Arch. exp. Path. Pharmak. **219**, 248—262 (1953).
REHN, N.O.: Effect of decentralisation on the content of catechol amines in the spleen and kidney of the cat. Acta physiol. scand. **42**, 309—312 (1958).
RICHARDSON, K.C.: The fine structure of autonomic nerve endings in smooth muscle of the rat vas deferens. J. Anat. (Lond.) **96**, 427—442 (1962).
ROSELL, S., AXELROD, J.: Relation between blockade of H^3-noradrenaline uptake and pharmacological actions produced by phenothiazine derivatives. Experientia (Basel) **19**, 318 to 319 (1963).
— SEDVALL, G.: Restoration of vasoconstrictor effects in reserpinized cats. Acta physiol. scand. **53**, 174—184 (1961).
ROSS, S.B., RENYI, A.L., BRUNFELTER, B.: Cocainesensitive uptake of sympathomimetic amines in nerve tissue. J. Pharm. Pharmacol. **20**, 283—288 (1968).
ROTH, R.H., STJÄRNE, L., v. EULER, U.S.: Factors influencing the rate of norepinephrine biosynthesis in nerve tissue. J. Pharmacol. exp. Ther. **158**, 373—377 (1967).
— STONE, E.A.: The action of reserpine on noradrenaline biosynthesis in sympathetic nerve tissue. Biochem. Pharmacol. **17**, 1581—1590 (1968).
RUTLEDGE, C.O., WEINER, N.: The effect of reserpine upon the synthesis of norepinephrine in the isolated rabbit heart. J. Pharmacol. **157**, 290—302 (1967).
RYD, G.: Protective effect of bretylium on noradrenaline stores in organs. Acta physiol. scand. **56**, 90—93 (1962).
SAMORAJSKI, T., MARKS, B.H., WEBSTER, E.J.: An autoradiographic study of the uptake and storage of norepinephrine-H^3 in tissues of mice treated with reserpine and cocaine. J. Pharmacol. exp. Ther. **143**, 82—89 (1964).
SCHMITERLÖW, C.G.: The formation *in vivo* of noradrenaline from 3:4-dihydroxyphenylserine (noradrenaline carboxylic acid). Brit. J. Pharmacol. **6**, 127—134 (1951).
SCHOTT, H.F., CLARK, W.G.: Dopa decarboxylase inhibition through the interaction of coenzyme and substrate. J. biol. Chem. **196**, 449—462 (1952).
SCHÜMANN, H.J.: Nachweis von Oxytyramin (Dopamin) in sympathischen Nerven und Ganglien. Naunyn-Schmiedeberg's Arch. exp. Path. Pharmak. **227**, 566—573 (1956).
— GROBECKER, H.: Nachweis und Lokalisation von α-Methyl-Noradrenalin in Meerschweinchenorganen nach Vorbehandlung mit α-Methyl-Dopa. Naunyn-Schmiedeberg's Arch. exp. Path. Pharmak. **247**, 279—298 (1964).
SEDVALL, G.: Noradrenaline storage in skeletal muscle. Acta physiol. scand. **60**, 39—50 (1964).
— KOPIN, I.J.: Influence of sympathetic denervation and nerve impulse activity of tyrosine hydroxylase in the rat submaxillary gland. Biochem. Pharmacol. **16**, 39—46 (1967).
SHAHAB, L., LISHAJKO, F., v. EULER, U.S.: Differentiated storage mechanism for noradrenaline and dopamine in the rabbit heart. Neuropharmacol. In press (1971).
SHORE, P.A., GIACHETTI, A.: Dual actions of guanethidine on amine uptake mechanisms in adrenergic neurons. Biochem. Pharmacol. **15**, 899—903 (1966).
SJOERDSMA, A., LOVENBERG, W., OATES, J.A., CROUT, J.R., UDENFRIEND, S.: Alterations in the pattern of amine excretion in man produced by a monoamine oxidase inhibitor. Science **130**, 225 (1959).
SOURKES, T.L.: Inhibition of dihydroxyphenylalanine decarboxylase by derivatives of phenylalanine. Arch. Biochem. **51**, 444—456 (1954).
— Substrate specificity of hydroxy-l-phenylalanine decarboxylases and related enzymes. Rev. canad. Biol. **14**, 49—63 (1955).
— DOPA decarboxylase: substrates, coenzyme, inhibitors. Pharmacol. Rev. **18**, 53—60 (1966).
— MURPHY, G.F., RABINOVITCH, A.: Conversion of DL-m-tyrosine to dopamine in the rat. Nature (Lond.) **189**, 577—578 (1961).
SPECTOR, S., GORDON, R., SJOERDSMA, A., UDENFRIEND, S.: End-product inhibition of tyrosine hydroxylase as a possible mechanism for regulation of norepinephrine synthesis. Mol. Pharmacol. **3**, 549—555 (1967).
— MELMON, K., LOVENBERG, W., SJOERDSMA, A.: The presence and distribution of tyramine in mammalian tissues. J. Pharmacol. exp. Ther. **140**, 229—235 (1963b).
— SJOERDSMA, A., UDENFRIEND, S.: Blockade of endogenous norepinephrine synthesis by α-methyl-tyrosine, and inhibitor of tyrosine hydroxylase. J. Pharmacol. exp. Ther. **147**, 86—95 (1965).
— — ZALTZMAN-NIRENBERG, P., LEVITT, M., UDENFRIEND, S.: Norepinephrine synthesis from tyrosine-C^{14} in isolated perfused guinea pig heart. Science **139**, 1299—1301 (1963a).
STITZEL, R.E., LUNDBORG, P.: Effect of reserpine and monoamine oxidase inhibition on the uptake and subcellular distribution of ^3H-noradrenaline. Brit. J. Pharmacol. **29**, 99—104 (1967).
STJÄRNE, L.: Studies of catecholamine uptake storage and release mechanisms. Acta physiol. scand. **62**, Suppl. 228 (1964).

STJÄRNE, L.: Studies of noradrenaline biosynthesis in nerve tissue. Acta physiol. scand. **67**, 441—454 (1966).

— HEDQVIST, P., LAGERCRANTZ, H.: Catecholamines and adenine nucleotide material in effluent from stimulated adrenal medulla and spleen. Biochem. Pharmacol. **19**, 1147—1158 (1970b).

— LISHAJKO, F.: Drug-induced inhibition of noradrenaline synthesis *in vitro* in bovine splenic nerve tissue. Brit. J. Pharmacol. **27**, 398—404 (1966).

— — Localization of different steps in noradrenaline synthesis to different fractions of a bovine splenic nerve homogenate. Biochem. Pharmacol. **16**, 1719—1728 (1967).

— — ROTH, R.H.: Regulation of noradrenaline biosynthesis in nerve tissue. Nature (Lond.) **215**, 770—772 (1967b).

— ROTH, R.H., BLOOM, F., GIARMAN, N.J.: Norepinephrine concentrating mechanisms in sympathetic nerve trunks. J. Pharmacol. exp. Ther. **171**, 70—79 (1970a).

— — GIARMAN, N.J.: Effect of desipramine on noradrenaline uptake into isolated nerve granules. Biochem. Pharmacol. **17**, 1464—1466 (1968).

— — LISHAJKO, F.: Noradrenaline formation from dopamine in isolated subcellular particles from bovine splenic nerve. Biochem. Pharmacol. **16**, 1729—1739 (1967a).

— WENNMALM, Å.: Quantitative estimation of secretion and reuptake of adrenergic transmitter in the rabbit heart. Acta physiol. scand. **81**, 286—288 (1971).

STRÖMBLAD, B.C.R., NICKERSON, M.: Accumulation of epinephrine and norepinephrine by some rat tissues. J. Pharmacol. exp. Ther. **134**, 154—159 (1961).

TAUGNER, G., HASSELBACH, W.: Über den Mechanismus der Catecholamin-Speicherung in den „chromaffinen Granula" des Nebennierenmarks. Naunyn-Schmiedeberg's Arch. Pharmak. exp. Path. **255**, 266—286 (1966).

THOENEN, H., HUERLIMAN, A., HAEFELY, W.: Wirkungen von Phenoxybenzamin, Phentolamin und Azapetin auf adrenergische Synapsen der Katzenmilz. Blockierung der α-adrenergischen Rezeptoren und Hemmung der Wiederaufnahme von neural freigesetztem Noradrenalin. Helv. Physiol. Acta **22**, 148—161 (1964a).

— — — The effect of sympathetic nerve stimulation on volume, vascular resistance and norepinephrine output in the isolated perfused spleen of the cat, and its modification by cocaine. J. Pharmacol. exp. Ther. **143**, 57—63 (1964b).

— MUELLER, R.A., AXELROD, J.: Transsynaptic induction of adrenal tyrosine hydroxylase. J. Pharmacol. exp. Ther. **169**, 249—254 (1969).

TISSARI, A.H., SCHÖNHÖFER, P.S., BOGDANSKI, D.G., BRODIE, B.B.: Mechanism of biogenic amine transport. II. Relationship between sodium and the mechanism of ouabain blockade of the accumulation of serotonin and norepinephrine by synaptosomes. Mol. Pharmacol. **5**, 593—604 (1969).

TITUS, E.O., SPIEGEL, H.E.: Effect of desmethylimipramine (DMI) on uptake of norepinephrine-7-H^3 (NE) in heart. Fed. Proc. **21**, 179 (1962).

TRENDELENBURG, U.: The supersensitivity caused by cocaine .J. Pharmacol. exp. Ther. **125**, 55—65 (1959).

— Modification of the effect of tyramine by various agents and procedures. J. Pharmacol. exp. Ther. **134**, 8—17 (1961).

— Supersensitivity and subsensitivity to sympathomimetic amines. Pharmacol. Rev. **15**, 225—276 (1963).

— Factors influencing the concentrations of catecholamines at the receptors. In: Handbook of Experimental Pharmacology, Section "Catecholamines". Eds. H. BLASCHKO and E. MUSCHOLL. Berlin-Heidelberg-New York: Springer 1971.

UDENFRIEND, S.: Tyrosine hydroxylase. Pharmacol. Rev. **18**, Part I, 43—51 (1966).

— Physiological regulation of noradrenaline biosynthesis. In: Ciba Foundation Study Group No 33 "Adrenergic neurotransmission", pp. 3—11. G.E.W. WOLSTENHOLME and M. O'CONNOR, Eds. London: J. & A. Churchill Ltd. 1968.

— CLARK, C.T., AXELROD, J., BRODIE, B.B.: Ascorbic acid in aromatic hydroxylation. I. A model system for aromatic hydroxylation. J. biol. Chem. **208**, 731—739 (1954).

— COOPER, J.R., CLARK, C.T., BAER, J.E.: Rate of turnover of epinephrine in the adrenal medulla. Science **117**, 663—665 (1953).

— WYNGAARDEN, J.B.: Precursors of adrenal epinephrine and norepinephrine *in vivo*. Biochim. biophys. Acta (Amst.) **20**, 48—52 (1956).

— ZALTZMAN-NIRENBERG, P.: On the mechanism of the norepinephrine release produced by α-methyl-meta-tyrosine. J. Pharmacol. exp. Ther. **138**, 194—199 (1962).

— — Norepinephrine and 3,4-dihydroxyphenethylamine turnover in guinea pig brain *in vivo*. Science **142**, 394—396 (1963).

— — NAGATSU, T.: Inhibitors of purified beef adrenal tyrosine hydroxylase. Biochem. Pharmacol. **14**, 837—845 (1965).

WEBER, E., MUSCHOLL, E.: Der Einfluß verschiedener Pharmaka auf die Elimination von α-Methyl-Noradrenalin aus der Perfusionsflüssigkeit des isolierten Kaninchenherzens. Naunyn-Schmiedeberg's Arch. exp. Path. Pharmak. **251**, 161 (1965).

WEGMANN, A., KAKO, K.: Particle-bound and free catecholamines in dog hearts and the uptake of injected norepinephrine. Nature (Lond.) **192**, 978 (1961).

WEIL-MALHERBE, H., WHITBY, L.G., AXELROD, J.: The uptake of circulating ^{3}H-norepinephrine by the pituitary gland and various areas of the brain. J. Neurochem. **8**, 55—64 (1961).

WEINER, N., RABADJIJA, M.: The effect of nerve stimulation on the synthesis and metabolism of norepinephrine in the isolated guinea-pig hypogastric nerve vas deferens preparation. J. Pharmacol. exp. Ther. **160**, 61—71 (1968).

— TRENDELENBURG, U.: The effect of cocaine and of pretreatment with reserpine on the uptake of tyramine-2-C^{14} and dl-epinephrine-2-C^{14} into heart and spleen. J. Pharmacol. exp. Ther. **137**, 56—61 (1962).

WEISS, P.: Self-renewal and proximo-distal convention in nerve fibres. Proc. Symposium "The effect of use and disuse on neuromuscular functions", held at Liblice near Prague, Sept. 1962. 171—183. E. GUTMAN and P. HNIK, Eds. Publi. House of the Czechoslovak Academy of Sciences (1963).

WEISSBACH, H., LOVENBERG, W., UDENFRIEND, S.: Enzymatic decarboxylation of α-methyl amino acids. Biochem. biophys. Res. Commun. **3**, 225—227 (1960).

WENNMALM, Å.: Maintenance of noradrenaline synthesis in rats after reserpine treatment. Acta physiol. scand. **73**, 523—526 (1968).

WESTFALL, T.C.: Uptake and exchange of catecholamines in rat tissues after administration of d- and l-adrenaline. Acta physiol. scand. **63**, 336—342 (1965).

WHITBY, L.G., AXELROD, J., WEIL-MALHERBE, H.: The fate of H^3-norepinephrine in animals. J. Pharmacol. exp. Ther. **132**, 193—201 (1961).

— HERTTING, G., AXELROD, J.: Effect of cocaine on the disposition of noradrenaline labelled with tritium. Nature (Lond.) **187**, 604—605 (1960).

WHITTAKER, V.P.: Catecholamine storage particles in the central nervous system. Pharmacol. Rev. **18**, Part I, 401—412 (1966).

WOLFE, D.E., POTTER, L.T., RICHARDSON, K.C., AXELROD, J.: Localizing tritiated norepinephrine in sympathetic axons by electron microscopic autoradiography. Science **138**, 440 to 442 (1962).

WURTMAN, R.J., KOPIN, I.J., HORST, D.W., FISCHER, J.E.: Epinephrine and organ blood flow: effects of hyperthyroidism cocaine and sympathetic denervation. Amer. J. Physiol. **207**, 1247—1250 (1964).

WYKES, A.A., LANDEZ, J.H.: Modification of the tissue norepinephrine and serotonin depleting action and toxic effects of decaborane-14 by pyridoxine hydrochloride and pyridoxal phosphate. Fed. Proc. **26**, No 2 (1967).

ZAIMIS, E., BERK, L., CALLINGHAM, B.: Morphological, biochemical and functional changes in the sympathetic nervous system of rats treated with NGF-antiserum. Nature (Lond.) **206**, 1221—1222 (1965).

ZWEIG, M., AXELROD, J.: Relationship between catecholamines and serotonin in sympathetic nerves of the rat pineal gland. J. Neurobiol. **1**, 87—97 (1969).

Chapter 7

The Synthesis, Uptake and Storage of Catecholamines in the Adrenal Medulla. The Effect of Drugs

L. STJÄRNE*

With 3 Figures

A. Synthesis

1. Formation of Adrenaline: N-methylation of Noradrenaline

The biosynthesis of noradrenaline in the adrenal medulla follows the same pathway as that described for sympathetic nerves (cf. Chapter by VON EULER, pp. 186). In fact, adrenal medulla has been the main tissue source for the isolation and purification of the enzymes catalyzing the three steps in the synthesis of noradrenaline from dietary tyrosine (FELLMAN, 1959; LEVIN et al., 1960; NAGATSU et al., 1964).

However, the adrenal medulla carries the synthesis sequence one step further and N-methylates noradrenaline to form adrenaline. This reaction was first described by BÜLBRING (1949), who was able to show by bioassay the formation of adrenaline on incubation of homogenates of cat or dog adrenal medulla with noradrenaline and ATP, using choline as methyl donor. In experiments with slices of bovine adrenal medulla KIRSHNER and GOODALL (1956) showed that S-adenosyl methionine served as methyl donor.

The enzyme responsible for the N-methylation of noradrenaline was later partially purified from adrenal glands of monkeys by AXELROD (1962), who found that it requires S-adenosyl methionine, that it is dependent on intact sulphydryl groups for activity and that it is specific for phenylethanolamines, with moderate preference for the naturally occurring laevorotatory stereoisomers, while not N-methylating phenylethylamines. It was thus named phenylethanolamine N-methyl transferase (PNMT) (AXELROD, 1966). Of the phenylethanolamines naturally occurring in the adrenal medulla it turned out that the O-methylated metabolites of the adrenal medullary hormones are, at least at higher concentrations (FULLER and HUNT, 1965), even better substrates for the enzyme than the hormones themselves. This fact has been utilized in a method for assay of the enzyme, in which normetanephrine is incubated with enzyme and ^{14}C-methyl-S-adenosylmethionine; the labelled metanephrine formed is then isolated by solvent extraction and measured radiometrically (AXELROD, 1962). Even secondary amines, such as adrenaline, can serve as substrates for the enzyme, with the introduction of a second methyl group on the nitrogen to form N-methyladrenaline, a tertiary amine which has been identified as normally occurring in the adrenal medulla from several species (AXELROD, 1960). Similarly, N-methyl-

* The review does not cover work published later than March 1970.

metanephrine has been found in human urine, both of normal subjects and, in elevated amounts, of patients suffering from phaeochromocytoma (ITOH et al., 1962).

Recent observations on this enzyme seem to provide one answer to the puzzling question why the adrenal medulla and cortex have fused to form one organ, the adrenal gland (cf. BLASCHKO, 1960). In studies of fetal adrenal medulla it was found that this tissue, which develops from the neural crest, is unable to methylate noradrenaline to form adrenaline (SHEPHERD and WEST, 1951; HÖKFELT, 1951) until it establishes intimate anatomical and circulatory contact with cortical tissue (ROFFI, 1964; BRUNDIN, 1965). The latter is mesodermal in origin and develops from the primitive genital ridge (cf. WILLIER, 1955). These observations, as well as the actual demonstration of adrenaline formation in noradrenaline-storing chromaffin cells *in vitro* induced by corticosteroids, suggest that adrenaline, but not noradrenaline, formation is glucocorticoid-dependent (COUPLAND, 1953; COUPLAND and MACDOUGALL, 1966). This is further supported by the finding in adult animals that the PNMT formation in adrenal medulla is depressed by hypophysectomy, and that this can be prevented by ACTH or glucocorticoid administration (WURTMAN and AXELROD, 1965), indicating that cortical hormones, which reach the medulla in high concentration *via* the portal system of the gland, control the formation of the enzyme.

Interestingly, noradrenaline is methylated to adrenaline in certain cases of phaeochromocytoma, where the tumour is not anatomically related to cortical tissue, and also in the sympathetic nerves of some non-mammalian species, in which the sympathetic neurotransmitter is adrenaline and not noradrenaline. This includes the frog, as shown by Otto Loewi, who was able to identify his "Accelerans-Stoff" from the classical experiments on the frog heart (LOEWI, 1921), with adrenaline (LOEWI, 1936). The remarkable point is that these N-methylating enzymes do not appear to require induction by steroid hormones. According to recent reports they are closely related, but not identical, to the PNMT derived from adrenal medulla (WURTMAN et al., 1968).

Several naturally occurring phenylethyl-and phenylethanolamines, as well as certain drugs, have been shown to inhibit PNMT (KRAKOFF and AXELROD, 1967). It is particularly interesting that tranylcypromine was found to be active in this respect, since it is also known to be a powerful inhibitor of MAO. Other MAO inhibitors, such as Pargyline and Nialamide, were relatively weak as inhibitors of the N-methyl transferase.

2. Role of Organelles in Synthesis

During the last few years there have been two different lines of thought on the extent to which the amine storage organelles are involved in the biosynthetic sequence from tyrosine to adrenaline (cf. Chapter by VON EULER, pp. 186). Studies of the subcellular distribution of the different enzymes led one group of workers to conclude that only the third step in the formation of noradrenaline, the β-hydroxylation of dopamine, proceeds in the vesicles (KIRSHNER, 1957), while all other enzymatic reactions take place outside them, in the cytoplasm (BLASCHKO et al., 1955; AXELROD, 1962; STJÄRNE, 1966; WEINER and RUTLEDGE, 1966; STJÄRNE and LISHAJKO, 1967; MUSACCHIO, 1968). However, in criticism of the earlier interpretation and also in the light of new evidence (NAGATSU et al., 1964), UDENFRIEND proposed the attractive hypothesis that all three steps leading from tyrosine to noradrenaline take place in one and the same organelle, possibly the amine storage vesicle, in which the different enzymes were assumed to be organized in an orderly sequence in a way analogous to the mitochondrial arrangement of enzymes involved in energy metabolism (UDENFRIEND, 1966a, 1968).

Although it is difficult to interpret centrifugation studies in terms of the subcellular distribution of different enzymes, the more recent evidence is in support of the earlier view. Thus of the enzymes involved in catecholamine synthesis, tyrosine hydroxylase (MUSACCHIO, 1968), dopa decarboxylase and PNMT all have a distribution profile with a minimum relative specific activity in the fractions which contain the amine storage vesicles, and a maximum relative specific activity in the non-particulate supernatant fractions, while the opposite holds true for dopamine β-hydroxylase (LADURON and BELPAIRE, 1968). Moreover, only this latter enzyme is characterized by a latency of action, supporting the interpretation that transport of dopamine formed outside the particles to the enzyme sites inside is a prerequisite for subsequent β-hydroxylation to form noradrenaline (BELPAIRE and LADURON, 1968). This is also in agreement with the observation that drugs such as reserpine, prenylamine and adrenergic α-receptor blocking agents (STJÄRNE and LISHAJKO, 1966), which depress uptake of amines, including dopamine, into the storage particles, inhibit catecholamine synthesis exclusively at the step of β-hydroxylation (KIRSHNER, 1962; STJÄRNE, 1966; WEINER and RUTLEDGE, 1966).

3. Rate of Synthesis in Adrenal Medulla, and Availability of Newly Formed Hormone for Secretion

The rate of catecholamine synthesis in the adrenal medulla has been a matter of dispute. After depleting the adrenaline stores of rat and rabbit adrenal glands with insulin HÖKFELT (1951) found that about one week was required for the restoration of the adrenaline content of the gland. In agreement with this, UDENFRIEND et al. (1953), determining the disappearance from the adrenals of catecholamines newly formed from radioactive precursors, arrived at a figure for the half-life of adrenal medullary hormones of the order of one week. However, this technique may give a too low estimate of the rate of hormone synthesis, as indicated by balance studies performed in various species, involving estimation or actual determination of amines secreted in response to stimulation, as well as of amines remaining in the stimulated gland and in the unstimulated contralateral gland used as a control. These techniques have, in the hands of some workers, given results indicating that the rate of synthesis is considerably accelerated by secretory stimulation and that the newly formed amines may even be preferentially secreted (HÖKFELT and MACLEAN, 1950; HOLLAND and SCHÜMANN, 1956; BYGDEMAN and EULER, 1958; BYGDEMAN et al., 1960). Other workers using similar techniques reported results suggesting the opposite conclusion, *viz.* no marked acceleration of synthesis resulting from short term splanchnic nerve stimulation (EADE and WOOD, 1958) or from secretion induced by injection of acetylcholine (BUTTERWORTH and MANN, 1957).

Recently the problem of rate of catecholamine synthesis in adrenal medulla was re-examined by collecting the venous effluent from the adrenal glands of cats and rabbits and determining the rate of secretion of amines newly formed from labelled tyrosine (HEMPEL and MÄNNL, 1969). It was found that the rate of formation of catecholamines from tyrosine was quite close to the resting secretion earlier reported by several workers. Newly formed amines accounted for about 10% of the total resting efflux, suggesting preferential release of newly formed amines during the "resting" conditions used, i.e. general anaesthesia and surgery. This may explain why estimation of turnover based on determination of resting amine efflux (cf. HEMPEL and MÄNNL, 1969) gives much lower figures (about 48 hours) than that based on the rate of disappearance of labelled amines from the gland (about 10 days, UDENFRIEND et al., 1953). This type of evidence strongly supports the concept of different functional pools of catecholamines in the adrenal medulla, with widely different rates of turnover (Udenfriend and Wyngaarden, 1956).

The availability of newly formed catecholamines in adrenal medulla for immediate secretion has recently been studied in the isolated perfused cat adrenal gland. It was observed that labelled catecholamines were secreted in response to injection of carbachol within 10 min after the start of infusion of labelled tyrosine. The specific activity of the noradrenaline secreted was about twice as high as the average specific activity of the noradrenaline in the adrenal gland, suggesting that not only resting secretion, but also that induced with carbachol preferentially involves newly formed amines (Stjärne, 1970a).

4. Regulation of Catecholamine Synthesis

The adrenal medulla is known to show considerable resistance to catecholamine depletion by neurogenically induced secretion (Hökfelt and McLean, 1950). Balance studies have already been discussed according to which the sum of amines secreted plus amines left in the stimulated gland considerably exceeds the calculated starting amine level of the gland (Hökfelt and McLean, 1950; Holland and Schümann, 1956; Bygdeman and Euler, 1958), indicating that neurogenically induced secretion accelerates catecholamine synthesis. Although there are reports to the contrary (Eade and Wood, 1958), the general concept of regulatory influence of neurogenically induced secretion on amine synthesis is supported by most of the experimental evidence. Thus repletion of the catecholamine store proceeds faster in the innnervated than in the denervated adrenal (Hökfelt, 1951; Kroneberg and Schümann, 1959), and amine synthesis in the adrenal medulla is accelerated when reflex secretion is induced, *e.g.* by injection of insulin (Bygdeman et al., 1960) or phenoxybenzamine (Dairman et al., 1968), by muscular exercise or by prolonged exposure to cold (Leduc, 1961; Gordon et al., 1966). While the turnover rate of catecholamines in the adrenal medulla is much slower than that in sympathetic nerves (Udenfriend, 1966a), it appears that in both types of tissue neurogenically induced secretion is a major factor in the local control of the rate of amine synthesis.

As already mentioned (Chapter by von Euler pp. 186) kinetic studies of the different steps in catecholamine synthesis from tyrosine, with partially purified enzyme preparations (Ikeda et al., 1965) as well as with whole tissue (Levitt et al., 1965), indicate that the rate-limiting step is the hydroxylation of tyrosine.

This is thus the main level at which one would expect regulation of synthesis to operate. Since it appears that the tissue level of tyrosine is normally so high that the enzyme is saturated with substrate (Udenfriend, 1966b), it seems that regulation might be exerted either by interference with availability of cofactor or by actual change in the amount of enzyme present. In fact both types of regulation have been demonstrated. Thus studies with partially purified enzyme *in vitro* (Nagatsu et al., 1964), or with homogenate fractions from adrenal medulla (Udenfriend et al., 1965), indicate that tyrosine hydroxylation can be inhibited by catechol derivatives, suggesting that catecholamine synthesis may be controlled by end product inhibition (Stjärne, 1966; Udenfriend, 1966a). Apparently this type of inhibition of tyrosine hydroxylation is not due to competition with substrate, but rather with the tetrahydrofolate cofactor (Ikeda et al., 1965). Since the hydroxylation of tyrosine seems to take place in the cytoplasm, outside the storage vesicles (cf. above A 2), the reaction is probably controlled by the concentration of "free" rather than of vesicle-bound catechols. This is supported by the studies, already quoted, of synthesis inhibition in sympathetic nerve tissue *in vitro*, according to which the concentration of free catecholamines in the suspension medium, but not that of granule-bound amine, distinctly controls the hydroxylation of tyrosine (STJÄRNE, 1966; STJÄRNE, unpublished). This concept is also in agreement with the observation that inhibition of MAO, resulting in increased levels of catecholamines, presumably both particle-bound and "free" (KOPIN, 1964), retards amine synthesis, at least in nerve tissue (NEFF and COSTA, 1966; SPECTOR et al., 1967).

Dopamine has been reported to be at least equally efficient (ROTH et al., 1968), or according to another author almost ten times as efficient, as inhibitor of tyrosine hydroxylation as noradrenaline (LADURON, 1969). Thus it appears conceivable that not only the ultimate end products of catecholamine synthesis, noradrenaline and/or adrenaline, but also dopamine formed in the cytoplasm may take part in the control of overall catecholamine formation by graded inhibition of the normally rate-limiting step: the hydroxylation of tyrosine (KOPIN and WEISE, 1968). However, it appears doubtful that cytoplasmic dopamine could play a "pivotal" role in the regulation of catecholamine synthesis (LADURON, 1969) in view of the fact that the concentration of this amine in the cytoplasm is even more efficiently limited by MAO than that of noradrenaline or adrenaline, which are less good substrates for this enzyme (WEINER, 1960).

End product inhibition operates less efficiently in homogenates of human phaeochromocytoma than in similar fractions from adrenal medulla from the same individual (ROTH et al., 1968). This might indicate tissue differences in the molecular properties of tyrosine hydroxylase, analogous to the differences in sensitivity to induction by steroids between PNMT from normal chromaffin tissue and tumours (WURTMAN et al., 1968) mentioned above. However, it appears more likely that the difference between normal and tumour tissue in sensitivity to product inhibition of tyrosine hydroxylation lies in the availability of cofactor. At any rate, it seems that inefficiency of the control of catecholamine synthesis in the tumour may be of major importance in determining its particular type of uncontrolled secretion (ROTH et al., 1968).

As has just been discussed, variation in the degree of end product inhibition of the rate-limiting hydroxylation of tyrosine is not the only mechanism whereby this reaction, and thus overall catecholamine synthesis, is affected by changes in the neurally induced secretory activity. Recently it was found that prolonged secretion from the adrenal medulla of the rat, for a period exceeding 12 hours, results in accelerated formation of tyrosine hydroxylase in the gland (THOENEN et al., 1969). The mechanism mediating this type of transsynaptic induction of the formation of enzyme protein is not clear as yet. But the implication seems to be that the impulse traffic in the secretory nerves controls the rate-limiting step in at least two different ways. Thus short-term variation in neurogenically induced secretion rapidly alters the degree of end product inhibition of tyrosine hydroxylation. More prolonged changes in the secretory activity further contribute to the control of this step, and thereby of overall catecholamine synthesis, by regulating the rate of ribosomal production of new tyrosine hydroxylase protein.

Additional mechanisms may also be of importance in regulating the hydroxylation of tyrosine. In nerve tissue it has been claimed that changes in the secretory activity alter the availability of cofactor for this reaction, or of substrate (SEDVALL and KOPIN, 1967), which may be regulated *via* a hypothetical tyrosine permease controlling tyrosine influx across the cell membrane (UDENFRIEND, 1966a), or *via* deflection of tyrosine into other metabolic routes, e.g. transamination (BARTHOLINI et al., 1970) or protein synthesis.

However, although it has become safely established that alterations of the rate of hydroxylation of tyrosine are of importance for the regulation of overall catecholamine synthesis, there are additional levels at which synthesis may be controlled, by changes in the level of "free" catecholamines or by the presence of drugs. Thus "free" catecholamines in the medium surrounding the specific vesicles may by competition limit the transport of dopamine formed extraneously to the vesicles to the sites of β-hydroxylation inside these organelles (Stjärne et al., 1967a; Roth et al., 1968; Laduron, 1969). It is not known to what extent this mechanism is rate-limiting in synthesis of noradrenaline and adrenaline under normal conditions. However, there is evidence, *in vitro* (Weiner and Rutledge, 1966; Stjärne and Lishajko, 1966) as well as *in vivo* (Randrup et al., 1963; Allegranza et al., 1965; Henning, 1966; Anden and Henning, 1968), that it may become rate-limiting after treatment with drugs such as reserpine, which blocks amine transport into the vesicles (Kirshner, 1962; Kirshner et al., 1963).

On the other hand, although there is evidence that reserpine may under certain circumstances block the synthesis of catecholamines at the β-hydroxylation step, it is equally well established that the inhibition of synthesis can be dissociated from, and is not nearly as strong, as the depression of the capacity for bulk amine storage (cf. Stjärne et al., 1967b). This is clearly demonstrated by the finding that repeated injections of low doses of reserpine in rats did not significantly alter the urinary excretion of either catecholamines or of VMA (3-methoxy-4-hydroxy mandelic acid), while strongly reducing the amine content of various tissues (Wennmalm, 1968). Moreover, the reported depression of the urinary excretion of catecholamines after a single high dose of reserpine (Anden and Henning, 1968) was apparent only for the initial period of 48—72 hours, and the excretion returned towards normal values while the catecholamine content of various tissues still remained very low. Interestingly, the time course of the inhibitory effect on amine synthesis paralleled that of depression of sympathetic neurotransmitter function, indicating that newly formed catecholamines are available for secretion and may sustain essentially normal function even when the total amine content of the stores is very low (cf. Stjärne, 1966).

Reserpine-induced inhibition of the β-hydroxylation of dopamine, may make this step rate limiting in noradrenaline and adrenaline synthesis, possibly as a function of the local dopamine/reserpine ratio in the extravesicular cytoplasm of sympathetic nerves and adrenal medulla (cf. Stjärne et al., 1967b). This may explain the lack of inhibition of noradrenaline formation in the adrenal medulla of reserpine-treated rabbits after administration of large amounts of DOPA (Bertler et al., 1961b): under these conditions the local concentration of free dopamine is abnormally high. Similar factors may account for the shift towards normal formation of noradrenaline in the brain of reserpine-treated rats which is induced by MAO inhibition; this too should raise the local dopamine/reserpine ratio (Glowinski et al., 1966).

In addition one should keep in mind the possibility that "free" noradrenaline even inside the storage particles, intravesicular but extragranular, may exert a regulatory influence on the β-hydroxylation of dopamine (Laduron, 1969). Although high concentrations of noradrenaline are required to demonstrate this type of inhibition, it might be physiologically relevant in view of the enormous catecholamine concentration in the storage particles, corresponding to 0.55 M if all the amines exist in free solution. However, this seems unlikely, for osmotic reasons and in view of the fact that the efflux of amines by diffusion is practically nil at 0° C, when the granule membrane has been shown to be permeable to catecholamines (Carlsson and Hillarp, 1958; Hillarp, 1959; Kirshner et al., 1966a).

5. Effect of Precursors

The rate of synthesis of adrenal medullary hormone, which has been found to increase on splanchnic nerve stimulation (cf. references above under A 4), can also be raised by intravenous administration of the precursor amino acid, DOPA (Bertler et al., 1960a). This intermediary metabolite does not seem normally to occur in the circulating blood (v. Studnitz, 1960). That administration of large amounts of DOPA to rabbits, even under resting conditions, results in rapid formation of dopamine and noradrenaline, was quoted as evidence that the rate-limiting step in catecholamine synthesis lies before the stage of decarboxylation (Bertler et al., 1960a). Even if administration of DOPA by-passes the hydroxylation of tyrosine, the step currently believed to be normally rate-limiting (Levitt et al., 1965), and thus does not lead to synthesis at physiological rates, the experiments provide evidence for the availability of newly formed amines for immediate secretion. The DOPA entering the chromaffin cells evidently becomes rapidly decarboxylated, and the dopamine formed almost equally rapidly enters the storage vesicles where it is to a large extent β-hydroxylated to noradrenaline. The rate of dopamine and noradrenaline formation was reported to be extremely high, corresponding to 30—50% per hour of the total catecholamine content of the tissue. The newly formed amines were to a large extent recovered from the particulate fraction which normally contains adrenaline only; however dopamine occurred in the soluble fraction to a higher extent than noradrenaline or adrenaline. Much of the noradrenaline formed was found to leave the particles in which it was synthesized, to be exposed to N-methylation in the cytoplasm. In the rabbit normally the specific amine storage vesicles store adrenaline exclusively; however, some of the noradrenaline formed was incorporated into the vesicles as such, and also retained as such for more than 24 hours. This may reflect the low turnover of the particle-bound amines of the adrenal medulla at rest; noradrenaline was only slowly released into the cytoplasm, methylated and re-bound as adrenaline (cf. Blaschko, 1959).

Interestingly, intravenous administration of dopamine was relatively inefficient in raising the intracellular content of dopamine in the adrenal gland as compared to injection of DOPA (Bertler et al., 1960a).

6. Inhibitors of Synthesis

Qualitatively the pharmacology of catecholamine synthesis in adrenal medulla is similar to that of synthesis in sympathetic nerves (cf. Section on Adrenergic Nerves). Quantitatively, however, there are important differences between nerve and chromaffin tissue. Thus, much higher dosage is generally required to bring about marked inhibitory effects on synthesis in the adrenal medulla. This is most likely mainly due to the much lower turnover of catecholamines in the adrenal medulla (cf. Udenfriend, 1966a).

Thus even inhibition of synthesis by α-methyltyrosine at the normally rate limiting step, that of tyrosine hydroxylation, does not alter the catecholamine content of the adrenal medulla at rest (Gordon et al., 1966). Only after turnover has been accelerated, e.g. by muscular exercise or exposure to cold, did the amine content of the adrenal medulla in the animals thus treated fall significantly.

In these pages, detailed discussion of mechanisms of action has been restricted to the inhibition of synthesis caused by reserpine only, since this drug has turned out to be of particular value as a pharmacological tool for elucidation of many aspects of the physiology of the sympatho-adrenal system, including amine synthesis (cf. above A 4). For a detailed presentation of other drugs affecting

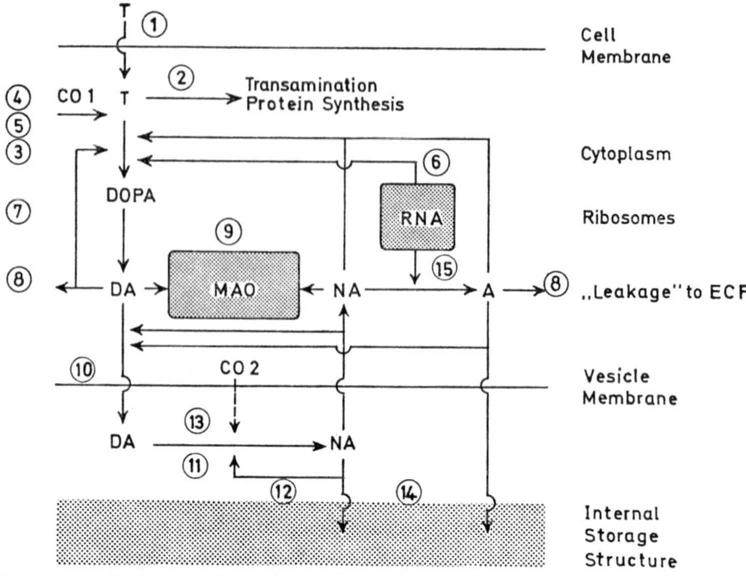

Fig. 1. Diagrammatic illustration of catecholamine synthesis and levels of physiological and pharmacological regulation. Figures below refer to diagram.

	Directly or indirectly affected by Secretory stimuli	"Drugs"
1. Availability of tyrosine. Controlled by "permease"?	?	— Phenylalanine
2. Deflection of tyrosine e.g. by transamination or to protein synthesis	?	?
3. Hydroxylation of tyrosine	+	— α-methyltyrosine
4. Availability of cofactor for tyrosine hydroxylase	?	?
5. Inhibition of hydroxylation of tyrosine by competition cofactor/"free" DA, NA, A	—	+ MAO inhibition
Factors which control concentration of "free" cytoplasmic amines, regulating steps 3,5 and 10, 11:		
"Removal "to storage vesicles (10)	+	— Reserpine
"Leakage" to ECF (8)	?	+ Tyramine
Deamination by MAO (9)	?	— MAO inhibition + Reserpine
6. Ribosomal synthesis of tyrosine hydroxylase	+	— Puromycin
7. Decarboxylation of DOPA	+ (?)	— Decaborane
10. Specific uptake of DA to DBO sites	+	— Reserpine
11. β-hydroxylation of DA	+	— Disulfiram
12. Product inhibition of β-hydroxylation of DA by "free", intravesicular but extragranular NA (?)	?	?
13. "Removal of cofactor for DBO	?	+ Disulfiram
14. Incorporation of NA, A (but not DA?) into internal storage structure	?	— Reserpine
15. Ribosomal synthesis of PNMT	+ (?)	+ Corticoids

Abbreviations and symbols:

T	— tyrosine	CO 1	— cofactor for tyrosine hydroxylase
DA, NA, A	— dopamine, noradrenaline, adrenaline	CO 2	— cofactor for DBO
ECF	— extracellular fluid	+	increased by
DBO	— dopamine β-hydroxylase	—	decreased by
PNMT	— phenylethanolamine N-methyl transferase	?	effect unknown

Drugs and other agents mentioned are typical examples. For details and references see the text in the Section on Synthesis, in this Chapter, and also in Section on Adrenergic Nerves, Chapter by von Euler, pp. 186.

catecholamine synthesis, in adrenal medulla as well as in sympathetic nerves, the reader is referred to the corresponding Section on Adrenergic Nerves in the Chapter by von Euler.

7. Diagrammatic Illustration of Catecholamine Synthesis and Levels of Physiological and Pharmacological Regulation

Synthesis in adrenal medulla is summarized diagrammatically in Fig. 1, in order to visualize the dynamics of catecholamine synthesis and the proposed levels of physiological and pharmacological control of this process. The Figure incorporates what has been discussed in the preceding pages.

B. Uptake

1. Uptake at the Cellular Level

While synthesis in the gland is the main mechanism whereby the catecholamine store of the adrenal medulla is built up, it appears for logical reasons necessary to consider the relative importance of another mechanism of net gain in amines, *viz.* uptake of preformed adrenaline and noradrenaline from the extracellular fluid.

a) Circulating Amines

In the early studies of the distribution of tracer amounts of radioactively labelled catecholamines it was found that the adrenal medulla is almost as efficient in accumulating the labelled material as tissues with the richest sympathetic innervation (Axelrod et al., 1959; Whitby et al., 1961). Since the absolute uptake was low in relation to the extremely high amounts of endogenous amine in this tissue, this mechanism for net gain of amine in adrenal medulla appears to be of negligible importance, quantitatively. However, the finding that uptake of circulating amines in adrenal medulla is blocked by cocaine indicates that the uptake mechanism in the medulla is qualitatively similar to that in sympathetic nerves (Campos and Crout, 1970).

The subcellular distribution of exogenous noradrenaline in the adrenal medulla of the rat was found to be initially different from that of exogenous adrenaline (Potter and Axelrod, 1963). Exogenous adrenaline was located mainly in the dense fractions containing the bulk of the catecholamines, whereas exogenous noradrenaline, during the early phase after the injection, was mainly recovered from a microsomal fraction. Later, 24 hours after injection, most of the radioactivity derived from the labelled noradrenaline injected appeared in the dense fractions, largely in form of adrenaline. It is at present difficult to evaluate this remarkable observation, since the difference in distribution of the two exogenous catecholamines is not matched by similar differences in endogenous amines, noradrenaline storing vesicles in adrenal medulla being if anything denser than those storing adrenaline (Eade, 1956, 1958; Schümann, 1957; Winkler, 1969). Moreover, the close similarity of the subcellular distribution of the enzyme dopamine β-hydroxylase and of endogenous adrenaline and noradrenaline (Oka et al., 1967a; Laduron and Belpaire, 1968; Viveros et al., 1969a) suggests that noradrenaline is not formed in microsomal particles, to be later transferred to the denser particles which store noradrenaline and/or adrenaline, but in the storage vesicles themselves, or in particles with very similar sedimentation properties. However, the interesting observation, which might have something to do with the finding in isolated particles *in vitro*, that noradrenaline is less efficiently, and more slowly, taken up than adrenaline (LADURON and BELPAIRE, 1968), certainly calls for reexamination of the problem.

b) Reuptake of Catecholamines Secreted

Studies of the secretion of catecholamines from cat adrenal medulla as a result of splanchnic nerve stimulation have led to the proposal that the amines secreted are to some extent recaptured by the secretory cells rather than being washed out into the general circulation (MARLEY and PATON, 1961). This would be an analogy with the sympathetic neuron, where a considerable proportion of the transmitter secreted as a result of previous nerve impulses, and still present in the immediate vicinity of the nerves, appears to be recaptured into the nerves and reused (PATON, 1960; STJÄRNE, 1964; BROWN, 1965; HAEFELY et al., 1965; GEFFEN, 1967; FOLKOW et al., 1968; HEDQVIST and STJÄRNE, 1969). It is particularly interesting that pretreatment of the cats with drugs such as phenoxybenzamine (KIRPEKAR and CERVONI, 1963) or cocaine (MARLEY and PATON, 1961) has been reported to increase the efflux of catecholamine from the adrenal medulla on subsequent splanchnic nerve stimulation, since phenoxybenzamine (BROWN and GILLESPIE 1957), or cocaine, alone (HUKOVIC and MUSCHOLL, 1962; THOENEN et al., 1964) or in combination with small amounts of alpha-blockers (HEDQVIST and STJÄRNE, 1969) strongly potentiate efflux of noradrenaline from sympathetically innervated tissues in response to nerve stimulation. However, the evidence that these drugs have such an action on secretion from the adrenal medulla in response to splanchnic nerve stimulation is conflicting (MARLEY and PATON, 1961; KIRPEKAR and CERVONI, 1963). Moreover, addition of phenoxybenzamine or cocaine to the perfusion medium, in concentrations highly efficient on transmitter release from the isolated spleen, did not affect the secretory response to acetylcholine and its analogues in the isolated perfused cat adrenal (STJÄRNE and HEDQVIST, 1970). Thus it seems that the available evidence does not support the concept of quantitatively relevant re-uptake into the adrenal medulla.

That the adrenal medulla does remove and retain circulating catecholamines to a limited extent seems logical in view of the close relationship, ontogenetically, of the chromaffin cell to the sympathetic neuron, the membrane of which has a powerful mechanism for trapping and concentrating extracellular catecholamines (HILLARP and MALMFORS, 1964; LINDMAR and MUSCHOLL, 1964). However, although this seems to be a property of the entire neuron, to some degree (NORBERG and HAMBERGER, 1964), the capacity of this transport mechanism is in fact more highly developed in the terminal regions of the axon than in its non-terminal parts (STJÄRNE et al., 1970b; HAMBERGER et al., 1970). One might thus assume that the common stem cell, which apparently has the potential to develop either into a chromaffin cell or into a sympathetic neuron, possesses in its plasma membrane a largely latent amine concentrating mechanism. The observations in adrenal medulla suggest that this latent capacity is not highly developed even in the mature adrenal medullary cell, as one might expect in view of the improbability that recapture of catecholamines, or uptake of circulating catecholamines from other sources, could be biologically advantageous (see BLASCHKO, 1968).

c) Functional Significance of Uptake of Circulating Catecholamines into Adrenal Medulla

If one assesses the quantitative aspects of uptake of preformed catecholamines from the extracellular fluid in relation to local synthesis it is interesting that intravenous administration to rabbits of the precursor amino acid DOPA is much more effective in raising the intracellular concentration in the adrenal medulla of dopamine, and thus also of noradrenaline and adrenaline, than intravenous injection of dopamine itself (BERTLER et al., 1960a). This probably reflects the relative inefficiency of amine transport across the membrane of adrenal medullary cells, which is apparently much more readily penetrated by the less polar precursor amino acid.

It seems likely that similar poor penetration of tyramine into the adrenal medullary cells, in contrast to relatively efficient transport into sympathetic neurons (TRENDELENBURG, 1963), might be part of the explanation of the observations made in several laboratories on the dramatic cardiovascular effects of intravenous injection of tyramine in the cat and dog that may occur in the complete absence of stimulation of secretion from the adrenal medulla (STRÖMBLAD, 1960; STJÄRNE, 1961; WEINER et al., 1962; ROBINSON, 1966). On the other hand the reports by other workers that tyramine at high concentration may induce an accelerated efflux of catecholamines from the isolated perfused adrenal gland (HAAG et al., 1961; ROBINSON, 1966) evidently indicate that a certain degree of tyramine penetration through the membrane of adrenal medullary cells can occur.

d) "False Hormones" in Adrenal Medulla

Observations analogous to those made with infusion of DOPA have been made with indole compounds. Thus on intravenous injection into rabbits, the precursor amino acid 5-hydroxytryptophan (5HTP) penetrates into the adrenal medullary cells and is rapidly converted to 5-hydroxytryptamine by decarboxylation(BERTLER et al., 1961). This shows that the adrenal medulla, as well as the sympathetic neuron (cf. KOPIN, 1968), is not completely specific for catecholamines. As pointed out, the main reason why the adrenal medulla contains catecholamines rather than indoleamines appears to be that the medulla is unable to form 5-HTP from its naturally occurring and circulating amino acid precursor, tryptophan, but can form DOPA from tyrosine; the reverse is obviously true for 5-hydroxytryptaminergic tissues (BERTLER et al., 1960b).

2. Uptake in Granules[1]

a) Methods

Since the adrenal glands receive less than one per cent of the cardiac output, and since their capacity to remove catecholamines from the circulation is not highly developed (cf. above), studies of the uptake of amines in the intracellular storage vesicles, under normal conditions as well as during exposure to drugs, have mainly been carried out *in vitro*.

The bovine adrenal gland has been the most convenient source of granule preparations for these studies, and has also been used extensively, but some work has also been done on the adrenal medulla of the sheep, the rabbit and the cat. The preparations used have often been semi-purified according to a method described by HILLARP (1958a), involving isolation of amine granules in isotonic sucrose media by differential centrifugation and removal of contaminating organelles,

1 The terms "chromaffin granules" or "nerve granules" for the amine storage particles in adrenal medulla and sympathetic nerves, respectively, have gained widespread acceptance, although in a strict sense the particles are vesicles, consisting of a membrane enveloping an internal structure (the "granule"). The terms "granules" and "storage vesicles" are used interchangeably in this chapter.

mainly mitochondria and lysosomes (see SMITH, 1968), from the pellet by swirling with sucrose. The subsequent incubations have been carried out in various buffered media, often based on isotonic sucrose, and usually under air or even under nitrogen. Radioisotope techniques have greatly facilitated the uptake studies. In experiments with drugs two different approaches have been used: Pretreatment of whole animals, mainly rabbits, *in vivo*, and study of the alterations induced in the properties of the isolated granules on subsequent incubation *in vitro*, or alternatively, addition of the drug to the medium *in vitro* for preincubation of the granules before the introduction of exogenous amines. The amines studied have included catecholamines, various sympathomimetic amines such as tyramine and even indolealkylamines.

b) Exchange versus Net Uptake

One major feature of the accumulation of exogenous adrenaline and noradrenaline in isolated adrenomedullary storage vesicles *in vitro* is that it does not imply net gain of vesicle-bound amines (TAUGNER and HASSELBACH, 1966; LISHAJKO, 1969a). However, this does not seem to apply to dopamine. LISHAJKO recently (1969a) reported distinct net uptake of this amine in particle suspensions from sheep adrenal medulla, where dopamine occurs in amounts corresponding to 2—3% of the total amines. In view of the striking differences, e.g. in spontaneous release and net uptake of dopamine, as compared to adrenaline and noradrenaline, the author concludes that he is dealing with a separate species of particles storing dopamine exclusively (LISHAJKO, 1968). There is so far no report of a successful separation of such particles from those containing noradrenaline and/or adrenaline, and an alternative interpretation will be proposed below (cf. Fig. 2).

However, for adrenaline and noradrenaline during incubation *in vitro* at or near body temperature, the uptake of amines only to a partial extent balances their "spontaneous" release (TAUGNER and HASSELBACH, 1966; LISHAJKO, 1969a). The uptake studies thus mainly deal with exchange of endogenous for exogenous amine. At temperatures close to 0°C no such exchange occurs, even after prolonged incubation in the presence of high concentrations (0.2 M) of exogenous catecholamines (CARLSSON and HILLARP, 1958).

c) Uptake at High Concentrations of Amine

While virtually no exchange of endogenous for exogenous catecholamines occurs at 0°C (HILLARP, 1959), it does so on incubation at a higher temperature. Thus considerable amounts of catecholamines as well as other amines, such as tyramine or octopamine, have been found to accumulate in bovine adrenal medullary granules on incubation at 31°C in isotonic media containing high concentrations (2—21 mM) of exogenous amines (CARLSSON and HILLARP, 1961; BERTLER et al., 1961a; SCHÜMANN and PHILIPPU, 1962). However, uptake of the exogenous amines did not lead to net gain of total amines. With tyramine this type of uptake represents exchange, based on displacement of the endogenous by exogenous amine (SCHÜMANN and PHILIPPU, 1962). The particular type of uptake involved at these high concentrations of exogenous amine in the incubation medium probably does not represent a true amine concentrating mechanism, judging from the observation that, although it is temperature-dependent, it does not require fortification of the medium with e.g. ATP and Mg^{++}, and that it is resistant to agents known to block specific amine transport, such as reserpine (CARLSSON and HILLARP, 1961).

d) ATP- and Mg^{++}-dependent Uptake

However, a true concentrating mechanism was discovered by CARLSSON et al. (1962) and by KIRSHNER (1962), who found that the inconspicuous uptake of exogenous catecholamines occurring at 30°—37°C at low (less than 0.5 mM) catecholamine concentrations in the medium, even in the absence of fortification, is strongly accelerated by the addition of ATP and Mg^{++} 2—5 mM to the incubation medium. This potentiation of uptake was found to have only moderate nucleotide specificity. Thus ITP, GTP and UTP were found to be nearly as active as ATP, while CTP was somewhat less, and ADP very much less, active and AMP completely inactive (KIRSHNER, 1962; CARLSSON et al., 1962, 1963; TAUGNER and HASSELBACH, 1966). Transphosphorylation was not ruled out, however. The metal requirement was not absolute either. Thus Mg^{++} could be replaced by Mn^{++} or by Co^{++}, but not by Ca^{++} (KIRSHNER, 1962; CARLSSON et al., 1963). The ATP-Mg^{++}-dependent uptake was found to be highly efficient at low amine concentrations, and was apparently saturated at 0.5 mM. However, the amounts of exogenous amine taken up did not exceed 10% of the endogenous catecholamines originally present in the granules (CARLSSON et al., 1963). The ATP-Mg^{++}-stimulated uptake process is strongly inhibited by low concentrations of reserpine (KIRSHNER, 1962; CARLSSON et al., 1962, 1963). It is highly temperature-dependent, with a Q_{10}, between 20° and 30°C, of 2.8 (KIRSHNER, 1962). Correction for the small uptake that occurs even in the presence of reserpine raised the Q_{10} value to 6 (KIRSHNER, 1962). The uptake process has been found to be moderately stereospecific, with some preference for the naturally occurring laevorotatory stereoisomers of adrenaline and noradrenaline (CARLSSON et al., 1963). Concerning the relative affinity of different catecholamines for the uptake mechanism the reports vary from no clear-cut difference in relative uptake of the three catecholamines (CARLSSON et al., 1963) to distinct preference for amines in the order dopamine/adrenaline/noradrenaline (LADURON and BELPAIRE, 1968). Interestingly, it is an amine entirely unrelated to chromaffin granules, 5-hydroxytryptamine, that has been found to show the highest affinity for this uptake mechanism (CARLSSON et al., 1963). Its uptake is strongly potentiated by ATP and Mg^{++} and inhibited by reserpine. At low concentrations in the medium the granules can accumulate as much as 60% of the 5-hydroxytryptamine present in the incubation medium, which would correspond to a calculated concentration gradient vesicles to medium of 1000/1, if the amines exist in free solution in the intravesicular water (CARLSSON et al., 1963).

In view of the proposed role of ATP in an intragranular amine storage complex it is of particular interest that uptake of ATP concomitantly with that of amines does not occur (KIRSHNER, 1962), or does not occur to nearly the same extent as that of amines, and is only slightly inhibited by reserpine (CARLSSON et al., 1963).

e) Other Amine Uptake Mechanisms

The uptake of tyramine evidently occurs only in part by the mechanism described above, since it is only slightly activated by ATP plus Mg^{++} and unaffected by reserpine (CARLSSON et al., 1963). The same holds true for other sympathomimetic amines such as metaraminol (LUNDBORG and STITZEL, 1967). These authors report that *in vitro* noradrenaline was taken up mainly by the ATP-Mg^{++}-dependent mechanism, which is inhibited by reserpine, while metaraminol uptake was entirely independent of ATP and Mg^{++}, and also reserpine resistant. α-Methylnoradrenaline was taken up by both mechanisms. These differences in amine uptake are parallelled by differences in their lipid solubility, suggesting that highly polar amines, such as noradrenaline, require specific transport to the interior of the storage vesicles, while less polar compounds may to a degree penetrate by diffusion.

f) Role of ATPase

While there has earlier been some controversy concerning the presence (Hillarp, 1958b) or absence (Fortier et al., 1959; Hagen and D'Iorio, 1965) of a specific ATPase in the amine storage vesicles, it has by now been established that purified chromaffin granule fractions show ATPase activity (Banks, 1965; Kirshner et al., 1966b). The enzyme has a relatively low specific activity when compared with that of mitochondria or microsomes, but shows specificity e.g. in requirement for Mg^{++} in contrast to the mitochondrial and microsomal enzymes, which are activated by Ca^{++} as well as by Mg^{++} (Banks, 1965). Interestingly, the ATPase of the chromaffin amine storage vesicles can be specifically and selectively inhibited by N-ethyl maleimide at concentrations which abolish amine uptake (Kirshner, 1965; Kirshner et al., 1966b). All of the ATPase activity of these particles was found to be restricted to the water-insoluble "membrane" protein (Banks, 1965), which also contained about 90% of the sulphydryl groups (Taugner and Hasselbach, 1968). By utilizing N-ethyl maleimide for blocking sulphydryl groups and ATP to protect the ATPase against this compound, and simultaneously studying catecholamine uptake and release and ATPase activity, Taugner and Hasselbach (1968) recently presented evidence which they interpret as indicating a mole per mole relationship between hydrolysis of ATP and uptake of catecholamines, one mole of ATP being split per mole of amine taken up.

3. Inhibitors of Uptake in Chromaffin Amine Storage Vesicles

As mentioned above the uptake studies deal with the balance between amine uptake and release, and normally essentially no net uptake occurs (Taugner and Hasselbach, 1966; Lishajko, 1969a). Thus the action of drugs will be reconsidered after the discussion of the characteristics of the amine storage mechanism (next section). However, at this stage the general features of drug effects on uptake of exogenous catecholamine will be briefly reviewed.

a) Inhibition of ATPase

The classical inhibitor of the ATP-Mg^{++}-dependent uptake of exogenous catecholamines into chromaffin amine storage vesicles, and still one of the most powerful known to date, is reserpine (Carlsson et al., 1962, 1963; Kirshner, 1962). This drug induces *in vivo* a profound and longlasting catecholamine depletion in the adrenal medulla (Holzbauer and Vogt, 1956; Carlsson et al., 1957b). In spite of the widespread awareness of the importance of this drug as a tool in catecholamine research, its exact mechanisms of action at the level of the granules still remain largely unknown. It is generally agreed that reserpine is highly active as inhibitor of amine uptake at very low concentrations, down to 10^{-8} M (Carlsson et al., 1962, 1963). It may be less generally appreciated that reserpine also inhibits "spontaneous" amine efflux, particularly in nerve granules (Euler and Lishajko, 1961) but also to some extent in adrenal medullary granules (Euler and Lishajko, 1961; Weil-Malherbe and Posner, 1963; Ferris et al., 1970). The inhibitory effects of reserpine are irreversible in the sense that they cannot be removed by washing (Carlsson et al., 1963). The degree of inhibition is highly dependent not only on the concentration of drug but also on the concentration of amines in the medium, suggesting competition at some level between reserpine and the amines (CARLSSON et al., 1963; JONASSON et al., 1964; STJÄRNE, 1964). The observation that reserpine causes 50% inhibition of amine uptake at a molar amine/drug ratio as high as 1000/1 has been quoted as evidence that it does not act at the binding sites, but rather at some bottleneck in the system, i.e. at some strategic transport step (STJÄRNE, 1964). Interestingly, reserpine has recently been found to cause a moderate degree of inhibition of the "transport ATPase" of purified chromaffin granules (TAUGNER and HASSELBACH, 1966); the degree of enzyme inhibition has been calculated to be reasonably well correlated to the blocking of catecholamine uptake. The possibility thus exists that at least part of the mechanism of action of reserpine on amine uptake consists in inhibition of a specific transport ATPase of the amine storage vesicles. However, other authors fail to find inhitory effects of reserpine on ATPase in amine storage vesicles (FERRIS et al., 1970).

The importance of ATPase for uptake of exogenous catecholamines is further supported by observations indicating that substances such as N-ethyl maleimide, known to inactivate various types of transport ATPase by binding to their SH-groups (HASSELBACH and SERAYDARIAN, 1966), strongly inhibit uptake of exogenous catecholamines into chromaffin granules (CARLSSON et al., 1963; KIRSHNER, 1965; TAUGNER and HASSELBACH, 1968). The degree of inhibition by N-ethyl maleimide of the specific Mg^{++}-activated ATPase in semipurified chromaffin amine storage vesicle fractions has been reported to be well correlated to the degree of blocking of ATP-Mg^{++}-dependent uptake of exogenous catecholamines into the vesicles (TAUGNER and HASSELBACH, 1968). In fact, these experiments have led to the conclusion that one mole of ATP is hydrolysed per mole of catecholamine taken up in the storage vesicles (TAUGNER and HASSELBACH, 1968).

Inhibition of a specific ATPase by removal of Mg^{++} may also well be the basis for the inhibitory action on amine uptake of chelating agents such as EDTA (KIRSHNER, 1962).

b) Competition for Inward Transport

The catecholamines themselves, interestingly in the order dopamine, adrenaline, noradrenaline (KIRSHNER, 1962), as well as various sympathomimetic amines, have been found to inhibit uptake of catecholamines into chromaffin amine storage vesicles (KIRSHNER, 1962; CARLSSON et al., 1963). The most potent inhibitor was found to be tyramine. Structure-effect relation studies indicate that removal or methoxylation of the ring hydroxyl group, as well as substitution of groups larger than methyl on the nitrogen, or addition of groups to the side chain, reduce the inhibitory effects (KIRSHNER, 1962). Interestingly, 5-hydroxytryptamine was found to be highly potent as inhibitor of catecholamine uptake into the vesicles (KIRSHNER, 1962; CARLSSON et al., 1963).

The apparent inhibitory action of sympathomimetic amines on the uptake of exogenous catecholamines seems to be an inhibition of uptake (KIRSHNER, 1962; CARLSSON et al., 1963) as well as a promotion of release (SCHÜMANN and PHILIPPU, 1961). The action of tyramine on catecholamine uptake is remarkable in view of the fact this amine seems to be taken up into the chromaffin storage vesicles by a different mechanism, not requiring ATP and Mg^{++} and not inhibited by reserpine (CARLSSON et al., 1963). However, the results probably imply that tyramine can be taken up by both ways (cf. LUNDBORG and STITZEL, 1967), and that it may therefore, in addition to competing with the endogenous catecholamines for binding sites in the interior of the storage granules (SCHÜMANN and PHILIPPU, 1961), also compete by occupying carrier sites of the ATP-Mg^{++}-dependent transport system (KIRSHNER, 1962; CARLSSON et al., 1963).

c) Block of Transport Sites

Several adrenoceptor blockers have been found to be moderately active as inhibitors of uptake of amines into chromaffin storage vesicles (Carlsson et al., 1963). This has led to the consideration of possible structural analogies between adrenoceptors and the specific sites of the ATP-Mg^{++}-dependent transport mechanism of the amine storage vesicles. However, in the experiments with isolated chromaffin granules the concentrations of these drugs required to produce reasonably complete block of uptake of amines were several orders of magnitude higher than those usually required to block adrenoceptors (Carlsson et al., 1963). Moreover, the finding that the effects of a drug such as phenoxybenzamine on amine uptake were reversible and could be washed out, as well as the failure of thiosulphate to abolish the amine transport blocking effect of phenoxybenzamine, have been regarded as indications that these substances may interfere with amine transport into chromaffin storage vesicles by a mechanism different from that by which they block adrenoceptors (Carlsson et al., 1963).

4. Diagrammatic Illustration of Catecholamine Uptake, and Levels of Drug Action

The Section on Uptake is summarized in Fig. 2, which proposes a model for uptake of the three catecholamines, and for mechanisms of physiological control and pharmacological interference. Whether or not the different compartments in this model exist in one single type of organelle, or in separate particles, is difficult to state with certainty at the present time. For instance it is possible that the adrenal medulla, which is known to contain cells capable of making adrenaline as well as cells unable to methylate noradrenaline and therefore storing this amine (Hillarp et al., 1954), in analogy with certain extra-adrenal tissues (Euler and Lishajko, 1957; Falk et al., 1959), may also contain specific cells making and storing dopamine only, as suggested by Lishajko (1968, 1969a). However, until such dopamine containing vesicles have been isolated and separated from those storing adrenaline and/or noradrenaline, the alternative interpretation should be considered, that the dopamine "granules" in fact, partly or totally, correspond to a separate dopamine compartment present in most or all adrenal medullary storage vesicles, as suggested by the close similarity in the subcellular distribution of dopamine β-hydroxylase and of noradrenaline and adrenaline in adrenal medulla (Kirshner, 1957; Oka et al., 1967a; Laduron and Belpaire, 1968; Viveros et al., 1969a). This compartment may well have capacity to store small amounts of dopamine.

Another difficulty is to define precisely at what level in the storage vesicles the ATPase might be located. The statement that it is "membrane-bound" might be taken as an indication that it is related to the unit membrane of the vesicles (Taugner and Hasselbach, 1966), in analogy with other types of ATPase. However, the experimental fact is simply that it is not water-soluble, and theoretically it might thus be located in the internal structure of the vesicles. This would make sense in view of the demonstrated permeability to catecholamines as well as to ATP of the membrane limiting the water space of the vesicles, at temperatures close to 0° C (Hillarp, 1959; Kirshner et al., 1966b). Whether or not metabolic processes make this membrane functionally impermeable at higher temperatures is still a matter of speculation.

With a distribution of ATPase in the interior of the vesicles it would follow that the promotion of amine uptake by hydrolysis of ATP would not be due to provision of energy for transport across membranes, but rather of energy to

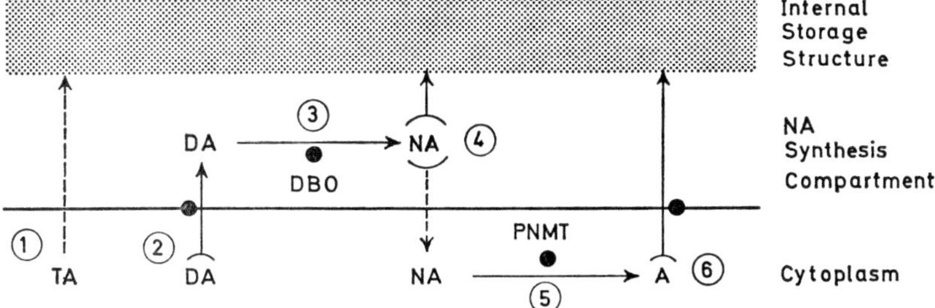

Fig. 2. Schematic diagram illustrating amine uptake in storage particles, and levels of drug action. Figures below refer to diagram.

1. *Passive uptake at high catecholamine concentrations — chief route for tyramine (TA):*
Characteristics:
Temperature dependent
Independent of fortification with, e.g. ATP and Mg^{++}
Not inhibited by reserpine
Physiological significance: Questionable
Pharmacological significance: Allows lipophilic amines (e.g. TA, MA) to reach binding sites in internal storage complex
"Affinity": MA > α-Me-NA > NA

2, 6. *Active (?), carrier-mediated (?) uptake at low (< 0.5 mM) amine concentrations:*

Characteristics:	*Implications:*
Temperature dependent, high Q_{10}	Enzymatic?
ATP-Mg^{++}-dependent, blocked by inhibition of ATPase	"Transport" ATPase? "Activation" ATPase?
Blocked by prenylamine	By blocking "activation" of storage complex?
Blocked by reserpine	By inhibition of ATPase? By blocking exchange? By competition for carrier?
Blocked by TA	By competition for carrier?
Specificity: Not completely specific for catecholamines, moderately stereospecific	
"Affinity": 5-HT > DA > A > NA	Separate DA carrier to protect synthesis?

Specifications:

2. *Carrier-mediated uptake of DA into NA "synthesis compartment" (carrier with preference for DA?)*
Physiological importance: "Protects" NA synthesis by trapping newly formed DA. Allows regulation of synthesis at this step, since uptake of DA will be limited by the concentration of "free" NA and A (which may be a function of the secretory activity)
Pharmacological importance: Synthesis of NA and A may be blocked at this step, by reserpine, TA.
3. *NA "synthesis compartment" — DA β-hydroxylation site:*
Moderate capacity for storage of DA — "DA compartment"?
NA formation limited by product inhibition?
4. *Carrier-mediated transport of NA*
Into internal storage structure — blocked by reserpine
To cytoplasm ("leakage") blocked by reserpine (less strongly)
5. *N-methylation of NA in cytoplasm*
6. *Carrier-mediated (different carrier?) uptake of A (and NA, 5-HT — but not DA?)*
Physiologically: Limited by spontaneous release of amines — no net uptake. *In vivo*, or *in vitro* in the presence of ATP and Mg^{++}: Release = Uptake
Pharmacologically: Blocked by reserpine, prenylamine, N-ethyl maleimide. Limited by competition with sympathomimetic amines such as TA.

Abbreviations:

DA, NA, A	— dopamine, noradrenaline, adrenaline
TA, 5-HT	— tyramine, 5-hydroxytryptamine
MA, α-Me-NA	— metaraminol, α-methylnoradrenaline
DBO	— dopamine β-hydroxylase
PNMT	— phenylethanolamine N-methyl transferase

For details and references see text in Section on Uptake

somehow activate the storage complex, allowing amine exchange (FERRIS et al., 1970). According to this hypothesis drugs may block uptake of amines by inhibition of ATPase (*e.g.* N-ethyl maleimide), by preventing the activation of the storage complex (*e.g.* prenylamine) or by blocking the amine exchange once the complex has been activated (*e.g.* reserpine).

C. Storage

For details concerning the biochemistry of adrenal chromaffin amine storage vesicles the reader is referred to the recent and excellent review by SMITH (1968).

1. Origin of Storage Vesicles

There seems to be every reason to assume that the chromaffin storage vesicles originate from the Golgi region of the endoplasmic reticulum (DE ROBERTIS and SABATINI, 1960). An interesting indication of this is the presence in purified chromaffin storage vesicles as well as in microsomes from adrenal medulla of a specific cytochrome of the b-type, called cytochrome b-559 (ICHIKAWA and YAMANO, 1965), which has no known functions in the storage particles. It seems that this compound is responsible for the bright pink colour of sedimented amine vesicles (SMITH, 1968).

2. Isolation of Chromaffin Amine Storage Vesicles

The experimental proof that the catecholamines of the adrenal medulla do not exist in free solution in the cytoplasm but are to a large extent stored in specific organelles was obtained by HILLARP et al., (1953) and by BLASCHKO and WELCH (1953), who after homogenization of the adrenal medulla in isotonic sucrose and removal of unbroken cells and nuclei by low speed centrifugation demonstrated that 70—80% of the amines in the low speed supernatant could be sedimented by centrifugation at higher rates.

However, it was realized from the very beginning that the chromaffin granules in the sediment obtained by this technique are heavily contaminated with other organelles such as mitochondria (BLASCHKO et al., 1955). Later experiments have shown that after initial centrifugation of the homogenate in isotonic sucrose for $6—10 \times 10^3$ g-min, subsequent centrifugation of this supernatant for $1.5—5 \times 10^5$ g-min produces a sediment of chromaffin granules contaminated mainly with mitochondria (BLASCHKO et al., 1955) and lysosomes (SMITH and WINKLER, 1966). These organelles are larger in size than the chromaffin storage vesicles, and have a "true" density relatively close to that of the vesicles (LADURON, 1969; LAGERCRANTZ et al., 1970b). Still, the amine storage vesicles separate to some extent from the other particles and form, after centrifugation in isotonic sucrose for $1.5—5 \times 10^5$ g-min, a distinctly pink bottom layer in the sediment. The brownish top layers of contaminating mitochondria and lysosomes can to a certain degree be removed by swirling with sucrose (BLASCHKO et al., 1955; HILLARP, 1958a). This simple technique for semi-purification of chromaffin granules has proved extremely valuable for preparative purposes, since the granules remain in an isotonic environment and are thus not exposed to osmotic shock.

A different approach to the isolation of chromaffin granules in relative purity in isotonic media was introduced by OKA et al. (1966a), who described a technique for purification of granules by serial filtration on filters of successively decreasing pore size. This technique has been reported to give granule preparations of high chemical (OKA et al., 1966a) and morphological purity (POISNER and TRIFARO, 1967).

The best methods for isolation of chromaffin granules of high purity are based on gradient centrifugation, mostly on sucrose gradients. However, these are not only density, but also osmolarity, gradients and thus expose the vesicles to hypertonic media. Restoration of isotonicity in the different fractions by dilution causes immediate and more or less complete osmotic lysis and depletion of the granules. This method can therefore be used only for analytical purposes. In sucrose gradients mitochondria equilibrate at the level of 1.1—1.3 M sucrose, lysosomes at about 1.6 M sucrose and the bulk of the chromaffin granules at about 1.8 M sucrose (BLASCHKO et al., 1957; SMITH and WINKLER, 1966). Thus in this system the granules show an apparent density considerably higher than that of the other organelles. However, when centrifuged on silica gradients, where the graded densities are not produced by increased concentrations of solute, but rather by differences in particle size (LAGERCRANTZ et al., 1970b), or on gradients made by mixing glycogen and sucrose (LADURON, 1969), the chromaffin granules can be made to equilibrate at different levels, depending on the chosen tonicity of the gradient. In an isotonic medium, 300 mosmol/l, the density of the granules, 1.12 g/cm^3, appears to be relatively close to that of the mitochondria, about 1.08 g/cm^3, (LADURON, 1969) while it is about 1.24 g/cm^3 in a strongly hypertonic medium, 900 mosmol/l, a tonicity in which the mitochondria form a band at a level corresponding to 1.17 g/cm^3 (LAGERCRANTZ et al. 1970b). It seems that the high apparent density of chromaffin granules on sucrose gradients is due to osmotically induced shrinking (cf. BEAUFAY et al., 1964). By sucrose density gradient centrifugation it is thus possible to utilize an artifactual difference in density for the purpose of isolation of pure chromaffin granules. It appears that this can be even more efficiently done on sucrose/D_2O gradients, if hypertonicity is accepted (LADURON, 1969; LAGERCRANTZ et al., 1970b), or alternatively on isotonic Ficoll/D_2O gradients (POISNER and TRIFARO, 1969).

3. Chemical Composition

The chromaffin amine storage vesicles have a water content ranging according to the different reports from 60 (KIRSHNER et al., 1966b) to 68.5 (HILLARP, 1959) % of their wet weight. Their sucrose space, in relation to total water, has been calculated to be only one third of that of mitochondria, while their relative osmotic space was found to be more than twice as large as that of mitochondria (LADURON, 1969). Catecholamines make up about 21% of their dry weight. Interestingly, this implies that the amine concentration in the granules is in the same range as that of protein, 35%, and lipid, 22% of the dry weight (HILLARP, 1960a), which makes it unlikely that the amines can be stored exclusively by binding to either protein or lipid (HILLARP, 1960a). However, the most striking feature about the chemical composition of the granules is their uniquely (BLASCHKO et al., 1956) high content of adenine nucleotides, mainly in the form of ATP (HILLARP et al., 1955; BLASCHKO et al., 1956; HILLARP, 1960b), which makes up 15% of their dry weight (HILLARP, 1960a). Characteristic about the ATP of the granules is firstly that it is metabolically almost inert, and therefore highly resistant to labelling (PRUSOFF et al., 1956; STJÄRNE et al., 1970a), and secondly that its concentration relative to catecholamines is maintained fairly constant at a level corresponding to a molar amine /ATP ratio close to 4/1 (FALCK et al., 1956; BLASCHKO et al., 1956) during various stages of amine depletion and repletion, both *in vivo* (CARLSSON and HILLARP, 1956; CARLSSON et al., 1957a; SCHÜMANN, 1958), and *in vitro* (HILLARP, 1958c; STJÄRNE, 1964), although certain exceptions to this general rule have also been reported (SCHÜMANN, 1958; BURACK et al., 1960). The relatively fixed molar ratio plus the metabolic inertness of the ATP have led to the proposition that the adenine nucleotides in the granules do not serve the purpose of storing metabolic energy, but rather that of providing negative charges to balance the positive charges of the catecholamines to maintain electroneutrality (Blaschko et al., 1956; Falck et al., 1956). In spite of considerable efforts it has proved difficult to demonstrate convincingly such an amine-ATP complex (Weiner and Jardetzky, 1964; Colburn and Maas, 1965). However, according to a recent report high concentrations of various amines, including catecholamines, form polymeric aggregates with ATP, of an apparent molecular weight of several thousand, which can be sedimented by high speed centrifugation (Berneis et al., 1969).

The proteins in the chromaffin granules include at least two with known enzymatic function, dopamine β-hydroxylase (Kirshner, 1957; Levin et al., 1960) and ATPase (Banks, 1965; Kirshner et al., 1966b). The former enzyme has recently been reported to occur in both soluble and insoluble form (Viveros et al., 1969b), while all of the ATPase activity occurs in the insoluble "membrane" protein fractions (Banks, 1965; Taugner and Hasselbach, 1968). Adenylate kinase activity has been reported in chromaffin granule fractions (Hillarp, 1958b), but according to recent observations this may well represent contamination (Lagercrantz et al., 1970a, b).

However, the bulk of the granule protein appears to lack enzymatic activity. The most striking feature about this structural protein is the high proportion of water-soluble material, estimated to from 63 (Helle and Serck-Hansen, 1969) to 77 (Hillarp, 1960b) % of the total protein. About 50% of this fraction has been found to consist of a highly acidic protein, or group of proteins, called chromogranins (Blaschko et al., 1967a), which appears to be specific for catecholamine storing particles in adrenal medulla (Blaschko and Helle, 1963; Helle, 1966a; Kirshner et al., 1966b), in phaeochromocytoma (Smith, 1968), and interestingly, in sympathetic nerves (Banks et al., 1969).

The antigenic properties of chromogranin, which form the basis for the immunological methods of assay of this protein, were originally described by Helle (1966b). About one-half of the water-insoluble protein in chromaffin storage particles has recently been found to consist of chromogranin-like material (Helle and Serck-Hansen, 1969). Thus it appears that chromogranin as well as dopamine β-hydroxylase (Viveros et al., 1969b) exists in the granules in two forms of different water solubility. Depending on the methods used the molecular weight has been variously estimated to 21—25000 (Helle, 1966; Kirshner et al., 1966b), 39000—40600 (Kirshner et al., 1966b; Kirshner and Kirshner, 1969), 75000—81200 (Blaschko et al., 1966; Smith and Winkler, 1967; Kirshner and Kirshner, 1969) or 150000—300000 (Helle and Serck-Hansen, 1969), suggesting different degrees of polymerization of subunits, possibly joined by disulphide bonds (Kirshner and Kirshner, 1969). The amino acid composition has been studied in various laboratories, and there is general agreement that the protein shows a large excess of acidic residues, mainly glutamic acid (Helle, 1966; Kirshner et al., 1966b; Smith and Winkler, 1967). The strikingly low content of cyst(e)ine indicates considerable flexibility (Smith and Winkler, 1967). The relatively high content of the helix-disrupting amino acid proline, as well as actual measurements of the hydrodynamic properties of purified chromogranin A have been interpreted as further indications of randomization of structure and high flexibility of conformation (Smith and Winkler, 1967). However, there is some disagreement as to the degree of randomization (Kirshner and Kirshner, 1969).

These strictly biochemical considerations have served as a basis for interesting proposals concerning mechanisms of storage and release of amines. Thus the postulated random coil characteristics of this protein imply that its hydrodynamic volume is determined by electrostatic repulsion between the excess of negatively charged amino acid residues, and that the volume will therefore be inversely related to the ionic strength of the medium (SMITH 1968). This implies contractility (LISHAJKO, 1970a), which may be physiologically relevant for amine release, since a shift in the physical state of catecholamines and ATP in the granules from a bound to a free ionized state would produce a considerable local rise in osmolarity (HILLARP and NILSON, 1954; CARLSSON and HILLARP, 1958; HILLARP, 1958a; LISHAJKO, 1970a). Another proposed implication of the random coil nature of chromogranin is that it should acquire gel form at low temperature, which may be the reason for the stability of the intragranular catecholamine storage complex and for the absence of exchange of exogenous for endogenous amines, at temperatures close to 0°C (HILLARP, 1959; SMITH, 1968).

Lipids make up 22% of the dry weight of the chromaffin storage vesicles (HILLARP, 1960a), which differ from other organelles such as mitochondria or microsomes in that they have a high cholesterol/phospholipid ratio and a uniquely high proportion of lysolecithin (BLASCHKO et al., 1967b). The presence of high amounts of lysolecithin in the amine storage vesicles is particularly interesting in view of its capacity to attack and destroy biological membranes. Lysolecithin might thus be critically involved in amine secretion. The evidence seems to be that the vesicles do not contain the enzyme required for synthesis of this type of lysolecithin, a phospholipase A_2, which however occurs in lysosomes. The lysolecithin in amine storage vesicles may thus be formed during the early history of the vesicles, in the Golgi region, where lysosomes are also formed (WINKLER and SMITH, 1968).

It may be relevant that the chromaffin storage particles contain about six times as much calcium per unit protein as do mitochondria (BOROWITZ et al., 1965). The presence of RNA in chromaffin granule fractions has been reported (HILLARP, 1958a; PHILIPPU and SCHÜMANN, 1963, 1964a), but the possibility that it might represent contamination does not appear to be ruled out.

4. Storage Complex

Although there are reasons to assume that at all times a certain small fraction of the catecholamines of chromaffin cells exist outside the specific storage vesicles, there is no doubt that the bulk of the amines is stored inside them. Little is known with certainty concerning the nature of the storage mechanism, by which the vesicles are able to maintain an enormous apparent amine concentration gradient to the surrounding cytoplasm.

a) Stability of Storage Complex at 0°C

The early observation that isolated chromaffin granules suspended in isotonic amine-free media maintain their catecholamine content at 0°C over a period of days (FALCK et al., 1956) indicates that the storage complex is not dependent on continuous supply of energy, at least not at low temperature. In view of the additional finding that the membrane of the storage vesicles is permeable to catecholamines (HILLARP, 1959; KIRSHNER et al., 1966a) as well as to ATP (KIRSHNER et al., 1966a), at 0°C, the conclusion has been reached that amines and ATP do not exist in the granules in a diffusible form (CARLSSON and HILLARP, 1958). This is further supported by the finding that little or no exchange of endogenous for exogenous catecholamines occurs at this temperature (Hillarp, 1959). The "storage complex hypothesis" thus postulates that the catecholamines are kept in the vesicles in a non-diffusible form by binding to equivalent amounts of ATP and some macromolecule, specific protein (Hillarp, 1958d) or RNA together with Ca^{++} and Mg^{++} (Holtz and Palm, 1966; Philippu and Schümann, 1966). The possibility has also been discussed that the storage complex is non-diffusible only at low temperature due to a change in the physical properties of the specific protein at 0° C, involving a transformation to gel form (Smith, 1968), or to the formation of large multimolecular aggregates of amines and ATP in the presence of divalent cations, at low temperature (Berneis et al., 1969), which might prevent outward diffusion of catecholamines and ATP as well as amine exchange.

However, although the storage complex is extremely stable in isotonic media at 0° C, it is readily disrupted by treatment known to damage the vesicle membrane such as freezing and thawing, lowering the pH, addition of detergents or exposure to hypotonic media (Hillarp and Nilson, 1954). In fact suspension in distilled water is a routine method for extraction of the granules (Hillarp, 1958a) which rapidly lose their soluble contents (Blaschko et al., 1956): catecholamine, ATP (Stjärne, 1964) and soluble protein (Lishajko, 1969a).

The evidence from experiments carried out at 0° C thus indicates that the stability of the storage complex is dependent on the integrity of the membrane of the vesicles, which at 0° C appears to constitute a diffusion barrier to macromolecules but not to smaller molecules such as catecholamines or ATP.

b) Osmotic Lysis

The osmotic effect is not dependent on the absolute tonicity, but on the relative tonicity of the medium *versus* that of the vesicles (Hillarp and Nilson, 1954). The effects of the osmotic shock, as judged by following the optical changes in the particle suspension (Hillarp and Nilson, 1954; Lishajko, 1970a), or by following catecholamine and ATP efflux (Stjärne, 1964), are strictly proportional to the osmolarity gradient involved and completed in a matter of minutes (Hillarp and Nilson, 1954; Stjärne, 1964; Lishajko, 1970a). The effects do not appear to be all-or-none in character, but allow reestablishment of equilibrium at a lower level (Hillarp and Nilson, 1954; Lishajko, 1970a). This has been interpreted as an indication of differences in osmotic resistance of different particles (Hillarp and Nilson, 1954). However, it may also reflect the reversibility of the effect of osmotic shock on the membrane of the vesicles. Osmotically induced swelling (Lishajko, 1970a), leads to over-distension and focal or diffuse "functional rupture" of the membrane. It appears that osmotic equilibrium is rapidly reestablished allowing sealing of the defects. In fact, particles exposed to such partial lysis appear to show essentially normal stability, as reflected in the rate of spontaneous amine release, and they even respond to ATP-Mg^{++} by accelerated amine uptake (Lishajko, 1970a).

It was recently reported that the effects of osmotic shock on isolated chromaffin storage vesicles are largely prevented when relatively low concentrations of Ca^{++} or Mg^{++}, 0.5—6 mM, are present in the medium (Lishajko, 1970a). Osmotic lysis was found to be normally accompanied by a fall in the refractive index of the particle suspension; this was interpreted as evidence of swelling of the particles. The inhibitory effect of the divalent ions was accompanied by a rise in the refractive index, reflecting contraction of the particles (Lishajko, 1970a). The mechanism of this protective effect appears to be that the ions by inducing contraction reduce the water space of the particles.

c) Stability of Storage Complex at Higher Temperature

At higher temperature suspensions of chromaffin granules in isotonic media undergo a gradual and largely parallel loss of catecholamines, ATP, soluble protein and even Ca^{++} and Mg^{++} (HILLARP, 1958c; PHILLIPPU and SCHÜMANN, 1964b; LISHAJKO, 1969a), at a rate progressively increasing with temperature (LISHAJKO, 1969a). In experiments at 31°C TAUGNER and HASSELBACH (1966) found that the catecholamine efflux occurred at a constant rate of 0.16% per min over 5 hours, and that it was independent of a 10-fold rise in the amine concentration of the medium. Studies of the uptake of labelled catecholamines added to the medium showed that the spontaneous release was partly balanced by uptake of amines, occurring at a rate of about 10% of the release. However, addition of ATP plus Mg^{++} to the medium completely prevented net loss of catecholamine from the granules. Studies with labelled amines in the incubation medium showed that the addition of ATP plus Mg^{++} had not altered the rate of spontaneous release, but had accelerated uptake by a factor of ten, so that uptake exactly balanced release. It should be mentioned that other authors, on the basis of the critical assumption that the amines in the vesicles represent a single homogeneous pool (cf. below, 4 i), maintain that the effect of ATP plus Mg^{++} is to decelerate amine release as well as to accelerate amine uptake (LISHAJKO, 1969a).

These results imply that, *in vitro* and possibly *in vivo*, maintenance of the integrity of the storage vesicles requires the presence of ATP and Mg^{++} in the medium. The store is preserved by balancing amine release and uptake, probably mainly by re-uptake of amines spontaneously "leaking" from the granules (EULER and LISHAJKO, 1967). If the catecholamine store is thus maintained, loss of ATP, protein and other soluble constituents is apparently prevented. In view of the fact that exogenous ATP does not exchange to any considerable extent with endogenous ATP, and certainly not in proportion to the exchange of catecholamines (CARLSSON et al., 1963), and since it seems highly unlikely that macromolecules rapidly move to and fro across intact unit membranes, the implication seems to be that release of catecholamines is normally dissociated from release of ATP and protein (cf. LISHAJKO, 1969a). Evidently the catecholamines stabilize the storage complex, and only when the amine deficit exceeds a critical level in time and magnitude do structural protein and ATP irreversibly leak out of the granules. This appears to be the main reason why net uptake of catecholamines does not occur in partially depleted chromaffin granules (TAUGNER and HASSELBACH, 1966; LISHAJKO, 1969a). Interestingly, nerve granules do not readily lose ATP on incubation, and net amine uptake is quite feasible in these granules (cf. EULER and LISHAJKO, 1967), indicating important differences in catecholamine storage in the two types of granule (cf. STJÄRNE, 1964).

d) Differences between Dopamine, Noradrenaline and Adrenaline Storage

In the preceding Section the general properties of the particles storing the bulk of the catecholamines in bovine adrenal medulla have been presented. However, it has recently been emphasized that there are important differences in the storage mechanisms for the three catecholamines (LISHAJKO, 1969a).

In sheep adrenal medulla, where dopamine corresponds to about 2% of the total catecholamines stored in particulate fractions, LISHAJKO (1968, 1969a) obtained evidence which he interpreted as indication that this dopamine is stored in separate particles containing dopamine only. However, the evidence is indirect and successful separation of such particles from those storing noradrenaline and adrenaline has not been reported. The "dopamine granules" were found to differ distinctly in two respects from the "adrenaline granules": they give off dopamine at a high rate, corresponding to a half-life of 22 min at 37 °C, or twice as rapidly as the "adrenaline granules" give up adrenaline, and they are, after partial depletion, capable of net uptake of dopamine, in the presence of ATP and Mg^{++}, when the dopamine concentration of the medium is raised. The reversibility of dopamine loss by spontaneous release suggests that it may not be accompanied by loss of ATP and soluble protein, in distinct contrast to the findings for noradrenaline and adrenaline storing particles, where it was concluded (cf. preceding Section) that an amine deficit interferes with the stability of the storage mechanism and leads to irreversible loss of ATP and protein. Thus the "dopamine granules" appear to behave much more like the nerve granules isolated from bovine splenic nerve trunk than like chromaffin granules in adrenal medulla. However, until "dopamine granules" have been separated from the other catecholamine storage vesicles the alternative interpretation must be considered, that the small amount of dopamine is stored in a separate "dopamine compartment" in vesicles mainly storing noradrenaline and/or adrenaline. This compartment might well be related to the enzyme dopamine β-hydroxylase, which has a subcellular distribution similar to that of adrenaline and noradrenaline (Kirshner, 1957; Oka et al., 1967a; Laduron and Belpaire, 1968; Viveros et al., 1969a). The high affinity of dopamine for uptake into chromaffin vesicles (Laduron and Belpaire, 1968), making net uptake feasible at a molar ratio of dopamine to noradrenaline and adrenaline of 0.05—0.2 (Lishajko, 1969a), suggests that uptake of dopamine is mediated by a specific dopamine carrier, for which the other catecholamines have a lower affinity but may compete and thus contribute to the regulation of overall synthesis of noradrenaline (cf. Fig. 2).

In isotonic media the spontaneous release of adrenaline follows a single exponential curve, whereas that of noradrenaline is biphasic, a rapid initial phase being followed by a slow one, largely parallel to the slope of the adrenaline curve (Oka et al., 1966b; Lishajko, 1969a). Interestingly, these differences were affected by alterations in the tonicity of the incubation medium. Thus in hypertonic media the release of both adrenaline and noradrenaline followed a single exponential curve, whereas in hypotonic media the release of adrenaline as well as of noradrenaline followed a biphasic curve (Lishajko, 1970a), suggesting differences in physical stability between the intragranular storage complexes for noradrenaline and those for adrenaline.

e) Importance of Medium for Stability

The question arises whether spontaneous amine release from the granules occurs *in vivo*, or represents an artifact, due to suspension of the particles in an unphysiological medium *in vitro*.

From this point of view it is interesting that the rate of spontaneous loss of amine, *e.g.* adrenaline, from isolated bovine adrenal medullary granules is different in different isotonic media. Thus the half-life at 37 °C and pH 7.5 in sucrose, potassium phosphate and potassium chloride was 110, 160 and 83 min, respectively (Lishajko, 1969a). However, incubation in press juice from the adrenal medulla, representing the natural environment of the vesicles, prolonged the half-life to 230 min. Similar prolongation was seen in various hypertonic media. The results are difficult to interpret, since the stabilizing effect of the press juice might be secondary to hypertonicity resulting from tissue damage. However, the alternative interpretation is that spontaneous release of amines *in vivo* may occur at a much slower rate than in most isotonic media *in vitro*.

f) Permeability of Vesicle Membrane. Role of ATPase in Amine Transport

The critical role of hydrolysis of ATP mediated by a specific ATPase in the presence of Mg^{++}, for maintaining the integrity of the catecholamine storage vesicles, at or close to body temperature, has been the main basis for the "active uptake" hypothesis for catecholamine storage (KIRSHNER, 1962; TAUGNER and HASSELBACH, 1966). According to this concept amine passage across the vesicle membrane at these temperatures represents active, carrier-mediated, transport. It is assumed that the vesicle membrane, which is permeable at 0°C to catecholamines as well as to ATP (HILLARP, 1959; KIRSHNER et al., 1966a), alters its permeability at higher temperature, when active metabolism occurs, to form an efficient barrier enclosing the stored amine (TAUGNER and HASSELBACH, 1966). However, this concept is based on indirect evidence only, and on the crucial assumption, that the "transport ATPase" operates at the level of the unit membrane of the vesicles (TAUGNER and HASSELBACH, 1968). This assumption may be correct, but the possibility remains that it is not; the alternative must still be considered that the membrane remains at all times permeable to catecholamines as well as to ATP, even at higher temperature. In that case the "transport ATPase' would operate at a different level, hydrolyzing ATP to mediate amine transport across some internal barrier in the vesicles (cf. STJÄRNE, 1964), or to somehow "activate" the storage complex so that amine exchange will be possible (FERRIS et al., 1970).

g) Ca^{++} as Promoter of Release: In vitro Models of Secretion by Exocytosis?

One crucial experiment to define the level of action of acetylcholine as trigger of secretion from the adrenal medulla is the testing of its direct effect on isolated chromaffin granules. In the very early stage of the work with isolated granules this experiment was done by BLASCHKO et al. (1955), who found that acetylcholine has no amine releasing action on the isolated storage vesicles.

This turned the interest to what might be regarded as the "second messenger" in stimulus-secretion coupling in the adrenal medulla, Ca^{++}, the presence of which at physiological concentrations is an obligatory requirement for the acetylcholine-induced secretion (cf. DOUGLAS, 1968).

The observed effects of Ca^{++} on isolated chromaffin granules are somewhat complex and confusing; they include facilitation as well as inhibition of amine release, depending on the circumstances.

As mentioned above, (C 4 b) Ca^{++} as well as Mg^{++} 6 mM cause the granules to shrink and inhibit the release of catecholamines, ATP and protein induced by osmotic shock (LISHAJKO, 1970a).

However, Ca^{++} 2.5 mM or higher was reported to accelerate the catecholamine release from isolated chromaffin granules incubated in sucrose media at 37°C for 60 min (PHILIPPU and SCHÜMANN, 1962). OKA et al. (1966b) reported that Ca^{++} even at 0.2 mM caused significant amine release from chromaffin granules purified by Millipore filtration. The same authors (OKA et al., 1967b) reported that Ca^{++} 0.5 mM induces structural changes in isolated chromaffin granules, leading to a progressive fall in optical density, which is known to imply swelling of the particles, and amine release. The effect was somewhat antagonized by Mg^{++}.

BANKS (1966) found no catecholamine releasing effects of Ca^{++} (2—5 mM) on isolated chromaffin granules incubated in sucrose media. However, he observed that Ca^{++} in sucrose (0.43 M)/KCl (150 mM) media slowed down (Ca^{++} 2.5 mM) or completely abolished (Ca^{++} 5 mM) the electrophoretic mobility of isolated chromaffin amine storage vesicles. He also observed that Ca^{++} at these concentrations induced clumping of the vesicles and concluded that Ca^{++} liberated during secretory stimulation, by abolishing the electrostatic repulsion might allow attachment of the negatively charged vesicles to the negatively charged interior aspect of the cell membrane, thus initiating the secretory events.

Quite recently LISHAJKO (1970c) described still another effect of Ca^{++} on isolated chromaffin granules. He found that Ca^{++} (2—6 mM) under specified conditions, including the presence of phosphate at concentrations from 3 mM (minimum) to 19 mM (optimum), induces rapid release of catecholamines, ATP and soluble protein from isolated bovine adrenal medullary granules. The effect was temperature-dependent, specific for Ca^{++}; Ba^{++} and Sr^{++} were inactive. The effect was antagonized by Mg^{++} (2 mM) and completely prevented by ATP (2 mM) plus Mg^{++} (2 mM). The releasing effect of Ca^{++} was rapid, essentially completed within 5 min, and it increased in proportion to the Ca^{++} concentration up to 6 mM when it resulted in complete depletion. The effect of Ca^{++} was potentiated by addition of RNA 1—6 g/ml; the threshold concentration of Ca^{++} was reduced to 0.3 mM. Release was apparently induced by calcium phosphate precipitate *in statu nascendi*. The effect could be obtained by adding freshly precipitated calcium phosphate to a granule suspension, but was lost by ageing of the precipitate.

Although it is difficult to evaluate the possible physiological significance of these observations, the fact that Ca^{++} and free phosphate, at concentrations which may possibly occur phasically and locally, *e.g.* close to the cell membrane during stimulation of chromaffin cells *in vivo*, induce a rapid and complete efflux of all the soluble components of catecholamine storage vesicles is intriguing, in view of the critical role of Ca^{++} for stimulus-secretion coupling *in vivo* (cf. DOUGLAS, 1968).

h) Cl^--dependent Acceleration of Spontaneous Release Induced by ATP plus Mg^{++}

Surprisingly, low concentrations of ATP and Mg^{++} may in certain media accelerate the spontaneous release of catecholamines (OKA et al., 1966b) as well as that of ATP and protein (POISNER and TRIFARO, 1967). This effect could be demonstrated in various ionic media but not in sucrose. Later experiments have shown that the apparent inhibitory effect of sucrose is due to absence of Cl^- ions, for which the reaction seems to have a relatively strict requirement (LISHAJKO, 1969b). This paradoxical effect of ATP shows a high nucleotide specificity (POISNER and TRIFARO, 1967; LISHAJKO, 1969b). The metal cofactor requirement seems to be largely the same as for the effect of higher concentrations of ATP promoting amine uptake (POISNER and TRIFARO, 1967).

The presence of ATPase activity in all kinds of secretory vesicles investigated, independently of the nature of the secretory material (cf. DOUGLAS, 1968), the crucial role of Ca^{++} in secretory events (cf. DOUGLAS, 1968) and the report that depolarization of plasma membranes causes liberation of bound ATP, which may thus become available for hydrolysis (ABOOD et al., 1962), led POISNER and TRIFARO (1967) to form an attractive hypothesis for the molecular events involved in stimulus-secretion coupling, based on the paradoxical effect of ATP plus Mg^{++} on catecholamine-ATP-protein release from isolated chromaffin granules incubated *in vitro*.

In this model it is assumed that the ATP released from the intragranular storage complex may, by a positive feed-back effect, accelerate the amine release originally initiated by the small amounts of ATP liberated from the plasma membrane (POISNER and TRIFARO, 1968). However, such an effect of granule-bound ATP would apply only to vesicles in which ATP is structurally involved in the storage complex. Moreover, it, may be questioned whether the ATP liberated from the plasma membrane by depolarization becomes available for hydrolysis inside the plasma membrane. Finally, since the assumption is that this secretory mechanism operates locally, close to the surface of the cell, it seems that such strictly localized acceleration of spontaneous release in a small population of vesicles — from a fraction of a per cent to one or two per cent per min (cf. TAUGNER and HASSELBACH, 1966; LISHAJKO, 1970a) — is insufficient to account for the secretion *in vivo*.

However, the proposition that ATP-Mg^{++}-stimulated acceleration of amine release from vesicles *in situ* may be a step in amine secretion from chromaffin tissue *in vivo* is supported by recent observations concerning similarities in inhibitory effects of certain drugs on amine release from isolated granules and on acetylcholine-induced secretion from perfused adrenal gland (FERRIS et al., 1970). But these pharmacological effects may be coincidental, and in that case the question still remains whether the spontaneous release of catecholamines from chromaffin granules as studied in various isotonic media *in vitro*, has any bearing on the secretory process *in vivo*. Secretion by exocytosis (cf. DOUGLAS, 1968) implies explosive, and according to recent reports all-or-none, discharge of the soluble contents of individual vesicles directly into the extracellular space (VIVEROS et al., 1969a). Such an event seems to be better mimicked *in vitro* by the osmotic lysis, or possibly by the calcium phosphate precipitation, experiments, since local damage to the vesicle membrane, possibly mediated by activation of its lysolecithin (BLASCHKO et al., 1967; DOUGLAS, 1968), appears to be a crucial event in physiologically induced secretion (cf. STJÄRNE, 1970b).

i) Homogeneity of Store

There can be little doubt that certain adrenal medullary cells manufacture noradrenaline only, while others have acquired the capacity to methylate noradrenaline and form adrenaline (HILLARP et al., 1954). In view of the demonstration in various tissues of specific dopamine storing cells (EULER and LISHAJKO, 1957; FALCK et al., 1959) it is not inconceivable that certain adrenal medullary cells are unable to β-hydroxylate dopamine, which may thus be stored in vesicles (EADE, 1958) specific for this amine (LISHAJKO, 1968), as already discussed. That dopamine may play a role as an independent adrenal medullary hormone, in addition to serving as precursor, has been supported by the demonstration of resting (HEMPEL and MÄNNL, 1969) as well as carbachol-induced secretion (LISHAJKO, 1970b) of small amounts of dopamine.

Different kinds of experimental evidence suggest that the catecholamine store of adrenal medulla is functionally compartmentalized, although it is difficult to state with certainty whether the compartments exist in the same or in different storage vesicles. In experiments where artifacts due to postmortal changes were carefully controlled, HILLARP (1960b) found ,in crude chromaffin granule fractions isolated from various species, an excess of catecholamines over adenine nucleotides, relative to the molar ratio of 4/1 expected if all amines are stored by salt-binding to nucleotides. He therefore postulated the existence of two functionally different amine "pools": a labile pool in storage vesicles of low density, deficient in adenine nucleotides, with a capacity of about 20% of the total store in the adrenal medulla; and a more stable pool in high-density vesicles, in which catecholamines appear to be stored in stoichiometric relationship to adenine nucleotides. Similar conclusions, that there are at least two different mechanisms of binding of catecholamines in storage vesicles, differing in amine/nucleotide ratio were reached on the basis of lysis experiments (Stjärne, 1964). This concept is supported by kinetic studies of uptake of labelled catecholamines by bovine adrenal medullary granules: the specific activity of the granule-bound amines, even after prolonged incubation, failed to equilibrate with that of the medium, but reached a quasi-stable level corresponding to about 20% equilibration (Taugner and Hasselbach, 1966). On subsequent incubation in amine-free medium the specific activity of the catecholamines appearing in the medium was initially lower than the mean specific activity of the preparation, only to rise gradually above that level, indicating lack of homogeneity of the amine pool labelled during the preceding incubation. This led Taugner and Hasselbach (1966) to the conclusion that the catecholamines exist in the storage vesicles in two separate and functionally different pools: One large one, containing 75—80% of the total amine, characterized by a slow exchange with exogenous catecholamines and probably binding amines in stoichiometric relationship to ATP, and one small pool of 20—25% of the total, not bound at all but requiring metabolic energy derived from continuous hydrolysis of ATP to be kept inside the vesicles.

While the evidence of heterogeneity of the catecholamine store in the vesicles appears convincing, the proposal that the amines in the small pool, corresponding to as much as 20—25% of the total, exist in free solution seems to be difficult to reconcile with the fact that 80% or more of the total amines of adrenal medulla can be recovered in the storage vesicles, after homogenization at 0°C in isotonic media, and are retained in them more or less indefinitely, in spite of the fact that the vesicle membrane is permeable to amines at this temperature (Hillarp, 1959; Kirshner et al., 1966b). Thus it may be necessary to postulate a three-compartment system: a very small pool of soluble amines; a labile pool with a high turnover, in which the amines are somehow bound, possibly to lipid (Euler, 1946, 1956; Stjärne, 1964); and a large, stable pool with a slow turnover, in which the amines are bound in stoichiometric relationship to ATP (cf. Stjärne, 1964). This idea is speculative, but appears to be supported by the high ratio, catecholamine/adenine nucleotide, observed in some cases of phaeochromocytoma (Schümann, 1960; Stjärne et al., 1964), implying that storage of large amounts of amine in vesicles is feasible even in the absence of a stoichiometric relation to adenine nucleotides.

5. Effects of Drugs

In a discussion of the effects of drugs (for a review see Holtz and Palm, 1966) on storage mechanisms it will be necessary to distinguish between pharmacological and biochemical aspects. Thus exogenous agents added *in vitro* in high concentration may exert actions on the storage vesicles which may be of biochemical interest although they have no immediate significance pharmacologically. *In vivo*, as already pointed out, the adrenal medulla is relatively resistant to the effect of drugs which have dramatic effects on the amine stores of sympathetic neurons.

a) Stabilizers

Some drugs, such as reserpine 10^{-6}M (Euler and Lishajko, 1961; Weil-Malherbe and Poisner, 1963), prenylamine 10^{-6}M to 5×10^{-5}M (Euler and Lishajko, 1968; Ferris et al., 1970) and certain phenothiazines 10^{-5}M (Weil-Malherbe and Posner, 1963), inhibit spontaneous release of amines from isolated chromaffin granules incubated *in vitro*, an effect much more marked in nerve granules (cf. Chapter by von Euler). Since the same drugs at higher concentrations accelerate amine release, Weil-Malherbe and Posner (1961), who had noted that this "protective" effect is pH-dependent, suggested that it is the cationic species of the drug which is responsible for the inhibition of release, while the unionized base promotes release. However, the promotion of release requires too high drug concentrations to appear specific, and at least in the case of prenylamine at 10^{-4}M concentration it rather has the character of unspecific damage, leading to lysis of the granules (Lundborg and Stitzel, 1968).

The recent observations already mentioned, of similarities between the inhibitory effects of drugs on amine release from isolated vesicles, and on acetylcholine-induced secretion from perfused adrenal glands (Ferris et al., 1970) suggest that studies of inhibition of amine release *in vitro* may be of pharmacological significance *in vivo*. Apart from that, the fact that spontaneous release of amines from the vesicles can be inhibited by drugs at low concentrations is of interest since it shows that this process, which has a high Q_{10} value and which is under certain conditions accelerated by ATP-Mg^{++} (Oka et al., 1966b; Poisner and Trifaro, 1967; Lishajko, 1969b), does not represent mere "leakage", due to damage of the storage particles, but is specific, enzyme-dependent and possibly carrier-mediated. The striking qualitative similarities between the inhibitory effects of various drugs on spontaneous or ATP-Mg^{++}-activated amine release and on amine uptake, not only in nerve granules (cf. Chapter by von Euler pp. 186), but also in chromaffin granules (Ferris et al., 1970), suggest that the two processes may be closely related (Ferris et al., 1970), possibly even coupled (Stjärne, 1964). In that case drugs might affect release by inhibition of the ATPase of the vesicles (*e.g.* N-ethyl maleimide), by preventing activation of the storage complex (*e.g.* prenylamine), or by blocking amine exchange in the activated complex (*e.g.* reserpine), possibly by competition for a postulated amine carrier (Stjärne, 1964).

b) Promoters of Release

Apart from the already mentioned promotion of release induced by Ca^{++} or by ATP- and Mg^{++} (see C 4 g, h) it appears that the only type of acceleration of release which can be induced *in vitro* without gross damage to the storage vesicles is that induced by certain indirectly acting sympathomimetic amines, such as tyramine (Schümann and Philippu, 1961). Although these agents seem to compete for the ATP-Mg^{++}-dependent transport system, they do not need to utilize such specific transport, but can apparently reach the intragranular storage complex by passive diffusion (Carlsson et al., 1963). Their mechanism of action is amine release by displacement, leading to accelerated efflux of catecholamines only, unaccompanied by ATP (Schümann and Philippu, 1961). According to the argument above it seems that tyramine can replace the catecholamines as stabilizers of the internal storage complex, preventing irreversible loss of ATP as well as of specific soluble protein.

c) Depleters

The vast majority of amine depleters *in vivo*, with a direct action on the storage vesicles, apparently act either by blocking re-uptake of preformed catecholamines given off from the storage complex, or by preventing uptake of dopamine and thus blocking synthesis of noradrenaline and adrenaline.

Certain drugs cause disproportionate depletion of catecholamines in adrenal medulla, with less effect on ATP. Thus in rats injection of 50 mg/kg of 6-aminonicotinic acid amide (Schacht et al., 1966) caused the initial molar ratio amines/ATP of about 4/1 to fall to 0.3. This effect is not unique — as a matter of fact,

A. Spontaneous Release :

B. Uptake:

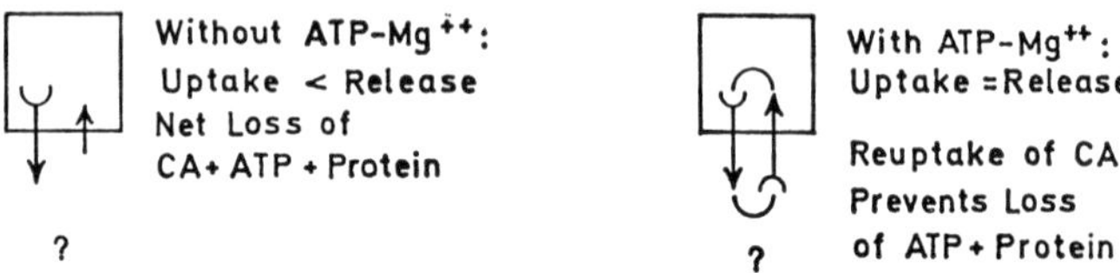

C. Pools :

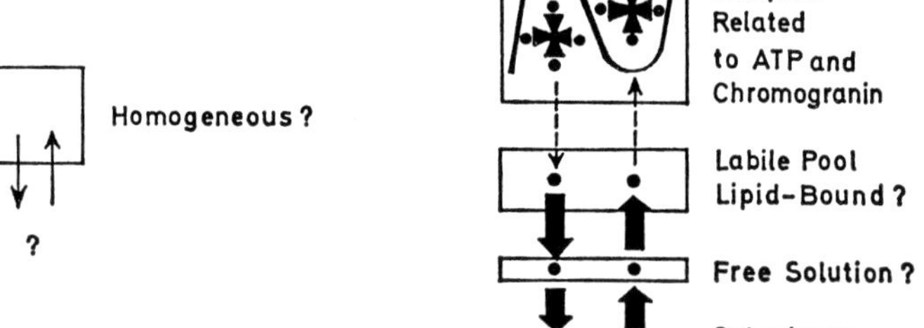

Fig. 3. Diagrammatic representation of dynamics of catecholamine storage.

A. *Spontaneous release:* "Leakage" — artifact due to damage? Or specific, possibly carrier-mediated transport?

Characteristics:

Involves CA, ATP and soluble protein. End result: Loss of all three, in stoichiometric amounts.

Occurs at constant rate, independent of external amine concentration.

High Q_{10} — enzymatic?

Accelerated by ATP-Mg^{++} in the presence of Cl^- — ATPase involved?

Antagonized by drugs:

Reserpine 10^{-8} M — By competition with amine for carrier? By blocking ATPase?

Prenylamine 10^{-6} M — By preventing "activation" of storage complex?

N-ethyl maleimide 10^{-5} M — By blocking ATPase.

Promoted by tyramine — By displacement.

B. *Uptake:* Closely related to release — coupled processes?

Characteristics:

Without ATP-Mg^{++} Uptake $= 0.1 \times$ Release

With ATP-Mg^{++} Uptake = Release

High Q_{10} — enzymatic?

Antagonized by drugs also (less strongly) blocking release:

Reserpine 10^{-8} M — By competition with amine for carrier? By blocking ATPase?

Prenylamine 10^{-6} M — By preventing "activation" of storage complex?

N-ethyl maleimide 10^{-5} M — By blocking ATPase.

One mole of ATP split per mole of amine taken up.

Function of ATP: To provide energy for transport across membranes? Or to "activate" storage complex?

Level of action: Unit membrane of vesicles? Internal barrier? Protein in storage complex?

Essentially an exchange mechanism; no net uptake because partial amine depletion leads to irreversible loss of "structural" ATP and protein.

CA act as stabilizers of the storage complex? Release of amines *precedes* that of ATP and protein (in isolated vesicles)? When amine re-uptake operates efficiently to balance release, ATP and protein release and loss are prevented.

C. *Pools:* Homogeneous store in vesicles? Heterogeneous?

Characteristics:

Deviation of CA/ATP molar ratio from 4/1 indicates that not all amines are bound together with stoichiometric amounts of ATP — Hillarp's "labile pool".

Lysis in the presence of trapping systems for amines and ATP leaving the granules shows an amine fraction relatively resistant to lysis, unrelated to ATP.

Kinetic studies indicate that only about 20—25% of the total particle-bound amines are rapidly exchangeable.

Question: Does this imply three compartments in dynamic equilibrium, of different capacities and turnover rates?

Abbreviation: CA — catecholamine(s)

there are some reports that even reserpine may, under certain circumstances, considerably depress the amine/ATP ratio of adrenomedullary granules (SCHÜMANN, 1958; BURACK et al., 1960). This becomes particularly interesting in view of the recent distinction between the effects of reserpine on catecholamines and on dopamine β-hydroxylase in adrenomedullary granules in rabbits, when reserpine was given to intact animals and to animals in which the adrenal gland was protected, by ganglionic blocking agents, against neurogenically induced secretion caused by reserpine (VIVEROS et al., 1969c). When reserpine depleted the adrenal gland by inducing neurogenic secretion there was a parallel loss of amines and of dopamine β-hydroxylase. However, when reserpine depleted the gland by a direct effect, presumably acting on the granules, the amine loss was selective, dopamine β-hydroxylase remaining unchanged.

6. Diagrammatic Representation of Dynamics of Catecholamine Storage

The details concerning mechanisms involved in catecholamine storage, as well as levels of action of various drugs, are still incompletely understood. An alternative model to the one presented in this chapter, for amine storage and for modes of action of several drugs, is discussed by HOLTZ and PALM (1966). In fact the different experimental observations seem as yet to be difficult to fit into any one single model, which could satisfactorily explain all the complex experimental data. Thus the Section on Adrenal Medulla is concluded by a brief diagrammatic review of a series of crucial aspects on catecholamine storage: The nature of the process of "spontaneous amine release"; mechanisms involved in promoting amine uptake; and the question of the homogeneity of the store in the chromaffin amine storage vesicles (Fig. 3).

References

ABOOD, L.G., KOKETSU, K., MIYAMOTO, S.: Outflux of various phosphates during membrane depolarization of excitable tissues. Amer. J. Physiol. **202**, 469—474 (1962).

ALLEGRANZA, A., BOZZI, R., BRUNO, A.: Urinary excretion of 5-hydroxyindoleacetic, homovanillic, and vanilmandelic acids in schizophrenics taking reserpine and chlorpromazine. J. nerv. ment. Dis. **140**, 207—214 (1965).

ANDÉN, N.-E., HENNING, M.: Effect of reserpine on the urinary excretion and the tissue levels of noradrenaline in the rat. Acta physiol. scand. **72**, 134—138 (1968).

AXELROD, J.: N-methyladrenaline, a new catecholamine in the adrenal gland. Biochem. biophys. Acta (Amst.). **45**, 614—615 (1960).

Axelrod, J.: Purification and properties of phenylethanolamine-N-methyl transferase. J. biol. Chem. **237**, 1657—1660 (1962).

— Methylation reactions in the formation and metabolism of catecholamines and other biogenic amines. Pharmacol. Rev. **18**, 95—113 (1966).

— Weil-Malherbe, H., Tomchick, R.: The physiological disposition of H^3-epinephrine and its metabolite metanephrine. J. Pharmacol. exp. Ther. **127**, 251—256 (1959).

Banks, P.: The adenosine-triphosphatase activity of adrenal chromaffin granules. Biochem. J. **95**, 490—496 (1965).

— An interaction between chromaffin granules and calcium ions. Biochem. J. **101**, 18c—20c (1966).

— Helle, K.B., Mayor, D.: Evidence for presence of a chromogranin-like protein in bovine splenic nerve granules. Molec. Pharmacol. **5**, 210—212 (1969).

Bartholini, G., Gey, K.F., Pletscher, A.: Enhancement of tyrosine transamination *in vivo* by catecholamines. Experientia (Basel) **26**, 980—981 (1970).

Beaufay, H., Jaques, P., Baudhuin, P., Sellinger, O.Z., Berthet, J., de Duve, C.: Tissue fractionation studies. Resolution of mitochondrial fractions from rat liver into three distinct populations of cytoplasmic particles by means of density equilibration in various gradients. Biochem. J. **92**, 184—205 (1964).

Belpaire, F., Laduron, P.: Tissue fractionation and catecholamines I. Latency and activation properties of dopamine-β-hydroxylase in adrenal medulla. Biochem. Pharmacol. **17**, 411—421 (1968).

Berneis, K.H., Pletscher, A., Da Prada, M.: Metal-dependent aggregation of biogenic amines: a hypothesis for their storage and release. Nature (Lond.) **224**, 281—283 (1969).

Bertler, Å., Hall, G., Hillarp, N.-Å., Rosengren, E.: Uptake of dopamine by the storage granules of the adrenal medulla *in vitro*. Acta physiol. scand. **52**, 167—170 (1961a).

— Hillarp, N.-Å., Rosengren, E.: Some observations on the synthesis and storage of catecholamines in the adrenaline cells of the suprarenal medulla. Acta physiol. scand. **50**, 124—131 (1960a).

— — — Effect of reserpine on the storage of new-formed catecholamines in the adrenal medulla. Acta physiol. scand. **52**, 44—48 (1961b).

— Rosengren, A.-M., Rosengren, E.,: *In vivo* uptake of dopamine and 5-hydroxytryptamine by adrenal medullary granules. Experientia (Basel) **16**, 418—419 (1960b).

Blaschko, H.: The development of current concepts of catecholamine formation. Pharmacol. Rev. **11**, 307—316 (1959).

— Storage of catechol amines. Ciba Foundation Symposium. In: "Adrenergic Mechanisms" pp. 61—62. Ed. by J.R. Vane, G.E.W. Wolstenholme and Maeve O'Connor. J. & A. Churchill Ltd. London: 1960.

— Catecholamines: Metabolism and storage. Recent Advances in pharmacology, pp. 135—153. Ed. by Robson and Stacey, 4th Edition. London: J. & A. Churchill Ltd. 1968.

— Born, G.V.R., D'Ioro, A., Eade, N.R.: Observations on the distribution of catecholamines and adenosine-triphosphate in the bovine adrenal medulla. J. Physiol. (Lond.) **133**, 548—557 (1956).

— Comline, R.S., Schneider, F.H., Silver, M., Smith, A.D.: Secretion of a chromaffin granule protein, chromogranin, from the adrenal gland after splanchnic stimulation. Nature (Lond.) **215**, 58—59 (1967a).

— Firemark, H., Smith, A.D., Winkler, H.: Lipids of the adrenal medulla: lysolecithin, a characteristic constituent of chromaffin granules. Biochem. J. **104**, 545—549 (1967b).

— Hagen, J.M., Hagen, P.: Mitochondrial enzymes and chromaffin granules. J. Physiol. (Lond.) **139**, 316—322 (1957).

— Hagen, P., Welch, A.D.: Observations on the intracellular granules of the adrenal medulla J. Physiol. (Lond.) **129**, 27—49 (1955).

— Helle, K.B.: Interaction of soluble protein fractions from bovine adrenal medullary granules with adrenaline and adenosine-triphosphatase. J. Physiol. (Lond.) **169**, 120P to 121P (1963).

— Smith, A.D., Winkler, H.: Untersuchungen an Eiweißfraktionen der chromaffinen Granula. Naunyn-Schmiedeberg's Arch. exp. Path. Pharmak. **253**, 23 (1966).

— Welch, A.D.: Localization of adrenaline in cytoplasmic particles of the bovine adrenal medulla. Naunyn-Schmiedeberg's Arch. exp. Path. Pharmak. **219**, 17—22 (1953).

Borowitz, J.L., Fuwa, K., Weiner, N.: Distribution of metals and catecholamines in bovine adrenal medulla subfractions. Nature (Lond.) **205**, 42—43 (1965).

Brown, G.L.: The Croonian Lecture, 1964. The release and fate of the transmitter liberated by adrenergic nerves. Proc. roy. Soc. B. **162**, 1—19 (1965).

— Gillespie, J.S.: The output of sympathetic transmitter from the spleen of the cat. J. Physiol. (Lond.) **138**, 81—102 (1957).

BRUNDIN, T.: Catecholamines in adrenals from fetal rabbits. Acta physiol. scand. **63**, 509—510 (1965).
BÜLBRING, E.: The methylation of noradrenaline by minced suprarenal tissue. Brit. J. Pharmacol. **4**, 234—244 (1949).
BURACK, W.R., WEINER, N., HAGEN, P.B.: The effect of reserpine on the catecholamine and adenine nucleotide contents of adrenal gland. J. Pharmacol. exp. Ther. **130**, 245—250 (1960).
BUTTERWORTH, K.R., MANN, M.: The release of adrenaline and noradrenaline from the adrenal gland of the cat by acetylcholine. Brit. J. Pharmacol. **12**, 422—426 (1957).
BYGDEMAN, S., v. EULER, U.S.: Resynthesis of catechol hormones in the cat's adrenal medulla. Acta physiol. scand. **44**, 375—383 (1958).
— — HÖKFELT, B.: Resynthesis of adrenaline in the rabbit's adrenal medulla during insulin-induced hypoglycemia. Acta physiol. scand. **49**, 21—28 (1960).
CAMPOS, H.R., CROUT, J.R.: Uptake of amines in the adrenal medulla. Fed. Proc. **29**, 545 Abs. (1970).
CARLSSON, A., HILLARP, N.-Å.: Release of adenosine triphosphate along with adrenaline and noradrenaline following stimulation of the adrenal medulla. Acta physiol. scand. **37**, 234—239 (1956).
— — On the State of the catechol amines of the adrenal medullary granules. Acta physiol. scand. **44**, 163—169 (1958).
— — Uptake of phenyl and indole alkylamines by the storage granules of the adrenal medulla *in vitro*. Med. exp. (Basel) **5**, 122—124 (1961).
— — HÖKFELT, B.: The concomitant release of adenosine triphosphate and catecholamines from the adrenal medulla. J. biol. Chem. **227**, 243—252 (1957a).
— — WALDECK, B.: A Mg^{++}-ATP dependent storage mechanism in the amine granules of the adrenal medulla. Med. exp. (Basel) **6**, 47—53 (1962).
— — — Analysis of the Mg^{++}-ATP dependent storage mechanism in the amine granules of the adrenal medulla. Acta physiol. scand. **59**, Suppl. 215, 1—38 (1963).
— ROSENGREN, E., BERTLER, Å., NILSSON, J.: Effect of reserpine on the metabolism of catecholamines. In: "Psychotropic Drugs", pp. 363—372. Ed. by S. GARATTINI and V. GHETTI. Amsterdam: Elsevier Publ. Co. 1957b.
COLBURN, R.W., MAAS, J.W.: Adenosine triphosphate-metal-norepinephrine ternary complexes and catecholamine binding. Nature (Lond.) **208**, 37—41 (1965).
COUPLAND, R.E.: On the morphology and adrenaline-noradrenaline content of chromaffin tissue. J. Endocr. **9**, 194—203 (1953).
— MACDOUGALL, J.D.B.: Adrenaline formation in noradrenalinestoring chromaffin cells *in vitro* induced by corticosterone. J. Endocr. **6**, 317—324 (1966).
DAIRMAN, W., GORDON, R., SPECTOR, S., SJOERDSMA, A., UDENFRIEND, S.: Increased synthesis of catecholamines in the intact rat following administration of α-adrenergic blocking agents. Molec. Pharmacol. **4**, 457—464 (1968).
DE ROBERTIS, E.D., SABATINI, D.D.: Submicroscopic analysis of the secretory process in the adrenal medulla. Fed. Proc. Suppl. **5**, 70—73 (1960).
DOUGLAS, W.W.: Stimulus-secretion coupling: the concept and clues from chromaffin and other cells. Brit. J. Pharmacol. **34**, 451—474 (1968).
DUNÉR, H.: The influence of the blood glucose level on the secretion of adrenaline and noradrenaline from the suprarenal. Acta physiol. scand. Suppl. 102, **28** (1953).
EADE, N.R.: Differential sedimentation of noradrenaline in homogenates of adrenal medullary granules. J. Physiol. (Lond.) **132**, 53—54P (1956).
— The distribution of the catechol amines in homogenates of the bovine adrenal medulla. J. Physiol. (Lond.) **141**, 183—192 (1958).
— WOOD, D.R.: The release of adrenaline and noradrenaline from the adrenal medulla of the cat during splanchnic stimulation. Brit. J. Pharmacol. **13**, 390—394 (1958).
EULER, U.S., v.: The presence of a substance with sympathin E properties in spleen extracts. Acta physiol. scand. **11**, 168—186 (1946).
— "Noradrenaline". Springfield, Ill.: Charles C. Thomas Publ. 1956.
— LISHAJKO, F.: Dopamine in mammalian lung and spleen. Acta physiol. pharmacol. neerl. **6**, 295—303 (1957).
— — Effect of reserpine on the release of catecholamines from isolated nerve and chromaffin cell granules. Acta physiol. scand. **52**, 137—145 (1961).
— — Reuptake and net uptake of noradrenaline in adrenergic nerve granules with a note on the affinity for l- and d-isomers. Acta physiol. scand. **71**, 151—162 (1967).
— — Observations on the actions of prenylamine (SegontinR) *in vivo* and on adrenergic transmitter granules. Biochemical Aspects of Prenylamine, Capri, 23.—24. X. 1967. In: "Biochimica Applicata". Ed. by F. CEDRANGOLO. **14**, Suppl. 1, 17—32 (1968).

Falck, B., Hillarp, N.-Å., Högberg, B.: Content and intracellular distribution of adenosine triphosphate in cow adrenal medulla. Acta physiol. scand. **36**, 360—376 (1956).
— — Torp, A.: A new type of chromaffin cells, probably storing dopamine. Nature (Lond.) **183**, 267—268 (1959).
Fellman, J.H.: Purification and properties of adrenal L-dopa decarboxylase. Enzymologia **20**, 366—375 (1959).
Ferris, R.M., Viveros, O.H., Kirshner, N.: Effects of various agents on the Mg^{2+}-ATP stimulated incorporation and release of catecholamines by isolated bovine adrenomedullary storage vesicles and on secretion from the adrenal medulla. Biochem. Pharmacol. **19**, 505—514 (1970).
Folkow, B., Häggendal, J., Lisander, B.: Extent of release and elimination of noradrenaline at peripheral adrenergic nerve terminals. Acta physiol. scand. Suppl. **307**, 1—38 (1968).
Fortier, A., Leduc, J., D'Iorio, A.: Biochemical composition of the chromaffin granules of the medulla. Rev. canad. Biol. **18**, 110—114 (1959).
Fuller, R.W., Hunt, J.M.: Substrate specificity of phenethanolamine N-methyl transferase. Biochem. Pharmacol. **14**, 1896—1897 (1956).
Geffen, L.B.: Noradrenaline storage, release, and inactivation in sympathetic nerves. Circulat. Res. **21**, Suppl. III, 57—61 (1967).
Glowinski, J., Iversen, L.L., Axelrod, J.: Storage and synthesis of norepinephrine in the reserpine-treated rat brain. J. Pharmacol. exp. Ther. **151**, 385—399 (1966).
Gordon, R., Spector, S., Sjoerdsma, A., Udenfriend, S.: Increased synthesis of norepinephrine and epinephrine in the intact rat during exercise and exposure to cold. J. Pharmacol. exp. Ther. **153**, 440—447 (1966).
Haag, H.W., Philippu, A., Schümann, H.J.: Freisetzung von Brenzcatechinaminen aus der isoliert durchströmten Nebenniere durch Tyramin und β-Phenyläthylamin. Experientia (Basel) **17**, 187—188 (1961).
Haefely, W., Hürlimann, A., Thoenen, H.: Relation between the rate of stimulation and the quantity of noradrenaline liberated from sympathetic nerve endings in the isolated perfused spleen of the cat. J. Physiol. (Lond.) **181**, 48—58 (1965).
Hagen, P., D'Iorio, A.: Studies with the ATPase of adrenal medulla. Canad. J.Biochem. **43**, 1633—1642 (1965).
Hamberger, B., Malmfors, T., Stjärne, L.: Histochemistry of NA uptake into bovine splenic nerve trunk. Acta physiol. scand. (in press) (1970).
Hasselbach, W., Seraydarian, K.: The role of sulfhydryl groups in calcium transport through the sarcoplasmic membranes of sceletal muscle. Biochem. Z. **345**, 159—172 (1966).
Hedqvist, P., Stjärne, L.: The relative role of recapture and of *de novo* synthesis for the maintenance of neuro-transmitter homeostasis in noradrenergic nerves. Acta physiol. scand. **76**, 270—283 (1969).
Helle, K.B.: Some chemical and physical properties of the soluble protein fraction of bovine adrenal chromaffin granules. Molec. Pharmacol. **2**, 298—310 (1966a).
— Antibody formation against soluble protein from bovine adrenal chromaffin granules. Biochim. biophys. Acta (Amst.) **117**, 107—110 (1966b).
— Serck-Hansen, G.: Chromogranin: the soluble and membrane-bound lipoprotein of the chromaffin granule. Pharmacol. Res. Communications **1**, 25—30 (1969).
Hempel, K., Männl, H.F.K.: Quantitative Analyse der Catecholamin-Biosynthese des Nebennierenmarks *in vivo* und Ruhesekretion neugebildeter Amine unter besondere Berücksichtigung des Dopamins. Naunyn-Schmiedeberg's Arch. Pharmak. **264**, 363—388 (1969).
Henning, M.: Urinary excretion of catecholamines after reserpine treatment. Acta physiol. scand. **68**, Suppl. 277 (1966).
Hillarp, N.-Å.: Isolation and some biochemical properties of the catechol amine granules in the cow adrenal medulla. Acta physiol. scand. **43**, 82—96 (1958a).
— Enzymic systems involving adenosinephosphates in the adrenaline and noradrenaline containing granules of the adrenal medulla. Acta physiol. scand. **42**, 144—165 (1958b).
— The release of catecholamines from the amine containing granules of the adrenal medulla. Acta physiol. scand. **43**, 292—302 (1958c).
— Adenosinephosphates and inorganic phosphate in the adrenaline and noradrenaline containing granules of the adrenal medulla. Acta physiol. scand. **42**, 321—332 (1958d).
— Further observations on the state of the catechol amines stored in the adrenal medullary granules. Acta physiol. scand. **47**, 271—279 (1959).
— Some problems concerning the storage of catecholamines in the adrenal medulla. In: "Adrenergic Mechanisms", pp. 481—486. Ed. by J.R. Vane, G.E.W. Wolstenholme and Maeve O'Connor. London: J. & A. Churchill Ltd. 1960a.
— Different pools of catecholamines stored in the adrenal medulla. Acta physiol. scand. **50**, 8—22 (1960b).

HILLARP, N.-Å., HÖKFELT, B., NILSON, B.: The cytology of the adrenal medullary cells with special reference to the storage and secretion of the sympathomimetic amines. Acta anat. (Basel) **21**, 155—167 (1954).
— LAGERSTEDT, S., NILSON, B.: The isolation of a granular fraction from the suprarenal medulla, containing the sympathomimetic catechol amines. Acta physiol. scand. **29**, 251—263 (1953).
— MALMFORS, T.: Reserpine and cocaine blocking of the uptake and storage mechanisms in adrenergic nerves. Life Sci. **3**, 703—708 (1964).
— NILSON, B.: The structure of the adrenaline and noradrenaline containing granules in the adrenal medullary cell with reference to the storage and release of the sympathomimetic amines. Acta physiol. scand. **31**, Suppl. 113, 79—107 (1954).
— — HÖGBERG, B.: Adenosine triphosphate in the adrenal medulla of the cow. Nature (Lond. **176**, 1032—1033 (1955).
HÖKFELT, B.: Noradrenaline and adrenaline in mammalian tisuues. Acta physiol. scand. **25**, Suppl. 92 (1951).
— MCLEAN, J.: The adrenaline and noradrenaline content of the suprarenal glands of the rabbit under normal conditions and after various forms of stimulation. Acta physiol. scand. **21**, 258—270 (1950).
HOLLAND, W.C., SCHÜMANN, H.J.: Formation of catechol amines during splanchnic stimulation of the adrenal gland of the cat. Brit. J. Pharmacol. **11**, 449—453 (1956).
HOLTZ, P., PALM, D.: Brenzkatechinamine und andere sympaticomimetische Amine. Biosynthese und Inaktivierung. Freisetzung und Wirkung. Ergebnisse der Physiologie, Biologischen Chemie und experimentellen Pharmakologie, Band 58. Berlin-Heidelberg-New York: Springer 1966.
HOLZBAUER, M., VOGT, M.: Depression by reserpine of the noradrenaline concentration in the hypothalamus of the cat. J. Neurochem. **1**, 8—11 (1956).
HUKOVIC, S., MUSCHOLL, E.: Die Noradrenalin-Abgabe aus dem isolierten Kaninchenherzen bei sympatischer Nervenreizung und ihre pharmakologische Beeinflussung. Naunyn-Schmiedeberg's Arch. exp. Path. Pharmak. **244**, 81—96 (1962).
ICHIKAWA, Y., YAMANO, T.: Cytochrome 559 in the microsomes of the adrenal medulla. Biochem. biophys. Res. Commun. **20**, 263—268 (1965).
IKEDA, M., LEVITT, M., UDENFRIEND, S.: Hydroxylation of phenylalanine by purified preparations of adrenal and brain tyrosine hydroxylase. Biochem. biophys. Res. Commun. **18**, 482—488 (1965).
ITOH, C., YOSHINAGA, K., SATO, T., ISHIDA, N., WADA, Y.: Presence of N-methylmetadrenaline in human urine and tumour tissue of phaeochromocytoma. Nature (Lond.) **193**, 477—478 (1962).
JONASSON, J., ROSENGREN, E., WALDECK, B.: Effects of some pharmacologically active amines on the uptake of arylalkylamines by adrenal medullary granules. Acta physiol. scand. **60**, 136—140 (1964).
KATZ, B.: The release of neural transmitter substances. Liverpool University Press, 1—60 (1969).
KIRPEKAR, S.M., CERVONI, P.: Effect of cocaine phenoxybenzamine and phentolamine on the catecholamine output from spleen and adrenal medulla. J. Pharmacol. exp. Ther. **142**, 59—70 (1963).
KIRSHNER, A.G., KIRSHNER, N.: A specific soluble protein from the catecholamine storage vesicles of bovine adrenal medulla. Biochim. biophys. Acta (Amst.) **181**, 219—225 (1969).
KIRSHNER, N.: Pathway of noradrenaline formation from dopa. J. biol. Chem. **226**, 821—825 (1957).
— Uptake of catecholamines by a particulate fraction of the adrenal medulla. J. biol. Chem. **237**, 2311—2317 (1962).
— The role of the membrane of chromaffin granules isolated from the adrenal medulla. In: "Pharmacology of Cholinergic and Adrenergic Transmission", pp. 225—233. Ed. by G.B. KOELLE, W.W. DOUGLAS and A. CARLSSON. Oxford: Pergamon Press 1965.
— GOODALL, M.C.: Biosynthesis of adrenaline and noradrenaline by adrenal slices. Fed. Proc. **15**, 110—111 (1956).
— HOLLOWAY, C., KAMIN, D.L.: Permeability of catecholamine granules. Biochim. biophys. Acta (Amst.) **112**, 532—537 (1966a).
— — SMITH, W.J., KIRSHNER, A.G.: Uptake and storage of catecholamines. In: "Mechanisms of release of biogenic amines". Ed. by U.S. v. EULER, S. ROSELL and B. UVNÄS. **5**, 109 to 123 (1966b).
— RORIE, M., KAMIN, D.L.: Inhibition of dopamine uptake *in vitro* by reserpine administered *in vivo*. J. Pharmacol. exp. Ther. **141**, 285—289 (1963).

KOPIN, I.J.: Storage and metabolism of catecholamines: the role of monoamine-oxidase. Pharmacol. Rev. **16**, 179—191 (1964).
— The influence of false adrenergic transmitters on adrenergic neurotransmission. In: "Adrenergic neurotramsmission". Ed. by G.E.W. WOLSTENHOLME and MAEVE O'CONNOR, pp. 95—103. Ciba Foundation Study Group No. 33. London 1968.
— WEISE, V.K.: Effect of reserpine and metaraminol on excretion of homovanillic acid and 3-methoxy-4-hydroxyphenylglycol in the rat. Biochem. Pharmacol. **17**, 1461—1464 (1968).
KRAKOFF, L.R., AXELROD, J.: Inhibition of phenylethanolamine-N-methyltransferase. Biochem. Pharmacol. **16**, 1384—1385 (1967).
KRONEBERG, G., SCHÜMANN, H.: Über die Bedeutung der Innervation für die Adrenalin-Synthese in Nebennierenmark. Experientia (Basel) **15**, 234—235 (1959).
LADURON, P.: Biosynthèse, localisation intracellulaire et transport des catécholamines. Mémoire présenté à l'Université Catholique de Louvain en vue de l'Obtention du Grade d'Agrégé de l'Enseignement supérieur. ed. Vander; Louvain 1—161 1969.
— BELPAIRE, F.: Tissue fractionation and catecholamines — II. Intracellular distribution patterns of tyrosine hydroxylase, dopa decarboxylase, dopamine-β-hydroxylase, phenylethanolamine N-methyltransferase and monoamine oxidase in adrenal medulla. Biochem. Pharmacol. **17**, 1127—1140 (1968).
LAGERCRANTZ, H., KUYLENSTIERNA, B., STJÄRNE, L.: On the origin of adenosine triphosphate in chromaffin granules. Experientia (Basel) **26**, 479—480 (1970a).
— PERTOFT, H., STJÄRNE, L.: Facts and artifacts in gradient centrifugation: Analysis of catecholamine granules. Acta physiol. scand. **78**, 561—566 (1970b).
LEDUC, J.: Catecholamine production and release in exposure and acclimation to cold. Acta physiol. scand. **53**, Suppl. 183 (1961).
LEVIN, E.Y., LEVENBERG, B., KAUFMAN, S.: The enzymatic conversion of 3,4-dihydroxyphenylethylamine to norepinephrine. J. biol. Chem. **235**, 2080—2086 (1960).
LEVITT, M., SPECTOR, S., SJOERDSMA, A., UDENFRIEND, S.: Elucidation of the rate-limiting step in norepinephrine biosynthesis in the perfused guinea-pig heart. J. Pharmacol. exp. Ther. **148**, 1—8 (1965).
LINDMAR, R., MUSCHOLL, E.: Die Wirkung von Pharmaka auf die Elimination von Noradrenalin aus der Perfusionsflüssigkeit und die Noradrenalinaufnahme in das isolierte Herz. Naunyn-Schmiedeberg's Arch. exp. Path. Pharmak. **247**, 469—492 (1964).
LISHAJKO, F.: Occurrence and some properties of dopamine containing granules in the sheep adrenal. Acta physiol. scand. **72**, 255—256 (1968).
— Release, reuptake and net uptake of dopamine, noradrenaline and adrenaline in isolated sheep adrenal medullary granules. Acta physiol. scand. **76**, 159—171 (1969a).
— Influence of chloride ions and ATP-Mg^{2+} on the release of catecholamines from isolated adrenal medullary granules. Acta physiol. scand. **75**, 255—256 (1969b).
— Osmotic factors determining release of catecholamines from isolated chromaffin cell granules. Acta physiol. scand. **79**, 64—75 (1970a).
— Dopamine secretion from the isolated perfused sheep adrenal. Acta physiol. scand. **79**, 405—410 (1970b).
— Releasing effect of calcium and phosphate on catecholamines, ATP, and protein from chromaffin cell granules. Acta physiol. scand. **79**, 575—584 (1970c).
LOEWI, O.: Über humorale Übertragbarkeit der Herznervenwirkung. Pflügers Arch. ges. Physiol. **189**, 239—242 (1921).
— Quantitative und qualitative Untersuchungen über den Sympaticusstoff. Pflügers Arch. ges. Physiol. **237**, 504—514 (1936).
LUNDBORG, P., STITZEL, R.: Uptake of biogenic amines by two different mechanisms present in adrenergic granules. Brit. J. Pharmacol. **29**, 342—349 (1967).
— — The effect of prenylamine on the subcellular distribution of biogenic amines. Biochemical Aspects of Prenylamine, Capri, 23.—24. X. 1967. In: "Biochimica Applicata". Ed. by F. CEDRANGOLO. **14**, Suppl. 1, 75—91 (1968).
MARLEY, E., PATON, W.D.M.: The output of sympathetic amines from the cat's adrenal gland in response to splanchnic nerve activity. J. Physiol. (Lond.) **155**, 1—27 (1961).
MUSACCHIO, J.M.: Subcellular distribution of adrenal tyrosine hydroxylase. Biochem. Pharmacol. **17**, 1470—1473 (1968).
NAGATSU, T., LEVITT, M., UDENFRIEND, S.: The initial step in norepinephrine biosynthesis. J. biol. Chem. **239**, 2910—2917 (1964).
NEFF, N.H., COSTA, E.: The influence of monoamine oxidase inhibition on catecholamine synthesis. Life Sci. **5**, 951—959 (1966).
NORBERG, K.-A., HAMBERGER, B.: The sympathetic adrenergic neuron. Acta physiol. scand. **63**, Suppl. 238 (1964).
OKA, M., KAJIKAWA, K., OHUCHI, T., YOSHIDA, H., IMAIZUMI, R.: Distribution of dopamine β-hydroxylase in subcellular fractions of adrenal medulla. Life Sci. **6**, 461—465 (1967a).

OKA, M., OHUCHI, T., YOSHIDA, H., IMAIZUMI, R.: The isolation of catecholamine storage granules from adrenal medulla by the membrane filter technique. Life Sci. **5**, 427—432 (1966a).

— — — — Selective release of noradrenaline and adrenaline from isolated adrenal medullary granules. Life Sci. **5**, 433—438 (1966b).

— — — — Structural changes in the catecholamine containing granules of adrenal medulla. Life Sci. **6**, 467—472 (1967b).

PATON, W.D.M.: Ciba Foundation Symposium. In: "Adrenergic Mechanisms", pp. 124—127. Ed. by J.R. VANE, G.E.W. WOLSTENHOLME and MAEVE O'CONNOR. London: J. & A. Churchill Ltd. 1960.

PHILIPPU, A., SCHÜMANN, H.J.: Der Einfluß von Calcium auf die Brenzcatechinaminfreisetzung. Experientia (Basel) **18**, 138—140 (1962).

— — Effect of ribonuclease on the ribonucleic acid, adenosinetriphosphate and catecholamine content of medullary granules. Nature (Lond.) **198**, 795—796 (1963).

— — Ribonucleaseaktivität isolierter Nebennierenmarkgranula. Experientia (Basel) **20**, 547—548 (1964a).

— — Die Bedeutung der divalenten Kationen für die Speicherung der Nebennierenmark-Hormone in den chromaffinen Granula. Naunyn-Schmiedeberg's Arch. exp. Path. Pharmak. **247**, 295—296 (1964b).

— — Über die Bedeutung der Calcium- und Magnesiumionen für die Speicherung der Nebennierenmarkhormone. Naunyn-Schmiedeberg's Arch. exp. Path. Pharmak. **252**, 339—359 (1966).

POISNER, A.M., TRIFARÓ, J.M.: The role of ATP and ATPase in the release of catecholamines from the adrenal medulla. I. ATP-evoked release of catecholamines, ATP, and protein from isolated chromaffin granules. Molec. Pharmacol. **3**, 561—571 (1967).

— — Release of catecholamines from isolated adrenal chromaffin granules by endogenous ATP. Molec. Pharmacol. **4**, 196—199 (1968).

— — The role of adenosine triphosphate and adenosine triphosphatase in the release of catecholamines from the adrenal medulla. III. Similarities between the effects of adenosine triphosphate on chromaffin granules and on mitochondria. Molec. Pharmacol. **5**, 294—299 (1969).

POTTER, L.T., AXELROD, J.: Subcellular localization of catecholamines in tissues of the rat. J. Pharmacol. exp. Ther. **142**, 291—298 (1963).

PRUSOFF, W.H., BLASCHKO, H., ORD, M.G., STOCKEN, L.A.: Incorporation of phosphorus-32 into adenosine triphosphate of adrenal chromaffin granules. Nature (Lond.) **190**, 354—355 (1961).

RANDRUP, A.A., RASMUSSEN, E.B., MUNKVAD, T.: Urinary excretion of 4-hydroxy-3-methoxymandelic acid: Effect of prolonged treatment of psychiatric patients with reserpine and chlorpromazine. In: "The Clinical Chemistry of Monoamines", pp. 215—216. Ed. by H. VARLEY and A.H. GOWENLOCK. Amsterdam: Elsevier Publishing Co. 1963.

ROBINSON, R.L.: Stimulation of the release of catecholamines from isolated adrenal glands by tyramine. J. Pharmacol. exp. Ther. **151**, 55—58 (1966).

ROFFI, J.: Dosage de l'adrénaline et de la noradrénaline dans les surrénales du foetus de lapin au cours de la gestation J. Physiol. (Paris) **56**, 434—435 (1964).

ROTH, R.H., STJÄRNE, L., LEVINE, R.J., GIARMAN, N.J.: Abnormal regulation of catecholamine in pheochromocytoma. J. Lab. clin. Med. **72**, 397—403 (1968).

SCHACHT, U., SCHULTZ, G., SENFT, G.: Catecholamin- und ATP-Gehalt der Nebennieren nach Gabe von 6-Aminonicotinsäureamid. Naunyn-Schmiedeberg's Arch. exp. Path. Pharmak. **253**, 355—363 (1966).

SCHÜMANN, H.J.: The distribution of adrenaline and noradrenaline in chromaffin granules from the chicken. J. Physiol. (Lond.) **137**, 318—326 (1957).

— Die Wirkung von Insulin und Reserpin auf den Adrenalin- und ATP-Gehalt der chromaffinen Granula des Nebennierenmarks. Naunyn-Schmiedeberg's Arch. exp. Path. Pharmak. **233**, 237—249 (1958).

— Hormon- und ATP-Gehalt des menschlichen Nebennierenmarks und des Phäochromocytomgewebes. Klin. Wschr. **38**, 11—13 (1960).

— PHILIPPU, A.: Untersuchungen zum Mechanismus der Freisetzung von Brenzcatechinaminen durch Tyramin. Naunyn-Schmiedeberg's Arch. exp. Path. Pharmak. **241**, 273 to 280 (1961).

— — Release of catechol amines from isolated medullary granules by sympathomimetic amines. Nature (Lond.) **193**, 890—891 (1962).

SEDVALL, G.C., KOPIN, I.J.: Acceleration of norepinephrine synthesis in the rat submaxillary gland *in vivo* during sympathetic nerve stimulation. Life Sci. **6**, 45—51 (1967).

SHEPHERD, D.M., WEST, G.B. Noradrenaline and the suprarenal medulla. Brit. J. Pharmacol. **6**, 665—674 (1951).

SMITH, A.D.: Biochemistry of adrenal chromaffin granules. In: A Symposium on the interaction of drugs and subcellular components in animal cells", pp. 239—292. Ed. by P.N. CAMPBELL. London: J. & A. Churchill Ltd. 1968.
— WINKLER, H.: The localization of lysosomal enzymes in chromaffin tissue. J. Physiol. (Lond.) **183**, 179—188 (1966).
— — Purification and properties of an acidic protein from chromaffin granules of bovine adrenal medulla. Biochem. J. **103**, 483—492 (1967).
SPECTOR, S., GORDON, R., SJOERDSMA, A., UDENFRIEND, S.: Endproduct inhibition of tyrosine hydroxylase as a possible mechanism for regulation of norepinephrine synthesis. Molec. Pharmacol. **3**, 549—555 (1967).
STJÄRNE, L.: Tyramine effects on catechol amine release from spleen and andrenals in the cat. Acta physiol. scand. **51**, 224—229 (1961).
— Studies of catecholamine uptake storage and release mechanisms. Acta physiol. scand. **62** Suppl. 228 (1964).
— Studies of noradrenaline biosynthesis in nerve tissue. Acta physiol. scand. **67**, 441—454 (1966).
— Preferential secretion of newly formed catecholamines: Comparison between sympathetic nerves and adrenal medulla. Progr. Brain Res. Elsevier. In press.
— Quantal or graded secretion of adrenal medullary hormone and sympathetic neurotransmitter. Bayer Symposium II. 1969. Springer Verlag 112—127 (1970b).
— v. EULER, U.S., LISHAJKO, F.: Catecholamines and nucleotides in phaeochromocytoma. Biochem. Pharmacol. **13**, 809—818 (1964).
— HEDQVIST, P.: Effects of cocaine and phenoxybenzamine on catecholamine secretion from cat spleen and adrenal medulla. To be published. (1970).
— — LAGERCRANTZ, H.: Catecholamines and adenine nucleotide material in effluent from stimulated adrenal medulla and spleen: a study of the exocytosis hypothesis for hormone secretion and neurotransmitter release. Biochem. Pharmacol. **19**, 1147—1158 (1970a).
— LISHAJKO, F.: Drug-induced inhibition of noradrenaline synthesis *in vitro* in bovine splenic nerve tissue. Brit. J. Pharmacol. **27**, 398—404 (1966).
— — Localization of different steps in noradrenaline synthesis to different fractions of a bovine splenic nerve homogenate. Biochem. Pharmacol. **16**, 1719—1728 (1967).
— — ROTH, R.H.: Regulation of noradrenaline biosynthesis in nerve tissue. Nature (Lond.) **215**, 770—772 (1967a).
— ROTH, R.H., LISHAJKO, F.: Noradrenaline formation from dopamine in isolated subcellular particles from bovine splenic nerve. Biochem. Pharmacol. **16**, 1729—1739 (1967b).
— — BLOOM, F., GIARMAN, N.J.: Norepinephrine concentrating mechanisms in sympathetic nerve trunks. J. Pharmacol. exp. Ther. **171**, 70—79 (1970b).
STRÖMBLAD, B.C.R.: Effect of denervation and of cocaine on the action of sympathomimetic amines. Brit. J. Pharmacol. **15**, 328—332 (1960).
STUDNITZ, W. v.: Methodische und klinische Untersuchungen über die Ausscheidung der 3-Methoxy-4-hydroxymandelsäure im Urin. Scand. J. clin. Lab. Invest. **12**, Suppl. 48 (1960).
TAUGNER, G., HASSELBACH, W.: Über den Mechanismus der Catecholamin-Speicherung in den „chromaffinen Granula" des Nebennierenmarks. Naunyn-Schmiedeberg's Arch. Pharmak. exp. Path. **255**, 266—286 (1966).
— — Die Bedeutung der Sulfhydryl-Gruppen für den Catecholamin-Transport der Vesikel des Nebennierenmarkes. Naunyn-Schmiedeberg's Arch. exp. Path. Pharmak. **260**, 58—79 (1968).
THOENEN, H., HÜRLIMANN, A., HAEFELY, W.: The effect of sympathetic nerve stimulation on volume, vascular resistance, and norepinephrine output in the isolated perfused spleen of the cat, and its modification by cocaine. J. Pharmacol. exp. Ther. **143**, 57—63 (1964).
— MUELLER, R.A., AXELROD, J.: Trans-synaptic induction of adrenal tyrosine. J. Pharmacol. exp. Ther. **169**, 249—254 (1969).
TRENDELENBURG, U.: Supersensitivity and subsensivity to sympathomimetic amines. Pharmacol. Rev. **15**, 225—276 (1963).
UDENFRIEND, S.: Biosynthesis of the sympathetic neurotransmitter norepinephrine. Harvey Lect. **60**, 57—83 (1966a).
— Tyrosine hydroxylase. Pharmacol. Rev. **18**, 43—51 (1966b).
— Physiological regulation of noradrenaline biosynthesis. Ciba Foundation Study Group No. 33. In: "Adrenergic Neurotransmission", pp. 95—103. Ed. by G.E.W. WOLSTENHOLME and MAEVE O'CONNOR. London 1968.
— COOPER, J.R., CLARK, C.T., BAER, J.E.: Rate of turnover of epinephrine in the adrenal medulla. Science **117**, 663—665 (1953).
— WYNGAARDEN, J.B.: Precursors of adrenal epinephrine and norepinephrine *in vivo.* Biochim. biophys. Acta (Amst.) **20**, 48—52 (1956).

UDENFRIEND, S., ZALTZMAN-NIRENBERG, P., NAGATSU, T.: Inhibitors of purified beef adrenal tyrosine hydroxylase. Biochem. Pharmacol. **14**, 837—845 (1965).
VIVEROS, O.H., ARQUEROS, L., KIRSHNER, N.: Quantal secretion from adrenal medulla all-or-none release of storage vesicle content. Science **165**, 911—913 (1969a).
— — — Mechanism of secretion from the adrenal medulla. V. Retention of storage vesicles membranes following release of adrenaline. Molec. Pharmacol. **5**, 342—349 (1969b).
WEIL-MALHERBE, H., POSNER, H.S.: The effect of drugs on the release of epinephrine from adrenomedullary particles *in vitro*. J. Pharmacol. exp. Ther. **140**, 93—102 (1963).
WEINER, N.: Substrate specificity of brain amine oxidase of several mammals. Arch. Biochem. **91**, 182—188 (1960).
— DRASKÓCZY, P.R., BURACK, W.R.: The ability of tyramine to liberate catecholamines *in vivo*. J. Pharmacol. exp. Ther. **137**, 47—55 (1962).
— JARDETZKY, P.: A study of catecholamine nucleotide complexes by nuclear magnetic resonance spectroscopy. Naunyn-Schmiedeberg's Arch. exp. Path. Pharmak. **248**, 308 to 318 (1964).
— RUTLEDGE, C.O.: The actions of reserpine on the biosynthesis and storage of catecholamines. In: "Mechanism of Release of Biogenic Amines". Ed. by U.S. v. EULER, S. ROSELL and B. UVNÄS, 307—318 1966.
WENNMALM, Å.: Maintenance of noradrenaline synthesis in rats after reserpine treatment. Acta physiol. scand. **73**, 523—526 (1968).
WHITBY, L.G., AXELROD, J., WEIL-MALHERBE, H.: The fate of H^3-norepinephrine in animals. J. Pharmacol. exp. Ther. **132**, 193—201 (1961).
WILLIER, B.H.: Ontogeny of endocrine correlation. In: "Analysis of development", pp. 574—619. Ed. by B.H. WILLIER, P.A. WEISS and V. HAMBURGER. Philadelphia: W.B. Saunders Co. 1955.
WINKLER, H.: Isolierung und Charakterisierung von chromaffinen Noradrenalin-Granula aus Schweine-Nebennierenmark. Naunyn-Schmiedeberg's Arch. Pharmak. exp. Path. **263**, 340—357 (1969).
WURTMAN, R.J., AXELROD, J.: Adrenaline synthesis: Control by the pituitary gland and adrenal glucocorticoids. Science **150**, 1464—1465 (1965).
— — VESELL, E.S., ROSS, G.T.: Species differences in inducibility of phenylethanolamine-N-methyltransferase. Endocrinology **82**, 584—590 (1968).

Chapter 8

Metabolic Degradation of Catecholamines. The Relative Importance of Different Pathways under Physiological Conditions and after Administration of Drugs

IRWIN J. KOPIN*

With 2 Figures

I. Introduction

The physiological importance of the catecholamines in the peripheral sympathetic nervous system had been well established by 1956 (VON EULER, 1956), and since that time impressive evidence for the importance of these compounds in the central nervous system has accumulated (GLOWINSKI and BALDESSARINI, 1966). When it was shown that only a small fraction of administered catecholamine is excreted unchanged (RICHTER, 1940; VON EULER and LUFT, 1951; VON EULER et al., 1953), it became important to understand the metabolic transformation and excretion products of these compounds.

SCHAYER et al. (1952, 1953) found that after administration of C^{14}-adrenaline to rats, five metabolic products could be separated using paper chromatography. Although almost all of the administered radioactivity could be recovered in the urine after administration of adrenaline labelled with C^{14} on the β-carbon, only about 50% was recovered when N-methyl-C^{14}-adrenaline had been administered (SCHAYER, 1951). After inhibition of monoamine oxidase (MAO) with iproniazid almost all of the N-methyl-C^{14} was recovered (SCHAYER et al., 1955). This provided the first direct evidence that MAO was involved in the metabolism of the catecholamines *in vivo*.

Although methylation of phenolic hydroxyl groups had been described (MACLAGLAN and WILKINSON, 1951), the chemical nature of the metabolic products of catecholamines remained unknown, however, until ARMSTRONG et al. (1957) demonstrated that 3-methoxy-4-hydroxymandelic acid (VMA) was the major metabolite of noradrenaline and SHAW et al. (1957) found that 3-methoxy-4-hydroxyphenylacetic acid (HVA) was a major metabolite of dihydroxyphenylalanine (DOPA). AXELROD (1957) and AXELROD et al. (1958) showed that O-methylation could precede deamination and that the O-methylated metabolites of catecholamines were also major excretion products of the administered labelled amines. It was apparent that there were two major routes for the metabolism of catecholamines, deamination and O-methylation. Other pathways such as conjugation with sulphate (BEYER and SHAPIRO, 1945) have also been described, but

* This chapter was written by IRWIN J. KOPIN, M.D. in his private capacity. No official support or endorsement by the U.S. Public Health Service is intended or should be inferred.

these do not appear to play a quantitatively important role in catecholamine metabolism.

Assessment of the relative roles of MAO and catechol-O-methyl transferase (COMT) in the metabolism of the catecholamines has been attempted using both physiological and biochemical approaches. The physiological methods are based on observing the alterations in responses induced by inhibitors of these enzymes; the biochemical methods examine directly the catecholamines and their metabolic products. Physiological methods are dependent primarily upon termination of the activity of the active compound and provide only indirect information about metabolism. The method is further complicated by processes such as transport which physically remove the agonist. Biochemical methods, on the other hand, provide direct information about the distribution and metabolic fate of the compounds but none about termination of activity. A combination of both methods or information obtained by use of both methods must be used to appraise accurately the roles of the various possible means of physically or enzymatically terminating the activity of catecholamines.

II. Metabolic Fate

1. Deamination by MAO

Deamination of amines by a liver enzyme was first noted over 40 years ago (HARE, 1928). It was subsequently observed that the enzyme MAO was present in many tissues and that adrenaline and noradrenaline were among the many compounds which are its substrates (BLASCHKO et al., 1937; PUGH and QUASTEL, 1937; RICHTER, 1937). BURN and ROBINSON (1952) reported that after chronic sympathetic denervation, levels of MAO were decreased in cat iris, nictitating membrane and blood vessels; and BURN (1953) assumed that deamination was the means of terminating the action of catecholamines *in vivo*. Although there has been some difficulty in convincingly repeating the observation that MAO levels are decreased after denervation (BURN et al., 1954; KOELLE and VALK, 1954), there is a decrease in the MAO content of the denervated salivary gland (STRÖMBLAD, 1956; SNYDER et al., 1965) and it is now generally agreed that MAO is present in adrenergic neurones.

The role of MAO in terminating the activity of the catecholamines was subject to evaluation when potent inhibitors of this enzyme were introduced (ZELLER and BARSKY, 1952). GRIESEMER et al. (1953) found that although iproniazid markedly potentiated and prolonged the actions of tyramine and phenylethylamine on the cat nictitating membrane, no potentiation of the action of adrenaline was observed. These observations were extended to other tissues and potentiation of the action of catecholamines was not found when MAO had been inhibited (CORNE and GRAHAM, 1957; FURCHGOTT et al., 1955; KAMIJO et al., 1955; RABHUN et al., 1954). Furthermore, inhibition of MAO did not slow the rate of disappearance of circulating administered catecholamines (CELANDER and MELLANDER, 1955; FRIEND et al., 1958) and had little effect on the urinary excretion of catecholamines (CORNE and GRAHAM, 1957; FRIEND et al., 1958). The release of noradrenaline into the venous blood leaving the cat spleen during sympathetic nerve stimulation was not altered by acute administration of MAO inhibitors (BROWN and GILLESPIE, 1957), but adrenergic blocking agents markedly increased the noradrenaline concentration in the effluent blood found during sympathetic stimulation. These observations suggested that the receptor has a role in inactivation of the released amine and that phenoxybenzamine, in preventing access to the receptor, interfered with the metabolism of the catecholamines. From these experiments it could be concluded that MAO was not responsible for terminating the action of catecholamines which were released during sympathetic stimulation or administered by injection.

From other experiments, however, it was apparent that MAO did have a role in the metabolism of the catecholamines. SCHAYER et al. (1953, 1955) showed that the half of the N-methyl-C^{14} adrenaline, which was normally lost, could be recovered from animals which had been pretreated with a MAO inhibitor. This important observation provided convincing evidence that this enzyme was responsible for removal of the N-methyl group. Furthermore, treatment with MAO inhibitors resulted in an elevation of levels of dopamine in brain and noradrenaline in brains and hearts of rabbits, rats and mice (SHORE et al., 1957; SPECTOR et al., 1958, 1960; PLETSCHER, 1961). In cats and dogs, however, MAO inhibitors failed to produce a rise in brain levels of noradrenaline (SPECTOR et al., 1960; VOGT, 1954, 1959). In these species, as well as in mice, cardiac noradrenaline levels are not increased by treatment with MAO inhibitors (MALING et al., 1962; SHARMAN et al., 1962); and in cat spleen, chronic treatment with a MAO inhibitor actually decreased levels of noradrenaline (DAVEY et al., 1963). Because treatment with MAO inhibitors prevents destruction of other amines such as tyramine, these compounds or their metabolic products may accumulate in the tissues and displace catecholamines (see chapter on Adrenergic False Transmitters by Muscholl). The alterations of levels of noradrenaline in tissues after treatment with MAO inhibitors must therefore be interpreted with caution; and even in species where inhibition of this enzyme does not elevate tissue levels of noradrenaline, a role for primary deamination of noradrenaline cannot be ruled out.

Deamination of noradrenaline (or adrenaline) by the action of MAO results in the formation of 3,4-dihydroxymandelic aldehyde (Fig. 1). This compound may then undergo further oxidation to 3,4-dihydroxymandelic acid or reduction to 3,4-dihydroxyphenylglycol. The latter two compounds have been found in tissues and in urine and have been demonstrated to be products of administered labelled catecholamines. Thus there is direct evidence that at least a portion of endogenous as well as exogenous catecholamines undergo deamination *in vivo*. When VMA was formed it was assumed that it was largely the product of O-methylation of 3,4-dihydroxymandelic acid.

2. O-Methylation by COMT

Shortly after ARMSTRONG et al. (1957) demonstrated that VMA was the major urinary metabolite of adrenaline, AXELROD (1957) showed that O-methylation was also a route of metabolism for adrenaline and noradrenaline. The metabolic products formed by O-methylation of these two amines are substrates for MAO so that VMA could be formed from catecholamines by O-methylation with subsequent deamination or by deamination and subsequent O-methylation (Fig. 1). COMT, the enzyme which transfers the methyl group from S-adenosylmethionine to a wide variety of catechols including those formed by deamination of the catecholamines (AXELROD, 1959), was found to be widely distributed in many tissues from a variety of species (AXELROD and TOMCHICK, 1958; AXELROD et al., 1959). Metanephrine and normetanephrine are relatively inactive (EVARTS et al., 1958) so that O-methylation is as effective a means for terminating the action of the catecholamines as is deamination.

The physiological role of COMT in terminating the action of administered or nerve impulse-released catecholamines has been assessed by using inhibitors of

COMT. Pyrogallol was known to potentiate the effects of administered catecholamines and was subsequently demonstrated to be a potent inhibitor of COMT (AXELROD and LAROCHE, 1959; BACQ et al., 1959). Other inhibitors of this enzyme

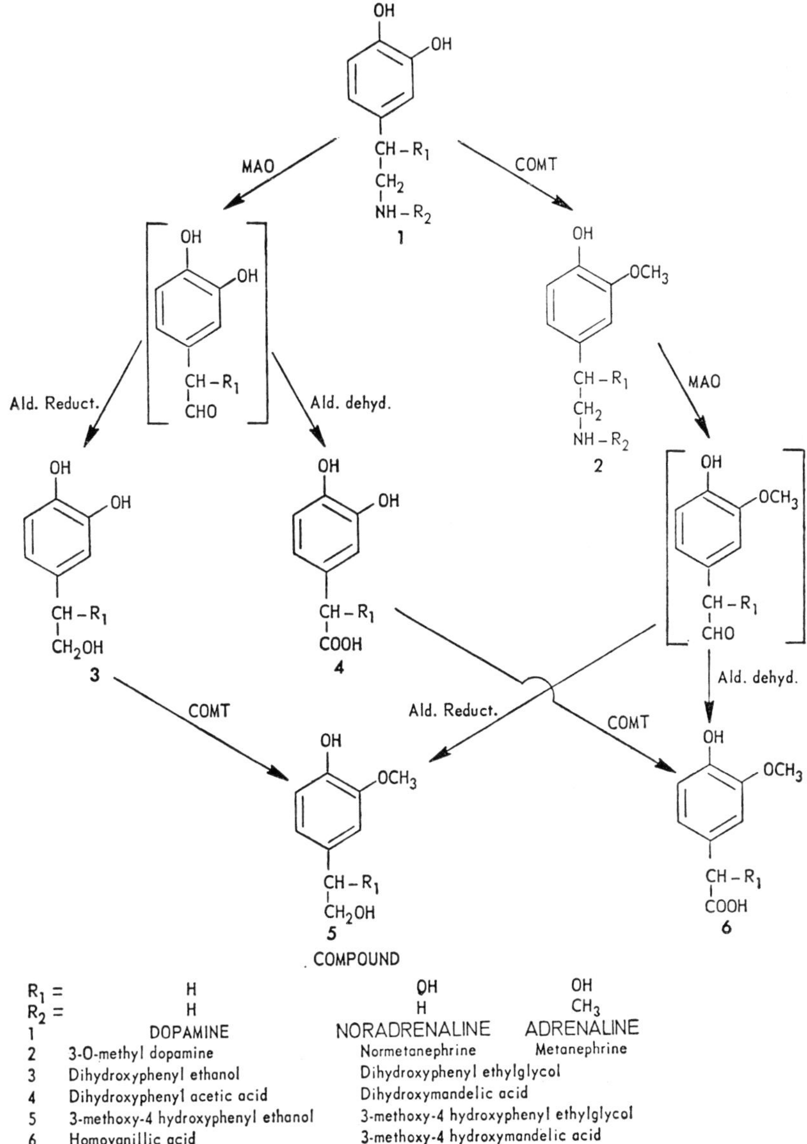

Fig. 1. Routes of metabolism of catecholamines. The enzymes are monoamine oxidase (MAO), catechol-O-methyl transferase (COMT), aldehyde dehydrogenase (Ald. dehyd.) and aldehyde reductase (Ald. Reduct.)

also prolong the actions of administered catecholamines (BELLEAU and BURBA, 1961), and in some tissues such inhibitors appear to prolong the effects of sympathetic nerve stimulation (WYLIE et al., 1960).

Recently Kalsner and Nickerson (1968, 1969a) introduced a new pharmacological method to assess the roles of O-methylation, deamination, and tissue uptake in terminating the action of amines on the rabbit aortic strip. They measure the rates of relaxation of a strip immersed in oil to prevent loss of active amine by diffusion into the surrounding medium. Under these conditions the residual contraction is an index of the concentration of the drug in the region of the receptor. Inhibition of MAO has little effect on the rate of relaxation, but when combined with cocaine (which inhibits neuronal amine uptake) or tropolone (to inhibit COMT) there is more marked prolongation of contraction than with these agents alone. Use of all three drugs markedly prolonged the contraction. From the relative magnitudes of the drug effects, Kalsner and Nickerson (1969b) conclude that COMT is the major means for terminating the effects of noradrenaline but that MAO provides an important alternative route of metabolic inactivation. Further studies using reserpine (Kalsner and Nickerson, 1969b) or haloalkylamines led to a modification of this conclusion. The major means of inactivation of noradrenaline in this preparation was attributed to removal of the catecholamine from the region of the receptor to non-neuronal sites where O-methylation is the major metabolic route and deamination an effective alternative. These studies show that in the rabbit aorta extraneuronal inactivation of exogenous catecholamines is the predominant means of terminating their activity. The role of an active process for extraneuronal inactivation was not apparent although the haloalkylamine did appear to block this means of inactivation to an extent equivalent to blocking both MAO and COMT.

There appears to be general agreement that physical inactivation, whether by reuptake into the neurone (Hertting and Axelrod, 1961) or by uptake into extraneuronal sites (Kalsner and Nickerson, 1969b), plays a greater role than enzymatic degradation in terminating the effects of both endogenous and exogenous catecholamines (see chapter 16 by Trendelenburg). Thus, inhibition of both COMT and MAO failed to potentiate the cardiovascular responses to intravenously administered catecholamines (Crout, 1961).

III. Use of Radioactive Catecholamines to Study Metabolic Routes

Radioactively labelled catecholamines provide a direct means for determining the fate of the exogenously administered compounds and have provided a valuable tool for the study of the physiological disposition and metabolism of these substances and for evaluating the effects of drugs on these processes. There are, however, limitations to such studies. In assessing the roles of MAO and COMT in the metabolism of the catecholamines, a distinction must be made between exogenously administered and endogenous compounds and differences in tissues and species must be considered. When labelled catecholamines are administered intravenously their distribution is determined largely by the distribution of the blood (Kopin et al., 1965; Wurtman et al., 1964). Adrenaline is synthesized mainly in the adrenal medulla and is discharged into the circulation. The metabolic fate of intravenously administered adrenaline would therefore be expected to parallel that of the endogenously formed and released catecholamine. Noradrenaline, however, is synthesized and stored in sympathetic nerve endings throughout the body and in the central nervous system. It may be metabolized, at least in part, in the tissue before reaching the circulation. Thus the fate of intravenously administered noradrenaline may not accurately reflect that of the endogenous catecholamines. A portion of administered noradrenaline is, however, taken up into sympathetic neurones where it is bound and appears to mix with the endogenously formed compound. This portion of the labelled catecholamine presumably is metabolized in the same manner as the endogenous amine.

As indicated above, the distribution of intravenously administered catecholamines is dependent on the distribution of the blood. Uptake of radioactive catecholamines into sympathetic neurones results in labelling of the endogenous stores, but such labelling is not uniform throughout the body since the distribution of the blood is not uniform. For example, in the rat, the heart receives a greater portion of the cardiac output than does the vas deferens. Since the heart receives, and takes up, a greater fraction of administered noradrenaline, the specific activity of the catecholamine in the heart is greater than that in the vas deferens (KOPIN et al., 1965). Labelled catecholamines do not penetrate the blood-brain barrier so that the amines in brain remain unlabelled. The overall metabolism of labelled noradrenaline which is mixed with endogenous stores will be more similar to the metabolism of the catecholamine in the tissues which receive the greater portion of the administered catecholamine and contain a high density of sympathetic nerve endings.

Dopamine is present in relatively low concentrations in peripheral tissues and is the major catecholamine only in certain regions of the brain (CARLSSON, 1959). Its role as an intermediate compound in the biosynthesis of noradrenaline has until relatively recently overshadowed its role as a central neurotransmitter (HORNYKIEWICZ, 1966). The metabolic fate of intravenously administered dopamine reflects the metabolism of the endogenously formed compound with distortions because of the same factors already considered for noradrenaline. Most endogenously formed dopamine does not reach the circulation. Dopamine is rapidly converted to noradrenaline; and except in certain regions of brain, tissue levels of this catecholamine are low. A portion of administered dopamine is taken up by sympathetic neurones where it is converted to noradrenaline. The tissue distribution of the exogenous labelled amine would be expected to be related to regional blood flow and sympathetic nerve density. Noradrenaline formed from the labelled dopamine would be highest in richly innervated regions which receive the greatest proportion of the cardiac output. In spite of these limitations,however, a good deal of valid information regarding the metabolic routes for degrading catecholamines has been obtained using isotopically labelled compounds.

1. Metabolism of Adrenaline

After adrenalectomy there is a marked decrease in urinary excretion of adrenaline but not of noradrenaline (VON EULER et al., 1954). Most adrenaline appears to originate in the adrenal medulla where it is synthesized, stored and probably not metabolized to a significant extent until discharged into the circulation. Thus, the fate of intravenously administered adrenaline-H^3 probably approximates that of the endogenous compound. A portion of the administered adrenaline will be converted by O-methylation to metanephrine. Part of the metanephrine formed is conjugated and excreted; part is deaminated. If the fraction of metanephrine which is conjugated and excreted can be determined, then the proportion of the administered catecholamine converted to adrenaline can be calculated. An estimate of this fraction of metanephrine excreted as a conjugate can be obtained by administering labelled metanephrine. This may be done as a separate experiment (LABROSSE et al., 1958), but to reduce variability and to determine the relative magnitudes of the pathways in a single experiment two isotopically labelled compounds may be used simultaneously (KOPIN, 1960).

Adrenaline-H^3 is administered with metanephrine-methoxy-C^{14}, and the various metabolites are isolated by column chromatography and solvent extraction. From the ratios of H^3/C^{14} in the various compounds, the proportion of adrenaline-H^3 converted to metanephrine may be calculated. Such studies have shown that in both man (Kopin, 1960) and rat (Kopin et al., 1961) about two-thirds of administered adrenaline is converted to metanephrine. In rats, when pyrogallol is used to block COMT, only about 11% of the administered adrenaline is O-methylated (Table I). MAO inhibition increases the pathway through metanephrine so that

Table I. *Fate of intravenously administered adrenaline-H^3 in the rat*

Treatment	Percent administered dose: Excreted in urine			
	Free	Conjugated	O-Methylated	Deaminated
Untreated	9	5	69	8
Iproniazid	10	4	82	1
Pyrogallol	27	5	17	29

From Kopin et al. (1961).

about four-fifths of the administered catecholamine is O-methylated. Clearly, direct O-methylation is the major metabolic route for exogenous adrenaline. Metanephrine, however, is extensively deaminated; O-methylated-deaminated products account for about one-third of the radioactive products recovered after injection of the labelled catecholamine.

2. Metabolism of Administered and Endogenous Noradrenaline

When tritiated noradrenaline is administered intravenously part of the radioactivity is rapidly excreted during the first 3 hours, after which the rate of excretion becomes slowed (Kopin and Gordon, 1963). During the first 3 hours about 70% of the tritium is excreted, about one-fourth as the unchanged catecholamine. Normetanephrine accounts for about 40% of the labelled metabolites although this amine can be further metabolized to VMA or MHPG, indicating that O-methylation is the major primary route for metabolic inactivation of the circulating catecholamine. In the whole mouse, Whitby et al. (1961) found that about 45% of administered noradrenaline-H^3 was recovered in the tissues 5 min after its administration. At this time all of the noradrenaline-H^3 had been inactivated and the catecholamine found in the tissues must have been in an inactive, presumably bound, form. The slow release of this bound noradrenaline-H^3 is the source of the radioactive compounds excreted after the initial rapid excretion is completed. Examination of the metabolites found in the urine during an interval after the products of initial metabolism of the administered amine has been excreted provides insight into the fate of the intraneuronally bound catecholamine (Kopin and Gordon, 1963). At this time about two-thirds of the excreted radioactivity is present as O-methylated, deaminated metabolites. The proportion of deaminated catechols is increased three-fold compared to the proportion of the radioactivity excreted as these compounds in the initial interval, and normetanephrine is only about one-third as important a metabolite (Table II). These findings suggested that deamination was the major route of metabolic inactivation of the catecholamine which had been retained in the nerve endings.

Table II.* *Metabolic fate of H^3-noradrenaline in the rat*

	0—3 hours after administration	10—13 hours after administration
Total excreted	70.2**	3.94**
Noradrenaline		
Free	23.2	1.20
Conjugated	3.1	5.20
Deaminated catechols		
Free	0.7	2.90
Conjugated	1.2	4.10
Normetanephrine		
Free	12.1	3.10
Conjugated	17.1	8.40
3-Methoxy-4-hydroxymandelic acid (VMA)	4.0	13.90
3-Methoxy-4-hydroxyphenylglycol	32.9	47.60
Total urinary tritium recovered in metabolite fractions	94.3	86.40

* From Kopin and Gordon (1963).
** Percentage of administered dose.

Rats received 100 μc (±) H^3-noradrenaline intravenously and urine was collected 0—3 hours after and 10—13 hours after and analyzed for tritiated metabolites. Results are mean values for seven experiments and are expressed as percentage of total radioactivity excreted during the collection period.

3. Effect of Drugs

The difference in the metabolic fate of intraneuronally and extraneuronally released noradrenaline is also apparent when drugs are used to deplete catecholamine stores. Tyramine administration results in partial depletion of noradrenaline stores and produces a marked sympathomimetic response as a consequence of the release of the catecholamine (Burn and Rand, 1958). The metabolic fate of catecholamine released by tyramine resembles closely that of the noradrenaline initially metabolized after intravenous administration. Comparison of the fate of noradrenaline administered after tyramine treatment with that released by tyramine suggests that over half the catecholamine released by the drug entered the systemic circulation unchanged and about 30% was O-methylated.

In contrast to the marked sympathetic response seen during release of noradrenaline by tyramine, depletion of catecholamine stores by reserpine although more complete than after tyramine is not associated with a sympathomimetic response. The metabolic products of the reserpine-released catecholamine are, like those of bound noradrenaline, mostly deaminated (Kopin and Gordon, 1962). It is apparent that during reserpine-induced catecholamine depletion most noradrenaline is deaminated within the neurone and only small amounts reach the circulation.

Similar studies with other drugs have related sympathomimetic activity to extraneuronal release of noradrenaline and subsequent O-methylation (Kopin and Gordon, 1963). Some drugs such as guanethidine and α-methyldopa appear to have actions intermediate between the extremes of tyramine and reserpine (Table III).

There are a number of factors which enter into the mechanism by which tyramine (or other sympathomimetic amines) results in extraneuronal release of noradrenaline. These amines can displace noradrenaline from its binding site in the synaptic vesicles; they may compete with the released catecholamine for MAO

(Smith, 1966) as well as for the transport site in the neuronal membrane which is important for reuptake of released catecholamines. Each of these actions serves to increase the portion of displaced amine which reaches extraneuronal sites and subsequent metabolism by COMT.

Table III. *Relation of mode to release to metabolic fate of noradrenaline*

	O-Methylation	Deamination
Nerve stimulation	+++	+
Sympathomimetic amines	+++	+
Intraneuronal depletion (Reserpine)	+	+++

The studies described above were performed in whole animals, but the results obtained are consistent with observations on the fate of catecholamines injected into the cerebral ventricles as well as those found in the isolated perfused heart. Glowinski and Axelrod (1965) showed that after labelling brain noradrenaline stores by intraventricular administration of the tritiated amine, both reserpine and amphetamine depleted the stores of the labelled compound. The metabolic products found in the brain after reserpine were mainly those produced by deamination, and there was a decrease in normetanephrine-H^3. After amphetamine, however, there was a striking increase in the O-methylated products. When these drugs were administered before injection of noradrenaline-H^3 there were similar changes in metabolic routes. These results suggested that amphetamine causes both release of the tritiated amine and inhibition of neuronal uptake. The primary extraneuronal metabolic route was O-methylation. Reserpine, which apparently has little effect on the neuronal membrane, blocks vesicular storage of the catecholamine so that it is susceptible to metabolism within the neurone, mainly by deamination.

In the isolated perfused rat heart, administered noradrenaline is metabolized by O-methylation (Kopin et al., 1962; Iversen et al., 1965); but in hearts from animals pretreated with reserpine, deamination is markedly increased although there appears to be little change in O-methylation. Isolated rat hearts perfused with tyramine released noradrenaline, but when reserpine is perfused the products of deamination of noradrenaline are released (Nash et al., 1964).

Noradrenaline is taken up into extraneuronal sites (Fischer et al., 1965) by a process which was described by Iversen (1965) as "Uptake$_2$". Although first noted at high concentrations of noradrenaline extraneuronal uptake does operate at low concentrations of catecholamines, but at low levels the amine is rapidly metabolized (Lightman and Iversen, 1969). When extraneuronal uptake of catecholamines is blocked by phenoxybenzamine, there is a striking decrease in formation of their O-methylated products although phenoxybenzamine does not block COMT (Eisenfeld et al., 1966, 1967). The results obtained using noradrenaline-H^3 to study directly the uptake and metabolism of this catecholamine are in total agreement with the inferences regarding the mechanisms for terminating the action of noradrenaline obtained from the studies of Kalsner and Nickerson (1969b) which were described above. They indicate that exogenous noradrenaline is removed from the region of the receptor by uptake into both neuronal and extraneuronal sites. The portion of catecholamine taken up into the neurone is stored in vesicles or destroyed by MAO, while that taken up extraneuronally is destroyed mainly by COMT. Only if COMT is inhibited does extraneuronal deamination play a major role in disposing of the catecholamine.

IV. Summary

The route of metabolic inactivation of the catecholamine depends upon the site of their release or uptake (Fig. 2). When endogenous catecholamines reach the circulation they are destroyed mainly by O-methylation in the liver and kidney. Physical inactivation by uptake either into the prejunctional neurone or into extraneuronal cells is the major means of terminating the action of noradrenaline.

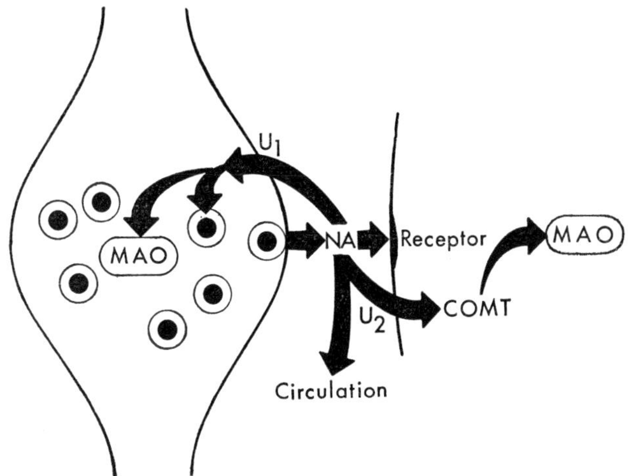

Fig. 2. Disposition of noradrenaline (NA) released from sympathetic nerve endings. Enzymes are abbreviated as in Fig. 1. See text for explanation of processes represented

When uptake into the neurone occurs, storage in the vesicles largely prevents destruction by MAO; but if this storage is blocked (e.g. by reserpine), deamination occurs. Uptake into extraneuronal sites results in metabolism by COMT. If COMT is blocked, extraneuronal MAO destroys the catecholamine. Thus deamination may occur both intra- and extraneuronally but O-methylation is mainly extraneuronal. Drugs which result in intraneuronal release permit destruction of the catecholamine by MAO, and unless this enzyme is blocked they cause depletion of catecholamine stores without a sympathomimetic response. Drugs which result in extraneuronal release elicit an indirect sympathomimetic response, and O-methylation is the primary route for metabolic inactivation of the released catecholamine.

References

Armstrong, M. D., McMillan, A., Shaw, K. N. F.: 3-Methoxy-4-hydroxy-D-mandelic acid, a urinary metabolite of norepinephrine. Biochim. biophys. Acta (Amst.) **25**, 422—423 (1957).

Axelrod, J.: O-Methylation of catechol amines *in vitro* and *in vivo*. Science **126**, 400—401 (1957).

— The metabolism of catechol amines *in vivo* and *in vitro*. Pharmacol. Rev. **11**, (Part 2), 402—408 (1959).

— Albers, R. W., Clemente, C. D.: Distribution of catechol-O-methyl transferase in the nervous system and other tissues. J. Neurochem. **5**, 68—72 (1959).

— Laroche, M. J.: Inhibitor of O-methylation of epinephrine and norepinephrine *in vitro* and *in vivo*. Science **130**, 800 (1959).

— Senoh, S., Witkop, B. B.: O-Methylation of catechol amines *in vivo*. J. biol. Chem. **233**, 697—701 (1958).

— Tomchick, R.: Enzymatic O-methylation of norepinephrine and other catechols. J. biol. Chem. **233**, 702—705 (1958).

Bacq, A.M., Gosselin, L., Dresse, A., Renson, J.: Inhibition of O-methyltransferase by catechol and sensitization to epinephrine. Science **130**, 453—454 (1959).
Belleau, B., Burba, J.: Tropolones: a unique class of potent noncompetitive inhibitors of S-adenosylmethionine-catechol methyltransferase. Biochim. biophys. Acta (Amst.) **54**, 195—196 (1961).
Beyer, K.H., Shapiro, S.H.: Excretion of conjugated epinephrine and related compounds. Amer. J. Physiol. **144**, 321—330 (1945).
Blaschko, H., Richter, D., Schlossman, H.J.: Inactivation of adrenaline. J. Physiol. (Lond.) **90**, 1—17 (1937).
Brown, G.L., Gillespie, J.S.: Output of sympathetic transmitter from the spleen of the cat. J. Physiol. (Lond.) **138**, 81—102 (1957).
Burn, J.H.: Mechanism of action of chemical substances at nerve endings. Acta physiol. scand. **29**, 40—49 (1953).
— Philpot, F.J., Trendelenburg, U.: Effect of denervation on enzymes in iris and blood vessels. Brit. J. Pharmacol. **9**, 423—429 (1954).
— Rand, M.J.: The action of sympathomimetic amines in animals treated with reserpine. J. Physiol. (Lond.) **144**, 314—346 (1958).
— Robinson, J.: Effect of denervation on amine oxidase in structures inervated by the sympathetic nerves. Brit. J. Pharmacol. **7**, 304—318 (1952).
Carlsson, A.: The occurrance, distribution, and physiological role of catecholamines in the nervous system. Pharmacol. Rev. **11**, 490—493 (1959).
Celander, O., Mellander, S.: Elimination of adrenaline and noradrenaline from circulating blood. Nature (Lond.) **176**, 973 (1955).
Corne, S.J., Graham, J.D.P.: Effect of inhibition of monoamine oxidase *in vivo* on administered adrenaline, noradrenaline, tyramine and serotonin. J. Physiol. (Lond.) **135**, 339—349 (1957).
Crout, J.R.: Effect of inhibiting both catechol-O-methyl transferase and monoamine oxidase on cardiovascular responses to norepinephrine. Proc. Soc. exp. Biol. (N.Y.) **108**, 482—484 (1961).
Davey, M.J., Farmer, J.B., Reinert, H.: The effects of nialamide on adrenergic function. Brit. J. Pharmacol. **20**, 121—134 (1963).
Eisenfeld, A.J., Axelrod, J., Krakoff, L.: Inhibition of the extraneuronal accumulation and metabolism of norepinephrine by adrenergic blocking agents. J. Pharmacol. exp. Ther. **156**, 107—113 (1966).
— Krakoff, L., Iversen, L.L., Axelrod, J.: Inhibition of the extraneuronal metabolism of noradrenaline in the isolated heart by adrenergic blocking agents. Nature (Lond.) **213**, 297—298 (1967).
Euler, U.S., von: Noradrenaline. Springfield, Illinois: Thomas 1956.
— Franksson, E., Hellstrom, J.: Adrenaline and noradrenaline output in urine after unilateral and bilateral adrenalectomy in man. Acta physiol. scand. **31**, 1 (1954).
— Luft, R.: Noradrenaline output in urine after infusion in man. Brit. J. Pharmacol. **6**, 286—288 (1951).
— — Sunden, T.: Excretion of urinary adrenaline in normals following intravenous infusion. Acta physiol. scand. **30**, 249—257 (1953).
Evarts, E.V., Gillespie, L., Fleming, T.C., Sjoerdsma, A.: Relative lack of pharmacological action of the 3-methoxy analogue of norepinephrine. Proc. Soc. exp. Biol. (N.Y.) **98**, 74—76 (1958).
Fischer, J.E., Kopin, I.J., Axelrod, J.: Evidence for extraneuronal binding of norepinephrine. J. Pharmacol. exp. Ther. **147**, 181—185 (1965).
Friend, G., Zileli, M.S., Hamilin, J.R., Reutter, F.W.: Effect of iproniazid on the inactivation of norepinephrine in the human. J. clin. exp. Psychotherap. **19**, 61—68 (1958).
Furchgott, R.F., Weinstein, P., Huebl, H., Bozorgmehri, P., Mensendiek, S.R.: Effect of inhibition of monoamine oxidase on response of rabbit aortic strips to sympathomimetic amines. Fed. Proc. **14**, 341—342 (1955).
Glowinski, J., Axelrod, J.: Effect of drugs on the uptake, release, and metabolism of H^3-norepinephrine in the rat brain. J. Pharmacol. **149**, 43—49 (1965).
— Baldessarini, R.J.: Metabolism of norepinephrine in the central nervous system. Pharmacol. Rev. **18**, 1201—1238 (1966).
Griesemer, E.C., Barsky, J., Dragstedt, C.A., Wells, J.A., Zeller, E.A.: Potentiating effect of iproniazid on the pharmacological actions of sympathomimetic amines. Proc. Soc. exp. Biol. (N.Y.) **84**, 699—701 (1953).
Hare, M.L.C.: Tyramine oxidase. I. A new enzyme system in liver. Biochem. J. **22**, 968—979 (1928).
Hertting, G., Axelrod, J.: Fate of tritiated noradrenaline at the sympathetic nerve-endings Nature (Lond.) **192**, 172—173 (1961).

HORNYKIEWICZ, O.: Dopamine (3-hydroxy-tyramine) and brain function. Pharmacol. Rev. **18**, 925—964 (1966).

IVERSEN, L.L.: The uptake of catecholamines at high perfusion concentrations in the rat isolated heart: a novel catecholamine uptake process. Brit. J. Pharmacol. **25**,18—33(1965).

— GLOWINSKI, J., AXELROD, J.: The uptake and storage of H^3-norepinephrine in the reserpine-pretreated rat heart. J. Pharmacol. exp. Ther. **150**, 173—183 (1965).

KALSNER, S., NICKERSON, M.: A method for the study of mechanisms of drug disposition in smooth muscle. Canad. J. Physiol. Pharmacol. **46**, 719—730 (1968a).

— — Disposition of norepinephrine and epinephrine in vascular tissue, determined by the technique of oil immersion. J. Pharmacol. exp. Ther. (1969a).

— — Effects of reserpine on the disposition of sympathomimetic amines in vascular tissue. Brit. J. Pharmacol. **35**, 394—405 (1969b).

KAMIJO, K., KOELLE, G.B., WAGNER, H.H.: Modification of the effects of sympathomimetic amines and of adrenergic nerve stimulation by 1-isonicotinyl-2-isopropylhydrazine (IIH) and isonicotinic acid hydrazide (INH). J. Pharmacol. exp. Ther. **117**, 213—227 (1955).

KOELLE, G.B., DET. VALK, A.: Physiological implications of the histochemical localization of monoamine oxidase. J. Physiol. (Lond.) **126**, 434—447 (1954).

KOPIN, I.J.: Technique for the study of alternative metabolic pathways: epinephrine metabolism in man. Science **131**, 1372—1374 (1960).

— AXELROD, J., GORDON, E.K.: The metabolic fate of H^3-epinephrine and C^{14}-metanephrine in the rat. J. biol. Chem. **236**, 2109—2113 (1961).

— GORDON, E.K.: Metabolism of norepinephrine-H^3 released by tyramine and reserpine. J. Pharmacol. **138**, 351—357 (1962).

— — Metabolism of administered and drug-released norepinephrine-7-H^3 in the rat. J. Pharmacol. **140**, 207—216 (1963).

— — HORST, W.D.: Studies of uptake of L-norepinephrine-C^{14}. Biochem. Pharmacol. **14**, 753—760 (1965).

— HERTTING, G., GORDON, E.K.: Fate of norepinephrine-H^3 in the isolated perfused rat heart. J. Pharmacol. exp. Ther. **138**, 34—40 (1962).

LABROSSE, E.H., AXELROD, J., KETY, S.S.: O-Methylation, the principal route of metabolism of epinephrine in man. Science **128**, 593—594 (1958).

LIGHTMAN, S., IVERSEN, L.L.: The role of Uptake_2 in the extraneuronal metabolism of noradrenaline in the isolated rat heart. Brit. J. Pharmacol. **37**, 638—649 (1969).

MACLAGLAN, N.F., WILKINSON, J.H.: Methylation of a phenolic hydroxyl group in the human body. Nature (Lond.) **168**, 251 (1951).

MALING, H.M., HIGHMAN, B., SPECTOR, S.: Neurologic, neuropathologic and neurochemical effects of prolonged administration of phenylisopropylhydrazine (JB 516) phenylisobutylhydrazine (JB 835) and other monoamine oxidase inhibitors. J. Pharmacol. exp. Ther. **137**, 334—343 (1962).

NASH, C.W., COSTA, E., BRODIE, B.B.: The actions of reserpine, guanethidine, and metaraminol on cardiac catecholamine stores. Life Sci. **3**, 441—449 (1964).

PLETSCHER, A.: Monoaminoxydase-Hemmer. Dtsch. med. Wschr. **86**, 647—657 (1961).

PUGH, C.E.M., QUASTEL, J.H.: Oxidation of aliphatic amines by brain and other tissues. Biochem. J. **31**, 286—291 (1937).

RABHUN, J., FEINBERG, S.M., ZELLER, E.A.: Potentiating effects of iproniazid on the action of some sympathomimetic amines. Proc. Soc. exp. Biol. (N.Y.) **87**, 218—220 (1954).

RICHTER, D.: Adrenaline and amine oxidase. Biochem. J. **31**, 2022—2028 (1937).

— Inactivation of adrenaline *in vivo* in man. J. Physiol. (Lond.) **98**, 361—374 (1940).

SCHAYER, R.W.: Metabolism of β-C^{14} DL-adrenaline. J. biol. Chem. **189**, 301—306 (1951).

— SMILEY, R.L., DAVIS, K.J., KOBAYASHI, Y.: Role of monoamine oxidase in noradrenaline metabolism. Amer. J. Physiol. **182**, 285—286 (1955).

— — KAPLAN, E.H.: Metabolism of adrenaline containing isotopic carbon (II). J. biol. Chem. **198**, 545—551 (1952).

— — KENNEDY, J.: Metabolism of epinephrine containing isotopic carbon (III). J. biol. Chem. **202**, 425—430 (1953).

SHARMAN, D.F., VANOV, S., VOGT, M.: Noradrenaline content in the heart and spleen of the mouse under normal conditions and after administration of some drugs. Brit. J. Pharmacol. **19**, 527—533 (1962).

SHAW, K.N.F., MCMILLAN, A., ARMSTRONG, M.D.: Metabolism of 3,4-dihydroxyphenylalanine. J. biol. Chem. **226**, 255—266 (1957).

SHORE, P.A., MEAD, A.R., KUNTZMAN, R.G., SPECTOR, S., BRODIE, B.B.: Physiological significance of monoamine oxidase in the brain. Science **126**, 1063—1064 (1957).

SMITH, C.B.: The role of monoamine oxidase in the intraneuronal metabolism of norepinephrine released by indirectly-acting sympathomimetic amines or by adrenergic nerve stimulation. J. Pharmacol. exp. Ther. **151**, 207—220 (1966).

SNYDER, S., FISCHER, J., AXELROD, J.: Evidence for the presence of monoamine oxidase in sympathetic nerve endings. Biochem. Pharmacol. **14**, 363—365 (1965).

SPECTOR, S., PROCKOP, D., SHORE, P.A., BRODIE, B.B.: Effect of iproniazid on brain levels of norepinephrine and serotonin. Science **127**, 704 (1958).

— SHORE, P.A., BRODIE, B.B.: Biochemical and pharmacological effects of monoamine oxidase inhibitors, iproniazid, l-phenyl-2-hydrazine propane (JB 516) and 1-phenyl-3-hydrazinobutane. J. Pharmacol. exp. Ther. **128**, 15—21 (1960).

STRÖMBLAD, B.L.R.: Supersensitivity and amine oxidase activity in denervated salivary glands. Acta physiol. scand. **36**, 137—153 (1956).

VOGT, M.: Concentration of sympathin in different parts of the central nervous system under normal conditions and after administration of drugs. J. Physiol. (Lond.) **123**, 451—481 (1954).

— Catechol amines in brain. Pharmacol. Rev. **11**, (Part 2), 483 (1959).

WHITBY, L.G., AXELROD, J., WEIL-MALHERBE, H.: The fate of H^3-norepinephrine in animals. J. Pharmacol. exp. Ther. **132**, 193—201 (1961).

WURTMAN, R.J., KOPIN, I.J., HORST, D.W., FISCHER, J.E.: Epinephrine and organ blood flow: effects of hyperthyroidism, cocaine and sympathetic denervation. Amer. J. Physiol. **207**, 1247—1250 (1964).

WYLIE, D.W., ARCHER, S., ARNOLD, A.: Augmentation of pharmacological properties of catecholamines by O-methyl transferase inhibitors. J. Pharmacol. exp. Ther. **130**, 239—244 (1960).

ZELLER, E.A., BARSKY, J.: *In vivo* inhibition of liver and brain by l-isonicotinyl-2-isopropyl-hydrazine. Proc. Soc. exp. Biol. (N.Y.) **81**, 459—461 (1952).

Chapter 9

The Classification of Adrenoceptors (Adrenergic Receptors). An Evaluation from the Standpoint of Receptor Theory[1]

Robert F. Furchgott

With 10 Figures

A. Introduction

A wide variety of tissues undergo a change of functional state on exposure to noradrenaline or adrenaline. Those molecular constituents of the effector cells of a tissue with which molecules of these catecholamines must first interact in order to produce a change of state — or response — of the tissue, are the so-called adrenoceptors (also commonly called adrenergic receptors). For convenience, we refer to noradrenaline, adrenaline and other agents which produce responses in tissues by interacting with adrenoceptors, as adrenergic agonists. An agent which specifically inhibits a response produced by an adrenergic agonist is referred to as adrenergic blocking agent or adrenergic antagonist.

Since adrenoceptors have not yet been isolated and chemically characterized, their classification depends on the application of pharmacological procedures in which selected adrenergic agonists and antagonists are used to reveal similarities or differences in the characteristics of different responses. This is an operational method for classification, in which the basic assumption is that similarities or differences in the characteristics of different responses reflect similarities or differences in the characteristics of the receptors mediating these responses.

The major emphasis in this chapter will be on a critical evaluation of the pharmacological procedures used for the characterization and classification of adrenoceptors, especially from the standpoint of current concepts of receptor theory. The chapter will not deal with speculation concerning the chemical nature of these receptors or the mechanisms by which the reaction between a specific type of receptor and an agonist initiates a change of state which leads ultimately to a response. Because of the limitations of space, a comprehensive review of the current status of classification of adrenoceptors mediating all recognized adrenergic responses in different tissues of different species is not possible here. For the most part, the responses considered will be those in mammalian tissues which have been most thoroughly investigated. Unfortunately, limited space has also

1 This work was supported in part by grants from the USPHS (HE-05237), the Life Insurance Medical Research Foundation, and the New York Heart Association.

made it necessary to omit citations of many papers which are just as relevant to the topics under discussion as those which have been cited.

B. Historical Background

As long ago as 1906 DALE, in his classical study of the influence of ergot alkaloids on the effects of adrenaline and sympathetic nerve stimulation, provided experimental evidence for two distinct classes of adrenoceptors. He found that excitatory or motor responses of various organs to adrenaline and nerve stimulation were "paralyzed" by the ergot alkaloids, whereas inhibitory responses were not. Indeed, an inhibitory response, not normally manifested by a given organ, was sometimes revealed after treatment with ergot alkaloids. His results were unequivocal for most smooth muscles. However, the reported ability of ergot alkaloids to block the excitatory effects of adrenaline and sympathetic nerve stimulation on mammalian heart was not clearly demonstrated (see NICKERSON, 1949, 1967).

Dale interpreted his results to mean that there were two distinct types of "sympathetic myoneural junctions" which were activated by adrenaline or sympathetic nerve stimulation, and that only the type responsible for motor effects was paralyzed by ergot alkaloids. He stated that "receptive substance for adrenaline", a term introduced in 1905 by LANGLEY, might be substituted for his own term of "sympathetic myoneural junction." In another early study in which adrenaline and related phenylethylamine derivatives were compared for potency in producing increases in blood pressure and responses in certain muscular organs, Dale concluded that "the myoneural junctions, or parts of myoneural junctions concerned with inhibition, are not identical in their affinities for chemical substances with those which are concerned with motor effects" (BARGER and DALE, 1910). Thus, the early work of Dale introduced two methods for differentiating types of adrenoceptors — namely, that of selective blockade by antagonists (i.e., the ergot alkaloids) and that of comparing the relative potencies of a series of sympathomimetic amines (adrenergic agonists).

In addition to certain ergot alkaloids, a fairly large number of other natural and synthetic compounds were subsequently found to block the motor responses but not the inhibitory responses to adrenaline and sympathetic nerve stimulation in most smooth muscles. By 1949, when NICKERSON reviewed the subject of "adrenergic blocking agents," it was generally agreed that most of these agents exerted their blockade by acting as reversible competitive antagonists at the receptor site mediating the motor response (referred to as "equilibrium blockade" by NICKERSON). However, NICKERSON (1949) pointed out that blockade by dibenamine and other related β-haloalkylamines, which he and his colleagues had begun to investigate, appeared to depend not on reversible competitive antagonism but rather on an inactivation of the receptor due to alkylation at its active site or a closely adjacent site (referred to as "non-equilibrium blockade"). Since the β-haloalkylamines produced essentially complete blockade of contractions of smooth muscles in response to adrenergic stimuli (adrenergic agonists or sympathetic nerve stimulation) without blocking the increase in rate and force of heart in response to the same stimuli, they clearly differentiated between the adrenoceptors mediating excitatory responses in smooth muscles and those mediating excitatory responses in heart. FURCHGOTT (1954) was able to demonstrate with isolated rabbit aortic strips that high concentrations of adrenergic agonists present during an incubation with dibenamine could selectively protect their own responses against the essentially irreversible blockade produced by dibenamine. He attributed this protection to reversible occupation of the active site of the adrenoceptor by the agonists, and concluded that dibenamine did indeed react covalently with this site to produce its blockade.

About the time that NICKERSON and coworkers were introducing the β-haloalkylamines as powerful new pharmacological tools for differentiating classes of adrenoceptors, AHLQUIST (1948) carried out his classical study on the differentiation of these receptors on the basis of the order of potency of a series of sympathomimetic amines in producing responses in each of a variety of sympathetically innervated effector organs or systems. The amines used by AHLQUIST were (1) adrenaline, (2) noradrenaline, (3) α-methyl-noradrenaline, (4) α-methyl-adrenaline, and (5) isoprenaline. He tested these amines in intact dogs, cats and rabbits, and on isolated tissues from these and other species. He found the relative potencies in descending order to be 1, 2, 3, 4, 5 for producing excitation of the smooth muscles of the peripheral blood vessels (vasoconstriction) nictitating membrane, uterus, ureter and *dilator pupillae*, and inhibition of the smooth muscle of intestine; but 5, 1, 4, 3, 2 for producing inhibition of the smooth muscles of blood vessels (vasodilation) and uterus, and excitation (increase in rate and force) of the heart. The two distinct orders of potencies led him to conclude that there were "two distinct types" of adrenoceptors mediating the responses which he studied, and he proposed calling the type associated with the first order *alpha*, and that with the second order, *beta*. Except for the inhibition of intestinal smooth muscle, all of the responses which he attributed to α-receptor activation were responses which could be successfully blocked by the adrenergic blocking agents known at that time, while all of the responses which he attributed to β-receptor activation were not susceptible to blockade by these agents.

In 1957 and 1958 the first reports were published on the pharmacology of the dichloro-analogue of isoprenaline (1-(3′,4′-dichlorophenyl)-2-isopropylaminoethanol). This compound, commonly referred to as DCI, was found to block both adrenergic inhibitory responses in a variety of smooth muscles (POWELL and SLATER, 1958) and adrenergic stimulatory responses in heart (MORAN and PERKINS, 1958) at concentrations which did not block adrenergic stimulatory responses in smooth muscles. The fact that blockade with DCI was selective for those responses which AHLQUIST had concluded were mediated by a common type of receptor, namely, the β-type, greatly strengthened his argument for two major types of receptors, and his *alpha* and *beta* classification soon came into general use. It now became customary to refer to classical adrenergic blocking agents as α-blocking agents.

With DCI available, FURCHGOTT (1959) re-examined the question of the classification of the adrenoceptor in intestine. In the isolated rabbit duodenum he found that the inhibitory effects of adrenaline or noradrenaline were not completely blocked by either DCI or by potent α-blocking agents (dibenamine or phentolamine), and postulated a third type of adrenoceptor for smooth muscle of intestine. However, this postulate was soon disproved when AHLQUIST and LEVY (1959), investigating motility of the dog small intestine *in situ*, showed that inhibition by adrenaline or noradrenaline could be successfully blocked by a combination of DCI and an α-blocking agent; inhibition by isoprenaline, by DCI alone; and inhibition by phenylephrine, by an α-blocking agent alone. Thus, it became apparent that both α- an β-receptors were present in intestine, and that activation of either type caused inhibition of motility. Shortly thereafter, FURCHGOTT (1960) obtained results on isolated rabbit intestine which were similar to those of AHLQUIST and LEVY on dog intestine.

Although FURCHGOTT (1960) agreed with the conclusion that both α- and β-receptors mediated relaxation of intestine, he noted that after blockade of α-receptors in rabbit duodenum (by dibenamine or phentolamine) noradrenaline was more potent than adrenaline. This order of potency was the reverse of that originally set forth by AHLQUIST for responses mediated by β-receptors, and introduced the possibility of different types of β-receptors in different smooth muscles. Using experimental conditions designed to exclude factors which could introduce quantitative errors in results, FURCHGOTT (1967) extended his work on the classification of adrenoceptors. On the basis of both the relative potencies of selected adrenergic agonists in producing specific responses in isolated tissues from rabbit and guineapig, and quantitative determinations of the affinities of specific competitive antagonists for receptors (pronethalol for β-receptors, and phentolamine for α-receptors), he concluded that in the limited number of tissues studied there was only one type of α-receptor, but at least three types of β-receptors. About the same time, LANDS and his colleagues had begun to publish the results of their investigations of the relative potencies of a large series of sympathomimetic amines in producing responses in both isolated tissues and in intact animals (LANDS et al., 1967a, b). On the basis of statistical comparisons of the potency series obtained for different responses, they concluded that there were two different types of β-receptors — which they termed β_1 and β_2 — and that these two types alone were sufficient to account for their results.

Further evidence for different types of β-receptors also was beginning to come out of experiments in which some of the newly developed β-blocking agents were being tested. For example, SALVADOR and coworkers (SALVADOR et al., 1964; BURNS et al., 1967) found that isopropylmethoxamine and butoxamine effectively blocked catecholamine-induced increases in plasma glucose, lactic acid and free fatty acid in anesthetized dogs, without blocking cardiac stimulatory effects. LEVY (1966) and MORAN (1967), using dogs and cats, respectively, found that butoxamine effectively blocked isoprenaline-induced vasodilitation but not cardiac stimulation and intestinal inhibition; and LEVY (1967) demonstrated the ability of this agent, in appropriate concentrations, to block isoprenaline-induced relaxation of the isolated rat uterus, but not that of the isolated rabbit jejunum. Butoxamine has been called a selective β-blocking agent. During the past several years still other selective β-blocking agents, as well as so-called selective β-agonists, have been introduced (see LEVY and WILKENFELD, 1970), and have proven useful in differentiating types of β-receptors.

In view of the growing evidence for different types of receptors within the general class of β-receptors, FURCHGOTT (1967) proposed a more general definition of a β-receptor. That definition, slightly modified to take into account the growing use of propranolol as an antagonist, follows: *a β-receptor is one which mediates a response pharmacologically characterized by: (1) a relative potency series in which isoprenaline > adrenaline > noradrenaline > phenylephrine, or isoprenaline > noradrenaline > adrenaline > phenylephrine; and (2) a susceptibility to specific blockade by either proprnaolol or pronethalol at relatively low concentrations.* For the purpose of this review this definition of a β-receptor will be used.

The definition of an α-receptor (AHLQUIST, 1966; FURCHGOTT, 1967) used in this review is as follows: *an α-receptor is one which mediates a response pharmacologically characterized by: (1) a relative potency series in which adrenaline > or = noradrenaline > phenylephrine > isoprenaline; and (2) a susceptibility to specific blockade by phentolamine, dibenamine or phenoxybenzamine at relatively low concentrations.*

C. Procedures for the Pharmacological Characterization and Classification of Adrenoceptors

I. General Comments

Two kinds of procedures are used for the characterization of adrenoceptors. In the first procedure the relative potencies (potency ratios) of a series of adrenergic agonists for eliciting a specific response in a test system are determined. In the second procedure the potency of an antagonist for blocking or inhibiting the response to a given agonist is determined. If the experimental conditions used are satisfactory (see below), then a finding for two different responses, of similar relative potencies for the series of agonists, and of a similar potency for the antagonist as a blocking agent, would indicate that the two responses are mediated by the same type of receptor. On the other hand, a finding of dissimilar relative potencies or of dissimilar potencies for the antagonist, or of both, would indicate mediation of the two responses by different types of receptors.

Since both the relative potencies of agonists and the potencies of selected antagonists are so different for responses mediated by α-receptors and β-receptors, respectively, in experiments used to determine whether a receptor responsible for a given response should be placed in the α- or β-class, conditions usually need not be controlled very rigorously. However, as will become apparent later, if experiments are to be used for the purpose of differentiating types of receptors within a single class, then the proper control of experimental conditions is of great importance.

In tests of relative potencies of agonists, the potency ratio of one to another is generally expressed by the reciprocal of the ratio of the doses or concentrations (expressed on a molar basis) for eliciting an equal response. The number of agonists compared varies with different studies. In the author's laboratory adrenaline, noradrenaline, isoprenaline and phenylephrine have constituted a highly satisfactory series.

With respect to the use of antagonists in differentiating adrenoceptors, it is well to point out that two types of antagonists are used, namely, the type which reversibly competes with an agonist for the receptor, and the type which inactivates receptors in an essentially irreversible manner. At present there are available antagonists of the former type for both α- and β-receptors; however, the only available antagonists of the latter type (e.g. haloalkylamines such as dibenamine and phenoxybenzamine) block α-receptors (as well as some non-adrenergic receptors) but not β-receptors. Reversible competitive antagonists have an advantage, because under proper experimental conditions, quantitative determinations of antagonistic potency permit an estimate of the affinity of the antagonist for a given receptor (see Section C.II. 2.). Such estimates are very useful in differentiating types of receptors within any one class. Irreversible antagonists of the haloalkylamine class are obviously very useful for differentiating α- from β-receptors, but up to the present they have not proven useful for differentiating types of receptors within the α-class.

II. Theoretical Concepts Related to the Procedures for Pharmacological Characterization

For a critical evaluation of the procedures used for characterizing receptors, and for an understanding of why certain experimental conditions are required in the proper application of those procedures, it is first necessary to consider some theoretical concepts relating drug-receptor interactions to response. In this section the equations introduced come from the so-called "occupation theory" of drug action. (Equations from the "rate theory" of PATON (1961) will not be used; but it should be noted that they would be formally similar for equilibrium situations). For derivations of the equations considered here, the reader is referred to ARIENS (1964), STEPHENSON (1956), FURCHGOTT (1964, 1966), SCHILD (1949), MACKAY (1966), and WAUD (1968).

1. Concepts Related to the Relative Potencies of Agonists

The first equation (FURCHGOTT, 1966) to be considered is essentially that proposed by STEPHENSON (1956) for an agonist acting on a specific type of receptor:

$$\frac{E_A}{E_m} = f(S) = f\left\{\varepsilon[\mathrm{RA}]\right\} = f\left\{\frac{e[\mathrm{RA}]}{[\mathrm{R_t}]}\right\} = f\left\{\frac{e[\mathrm{A}]}{K_A + [\mathrm{A}]}\right\}. \tag{1}$$

Here, E_A is the response to agonist A; E_m is the maximal response possible with the effector (test preparation); S is the stimulus; [RA] is the concentration of receptor-agonist complex; ε is the intrinsic efficacy of RA for eliciting a stimulus; $[\mathrm{R_t}]$ is the total concentration of receptor; [A] is the concentration of free agonist in the region of the receptors in equilibrium with [RA]; K_A is the dissociation constant (inverse of affinity constant) of RA; e is efficacy.

The relative response E_A/E_m is some function of S (the product of ε and RA). The function is considered a monotonous one, but is not otherwise defined. The efficacy term, e of STEPHENSON (1956) is the product of ε and $[\mathrm{R_t}]$. (The modified, but not the original intrinsic activity term, α, of ARIENS is equivalent to e (VAN ROSSUM and ARIENS, 1962). K_A is equal to $[\mathrm{R}]\cdot[\mathrm{A}]/[\mathrm{RA}]$ at equilibrium, where [R] is the concentration of free receptor.

The following are the principal assumptions made in the derivation of equation (1) and in its application to experimental data obtained with isolated biological test preparations:

(a) Response E_A of the test preparation is the result of agonist A reacting with only one type of receptor. The reaction is a reversible bimolecular one governed by the law of mass action, and is characterized by a specific dissociation constant K_A for a specific receptor-agonist complex.

(b) In the case of different agonists acting individually on the same type of receptor in the same test preparation, the function relating response to stimulus is independent of the particular agonist, and equal responses will be elicited by different agonists when they produce equal stimuli (not necessarily when they occupy an equal fraction of the receptors, unless their efficacies are equal).

(c) When a response is measured, the concentration of the free agonist in the region of the receptors is in thermodynamic equilibrium with both agonist combined with receptors, and with free agonist in the bathing or perfusion solution.

Equation (1) cannot be directly applied for determining K_A or efficacy values from concentration response data, because the function f is not defined. The maximum response (E_{Am}) to a given agonist would be approached as [A], and consequently $[\mathrm{R_A}]/[\mathrm{R_t}]$ is increased. If $[\mathrm{RA}]/[\mathrm{R_t}]$ has to reach its absolute maximum of 1 (i.e., saturation of receptors) before an essentially maximal response occurs, then for two different agonist with different efficacies a lower maximal response would be obtained with the one with lower efficacy. The agonist with the lower efficacy is termed a "partial agonist" (STEPHENSON, 1956) relative to the one with higher efficacy. Theoretically, in systems where E_m is practically attained when $[\mathrm{R_A}]/[\mathrm{R_t}]$ is $\ll 1$, an agonist with lower efficacy might give a maximal response insignificantly different from that given by one with higher efficacy.

Experimental evidence for such systems (systems with "spare receptors" or "receptor reserve") has been obtained in the case of responses of certain preparations to muscarinic agonists (STEPHENSON, 1956; ARIENS, 1964; FURCHGOTT, 1966; FURCHGOTT and BURSZTYN, 1967), but not in the case of responses to adrenergic agonists.

It is apparent from equation (1) that the relative potencies of a series of agonists (based on doses to produce an equal response) will be the same as their relative affinities for a given type of receptor (reciprocals of their K_A values) only when their efficacies are equal. According to a preliminary report of BESSE and FURCHGOTT (1967), this appears to be the situation for adrenaline, noradrenaline and phenylephrine acting on α-receptors in isolated rabbit aortic strips. It should be noted, however, that for each of these agonists on this preparation the estimated K_A value was only about one-tenth of the ED_{50} value, so that half-maximal response appeared to occur with only about 10% occupation of receptors.

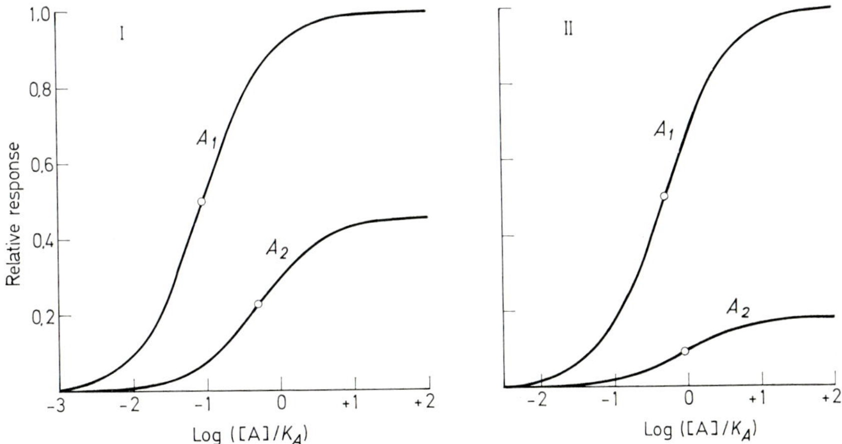

Fig. 1. Hypothetical log concentration-response curves for a strong agonist, A_1, and a partial agonist, A_2, acting on the same type of receptor in two effector systems (I and II). A smaller fraction of the total receptors has to be occupied by A_1 in I than in II to give the same fractional response. In both effector systems the relative efficacy of A_2 to A_1 is 0.1. For convenience of comparison, both agonists have been assigned the same K_A value for the receptor. ED_{50} values are indicated by circles on each curve

In the comparison of agonists with high and essentially equal efficacies, the relative potencies of the agonists should be the same for all responses mediated by the same specific type of receptor, regardless of the test preparation, provided that experimental conditions are satisfactory. However, even with satisfactory conditions, a comparison of the potency of an agonist with low efficacy (partial agonist) to that of one with high efficacy (strong agonist) in different preparations poses problems. This is apparent from Fig. 1, in which are plotted theoretical curves for the same strong agonist and partial agonist on two different preparations. In each case the relative potency of the partial agonist will depend on the degree of response measured, and in the two different cases it will be different, even for the same degree of response (relative to the maximum with the strong agonist). Using individual ED_{50} values for individual agonists still results in different relative potencies with the two preparations.

2. Concepts Related to Reversible Competitive Antagonism

The following equation is the modification of equation (1) for the case of reversible competitive antagonism:

$$\frac{E'_A}{E_m} = f(S') + f\{\varepsilon[\mathrm{RA'}]\} = f\left\{\frac{e[\mathrm{RA'}]}{[\mathrm{R_t}]}\right\} = f\left\{\frac{e[\mathrm{A'}]}{K_A(1+[\mathrm{B}]/K_B)+[\mathrm{A'}]}\right\}. \tag{2}$$

Here, [B] is the concentration of antagonist in equilibrium with the receptor, K_B is the dissociation constant of the receptor-antagonist complex, and all other terms are as in equation (1), but with a 'mark to indicate the presence of the competitive antagonist. If E'_A is set equal to E_A of equation (1) (that is, equal responses with and without B present), then one can obtain from the two equations:

$$\frac{[\mathrm{A'}]}{[\mathrm{A}]} - 1 = \frac{[\mathrm{B}]}{K_B}, \tag{3}$$

where [A′]/[A] is the ratio of concentrations of agonist giving an equal response in the presence and in the absence of the antagonist, respectively. This ratio is commonly referred to as the "dose ratio" and will henceforth be designated as *dr*. Equation (3) when put in logarithmic form becomes:

$$\log(dr - 1) = \log[\mathrm{B}] - \log K_B. \tag{4}$$

Equation (4) is sometimes written in the form originally introduced by SCHILD (1949):

$$\log(x - 1) = \log 1/K_B - pA_x, \tag{5}$$

where x is the dose ratio and pA_x is the negative logarithm of the concentration of antagonist required to give that dose ratio.

The assumptions involved in the derivation of these equations for competitive antagonism, and in their application to experimental data obtained with isolated test preparations, are assumptions (a) through (c) already listed with respect to equation (1) and, in addition, the following:

(d) The antagonist B combines reversibly with the same type of receptor as does A, in a bimolecular reaction in accord with the law of mass action, and this reaction is characterized by a specific dissociation constant K_B for a specific receptor-antagonist complex (RB).

(e) The agonist A cannot combine with RB, nor can B combine with RA.

(f) RB produces no response itself (efficacy of zero), and B alters the response to A only by competing with A for occupancy of receptors of this type.

(g) When a response to A is measured, the concentration of free B in the region of the receptors is in thermodynamic equilibrium with both B combined with receptors and with free B in the bathing or perfusion medium.

(h) Both in the absence and presence of B, response is the same when the concentration of receptor-agonist complex is the same.

Equation (3) or its logarithmic forms can be used for determining K_B. Equation (3) states that a plot of $(dr-1)$ against [B] should give a straight line from the origin with a slope of $1/K_B$; equations (4) and (5) state that a plot of $\log(dr-1)$ against log [B] or pA_x should give a straight line with a slope of 1 or −1, respectively; and that when $\log(dr-1)$ is zero (when dr equals 2), [B] is equal to K_B. Obviously, if all assumptions are valid, pA_2 is equal to $-\log K_B$. Also, it is apparent from equation (4) that for any concentration of B, the log concentration-response curve of an agonist should shift in a parallel fashion to the right on the log concentration axis, with the shift being given by $\log([\mathrm{B}]/K_B+1)$. As first pointed out by SCHILD (1947), pA values (or K_B values) for a given antagonist acting on a specific receptor in a given preparation, should be the same regardless of the agonist used; and pA values (or K_B values) for a given antagonist acting on the same type of receptor in two different preparations should be the same. Thus, the determination of pA or K_B values provides a powerful method for both classifying agonists according to the receptors on which they act, and for classifying receptors on which a given agonist acts.

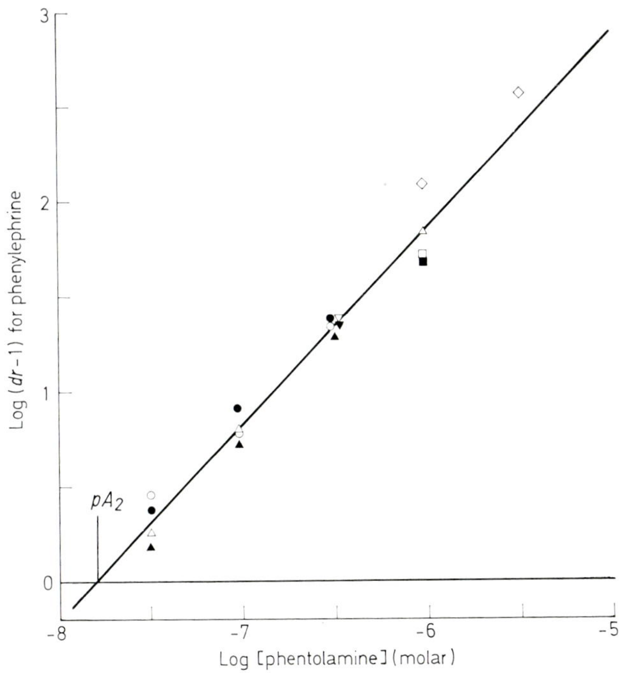

Fig. 2. Plot of log (dr—1) against log [antagonist] for phentolamine-phenylephrine antagonism on isolated strips of thoracic aorta from reserpine-treated rabbits. Krebs-bicarbonate solution at 37° C, containing propranolol (0.1 μg/ml). Strips pre-treated with iproniazid (100 μg/ml) for 20 min to block MAO. Exposure to phentolamine, 60 min. Each symbol represents results from one experiment with one or more strips from the same aorta. Fitted regression line has a slope of 1.06, and gives a pA_2 of 7.8 (equivalent to a K_B of 1.58×10^{-8} M). Average K_B calculated from individual points is 1.44 ± 0.08 M $\times 10^{-8}$ M

For accurate determinations of pA_2 or K_B it is desirable to obtain dose-response curves for the agonist over a wide range of antagonist concentrations (Arunlakshana and Schild, 1959). In Fig. 2 is shown a plot of log (dr—1) against log [B] for phentolamine-phenylephrine antagonism on isolated rabbit aortic strips, based on data obtained over a 100-fold range of phentolamine concentrations. The slope of the straight line fitting the points is not significantly different from 1. If a plot of (dr—1) against [B] does not give a straight line, or if a plot of log (dr—1) against log [B] does not give a straight line with a slope of 1, then either the theoretical assumptions on which the equations are based are wrong, or experimental conditions are not satisfactory for application of the equations. Although alternate theories have been proposed to explain log-log plots with slopes less than 1 (especially that a stimulus results only after two agonist molecules have combined with a receptor to give RA_2; see Wenke et al., 1967), the author believes that most of these low slopes result from unsatisfactory experimental conditions (see Section III.C.5.b).

3. Concepts Related to Irreversible Antagonism

In the case of antagonism in which the antagonist inactivates receptors in an essentially irreversible manner (as in the case of certain haloalkylamines acting on α-receptors and some non-adrenergic receptors), the following modification of equation (1) applies (FURCHGOTT, 1966):

$$\frac{E_A^*}{E_m} = f(S^*) = f\left\{\varepsilon[\mathrm{RA}^*]\right\} = f\left\{\frac{eq[\mathrm{RA}^*]}{q[\mathrm{R_t}]}\right\} = f\left\{\frac{eq[\mathrm{A}^*]}{K_A + [\mathrm{A}^*]}\right\}. \tag{6}$$

Here, q is the fraction of the original $[\mathrm{R_t}]$ which is not inactivated (still activatable by the agonist) following treatment with the antagonist, and all other terms are as in equation (1), but with an * mark to indicate that an irreversible antagonist has acted on the system. If q is sufficiently above zero to permit some response to A, and if a response E_A^* is equal to E_A of equation (1), then one can obtain from the equations (6) and (1):

$$\frac{1}{[\mathrm{A}]} = \frac{1-q}{qK_A} + \frac{1}{q[\mathrm{A}^*]}. \tag{7}$$

The assumptions involved in the derivation of these equations for irreversible antagonism, and in their application to experimental data obtained with isolated test preparations, are assumptions (a) through (c) already listed with respect to equation (1), and, in addition, the following:

(i) The antagonist alters the response to the agonist only by reducing the concentration of receptors which can be activated by the agonist.

(j) During the period over which the agonist is tested to obtain concentration-response data following action of the antagonist (after washout of antagonist in isolated preparations), the fraction of receptors still activatable (q) remains essentially constant.

(k) Both before and after irreversible inactivation of a fraction of receptors, response is the same when the concentration of receptor- agonist complex is the same (i.e., the intrinsic efficacy ε of the remaining receptors is the same as that for the original population of receptors.)

Equation (7) states that a plot of reciprocals of equi-effective concentrations of agonists before and after fractional receptor inactivation should give a straight line for which the slope is $1/q$, the ordinate intercept is $(1-q)/qK_A$, and K_A is (slope—1)/intercept. With K_A values known for two agonists acting on the same receptor, it is then possible to calculate the relative efficacy of one agonist to the other in interactions with that receptor (FURCHGOTT, 1966). Equation (7) (or a rearrangement of it) has been applied in several instances in attempt to obtain the K_A values of different agonists acting on muscarinic receptors (e.g., FURCHGOTT, 1966; FURCHGOTT and BURSZTYN, 1967); and to obtain relative efficacies of these agonists. The equation has been applied in a preliminary study by BESSE and FURCHGOTT (1967 and unpublished) in an attempt to obtain K_A values and relative efficacies of adrenergic agonists acting on α-receptors in aortic strips. Figure 3 is from one of their experiments.

It might first appear that q values obtained for α-receptors in different preparations subjected to a fixed concentration of an agent like dibenamine for a fixed time of exposure, could be used for differentiating types of α-receptors. However, differences in accessibility of receptors in different preparations to the alkylating ethyleneimmonium intermediate of the haloalkylamine would be difficult to control and could give misleading results. More promising for differentiating types of α-receptors would be a comparison of K_A values obtained for one or more agonists in different preparations. However, the validity of the method for obtaining K_A values for agonists reacting with α-receptors needs further testing before such a comparison is attempted.

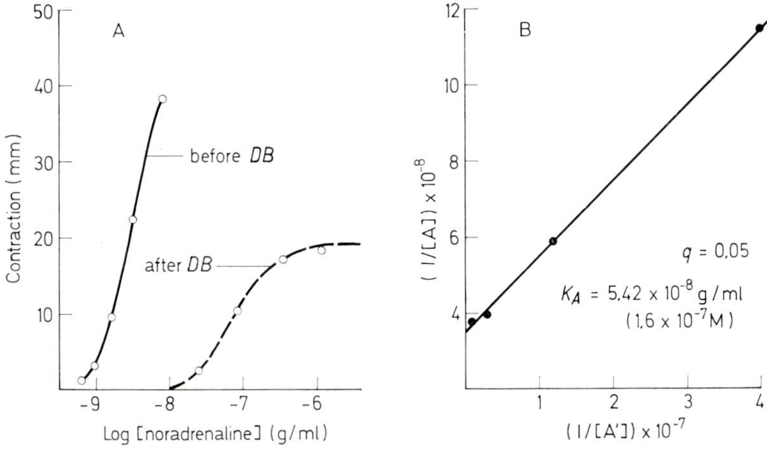

Fig. 3 A and B. Experiment to determine apparent K_A value for the reaction of (—)-noradrenaline with the α-receptor of the rabbit aortic strip. Krebs-bicarbonate solution at 37° C, containing cocaine (10 μg/ml) and propranolol (1 μg/ml). A: response as a function of noradrenaline concentration (as the bitartrate) before and after exposure of the strip to dibenamine *(DB)* (0.3 μg/ml for 15 min). B: plot of reciprocals of equiactive concentrations of noradrenaline before and after dibenamine treatment. Slope and intercept of line were used to calculate fraction of receptors still active *(q)* and apparent K_A, as indicated in text. Dashed curve in A is theoretical curve constructed on the basis of q, K_A, and the control curve (from BESSE and FURCHGOTT, unpublished results)

III. Experimental Conditions and their Control

1. Desired Optimal Conditions

In view of the assumptions made in the application of the equations of receptor theory to the interpretation of data obtained in experiments designed to characterize adrenoceptors, FURCHGOTT (1970) made a list of what he considered to be optimal conditions for such experiments on isolated tissues. That list, modified slightly and extended to include the possible use of irreversible antagonists, is given in Table 1. The "external solution" refers either to a bathing or perfusing solution. It is assumed that the tissue remains in good physiological condition throughout an experiment; that factors such as oxygenation, pH, and temperature are satisfactorily maintained. With our growing awareness of those conditions which are undesirable and the development of means to control them, it now appears feasible to bring actual conditions close to the optimal ones in experiments on a number of isolated tissue preparations (FURCHGOTT, 1968).

Obviously, the desired conditions listed in Table 1 cannot be approached in experiments on the intact animal. In the intact animal, the investigator is faced with a multitude of experimental variables which are very difficult and often impossible to control. Among the more important of these are the distribution and disposition patterns in the body of the administered drugs, the occurrence of responses which are the resultant of actions of a single drug on more than one kind of organ or tissue, and the modification of the response of a single organ or tissue as a result of nervous reflexes or humoral "feed-back" mechanisms. The possibility

Table 1. *Optimal conditions in experiments for the pharmacological characterization of adrenoceptors in isolated tissues*

1. The response of the tissue preparation to an agonist should be due solely to the direct action of the agonist on one type of receptor. It should not be the resultant of actions on more than one type of receptor, nor should it be due even partially to indirect action (e.g., release of endogenous noradrenaline).

2. The altered sensitivity to an agonist in the presence of a competitive antagonist should be due solely to competition between the antagonist and the agonist for the receptor. The altered sensitivity after treatment with an irreversible antagonist should be due solely to inactivation of the receptor.

3. The response following the addition of a given dose of agonist should be measured at the maximal level reached. In the most suitable tissues, this maximal level is maintained for a reasonable length of time.

4. In the case of either an agonist or competitive antagonist, the free concentration in the external solution should be maintained at a steady level at the time a response is measured, and should be known. In the case of an irreversible antagonist, the concentration in the solution should be essentially zero during the measurement of responses.

5. In the case of either an agonist or competitive antagonist, the concentration in the region of the receptors should be in diffusion-equilibrium with that in the external solution at the time a response is measured. To meet this condition, the rate of removal of drug from this region due to enzymic action, transport into cells, and binding should be negligible compared with the rate due to diffusion back to the outside solution. In the case of an irreversible antagonist, the fraction of receptors which is not inactivated should remain constant over the total period during which responses are measured.

6. The experimental design should include proper controls to permit measurements of, and corrections for, any changes in sensitivity of the tissue preparation to agonists during the course of an experiment that are not due to addition of an antagonist.

of multiple actions of agonists, and "feed-back" mechanisms giving misleading results, has been especially stressed in the case of *in vivo* studies on metabolic responses to adrenergic agonists (e.g., see HIMMS-HAGEN, 1967, 1970; HORNBROOK, 1970).

When agonists are injected in single doses in whole animal experiments, measurements of response cannot be made under equilibrium or steady-state conditions, since the concentration of agonist in a given tissue will rise and then fall, often within a short period. In tests of the relative potencies of various agonists for eliciting different responses *in vivo*, the best that can be hoped for is that the fraction of the injected dose reaching a specific responding tissue will remain constant for all doses of all the agonists being compared, and the time-course of the concentration transient will also remain constant. However, varying patterns of distribution and disposition of different agonists make this situation unlikely in most cases when injections are used. If injections are made into the artery directly supplying blood to a responding tissue, control of the doses of agonists reaching the tissue can be fairly accurate. When an antagonist is injected, the concentrations present in different responding tissues are also unknown, may vary from one tissue to another at any one time, and may vary in a single tissue over the period of time during which various doses of an agonist are tested.

Despite the disadvantages of *in vivo* testing as compared to *in vitro* testing, experiments on whole animals have been helpful, ever since the pioneer studies of DALE, in the general classification of adrenoceptors mediating various responses; and in recent years they have provided some of the evidence for more than one type of β-receptor. However, for more refined and exact characterization and differentiation of types of receptors in any one class, experiments with isolated tissue preparations are required.

Unfortunately, in many experiments carried out on isolated tissues for the purpose of characterizing adrenoceptors mediating responses, the experimental conditions have not been satisfacoty — that is, they have diverged too much from the desired optimal conditions. The following sections will deal with commonly encountered unsatisfactory conditions, giving selected examples from the literature of how these conditions have led or could lead to wrong conclusions, and what means have been used in attempts to control these conditions.

2. Changes in Sensitivity to Agonists not Due to Treatment with Antagonists

Changes in sensitivity of isolated tissue preparations to agonists during an experiment are not uncommon. Sensitivity changes often occur during the preliminary "equilibration" period for a tissue preparation, as in the case of the rabbit aortic strip (FURCHGOTT and BHADRAKOM, 1953) and the guinea-pig *vas deferens* (NEDERGAARD and WESTERMANN, 1968), both of which show a gradually developing, marked increase in sensitivity to adrenergic agonists for the first 1 or 2 hours after being mounted in a muscle chamber. In very long experiments it is not uncommon to encounter a late spontaneous decrease in sensitivity to agonists, probably arising from some physiological deterioration of the preparation.

Some sensitivity changes are obviously related to changes in the "basal" functional state of the test preparation over the course of an experiment (e.g., changes in tone and amplitude of contraction of intestinal segments or change in spontaneous rate or amplitude of isolated atria). Needless to say, a preparation whose "basal" functional state remains essentially constant throughout an experiment is the preferred type of preparation. In the case of isolated segments of rabbit duodenum, atropine (10^{-6} M) in the bathing solution is sometimes helpful in stabilizing both contractile activity and sensitivity to adrenergic agonists (FURCHGOTT, 1960). In experiments of long duration on guinea-pig atria or cat papillary muscle, both the basal contraction amplitude and sensitivity to adrenergic agonists are much better maintained when the temperature of the bathing solutions is 32.5° C (BLINKS, 1967).

A change in basal functional state of the test preparation is very likely to alter the relative potency of a partial agonist as compared to a strong agonist. For example, for relaxing isolated strips of guinea-pig trachea, the potency ratio of phenylephrine (a partial agonist) to isoprenaline (a strong agonist) is greater at low levels than at high levels of initial contraction of the strip (contraction controlled by additions of carbamylcholine); and at very low levels of initial contraction phenylephrine may produce essentially complete relaxation, thus giving the false impression that it is a "full" rather than partial agonist (FURCHGOTT, unpublished results).

The possibility of changes in sensitivity of a test preparation to agonists during the course of an experiment should always be considered as a possible source of error in experiments for comparison of potencies. In the case of the comparison of potencies of different agonists on a single preparation, the experimental design should allow detection of and correction for changes in sensitivity occurring during testing. FURCHGOTT (1967) has recommended a "bracketing" procedure in which concentration-response data for the standard agonist are always obtained both before and after obtaining such data for another agonist.

In the case of studies on competitive antagonism it is always best if one can use a "paired control" preparation to correct for any sensitivity change not caused by the antagonist in the experimental preparation. This is possible when two or more well matched preparations can be obtained from a single organ (such as strips from an artery, gut, trachea or left atrium). The control preparation is treated exactly like the experimental except that it receives no antagonist. Any displacement of the log concentration-response curve of the control preparation is subtracted from the displacement of the curve of the experimental preparation, and the difference is taken as the displacement due to action of the antagonist. Furchgott (1967, 1970) and Patil (1969) have reported examples of this type of correction for change of sensitivity in studies of competitive antagonism in the case of several tissue preparations. In the case of the isolated left atrium of the guinea-pig, the estimated K_B of the competitive antagonist tested was sometimes appreciably altered by application of the correction (Furchgott, 1967).

In studies on competitive antagonism where "paired control" preparations are not available, a sufficient number of unpaired control experiments (with no antagonist added) should be performed to obtain a statistically valid estimate of any change in sensitivity which should be used in corecting the change found in experiments with the antagonist.

Decreases in sensitivity to an agonist following continuous or continual exposures of an isolated preparation to the agonist is not an uncommon phenomenon. Causes of agonist-induced desensitization are not clear in most cases, and speculation about causes need not be considered here. Desensitization to one agonist producing its response by acting on a specific receptor is accompanied by desensitization to other agonists acting on the same receptor. Desensitization due to exposure to an agonist is usually most striking when the preparation is exposed to high concentrations producing maximal or near maximal responses. Although the onset of desensitization may not always be apparent during the actual exposure (as manifested by a decline of response with time), the desensitized state is revealed when smaller concentrations of agonist are retested after washout of the high concentrations. In the case of rabbit aortic strips, exposure to 10^{-5} g/ml adrenaline markedly reduced sensitivity to subsequent additions of this agonist in the range of 10^{-9} to 10^{-8} g/ml, and recovery of sensitivity was usually incomplete even 2 hours after the exposure (Furchgott and Bhadrakom, 1953).

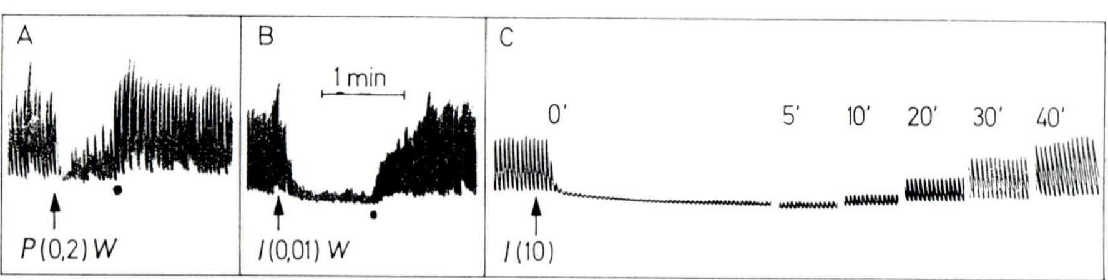

Fig. 4A—C. Inhibition of spontaneous contraction of rabbit duodenal segments produced by phenylephrine *(P)*, an α-agonist, and by isoprenaline *(I)*, a β-agonist. Krebs-bicarbonate solution at 37° C. Concentrations in μg/ml of the hydrochloride salts. Same segment used in A and B. A: rapid response to phenylephrine, followed by developing desensitization prior to wash *(W)*. B: slower response to isoprenaline, with no detectable desensitization prior to wash. C: gradual desensitization to isoprenaline during a 40-min continuous exposure to a high concentration. After 50 min (not shown in record), addition of another 10 μg/ml of isoprenaline caused no inhibition

In some preparations the occurence of agonist-induced desensitization may be apparent during an exposure to the agonist, as evidenced by a decrease of the response after it has reached a maximal level during the exposure. In some cases the decrease is gradual, as in that of the inhibitory response of the isolated rabbit intestine exposed to a high concentration of isoprenaline (Fig. 4C). In other cases it may be quite fast, with response reaching a peak and then "fading" in less than a minute after addition of the agonist. Well-known examples of responses exhibiting a rapid fade are the contraction of guinea-pig *vas deferens* caused by α-receptor agonists (e.g., see NEDERGAARD and WESTERMANN, 1968) and the relaxation of intestinal segments caused by the same agonists (e.g., see BOWMAN and HALL, 1970; and Fig. 4A).

In test systems in which the occurrence of desensitization (or accommodation) is apparent during an exposure to a single addition of an agonist, it is unwise to obtain data for concentration-response curves of the agonist by the method of cumulative additions, since desensitization will also be cumulative. In such systems it is safer to use separate additions of agonist, with each addition followed by a washout period sufficiently long for recovery of sensitivity. In test systems in which there is long-lasting desensitization following exposures to concentrations of agonists giving near maximal responses, but not to lower concentrations giving low to intermediate responses, it is often preferable to obtain data with the lower concentrations only, both for the purpose of estimating relative potencies of agonists and for estimating the potencies of antagonists.

3. Responses Complicated by an Indirect Action of the Agonist

It is now well recognized that a large number of sympathomimetic amines produce all or part of their effects indirectly by releasing noradrenaline from adrenergic nerve terminals — with the released noradrenaline then acting on adrenoceptors. Since this subject is comprehensively reviewed by TRENDELENBURG in Chapter 9 of this volume, the reader should refer to that chapter for a discussion of the separation of different sympathomimetic amines into directly-acting, indirectly-acting, and mixed-acting groups. However, it is well to recall here the two principal methods presently used to eliminate indirect actions: namely, (a) postganglionic sympathetic denervation of the tissue to be studied (resulting in degeneration of nerve terminals), and (b) appropriate pretreatment with reserpine of the animal whose tissues are to be studied. Pretreatment with reserpine, which depletes the stores of noradrenaline in nerve terminals, is the method most often used, because it is technically so much simpler than denervation. However, denervation has the added advantage of eliminating neuronal uptake of adrenergic agonists (see Section C.III. 5.).

Certainly, in comparisons of the relative potencies of a series of adrenergic agonists for the purpose of characterizing types of adrenoceptors, only directly-acting agonists should be employed. If one or more mixed-acting agonists are included in the series, then testing should be carried out on denervated preparations or preparations from reserpine-treated animals, so that response is only the result of direct action. Even when all agonists in a series are thought to be directly-acting, it is a good precaution to carry out some of the testing of relative potencies on preparations from reserpine-treated animals. This is so because an agonist which may be exclusively directly-acting on one kind of preparation may be mixed-acting on another. For example, dopamine appears to elicit contractions in normal rabbit aortic strips by direct action only (BESSE and FURCHGOTT, unpublished), but produces part of its inotropic response in normal guinea-pig atria by indirect action (PALM et al., 1967).

Even if an amine which has a definite component of indirect action still produces some response in a preparation depleted of endogenous noradrenaline, this does not necessarily mean that the response is due to direct action on an adrenoceptor, since it may be due to action on some other type of receptor (see Section III,C,4). To determine whether a response to an agonist in a reserpine-treated or denervated preparation is really due to a direct action on an adrenoceptor, a comparison should be made of the pA_2 (or K_B) of an appropriate reversible competitive antagonist acting against the agonist in question and against a known directly-acting adrenergic agonist. In a comparison of this type on the reserpine-pretreated rabbit aortic strip, it was found that much lower pA_2 values (or much higher K_B values) were obtained for phentolamine against amphetamine and tyramine than against phenylephrine — indicating that the direct actions of amphetamine and tyramine in this preparation are on some receptor (or receptors) other than the α-receptor (KOHLI, 1968; FURCHGOTT, 1970).

4. Responses which are the Resultant of Actions of an Agonist on More than One Type of Receptor

a) Actions on Both α- and β-Receptors

Errors in characterizing adrenoceptors pharmacologically have sometimes been made because the responses measured, in the case of one or more of the agonists being tested, have been the resultant of actions on more than one type of receptor. It has been appreciated for many years that certain smooth muscles, such as those of the resistance vessels in certain vascular beds, and those of the uterus in some species of mammals, contain both "motor" α- and "inhibitory" β-adrenoceptors (see Section I). In recent years, largely as a result of the availability of newer blocking agents, the presence of both α- and β-receptors has been revealed in many tissues which had previously been thought to contain only one type of receptor. Some of those tissues in which α-receptors have been revealed in the presence of "dominant" β-receptors are guinea-pig lung and trachea (NAGASAKA et al., 1964; PERSSON and JOHNSON, 1970), rat uterus (BRODY and DIAMOND, 1967); and guinea-pig and rabbit atria (GOVIER et al., 1966; BENFEY and VARMA, 1967; GOVIER, 1968). Examples of tissues in which β-receptors have been revealed in the presence of dominant α-receptors are the cat nictitating membrane (SMITH, 1963) and the mouse spleen (IGNARRO and TITUS, 1968).

Although in most test systems the responses to α- and β-receptor activation are in opposite directions, they are in the same direction in some systems. The best known examples of responses in the same direction are in the case of inhibition of a variety of intestinal smooth muscle preparations from different species, including man (e.g., see AHLQUIST and LEVY, 1959; FURCHGOTT, 1960; KOSTERLITZ and WATT, 1965; BENNETT, 1965). However, it should be noted that the mechanism of inhibition appears to be different for the intestinal α- and β-receptors (JENKINSON and MORTON, 1967; BÜLBRING and TOMITA, 1969; BOWMAN and HALL, 1970).

Another example of α- and β-receptors mediating responses in the same direction was discovered by GOVIER (1968) in an investigation of adrenergic agonists and antagonists on the isolated left atrium of the guinea-pig. Although the positive inotropic response evoked by all concentrations of adrenaline or noradrenaline appeared to be due principally to β-receptor activation, the response evoked by low concentrations of phenylephrine (a strong agonist for α-receptors but a very weak partial agonist for β-receptors) appeared to be due mainly to α-receptor activation. Interestingly enough, changes in the relative refractory period of atrial preparations brought about by activation of the two types of receptors are in opposite directions — lengthening with α-activation and shortening with β-activation (GOVIER et al., 1966; BENFEY and VARMA, 1967).

Frog heart also appears to have both α- and β-receptors for the mediation of positive inotropic responses. Whether activation of the α- or β-type contributes more to the response evoked by adrenaline or noradrenaline depends on whether the frog is a winter or summer frog, and on the temperature of the experiment. KUNOS and SZENTIVANYI (1968) and BUCKLEY and JORDAN (1970), in studies with α- and β-blocking agents, showed α-receptor activation to be dominant at low temperatures and β-receptor activation at high temperatures.

With any test preparation in which preliminary experiments indicate the existence of both α- and β-receptors, it is important that one type of receptor be effectively blocked when definitive experiments are carried out to determine the relative potencies of agonists on the other type. In experiments to determine the pA_2 or K_B of a competitive antagonist on one type of receptor, the preferred kind of agonist to use is one which has a much higher potency for activating the type of receptor under study in comparison to the other type present (e.g., phenylephrine in the case of α-receptors, and isoprenaline in the case of β-receptors). However, even when such a "selective" agonist is used, it is a worthwhile precaution to block the other type of receptor, especially when high concentrations of the agonist are required to compete with the antagonist. Satisfactory blockade of α-receptors can usually be obtained by adding 0.1—1.0 μg/ml of phentolamine to the bathing solution, or by pretreating the preparation with 1.0 μg/ml of dibenamine or 0.1 μg/ml of phenoxybenzamine for 20—30 min (FURCHGOTT, 1967). If phenoxybenzamine is used at a sufficiently high concentration in the pretreatment (from 1.0—30 μg/ml, depending on the preparation), it has the added advantage of blocking uptake mechanisms which remove adrenergic agonists from the region of the receptors (see Section III,C,5). For blocking β-receptors when α-receptors are under study, various competitive antagonists have been used, with propranolol probably being the most common in recent years. FURCHGOTT (1970) found that after β-receptors of the rabbit aortic strip were blocked with propanolol (0.1 to 1 μg/ml), the relative potency of adrenaline to noradrenaline increased from 0.8 to 1.2. Apparently, the lower relative potency in the absence of propranolol resulted from the much higher potency of adrenaline for activating the "subordinate" β-receptors in the preparation.

In using so-called selective blocking agents for the purpose of limiting the actions of adrenergic agonists to only one type of adrenoceptor, it must be remembered that many of these agents, especially when used in high concentrations, are likely to exert other actions, some of which can give misleading results. These other actions will be discussed in Section III,C,6. However, it may be well to point out at this time that many of the commonly employed, potent β-blocking agents, at concentrations about 100- to 1000-fold greater than those required for detectable blockade of β-receptors, begin to produce detectable blockade of α-receptors (MAZURKIEWICZ-KWILECKI, 1968; GULATI et al., 1969); and such high concentrations have often been exceeded by investigators when using these agents in attempts to block β-receptors selectively.

b) Actions Other than Those on α- or β-Receptors

In addition to the rather common problem of a response to an adrenergic agonist being the resultant of its actions on both α- and β-receptors, there is also the occasional problem of an action at sites which cannot be characterized as either α- or β-receptors. For example, MANLEY and LAWSON (1968), on the basis of a comparison of the ability of propranolol to block the vasodilating effect of isoprenaline, nylidrine and isoxsuprine in the dog hind limb, concluded that the last two agents (both of which are oxedrines with bulky N-substituents) owed much of their effect to actions at a site (or sites) other than the β-receptor. Indeed, vasodilation by isoxsuprine was hardly reduced by a dose of propranolol which almost completely blocked vasodilation by equi-active doses of isoprenaline.

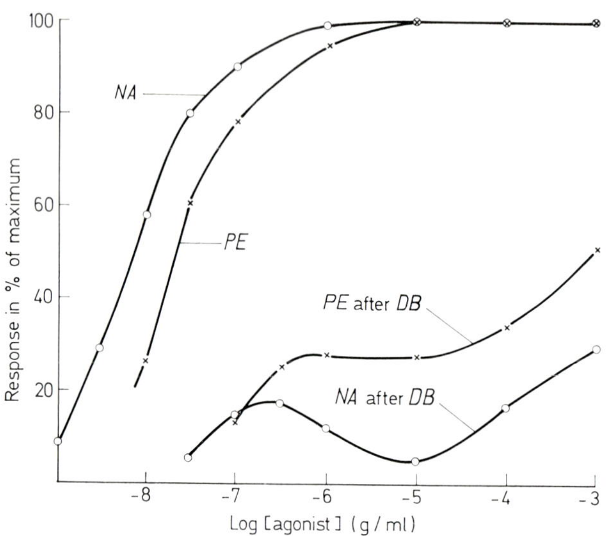

Fig. 5. Concentration-response curves for (—)-noradrenaline *(NA)* and (—)-phenylephrine *(PE)* on the rabbit aortic strip before and after irreversible blockade of a fraction of the α-receptors with dibenamine *(DB)*. Krebs-bicarbonate solution at 37° C. Concentrations in terms of the bitartrate of noradrenaline and the hydrochloride of phenylephrine. Strips from different rabbits. Exposure to dibenamine (1 μg/ml), 5 min. Decrease of response (relaxation) at intermediate concentrations of noradrenaline after dibenamine can be attributed to activation of β-receptors. Second rising phase of curves with both amines in very high concentration range is considered to be the result of an action on some kind of receptor other than the α-receptor responsible for the first rising phase

Additional actions of adrenergic agonists have sometimes been noted when unusually high concentrations of these agents have been used. For example, quantitative studies of the antagonism of phentolamine to various agonists for the α-receptor in rabbit aortic strips (from reserpine-treated animals) have provided evidence that ephedrine, a partial agonist for the α-receptor, produces part of its contractile response at very high concentrations by an action at some site other than the α-receptor (KOHLI, 1968; FURCHGOTT, 1970). Some evidence that even strong α-agonists like noradrenaline and phenylephrine, at very high concentrations, may stimulate contraction in aortic strips by a action on a second site, has been obtained in experiments in which a marked but incomplete irreversible blockade of α-receptors has first been achieved by pretreatment of the strips with dibenamine. Concentration-response curves from two experiments of this type are shown in Fig. 5. The curves show two distinct rising phases. The first phase is due to an action of the agonist on the well characterized α-receptor, but the second phase in the very high concentration range may well be due to action at another site. (Further treatment of the strip with dibenamine will completely block contractions, even at very high concentrations of the agonists, but this agent is known to be able to block receptors other than α-receptors (FURCHGOTT, 1966).)

An unusual example of a response to an adrenergic agonist being complicated by an action on a receptor other than an adrenoceptor was encountered in an investigation of the relative potencies of agonists for relaxing tracheal strips from reserpine-treated guinea-pigs (FURCHGOTT, 1970). The strips were pretreated with dibenamine to block α-receptors, and carbamylcholine was used in the bathing solution to produce a moderate level of tonic contraction. On this preparation two partial agonists for β-receptors, phenylephrine and synephrine (sympatol), gave log concentration-response curves for relaxation which showed two distinct falling phases, with the second phase becoming obvious at very high concentrations (>0.1 mg/ml). By using atropine in the bathing solution at a concentration of 10^{-7} M (about 200 times its K_B for the muscarinic receptor) and increasing the concentration of carbamylcholine as required to produce the same level of tonic contraction, it was possible to eliminate the second phase of relaxation elicited by phenylephrine and synephrine. It was concluded that only the first phase of the relaxation curves produced by these agonists was due to activation of β-receptors, and that the second phase was the result of their capacity at very high concentrations to compete with carbamylcholine for muscarinic receptors. In the same study, on the basis of experiments using propranolol as well as atropine, it was concluded that all relaxation produced by ephedrine (D(—) or racemic) on reserpine-pretreated strips initially contracted by carbamylcholine or methacholine, was due to competition by the ephedrine for the muscarinic receptors. When ephedrine reacted with β-receptors, it exerted no agonistic action, but only acted as a competitive antagonist to true agonists. It is also likely, in the study of FARMER and COLEMAN (1970) on relaxation of isolated guinea-pig trachea contracted by transmural electrical stimulation, that the second and steeper phase of the log dose-response curve obtained with phenylephrine was also due to its competing at high concentrations for the muscarinic receptors acted on by endogenous acetylcholine released by the electrical stimulation.

The phenomenon of autoinhibition— that is, a decrease in response with increase in concentration of agonist above a concentration giving a maximal response — has been reported with adrenergic agonists in a few test systems in which it is unlikely that a combination of activation of α- and β-receptors was responsible for the phenomenon. TRENDELENBURG et al. (1963), investigating changes in spontaneous rate of isolated atria from reserpine-treated guinea-pigs, found striking autoinhibition in the case of several sympathomimetic amines — with the descending limbs of log concentration-response curves often showing a net decrease below the basal rate. Not only was autoinhibition found in the case of partial agonists for the β-receptor of the atrial pacemaker, such as phenylephrine and sympatol, but also in the case of noradrenaline at extremely high concentrations (2 μg/ml depressing the rate to the basal level).

Autoinhibition has frequently been reported in the case of the lipolytic response of isolated adipose tissue of the rat to catecholamines (e.g., see ČERNOHORSKÝ et al., 1967; FASSINA, 1967). HIMMS-HAGEN (1970) has proposed that autoinhibition in this system is caused by an activation of α-receptors by the amines at higher concentrations, which produces an effect which is opposed to that produced by activation of β-receptors (i.e., activation of α-receptors decreases lipolysis by inhibiting the formation of the mediating cyclic AMP). However, convincing experimental evidence in support of this hypothesis is presently not available. Recently, ALLEN et al. (1969), investigating the lipolytic response of isolated fat cells of the rat to isoprenaline, adrenaline and noradrenaline, found not only the usual autoinhibition as the concentration was increased to about 10 μM, but also a second phase of stimulation followed by a second phase of autoinhibition as the concentration was increased further. Propranolol antagonized the first phase of lipolytic stimulation but not the second; and the α-blocking agent phentolamine at a very high concentration (10^{-4} M) appeared to partially block the first phase in a noncompetitive manner, but had very little effect on the second phase. Certainly, the complex "double-humped" log concentration-response curve of ALLEN and coworkers must reflect other actions of the adrenergic agonists in addition to their recognized action on the β-receptor of the fat cells.

A special type of second action of an agonist, which influences the degree of response produced, is that which is sometimes encountered when a racemic mixture of an agonist is used. For example, the maximal contraction obtainable with racemic isoprenaline is significantly less than that with (—)-isoprenaline on rabbit aortic strips (FURCHGOTT, 1955) and rat vas deferens (ARIËNS, 1967). ARIËNS demonstrated that the lower maximum was caused by the (+)-isomer of the racemate competing as an antagonist for the α-receptor which is stimulated by the (—)-isomer. A similar situation has been demonstrated in the case of racemic ephedrine acting on α-receptors of aortic strips, where the (—)-isomer is an active partial agonist and the (+)-isomer is a competitive antagonist (LAPIDUS et al., 1967). Findings such as these should make the investigator wary of the possibility of competitive antagonism between stereoisomers in racemates, especially when high concentrations are required to produce responses.

5. Removal of the Agonist from the Region of the Receptor

a) Removal Processes and their Influence on Relative Potencies of Agonists

In the ideal test system for pharmacologically characterizing receptors, the concentration of the free agonist in the region of the receptors at the time a response is measured should be in thermodynamic equilibrium with both agonist bound to receptors and with free agonist in the bathing or perfusing solution. If there is some active process (or processes) in the tissue preparation which continuously removes the agonist from the region of the receptors, then equilibrium cannot be achieved, even though an essentially steady-state condition may be (FURCHGOTT, 1955; WAUD, 1969). The extent to which the concentration in the region of the receptors falls short of being at equilibrium will depend on the rate of removal of the agonist from the region of the receptors (sometimes called the "biophase") by this process (or processes) as compared to the rate of diffusion of the agonist from that region back into the bathing or perfusing solution (sometimes called the "aqueous phase"). Obviously, if the rate of removal differs for different agonists being compared for potency in a test system, the relative potencies of those agonists which are removed most rapidly will be underestimated.

In Chapter 15 of this volume TRENDELENBURG has discussed in detail the nature of the different processes which remove noradrenaline and related adrenergic agonists in tissues, and therefore only a brief discussion of these processes will be presented here to serve as a background for the remainder of this section.

Recognized removal processes include both transport of the agonist into cells (uptake processes) and enzymic inactivation. (Removal also may result from adsorption at binding sites in the tissue, but such a process will be self-limiting once the bound agonist comes to equilibrium with free agonist). Active transport into adrenergic nerve terminals appears to be the dominant removal process for noradrenaline and adrenaline in many tissues when they are exposed to low concentrations of these agonists. This active transport has been called Uptake_1 by IVERSEN (1966). In some tissues a second uptake process becomes evident at concentrations of noradrenaline and adrenaline above those which essentially saturate the $Uptake_1$ process, and has been called the $Uptake_2$ process by IVERSEN. It now appears that $Uptake_2$ involves transport of the agonist into non-neuronal cells of the responding tissue. Rather selective inhibitors of $Uptake_1$ (e.g., cocaine and desipramine) and $Uptake_2$ (e.g., normetanephrine) are known. Phenoxybenzamine is a potent inhibitor of both uptake processes. It is worth noting that inhibition of uptake by cocaine is of a reversible competitive type; whereas inhibition of uptake by phenoxybenzamine is essentially irreversible (FURCHGOTT, 1966).

The two recognized enzymes which can inactivate adrenergic agonists, if the latter have appropriate chemical structures, are monoamine oxidase (MAO) and catechol-O-methyltransferase (COMT). It does not appear that MAO, an intracellular enzyme, has a primary role in removing noradrenaline from the region of the receptors, since inhibition of MAO does not potentiate the response to this amine in normal isolated tissues. However, intracellular MAO can deaminate noradrenaline taken up into adrenergic nerves and other cells if the intracellular storage and binding capacity for the amine in these cells is exceded.

COMT may contribute to removal of catecholamines from the region of the receptors, but its relative importance compared to uptake processes will depend on the tissue and the catecholamine. Recent evidence indicates that COMT is an intracellular enzyme in non-neuronal cells, and that a membrane transport system is required for movement of catecholamines into these cells. Since the agents which block access of noradrenaline to COMT also reduce the amounts of this catecholamine accumulated extraneuronally, it appears that the membrane transport mechanism allowing catecholamines to gain access to COMT may well be the $Uptake_2$ mechanism.

Neuronal uptake ($Uptake_1$) appears to be the principal mechanism for removing noradrenaline in isolated guinea-pig left atria, since the increase in sensitivity to this amine in this preparation produced by cocaine (about 30-fold) is essentially the same as that produced by phenoxybenzamine (FURCHGOTT et al., 1963). In the same preparation cocaine produces no significant increase in sensitivity to isoprenaline, whereas phenoxybenzamine produces a small increase (1.5 to2-fold) (FURCHGOTT, 1967). This finding indicates a lack of effective removal of isoprenaline by neuronal uptake (a conclusion supported by chemical and pharmacological findings of others), and possibly some removal by the $Uptake_2$ mechanism. In the case of guinea-pig isolated trachea, the pharmacological and chemical findings of FOSTER (1967, 1968, 1969) indicate that both $Uptake_1$ and $Uptake_2$ are active in the removal of noradrenaline, with the former being dominant. In this preparation, maximal sensitization to noradrenaline produced by cocaine or desipramine was 30 to 40-fold, while that produced by phenoxybenzamine was about 80-fold. On the other hand, Foster's findings indicate that the $Uptake_2$ mechanism is the only important one for removing isoprenaline in trachea. Sensitivity to this catecholamine could be increased about 20-fold with phenoxybenzamine and over 10-fold with normetanephrine, but not at all with cocaine or desipramine.

The influence of inhibiting neuronal uptake on the relative potencies of noradrenaline, adrenaline, isoprenaline and phenylephrine for responses mediated by β-receptors in selected isolated tissues from rabbit and guinea-pig are shown in Table 2 (FURCHGOTT, 1967). Cocaine was used as the inhibitor in the smooth muscle preparations, and phenoxybenzamine in the cardiac preparations. In all the preparations except rabbit aorta and rabbit duodenum, inhibition of neuronal uptake significantly altered the measured relative potencies of the series of agonists; and at the same time considerably increased the sensitivity to noradrenaline, the reference agonist (about 5 to 25 times, depending on the preparation). In these preparations sensitivity was also increased to adrenaline (but less than to noradrenaline) and slightly increased to phenylephrine. Sensitivity to isoprenaline was only increased in atria pretreated with phenoxybenzamine, and then only slightly. Thus, in all of these preparations neuronal uptake apparently caused a considerable error in the estimation of potencies. In the case of rabbit aorta and rabbit duodenum, the rate of neuronal uptake from the region of the receptors was apparently too low — as evidenced by less than a two-fold sensitization to noradrenaline after cocaine — to have much influence on measured relative potencies.

In the experiments with rabbit and guinea-pig atria (Table 2), phenoxybenzamine was used for the purpose of blocking neuronal uptake, but in view of recent findings (see above), it was probably blocking extraneuronal uptake as well. If extraneuronal as well as neuronal uptake had also been blocked in the other preparations, the relative potencies in some cases may have been further altered, and closer to the true relative potencies of the agonists at the receptor level. It seems likely that this would have been the case for guinea-pig trachea, in which there appears to be an effective extraneuronal uptake system for isoprenaline (FOSTER, 1967, 1968, 1969).

KAUMANN (1968) showed that inhibition of COMT caused a six-fold increase in sensitivity of cat papillary muscle to isoprenaline, and concluded that inactivation by COMT is the major process for removal of this catecholamine in this tissue. In rabbit aortic strips, both uptake and inactivation by COMT appear to contribute to the removal of noradrenaline and adrenaline from the region of the receptors (KALSNER and NICKERSON, 1969a; LEVIN and FURCHGOTT, 1970). To explain the capacity of both cocaine and a COMT inhibitor (4-tropolone acetamide) to potentiate moderately the response to noradrenaline (or adrenaline), whether or not the other agent was already present, LEVIN and FURCHGOTT (1970) postulated that neuronal uptake is the dominant mechanism for removing noradrenaline in the region of the smooth muscle cells of the aortic media close to the adventitia (where innervation is rich), while O-methylation is the dominant mechanism in the region of cells more distant from the adventitia.

For a generalized block of uptake processes in test preparations in which the pharmacological characteristics of β-receptors are under study, an appropriate pretreatment with phenoxybenzamine is recommended. Such a pretreatment has the added advantage of blocking α-receptors in the preparation. However, since phenoxybenzamine and related haloalkylamines can also release endogenous catecholamines in some tissues (FURCHGOTT and KIRPEKAR, 1963), preparations from reserpine-treated animals are preferable when these agents are used as blockers.

There is no single agent known to block both neuronal and extraneuronal uptake effectively without having some action on α-receptors (either blockade or stimulation). Recent work with GD 131 (N-cyclohexyl-methyl-N-ethyl-β-chloroethylamine), indicates that an appropriate pretreatment with this haloalkylamine can effectively block extraneuronal uptake in aortic strips before it effectively blocks α-receptors (KALSNER and NICKERSON, 1969b; LEVIN and FURCHGOTT, 1970); but unfortunately, the more intense pretreatment with GD 131 necessary to block neuronal uptake also blocks α-receptors.

It should be remembered that agents which are used to block removal processes often have additional actions which may interfere with proper testing of agonists and antagonists, and these actions should be recognized and avoided, if possible. Some of these actions may be exerted on the adrenoceptors under study, either directly or indirectly (by the release of endogenous catecholamine). Other inter-

Table. 2. *Relative potencies of adrenergic agonists for responses mediated by β-receptors before and after treatment to block uptake mechanism of adrenergic nerve terminals*

Tissue[a]	Response Measured	Treatment to Block Uptake[b]	Relative Potencies[c]			
			ISO	A	N	PE
Rabbit thoracic aorta (α-receptors blocked)	Relaxation of acetylcholine contraction	None	130	65	1	0.2
		Cocaine 10^{-5} g/ml	~130	65	1	0.1
Rabbit stomach muscle (α-receptors blocked)	Relaxation of carbamylcholine contraction	None	10	2.5	1	~ .003
		Cocaine 10^{-5} g/ml	2.5	1.2	1	~ .003
Rabbit left atrium (frequency 1/sec)	Increase in amplitude of contraction	None	70	1.3	1	
		PBZ 3×10^{-5}, 20 min	3.5	0.5	1	
Rabbit duodenum (α-receptors blocked)	Decrease in amplitude of contraction	None	3.5	0.3	1	< .01
		Cocaine 10^{-5} g/ml	1.5	0.2	1	< .01
Guinea-pig trachea (α-receptors blocked)	Relaxation of carbamylcholine contraction	None	160	25	1	0.2
		Cocaine 10^{-5} g/ml	47	12	1	0.06
Guinea-pig duodenum (α-receptors blocked)	Relaxation of carbamylcholine contraction	None	20	1	1	
		Cocaine 10^{-5} g/ml	3	0.5	1	
Guinea-pig left atrium (frequency 1/sec)	Increase in amplitude of contraction	None	70	1.2	1	< .1
		Cocaine 10^{-5} g/ml or PBZ 10^{-5}, 20 min	4.0	0.5	1	< .01

[a] All tissues were in Krebs bicarbonate solution at 37° C. *Alpha*-receptors were blocked by adequate pretreatment of the tissues with dibenamine or phenoxybenzamine (PBZ) or by having 10^{-6} to 10^{-7} g/ml of phentolamine in the Krebs solution. Strips of rabbit stomach muscle were from the fundic region. (From FURCHGOTT, 1967)

[b] PBZ, phenoxybenzamine

[c] ISO, isoprenaline; A, adrenaline; N, noradrenaline; PE, phenylephrine

fering actions are less specific. For example, cocaine in excessively high doses depresses all muscle preparations, and the COMT inhibitor, pyrogallol, is toxic to a number of tissues.

b) Influence of Removal Processes on Potencies of Competitive Antagonists

BLINKS (1967) and FURCHGOTT (1967) independently found with the isolated guinea-pig left atrium that a competitive β-antagonist produced a smaller displacement of the log [agonist]-response curve to the right when the agonist was noradrenaline than when it was isoprenaline. Using the agonist dose ratio (*dr*) obtained in experiments with 1.13 μM pronethalol for calculation of K_B values (see equation 3 in Section III,B,2), FURCHGOTT found the calculated value when noradrenaline was the agonist to be about 5 to 10 times higher than that when

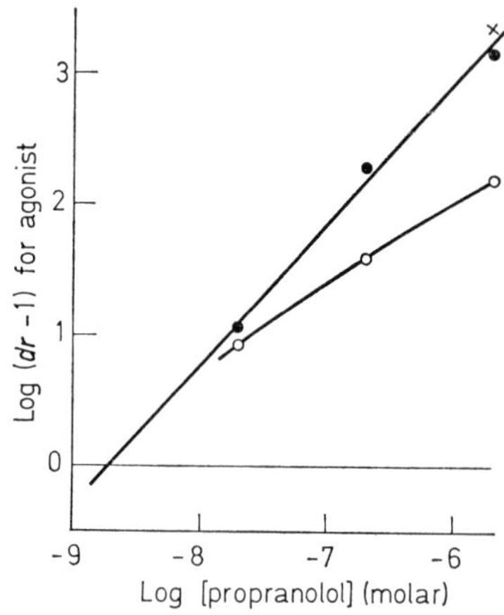

Fig. 6. Plot of log (*dr*—1) against log [antagonist] for propranolol-isoprenaline antagonism and propranolol-noradrenaline antagonism in the isolated left atrium of the guinea-pig. Response measured was increase in force of contraction. Krebs-bicarbonate solution at 32.5° C. Exposure to propranolol, 60 min. ● isoprenaline as agonist (1 experiment); ○ noradrenaline as agonist (1 experiment); × noradrenaline as agonist in presence of 2×10^{-5} M cocaine (mean of 6 or more experiments). Plotted points in the figure were calculated from ED_{50} values for the agonists in the presence and absence of propranolol. These ED_{50} values were estimated from the published log concentration-response curves of BLINKS (1967)

isoprenaline was the agonist. Figure 6 shows the result of BLINKS in a plot of log (*dr*—1) against log [propranolol]. It will be noted that the slope of the curve with isoprenaline as the agonist is essentially unity, as expected from receptor theory; but the slope with noradrenaline as the agonist is definitely less than unity — reflecting the smaller displacement of the log [noradrenaline]-response curve. Both BLINKS and FURCHGOTT attributed the smaller displacement to an influence of the neuronal uptake process, since the displacement with noradrenaline as the agonist could be made equal to that with isoprenaline by blocking the neuronal uptake process with cocaine. FURCHGOTT considered that the smaller displacement of the log [noradrenaline]-response curve by the antagonist in the absence of cocaine was due to blockade of the uptake process by the antagonist itself, with this blockade tending to potentiate the response to noradrenaline and thus partially counteract the effect of blockade of the β-receptors. BLINKS also considered such a possibility; however, he also proposed that the high concentrations of noradrenaline required in the presence of the antagonist might tend to saturate ("swamp") the uptake process and so diminish its effectiveness in limiting the concentration of noradrenaline in the region of the receptors. It now seems likely in the case of both propranalol-noradrenaline and pronethalol-noradrenaline antagonism in the guinea-pig atrium that this latter proposal of BLINKS best explains the divergence of experimental results from the predictions of receptor theory. Although both of these antagonists have been shown to inhibit uptake (IVERSEN, 1966; FOO et al., 1968), the concentrations required for effective inhibition are considerably higher than those which are required for effective competitive blockade of β-receptors of the guinea-pig atrium.

On isolated guinea-pig tracheal chains, noradrenaline is also antagonized less than isoprenaline by equivalent concentrations of propranolol (smaller shift of log [agonist]-relaxation response curve) (FOSTER, 1966; MOORE and O'DONNELL, 1970). MOORE and O'DONNELL attributed the difference to an influence of neuronal uptake, since noradrenaline, in the presence of cocaine, was antagonized by propranolol to the same extent as was isoprenaline. Moreover, the slope of the log (*dr*—1) — log [propranolol] curve for noradrenaline, which was 0.77 without cocaine, approached the theoretical value of 1.0 in the presence of this blocker of neuronal uptake. MOORE and O'DONNELL also found cocaine to have a similar effect on the pattern of antagonism for LB46 (4-(2-hydroxy-3-isopropylamino-propoxy)-indole), a β-antagonist several times more potent than propranolol.

The results of LANGER and TRENDELENBURG (1969) on noradrenaline-phentolamine antagonism in the isolated nictitating membrane are shown in Fig. 7. The slope of the log (*dr*—1) — log [phentolamine] curve for the denervated membrane is close to unity, in good agreement with receptor theory; but the slope of the curve for the normal membrane is about 0.3 for lower concentrations of phentolamine and only approaches unity at the higher concentrations. The divergence of the experimental data obtained on the normal membrane from the prediction of receptor theory was attributed to the operation of the saturable neuronal uptake system for noradrenaline in this preparation, since a similar divergence could be shown when hypothetical log concentration-response curves were constructed on the basis of a "model" for a saturable uptake system operating on an agonist in the presence of a competitive antagonist (LANGER and TRENDELENBURG, 1969; WAUD, 1969). (For further discussion of this "model" and its predictions about the influence of a saturable uptake system on the slopes of log dose-response curves, the reader is referred to Chapter 15 by TRENDELENBURG in this volume).

If the first three plotted points on the curve for the normal membrane in Fig. 7 are used to calculate K_B values for phentolamine, the calculated values increase progressively. Moreover, if only that part of the curve fitting the points for the two highest concentrations of phentolamine (where slope is close to unity) is extrapolated downward, it gives an estimated pA_2 of 6.0 for this antagonist — in contrast to a pA_2 of 7.15 estimated from the full linear curve in the case of the denervated membrane. When methoxamine, rather than noradrenaline, was used as the agonist, the slope of the log (*dr*—1)— log [phentolamine] curve was close to unity in the normal as well as in the denervated membrane (TRENDELENBURG et al., 1970). This is what would be predicted on the basis of the saturable uptake model, since methoxamine is an α-agonist which is not removed by neuronal uptake.

From the various examples already cited in this section, it is clear that the operation of a saturable uptake process for an agonist can result in erroneously low estimates of pA_2 values and erroneously high estimates of K_B values for the competitive antagonist used against the agonist. When a curve for log (dr—1) against log [antagonist] has a slope which is significantly lower than unity, consideration should always be given to the possibility that a saturable removal process for the agonist is responsible for this deviation from the prediction of

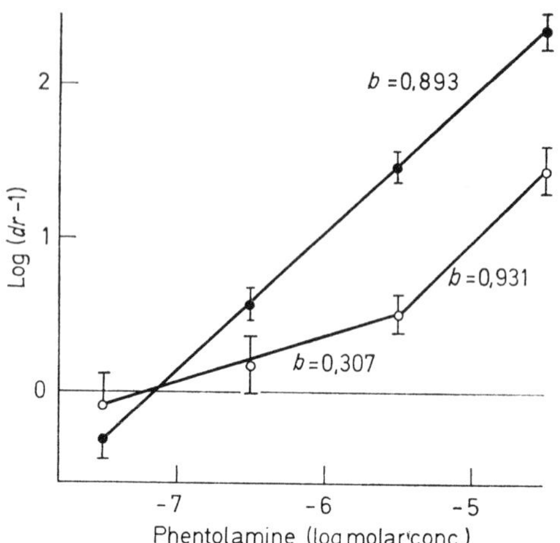

Fig. 7. Plot of log (dr—1) against log [antagonist] for phentolamine-noradrenaline antagonism on the isolated nictitating membrane of the cat. Krebs-bicarbonate solution at 37° C. Exposure to phentolamine, 15 min. Shown are means (± S.E. as bars) for 4—5 experiments per group. ● denervated nictitating membrane; ○ normal nictitating membrane. b indicates slope. Slopes for normal membrane were calculated for the three lowest concentrations and for the two highest concentrations of phentolamine. (Reprinted from LANGER and TRENDELENBURG (1969), with permission of the authors and publisher)

receptor theory. Before citing other examples from the literature of curves of this type with low slopes, it is well to derive an equation for the saturable uptake model system which will permit us to construct hypothetical log (dr—1) — log [antagonist] curves, with which actual experimental curves can be compared.

To derive the desired equation, we begin with two basic equations for the saturable uptake model under steady-state conditions. These two equations, which are similar to those of WAUD (1969) but with some change of symbols, are:

$$U = k\,([\mathrm{A_a}] - [\mathrm{A_b}]), \tag{8}$$

where U is rate of uptake, $[\mathrm{A_a}]$ is the concentration of agonist in the external solution, $[\mathrm{A_b}]$ the concentration in the biophase (i.e., region of receptors and uptake system), and k is a diffusion coefficient for flow of the agonist between external solution and biophase (inverse of WAUD' resistance term, R); and

$$U = \frac{U_m\,[\mathrm{A_b}]}{[\mathrm{A_b}] + K_{AU}}, \tag{9}$$

where U_m is the maximal rate of uptake when the system is saturated, and K_{AU} is the constant characterizing the saturable system (Michaelis-Menten type of kinetics). It is assumed that removal of agonist from the biophase by any process other than that of the specified uptake system is negligible in comparison to removal by diffusion back into the external solution (given by $k\,[\mathrm{A_b}]$).

Combining equations (8) and (9) gives:

$$\frac{[\mathrm{A_b}]}{[\mathrm{A_a}]} = \frac{[\mathrm{A_b}] + K_{AU}.}{[\mathrm{A_b}] + K_{AU} + U_m/k}\,. \tag{10}$$

Before continuing, a few comments should be made about this equation. It can be seen that when $[A_b] \ll K_{AU}$, the ratio of $[A_b]/[A_a]$ will be given by $K_{AU}/(K_{AU}+U_m/k)$. For example, if U_m/k is 24 times K_{AU}, then the ratio will be 1/25. In this situation total block of uptake (U_m reduced to zero) will raise the ratio to 1, and cause a 25-fold increase in sensitivity to the added agonist. On the other hand, when $[A_b] \gg K_{AU}$ (i.e., the uptake system is essentially saturated), $[A_b]/[A_a]$ will be essentially 1, and blockade of uptake will no longer cause an increase in sensitivity to the agonist. LANGER and TRENDELENBURG (1969) call the region in which $[A_b] \ll K_{AU}$, Region I; that in which $[A_b] \gg K_{AU}$, Region III; and that in between, Region II.

The final desired equation is derived from equation 10 and equation 3 (Section III,B,2). It is first appropriate to rewrite equation 3 as:

$$[A_b]/[A_b]_o = (1 + [B]/K_B), \tag{11}$$

with $[A_b]$ and $[A_b]_o$ representing the concentrations of agonist required in the region of the receptors to give equal $[RA]/[R_t]$ values, and hence equal responses, in the presence and absence of the antagonist, respectively. Combining this equation with equation 10, and rearranging, gives:

$$[A_a] = [A_b]_o (1 + [B]/K_B) \left\{ 1 + \frac{\dfrac{U_m}{k \cdot K_{AU}}}{1 + \dfrac{[A_b]_o (1 + [B]/K_B)}{K_{AU}}} \right\}. \tag{12}$$

This equation allows the calculation of equi-active relative concentrations of agonist in the external solution (i.e., $[A_a]$ relative to $[A_b]_o$) for any value of $[B]/K_B$, provided values are given to the two constant terms, $U_m/k \cdot K_{AU}$ and $[A_b]_o/K_{AU}$. Thus, the dose ratio (*dr*) for A_a may be obtained for different values of $[B]/K_B$ and used for plotting theoretical curves for log (*dr*—1) against log ($[B]/K_B$).

Figure 8 shows a series of curves obtained with equation 12, when $U_m/k \cdot K_{AU}$ is set at 24, and $[A_b]_o/K_{AU}$ is varied from .01 to 100. (The value of 24 for $U_m/k \cdot K_{AU}$ is not unreasonable, for it permits a 25-fold increase in sensitivity to $[A_a]$ as a result of complete block of uptake if initially $[A_b] \ll K_{AU}$ — an increase often exceeded experimentally in the case of noradrenaline following block of neuronal uptake in certain tissues). The degree of saturation of the uptake system in the absence of antagonist depends on the value of $[A_b]_o/K_{AU}$ (see equation 9). From Fig. 8 it is apparent that when $[A_b]_o/K_{AU}$ is 100 or greater, the slope of the whole curve is essentially 1, and the estimated pA_2 value is very little different from the true pA_2 obtained from the "control" curve representing no uptake process. When $[A_b]_o/K_{AU}$ is 10 or 1, most of the curve still has a slope close to 1, but a pA_2 value estimated from extrapolation of the linear portion of the curve is significantly less than the true pA_2 (by about 0.5 and 1.0 log units, respectively). A situation of this kind might possibly account for the results of FOSTER (1966) on propranolol-noradrenaline antagonism in guinea-pig trachea; for he obtained a curve with a slope close to unity, yet his estimate of the pA_2 for propranolol was considerably lower than estimates made by others.

When $[A_b]_o/K_{AU}$ is 0.316, the average slope of the curve over the lower range of log $[B]/K_B$ (from 0—2) is only about 0.5, but in the higher range the slope approaches 1. This curve is very similar in its characteristics to the experimental curve of LANGER and TRENDELENBURG (1969) for phentolamine-noradrenaline antagonism in the isolated nictitating membrane (Fig. 7). When $[A_b]/K_{AU}$ is 0.1 or less, the slope of the curve is triphasic: beginning close to 1, then decreasing over an intermediate range of log $[B]/K_B$ (the lower $[A_b]_o/K_{AU}$, the higher is this range), and finally increasing again to 1. The lower portion of such a curve would give a fairly accurate estimate of the pA_2 (or K_B), but estimates of pA_2 (or K_B) based on extrapolation of selected upper portions of the curve would obviously be in error. It might be noted that the curve for $[A_b]_0/K_{AU}$ set at 0.01,

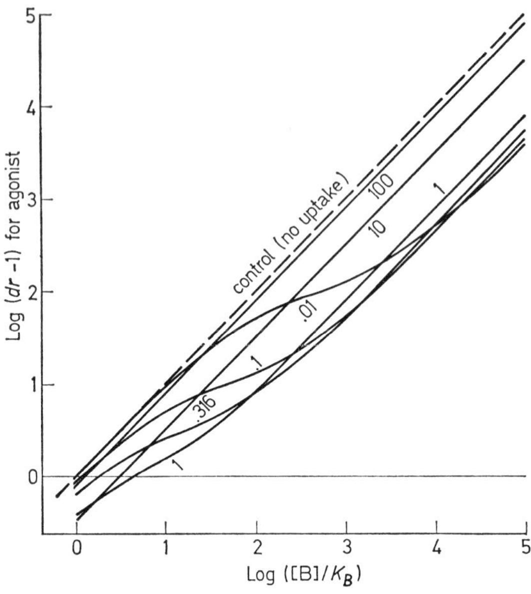

Fig. 8. Theoretical curves for log (dr—1) as a function of log ($[B]/K_B$) (constructed with the use of Equation 12) for a model system with a saturable uptake process for removing the agonist from the region of the receptors. For all curves $U_m/k \cdot K_{AU}$ set at 24. Values for $[A_b]_0/K_{AU}$ are shown next to corresponding curves. (See text for further details)

over the range of log $[B]/K_B$ from 1—3, closely resembles the experimental curve in Fig. 6, based on BLINKS' data for propranolol-noradrenaline antagonism in guinea-pig left atrium.

In some investigations on isolated tracheal preparations, data on the antagonism of various β-blocking agents toward isoprenaline have fitted log (dr—1) — log [antagonist] curves with slopes close to 1 (e.g., see MOORE and O'DONNELL (1970) and CHAHL and O'DONNELL (1967) for guinea-pig trachea); but in other investigations such data have better fitted curves with slopes significantly lower than 1 (e.g., see PATIL (1968) and LEVY and WASSERMAN (1970) for guinea-pig trachea, and BRISTOW et al. (1970) for rabbit trachea). PATIL found slopes ranging from 0.46—0.75 in the case of seven different moderately potent antagonists, and slopes approaching 1 only in the case of two very weak antagonists. Figure 9 illustrates Patil's findings with the stereoisomers and desoxy analogue of sotalol (MJ 1999; 4-(2-isopropylamino-1-hydroxyethyl) methanesulfonanilide). BRISTOW et al. found slopes ranging from 0.5—0.8 in the case of three different antagonists.

Since FOSTER (1967, 1968, 1969) has presented evidence that isoprenaline is removed by an active uptake process, probably extraneuronal, in guinea-pig trachea, the question arises whether all of the lower slopes obtained in the studies cited above can be explained by an increasing saturation of the uptake sites by isoprenaline with increasing concentrations of this agonist. This explanation is not sufficient, since it would demand that all log (dr—1) — log [antagonist] curves should have the same slope, regardless of the antagonist used. To explain the variations in slope found with different antagonists, it is proposed that they reflect the influence of competitive blockade of the uptake sites by some of the antagonists used to block β-receptors. Just as equation 12 was derived for a

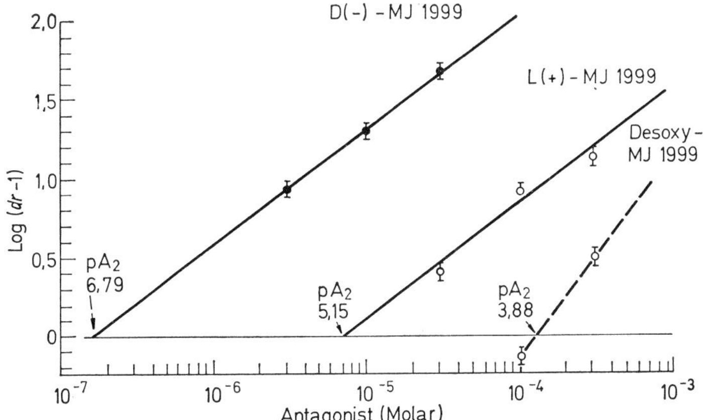

Fig. 9. Plot of log (dr—1) against log [antagonist] for antagonism between (—)-isoprenaline and (—)-MJ 1999 (●—●), (+)-MJ 1999 (O—O) and desoxy-MJ 1999 (O- - -O) on the isolated tracheal chain of the guinea-pig. Krebs-bicarbonate solution at 37.5° C, containing methacholine (10^{-7} M) to produce initial tone. Exposure to antagonist, 30 min. Shown are means ($\pm$ S.E. at bars). Slopes of regression lines for (—)-MJ 1999, (+)-MJ 1999 and desoxy-MJ 1999 are 0.72, 0.73, and 1.23, respectively. (Reprinted from PATIL (1968), with permission of the author and publisher)

model system with a saturable uptake process for the agonist, a more complex equation can be derived for a model system in which the antagonist competes with the agonist for uptake sites, as well as for receptor sites. The equation is:

$$[A_a] = [A_b]_o\,(1 + [B]/K_B)\left\{1 + \frac{\dfrac{U_m}{k \cdot K_{AU}}}{1 + \dfrac{[A_b]_o\,(1 + [B]/K_B)}{K_{AU}} + \dfrac{[B]}{K_B} \cdot \dfrac{K_B}{K_{BU}}}\right\}. \tag{13}$$

In this equation K_{BU} is the dissociation constant of the uptake site-antagonist complex. It is assumed that the antagonist which competes with the agonist for uptake sites is not itself effectively removed by the uptake process.

Figure 10 shows a series of curves obtained with equation 13 when $U_m/k \cdot K_{AU}$ is set at 24, $[A_b]_o/K_{AU}$ is set at .01, and K_B/K_{BU} is varied from .001—100. It is apparent from this figure that the slope of the curve can vary greatly, depending on the value of K_B/K_{BU}. This constant term, in effect, gives the ratio of the affinities of the antagonist for the uptake sites and the receptor sites, respectively. When this ratio is higher than 1, the initial slope of the curve (at the level of log (dr—1) equal zero) is even greater than 1, and the estimated pA_2 value would be much lower than the true pA_2 value. When K_B/K_{BU} is 1, the slope of the curve is essentially 1 throughout, but the estimate of pA_2 is still low (by 1.4 units), and that of K_B is too high. When K_B/K_{BU} is decreased below 1, the initial slope of the curve begins to decrease, reaching a level somewhat below 0.5 when K_B/K_{BU} is set at .316. As K_B/K_{BU} becomes very low (.001 or less), the antagonist no longer successfully competes with the agonist for the uptake sites, and the shape of the curve is determined by increasing saturation of the uptake sites by the agonist alone.

It is interesting to compare the experimental results of PATIL, shown in Fig. 9, with the theoretical curves of Fig. 10. With proper alignment of the abscissa scales of the two figures, there is a reasonably good fit of the plotted points for D(—)-MJ 1999 on the curve where K_B/K_{BU} is 0.001; those points for L(+)-MJ 1999 on the curve where K_B/K_{BU} is 0.03; and those points for desoxy-MJ 1999 on the curve where K_B/K_{BU} is 2.

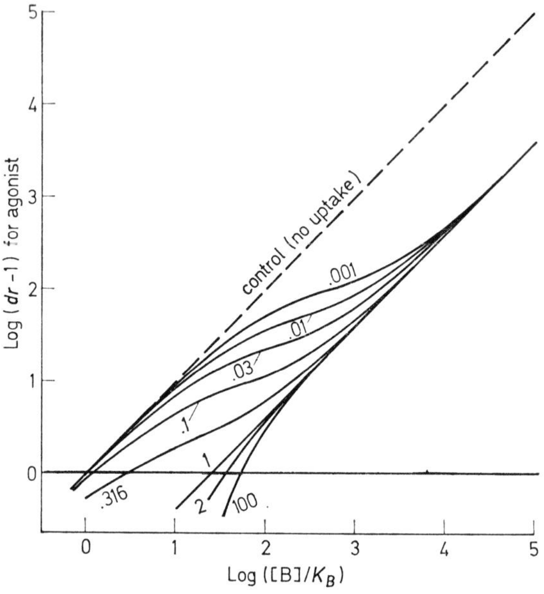

Fig. 10. Theoretical curves for log (dr—1) as a function of log ([B]/K_B) (constructed with the use of Equation 13) for a model system with a saturable uptake process which removes the agonist from the region of the receptors, and which can be competitively inhibited by the antagonist. $U_m/k \cdot K_{AU}$ was set at 24, and $[A_b]_o/K_{AU}$ was set at 0.01. Values for K_B/K_{BU} are shown next to corresponding curves. (See text for further details)

WENKE et al. (1967), in an investigation of antagonism between isoprenaline and various competitive antagonists on the lipolytic response in isolated fat cells of the rat, obtained results not unlike those of PATIL (1968) and BRISTOW et al. (1970) in their studies on isolated trachea. A plot of the data of WENKE and co-workers in the form of log (dr—1) against log [antagonist] gives best-fitting curves for the various antagonists used that vary in slope from about 0.5 to a little greater than 1. These workers attempted to explain their results on the basis of a trimolecular reaction between isoprenaline and the β-receptor (to form RA_2), and either a bimolecular or a trimolecular reaction between the antagonist and the receptor (to give either RB or RB_2), depending on the antagonist used. However, it appears to this reviewer that a more reasonable explanation of these results on rat fat cells is the same as that proposed to explain the results of the other workers on trachea: namely, that they reflect competition of certain of the antagonists with isoprenaline for a saturable uptake mechanism as well as for β-receptors. Perhaps a saturable uptake mechanism also accounts for the observation of WENKE et al. (1967) on the steeper log concentration-lipolytic response curves for catecholamines than for corresponding oxedrines. These workers hypothesized that the difference was due to the formation of an RA_2 complex with catecholamines, in contrast to an RA complex with oxedrines. However, a simpler explanation is that the catecholamines, but not the oxedrines, were removed by an active saturable uptake process (or processes); for such a situation could lead to relatively steeper curves for the former compounds (LANGER and TRENDELENBURG, 1969).

Returning to equations 12 and 13, it is apparent that the value of the term $U_m/k \cdot K_{AU}$ determines the potential maximal deviation that will occur in a family of curves with respect to the "control" curve representing no effective uptake process. For example, if this term were 1.0 (rather than 24, as in the illustrations given), then deviations for all curves would be small, and any curve would give a fairly close estimate of the true pA_2 or K_B value.

It is also apparent from equation 13 that if K_B/K_{BU} is considerably greater than 1 (indicating considerably greater affinity of antagonist for uptake sites than for receptor sites) and if $[A_b]_0/K_{AU}$ is considerably less than 1, increasing the concentration of antagonist will first reduce the dose ratio of the agonist below 1 before raising it progressively above 1. In this situation the antagonist will behave as a potentiating agent at lower concentrations, and as a blocking agent at higher ones. Experimental results which may reflect this situation have been reported in the case of the interaction between adrenaline (or noradrenaline) and ergotamine on the perfused rabbit ear (JANG, 1941), on the cat nictitating membrane *in situ*, and on the perfused cat spleen (SALZMANN et al., 1968); between adrenaline (or noradrenaline) and DCI on the isolated, cat splenic strip (BICKERTON, 1963); between isoprenaline and H 35/25 (1(4'-methylphenyl)-2-isopropylamino-propanol) on the isolated, rabbit right atrium (BRISTOW et al., 1970); and between noradrenaline and phenylephrine (a very weak partial agonist used as an antagonist) on the isolated left atrium from the reserpine-treated guinea-pig (FURCHGOTT, 1967).

The main conclusion to be drawn from the experimental findings and theoretical concepts presented in this section is that in any tissue preparation which has an active saturable removal process (or processes) for the agonist being tested, the experimental estimations of pA_2 or K_B values of an antagonist tested against the agonist may be in considerable error. To avoid this possibility it is necessary to block effectively the removal process (or processes) with some other agent (or agents) throughout the course of testing. Finally, it should also be noted that although the removal process has generally been referred to as an uptake process in this section, it might in some cases be an enzymic process for inactivation of the agonist. If such were the case, U_m would represent the maximal rate of enzymic inactivation rather than the maximal rate of a transport process for uptake of the agonist.

6. Modification of the Response to the Agonist by Actions of an Antagonist at Sites other than the Receptor

When data on agonist-antagonist interactions are analyzed with the use of equations from receptor theory, a basic assumption is that the antagonist alters sensitivity of the test system to the agonist solely by reacting with the receptor for the agonist. If the antagonist exerts other actions which modify the response to the agonist, it is important to recognize their existence; and, if possible, to modify experimental conditions so as to eliminate them.

One kind of other action, already discussed fully in the preceding section, is that in which the antagonist inhibits the effectiveness of an active saturable removal process for the agonist — either directly or indirectly. This kind of action can result in an erroneously low pA_2 value and an erroneously high K_B value for the antagonist. To avoid this kind of action, the removal process for the agonist should be effectively blocked by some means (see Section III,C,5,a) before tests on antagonism are carried out.

Another kind of undesirable action sometimes exerted by antagonists is a generalized depression of function of the responding tissue. This type of action is commonly encountered with β-blocking agents when they are used in excessively high concentrations on a variety of muscular tissues. For example, BLINKS (1967 and personal communication) has found that all of a large variety of β-blocking agents which he has tested on isolated cardiac preparations, directly depress contractility and spontaneous rate if certain concentrations are exceeded. In some cases the minimal concentration for onset of direct depression is not greatly above that for demonstrable competitive antagonism. The direct depression exerted by β-blocking agents may in some instances be the result of their local anesthetic or quinidine-like action — an action which is also thought to play a role in the anti-arrhythmic effects of these agents (e.g., see SOMANI and LUM, 1965; LUCCHESI et al., 1967). On spontaneously contracting smooth muscles, β-blocking agents can also directly depress contractile activity when they are used in too high a concentration (FURCHGOTT, 1960 and unpublished results).

Some β-antagonists at low concentrations have been found to behave as partial agonists on certain test preparations. For example, DCI exhibits some sympathomimetic activity on isolated cardiac preparations from reserpine-treated as well as normal animals (FLEMING and HAWKINS, 1960; FURCHGOTT, 1959); and some of the newer β-antagonists exhibit similar activity, but to a lesser degree (BLINKS, 1967). On isolated rat fat cells, DCI and β-hydroxy-N-t-butyl-2,4-dichlorophenethylamine, but not propranolol, act as partial agonists for the lipolytic response (FAIN, 1967). On the same tissue, pronethalol has been shown to be a weak partial agonist for the synthesis of cyclic AMP, as well as an antagonist to activation of this synthesis by catecholamines (BUTCHER et al., 1968). DAVIS (1970) has recently reported that several β-blocking agents — including DCI, sotalol, INPEA and pronethalol, but not propranolol — exhibit weak intrinsic sympathomimetic activity on the isolated guinea-pig taenia coli, as evidenced by a hyperpolarization of the cell membrane (α-effect) and an abolition of spontaneous spike discharge (β-effect ?).

In testing for partial agonistic action of antagonists, it is important to use tissues from reserpine-treated animals to avoid the possibility of a sympathomimetic response being mediated indirectly by release of noradrenaline.

In some instances adrenergic antagonists produce stimulatory effects which cannot be attributed either to release of noradrenaline or to a partial agonistic activity of these agents on adrenoceptors. Examples of effects of this kind are the stimulation of contraction of vascular and uterine smooth muscle by ergotamine (ROTHLIN and CERLETTI, 1949), and the enhancement of tone and amplitude of phasically contracting strips of uterus or intestine by phentolamine (LEVY and TOZZI, 1963; FURCHGOTT, unpublished results).

In some isolated tissue preparations evidence has been obtained that β-antagonists can also act as competitive antagonists for α-receptors (e.g., DCI on rabbit aorta, WURZEL et al., 1963; DCI on cat spleen, BICKERTON, 1963; propranolol on rabbit aorta, KOHLI and LING, 1967; several different β-antagonists on rabbit aorta, MAZURKIEWICZ-KWILECKI, 1968, and GULATI et al., 1969). From a quantitative standpoint, the results of GULATI et al. are the most useful, since they used each β-antagonist over a small concentration range which did not extend into the high range in which responses to the α-agonists (noradrenaline and methoxamine) would have been reduced because of direct depression or a non-competitive type of antagonism. They were able to obtain plots of log $(dr—1)$ against log [antagonist] which fitted straight-line curves with slopes close to unity reasonably well. Their estimated pA_2 values for β-antagonists acting on the α-receptor were 5.17 for propranolol, 5.51 for pronethalol, 3.9 for D(—)-INPEA, 5.3 for DCI, and 3.98 for L(+)-INPEA. In the case of the first three antagonists, the pA_2 values are anywhere from 2—3 units smaller than the respective pA_2 values for the same antagonists acting on β-receptors in kitten atrial strips or guinea-pig trachea — indicating about one-hundredth to one-thousandth as great an affinity of the antagonists for the α-receptor. In the case of DCI, the pA_2 value would indicate about one-twentieth as great an affinity for the α-receptor.

Evidence that β-antagonists also have some affinity for α-receptors in the rat *vas deferens* has been provided by PATIL et al. (1968), who showed that a number of these agents, at appropriately high concentrations, could partially protect against the irreversible blockade by dibenamine of the stimulatory response to noradrenaline. They attributed this protection to reversible occupation of the α-receptors by the β-antagonists (see FURCHGOTT, 1954).

If β-antagonists, at sufficiently high concentrations, can effectively compete for α-receptors, what consequence would this have in experiments for characterizing α-receptors in which a β-antagonist was purposely used to block β-receptors? In the case of experiments to determine the relative potencies of a series of α-agonists, competitive blockade of the α-receptors by the β-antagonist would not be expected to alter the relative potencies, since the sensitivity to each agonist would be reduced to the same extent. However, in the case of experiments to obtain the pA_2 or K_B value of a known competitive antagonist for the α-receptor, the presence of a β-blocker at a concentration approaching or exceeding its own dissociation constant for the α-receptor would lead to erroneous results. The reason for this is apparent in the equation from receptor theory which applies to the dose ratio (dr) of an agonist for equal responses when the agonist is tested in the presence of a fixed concentration of one competitive antagonist, B_1, both before and after the addition of a second competitive antagonist, B_2:

$$(dr—1) = \frac{[B_2]}{K_{B2}\,(1+[B_1]/K_{B1})}\,. \tag{14}$$

Here, K_{B1} and K_{B2} are the respective dissociation constants of the two antagonists for the same receptor. Putting the equation in logarithmic form gives:

$$\log\,(dr—1) = \log\,[B_2] - \log\,K_{B2}\,(1+[B_1]/K_{B1}). \tag{15}$$

Thus, it can be seen that an estimate of K_{B2} from the $(dr—1)$ at any value of $[B_2]$ would be too high by the multiplication factor $(1+[B_1]/K_{B1})$; and even though a plot of log $(dr—1)$ against log $[B_2]$ would give a straight line with slope of 1, an estimate of pA_2 (that is, $-\log K_{B2}$) from the plot would give a value which was too low by an increment equal to $\log\,(1+[B_1]/K_{B1})$.

Competition of a β-antagonist for α-receptors probably accounts in large part of the relatively low pA_2 value of 7.07 obtained by URQUILLA et al. (1970) for phentolamine as an α-antagonist to noradrenaline in the rabbit aortic strip — a value about one unit less than that obtained by FURCHGOTT (1967). To block β-receptors URQUILLA et al. used 4×10^{-5} M propranolol in the bathing solution. On the basis of the pA_2 value found by GULATI et al. (1969) for propranolol acting on the α-receptor in the aortic strip, namely, 5.16 (equivalent to a K_B of 6.75×10^{-6} M), this concentration of propranolol would have resulted in a $[B_1]/K_{B1}$

of 5.9, and therefore would have led to an error of about —0.8 in the estimated pA_2 for phentolamine. URQUILLA et al. suggested that their low pA_2 value was the result of the rather short exposure (10 min) to phentolamine used by them; but the calculation given above would indicate that the propranolol present, rather than the exposure time, was the main contributing factor.

Blockade of non-adrenergic receptors by adrenergic antagonists also occurs. The results of MAZURKIEWICZ-KWILECKI (1968) on interactions between 5-hydroxytryptamine and β-antagonists on rabbit aortic strips indicate that propranolol, Kö 592 (1-(3-methylphenoxy)-2-hydroxy-3-isopropylaminopropane) and INPEA competitively block the receptor for this amine, prior to producing a non-competitive blockade. Competitive blockade of receptors for acetylcholine and for histamine in the guinea-pig ileum by propranolol, pronethalol, sotalol (MJ 1999) and 1-isopropylamino-2-hydroxy-3-(o-allyloxy-phenoxy) propane (Ciba 39089 Ba) has been reported by RAPER and WALE (1968). On the basis of estimated pA_2 values these workers concluded that the affinity of each β-antagonist was greater for β-receptors (of guinea-pig atria) than for the other receptors; but in some instances it was not very much greater. With regard to α-antagonists, it has been recognized for many years that many of them also block non-adrenergic receptors (see FURCHGOTT, 1955). In rabbit aortic strips phentolamine, as a competitive antagonist, has about one-tenth the affinity for the 5-hydroxytryptamine receptor as for the α-receptor; and dihydroergotamine actually has a higher affinity for the former receptor. In addition, dibenamine and phenoxybenzamine irreversibly block the 5-hydroxytryptamine receptor as readily as the α-receptor, and in sufficient concentrations also irreversibly block the histamine and acetylcholine receptors.

In general, the concomitant blockade of a non-adrenergic receptor and an adrenoceptor by an adrenergic antagonist would not be expected to influence the results of an experiment in which the antagonist was being used to characterize the adrenoceptor. However, if the basal functional state of the tissue preparation used were partly determined by the action of either an endogenous or exogenous agonist acting on the non-adrenergic receptor, then blockade of that receptor could lead to erroneous results.

Potent α-antagonists do not appear to interact directly with β-receptors (NICKERSON, 1967). However, on some tissues some of these agents, when used at very high concentrations, do produce non-competitive or non-specific blockade of β-receptor-mediated responses. For example, on isolated strips of rabbit duodenum, dihydroergotamine (DHE), at a concentration about 1000 times greater than that needed to first show competitive blockade of α-receptors (about 10^{-8} M), does begin to block catecholamine-induced relaxation mediated by β-receptors (FURCHGOTT, 1960, and unpublished results). This blockade, however, is not competitive in nature. DHE in relatively high concentrations has also been shown to block a number of other responses that are considered to be mediated by β-receptors. Among these responses are adrenaline-induced relaxation in rat uterus (LEVY and TOZZI, 1963); catecholamine-induced lipolysis in rat fat cells (BROOKER and CALVERT, 1967; FAIN, 1970); and adrenaline-induced release of glucose in perfused rat liver (NORTHROP, 1968) and in rabbit liver slices (CHAN and ELLIS, 1969). Again, it appears likely that in all of these systems the blockade is not competitive and is the result of an action by DHE at some step beyond the β-receptor. In this regard, it is noteworthy that NORTHROP found that the concentration of DHE which inhibited the release of glucose by adrenaline, also inhibited the release of glucose by cyclic AMP. Several workers have also reported that phentolamine, at concentrations much higher than those required for blockade of α-receptors, inhibits catecholamine-induced lipolysis in rat fat cells in a non-competitive manner (see FAIN, 1967).

7. Lack of Equilibrium Conditions for Agonist or Antagonist at the Time a Response is Measured

Even if active removal processes in a tissue preparation are not significantly influencing the concentration of a drug in the region of the receptors (see Section C.III.5.), the question arises whether this concentration is essentially in equilibrium with the concentration of drug in the external solution (bathing or perfusion fluid) at the time a response is measured. In the case of an agonist, the time-course of the response may provide presumptive evidence for or against attainment of equilibrium at the time of measurement of the response. If the response of the test preparation, following its initial rise after addition of the agonist, remains at an essentially steady level for at least several minutes, it is likely that the agonist has attained equilibrium. However, if the response is characterized by a rapidly developed transient peak, followed by a rapid decline (fade), it is unlikely that the time between addition of agonist and the peak is sufficient for attainment of equilibrium. With preparations exhibiting this type of response (see Section C.III.2.), it can only be hoped that when a measurement of response is made — usually at the peak — the ratio of the concentration of agonist in the region of the receptors to that in the external solution is the same for all agonists and all concentrations of agonists tested.

In the case of a competitive antagonist, retesting of the agonist at selected time intervals after addition of the antagonist provides a means of judging whether the antagonist has attained equilibrium. Equilibrium is indicated when there is no further displacement of the concentration-response curve for the agonist (corrected for any displacement not due to the antagonist, as discussed in Section C.III.2.). Unfortunately, the time required for full displacement is usually very long for potent competitive antagonists on most test preparations. The theoretical basis for this slow approach to final equilibrium is a controversial matter (see FURCHGOTT, 1964; RANG, 1966; THRON and WAUD, 1968); but the fact remains that many minutes, or even hours, may be required. In rabbit aortic strips, equilibration of dihydroergotamine appears to be somewhat incomplete even in 2 hours; and equilibration of phentolamine appears to be only about one-half complete in 30 min, and essentially complete in 90 min (FURCHGOTT, 1955; FURCHGOTT, 1967). FURCHGOTT (1967) has reported that approximately 1 hour is required for attainment of apparent equilibrium with pronethalol in a variety of tissues. Also, POTTER (1967), in careful kinetic experiments on propranolol antagonism of β-receptors in guinea-pig atria, estimated that 90 min were required for this antagonist to attain about 98% of equilibrium.

Obviously, if the concentration of a competitive antagonist in the region of the receptors is considerably short of its equilibrium level at the time when the agonist is retested, this will tend to make the estimated K_B too high and the estimated pA_2 too low. For this reason, it is preferable to allow the competitive antagonist to come essentially to equilibrium before retesting of the agonist. Since, from a practical standpoint, this is not always possible, the time of exposure to the antagonist should always be indicated, along with reported K_B values or pA_2 values.

8. Loss of Free Drug from the External Solution

In all experiments designed to pharmacologically characterize adrenoceptors in tissue preparations, values for the concentrations of drugs (both agonists and antagonists) in the medium (external solution) are used in the final calculations. Actually, the concentration of a drug in the medium is rarely measured directly; it is simply estimated by dividing the amount of added drug by the total volume of the medium to which it is added. If the volume of the medium is very much larger than the volume of the isolated tissue preparation (e.g., $> 100\times$), this estimated value is probably close enough to the true value to cause no serious error. However, if the volume of the medium is not considerably larger than the tissue volume, there is the possibility that the estimated value of the concentration of the drug in the medium is too high, since removal of the drug by the tissue (due to diffusion, adsorption, active uptake or enzymic alteration) may be appreciable. Even when the volume of the medium is very large relative to the tissue preparation, there may be some loss of drug from the medium due to adsorption by the tissue or by surfaces of the organ chamber or perfusing apparatus. Loss by adsorption probably would not be significant in most systems, but it should be considered as a possibility whenever extremely low concentrations of drugs are used. If the medium contains appreciable added protein — for example, serum albumin as in the case of studies on free fatty acid release from fat cells — then the possibility of binding of added drugs by the protein has to be considered.

In some instances, there may be a loss of drug from the medium due to chemical reactions. An example of this would be the oxidation of catecholamines added to an oxygenated medium in which there are traces of heavy metals which catalyze the reaction. A commonly used method for largely eliminating the oxidation of catecholamines in oxygenated media is the addition of the heavy metal-chelating agent, disodium-EDTA (ethylene-diamine tetraacetic acid) at a final concentration of about 10^{-5} g/ml (FURCHGOTT, 1955).

D. Present Status of Classification of Adrenoceptors

I. General Comments

As pointed out in the Introduction, a survey of all the literature concerned with the classification of adrenoceptors mediating responses in all kinds of effector organs or tissues in all species of animals is beyond the scope of this review. In general, as far as the author is aware, the present pharmacological evidence is consistent with the following statements concerning adrenoceptors for functional responses in mammalian smooth muscles and heart: (a) α-receptors mediate contraction in all smooth muscles except those of the non-sphincter regions of the intestinal tract, in which they mediate relaxation; (b) β-receptors mediate relaxation in all smooth muscles, including those of the intestinal tract; (c) β-receptors mediate positive chronotropic responses, positive inotropic responses, improved atrioventricular conduction, and automaticity (in non-pacemaker cells) of the heart. A few possible exceptions to these general statements have appeared in the literature. For example, MUNRO (1953) found that adrenaline and noradrenaline caused contraction of the longitudinal muscle of the extreme ends of the fetal guinea-pig small intestine (indicating an α-receptor). REDDY and MORAN (1968) found that high doses of isoprenaline produced a contraction of smooth muscle of the sphincter regions of the rabbit gastrointestinal tract, which were blocked by DCI but not by phentolamine (indicating a β-receptor). KABELA et al. (1969) showed that the initial transient decrease in coronary flow (interpreted as vasoconstriction) of the perfused dog heart caused by catecholamines had all the pharmacological characteristics of a response mediated by β-receptors. Finally, as already noted in Section III, there is evidence that α-receptors mediate a small part of the total positive inotropic response to catecholamines in guinea-pig atria (GOVIER, 1968).

With respect to a wide variety of other responses in mammalian species, the reader is referred to the following reviews for discussions of evidence for the accompanying classifications: BOWMAN and NOTT (1969) on β-receptors in skeletal muscle for enhancement of contraction of fast muscles, inhibition of contraction of slow muscles and hyperpolarization of the cell membrane, and α-receptors (probably presynaptic) for enhancement of neuromuscular transmission; VOLLE (1969) on β-receptors in autonomic ganglia for postsynaptic depolarization and facilitation of transmission, and α-receptors for postsynaptic hyperpolarization and inhibition of transmission; MAYER (1970) on β-receptors in heart for metabolic responses, including an increase in cyclic AMP and responses causally related to this increase (e.g., activation of phosphorylase and glycogenolysis); BRODY and MCNEILL (1970) on β-receptors in skeletal muscle and some smooth muscles for an increase in cyclic AMP and related metabolic responses; HORNBROOK (1970) on β-receptors in liver for an increase in cyclic AMP and related metabolic responses, and α-receptors (but with less certainty) for an increase in K^+ and Ca^{++} efflux; FAIN (1970) and HIMMS-HAGEN (1970) on β-receptors in adipose tissue for an increase in cyclic AMP and related metabolic responses, including lipolysis; ROBISON et al. (1967) on β-receptors in cyclase-containing particulate fractions from heart, skeletal muscle, liver and fat cells for activation of synthesis of cyclic AMP; ASHMORE (1970) for α-receptors in pancreas for inhibition of insulin secretion, and β-receptors for enhancement of secretion; JENKINSON and MORTON (1967) on α-receptors in intestinal smooth muscles for increasing membrane permeability to K^+ and causing hyperpolarization; DANIEL et al. (1970) on both α- and β-receptors in many tissues for altering membrane properties, as reflected in changes of resting potential, ion fluxes, ion transport, etc.; FÜLGRAFF et al. (1969) for β-receptors in kidney for antidiuresis.

Adrenoceptors mediating some responses have not been successfully classified as either *alpha* or *beta*. This is particularly true in the case of responses in, or stemming from actions in, the central nervous system. Part of the difficulty here lies in the major technical and interpretive problems associated with CNS studies. However, even when microelectrodes are used to measure electrical activity in single neurons to which drugs are delivered by electrophoresis from micropipettes, the responses (usually inhibition, but sometimes excitation) usually do not have the pharmacological characteristics associated with α- or β-receptor-mediated responses (BLOOM and GIARMAN, 1968; CURTIS and CRAWFORD, 1969). Only occasionally is there fair evidence that an inhibitory response (as in some neurons of the olfactory bulb) is mediated by β-receptors (SALMOIRAGHI, 1966).

Some controversy also exists as to the type of receptor which mediates metabolic responses in rat liver, and also possibly in human liver (ELLIS et al., 1967). Metabolic responses in the rat liver, unlike in livers of other species of laboratory mammals, are much more sensitive to adrenaline, and often even to noradrenaline, than to isoprenaline, and are usually only partially blocked by β-antagonists. Nevertheless, HORNBROOK (1970), on the basis of recent evidence, believes the receptor involved is more of a β- than an α-type, as has been somtimes stated.

As noted in Section II, pharmacological evidence for different types of receptors within the general class of β-receptors has recently begun to accumulate. In the following sections the evidence for different types of receptors within both the β-class and the α-class will be examined critically. For the most part, consideration will be given to results obtained on isolated tissue preparations rather than on intact animals, because of the difficulties of obtaining uncomplicated results on the latter (see Section C.III.1.). Nevertheless, it should be noted that some o the results which have first indicated different types of β-receptors have come from experiments on intact animals (e.g., see LANDS et al., 1966; LEVY, 1966; DUNLOP and SHANKS, 1968; MORAN, 1967).

II. ß-Receptors

1. The Proposal for Two Types - β_1 and β_2

LANDS, ARNOLD and their colleagues have determined the potencies of a number of related catecholamines (isoprenaline, adrenaline, noradrenaline, α-methylnoradrenaline, α-ethylnoradrenaline, and a number of N-substituted derivatives of the last three compounds) for producing a variety of "*beta*" responses in both isolated tissues and in intact animals (LANDS et al., 1967a, 1967b, 1969; ARNOLD et al., 1968; ARNOLD and MCAULIFF, 1968, 1969; ARNOLD and SELBERIS, 1968). After first normalizing the potencies of all amines relative to that of isoprenaline in the case of each response, and then taking the logarithms of the resulting relative potencies, they made statistical comparisons of the resulting sets of log relative potencies. A compilation of some of the correlation coefficients which they obtained are shown in Table 3. On the basis of the degree of correlation between paired sets of relative potencies, they were able to divide the responses investigated into two groups. Within any one of these groups the correlation coefficient was greater than 0.9 for a comparison of any pair of sets. The responses within the first group included increase in rate and increase in force of the perfused rabbit heart, lipolysis in rat and guinea-pig adipose tissue, inhibition of rabbit small intestine, and calorigenesis in the intact rat. The responses within the second group included vasodepression in the intact dog, bronchodilation in the perfused guinea-pig lung, inhibition of the rat uterus, facilitation of contraction of the rat diaphragm, elevation of blood lactic acid in the rat and in the dog (considered to reflect glycogenolysis in skeletal muscle), and elevation of blood glucose in the dog. When a set of relative potencies for any response in the first group was compared with a set for any response in the second group, correlation was poor (ranging from 0—0.57). Because of the good correlation within any one group, LANDS and co-workers concluded that all responses in the first group were mediated by one type of β-receptor, termed β_1; and all responses in the second group by a second type, termed β_2. These workers even extended this approach to responses in non-mammalian species (LANDS et al., 1969), classifying the β-receptor for stimulation of chicken heart as a β_1-type, but that for inhibition of the chicken rectal caecum and for stimulation of frog heart as a β_2-type.

The experimental evidence on which LANDS, ARNOLD and co-workers based their differentiation of β-receptors into two distinct types is open to some criticism. Four of the responses were measured in whole animals, in which a number of uncontrolled factors may have influenced the degree of response. Even when isolated preparations were used, very few special precautions were taken to avoid unfavorable experimental conditions. The precaution of blocking α-receptors was taken only in experiments on isolated rabbit intestine and when adrenaline was tested for vasodepression in the dog. No precautions were taken to avoid the possible release of endogenous noradrenaline, or to block active removal processes for agonists. Moreover, despite the high correlation coefficients reported for comparisons within one of the two groups of responses, a close scrutiny of the actual relative potencies sometimes reveals differences between two relative potencies series which would hardly be expected with receptors of exactly the same type. Of course there is the possibility that if measures had been taken to

Table 3. *Comparison of relative potencies of a series of catecholamines for producing different responses mediated by β-receptors (selected results of Lands, Arnold and coworkers)*

Responses for which log relative potencies of agonists were compared	No. of agonists	Correlation coefficient	Conclusion about types of receptors compared
Rabbit heart force/rabbit heart rate	12	0.923	β_1/β_1 [1]
Rat adipose tissue lipolysis/rabbit heart rate	12	0.916	β_1/β_1 [1]
Rabbit jejunum inhibition[a]/rabbit heart rate	11	0.982	β_1/β_1 [1]
Guinea-pig ad. t. lipolysis/rat ad. t. lipolysis	7	0.98	β_1/β_1 [2]
Rat calorigenesis/other β_1-responses (combined)[b]	5	0.93	β_1/β_1 [3]
Dog vasodepression/guinea-pig bronchodilation[c]	15	0,957	β_2/β_2 [4]
Rat uterus inhibition/g.p. bronchodilation	12	0.93	β_2/β_2 [1]
Rat diaphragm contraction[d]/g. p. bronchodilation	8	0.957	β_2/β_2 [1]
Rat muscle glycogenolysis[e]/g. p. bronchodilation	7	0.971	β_2/β_2 [5]
Rat diaphragm contraction/rat uterus inhibition	8	0.905	β_2/β_2 [1]
Rat muscle glycogenolysis/rat ad. t. lipolysis	9	0.061	β_2/β_1 [5]
Guinea-pig ad. t. lipolysis/g. p. bronchodilation	6	0.02	β_1/β_2 [2]
Dog vasodepression/rabbit heart stimulation	15	0.312	β_2/β_1 [4]

[a] *Alpha*-receptors blocked with phentolamine.
[b] Median values for all other responses classified as β_1.
[c] Antagonism to histamine bronchoconstriction in perfused guinea-pig lung.
[d] Enhancement of twitch height in curarized diaphragm treated with high KCl.
[e] Based on increase in blood lactic acid in intact rats.

References: 1. Lands et al., 1967b; 2. Arnold and McAuliff, 1968; 3. Arnold and McAuliff, 1969; 4. Lands et al., 1967a; Arnold and Selberis, 1968.

make the experimental conditions more suitable, the correlations might have been even better than those actually reported. Further consideration of the proposal for β_1- and β_2-types of receptors will be included in the following section.

2. Evidence for Multiple Sub-types of ß-Receptors

Table 4 contains selected results from a number of investigations on the pharmacological characterization of responses mediated by β-receptors in a variety of isolated tissues. The results were selected on the following bases: (a) that they came from experiments in which appropriate special precautions were taken to control at least some of the conditions which might lead to erroneous results; or (b) that they came from experiments in which no, or insufficient, special precautions were taken, but are nevertheless, useful for making some interesting comparisons.

The results in category (a) are indicated by italicized figures in the table, and will be considered first. However, before considering them, several comments should be made. First, with respect to isoprenaline, the (—)-isomer would undoubtedly have essentially twice the potency of the racemic compound for the same response. Secondly, since phenylephrine is a partial agonist relative to the other agonists listed, a comparison of its relative potencies for different responses may not always be meaningful for receptor differentiation (see Section C.II.1.). Thirdly, there is the possibility that the pA_2 values for antagonists acting against isoprenaline in the case of tracheal preparations may be somewhat too low because of the influence of an active removal process for isoprenaline in these preparations (see Section III,C,5,a). Finally, there is the question of what quantitative differences in equivalent data for two respon-

Table 4. *Relative potencies of agonists and pA_2 values of competitive antagonists for responses mediated by β-receptors in isolated tissues*

Species Tissue and response	Relative potencies of agonists[a]						pA_2 values of antagonists against isoprenaline[a]					
	(—)I	(±)I	(—)A	(—)NA	(—)PE	Ref.	PNL	PPL	Sotalol	INPEA	PRTL	H 35/25
Rabbit												
Thoracic aorta, relaxation		130	65	1	<0.1	[1][bcd]	7.47 [1][bce]	8.98 [2][ef]			3.89 [2]	6.83 [2][ef]
Left atrium, ↑ force		3.5	0.5	1		[1][bg]	7.13 [1]					
Right atrium, ↑ rate								8.8 [2][e]			6.91 [2][ef]	6.40 [2][ef]
Trachea, relaxation								8.8 [2][ef]			5.98 [2][ef]	5.80 [2][ef]
Small intestine, longitudinal muscle, relaxation		1.5	0.2	1	<0.01	[1][bcd]	6.34 [1][ce]	6.8 [15][eg]			5.9 [3][h]	
Stomach fundus, circular muscle, relaxation		2.5	1.2	1	<0.01	[1][bcd]	6.25 [1][ce]	6.89 [2][ef]			<3.5 [2][ef]	6.71 [2][ef]
Guinea-pig												
Left atrium, ↑ force		5.0	0.5	1	<0.001	[1][bg]	7.13 [1][be]	8.8 [4][i]			7.3 [3][h]	
Right atrium ↑ rate	15		0.45	1		[5][dfj]		8.6 [6]	6.21 [5][efk]	6.81 [5][f]	7.25 [5][f]	
											6.43 [5][ef]	
Trachea, relaxation	74		9	1		[5][dfj]		8.7 [3][h]	7.46 [5][efk]	7.12 [5][f]	5.54 [5][ef]	
		47	12	1	0.06[l]	[1][bcd]	7.51 [1][bce]	8.7 [15][bce]				
Small intestine, longitudinal muscle, relaxation		3	0.5	1		[1][bcd]	7.02 [1][ce]					
Adipose tissue, lipolysis	14		0.34	1		[7]						
Vas deferens, relaxation								8.9 [3][dh]			6.8 [3][dh]	
Cat												
Left atrium, ↑ force							7.4 [4][i]	8.8 [4][i]				
Right atrium, ↑ rate								8.5 [4][i]				
Rat												
Uterus, relaxation	500		103	1		[7]		8.5 [3][h]			5.0 [3][h]	
Adipose tissue, lipolysis	6		0.7	1		[8]	~5.4 [8][h]	6.75 [9][h]		6.32 [9][h]		
Bovine												
Trachea (calf), relaxation		40	10	1		[10]	~7.0 [10][h]	~8.2 [10][h]				
Iris sphincter, relaxation		30		1	0.1	[5, 11]		<6.0 [11][em]	6.6 [11][em]			
Dog												
Small skeletal muscle artery, relaxation		≫1	>1	1		[12][n]						
Small coronary artery, relaxation		3	0.1	1		[12][n]						

(Continuation of Table 4)

Species Tissue and response	Relative potencies of agonists[a]						pA₂ values of antagonists against isoprenaline[a]					
	(—)I	(±)I	(—)A	(—)NA	(—)PE	Ref.	PNL	PPL	Sotalol	INPEA	PRTL	H35/25
Mouse												
Spleen, relaxation		≫1	>1	1		[13][n]			8.5 [13][n]			
Human												
Bronchus, circular muscle, relaxation		*140*	*110*	*1*		[14][do]						
Stomach, lower body longitudinal muscle, relaxation		*3.8*	*2.7*	*1*	*0.07*	[14][do]						
Duodenum, longitudinal muscle, relaxation		*3*	*0.6*	*1*	*0.001*	[14][do]						
Colon, longitudinal muscle, relaxation		*5*	*3*	*1*	*0.08*	[14][do]						
Colon, circular muscle, relaxation		*2*	*6*	*1*	*0.2*	[14][do]						

Abbreviations: (—)I, (—)-isoprenaline; (±)I, racemic isoprenaline; (—)A, (—)-adrenaline; (—)NA, (—)-noradrenaline; (—)PE, (—)-phenylephrine; PNL, pronethalol; PPL, propranolol; INPEA, (—)-1-(4-nitrophenyl)-2-isopropylaminoethanol; PRTL, practolol, 4(2-hydroxy-3-isopropylamino-propoxy)acetanilid; H 35/25, 1-(4-methylphenyl)-2-isopropylaminopropanol.

[a] All preparations were in Krebs-bicarbonate solution or closely related physiologic salt solutions. Temperature was 37—38° C unless otherwise indicated. Duration of exposure to antagonist prior to retesting agonist was 45 min or longer unless otherwise indicated. Where a pA_2 value was not given in cited reference, it was calculated from a K_B value or from tabulated or plotted data included in reference. [b] Tissue from reserpine-pretreated animals. [c] Dibenamine used to block α-receptors. [d] Cocaine used to block neuronal uptake mechanism. [e] Corrected for sensitivity change of control preparation. [f] Phentolamine used to block α-receptors. [g] Phenoxybenzamine used to block α-receptors and uptake mechanisms. [h] exposure time to antagonist not given. [i] Temperature of 32.5° C. [j] Tropolone used to block COMT. [k] Levorotatory isomer. [l] Relative potency of PE is less at high levels of contraction. [m] 30 min exposure to antagonist. [n] Phenoxybenzamine used to block α-receptors. [o] Thymoxamine used to block α-receptors.

References: 1. Furchgott, 1967; 2. Bristow, et al. 1970; 3. Farmer and Levy, 1970; 4. Blinks, 1967; 5. Buckner and Patil (1971); 6. Potter, 1967; 7. Lands et al., 1967b; 8. Brooker and Calvert, 1967; 9. Fassina, 1967; 10. Ariëns, 1967; 11. Patil, 1969; 12. Bohr, 1967; 13. Ignarro and Titus, 1968; 14. Hedges and Turner, 1969; 15. Furchgott (unpublished results).

ses, obtained under close to optimal experimental conditions, are required for the conclusion that the responses are mediated by different "types" of receptors. It is suggested that a greater than three-fold difference, in the case of the relative potencies for the same agonist, or a difference of greater than 0.5 in the case of the pA_2 values for the same antagonist (equivalent to a greater than three-fold difference in K_B), should be considered preliminary evidence for different types of receptors, and that a combination of two or more such differences should be considered as strong evidence.

The results in Table 4 for isolated tissue from the rabbit indicate that the responses of aorta, left atrium (force or rate), trachea, small intestine and stomach may all be mediated by different types of β-receptors. They also indicate that some types may be more closely related than others (e.g., the receptors for atrial stimulation and intestinal relaxation in contrast to receptors for aortic relaxation. LANDS and co-workers (see Section D.II.1.) concluded that receptors for cardiac stimulation and for intestinal relaxation were both of the same type, β_1. On the basis of the relative potencies of the agonists shown in Table 4, the receptors for increase in atrial force and for intestinal relaxation in the rabbit could well be of the same type; however, the considerable difference in the pA_2 values for pronethalol differentiate the two. Also, the pA_2 values for practolol and for propranolol differentiate the receptor for increase in atrial rate from that for intestinal relaxation. LANDS and co-workers concluded that receptors for relaxation of trachea and blood vessels were both of the same type, β_2. Yet, the results of BRISTOW et al. (1969) (ref. 2 of Table 4) clearly show a marked difference in the pA_2 values for practolol in the case of rabbit trachea and aortic strip. The pA_2 values for practolol, as well as the relative potency values for adrenaline, differentiate the receptors for intestinal relaxation and stomach fundic muscle relaxation, respectively.

In the case of guinea-pig tissues, the data in Table 4 clearly differentiate the receptors mediating the increase in atrial force or rate from those for tracheal relaxation. On the basis of the relative potencies for agonists and the pA_2values for pronethalol, the receptors for increases in atrial force and intestinal relaxation in this species appear to be of a similar type; however, further testing with other agonists and antagonists under proper conditions is needed to establish this firmly. The relative potencies of agonists for lipolysis of guinea-pig adipose tissue are almost identical with those for increases in atrial rate, but pharmacological characterization of the former response under properly controlled conditions and with selected antagonists is needed for a more complete comparison. The data presented here for the guinea-pig are consistent with the β_1- and β_2-typing of LANDS and co-workers (see Section D.I.), but they are too limited to rule out conclusively the existence of more than two types of β-receptors. It might be noted that TAKAGI and TAKAYANAGI (1970), on the basis of pA_2 values obtained for practalol and other antagonists, concluded that the receptors for guinea-pig atrial stimulation and taenia coli relaxation are similar to each other, but different from those for tracheal relaxation. (Their pA_2 values are not included in Table 4 because they are all considerably lower than comparable values reported by others, and the experimental conditions are unspecified). Also, the so-called selective β-agonists (e.g., salbutamol, soterenol and trimetoquinol) have been demonstrated in *in vitro* studies to have a much higher relative potency for tracheal relaxation than for atrial stimulation (FARMER et al., 1970).

In the case of the rat, none of the experiments on isolated tissues of which the author is aware have been carried out with adequate special precautions. Nevertheless, the results in Table 4 leave little doubt that the receptors in uterus and adipose tissue are of different types. Also, the pA_2 values reported by TAKAGI and TAKAYANAGI (1970) (not included in the table for reasons given in the preceding paragraph) for three antagonists acting on rat uterus and rat fundus, provide preliminary evidence for different types of β-receptors mediating relaxation in these preparations.

In the case of bovine tissues, the type of β-receptor in the iris sphincter appears different from that in trachea, in view of the unusually low pA_2 for propranolol found by PATIL (1969) with the former preparation. In the case of the dog, the striking finding of BOHR (1967) on the markedly different relative potency series for agonists in the case of a small coronary artery as compared to a small skeletal muscle artery, is strong evidence for different types of β-receptors in these two blood vessels.

In the case of isolated human smooth muscles, the relative potencies of agonists found by HEDGES and TURNER (1969) (ref. 14 of Table 4) provide evidence that β-receptors in the various smooth muscles of the gastrointestinal tract may be of several types. However, this evidence is preliminary (only 1—4 specimens of each preparation tested); and there is the possibility that in some of their preparations the thymoxamine (2 μg/ml) used did not completely block a relaxing effect resulting from the actions of adrenaline and phenylephrine on α-receptors.

It is noteworthy that the pA_2 value for sotalol is much higher in the case of mouse spleen (8.5) than in the case of any other smooth muscle preparation listed in Table 4 (6.6—7.46). It is also noteworthy that the pA_2 values for pronethalol and propranolol in the case of rat adipose tissue are much lower than the respective values for these antagonists in the case of atria from other species — especially since the receptors for lipolysis and cardiac stimulation are both classified as β_1-types by LANDS and colleagues (see Section D.II.1.). However, a number of factors may have contributed to the lowness of the pA_2 values in the case of adipose tissue. Among the possible contributing factors are: the species difference; the influence of a saturable removal process for the agonist used (see Section C.III.5.b); and a high degree of binding of the antagonist by the serum albumin employed in the bathing solution in studies on lipolysis.

III. α-Receptors

VAN ROSSUM (1965) compared the relative potencies of a large series of adrenergic agonists, and the pA_2 values of a large series of antagonists (acting against noradrenaline) on the isolated rat *vas deferens* (contraction) and the rabbit jejunum (initial rapid relaxation). He found significant differences between the two preparations both with respect to the relative potencies of a number of the individual agonists, and with respect to the pA_2 values of a number of the individual antagonists, and concluded that the α-receptors mediating the two responses were of different types. Unfortunately, he did not take many of the important precautions which are so necessary to ensure satisfactory conditions for pharmacological characterization of receptors. For this reason, his results can only be considered suggestive, rather than conclusive. It would also have been preferable in a study such as his to use two preparations from a single species.

BEVAN and OSHER (1965), in a study of the relative potencies of nine different adrenergic agonists for eliciting contraction of helical strips of isolated blood vessels of the rabbit, did provide a number of comparisons suggesting that α-receptors in both the anterior mesenteric artery and the inferior vena cava, differed somewhat in characteristics from the receptors in thoracic aorta and pulmonary artery. They used DCI to block β-receptors in some experiments. Unfortunately, however,

Table 5. *Relative potencies of agonists and pA_2 values of competitive antagonists for responses mediated by α-receptors in isolated tissues*

Species Tissue and response	Relative potencies of agonists[a]					pA_2 values for antagonist against PE or another agonist[a]	
	(—)A	(—)NA	(—)PE	I	Ref.	PTA	DHE
Rabbit							
Thoracic aorta, contraction	*1.2*	*1*	*0.2*	~*0.01*[b]	[1][cde]	*7.83* [1][cdfg]	8.3 [2][f]
Duodenum, longitudinal muscle, relaxation	2	1	0.25	<0.1	[3][ih]	*8.13* [3][f]	>8.0 [4][f]
Stomach fundus circular muscle, contraction	~1	1	0.25	<0.01	[3]	*8.03* [3][f]	
Guinea-pig							
Vas deferens, contraction	~1	1		<0.05	[5][c]		
Taenia coli, relaxation	~5	1		~0.005	[6]		
Trachea, contraction	2.3	1			[7][d]		
Left atrium, ↑ force						*7.9* [8][i]	
Rat							
Vas deferens, contraction	2	1	0.3	~0.04[b]	[9]	7.0 [9][jk]	
Seminal vesicle, contraction	3.6	1	0.33	<0.002	[10]		
Cat							
Spleen, contraction	6.5	1		~0.01	[11]	*6.45* [12][kmn]	
Nictitating membrane, contraction	*1.8*	*1*	*0.4*		[13][n]	*7.15* [13][kno] *7.42* [14][nop]	
Dog							
Saphenous vein, contraction	2	1		~0.01	[15]		

(Continuation of Table 5)

Species Tissue and response	Relative potencies of agonists[a]					pA_2 values for antagonist against PE or another agonist[a]	
	(—)A	(—)NA	(—)PE	I	Ref.	PTA	DHE
Mouse							
Spleen, contraction	*3*	*1*		*~0.01*	[16][l]	*8.26* [16][kl]	
Human							
Saphenous vein, contraction	*4*	*1*	*0.08*	*0.005*	[17][de]		
Popliteal artery, contraction	*4*	*1*	*0.2*		[17][de]		
Oesophagus, lower third, circular muscle, contraction	*5*	*1*	*0.2*		[17][de]		
Ileum longitudinal muscle, relaxation	*5*	*1*	*0.2*	*0.005*	[17][de]		
Colon longitudinal muscle, relaxation	*3—10*	*1*	*0.2*	*0.03—0.003*	[17][de]		
Bladder detrusor muscle, contraction	*2*	*1*	*0.3*		[17][de]		

Abbreviations: (—)A, (—) adrenaline; (—)NA, (—)-noradrenaline; (—)PE, (—)-phenylephrine; I, (±)-isoprenaline; PTA, phentolamine; DHE, dihydroergotamine.

[a] All preparations were in Krebs-bicarbonate solution or closely related physiologic salt solutions. Temperature was 37—38° C unless otherwise indicated. Duration of exposure to antagonist prior to retesting agonist was 45 min or longer unless otherwise indicated. Where a pA_2 value was not given in cited reference, it was calculated from a K_B value or from tabulated or plotted data included in reference. [b](—)-isoprenaline used. [c] Tissue from reserpine treated animal. [d] Propranolol used to block β-receptors. [e] Cocaine used to block neuronal uptake mechanism. [f] Corrected for sensitivity change of control preparation. [g] Pre-incubation with iproniazid to block MAO. [h] DCI used to block β-receptors. [i] Pronethalol used to block β-receptors. [j] Exposure time to antagonist not given. [k] NA used as agonist for pA_2 determination. [l] Sotalol used to block β-receptors. [m] 5-min exposure to antagonist. [n] Chronically denervated preparation. [o] 15-min exposure to antagonist. [p] Methoxamine used as agonist for pA_2 determination.

References: 1. Furchgott, 1970; 2. Furchgott, 1955; 3. Furchgott, 1967; 4. Furchgott (unpublished results); 5. Nedergaard and Westermann, 1968; 6. Weisbrodt et al., 1969; 7. Persson and Johnson, 1970; 8. Govier, 1968; 9. van Rossum, 1965; 10. Miller, 1967; 11. Bickerton, 1963; 12. Green and Fleming, 1968; 13. Langer and Trendelenburg, 1969; 14. Trendelenburg et al., 1970; 15. Guimaraes and Osswald, 1969; 16. Ignarro and Titus, 1968; 17. Coupar and Turner, 1969.

they took no precautions to block uptake processes or to prevent release of endogenous noradrenaline, and therefore it would be premature to consider their results as conclusive evidence for different types of α-receptors in rabbit blood vessels.

Table 5 contains selected results from a number of investigations on the pharmacological characterization of responses mediated by α-receptors in a variety of isolated tissues. The bases for selection of results were the same as those used for selection of results in Table 4. Again, results which came from experiments in which appropriate special precautions were taken to control some important experimental conditions are indicated by italicized figures in the table. In this table, the uniformly low relative potency figures for isoprenaline are not of much use for quantitative comparisons. This is so because this potent β-agonist may well have given responses which were the resultant of its actions on both β- and α-receptors, even when β-antagonists were employed to block the former receptors.

In the case of the rabbit, the relative potencies of the agonists and the pA_2 values for phentolamine and DHE (Table 5) are all consistent with there being only one type of α-receptor mediating contraction of the aorta, contraction of the fundus muscle and relaxation of the duodenum.

In the case of the human, the data of COUPAR and TURNER (1969) on the relative potencies of agonists (ref. 17 of Table 5) are also consistent with there being only one type of α-receptor mediating responses in a variety of vascular, gastrointestinal and urinary bladder smooth muscle preparations. Some of the small discrepancies in potency ratios could be the result of insufficient testing (only 1—4 specimens used for each preparation); or could reflect some "breakthrough" activation of β-receptors (especially by isoprenaline and adrenaline) in some preparations, despite the presence of 0.5 μg/ml of propranolol.

The limited data in Table 5 on guinea-pig and rat smooth muscle preparations come mainly from experiments in which conditions for testing were inadequately controlled. Nevertheless, they are not inconsistent with the postulate of a single type of α-receptor mediating the responses shown for any one of these species.

In the case of the two tissues from the cat, the higher potency ratio of adrenaline to noradrenaline in the spleen than in the denervated nictitating membrane may be due to the influence of the neuronal uptake process present in the former preparation only. The lower pA_2 value for phentolamine in the spleen than in the nictitating membrane is more difficult to fault. At first, it might be thought that this difference is due to the shorter exposure time to phentolamine used in the experiments on the spleen (5 min as compared to 15 min); however, GREEN and FLEMING (1968) point out that they obtained no significant increase in the pA_2 in normal spleen when the exposure time was increased from 5 to 20 min. Nevertheless, further work is required on the pharmacological characterization of the adrenergic responses of the splenic and the nictitating membrane smooth muscle (preferably from the very same cats) before a conclusion can be reached on whether the two preparations have the same or different types of α-receptors.

In comparing data for the various tissue preparations from the different species represented in Table 5, it is surprising how similar the relative potencies for the four agonists are in the case of all preparations from all species. Also noteworthy is the closeness of the pA_2 values for phentolamine in the case of preparations from the rabbit, guinea-pig and mouse. It seems likely that the pA_2 values for phentolamine in the case of both preparations from the cat would have been higher if longer exposure periods had been employed (thereby ensuring a closer approach to equilibrium of the antagonist in the tissues). The pA_2 value of 7.0 reported by VAN ROSSUM (1965) for phentolamine in the case of the rat vas deferens is very likely too low as a result of unsatisfactory experimental conditions. His reported pA_2 value for this same antagonist on rabbit intestine was only 6.3, in contrast to the value of 8.13 obtained in the present author's laboratory.

Additional strong evidence for the similarity of α-receptors mediating responses in different tissues comes from the recent determinations by PATIL et al. (1971) of the potency ratio for (—)-noradrenaline to (+)-noradrenaline. When cocaine, sotalol and tropolone were present, the ratio was almost identical (approximately 300:1) in the case of "α-responses" in rabbit aorta, vena cava, spleen and ileum, and rat vas deferens and seminal vesicle. In distinct contrast, the ratio varied considerably in the case of "β-responses" in a variety of tissues, even when cocaine, phentolamine and tropolone were present.

IV. Conclusions

A large number of experiments have now definitely shown that all β-receptors are not of the same type. The proposal by LANDS, ARNOLD and coworkers that β-receptors are of two distinct types — termed by them β_1 and β_2 — is an interesting one, and their evidence for such a division is rather impressive (Section D.II.1.). However, the results of a limited number of experiments in which special precautions have been taken to insure desirable conditions for testing, have already shown that in a single species some receptors assigned to either the β_1-subclass or the β_2-subclass, respectively, do exhibit significant quantitative differences in certain pharmacological characteristics (Section D.II.2). These results do not rule out the possibility that there are two major subclasses of β-receptors, with the receptors in each subclass having somewhat similar, but not necessarily identical, pharmacological characteristics. Nevertheless, they do suggest caution in accepting the proposal for two major subclasses. Only future experiments, properly designed and controlled, can settle the question of whether there are two or more distinct subclasses of β-receptors, and whether it is possible and practical to further subdivide receptors in any one subclass into different groups on the basis of extremely similar, if not identical, pharmacological characteristics.

In the case of α-receptors, the evidence to date is not inconsistent with there being only one type in any one species; and extremely similar types among different species. However, there has been considerably less investigation of the pharmacological characteristics of responses mediated by α-receptors in different tissues in comparison to responses mediated by β-receptors. Therefore, the conclusion that all α-receptors are of a single type is highly tentative, and will have to be tested in future experiments. In such experiments it will be well to quantify the potencies of a number of other competitive antagonists, in addition to phentolamine, for blocking different responses mediated by α-receptors.

Finally, it should again be emphasized that the differentiation of receptors is an operational procedure based on the pharmacological characterization of responses mediated by the receptors. With this in mind, the question arises whether different types of β-receptors, as defined by this procedure, differ in their chemical constitution. One possibility is that they do. The other possibility is that all β-receptors, at least in any one species, are identical molecules, but that their properties are influenced by their interactions with surrounding molecules in the macromolecular structures, such as cell membranes, in which they are located or "embedded". If these macromolecular structures vary somewhat in composition from one effector system to another, then this variation may sufficiently alter the properties of the "embedded" β-receptors for interactions with agonists and antagonists, so as to cause the quantitative differences in pharmacological characteristics observed in experiments on different effector systems.

References

AHLQUIST, R.P.: A study of the adrenotropic receptors. Amer. J. Physiol. **153**, 586—600 (1948).
— The adrenergic receptor. J. pharm. Sci. **55**, 359—367 (1966).
— LEVY, B.: Adrenergic receptive mechanism of canine ileum. J. Pharmacol. exp. Ther. **127**, 146—149 (1959).
ALLEN, D.O., HILLMAN, C.C., ASHMORE, J.: Studies on a biphasic lipolytic response to catecholamines in isolated fat cells. Biochem. Pharmacol. **18**, 2233—2240 (1969).
ARIËNS, E.J.: Molecular Pharmacology, Vol. 1. New York: Academic Press 1964.
— The structure-activity relationships of *beta* adrenergic drugs and *beta* adrenergic blocking drugs. Ann. N.Y. Acad. Sci. **139**, 606—631 (1967).
ARNOLD, A., MCAULIFF, J.P.: Guinea-pig adipose tissue responsiveness to catecholamines, Experientia (Basel) **24**, 436 (1968).
— — Correlation of calorigenesis with other β-l receptor mediated responses to catecholamines. Arch. int. Pharmacodyn. **179**, 381—387 (1969).
— — COLELLA, D.F., O'CONNOR, W.V., BROWN, JR., Th.G.: The β-2 receptor mediated glycogenolytic responses to catecholamines in the dog. Arch. int. Pharmacodyn. **176**, 451—457 (1968).
— SELBERIS, W.H.: Activities of catecholamines on the rat muscle glycogenolytic (β-2) receptor. Experientia (Basel) **24**, 1010—1011 (1968).
ARUNLAKSHANA, O., SCHILD, H.O.: Some quantitative uses of drug antagonists. Brit. J. Pharmacol. **14**, 48—58 (1959).
ASHMORE, J.: Insulin and adrenergic receptors. Fed. Proc. **29**, 1386—1387 (1970).
BARGER, G., DALE, H.H.: Chemical structure and sympathomimetic action of amines. J. Physiol. (Lond.) **51**, 19—59 (1910).
BENFEY, B.G., VARMA, D.R.: Interactions of sympathomimetic drugs, propranolol and phentolamine, on atrial refractory period and contractility. Brit. J. Pharmacol. **30**, 603—611 (1967).
BENNETT, A.: A pharmacological investigation of human isolated ileum. Nature (Lond.) **208**, 1289—1291 (1965).
BESSE, J., FURCHGOTT, R.F.: Dissociation constants and relative efficacies of agonists acting on adrenergic α-receptors. Fed. Proc. **26**, 401 (1967).
BEVAN, J.A., OSHER, J. V.: Relative sensitivity of some large blood vessels of the rabbit to sympathomimetic amines. J. Pharmacol. exp. Ther. **150**, 370—374 (1965).
BICKERTON, R.K.: The response of isolated strips of cat spleen to sympathomimetic drugs and their antagonists. J. Pharmacol. exp. Ther. **142**, 99—110 (1963).
BLINKS, J.R.: Evaluation of the cardiac effects of several *beta* adrenergic blocking agents. Ann. N.Y. Acad. Sci. **139**, 673—685 (1967).
BLOOM, F.E., GIARMAN, N.J.: Physiologic and pharmacologic considerations of biogenic amines in the nervous system. Ann. Rev. Pharmacol. **8**, 229—258 (1968).
BOHR, D.F.: Adrenergic receptors in coronary arteries. Ann. N.Y. Acad. Sci. **139**, 799—807 (1967).
BOWMAN, W.C., HALL, M.T.: Inhibition of rabbit intestine mediated by α- and β-adrenoceptors. Brit. J. Pharmacol. **38**, 399—415 (1970).
— NOTT, M.W.: Actions of sympathomimetic amines and their antagonists on skeletal muscle. Pharmacol. Rev. **21**, 27—72 (1969).
BRISTOW, M., SHERROD, T.R., GREEN, R.D.: Analysis of *beta* receptor drug interactions in isolated rabbit atrium, aorta, stomach and trachea. J. Pharmacol. exp. Ther. **171**, 52—61 (1970).
BRODY, T.M., DIAMOND, J.: Blockade of the biochemical correlates of contraction and relaxation in uterine and intestinal smooth muscle. Ann. N.Y. Acad. Sci. **139**, 772—780 (1967).
— MCNEILL, J.H.: Adrenergic receptors for metabolic responses in skeletal and smooth muscles. Fed. Proc. **29**, 1375—1378 (1970).
BROOKER, W.D., CALVERT, D.N.: Blockade of catecholamine mediated release of free fatty acids from adipose tissue *in vitro*. Arch. int. Pharmacodyn. **169**, 117—130 (1967).
BUCKLEY, G.A., JORDAN, C.C.: Temperature modulation of α- and β-adrenoceptors in the isolated frog heart. Brit. J. Pharmacol. **38**, 394—398 (1970).

BUCKNER, C.K., PATIL, P.N.: Steric aspects of adrenergic drugs. XVI. Beta-adrenergic receptors of guinea-pig atria and trachea. J. Pharmacol. exp. Ther. **176**, 634—649 (1971).
BÜLBRING, E., TOMITA, T.: Suppression of spontaneous spike generation by catecholamines in the smooth muscle of the guinea-pig taenia coli. Proc. roy. Soc. B. **172**, 103—119 (1969).
BURNS, J.J., SALVADOR, R.A., LEMBERGER, L.: Metabolic blockade by methoxamine and its analogs. Ann. N.Y. Acad. Sci. **139**, 833—840 (1967).
BUTCHER, R.W., BAIRD, C.E., SUTHERLAND, E.W.: Effects of lipolytic and antilipolytic substances on adenosine 3,'5'-monophosphate levels in isolated fat cells. J. biol. Chem. **243**, 1705—1712 (1968).
CERNOHORSKÝ, M., CEPELIK, J., LINCOVÁ, D., WENKE, M.: Comparison of lipomobilizing effects of norepinephrine and phenyl-t-butyl-noroxedrine *in vitro*. Arch. int. Pharmacodyn. **165**, 45—52 (1967).
CHAHL, L.A., O'DONNELL, S.R.: The interaction of cocaine and propranolol with catecholamines on guinea-pig trachea. Europ. J. Pharmacol. **2**, 77—82 (1967).
CHAN, P.S., ELLIS, S.: Dihydroergotamine antagonism of glucose release by rabbit liver slices induced by catecholamines, glucagon and 3',5'-AMP. Fed. Proc. **28**, 742 (1969).
COUPAR, I. M., TURNER, P.: Relative potencies of sympathetic amines in human smooth muscle. Brit. J. Pharmacol. **36**, 213P—214P (1969).
CURTIS, D.R., CRAWFORD, J.M.: Central synaptic transmission — microelectrophoretic studies. Ann. Rev. Pharmacol. **9**, 209—240 (1969).
DALE, H.H.: On some physiological actions of ergot. J. Physiol. (Lond.) **34**, 163—206 (1906).
DANIEL, E.F., PATON, D.M., TAYLOR, G.S., HODGSON, B.J.: Adrenergic receptors for catecholamine effects on tissue electrolytes. Fed. Proc. **29**, 1410—1425 (1970).
DAVIS, W.G.: The effects of beta adrenoceptor blocking agents on the membrane potential and spike generation in the smooth muscle of guinea-pig taenia coli. Brit. J. Pharmacol. **38**, 12—19 (1970).
DUNLOP, D., SHANKS, R.G.: Selective blockade of adrenoceptive beta receptors in the heart. Brit. J. Pharmacol. **32**, 201—218 (1968).
ELLIS, S., KENNEDY, B.L., EUSEBI, A.J., VINCENT, N.H.: Autonomic control of metabolism. Ann. N.Y. Acad. Sci. **139**, 826—832 (1967).
FAIN, J.N.: Adrenergic blockade of hormone-induced lipolysis in isolated fat cells. Ann. N.Y. Acad. Sci. **139**, 879—890 (1967).
— Dihydroergotamine, propranolol and the *beta* adrenergic receptors of fat cellls. Fed. Proc. **29**, 1402—1407 (1970).
FARMER, J.B., COLEMAN, R.A.: A new preparation of the isolated intact trachea of the guinea-pig. J. Pharm. Pharmacol. **22**, 46—50 (1970).
— LEVY, G.P.: Differentiation of β-adrenoreceptors by the use of blocking agents. J. Pharm. Pharmacol. **22**, 145—146 (1970).
— KENNEDY, I., LEVY, G.P., MARSHALL, R.J.: A comparison of the β-adrenoreceptor stimulant properties of isoprenaline, with those of orciprenaline, salbutamol, soterenol and trimetoquinol on isolated atria and trachea of the guinea-pig. J. Pharm. Pharmacol. **22**, 61—63 (1970).
FASSINA, G.: Effects of two beta-adrenergic blocking agents, propranolol and INPEA, on lipid metabolism. Arch. int. Pharmacodyn. **166**, 281—293 (1967).
FLEMING, W.W., HAWKINS, D.F.: The actions of dichloroisoproterenol in the dog heart-lung preparation and the isolated guinea-pig atrium. J. Pharmacol. exp. Ther. **129**, 1—10 (1960).
FOO, J.W., JOWETT, A., STAFFORD, A.: The effects of some β-adrenoreceptor blocking drugs on the uptake and release of noradrenaline by the heart. Brit. J. Pharmacol. **34**, 141—147 (1968).
FOSTER, R.W.: The nature of the adrenergic receptors of the trachea of the guinea-pig. J. Pharm. Pharmacol. **18**, 1—12 (1966).
— The potentiation of the responses to noradrenaline and isoprenaline of the guinea-pig isolated tracheal chain preparation by desipramine, cocaine, phentolamine, phenoxybenzamine, guanethidine, metanephrine and cooling. Brit. J. Pharmacol. **31**, 466—482 (1967).
— A correlation between inhibition of the uptake of ^{3}H from (±)-^{3}H-noradrenaline and potentiation of the responses to (—)-noradrenaline in the guinea-pig isolated trachea. Brit. J. Pharmacol. **33**, 357—367 (1968).
— An uptake of radioactivity from (±)-^{3}H-isoprenaline and its inhibition by drugs which potentiate the responses to (—)-^{3}H-isoprenaline in the guinea-pig isolated trachea. Brit. J. Pharmacol. **35**, 418—427 (1969).
FÜLGRAFF, G., HEIDENREICH, O., HEINTZE, K., OSSWALD, H.: Die Wirkung von α- und β-Sympathomimetica und Sympatholytica auf die renale Exkretion und Resorption von Flüssigkeit und Elektrolyten in Ausscheidungs- und Mikropunktionsversuchen an Ratten. Naunyn-Schmiedebergs Arch. Pharmak. exp. Path. **262**, 295—308 (1969).

FURCHGOTT, R.F.: Dibenamine blockade in strips of rabbit aorta and its use in differentiating receptors. J. Pharmacol. exp. Ther. **111**, 165-284 (1954).
— The pharmacology of vascular smooth muscle. Pharmacol. Rev. **7**, 183—265 (1955).
— The receptors for epinephrine and norepinephrine (adrenergic receptors). Pharmacol. Rev. **11**, 429—441 (1959).
— Receptors for sympathomimetic amines. Receptors for sympathomimetic amines. In: Ciba Foundation Symposium on adrenergic mechanisms, pp. 246—252. Ed. by J. R. VANE, G.E.W. WOLSTENHOLME and C.M. O'CONNOR. Boston: Little, Brown 1960.
— Receptor mechanisms. Ann. Rev. Pharmacol. **4**, 21—50 (1964).
— The use of β-haloalkylamines in the differentiation of receptors and in the determination of dissociation constants of receptoragonist complexes. In: Advances in drug research, Vol. 3, pp. 21—55. Ed. by HARPER and A.B. SIMMONDS. London: Academic Press 1966.
— The pharmacological differentiation of adrenergic receptors. Ann. N.Y. Acad. Sci. **139**, 553—570 (1967).
— A critical appraisal of the use of isolated organ systems for the assessment of drug action at the receptor level. In: Importance of fundamental principles in drug evaluation, pp. 277—298. Ed. by D.H. TEDESCHI and R.E. TEDESCHI. New York: Raven Press 1968.
— Pharmacological characteristics of adrenergic receptors. Fed. Proc. **29**, 1352—1361 (1970).
— BHADRAKOM, S.: Reactions of strips of rabbit aorta to epinephrine, isoproterenol, sodium nitrite and other drugs. J. Pharmacol. exp. Ther. **108**, 129—143 (1953).
— BURSZTYN, P.: Comparison of dissociation constants and of relative efficacies of selected agonists acting on parasympathetic receptors. Ann. N.Y. Acad. Sci. **144**, 882—899 (1967).
— KIRPEKAR, S.M.: Competition between β-haloalkylamines and norepinephrine for sites in cardiac muscle. Proc. First Intern. Pharmacol. Meeting. Vol. **7**, 339—350. Oxford: Pergamon 1963.
— — RIEKER, M.S., SCHWAB, A.: Actions and interactions of norepinephrine, tyramine and cocaine on aortic strips of rabbit and left atria of guinea-pig and cat. J. Pharmacol. exp. Ther. **142**, 39—58 (1963).
GOVIER, W.C.: Myocardial *alpha* adrenergic receptors and their role in the production of a positive inotropic effect by sympathomimetic agents. J. Pharmacol. exp. Ther. **159**, 82—90 (1968).
— MOSAL, N.C., WHITTINGTON, P., BROOM, A.H.: Myocardial *alpha* and *beta* adrenergic receptors as demonstrated by atrial functional refractory period changes. J. Pharmacol. exp. Ther. **154**, 255—263 (1966).
GREEN, R.D., III, FLEMING, W.W.: Analyiss of supersensitivity in the isolated spleen of the cat. J. Pharmacol. exp. Ther. **162**, 254—262 (1968).
GUIMARAES, S., OSSWALD, W.: Adrenergic receptors in the veins of the dog. Europ. J. Pharmacol. **5**, 133—140 (1969).
GULATI, O.D., GOKHALE, S.D., PARIKH, H.M., UDWADIA, B.P., KRISHNAMURTY, V.S.R.: Evidence for a sympathetic *alpha* receptor blocking action of *beta* receptor blocking agents. J. Pharmacol. exp. Ther. **166**, 35—43 (1969).
HEDGES, A., TURNER, P.: Beta-receptors in human isolated smooth muscle. Brit. J. Pharmacol. **37**, 547P—548P (1969).
HIMMS-HAGEN, J.: Sympathetic regulation of metabolism. Pharmacol. Rev. **19**, 367—461 (1967).
— Adrenergic receptors for metabolic responses in adipose tissue. Fed. Proc. **29**, 1388—1401 (1970).
HORNBROOK, K.R.: Adrenergic receptors for metabolic responses in the liver. Fed. Proc. **29**, 1381—1385 (1970).
IGNARRO, L.J., TITUS, E.: The presence of antagonistically acting *alpha* and *beta* adrenergic receptors in the mouse spleen. J. Pharmacol. exp. Ther. **160**, 72—80 (1968).
IVERSEN, L.L.: The uptake and storage of noradrenaline in sympathetic nerves. Cambridge: Cambridge University Press 1966.
JANG, C.-S.: The potentiation and paralysis of adrenergic effect by ergotamine and other substances. J. Pharmacol. exp. Ther. **71**, 87—94 (1941).
JENKINSON, D.H., MORTON, I.K.M.: Adrenergic blocking drugs as tools in the study of the actions of catecholamines on the smooth muscle membrane. Ann. N.Y. Acad. Sci. **139**, 762—771 (1967).
KABELA, E., JALIFE, J., PEON, C., CROS, L., MENDEZ, R.: The adrenergic receptors of the coronary circulation in the isolated dog heart. Arch. int. Pharmacodyn. **181**, 328—342 (1969).
KALSNER, S., NICKERSON, M.: Disposition of norepinephrine and epinephrine in vascular tissue, determined by the technique of oil immersion. J. Pharmacol. exp. Ther. **165**, 152—165 (1969a).
— — Effects of a haloalkylamine on responses to and disposition of sympathomimetic amines. Brit. J. Pharmacol. **35**, 440—455 (1969b).

KAUMANN, A.J.: Supersensitivity to exogenous and endogenously released norepinephrine after COMT inhibition and cocaine. Fed. Proc. **27**, 711 (1968).

KOHLI, J.D.: Receptors for sympathomimetic amines in the rabbit aorta: Differentiation by specific antagonists. Brit. J. Pharmacol. **32**, 273—279 (1968).

— LING, G.M.: *Alpha*-adrenergic blocking action of propranolol. J. Pharm. Pharmacol. **19**, 629—631 (1967).

KOSTERLITZ, H.W., WATT, A.J.: Adrenergic receptors in the guinea-pig ileum. J. Physiol. (Lond.) **177**, 11P—12P (1965).

KUNOS, G., SZENTIVANYI, M.: Evidence favouring the existence of a single adrenergic receptor. Nature (Lond.) **217**, 1077—1078 (1968).

LANDS, A.M., ARNOLD, A., MCAULIFF, J.P., LUDUENA, F.P., BROWN, T.G.: Differentiation of receptor systems activated by sympathomimetic amines. Nature (Lond.) **214**,597—598 (1967a).

— GROBLEWSKI, G.E., BROWN, T.G.: Comparison of the action of isoproterenol and several related compounds on blood pressure, heart and bronchioles. Arch. int. Pharmacodyn. **161**, 68—75 (1966).

— LUDUENA, F.P., BUZZO, H.J.: Differentiation of receptors responsive to isoproterenol. Life Sci. **6**, 2241—2249 (1967b).

— — — Adrenotrophic β-receptors in the frog and chicken. Life Sci. **8**, 373—382 (1969).

LANGER, S.Z., TRENDELENBURG, U.: The effect of a saturable uptake mechanism on the slopes of dose-response curves for sympathomimetic amines and on the shifts of dose-response curves produced by a competitive antagonist. J. Pharmacol. exp. Ther. **167**, 117—142 (1969).

LANGLEY, J.N.: On the reaction of cells and of nerve-endings to certain poisons, chiefly as regards the reaction of striated muscle to nicotine and to curare. J. Physiol. (Lond.) **33**, 374—413 (1905).

LAPIDUS, J.B., TYE, A., PATIL, P.N.: Steric aspects of adrenergic drugs. VII. Certain pharmacological actions of D(—)-pseudoephedrine. J. pharm. Sci. **56**, 1125—1130 (1967).

LEVIN, J.A., FURCHGOTT, R.F.: Interactions between potentiating agents of adrenergic amines in rabbit aortic strips. J. Pharmacol. exp. Ther. **172**, 320—331 (1970).

LEVY, B.: The adrenergic blocking activity of N-tert.-butylmethoxamine (butoxamine). J. Pharmacol. exp. Ther. **151**, 413—422 (1966).

— Selective *beta* receptor blockade in rat smooth muscle. Arch. int. Pharmacodyn. **170**, 418—427 (1967).

— TOZZI, S.: The adrenergic receptive mechanism of the rat uterus. J. Pharmacol. exp. Ther. **142**, 178—184 (1963).

— WASSERMAN, M.: 1-isopropylamino-3-(4-indanoxy)-2-propanol HCl: a potent β-adrenoceptor antagonist. Brit. J. Pharmacol. **39**, 139—148 (1970).

— WILKENFELD, B.E.: Selective interactions with *beta* adrenergic receptors. Fed. Proc. **29**, 1362—1364 (1970).

LUCCHESI, B.R., WHITSITT, L.S., STICKNEY, J.I.: Antiarrhythmic effects of *beta* adrenergic blocking agents. Ann. N.Y. Acad. Sci. **139**, 940—951 (1967).

MACKAY, D.: The mathematics of drug-receptor interactions. J. Pharm. Pharmacol. **18**, 201—222 (1966).

MANLEY, E.S., LAWSON, J.W.: Effect of beta adrenergic receptor blockade on skeletal muscle vasodilatation produced by isoxsuprine and nylidrin. Arch. int. Pharmacodyn. **175**, 239—250 (1968).

MAYER, S.E.: Adrenergic receptors for metabolic responses in the heart. Fed. Proc. **29**, 1367—1372 (1970).

MAZURKIEWICZ-KWILECKI, I.M.: Antagonistic effects of β-adrenergic blocking agents on responses to adrenaline in vascular smooth muscle. Arch. int. Pharmacodyn. **174**, 199—209 (1968).

MILLER, J.W.: Adrenergic receptors in the myometrium. Ann. N.Y. Acad. Sci. **139**, 788—798 (1967).

MOORE, G.E., O'DONNELL, S.R.: A potent β-adrenoreceptor blocking drug: 4-(2-hydroxy-3-isopropylaminopropoxy)indole. J. Pharm. Pharmacol. **22**, 180—188 (1970).

MORAN, N.C.: The development of *beta* adrenergic blocking drugs: A retrospective and prospective evaluation. Ann. N.Y. Acad. Sci. **139**, 649—660 (1967).

— PERKINS, M.E.: Adrenergic blockade of the mammalian heart by a dichloro analogue of isoproterenol. J. Pharmacol. exp. Ther. **124**, 223—237 (1958).

MUNRO, A.F.: The effect of adrenaline and noradrenaline on the activity of isolated preparations of the gut from the foetal guinea-pig. Brit. J. Pharmacol. **8**, 38—41 (1953).

NAGASAKA, M., BOUCKAERT, J., DE SCHAEPDRYVER, A.F., HEYMANS, C.: Adrenergic constriction in isolated guinea-pig lung revealed by Nethalide. Arch. int. Pharmacodyn. **149**, 237—242 (1964).

NEDERGAARD, O.A., WESTERMANN, E.: Action of various sympathomimetic amines on the isolated stripped vas deferens of the guinea-pig. Brit. J. Pharmacol. **34**, 475—483 (1968).
NICKERSON, M.: The pharmacology of adrenergic blockade. Pharmacol. Rev. **1**, 27—101 (1949).
— New developments in adrenergic blocking drugs. Ann. N.Y. Acad. Sci. **139**, 571—579 (1967).
NORTHROP, G.: Effects of adrenergic blocking agents on epinephrine- and 3',5'-AMP-induced responses in the perfused rat liver. J. Pharmacol. exp. Ther. **159**, 22—28 (1968).
PALM, D., LANGENECKERT, W., HOLTZ, P.: Bedeutung der N- und β-Methylierung für die Affinität von Brenzcatechinaminen zu den adrenergischen Receptoren. Naunyn-Schmiedeberg's Arch. Pharmak. exp. Path. **258**, 128—149 (1967).
PATIL, P.N.: Steric aspects of adrenergic drugs. VIII. Optical isomers of *beta* adrenergic receptor antagonists. J. Pharmacol. exp. Ther. **160**, 308—314 (1968).
— Adrenergic receptors of the bovine iris sphincter. J. Pharmacol. exp. Ther. **166**, 299—307 (1969).
— PATEL, D.G., KRELL, R.D.: Steric aspects of adrenergic drugs. XV. Use of isomeric-activity-ratio as a criterion to differentiate adrenergic receptors. J. Pharmacol. exp. Ther. **176**, 622—633 (1971).
— TYE, A., MAY, C., HETEY, S., MIYAGI, S.: Steric aspects of adrenergic drugs. XI. Interactions of dibenamine and *beta* adrenergic blockers. J. Pharmacol. exp. Ther. **163**, 309—319 (1968).
PATON, W.D.M.: A theory of drug action based on the rate of drug-receptor combination. Proc. roy. Soc. B. **154**, 21—69 (1961).
PERSSON, H., JOHNSON, B.: Adrenergic receptors in the guinea-pig trachea and lung. Acta pharmacol. (Kbh.) **28**, 49—56 (1970).
POTTER, L.T.: Uptake of propranolol by isolated guinea-pig atria. J. Pharmacol. exp. Ther. **155**, 91—100 (1967).
POWELL, C.E., SLATER, I.H.: Blocking of inhibitory adrenergic receptors by a dichloro analogue of isoproterenol. J. Pharmacol. exp. Ther. **122**, 480—488 (1958).
RANG, H.P.: The kinetics of action of acetylcholine antagonists in smooth muscle. Proc. roy. Soc. B. **164**, 488—510 (1966).
RAPER, C., WALE, J.: Specificity of β-receptor antagonists. Europ. J. Pharmacol. **3**, 279—281 (1968).
REDDY, V., MORAN, N.C.: An evaluation of the adrenergic receptor types in isolated segments of the small intestine of the rabbit. Arch. int. Pharmacodyn. **176**, 326—336 (1968).
ROBISON, G.A., BUTCHER, R.W., SUTHERLAND, E.W.: Adenyl cyclase as an adrenergic receptor. Ann. N.Y. Acad. Sci. **139**, 703—723 (1967).
ROTHLIN, E., CERLETTI, A.: Untersuchungen über die Kreislaufwirkung des Ergotamin. Helv. physiol. pharmacol. Acta **7**, 333—370 (1949).
SALMOIRAGHI, G.C.: Central adrenergic synapses. Pharmacol. Rev. **18**, 717—726 (1966).
SALVADOR, R.A., COLVILLE, K.I., APRIL, S.A., BURNS, J.J.: Inhibition of lipid mobilization by N-isopropyl methoxamine. J. Pharmacol. exp. Ther. **144**, 172—180 (1964).
SALZMANN, R., PACHA, W., TAESCHLER, M., WEIDMANN, H.: The effect of ergotamine on humoral and neuronal actions in the nictitating membrane and the spleen of the cat. Naunyn-Schmiedeberg's Arch. Pharmak. exp. Path. **261**, 360—378 (1968).
SCHILD, H.O.: The use of drug antagonists for the identification and classification of drugs. Brit. J. Pharmacol. **2**, 251—258 (1947).
— pA_x and competitive drug antagonism. Brit. J. Pharmacol. **4**, 277—280 (1949).
SMITH, C.B.: Relaxation of the nictitating membrane of the spinal cat by sympathomimetic amines. J. Pharmacol. exp. Ther. **142**, 163—170 (1963).
SOMANI, P., LUM, B.K.B.: The antiarrhythmic actions of beta-adrenergic blocking agents. J. Pharmacol. exp. Ther. **147**, 194—204 (1965).
STEPHENSON, R.P.: A modification of receptor theory. Brit. J. Pharmacol. **11**, 379—393 (1956).
TAKAGI, K., TAKAYANAGI, I.: Beta-adrenergic receptors in various organs. Jap. J. Pharmacol. **20**, 92—101 (1970).
THRON, C.D., WAUD, D.R.: The rate of action of atropine. J. Pharmacol. exp. Ther. **160**, 91—105 (1968).
TRENDELENBURG, U., DE LA SIERRA, B.G.A., MUSKUS, A.: Modification by reserpine of the response of the atrial pacemaker to sympathomimetic amines. J. Pharmacol. exp. Ther. **141**, 301—309 (1963).
— MAXWELL, R.A., PLUCHINO, S.: Methoxamine as a tool to assess the importance of intraneuronal uptake of l-norepinephrine in the cat's nictitating membrane. J. Pharmacol. exp. Ther. **172**, 91—99 (1970).

Urquilla, P.R., Stitzel, R.E., Fleming, W.W.: The antagonism of phentolamine against exogenously administered and endogenously released norepinephrine in rabbit aortic strips. J. Pharmacol. exp. Ther. **172**, 310—319 (1970).

Van Rossum, J.M.: Different types of sympathomimetic α-receptors. J. Pharm. Pharmacol. **17**, 202—216 (1965).

— Ariëns, E.J.: Receptor-reserve and threshold-phenomena. Arch. int. Pharmacodyn. **136**, 385—413 (1962).

Volle, R.L.: Ganglionic transmission. Ann. Rev. Pharmacol. **9**, 135—146 (1969).

Waud, D.R.: Pharmacological receptors. Pharmacol. Rev. **20**, 49—88 (1968).

— A quantitative model for the effect of a saturable uptake on the slope of the dose-response curve. J. Pharmacol. exp. Ther. **167**, 140—142 (1969).

Weisbrodt, N.W., Hug, C.C., Jr., Bass, P.: Separation of the effects of *alpha* and *beta* adrenergic receptor stimulation on taenia coli. J. Pharmacol. exp. Ther. **170**, 272—280 (1969).

Wenke, M., Lincová, D., Cepelík, J., Cernohorský, M., Hynie, S.: Some aspects of the action of *beta* adrenergic blocking drugs on adrenergic lipid mobilization. Ann. N.Y. Acad. Sci. **139**, 860—878 (1967).

Wurzel, M., Pruss, T.P., Koppanyi, T., Maengwyn-Davies, G.D.: Dichloroisoproterenol blockade of the rabbit aortic strip. Arch. int. Pharamcodyn. **141**, 153—162 (1963).

Chapter 10

Classification of Sympathomimetic Amines

U. Trendelenburg

With 5 Figures

I. Introduction

Long before the mechanism of action of the indirectly acting sympathomimetic amines was understood, it was clear that the amines of this group differ pharmacologically. For instance, while cocaine potentiates the effects of adrenaline (Fröhlich and Loewi, 1910) it antagonizes the effects of tyramine (Tainter and Chang, 1927). A parallel to this "cocaine paradox" was observed after chronic sympathetic denervation, a procedure which potentiates the effects of adrenaline and antagonizes those of tyramine (Burn and Tainter, 1931; Bülbring and Burn, 1938).

In 1932 Burn was the first to suggest that storage sites of the adrenergic transmitter might be involved in the action of tyramine, since the effect of tyramine on the perfused hind leg of the dog was restored after infusions of adrenaline into preparations which had lost their responsiveness to tyramine. However, this explanation of the mode of action of tyramine was dropped in favor of another hypothesis (Bülbring and Burn, 1938). A careful quantitative comparison of the effects of chronic sympathetic denervation and of cocaine on responses to a large series of sympathomimetic amines (Fleckenstein and Burn, 1953; Fleckenstein and Bass, 1953; Fleckenstein and Stöckle, 1955) led Fleckenstein (1953) to subdivide sympathomimetic amines into three groups: the "directly acting" amines (assumed to act directly on the adrenoceptors of effector organs), an "intermediate group" (thought to owe its action partly to a direct effect, partly to an action on the adrenergic neurone), and the "neuro-sympathomimetic amines" (effective only in the presence of functionally intact adrenergic nerve endings). As one possibility it was suggested that neuro-sympathomimetic amines might release the transmitter from adrenergic nerve endings.

Conclusive evidence for the release of noradrenaline by tyramine (and similar drugs) was obtained in subsequent years. A decisive step was the discovery of the noradrenaline-depleting action of reserpine (Carlsson et al., 1957; Paasonen and Krayer, 1957; Burn and Rand, 1957) and the demonstration that tyramine lost its effectiveness after depletion of the noradrenaline stores by reserpine (Carlsson et al., 1957; Burn and Rand, 1958). Burn and Rand (1958) were the first to use pretreatment with reserpine as an experimental tool for distinguishing various directly acting amines from those which act through the release of the transmitter (*i.e.*, the indirectly acting ones). With the help of radioactively labeled noradrenaline and of newly developed fluorimetric methods for the determination of noradrenaline, the mode of action of tyramine was then established by contributions from many laboratories.

Thus, it became evident that some sympathomimetic amines (*i.e.*, the directly acting ones) interact with the α- or β-receptors of the effector organs, while others (*i.e.*, the indirectly acting amines) exert their actions through the release of the stored transmitter. Several attempts were made to classify sympathomimetic amines (FLECKENSTEIN and BURN, 1953; FLECKENSTEIN and BASS, 1953; FLEKKENSTEIN and STÖCKLE, 1955; BURN and RAND, 1958; MAXWELL et al., 1959b; HOLTZ et al., 1960; SCHMITT and SCHMITT, 1960; LIEBMAN, 1961; MARLEY, 1962; TRENDELENBURG et al., 1962a; TRENDELENBURG et al., 1962b; SCHMIDT and FLEMING, 1963; TRENDELENBURG et al., 1963) most of which have been reviewed earlier (TRENDELENBURG, 1963). Two main conclusions can be drawn from these attempts. First, sympathomimetic amines do not fall into just two groups; they cover the whole spectrum that reaches from purely directly acting amines to the purely indirectly acting ones. Second, a classification of amines derived from a study of one organ or system does not necessarily apply to other organs or systems; or in other words, there are organ differences, and there may well be species differences.

It is the aim of this review to discuss the factors which determine to what extent an amine exerts its effects directly and/or indirectly. For a better understanding of these factors, the mode of action of the indirectly acting amines will be discussed briefly. Since most of the work has been carried out with tyramine, this agent may be regarded as the prototype of the indirectly acting sympathomimetic amines.

The adrenergic neurone has two uptake mechanisms for agents related to noradrenaline, one in the neuronal cell membrane, the other in storage vesicles. In order to avoid confusion, in this review the uptake across the neuronal membrane will be referred to as "membranal uptake", while "vesicular uptake" refers to the uptake from the cytoplasm into storage vesicles.

II. The Mode of Action of Tyramine

In most adrenergically innervated tissues tyramine has very weak direct actions on α-receptors and even weaker effects on β-receptors. Uptake by adrenergic nerves occurs through the cocaine-sensitive uptake of the neuronal cell membrane (ROSS and RENYI, 1966a; COMMARATO et al., 1969). Tyramine is a good substrate of intraneuronal monoamine oxidase (MAO), the activity of which reduces the concentration of cytoplasmic tyramine; this is indicated by the pronounced potentiation of the indirect effects of tyramine after block of MAO (SMITH, 1966). From the cytoplasm tyramine is taken up by the storage vesicles; the mechanism involved is not the ATP-Mg^{++}-activated uptake which transports noradrenaline and adrenaline (CARLSSON et al., 1963; LUNDBORG, 1966).

Inside the vesicles two events take place. Endogenous noradrenaline is displaced from vesicular binding sites, and tyramine is converted by dopamine β-hydroxylase to octopamine. It is unlikely that the second event is a precondition for the first, since block of dopamine β-hydroxylase by disulfiram does not prevent the indirect effects of tyramine (MUSACCHIO et al., 1966).

The noradrenaline displaced from vesicular storage sites has to pass through the cytoplasm before reaching the extracellular space; hence, some of the displaced noradrenaline is deaminated intraneuronally. This view is based on the observation that pretreatment with α-methyl-dopa (and the consequent formation of the false transmitter, α-methyl-noradrenaline, which is not a substrate of MAO) potentiates the indirect effects of tyramine, although the potency of α-methylnoradrenaline equals that of noradrenaline in the tissue under study (isolated guinea-pig atria) (SMITH, 1966). The amounts of noradrenaline which finally escape from the neuron are very small (LINDMAR and MUSCHOLL, 1961; WEINER et al., 1962); nevertheless, they cause pronounced sympathomimetic effects, since tyramine prevents the re-uptake of the released transmitter (LINDMAR and MUSCHOLL, 1965).

Part of the intravesicular tyramine is converted to octopamine. Since at least two hydroxyl groups are required for intravesicular binding (MUSACCHIO et al., 1965) octopamine is bound in vesicles while tyramine is not. As a consequence, octopamine is well retained by adrenergically innervated tissues, while tyramine is lost quite rapidly (LEE et al., 1967; COMMARATO et al., 1969). The intraneuronal tyramine and octopamine are responsible for two phenomena which are typical for indirectly acting amines: tachyphylaxis and the formation of a false transmitter. Tachyphylaxis develops on repeated administration of tyramine and is accompanied by a reduction in the release of noradrenaline (AXELROD et al., 1962) because tyramine then releases a mixture of the transmitter plus tyramine and/or octopamine (PÖCH and KOPIN, 1966; LEE et al., 1967). Apparently, tyramine acts on a small compartment of the noradrenaline stores, since pronounced tachyphylaxis is observed without any measurable decline in the total noradrenaline content of the tissue (LEE et al., 1967; WAKADE et al., 1970). The vesicle-bound octopamine behaves like a false transmitter and is released by nerve stimulation (KOPIN et al., 1965).

An important aspect of the action of tyramine concerns the size of the noradrenaline compartment on which the indirectly acting amine acts. As mentioned above, moderate doses of tyramine do not deplete the noradrenaline stores and thus seem to act on a small compartment. Moreover, when tachyphylaxis to tyramine is abolished by an exposure of the tissue to noradrenaline, only the first response to tyramine is restored to nearly normal; tachyphylaxis is quickly reestablished to subsequent administrations of tyramine (WAKADE et al., 1970). The small size of the noradrenaline compartment involved in responses to tyramine is also demonstrated by experiments with reserpine-pretreated guinea-pig atria whose response to tyramine is restored to nearly normal by an exposure to noradrenaline. A restoration of the effect to 70% of normal is obtained when the noradrenaline content of the tissue rises from 1.1 to 2.2% of normal (CROUT et al., 1962). As with tachyphylaxis to tyramine (in normal atria), the refilling of noradrenaline stores restores the response to only one administration of tyramine; the response to subsequent administrations of tyramine declines (TRENDELENBURG and CROUT, 1964). All these findings are in agreement with the view that a very small compartment of the total noradrenaline store is involved in responses to tyramine as well as in the phenomena of restoration of responses to tyramine after tachyphylaxis or pretreatment with reserpine.

Very high doses of tyramine seem to affect a larger compartment, since they are able to produce partial depletion of the noradrenaline stores (WEINER et al., 1962).

There has not been any corroboration of the claim that tyramine acts on specific tyramine receptors (VARMA et al., 1964), neither has supporting evidence been obtained for the view that though tyramine acts on adrenoceptors, the presence of noradrenaline or a closely related amine acting as a catalyst is required (MURNAGHAN, 1965).

While several schemes can be envisaged to account for the compartments of the noradrenaline stores, a simple model suggested by CROUT (1964) may be the most useful. According to this model the population of storage vesicles and of binding sites is homogeneous. The decisive factor is the distance of the storage vesicles from the cell membrane. Because of the very high rate of uptake of tyramine through the cell membrane, the peripherally located vesicles should be exposed to a very high concentration of tyramine. The concentration gradient towards the centre of the varicosity should be accentuated by the deamination of cytoplasmic tyramine by mitochondrial MAO. According to this view, tyramine reaches only a small compartment of the total store, that in the peripherally located vesicles; the transmitter would be displaced from vesicles in the vicinity of the cell membrane, where deamination of the displaced transmitter would play a minor role. Very high doses of tyramine, on the other hand, would also affect the more centrally located vesicles. This view is attractive because the size of the compartment would be determined by the dose of the releaser, by the rate of uptake and by the activity of intraneuronal MAO. Or in other words, depleting effects need not be regarded as being qualitatively different from noradrenaline-releasing effects.

It is quite possible that the events summarized here may be modified in tissues in which the adrenergic nerves have unusual properties. For instance, BARNETT et al. (1969) found the indirect effects of tyramine on the isolated vas deferens of the rat to be cocaine-resistant. Apparently, the membranal uptake of this organ differs from that of others.

Recent experiments with cocaine and cocaine-like agents revealed new facts. While cocaine competitively antagonizes the retention of tyramine in rat brain slices as well as the deamination of the amine and the synthesis of octopamine, desipramine depresses the synthesis of octopamine much more than the retention as well as the deamination of tyramine (STEINBERG and SMITH, 1970). Thus, while cocaine seems to have one site of action (the uptake across the neuronal membrane), desipramine appears to antagonize the vesicular uptake of tyramine as well. On the isolated human umbilical artery the effect of tyramine is potentiated by cocaine rather than antagonized. Since this preparation develops tachyphylaxis to tyramine, and since noradrenaline restores responses of tachyphylactic arteries to tyramine, GULATI and KELKAR (1971) suggest that extraneuronal noradrenaline may be the mediator of the effect of tyramine on this nerve-free preparation.

III. Experimental Approaches to the Classification

Three different designs of experiments have been used in attempts to classify sympathomimetic amines. Though useful information has been obtained with all three, pretreatment with reserpine yields the most reliable quantitative information. However, even this method presents problems.

a) Cocaine

As mentioned above, cocaine tends to potentiate the directly acting amines, while it antagonizes the indirectly acting ones. However, two complicating factors are encountered in experiments with cocaine:

1. Cocaine has sympathomimetic actions, *i.e.*, it causes a contraction of the cat's nictitating membrane and it has a positive chronotropic effect on isolated guinea-pig atria (TRENDELENBURG, 1968). These sympathomimetic effects seem to be due to the release of noradrenaline from the stores; or in other words, cocaine has indirect effects. The noradrenaline-releasing effect of cocaine results in a false baseline for dose-response curves for sympathomimetic amines; hence, determinations of the potency of amines in the presence of cocaine are not accurate. They are accurate only when the indirect effects of cocaine have been abolished by pretreatment with reserpine (TRENDELENBURG, 1968).

2. Cocaine potentiates only those directly acting amines which are taken up. Directly acting amines which are not taken up (*e.g.*, isoprenaline — HERTTING, 1964; methoxamine — TRENDELENBURG et al., 1970) cannot be expected to be

potentiated by cocaine. However, failure by cocaine to alter the sensitivity of an organ to an amine does not necessarily indicate that the amine is a directly acting one which is not taken up by adrenergic nerve endings. It might as well be an amine which is taken up and which has both direct and indirect effects; cocaine may fail to cause a change in sensitivity to the amine, because the supersensitivity to the direct effects masks the subsensitivity to the indirect ones. Thus, in the absence of information on uptake, results with cocaine may lead to errors in classification.

b) Denervation

As with cocaine, indirect effects may be masked by the supersensitivity to direct ones of those amines which are taken up. Moreover, further possible complications have to be considered:

1. Spinal cats have rather high levels of circulating catecholamines (LANGER et al., 1967); these cause a contraction of the denervated but not of the normal nictitating membrane of the cat (LANGER, 1966). This unilateral tone distorts dose-response curves and falsifies ED50's (LANGER et al., 1967). This problem can be avoided by the use of pithed cats which lack tone of the denervated nictitating membrane.

2. When the interval between denervation and the experiment is increased beyond 3 days, the nictitating membrane acquires a second type of supersensitivity which is unrelated to nerve endings. This nonspecific, postjunctional type of supersensitivity resembles that seen after decentralization (preganglionic denervation) and is equally pronounced for directly and indirectly acting amines (TRENDELENBURG, 1963). It is equally pronounced for amines which are taken up and for those which are not (PLUCHINO and TRENDELENBURG, 1968; TRENDELENBURG et al., 1970). In order to avoid these changes in sensitivity which are not related to changes in adrenergic nerve endings, experiments with denervated preparations should be carried out before the decentralization-type of supersensitivity develops.

c) Pretreatment with Reserpine

Pretreatment with reserpine depletes the noradrenaline stores and thus abolishes the indirect effects of sympathomimetic amines (BURN and RAND, 1958). Since this pretreatment does not affect the membranal uptake (LINDMAR and MUSCHOLL, 1964), the disadvantages of cocaine and denervation (*i.e.*, the potentiation of those amines which are taken up) are largely avoided. However, pretreatment with reserpine is not without difficulties. For instance, the dose of reserpine required for adequate depletion of the noradrenaline stores may differ very much from organ to organ (LEE, 1967); hence, the adequacy of the pretreatment should be determined. Moreover, the schedule of pretreatment is of importance, since prolonged pretreatment results in the appearance of the decentralization-type of supersensitivity (FLEMING and TRENDELENBURG, 1961). Unfortunately, there are pronounced organ differences with regard to the duration of the pretreatment required to produce this postjunctional supersensitivity. For instance, in spinal cats there is no change in the sensitivity of the nictitating membrane to (—)-noradrenaline 24 hours after a single dose of reserpine, while both blood pressure and heart rate exhibit some supersensitivity (FLEMING and TRENDELENBURG, 1961). On the other hand, large doses of reserpine can cause postjunctional depressant effects which are unrelated to the depletion of the noradrenaline stores (FLEMING and TRENDELENBURG, 1961; WESTFALL and FLEMING, 1968). Hence, it is necessary to select for each organ an optimal pretreatment schedule, *i.e.*, one which combines pronounced depletion of the noradrenaline stores with minimal changes in sensitivity.

Irrespective of the method used for classification, another problem lies in the determination of the potency of the direct effects. Incomplete abolition of the indirect effects (because of inadequate doses of cocaine or reserpine, or because of incomplete denervation) would lead to false values for direct effects. On the other hand, some unquestionably direct effects have been demonstrated for most indirectly acting amines, although the nature of these effects has not been established in all cases. Since indirectly acting amines lose most of their potency after pretreatment with reserpine (or after denervation or cocaine), it is quite possible that the remaining weak direct effects are due to an action on receptors other than the α- or β-receptors. For instance, some sympathomimetic amines have been found to act on 5-hydroxytryptamine receptors of various tissues (INNES and KOHLI, 1969). Another complicating factor arises from the possibility that indirectly acting amines might exert other indirect effects which are not mediated by adrenergic nerves. Tyramine, for instance, is able to release histamine (VANDERIPE and KAHN, 1964; GROBECKER et al., 1966; MAJ and LANGWINSKI, 1966). Finally, high concentrations of indirectly acting amines may exert non-specific depressant effects on certain tissues which prevent the detection of weak stimulant effects; this is seen with isolated guinea-pig atria (TRENDELENBURG et al., 1963; TSAI et al., 1969). These considerations demonstrate the difficulties encountered in the exact quantitative determination of the weak direct potency of predominantly indirectly acting amines.

KALSNER (1970) observed another effect of tyramine which is unrelated to the properties of the amine enumerated above. Tyramine potentiates the effects of histamine on rabbit aortic strips by preventing the metabolism of the latter by imidazole-N-methyl transferase.

IV. Factors Determining the Magnitude of Direct and of Indirect Effects

The terms "directly" and "indirectly acting sympathomimetic amines" are unfortunate in so far as they imply qualitative differences between the two groups. However, we have to consider quantitative differences. As described for tyramine (see section II), a series of events leads to the release of endogenous noradrenaline, and the mechanisms involved in these events are those which normally handle the natural transmitter (or its precursor, dopamine). Hence, any differences between the actions of noradrenaline (the prototype of the directly acting amines) and tyramine (the indirectly acting amine) are quantitative rather than qualitative. As a corollary, any classification of amines should be based on quantitative considerations. Sympathomimetic amines should be regarded as a group of agents which share certain basic properties but which may differ quantitatively in their affinities to the various mechanisms involved.

As a broad generalization, it may be stated that direct effects of an amine should be expected to predominate whenever the affinity of the amine to the adrenoceptors is high, while a low affinity to the receptors should favour the appearance of indirect effects. It should be realized that many sympathomimetic amines may well be able to release endogenous noradrenaline without exerting any indirect effects; their direct effects may occur with concentrations which fail to cause any substantial release of the transmitter. Adrenaline may be regarded as an extreme example, since its affinity to α- and β-receptors is usually greater than that of (—)-noradrenaline. Although (—)-adrenaline is taken up by the adrenergic nerve endings, and although it exchanges with endogenous noradrenaline (*i.e.*, it releases the transmitter) (STRÖMBLAD and NICKERSON, 1961), the noradrenaline-releasing action of adrenaline does not result in an indirect action; the amounts of released noradrenaline are too small, and the potency of the released transmitter is less than that of the releaser. Similar arguments apply to exogenous noradrenaline which is also known to exchange with endogenous transmitter. Hence, it is clear that the ability to release noradrenaline is not unique for the indirectly acting amines. However, of great importance are the quantitative relationships between affinity to the receptors and ability to release noradrenaline.

From the description of the mode of action of tyramine (section II), the following factors emerge as being able to influence this relationship between affinity to adrenoceptors and ability to release endogenous noradrenaline:

1. Affinity to α- and β-receptors.
2. Morphology of the synaptic region.
3. Affinity to the membranal (cocaine-sensitive) uptake mechanism (as a determinant of rate of uptake of the amine as well as of its ability to prevent the re-uptake of the released noradrenaline).
4. Affinity to intraneuronal MAO.
5. Affinity to vesicular uptake mechanisms.
6. Affinity to vesicular binding sites.

These factors will be discussed below. In this discussion, the term "direct effect" or "potency of direct effect" refers to observations made in reserpine-pretreated animals or preparations. Very occasionally (and only when evidence with reserpine-pretreated preparations is not available) an indirect action will be inferred from experiments which show that cocaine or sympathetic denervation greatly antagonized the sympathomimetic effects of an amine.

1. Affinity to α- and β-Receptors

It is customary to determine relative affinities of amines to receptors by measurements of their relative potencies. However, relative potencies depend not only on the affinity to adrenoceptors but also on mechanisms of inactivation, the importance of which differs from amine to amine and also from organ to organ (see Chapter 16 of this handbook). The profound influence of mechanisms of inactivation on relative potencies may be illustrated by one example: on the isolated normal nictitating membrane of the cat the directly acting amine, (±)-methoxamine (which is a substrate neither of COMT nor of MAO, and which is not taken up), is 16 times more potent than (—)-noradrenaline; after denervation (which removes uptake as a mechanism of inactivation) the two amines are about equipotent; after additional block of COMT (—)-noradrenaline is about 6 times more potent than methoxamine; (TRENDELENBURG et al., 1970; TRENDELENBURG et al., 1971). Thus, elimination of two mechanisms of inactivation changed relative potencies by a factor of nearly 100. For this reason, relative potencies should be determined after block of all mechanisms of inactivation if one desires to obtain exact values for affinity to receptors. However, such studies have not been done for larger series of sympathomimetic amines; consequently, the following considerations are based on experiments in which no attempt has been made to abolish mechanisms of inactivation. However, reference is made only to results obtained after pretreatment with reserpine so that only the direct effects of amines are considered.

In this brief account only a few points will be made which are relevant to amines which represent relatively minor modifications of the basic phenylethylamine structure and which have been used extensively in pharmacological work.

Table 1. *Relative potencies (for direct effects) of sympathomimetic amines after intravenous injection to cats*

change in structure	amine	n.m.[a]	h.r.[b]	iris[c]	amine	n.m.[a]	h.r.[b]	iris[c]
none	(—)-adrenaline	0	0	0	(—)-noradrenaline	0.73	0.23	1.18
no β-OH	epinine	1.60[d]	—	2.26	dopamine	1.86	2.59	2.60
no para-OH	(—)-phenylephrine	0.57	2.30	2.31	(±)-norphenylephrine[e]	1.67	2.49	—
no meta-OH	(±)-synephrine[e]	2.04	3.08	2.91	(±)-norsynephrine[e]	2.36	2.82	—
α-CH_3	(±)-α-methyl-adrenaline[e]	1.90[d]	—	—	(±)-α-methyl-noradrenaline[e]	1.53[d]	—	2.17
α-CH_3 and no β-OH	α-methyl-epinine	—	—	—	(±)-α-methyl-dopamine	2.08	1.74	—
α-CH_3 and no para-OH	(±)-m-OH-ephedrine[e]	2.12	2.89	—	(±)-metaraminol[e]	1.83	2.84	—
α-CH_3 and no meta-OH	(±)-p-OH-ephedrine[e]	2.63	3.44	—	(±)-p-OH-phenylpropanolamine[e]	2.55	3.25	—

Shown are log ratios of equieffective doses (in moles/kg) "amine under study/(—)-adrenaline"; figures represent negative log potency relative to that of (—)-adrenaline.

[a] nictitating membrane after pretreatment with reserpine; values are based on ED50's; taken from Trendelenburg et al. (1962a) and Tsai et al. (1967).

[b] heart rate after pretreatment with reserpine; values are based on ED50's; taken from Trendelenburg et al. (1962a) and Tsai et al. (1967).

[c] threshold doses for mydriasis; taken from Marley (1962).

[d] calculated from equieffective doses (about equivalent to the ED20) obtained by Fleckenstein and Bass (1953) in animals *not* pretreated with reserpine.

[e] values were obtained for the racemate; if only the (—)-isomer is active, values should be reduced by 0.3.

a) *α-Receptors.* With (—)-adrenaline as the reference substance, relative potencies for various amines are presented in Table 1 for the nictitating membrane of the cat. The following points emerge from this summary. The introduction of an α-methyl group decreases potency, as does the omission of a β-OH group. Of the two phenolic hydroxyl groups, the one in meta-position is far more important for a high potency than the para-OH group. Not shown in the table are the well known facts that an increase in the N-substitution beyond the methyl group of adrenaline causes a pronounced decline in potency, as does O-methylation.

b) *β-Receptors.* As for α-receptors, the relative importance of the hydroxyl groups for potency decreases meta-OH>β-OH>para-OH. However, the introduction of an N-isopropyl group (isoprenaline) increases rather than decreases potency.

More important for the present discussion are differences in the effect of any given substitution on affinities to α- and β-receptors. For instance, loss of any hydroxyl group results in a decrease in α-activity on the nictitating membrane, which is consistently smaller than the corresponding loss in β-activity (heart rate, Table 1). The results of Table 1 demonstrate clearly that relative potencies do not show the same pattern in three organs of the cat. Phenylephrine, for instance, has a relative potency 55 times higher on the nictitating membrane than on the iris, while metaraminol has a relative potency 10 times higher on the nictitating membrane than on heart rate (Table 1).

An indirect effect of an amine should become evident when two conditions are fulfilled: the direct action of the amine should be weak (*i.e.*, it should have a low potency), and the amine should be able to enter the neurone to release the transmitter. If it is assumed that the adrenergic nerves of various cat organs have rather similar properties, it follows that a decrease in potency should increase the probability of an indirect effect to become evident. This is true for both, (—)-phenylephrine and metaraminol. While (—)-phenylephrine has a direct action on the nictitating membrane (TRENDELENBURG et al., 1962a), it has some indirect effects on the iris (MARLEY, 1962). While metaraminol has direct effects on the nictitating membrane, it has some indirect ones on the heart (TRENDELENBURG et al., 1962b; STONE et al., 1966).

Further evidence for the view that the magnitude of indirect effects is inversely related to the potency of the direct effects is obtained from five earlier series of experiments in which a variety of amines were classified on the cat nictitating membrane, cat heart rate (TRENDELENBURG et al., 1962a; TSAI et al., 1967), the iris of the cat (MARLEY, 1962), the isolated ileum of the rabbit (SCHMIDT and FLEMING, 1963) and the isolated rat vas deferens (PATIL et al., 1967a, 1967b). As shown in Figs. 1—5, all series of experiments show that indirect effects (measured for equal responses as negative log molar dose, or concentration, without reserpine minus negative log molar dose after reserpine) appear only when potency falls to a certain level. Moreover, for many (but not for all) amines, there is a reasonable correlation between potency and magnitude of indirect effects. It should be realized, that many amines with very pronounced indirect effects are not included, since the ED50 of their direct effects cannot be determined with accuracy whenever their direct effects are very weak. Some details of the results presented in Figs. 1—5 will be discussed below. It seems to be justified to state that indirect effects appear only when amines have a low affinity to the adrenoceptors, and that, because of the structure action relationships for each type of receptor,the degree of indirect effect may well vary from organ to organ.

Adrenoceptors are stereospecific; of the compounds which carry a hydroxyl group on the β-carbon atom those belonging to the (—)-series have a higher potency for their direct effects than their enantiomers. If there is a relation between potency and magnitude of indirect effects, (+)-isomers should have more pronounced indirect effects than their (—)-isomers. The experimental evidence is in agreement with this postulate. On the nictitating membrane of the cat both

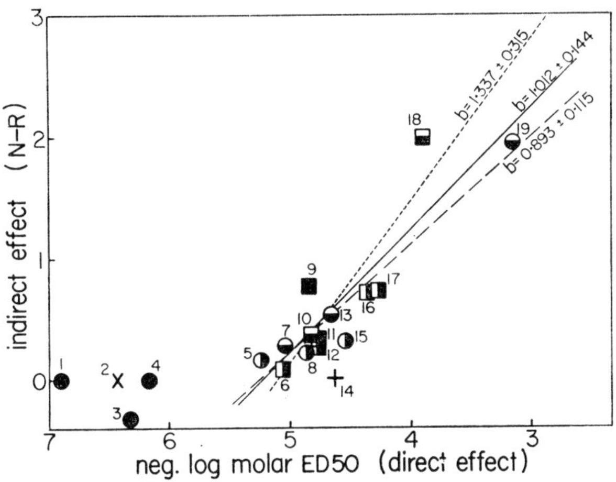

Fig. 1. Relation between potency of direct effect and magnitude of indirect effect of various sympathomimetic amines on the nictitating membrane of the cat. Ordinate: magnitude of indirect effect (neg. log molar ED50 normal — neg. log molar ED50 after reserpine). Abscissa: neg. log molar ED50 after pretreatment with reserpine (i.e., potency of direct effect). For identification of the 19 amines see Table 2. Symbols: circles: phenylethylamine derivatives with no α-CH_3 group, with N-substitution not greater than CH_3, and not O-methylated; squares: same but with an α-CH_3 group; x: O-methylated amines; +: amines with N-substituents greater than CH_3. Filled symbols refer to (—)-isomers (with regard to β-carbon); open symbols to (+)-isomers; vertically divided half filled symbols to racemates; horizontally divided half filled symbols to amines which lack the asymmetric β-carbon. Solid line: common regression line for all circles and squares with neg. log molar ED50 of less than 5.4. Upper broken line: regression for α-methylated amines (squares); lower broken line: regression line for non-methylated amines (circles). Given are regression coefficients ± S.E. Results were taken from TRENDELENBURG et al. (1962a) and TSAI et al. (1967)

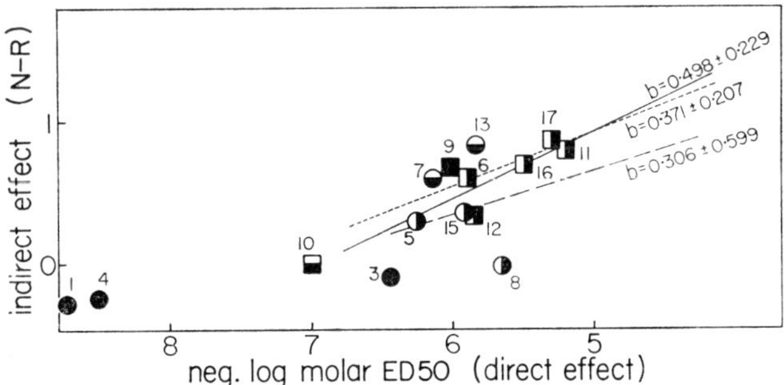

Fig. 2. Relation between potency of direct effect and magnitude of indirect effect of various sympathomimetic amines on the cardiac pacemaker of the cat. Ordinate: magnitude of indirect effect (neg. log molar ED50 normal — neg. log molar ED50 after reserpine). Abscissa: neg. log molar ED50 after pretreatment with reserpine (i.e., potency of direct effect). For identification of the 15 amines see Table 2. Symbols and regression lines as in Fig. 1. Regression lines were calculated for amines with neg. log molar ED50 of less than 6.6. Results were taken from TRENDELENBURG et al. (1962a) and TSAI et al. (1967)

isomers of noradrenaline and adrenaline have direct effects, but of phenylephrine only the (+)-isomer has some indirect effects (TYE et al., 1967b). On the vas deferens of the rat both isomers of noradrenaline and adrenaline have direct effects, but of α-methyl-noradrenaline, metaraminol, phenylephrine and synephrine only the (+)-isomers have some indirect effects, while the (—) isomers are

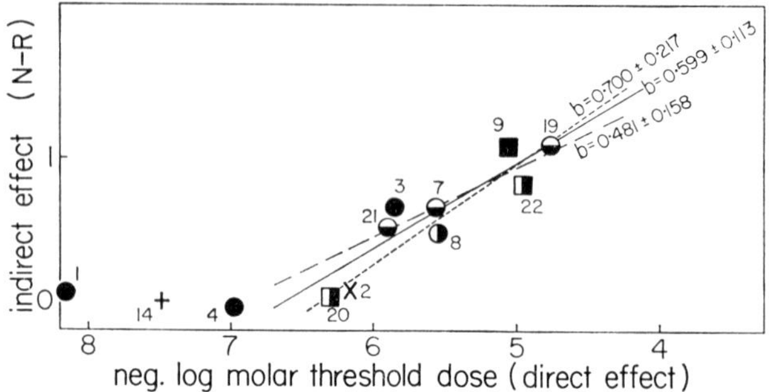

Fig. 3. Relation between potency of direct effect and magnitude of indirect effect of various sympathomimetic amines on the iris of the cat. Ordinate: magnitude of indirect effect (neg. log molar threshold dose normal — neg. log molar threshold dose after reserpine). Abscissa: neg. log molar threshold dose after pretreatment with reserpine (i.e., potency of direct effect). For identification of the 12 amines see Table 2. Symbols and regression lines as in Fig. 1. Regression lines were calculated for amines with neg. log molar threshold doses of less than 6.4. Results were taken from MARLEY (1962)

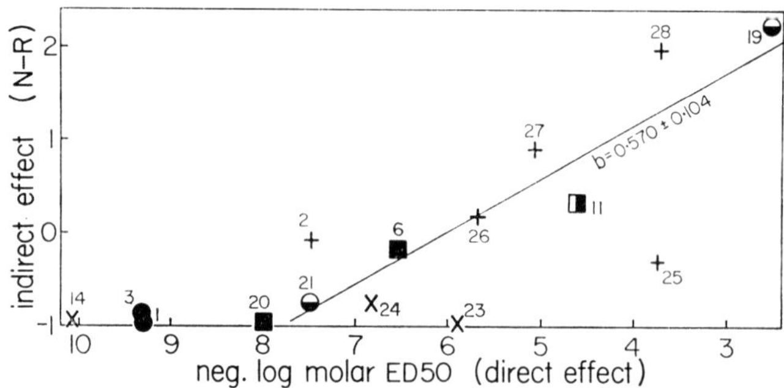

Fig. 4. Relation between potency of direct effect and magnitude of indirect effect of various sympathomimetic amines on the isolated rabbit ileum. Ordinate: magnitude of indirect effect (neg. log molar ED50 normal — neg. log molar ED50 after reserpine). Abscissa: neg. log molar ED50 after pretreatment with reserpine (i.e., potency of direct effect). For identification of the 15 amines see Table 2. Symbols and common regression line as in Fig. 1. The common regression line was calculated for amines with neg. log molar ED50 of less than 7.6. Results were taken from SCHMIDT and FLEMING (1963). Negative values for indirect effects of the most potent amines indicate that this tissue developed supersensitivity to the direct effects of amines

directly acting; (—)-octopamine has some direct and some indirect effects, but (+)-octopamine has very pronounced indirect effects (PATIL et al., 1967a, 1967b). A study of the four isomers of ephedrine showed the same reciprocity between potency of direct effects and magnitude of indirect effects (TYE et al., 1967a).

The indirect effects of (+)-isomers indicate that some uptake must take place, but the rate of uptake must not necessarily be as high as that for (—)-isomers. Although it is correct to state that the indirect effects of (+)-isomers are more pronounced than those of the corresponding (—)-isomers, their overall potency (*i.e.*, the sum of their direct and indirect action as determined on organs not pretreated with reserpine) is lower than that of the (—)-isomers. Evidently, (+)-isomers lose more in direct potency than they gain in indirect action (TYE et al., 1967a; PATIL et al., 1967a, 1967b). However, this general rule is not without exceptions (see below and Fig. 5).

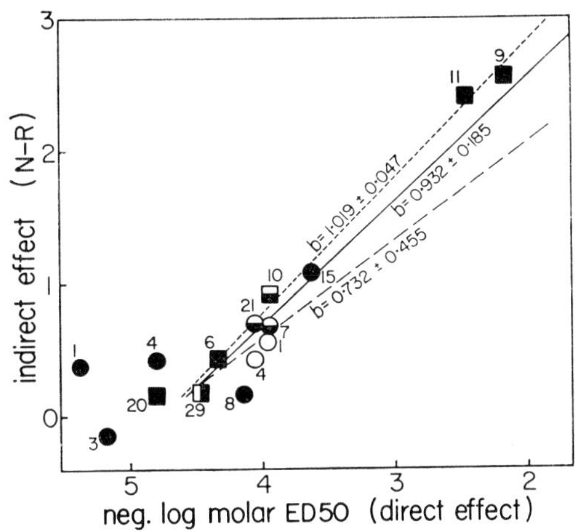

Fig. 5. Relation between potency of direct effect and magnitude of indirect effect of various sympathomimetic amines on the isolated rat vas deferens. Ordinate: magnitude of indirect effect (neg. log molar ED50 normal — neg. log molar ED50 after reserpine). Abscissa: neg. log molar ED50 after pretreatment with reserpine (i.e., potency of direct effect). For identification of the 15 amines see Table 2. Symbols and regression lines as in Fig. 1. Regression lines were calculated for amines with neg. log molar ED50 of less than 4.6. Results were taken from PATIL et al. (1967a, 1967b) and PATIL and JACOBOWITZ (1968). The positive values for indirect effects of highly potent amines indicate that pretreatment with reserpine decreased the sensitivity of the tissue; it is unlikely that in this tissue amines like (—)-adrenaline and (—)-noradrenaline have an indirect effect

Table 2. *Identification of amines shown in Figures 1—5*

1 adrenaline	11 phenylpropanolamine	21 epinine
2 (±)-methoxamine	12 *m*-OH-ephedrine	22 pholedrine
3 phenylephrine	13 *m*-OH-phenylethylamine (metatyramine)	23 isoxsuprine
4 noradrenaline	14 isoproterenol	24 dichloroisoproterenol
5 norphenylephrine	15 octopamine	25 methoxytyramine
6 metaraminol	16 *p*-OH-phenylpropanolamine	26 metanephrine
7 dopamine	17 *p*-OH-ephedrine	27 normetanephrine
8 synephrine	18 (+)-amphetamine	28 methoxyphenamine
9 ephedrine	19 tyramine	29 *α*-methyl-adrenaline
10 (±)-*α*-methyl-dopamine	20 *α*-methyl-noradrenaline	

2. The Morphology of the Synaptic Region

The importance of the morphology of adrenergic synapses has become evident only quite recently. Detailed studies of the influence of morphology on the classification of amines are not yet available. Hence, only three examples are given.

The artery of the rabbit ear shares with many other blood vessels a type of adrenergic innervation of its muscle which is characterized by a wide gap between nerve endings (which are found at the adventitio-medial border) and the smooth muscle cells (in the media). Thus, amines administered into the lumen of the blood vessel can reach the smooth muscle cells before coming into contact with the adrenergic nerve endings, *i.e.*, the sites of uptake and of release of noradrenaline. As a result of this anatomical arrangement, tyramine has been found to have pronounced direct and weak indirect effects when administered intraluminally (DE LA LANDE and WATERSON, 1968). Extraluminal administration of tyramine, on the other hand, leads to a situation where the amine has to pass the adrenergic nerve endings before it reaches the smooth muscle cells of the media. Therefore, extraluminally applied tyramine has weak direct and pronounced indirect effects (DE LA LANDE and WATERSON, 1968).

The smooth muscle of the cat's nictitating membrane differs from vascular smooth muscle in having a dense adrenergic innervation which is in close contact with most of the smooth muscle cells (VAN ORDEN et al., 1967). The medial smooth muscle of the membrane has a denser adrenergic innervation than the inferior muscle, although the two muscles seem to be very similar in all other respects (TRENDELENBURG et al., 1969). The relative potency of tyramine (in relation to that to noradrenaline) is higher for the medial than for the inferior muscle. It is very likely that these differences in relative potencies are related to differences in density of adrenergic innervation (TRENDELENBURG et al., 1969).

In rabbit aortic strips phentolamine is much more effective against responses to tyramine and nerve stimulation than against responses to exogenous noradrenaline (URQUILLA et al., 1970). It is very likely that the asymmetry of the adrenergic innervation is responsible for this observation, since the release of the transmitter from the nerve endings (at the medio-adventitial border) must generate a very steep concentration gradient from the nerve terminals to the smooth muscle; for exogenous noradrenaline the concentration gradient must be reversed.

These three examples may serve as illustrations of the possibility that the morphology of adrenergic synapses may well influence the relation between the direct effects of an amine on adrenoceptors and its ability to release noradrenaline.

3. Affinity to the Membranal Uptake Mechanism

For the indirect effects of tyramine-like drugs uptake through the neuronal membrane is important for two different reasons: the amine has to be taken up in order to reach the storage sites of the transmitter, and it also may competitively antagonize the re-uptake of the released transmitter. Although both actions involve the same mechanism, it does not follow that there must be a close parallelism between rate of uptake of the amine and its ability to prevent the re-uptake of noradrenaline. Though it may be assumed that an amine is hardly taken up if its ability to impair the uptake of noradrenaline is very poor, the reverse is not necessarily true. It is indeed conceivable that an agent is a potent inhibitor of the uptake of noradrenaline without being taken up itself at a high rate. For this reason, experimental determination of the "affinity of an amine to the uptake mechanism", by determining its ability to prevent the uptake of noradrenaline, is not necessarily an index of the rate of uptake of that amine. This fact should be borne in mind, since most experiments that deal with "affinity to the uptake mechanism" are indeed based on determination of the ability to prevent the uptake of noradrenaline (or a related amine).

Methods. A discussion of the structure-action relationship of the mechanism of uptake through the neuronal membrane is made difficult by the fact that most studies also involve vesicular uptake and vesicular binding. This is true for all studies in which the accumulation of an amine in the tissue is determined. Since the structural requirements for membranal uptake differ from those for vesicular uptake and vesicular binding, relative rates of accumulation do not necessarily reflect relative rates of membranal uptake. For instance, when the accumulation of an amine in the tissue is poor, one cannot be certain whether this is due to a low rate of membranal or of vesicular uptake; in the latter case, the amine might well be metabolized intraneuronally instead of being stored. These difficulties are avoided when arterio-venous differences are determined in organs perfused with low concentrations of amines. According to LINDMAR and MUSCHOLL (1964) this difference is a reliable measure of membranal net uptake which is not influenced by intraneuronal events (such as block of vesicular uptake by reserpine or block of intraneuronal MAO). Although this method is optimal for determinations of relative rates of membranal net uptake, it has not been used extensively.

Stereospecificity. Earlier studies failed to establish beyond doubt whether the membranal uptake is stereospecific (MAICKEL et al., 1963; KOPIN and BRIDGERS, 1963; IVERSEN, 1963). Recent determinations of arterio-venous differences in perfused rabbit heart showed clearly that the membranal uptake of this organ is not stereospecific (DRASKÓCZY and TRENDELENBURG, 1968). However, this finding cannot be extended to other organs or species, since JARROT and IVERSEN (personal communication), using the same method, found stereospecificity for the membranal uptake of rat but not of guinea-pig hearts. Thus, stereospecificity of the membranal uptake cannot be assumed to exist in organs (or species) which have not yet been studied. Moreover, because of the observed differences with regard to stereospecificity, it is quite possible that there are other species-dependent differences in the structural requirements for optimal uptake.

Affinity. Affinity constants for membranal uptake were obtained by IVERSEN (1967) by determining those concentrations of various amines which reduced the uptake of ($\pm$)-noradrenaline-H^3 (10 ng/ml) in the rat heart by 50%. From results with about 50 amines, the following conclusions can be drawn. Affinity was increased by the introduction of hydroxyl groups in meta- or para-position (with little difference between the two) or by α-methylation. Affinity was decreased, on the other hand, by β-hydroxylation, by substitution of the nitrogen or by O-methylation. With the experimental design used for this study, one cannot be certain that the amines have only one site of action, the membranal uptake mechanism. It is quite possible that those amines which are taken up then compete with noradrenaline for vesicular uptake (and possibly for vesicular binding). The effectiveness of this additional competition may then well depend on the intraneuronal fate of these amines, *i.e.*, on MAO.

MUSCHOLL and WEBER (1965) carried out a similar study but determined arterio-venous differences in rabbit hearts perfused with 10 ng/ml of α-methylnoradrenaline. With eight amines they found rather similar structure-action relationships: the affinity was increased by the introduction of a meta-OH group or by α-methylation, while β-hydroxylation decreased affinity. Since intraneuronal events do not influence results obtained with this method (see above), it may be concluded that the structure-action relationships observed by IVERSEN (1967) and by MUSCHOLL and WEBER (1965) are indeed related to the uptake by the axonal membrane. However, there is an interesting quantitative difference between the two studies in that (—)-metaraminol and (+)-amphetamine were 1440 and 610 times more potent than β-phenylethylamine in IVERSEN's study, and 750 and 230 times in that of MUSCHOLL and WEBER (1965). Although this may be due to a species difference, it is also possible that the high potency observed by IVERSEN (1967) was partly due to multiple sites of action of these amines (*i.e.*, actions on vesicular uptake and possibly on vesicular binding).

Carlsson and Waldeck (1966) pretreated mice with tyramine-C^{14} to induce the synthesis of octopamine-C^{14} in their hearts. A fixed dose of various amines was then injected to determine their ability to deplete the newly synthesized octopamine. It is evident that structural requirements for vesicular uptake (and possibly for vesicular binding) must have influenced results, since the depletion of the octopamine involved entry of the releasing amines into the storage vesicles. The structural requirements for depletion of octopamine were rather similar to those observed in the studies mentioned above: effectiveness was increased by the introduction of phenolic hydroxyl groups (meta-OH>para-OH); N-methylation had little effect, and O-methylation or the introduction of larger radicals at the nitrogen decreased effectiveness. There is one interesting difference in that β-hydroxylation increased effectiveness in depleting octopamine but reduced uptake (see above). It is possible that the increase in affinity to the vesicular binding sites caused by β-hydroxylation more than balances the decrease in membranal uptake.

Lack of uptake. As pointed out, a low affinity to the membranal uptake mechanism (as determined in the studies discussed above) may well indicate a lack of uptake of the amine. For instance, both Iversen (1967) and Carlsson and Waldeck (1966) obtained a low affinity constant for isoprenaline. This is in good agreement with the lack of accumulation of isoprenaline in adrenergically innervated organs (Hertting, 1964; Ross and Renyi, 1966b; Draskóczy and Trendelenburg, 1970). With isoprenaline one can be certain that lack of accumulation in adrenergic nerve endings is not due to an inability to enter the storage vesicles, since isoprenaline is taken up and retained by isolated vesicles obtained from bovine splenic nerve (von Euler and Lishajko, 1967). Since this amine is not a substrate of MAO, lack of accumulation in adrenergic nerves must be due to lack of membranal uptake.

The affinity constant for methoxamine is even lower than that for isoprenaline (Iversen, 1967) and methoxamine is not accumulated in adrenergic nerve endings (Trendelenburg et al., 1970). The lack of uptake of isoprenaline and of methoxamine is of interest, since it appears that the structural requirements for membranal uptake are quite different from those for optimal effectiveness on either α- or β-receptors.

Specificity of uptake. When O-methylated amines and amines with large substituents on the nitrogen are omitted from the discussion, it appears that the specificity of the uptake mechanism is not very high for the large number of amines which differ in phenolic and β-hydroxyl and in α- and N-methyl groups. This is evident from the results presented in Figs. 1—5. If rates of membranal uptake (and of vesicular uptake) were identical for all amines, a strictly linear relationship between potency and magnitude of indirect effect should ensue. In all five systems (Figs. 1—5) the relationship was not strictly linear. Amines below the regression lines must be assumed to have lower rates of membranal and/or vesicular uptake than those above the lines. For Figs. 1, 2, 3 and 5 there is good agreement with the affinity constants of Iversen (1967) in so far as indirect effects appear only with those amines whose affinity constants are not excessively low. The results presented in Fig. 4 are puzzling as some O-methylated amines (*e.g.* normetanephrine and metanephrine) have indirect effects, although they have very little affinity to the uptake mechanism(s) according to Iversen (1967) and Carlsson and Waldeck (1966). However, it cannot be ruled out that the adrenergic nerve endings in the rabbit ileum differ from others in being able to take up these amines.

The *erythro* configuration of α-methylated phenylethanolamines has a much higher affinity to α- and β-receptors than the corresponding *threo* configuration

(MUSCHOLL and SPRENGER, 1966; TYE et al., 1967a; WALDECK, 1967; PATIL and JACOBOWITZ, 1968). On the other hand, the racemates of the diastereomers are rather similar with regard to uptake (MUSCHOLL and SPRENGER, 1966; WALDECK, 1967) and to magnitude of indirect effects (TYE et al., 1967a; PATIL and JACOBOWITZ, 1968). This seems to provide another example for differences between affinity to receptors and to the uptake mechanism.

Lipid solubility. An increase in the lipid solubility of an amine might enable the agent to penetrate the neuronal or vesicular membrane without the help of the cocaine-sensitive membranal or the reserpine-sensitive vesicular uptake. A decrease in the number of phenolic or β-hydroxyl groups increases lipid-solubility and thus leads to an accumulation of the amine not antagonized by cocaine. This has been shown for (+)-amphetamine (ROSS and RENYI, 1966a, 1966b; THOENEN et al., 1968), phenylpropanolamine and phenylethanolamine (ROSS et al., 1968) as well as for ephedrine (JACQUOT et al., 1969). On the other hand, the indirect effects of (+)-amphetamine, phenylpropanolamine and (—)-ephedrine are antagonized by cocaine (FLECKENSTEIN and STÖCKLE, 1955; TRENDELENBURG et al., 1962b). This seeming contradiction may be resolved by two considerations. First, if a lipid-soluble amine is able to penetrate the cell membrane of neurones, it can be expected to penetrate the membranes of smooth or cardiac muscle as well. Thus, accumulation in any adrenergically innervated tissue may occur mainly in extraneuronal tissues with the consequence that the small contribution by the cocaine-sensitive uptake of the neuronal membrane is masked. Second, the noradrenaline-releasing or indirect effect of these amines may well depend on a high rate of uptake which is achieved only with the help of the membranal uptake mechanism. After cocaine the rate of uptake may be too slow for the build-up of those high concentrations in the immediate neighborhood of the peripherally located vesicles which are required for the release of the transmitter into the extracellular space. In other words, when the cocaine-sensitive uptake does not operate, lipid-soluble amines may behave like reserpine, which is able to deplete the stores without causing any substantial release of the transmitter into the extracellular space.

The hypotensive effect of isoprenaline is reversed to a pressor response if the amine is administered after an injection of pilocarpine (HAMILTON, 1971). Since this pressor response to isoprenaline is abolished by cocaine or guanethidine and since it is not observed after pretreatment with reserpine, it may represent an indirect effect. If this is true, the presence of cholinomimetic drugs seems to cause drastic changes in the properties of the neuronal uptake mechanism.

4. Role of Intraneuronal MAO

Since α-methylated amines cannot be deaminated after their uptake into the cytoplasm (because they are not substrates of MAO) their indirect effects might be expected to be stronger than those of the parent amines. Earlier observations seemed to confirm this postulate (TSAI et al., 1967), but it was not realized that an increase in indirect effects may also be due to a decrease in potency (see Figs. 1—5). Since α-methylation decreases the potency of direct effects (see section IV, 1), the problem requires re-investigation. Although other factors (stereospecificity of uptake, the importance of the other substituents, the steric position of the α-methyl group) also exert their influence, the results of Figs. 1, 2, and 5 show that the α-methylated amines tend to lie above the common regression line; or in other words, they seem to have more pronounced indirect effects even when changes in potency are accounted for. Unfortunately, various amines with very pronounced indirect effects do not appear in these figures, because their direct effects were too small for determinations of meaningful ED50's.

A small degree of stereospecificity of MAO has been reported (PRATESI and BLASCHKO, 1959; GIACHETTI and SHORE, 1966).

5. Affinity to Vesicular Uptake Mechanisms

Vesicular uptake has a high degree of stereospecificity (CARLSSON et al., 1963, for medullary vesicles; VON EULER and LISHAJKO, 1964; STJÄRNE and VON EULER, 1966, for nerve vesicles); this contributes to the low potency of (+)-isomers on innervated organs (*i.e.*, the sum of their direct and indirect effects) (PATIL et al., 1967a, 1967b).

Nerve vesicles have two uptake mechanisms: a reserpine-sensitive uptake which is activated by ATP-Mg^{++} and which is responsible for the uptake of noradrenaline and adrenaline, and a reserpine-resistant uptake which is not activated by ATP-Mg^{++} and which seems to be responsible for the accumulation of a variety of amines (CARLSSON et al., 1963). Since tyramine enters the vesicles by the reserpine-resistant route (CARLSSON et al., 1963), it must be concluded that this mode of uptake is adequate for the indirect effects of amines.

Vesicular uptake, as a whole, seems to be considerably less specific than membranal uptake. For instance, isolated nerve vesicles take up isoprenaline at a high rate (VON EULER and LISHAJKO, 1967), although this amine has a very low affinity to the membranal uptake mechanism.

6. Affinity to Vesicular Binding Sites

Storage vesicles seem to be able to retain amines only when they are either catechols or β-hydroxylated (MUSACCHIO et al., 1965). Results obtained by NASH et al. (1968) indicate that affinity to the binding sites may be a determinant of the releasing effect of indirectly acting amines. For catecholamines with a β-OH group, the authors observed a parallelism between releasing ability and affinity to the membranal uptake mechanism (as determined by IVERSEN, 1963). For dopamine, tyramine and phenylethylamine, however, the ability to release noradrenaline was smaller than expected from their affinities to the membranal uptake mechanism. Apparently, for amines which are neither catechols nor β-hydroxylated, there is a limiting factor in addition to membranal uptake; the rate of exchange at vesicular storage sites may well be involved.

A high affinity to vesicular storage sites, on the other hand, does not seem to be a prerequisite for an indirect action. For instance, tyramine (rather than its β-hydroxylated metabolite, octopamine) seems to be involved in the displacement of noradrenaline from storage sites, since the indirect effects of tyramine are not antagonized by block of dopamine β-hydroxylase; however, tyramine is not retained by storage vesicles (MUSACCHIO et al., 1965; KOPIN et al., 1965).

V. Various Agents with Indirect Actions

In the following a few agents (or groups of agents) which differ in structure and/or mode of action from the phenylethylamines will be discussed.

a) Aliphatic Amines

The sympathomimetic effectiveness of aliphatic amines increases with increasing lenght of the aliphatic chain to reach an optimum with *n*-hexylamine; longer chains result in amines with decreased pressor effectiveness (BARGER and DALE, 1910). These sympathomimetic effects seem to be predominantly indirect, since they are strongly reduced or abolished after pretreatment with reserpine or after the administration of cocaine (HOLTZ and PALM, 1965). The similarity of their mode of action with that of tyramine is also indicated by the finding that the aliphatic amines (like tyramine) displace catecholamines from isolated adrenal medullary vesicles (EADE, 1957).

In one respect these amines differ quantitatively from tyramine: although their rate of deamination by MAO is lower than that of tyramine, their potentiation by an inhibitor of MAO is greater than that of tyramine. HOLTZ and PALM (1965) suggested that the high lipid solubility of the aliphatic amines enabled them to reach those vesicles which are located in the centre of varicosities. Thus, the deamination of the released transmitter may play a greater role in the metabolism of the displaced transmitter than after tyramine which may be assumed to act predominantly on the more peripherally located vesicles (see section B). According to this view, the potentiating effect of inhibitors of MAO is to a considerable part exerted on the displaced transmitter rather than on the releaser itself.

b) Aldehydes

In adrenalectomized spinal cats acetaldehyde, propionaldehyde and butyrylaldehyde cause pressor responses as well as contractions of the nictitating membrane which are not antagonized by ganglion blockers but abolished by pretreatment with reserpine; cocaine potentiated rather than antagonized these effects (EADE, 1959). The positive chronotropic and inotropic response of isolated guinea-pig atria to acetaldehyde was antagonized by propranolol and by pretreatment with reserpine (WALSH et al., 1969). Hence, these aldehydes have indirect effects, though the cocaine-sensitive uptake does not seem to be involved.

c) α-Receptor Blocking Agents

Various agents of this group exert sympathomimetic effects which are either direct or indirect. Ergotamine (SALZMANN et al., 1968), and tolazoline (HOSZOWSKA-OWCZAREK et al., 1968) have a direct stimulant effect on the α-receptors of the cat's nictitating membrane as indicated by the observation that the response was reduced by other α-receptor blocking agents but not by pretreatment with reserpine.

Indirect effects have been described for dibenamine, phentolamine and chlorpromazine which exert a positive chronotropic effect in cats whose cardiovascular reflexes have been eliminated by spinalization or by the use of ganglion-blocking agents; the response was absent after pretreatment with reserpine (BENFEY and VARMA, 1962).

For a series of β-haloalkylamines (including dibenamine and phenoxybenzamine) FURCHGOTT and KIRPEKAR (1963) reported a positive inotropic and chronotropic effect on isolated guinea-pig atria which was absent after pretreatment with reserpine and which was restored by incubation of reserpine-pretreated atria with (—)-noradrenaline. Hand in hand with these indirect effects a potentiation of the effect of (—)-noradrenaline was observed. Apparently, the β-haloalkylamines resemble tyramine in so far as they are able to release noradrenaline and to prevent the uptake of the released transmitter. However, they seem to differ from tyramine in that their indirect effects on rat atria are not antagonized by cocaine (CHANG, 1968).

d) Cocaine

Cocaine is well known to cause various sympathomimetic effects (pressor response, contraction of nictitating membrane) which are not observed in animals pretreated with reserpine. The sympathomimetic effects of cocaine are potentiated by block of MAO (MAENGWYN-DAVIES and KOPPANYI, 1966). On isolated guinea-pig atria cocaine has positive and negative chronotropic effects; the positive effects are enhanced by pretreatment with an inhibitor of MAO (pargyline), antagonized by propranolol and abolished after pretreatment with reserpine (TRENDELENBURG, 1968). These observations indicate that cocaine is not only able to prevent the uptake of noradrenaline but also to release the transmitter. The amounts involved in this release seem to be quite small, but the responses are considerable because of the pronounced increase in sensitivity to noradrenaline.

e) Methylphenidate

The weak sympathomimetic effects of methylphenidate seem to be indirect, since the contraction of the cat's nictitating membrane elicited by this agent is absent after chronic sympathetic denervation (MAXWELL et al., 1959a) and since the mydriatic effect of methylphenidate is abolished by pretreatment with reserpine (MARLEY, 1962). It is of interest that methylphenidate shares with cocaine not only the ability to prevent the uptake of noradrenaline and thus to potentiate the effects of the latter (MAXWELL et al., 1966), but also that of releasing small amounts of noradrenaline.

f) Adrenergic Neurone Blockers

The sympathomimetic effects of bretylium on isolated guinea-pig atria are antagonized by cocaine or dichloroisoprenaline, and abolished after pretreatment with reserpine; responses of reserpine-pretreated preparations are restored by an incubation with adrenaline, noradrenaline, dopamine or L-dopa (FURCHGOTT and KIRPEKAR, 1960; BHAGAT and SHIDEMAN, 1963; KIRPEKAR and FURCHGOTT, 1964). Sympathetic denervation of guinea-pig atria abolishes the effect of bretylium which is not restored by an incubation with noradrenaline (KIRPEKAR and FURCHGOTT, 1964). Similar indirect effects of this agent were observed for rabbit aortic strips (KIRPEKAR and FURCHGOTT, 1964).

Xylocholine (TM10) likewise exerts sympathomimetic effects on isolated atria of various species (TRENDELENBURG, 1960).

g) Noradrenaline-Depleting Agents

Reserpine: Under most experimental conditions the noradrenaline-releasing action of reserpine is weak in spite of its pronounced noradrenaline-depleting effects. Unequivocal pressor responses to the acute injection of reserpine are observed only after cocaine (HORITA, 1958; VALDECASAS et al., 1958). On the other hand, the heart-lung preparation of the dog responds to the acute injection of reserpine with a pronounced tachycardia (PAASONEN and KRAYER, 1958); this is an indirect effect, since it is prevented by pretreatment with reserpine (PAASONEN and KRAYER, 1958) or with other reserpine-like alkaloids (LIEBMAN et al., 1962). The indirect effects of reserpine on the heart-lung preparation of the dog differ from those of tyramine in so far as a noradrenaline infusion into a reserpine-pretreated preparation restores the effects of the latter but not of the former (MUSKUS, 1964); moreover cocaine antagonizes the indirect effects of tyramine but not those of reserpine (PLUCHINO et al., 1969).

The indirect effect of an acute administration of reserpine can be shown in isolated guinea-pig atria as well, but most of the response is masked by a direct negative chronotropic effect. In this preparation the positive chronotropic effect of reserpine is greatly increased after block of MAO (by pargyline), it is antagonised by propranolol and absent after pretreatment with reserpine. Parallel determinations of the noradrenaline-depleting action of reserpine indicate that the release is accompanied by a small degree of depletion; apparently only a very small fraction of the noradrenaline lost from the stores is released into the extracellular space (BRIMIJOIN and TRENDELENBURG, 1971). Since reserpine does not impair the re-uptake of released noradrenaline, its sympathomimetic effects are small. An intravenous injection of reserpine does not cause any appreciable rise in the noradrenaline content of the venous coronary blood, even if the dose is high enough to deplete the heart of 65% of its noradrenaline within 4 hours (HARRISON et al., 1963).

These observations indicate that reserpine enters the stores of adrenergic nerves independently of the cocaine-sensitive uptake. It is likely that the rate of entry is low (as compared to that of tyramine) with the result that the noradrenaline-releasing effects of this drug are weak. Most of the depleted transmitter is deaminated before leaving the neurone.

Guanethidine. The indirect effects of guanethidine are much more pronounced than those of reserpine. It is likely that two factors account for this difference. First, guanethidine is taken up by the cocaine-sensitive route of uptake, since its accumulation by the heart is decreased by prior treatment with cocaine, tyramine or imipramine (LINDMAR and MUSCHOLL, 1966) and since cocaine and protriptyline partly antagonize the positive chronotropic response of the heart-lung preparation to guanethidine (PLUCHINO et al., 1969). Second, unlike reserpine, guanethidine potentiates responses to noradrenaline (KRAYER et al., 1962), presumably by an impairment of uptake. These two properties of guanethidine lead to the appearance of easily detectable indirect effects (blood pressure: KADZIELAWA, 1962; isolated rat atria: BHAGAT and SHIDEMAN, 1963) and increases in venous plasma levels of noradrenaline are readily observed on intraarterial injection into the spleen (HERTTING et al., 1962) or in coronary vein blood after intravenous injection (HARRISON et al., 1963).

It is of interest to note that guanethidine takes an intermediate position between the extremes, tyramine and reserpine: it is tyramine-like in that responses of reserpine-pretreated preparations to guanethidine are restored by an exposure to noradrenaline (BHAGAT and SHIDEMAN, 1963; MUSKUS, 1964), while it is reserpine-like in causing depletion of noradrenaline stores as well as in being able to cause some indirect effects even after pretreatment with cocaine or protriptyline (PLUCHINO et al., 1969). It is tempting to speculate that the tyramine-like effects of guanethidine depend mainly on the high rate of uptake achieved by the cocaine-sensitive route, while its reserpine-like effects can be exerted when the rate of uptake is quite low.

h) Monoamine Oxidase Inhibitors

Many members of this group have sympathomimetic effects. These can be either direct, *i.e.*, resistant to pretreatment with reserpine but sensitive to the appropriate sympatholytic agent (examples: tranylcypromine and harmaline) or indirect, *i.e.*, abolished by pretreatment with reserpine (examples: phenelzine, pheniprazine, pargyline, phenylcyclopropylamine) (LEE et al., 1961; TSAI and FLEMING, 1965). An exposure of reserpine-pretreated preparations to noradrenaline restores the effects of the indirectly acting MAO inhibitors (LEE et al., 1961). The possible antagonism by cocaine does not seem to have been studied.

i) Nicotinic Agents

The action of most nicotinic drugs on adrenergic nerve endings is exerted through hexamethonium-sensitive nicotine receptors which are probably located in the cell membrane. This site and mode of action will not be discussed here. However, for one member of this group tyramine- and bretylium-like effects have been described. On isolated atria of rats, dimethyl-phenylpiperazinium (DMPP) exerts sympathomimetic effects which are not antagonized by hexamethonium (while those of nicotine are), but blocked by either dichloroisoprenaline or pre-treatment with reserpine. Responses were tyramine-like in so far as an exposure of reserpine-pretreated atria to noradrenaline restored their response to DMPP (but not to nicotine). This seems to be a species-dependent phenomenon, since DMPP was partly antagonized by hexamethonium on guinea-pig atria (LINDMAR, 1962). On the Finkleman preparation of the rat intestine DMPP is bretylium-like, *i.e.*, the inhibition of the response to postganglionic sympathetic stimulation is resistant to hexamethonium, while it is reversed by dopamine and (+)-amphetamine (BIRMINGHAM and WILSON, 1965).

On the rabbit pulmonary artery the indirect effects of nicotine are antagonized by cocaine and desipramine (SU and BEVAN, 1970). The authors consider it possible that uptake of nicotine by the cocaine-sensitive uptake mechanism may be involved in the indirect effects of nicotine.

k) 5-Hydroxytryptamine

Recent evidence indicates that 5-hydroxytryptamine is accumulated by adrenergic nerve endings and that cocaine antagonizes this accumulation (THOA et al., 1969). Hence, it is not surprising that indirect sympathomimetic effects of 5-hydroxytryptamine have been described. An analysis on the isolated nictitating membrane showed that low concentrations of 5-hydroxytryptamine caused predominantly direct effects resulting in a very flat dose-response curve; high concentrations (of > 1 μg/ml) caused additional indirect effects producing a steep dose-response curve. The latter (but not the former) were antagonized by pre-treatment with reserpine, by denervation, by cocaine and by a competitive α-receptor antagonist, phentolamine; like those of tyramine, they are potentiated by pretreatment with an inhibitor of MAO, pargyline (PLUCHINO, 1972). Moreover, tachyphylaxis develops to 5-hydroxytryptamine as it develops to tyramine; muscles made tachyphylactic to one of these agents are also tachyphylactic to the other.

In isolated strips of the cat spleen, on the other hand, 5-hydroxytryptamine has only indirect effects which are antagonized by the procedures mentioned above (INNES, 1962; PLUCHINO, 1972).

Although there is not enough evidence available for a detailed analysis of the indirect effects of 5-hydroxytryptamine, it is suggested that they may be demonstrable in those organs in which its direct effects are weak. In this respect 5-hydroxytryptamine does not differ from the classical sympathomimetic amines.

l) 6-Hydroxydopamine

This amine is taken up and retained by adrenergic neurons and leads to their degeneration (THOENEN and TRANZER, 1968). Very soon after the *in vivo* administration of 6-hydroxydopamine, noradrenaline is released from the isolated cat heart (HAEUSLER, 1971). While the release of the transmitter by nerve impulses is dependent on the presence of calcium ions, that by tyramine is not (LINDMAR et al., 1967; THOENEN et al., 1969). It is of interest that the 6-hydroxydopamine-induced release of noradrenaline is calcium-dependent (HAEUSLER, 1971). Apparently, the indirect effect of this amine is unlike that of tyramine; the noradrenaline-releasing effect of 6-hydroxydopamine may well be related to the chemical denervation caused by this agent.

VI. Conclusions

Each sympathomimetic amine should be regarded as potentially able to exert both direct and indirect effects. Its overall effects in any given organ or system (*i.e.*, the classification of the amine) depends on the affinity of the amine to the receptors, to the uptake mechanisms, on its ability to impair the re-uptake of the released transmitter as well as on the factors which influence the concentration of amines at the receptors (such as the morphology of the synaptic region). Because of the marked differences in structural requirements for optimal effects on receptors and for optimal uptake through the neuronal or vesicular membrane, it is impossible to develop a classification that holds true for all organs or systems.

A short discussion of the indirect effects of other agents has been included in this review. A consideration of these agents is of interest, since they may serve as an illustration of the multitude of agents which can (by various means) enter adrenergic nerve endings and (by various mechanisms) release noradrenaline. It is also of interest to note that there is hardly an agent that exerts only one action. The discussion may serve to reemphasize the fact that our labels ("inhibitor of uptake", "noradrenaline-depleting agent", "adrenergic neurone blocker" etc.) merely describe the most prominent effect of these agents. In most cases they are able to exert a multitude of effects within the complicated system of adrenergic nerve endings. Directly relevant to this review is the fact that the ability to release noradrenaline is shared by many agents of very diverse chemistry and pharmacology.

References

AXELROD, J., GORDON, E., HERTTING, G., KOPIN, I.J., POTTER, L.T.: On the mechanism of tachyphylaxis to tyramine in the isolated rat heart. Brit. J. Pharmacol. **19**, 56—63 (1962).

BARGER, G., DALE, H.H.: Chemical structure and sympathomimetic action of amines. J. Physiol. (Lond.) **41**, 19—59 (1910).

BARNETT, A., STAUB, M., SYMCHOWICZ, S.: The effect of cocaine and imipramine on tyramine-induced release of noradrenaline-^{3}H from the rat vas deferens in vitro. Brit. J. Pharmacol. **36**, 79—84 (1969).

BENFEY, B.G., VARMA, D.R.: Studies on the cardiovascular actions of antisympathomimetic drugs. Int. J. Neuropharmacol. **1**, 9—12 (1962).

BHAGAT, B., SHIDEMAN, F.E.: Mechanism of the positive inotropic response to bretylium and guanethidine. Brit. J. Pharmacol. **20**, 56—62 (1963).

BIRMINGHAM, A.T., WILSON, A.B.: An analysis of the blocking action of dimethylphenylpiperazinium iodide on the inhibition of isolated small intestine produced by stimulation of the sympathetic nerves. Brit. J. Pharmacol. **24**, 375—386 (1965).

BRIMIJOIN, S., TRENDELENBURG, U.: Reserpine-induced release of norepinephrine from isolated spontaneously beating guinea-pig atria. J. Pharmacol. exp. Ther. **176**, 149—159 (1971).

BÜLBRING, E., BURN, J.H.: The action of tyramine and adrenaline on the denervated nictitating membrane. J. Physiol. (Lond.) **91**, 459—473 (1938).

BURN, J.H.: The action of tyramine and ephedrine. J. Pharmacol. exp. Ther. **46**, 75—95 (1932).

— RAND, M.J.: Reserpine and adrenaline in arterial walls. Lancet **273**, 1097 (1957).

— — The action of sympathomimetic amines in animals treated with reserpine. J. Physiol. (Lond.) **144**, 314—336 (1958).

— TAINTER, M.L.: An analysis of the effect of cocaine on the action of adrenaline and tyramine. J. Physiol. (Lond.) **71**, 169—193 (1931).

CARLSSON, A., HILLARP, N.-Å., WALDECK, B.: Analysis of the Mg^{++}-ATP dependent storage mechanism in the amine granules of the adrenal medulla. Acta physiol. scand. **59**, Suppl. 215, 38pp (1963).

CARLSSON, A., ROSENGREN, E., BERTLER, Å., NILSSON, J.: Effect of reserpine on the metabolism of catechol amines. Psychotropic drugs, pp. 363—372. Amsterdam-London-New York-Princeton: Elsevier Publishing Co. 1957.

— WALDECK, B.: Structure-activity relationships for release of ^{14}C-octopamine from adrenergic nerves by phenylethylamines. Acta pharmacol. (Kbh.) **24**, 255—262 (1966).

CHANG, P.: Sympathomimetic actions of phenoxybenzamine on rat heart. Europ. J. Pharmacol. **4**, 240—245 (1968).

COMMARATO, M.A., BRODY, T.M., MCNEILL, J.H.: The effect of various drugs on the uptake and metabolism of tyramine-H^3 in the rat heart. J. Pharmacol. exp. Ther. **167**, 151 to 158 (1969).

CROUT, J.R.: The uptake and release of H^3-norepinephrine by the guinea-pig heart in vivo. Naunyn-Schmiedeberg's Arch. exp. Pathol. Pharmakol. **248**, 85—98 (1964).

— MUSKUS, A.J., TRENDELENBURG, U.: Effect of tyramine on isolated guinea-pig atria in relation to their noradrenaline stores. Brit. J. Pharmacol. **18**, 600—611 (1962).

DE LA LANDE, I.S., WATERSON, J.G.: The action of tyramine on the rabbit ear artery. Brit. J. Pharmacol. **34**, 8—18 (1968).

DRASKÓCZY, P.R., TRENDELENBURG, U.: The uptake of l- and d-norepinephrine by the isolated perfused rabbit heart in relation to the stereospecificity of the sensitizing action of cocaine. J. Pharmacol. exp. Ther. **159**, 66—73 (1968).

— — Intraneuronal and extraneuronal accumulation of sympathomimetic amines in the isolated nictitating membrane of the cat. J. Pharmacol. exp. Ther. **174**, 290—306 (1970).

EADE, N.R.: The release of catechol amines from isolated chromaffin granules. Brit. J. Pharmacol. **12**, 61—65 (1957).

— Mechanism of sympathomimetic action of aldehydes. J. Pharmacol. exp. Ther. **127**, 29—34 (1959).

VON EULER, U.S., LISHAJKO, F.: Uptake of l- and d-isomers of catecholamines in adrenergic nerve granules. Acta physiol. scand. **60**, 217—222 (1964).

— — The uptake of isoprenaline in nerve granules. Int. J. Neuropharmacol. **6**, 431—434 (1967).

FLECKENSTEIN, A.: Über Neuro-Sympathomimetica. Verhandl. der Deutschen Ges. f. inn. Med., 59. Kongress, 1953, p. 17—22.

— BASS, H.: Zum Mechanismus der Wirkungsverstärkung und Wirkungsabschwächung sympathomimetischer Amine durch Cocain und andere Pharmaka. I. Die Sensibilisierung der Katzen-Nickhaut für Sympathomimetica der Brenzkatechin-Reihe. Naunyn-Schmiedeberg's Arch. exp. Pathol. Pharmakol. **220**, 143—156 (1953).

— BURN, J.H.: The effect of denervation on the action of sympathomimetic amines on the nictitating membrane. Brit. J. Pharmacol. **8**, 69—78 (1953).

— STÖCKLE, D.: Zum Mechanismus der Wirkungsverstärkung und Wirkungsabschwächung sympathomimetischer Amine durch Cocain und andere Pharmaka. II. Die Hemmung der Neuro-Sympathomimetica durch Cocain. Naunyn-Schmiedeberg's Arch. exp. Pathol. Pharmakol. **224**, 401—415 (1955).

FLEMING, W.W., TRENDELENBURG, U.: Development of supersensitivity to norepinephrine after pretreatment with reserpine. J. Pharmacol. exp. Ther. **133**, 41—51 (1961).

FRÖHLICH, A., LOEWI, O.: Untersuchungen zur Physiologie und Pharmakologie des vegetativen Nervensystems. II. Mitteilung: Über eine Steigerung der Adrenalinempfindlichkeit durch Cocain. Naunyn-Schmiedeberg's Arch. exp. Pathol. Pharmakol. **62**, 159—169 (1910).

FURCHGOTT, R.F., KIRPEKAR, S.M.: Release of catecholamines in heart by β-haloalkylamines and by bretylium. Pharmacologist **2**, 93 (1960).

— — Competition between β-haloalkylamines and norepinephrine for sites in cardiac muscle. Proceedings of the First International Pharmacological Meeting, vol. 7, pp. 339—350. Oxford: Pergamon Press 1963.

GIACHETTI, A., SHORE, P.A.: Optical specificity of monoamine oxidase. Life Sci. **5**, 1373—1378 (1966).

GROBECKER, H., HOLTZ, P., JONSSON, J.: Über die Wirkung des Tyramins auf den isolierten Darm. Naunyn-Schmiedeberg's Arch. exp. Pathol. Pharmakol. **255**, 491—509 (1966).

GULATI, O.S., KELKAR, V.V.: Effect of tyramine on human umbilical artery in vitro. Brit. J. Pharmacol. **42**, 155—158 (1971).

HAEUSLER, G.: Early pre- and postjunctional effects of 6-hydroxydopamine. J. Pharmacol. exp. Ther. **178**, 49—62 (1971).

HAMILTON, T.C.: Modification of the vascular response to isoprenaline by cholinomimetic drugs. Brit. J. Pharmacol. **42**, 254—262 (1971).

HARRISON, D.C., CHIDSEY, C.A., GOLDMAN, R., BRAUNWALD, E.: Relationships between the release and tissue depletion of norepinephrine from the heart by guanethidine and reserpine. Circulat. Res. **12**, 256—263 (1963).

HERTTING, G.: The fate of ^{3}H-isoproterenol in the rat. Biochem. Pharmacol. **13**, 1119—1128 (1964).
— AXELROD, J., PATRICK, R.W.: Actions of bretylium and guanethidine on the uptake and release of (^{3}H)-noradrenaline. Brit. J. Pharmacol. **18**, 161—166 (1962).
HOLTZ, P., OSSWALD, W., STOCK, K.: Über die Beeinflussung der Wirkungen sympathicomimetischer Amine durch Cocain und Reserpin. Naunyn-Schmiedeberg's Arch. exp. Pathol. Pharmakol. **239**, 14—28 (1960).
— PALM, D.: Über den Mechanismus der sympathicomimetischen Wirkungen einiger aliphatischer Amine. Naunyn-Schmiedeberg's Arch. exp. Pathol. Pharmakol. **251**, 144—158 (1965).
HORITA, A.: A vasopressor response to reserpine in the cocainized dog. J. Pharmacol. exp. Ther. **122**, 474—479 (1958).
HOSZOWSKA-OWCZAREK, A., LANGER, S.Z., DJORDJEVIC, N., DE SCHAEPDRYVER, A.F.: Stimulant action of tolazoline on the nictitating membrane of the pithed cat. Arch. int. Pharmacodyn. **174**, 135—143 (1968).
INNES, I.R.: An action of 5-hydroxytryptamine on adrenaline receptors. Brit. J. Pharmacol. **19**, 427—441 (1962).
— KOHLI, J.D.: Excitatory action of sympathomimetic amines on 5-hydroxytryptamine receptors of gut. Brit. J. Pharmacol. **35**, 383—393 (1969).
IVERSEN, L.L.: The uptake of noradrenaline by the isolated perfused rat heart. Brit. J. Pharmacol. **21**, 523—537 (1963).
— The uptake and storage of noradrenaline in sympathetic nerves, 253 pages. Cambridge, England: Cambridge University Press 1967.
JACQUOT, C., BRALET, J., COHEN, Y., VALETTE, G.: Fixation de la dl-ephedrine-^{14}C par le coeur isolé perfusé de rat. Biochem. Pharmacol. **18**, 903—914 (1969).
KADZIELAWA, K.: Mechanism of action of guanethidine. Brit. J. Pharmacol. **19**, 74—84 (1962).
KALSNER, S.: Effects of tyramine on responses to and inactivation of histamine in aortic strips. J. Pharmacol. exp. Ther. **175**, 489—495 (1970).
KIRPEKAR, S.M., FURCHGOTT, R.F.: The sympathomimetic action of bretylium on isolated atria and aortic smooth muscle. J. Pharmacol. exp. Ther. **143**, 64—76 (1964).
KOPIN, I.J., BRIDGERS, W.: Differences in d- and l-norepinephrine-H^3. Life Sci. **2**, 356—362 (1963).
— FISCHER, J.E., MUSACCHIO, J.M., HORST, W.D., WEISE, V.K.: "False neurochemical transmitters" and the mechanism of sympathetic blockade by monoamine oxidase inhibitors. J. Pharmacol. exp. Ther. **147**, 186—193 (1965).
KRAYER, O., ALPER, M.H., PAASONEN, M.K.: Action of guanethidine and reserpine upon the isolated mammalian heart. J. Pharmacol. exp. Ther. **135**, 164—173 (1962).
LANGER, S.Z.: Presence of tone in the denervated and in the decentralized nictitating membrane of the spinal cat and its influence on determinations of supersensitivity. J. Pharmacol. exp. Ther. **154**, 14—34 (1966).
— DRASKÓCZY, P.R., TRENDELENBURG, U.: Time course of the development of supersensitivity to various amines in the nictitating membrane of the pithed cat after denervation or decentralization. J. Pharmacol. exp. Ther. **157**, 255—273 (1967).
LEE, F.L.: The relation between norepinephrine content and response to sympathetic nerve stimulation of various organs of cats pretreated with reserpine. J. Pharmacol. exp. Ther. **156**, 137—141 (1967).
— WEINER, N., TRENDELENBURG, U.: The uptake of tyramine and formation of octopamine in normal and tachyphylactic rat atria. J. Pharmacol. exp. Ther. **155**, 211—222 (1967).
LEE, W.C., SHIN, Y.H., SHIDEMAN, F.E.: Cardiac activities of several monoamine oxidase inhibitors. J. Pharmacol. exp. Ther. **133**, 180—185 (1961).
LIEBMAN, J.: Modification of the chronotropic action of sympathomimetic amines by reserpine in the heart-lung preparation of the dog. J. Pharmacol. exp. Ther. **133**, 63—69 (1961).
— MUSKUS, A.J., WAUD, D.R.: The depletion of norepinephrine stores in the heart of the dog by reserpinetype alkaloids. J. Pharmacol. exp. Ther. **136**, 76—79 (1962).
LINDMAR, R.: Die Wirkung von 1,1-Dimethyl-4-Phenyl-Piperazinium-Jodid am isolierten Vorhof im Vergleich zur Tyramin- und Nicotinwirkung. Naunyn-Schmiedeberg's Arch. exp. Pathol. Pharmakol. **242**, 458—466 (1962).
— LÖFFELHOLZ, K., MUSCHOLL, E.: Unterschiede zwischen Tyramin und Dimethylphenylpiperazin in der Ca^{++}-Abhängigkeit und im zeitlichen Verlauf der Noradrenalin-Freisetzung am isolierten Kaninchenherzen. Experientia (Basel) **23**, 933—934 (1967).
— MUSCHOLL, E.: Die Wirkung von Cocain, Guanethidin, Reserpin, Hexamethonium, Tetracain und Psicain auf die Noradrenalin-Freisetzung aus dem Herzen. Naunyn-Schmiedeberg's Arch. exp. Pathol. Pharmakol. **242**, 214—227 (1961).

Lindmar, R., Muscholl, E.: Die Wirkung von Pharmaka auf die Elimination von Noradrenalin aus der Perfusionsflüssigkeit und die Noradrenalinaufnahme in das isolierte Herz. Naunyn-Schmiedeberg's Arch. exp. Pathol. Pharmakol. **247**, 469—492 (1964).
— — Die Verstärkung der Noradrenalin-Wirkung durch Tyramin. Naunyn-Schmiedeberg's Arch. exp. Pathol. Pharmakol. **251**, 122—133 (1965).
— — Der Einfluß von Pharmaka auf die Aufnahme von Guanethidin in das Herz. Naunyn-Schmiedeberg's Arch. exp. Pathol. Pharmakol. **253**, 67 (1966).
Lundborg, P.: Uptake of metaraminol by the adrenal medullary granules. Acta physiol. scand. **67**, 423—429 (1966).
Maengwyn-Davies, G.D., Koppanyi, T.: Cocaine tachyphylaxis and effects on indirectly-acting sympathomimetic drugs in the rabbit aortic strip and in splenic tissue. J. Pharmacol. exp. Ther. **154**, 481—492 (1966).
Maickel, R.P., Beaven, M.A., Brodie, B.B.: Implications of uptake and storage of norepinephrine by sympathetic nerve endings. Life Sci. **2**, 953—958 (1963).
Maj, J., Langwinski, R.: Hypotensive action of tyramine in cats. J. Pharm. Pharmacol. **18**, 820—821 (1966).
Marley, E.: Action of some sympathomimetic amines on the cat's iris, in situ or isolated. J. Physiol. (Lond.) **162**, 193—211 (1962).
Maxwell, R.A., Plummer, A.J., Povalski, H., Schneider, F., Coombs, H.: A comparison of some of the cardiovascular actions of methylphenidate and cocaine. J. Pharmacol. exp. Ther. **126**, 250—257 (1959a).
— Povalski, H., Plummer, A.J.: A differential effect of reserpine on the pressor amine activity and its relationship to other agents producing this effect. J. Pharmacol. exp. Ther. **125**, 178—183 (1959b).
— Wastila, W.B., Eckhardt, S.B.: Some factors determining the response of rabbit aortic strips to dl-norepinephrine-7-H^3 hydrochloride and the influence of cocaine,guanethidine and methylphenidate on these factors. J. Pharmacol. exp. Ther. **151**, 253—261 (1966).
Murnaghan, M.F.: Potentiation of tyramine responses by nor-sympathomimetic amines in the reserpine-pretreated cat. Arch. int. Pharmacodyn. **155**, 332—355 (1965).
Musacchio, J.M., Bhagat, B., Jackson, C.J., Kopin, I.J.: The effect of disulfiram on the restoration of the response to tyramine by dopamine and a-methyl-DOPA in the reserpine-treated cat. J. Pharmacol. exp. Ther. **152**, 293—297 (1966).
— Kopin, I.J., Weise, V.K.: Subcellular distribution of some sympathomimetic amines and their beta-hydroxylated derivatives in the rat heart. J. Pharmacol. exp. Ther. **148**, 22—28 (1965).
Muscholl, E., Sprenger, E.: Vergleichende Untersuchungen der Blutdruckwirkung, Aufnahme und Speicherung von Dihydroxyephedrin (a-Methyladrenalin) und Dihydroxypseudoephedrin. Naunyn-Schmiedeberg's Arch. exp. Pathol. Pharmakol. **254**, 109—124 (1966).
— Weber, E.: Die Hemmung der Aufnahme von a-Methylnoradrenalin in das Herz durch sympathomimetische Amine. Naunyn-Schmiedeberg's Arch. exp. Pathol. Pharmakol. **252**, 134—143 (1965).
Muskus, A.J.: Evidence for different sites of action of reserpine and guanethidine. Naunyn-Schmiedeberg's Arch. exp. Pathol. Pharmakol. **248**, 498—513 (1964).
Nash, C.W., Wolff, S.A., Ferguson, B.A.: Release of tritiated noradrenaline from perfused rat hearts by sympathomimetic amines. Canad. J. Physiol. Pharmacol. **46**, 35—42 (1968).
Paasonen, M.K., Krayer, O.: Effect of reserpine upon the mammalian heart. Fed. Proc. **16**, 326 (1957).
— — The release of norepinephrine from the mammalian heart by reserpine. J. Pharmacol. exp. Ther. **123**, 153—160 (1958).
Patil, P.N., Jacobowitz, D.: Steric aspects of adrenergic drugs. IX. Pharmacologic and histochemical studies on isomers of cobefrin (a-methylnorepinephrine). J. Pharmacol. exp. Ther. **161**, 279—295 (1968).
— Lapidus, J.B., Tye, A.: Steric aspects of adrenergic drugs. I. Comparative effects of DL isomers and desoxy derivatives. J. Pharmacol. exp. Ther. **155**, 1—12 (1967a).
— — Campbell, D., Tye, A.: Steric aspects of adrenergic drugs. II. Effects of DL isomers and desoxy derivatives on the reserpine-pretreated vas deferens. J. Pharmacol. exp. Ther. **155**, 13—23 (1967b).
Pluchino, S.: Direct and indirect effects of 5-hydroxytryptamine and tyramine on cat smooth muscle. Naunyn-Schmiedeberg's Arch. Pharmak. in press (1972).
— Muskus, A.J., Pluchino, R.: The mechanism of action of guanethidine on the isolated mammalian heart. J. Pharmacol. exp. Ther. **170**, 44—49 (1969).
— Trendelenburg, U.: The influence of denervation and of decentralization on the *alpha* and *beta* effects of isoproterenol on the nictitating membrane of the pithed cat. J. Pharmacol. exp. Ther. **163**, 257—265 (1968).

Pöch, G.R., Kopin, I.J.: The role of octopamine in tachyphylaxis to tyramine. Biochem. Pharmacol. **15**, 210—212 (1966).

Pratesi, P., Blaschko, H.: Specificity of amine oxidase for optically active substrates and inhibitors. Brit. J. Pharmacol. **14**, 256—260 (1959).

Ross, S.B., Renyi, A.L.: Uptake of tritiated tyramine and (+)-amphetamine by mouse heart slices. J. Pharm. Pharmacol. **18**, 756—757 (1966a).

— — Uptake of some tritiated sympathomimetic amines by mouse brain cortex slices in vitro. Acta pharmacol. (Kbh.) **24**, 297—309 (1966b).

— — Brunfelter, B.: Cocaine-sensitive uptake of sympathomimetic amines in nerve tissue. J. Pharm. Pharmacol. **20**, 283—288 (1968).

Salzmann, R., Pacha, W., Taeschler, M., Weidmann, H.: The effect of ergotamine on humoral and neuronal actions in the nictitating membrane and the spleen of the cat. Naunyn-Schmiedeberg's Arch. exp. Pathol. Pharmakol. **261**, 360—378 (1968).

Schmidt, J.L., Fleming, W.W.: The structure of sympathomimetics as related to reserpine induced sensitivity changes in the rabbit ileum. J. Pharmacol. exp. Ther. **139**, 230—237 (1963).

Schmitt, H., Schmitt, H.: Modification des effects des amines sympathicomimétiques sur la pression artérielle et la membrane nictitante par la réserpine. Arch. int. Pharmacodyn. **125**, 30—47 (1960).

Smith, C.B.: The role of monoaminoxidase in the intraneuronal metabolism of norepinephrine released by indirectly-acting sympathomimetic amines or by adrenergic nerve stimulation. J. Pharmacol. exp. Ther. **151**, 207—220 (1966).

Steinberg, M.I., Smith, C.B.: Effects of desmethylimipramine and cocaine on the uptake, retention and metabolism of H^3-tyramine in rat brain slices. J. Pharmacol. exp. Ther. **173**, 176—192 (1970).

Stjärne, L., von Euler, U.S.: Stereospecificity of amine uptake mechanism in nerve granules. J. Pharmacol. exp. Ther. **150**, 335—340 (1966).

Stone, C.A., Stavorski, J.M., Ludden, C.T., Wenger, H.C., Torchiana, M.L.: Some direct and indirect sympathomimetic actions of metaraminol. Arch. int. Pharmacodyn. **161**, 49—60 (1966).

Strömblad, B.C.R., Nickerson, M.: Accumulation of epinephrine and norepinephrine by some rat tissues. J. Pharmacol. exp. Ther. **134**, 154—159 (1961).

Su, C., Bevan, J.A.: Blockade of the nicotine-induced norepinephrine release by cocaine, phenoxybenzamine and desipramine. J. Pharmacol. exp. Ther. **175**, 533—540 (1970).

Tainter, M.L., Chang, D.K.: The antagonism of the pressor action of tyramine by cocaine. J. Pharmacol. exp. Ther. **30**, 193—207 (1927).

Thoa, N.B., Eccleston, D., Axelrod, J.: The accumulation of C^{14}-serotonin in the guinea-pig vas deferens. J. Pharmacol. exp. Ther. **169**, 68—73 (1969).

Thoenen, H., Hürlimann, A., Haefely, W.: Mechanism of amphetamine accumulation in the isolated perfused heart of the rat. J. Pharm. Pharmacol. **20**, 1—11 (1968).

— — — Cation dependence of the noradrenaline-releasing action of tyramine. Europ. J. Pharmacol. **6**, 29—37 (1969).

— Tranzer, J.P.: Chemical sympathectomy by selective destruction of adrenergic nerve endings with 6-hydroxydopamine. Naunyn-Schmiedeberg's Arch. exp. Path. Pharmak. **261**, 271—288 (1968).

Trendelenburg, U.: The action of histamine and 5-hydroxytryptamine on isolated mammalian atria. J. Pharmacol. exp. Ther. **130**, 450—460 (1960).

— Supersensitivity and subsensitivity to sympathomimetic amines. Pharmacol. Rev. **15**, 225—276 (1963).

— The effect of cocaine on the pacemaker of isolated guinea-pig atria. J. Pharmacol. exp. Ther. **161**, 222—231 (1968).

— Crout, J.R.: The norepinephrine stores of isolated atria of guinea pigs pretreated with reserpine. J. Pharmacol. exp. Ther. **145**, 151—161 (1964).

— Draskóczy, P.R., Pluchino, S.: The density of adrenergic innervation of the cat's nictitating membrane as a factor influencing the sensitivity of the isolated preparation to l-norepinephrine. J. Pharmacol. exp. Ther. **166**, 14—25 (1969).

— Gomez Alonso de la Sierra, B., Muskus, A.: Modification by reserpine of the response of the atrial pacemaker to sympathomimetic amines. J. Pharmacol. exp. Ther. **141**, 301 to 309 (1963).

— Höhn, D., Graefe, K.H., Pluchino, S.: The influence of block of catechol-O-methyl transferase on the sensitivity of isolated organs to catecholamines. Naunyn-Schmiedeberg's Arch. Pharmak. **271**, 59—92 (1971).

— Maxwell, R.A., Pluchino, S.: The importance of the intraneuronal uptake in the cat's nictitating membrane as assessed with methoxamine, a sympathomimetic amine which is not taken up by adrenergic nerves. J. Pharmacol. exp. Ther. **172**, 91—99 (1970).

Trendelenburg, U., Muskus, A., Fleming, W.W., Gomez Alonso de la Sierra, B.: Modification by reserpine of the action of sympathomimetic amines in spinal cats; a classification of sympathomimetic amines. J. Pharmacol. exp. Ther. **138**, 170—180 (1962a).

— — — — Effect of cocaine, denervation and decentralization on the response of the nictitating membrane to various sympathomimetic amines. J. Pharmacol. exp. Ther. **138**, 181—193 (1962b).

Tsai, T.H., Fleming, W.W.: Sympathomimetic actions of monoamine oxidase inhibitors in the isolated nictitating membrane of the cat. Biochem. Pharmacol. **14**, 369—371 (1965).

— Langer, S.Z., Trendelenburg, U.: Effects of dopamine and α-methyl-dopamine on smooth muscle and on the cardiac pacemaker. J. Pharmacol. exp. Ther. **156**, 310—324 (1967).

— Wendt, R.L., McGrath, W.R.: The negative chronotropic effect of tyramine on isolated guinea-pig atria. J. Pharmacol. exp. Ther. **168**, 290—294 (1969).

Tye, A., Baldesberger, R., Lapidus, J.B., Patil, P.N.: Steric aspects of adrenergic drugs. VI. Beta adrenergic effects of ephedrine isomers. J. Pharmacol. exp. Ther. **157**, 356—362 (1967a).

— Patil, P.N., Lapidus, J.B.: Steric aspects of adrenergic drugs. III. Sensitization by cocaine to isomers of sympathomimetic amines. J. Pharmacol. exp. Ther. **155**, 24—30 (1967b).

Urquilla, P.R., Stitzel, R.E., Fleming, W.W.: The antagonism of phentolamine against exogenously administered and endogenously released norepinephrine in rabbit aortic strips. J. Pharmacol. exp. Ther. **172**, 310—319 (1970).

Valdecasas, F.G., Salva, J.A., Cuenca, E.: Effect of reserpine on the blood pressure of the spinal cat treated with inhibitors of amino-oxydase. Arzneimittel-Forsch. **8**, 655—656 (1958).

Vanderipe, D.R., Kahn, J.B.: The mechanism of the vasodepressor response to tyramine in dogs. J. Pharmacol. exp. Ther. **145**, 292—298 (1964).

Van Orden, L.S. III, Bensch, K.G., Langer, S.Z., Trendelenburg, U.: Histochemical and fine structural aspects of the onset of denervation supersensitivity in the nictitating membrane of the spinal cat. J. Pharmacol. exp. Ther. **157**, 274—283 (1967).

Varma, D.R., Gillis, R.A., Benfey, B.G.: Reserpine as an antagonist of tyramine. J. Pharmacol. exp. Ther. **144**, 181—185 (1964).

Wakade, A.R., Cervoni, P., Furchgott, R.F.: Tyramine tachyphylaxis and the interaction of tyramine and bretylium in the guinea-pig isolated left atrium. J. Pharmacol. exp. Ther. (in press).

Waldeck, B.: On the interaction of threo-^{3}H-α-methylnoradrenaline with the uptake and storage mechanisms of the adrenergic neuron. Europ. J. Pharmacol. **2**, 208—213 (1967).

Walsh, M.J., Hollander, P.B., Truitt, E.B., jr.: Sympathomimetic effects of acetaldehyde on the electrical and contractile characteristics of isolated left atria of guinea pigs. J. Pharmacol. exp. Ther. **167**, 173—186 (1969).

Weiner, N., Draskóczy, P.R., Burack, W.R.: The ability of tyramine to liberate catecholamines *in vivo*. J. Pharmacol. exp. Ther. **137**, 47—55 (1962).

Westfall, D.P., Fleming, W.W.: The sensitivity of the guinea-pig pacemaker to norepinephrine and calcium after pretreatment with reserpine. J. Pharmacol. exp. Ther. **164**, 259—269 (1968).

Chapter 11

Effects of Catecholamines on Metabolism*

JEAN HIMMS-HAGEN**

With 10 Figures

A. Introduction

The topic of the metabolic effects of catecholamines is one of interest to pharmacologists, physiologists and biochemists alike. From the reviewer's point of view the definition of the term "metabolic" is important in determining the scope of the review. This term is generally defined by biochemists as including "all chemical processes within cells and tissues that are concerned with their building up and breaking down and in their functional operation" (WEST et al., 1966). Such a broad definition clearly encompasses both the traditional pharmacological and the traditional metabolic effects of the catecholamines. Indeed, the distinction between metabolic actions and other actions of catecholamines, once so clear, is now becoming less definite as more is becoming known about the molecular nature of the pharmacological effects of the catecholamines. On the one hand, the concept that adenyl cyclase may be very closely associated with the adrenergic receptor, first clearly formulated by ROBISON, BUTCHER and SUTHERLAND (1967) has opened up the possibility that all effects of catecholamines may ultimately be described in biochemical terms. On the other hand, the *second messenger* concept, which originally arose from the studies of SUTHERLAND and his colleagues of the metabolic effects of the catecholamines (see SUTHERLAND et al., 1965; ROBISON et al., 1968) is now clearly applicable to all cells, whether they are

Abbreviations used are:

cAMP: cyclic AMP; cyclic 3′,5′-AMP; adenosine 3′,5′-monophosphate.
dBcAMP: dibutyryl cyclic AMP; N^6-$O^{2'}$-dibutyryl cyclic AMP (dBcAMP is a synthetic analogue of cAMP; it differs from it in that it may enter cells more readily that cAMP itself and, in some tissues, is less susceptible to hydrolysis by cAMP phosphodiesterase).
FFA: free fatty acids
HIOMT: hydroxyindole-O-methyltransferase
5-HTP: 5-hydroxytryptophan
OMP: orotidylic acid; orotidine 5′-monophosphate
aGP: glycerol-3-phosphate
FDP: fructose-1,6-diphosphate
F6P: fructose-6-phosphate
G1P: glucose-1-phosphate
G6P: glucose-6-phosphate
UDPG: uridine diphosphate glucose
PEP: phosphoenolpyruvic acid
TCA cycle: tricarboxylic acid cycle
PGE_1: prostaglandin E_1
2,4-DNP: 2,4-dinitrophenol
SAM^+: S-adenosylmethionine
FCCP: carbonyl cyanide p-trifluoromethoxyphenylhydrazone

* Unpublished work described in this review was supported by a grant from the Medical Research Council of Canada.
** Associate of the Medical Research Council of Canada.

sensitive to catecholamines or not; it provides an explanation of one of the ways in which the complex intracellular regulatory machinery of any cell can receive information from and thus be regulated by its environment. Thus, the effects of catecholamines comprise only one aspect of the general area of the interaction of certain hormones with their specific target cells via the adenyl cyclase system.

Table 1. *Regulation of metabolic processes*

I. INTRACELLULAR REGULATION

[Factors influencing the rates of enzyme-catalyzed reactions]

1. *Substrate concentration:* depends on
   - a) rate of formation
   - b) rate of entry
   - c) rate of removal
2. *Enzyme concentration:* depends on
   - a) rate of synthesis
   - b) rate of degradation
   - c) rate of formation from precursor
     - (i) irreversible
     - (ii) reversible
3. *Enzyme activity:* depends on
   - a) concentration of stimulators
   - b) concentration of inhibitors

II. INTERCELLULAR REGULATION

[Factors integrating the metabolic activities of cells in different tissues: these factors act entirely through the mechanisms listed in I]

1. Endocrine system
2. Nervous system

Before discussing the metabolic effects of the catecholamines it is desirable to consider briefly the general mechanisms of regulation of intracellular metabolic processes; it is only via these mechanisms that catecholamines can exert any influence upon the metabolism of cells. Table 1 gives an outline of the processes involved in regulation of metabolism in mammalian cells. Because metabolic pathways are simply sequences of enzyme-catalyzed reactions it is obvious that they are regulated by factors that influence the rates of such reactions, namely, concentrations of both substrate and enzyme and activity of enzyme. Changes in substrate concentration can be brought about by changes in its rate of formation within the cell or by changes in its rate of entry from outside the cell. Changes in amount of enzyme can be brought about by an increase or decrease in its rate of synthesis or in its rate of degradation. The terms *induction* and *repression* are used to describe an increase and a decrease respectively in rate of synthesis of enzyme without, however, implying any specific mechanism for the change in rate but only that such a change does occur. The formation of enzyme from a precursor can be either reversible or irreversible. Best known examples of the latter, activation of digestive enzymes and activation of the enzymes involved in blood coagulation, actually occur *extra*cellularly and this irreversible process does not appear to be an important mechanism of *intra*cellular regulation. The reversible transformation of enzymes from less active to more active forms is an important intracellular regulatory mechanism; these enzymes are principally those that either utilize or synthesize storage material in cells. Changes in enzyme activity can be brought about by changes in concentration of stimulatory compounds or of inhibitory compounds[1].

Integration of the metabolic activities of the cells of different organs is brought about by the endocrine and nervous systems. These act only through the basic intracellular regulatory mechanisms noted above. Thus, the catecholamines, whose integrative action on metabolic activities can be included under both endocrine and nervous systems, act primarily by altering (either increasing or decreasing in an unknown fashion) the catalytic activity of a cell membrane enzyme, adenyl cyclase. The product of this enzyme, cyclic AMP, is a stimulatory compound for a variety of enzymes in different cells. If the enzyme whose activity is stimulated is one which transforms one form of an enzyme to another, then the relative proportions of the latter enzyme in the two forms will change. This will in turn lead to a change in the breakdown or synthesis of storage material; hence the rate of production of substrates for other enzymes will also change. Cyclic AMP is also known to influence the rate of synthesis of certain enzymes, although the mechanism of this action is entirely unknown. Cyclic AMP also influences the transport of materials across membranes; again the mechanism of action is not understood. The hypothesis that *all* intracellular effects of cAMP are mediated by stimulation of specific protein kinases (Kuo and Greengard, 1969a, b) provides a useful framework within which to study these effects of cAMP, but for the most part the nature of and the physiological substrates for these protein kinases are unknown.

In some cells the regulation of metabolic processes proceeds primarily in accordance with the needs of the cell in which it occurs: skeletal muscle is a good example of this kind of cell. In other cells the regulation of metabolic processes proceeds predominantly in accordance with the needs of other tissues; the liver and the white adipose tissue are good examples of this kind of cell. The effects of the catecholamines on metabolic processes in these two types of cell are somewhat different. In the first type of cell the effect of the catecholamine may at first sight appear rather superfluous because the cell itself is capable of directing its metabolism in much the same way without the aid of the catecholamines. In the second type of cell the catecholamines may actually call forth the function of the cell; under the influence of the catecholamines the liver and white adipose tissue deliver substrates to other tissues whether the latter need them or not. In all cells the effect of the catecholamines is to shift the balance in a pre-existing closely regulated system of metabolic pathways. Such a shift in balance has repercussions throughout the metabolic machinery of the cell. For this reason the metabolic effects of the catecholamines may appear exceedingly complex, particularly in those tissues, such as liver, that have a very complex metabolic machinery; practically every metabolic process existing in the cell is influenced in one way or another as a consequence of the action of the catecholamines.

The rather large number of catecholamine-sensitive tissues compared with the small number of tissues that usually respond to any one hormone makes the understanding of the effects of catecholamines an important goal in endocrinology.

---

1 The term *activation* will be used to describe the increase in catalytic activity that results when a less active form of an enzyme is transformed in an enzyme-catalyzed reaction to a more active enzyme species. The increase in catalytic activity which happens when a single enzyme species is exposed to a stimulatory compound other than an enzyme, sometimes referred to as allosteric activation, will be referred to in this review as *stimulation* to distinguish it from the process of activation defined above. The transformation of a more active species of an enzyme back to a less active form, also enzyme-catalyzed, will be referred to as *inactivation*. The reduction in catalytic activity of a single enzyme species by an inhibitory compound will be referred to as *inhibition*.

The multiplicity of tissues that respond to catecholamines also makes the understanding of their effects much more difficult than it otherwise would be because of the necessity of understanding in detail the metabolic and functional processes and their regulation for each individual tissue.

In this essay a survey will be given of current knowledge of metabolic and other processes in the catecholamine-sensitive tissues, of the consequences of the stimulation of the tissues by the catecholamines and of how the stimulation by the catecholamines relates to the functioning of the tissues in the intact animal. This last is not always possible. In at least two catecholamine-sensitive tissues whose adenyl cyclase has been demonstrated to be stimulated by catecholamines (brain and red blood cells) there is no known function for this response. The metabolic effects of catecholamines and of stimulation of the sympathetic nervous system in intact animals (hyperglycemic effect, fatty acid mobilizing effect, calorigenic effect) will be touched on only briefly. This topic has been reviewed fairly recently (HIMMS-HAGEN, 1967) and although a considerable literature on this topic has accumulated in the last few years no fundamentally new concepts have been developed. In particular, both the calorigenic effect of the catecholamines and the marked enhancement of this calorigenic effect that occurs in animals that have been adapted to cold are still very poorly understood.

The problem of the nature of the adrenergic receptor will also be discussed rather briefly. In the last few years the study of the nature of the receptor has changed to some extent from the traditional pharmacological approach. This approach, which used the kinetics of the relationship between response and catecholamine concentration, the responses to analogues of catecholamines and the inhibition of responses by blocking agents, led to the development, over 20 years ago, of the α- and β-adrenergic receptor concept, a concept recently modified to α-, β_1- and β_2-adrenergic receptors but otherwise still very much in use. The newer approach, currently in use in a number of laboratories, emphasizes rather the structure of the cell membrane that contains the receptor(s) and the interrelationship between the different structures in the cell membrane. This approach is still in its infancy, limited largely by the availability of suitable techniques for the study of the function and structure of membrane components. However, it appears likely that future developments of the receptor theory will occur in this area. The new technique described by BARRNETT and co-workers (REIK et al., 1970) for the cytochemical visualization of adenyl cyclase should provide much needed information on the location of this receptor-associated enzyme. For example, in tissues with a heterogeneous cell population (such as liver), in tissues for which differential centrifugation gives ambiguous results (such as heart and muscle), and in tissues too small to be studied in any other way (such as the pineal gland), this technique should permit the resolution of certain questions such as the number of different hormone-sensitive adenyl cyclases in any one cell type, and the exact cellular location of the postulated receptor in tissues where the enzyme is apparently associated with intracellular structures.

B. Effects of Catecholamines on Metabolism and Function of Individual Tissues

I. Liver

The catecholamines can modify the metabolism of carbohydrates, lipids and proteins in the liver and can, moreover, modify the synthesis of certain enzymes

Table 2. *Metabolic processes in liver that are altered by catecholamines and/or cAMP*

Carbohydrate Metabolism	increased glycogenolysis decreased glycogenesis increased gluconeogenesis
Lipid Metabolism	decreased lipid secretion increased lipolysis increased fatty acid oxidation increased ketogenesis
Protein Metabolism	increased proteolysis increased urea production (increased gluconeogenesis) increased synthesis of certain enzymes: 1. tyrosine transaminase 2. serine dehydratase 3. phosphoenolpyruvate carboxykinase
Cation Metabolism	loss of potassium loss of calcium

(Table 2). The metabolic effects of the catecholamines on liver are qualitatively the same as those of glucagon. In fact, in most studies of hormonal regulation of metabolic processes in isolated liver, glucagon has been used as the stimulating agent and the extent to which cAMP or dBcAMP mimics its action has been studied. It has not yet been demonstrated for many of the effects of cAMP listed in Table 2 that they are shared by the catecholamines. The relative lack of information about effects of catecholamines on the liver is due largely to technical problems that arise when these compounds are used in the perfused liver preparation: both adrenaline and noradrenaline cause marked vasoconstriction (NORTHROP and PARKS, 1964; SOKAL et al., 1964). The effects of the resulting anoxia of the liver tissue may overshadow the metabolic action of the catecholamines, and the catecholamines may not reach all regions of the liver. Although the use of phentolamine to prevent the decrease in blood flow (SOKAL et al., 1964; HEIMBERG and FIZETTE, 1963) can permit metabolic effects to occur in the absence of vasoconstriction, the possible inhibitory effect of the α-adrenergic blocking agents on some of the metabolic effects of the catecholamines or on some of the actions of the cAMP must also be considered in such experiments. In the discussion that follows, the actions of glucagon and cAMP will be considered together with the actions of the catecholamines, and those instances in which the actions of the cyclic nucleotide have not yet been demonstrated to be shared by the catecholamines will be pointed out (Fig. 1).

a) Adenyl Cyclase

Adenyl cyclase was first discovered in preparations of liver as was also its responsiveness to the catecholamines and its important role in mediating the actions of catecholamines on liver. The history of its discovery and the earlier descriptions of its properties have been reviewed by SUTHERLAND and ROBISON (1966), by SUTHERLAND and RALL (1960) and by ROBISON, BUTCHER and SUTHERLAND (1968). Cyclic AMP phosphodiesterase, which breaks down cAMP, is also present in liver but although small changes in the amount of this enzyme can occur in intact rats in response to dietary or hormonal treatment (SENFT et al., 1968a and b) it seems unlikely that modification of its activity plays a significant role in the effects of hormones on the liver.

The adenyl cyclase of broken cell preparations of liver can be stimulated by catecholamines (MURAD et al., 1962) and by glucagon (MAKMAN and SUTHERLAND,

1964). Early observations indicated that the maximum obtainable stimulation of adenyl cyclase by glucagon *in vitro* was very much greater than the maximum stimulation by adrenaline (MAKMAN and SUTHERLAND, 1964); this is also the case in the perfused liver, where the accumulation of cAMP after glucagon is very much greater than that brought about by adrenaline, noradrenaline or isopropylnoradrenaline (EXTON and PARK, 1968a). There are two explanations for this. Firstly, the adrenaline-responsive system is very much more labile than the glucagon-responsive system. Although adenyl cyclase of a homogenate of liver is equally responsive to adrenaline and to glucagon (BITENSKY et al., 1968, 1970) washing of the particulate fraction from such a homogenate, or even dilution of the homogenate, results in considerable reduction or even complete and irreversible loss of the response to adrenaline but does not alter the response to glucagon (BITENSKY et al., 1968). This difference may explain the report of a glucagon-specific adenyl cyclase in rat liver (POHL et al., 1969). The reason for the greater lability of the adrenaline-responsive system is not clear. One possible explanation could be the loss, by washing or by dilution, of some factor such as calcium (BITENSKY et al., 1968). The adenyl cyclase of liver membranes prepared and washed in a calcium-containing medium shows a greater response to adrenaline than to glucagon (MARINETTI et al., 1969) and the recovery of membranes containing adenyl cyclase is also improved by calcium (RAY, 1970); moreover, calcium is essential for the effect of adrenaline but depresses the response to glucagon (MARINETTI et al., 1969). Also, adenyl cyclases in different cells of the liver have different hormone sensitivities. Recent evidence for this is provided by the cytochemical demonstration of adenyl cyclase sensitive to catecholamine (isopropylnoradrenaline) in the plasma membrane of hepatocytes but not of reticuloendothelial cells and of glucagon-sensitive adenyl cyclase in plasma membranes of *both* hepatocytes and reticuloendothelial cells (REIK et al., 1970): adenyl cyclase in both cell types was stimulated by fluoride.

It is not possible at present to distinguish between the presence of more than one type of adenyl cyclase in the liver cell membrane and the presence of a single type of adenyl cyclase associated with more than one type of regulatory unit (ROBISON et al., 1967) or discriminator unit (BÄR and HECHTER, 1969). The different discriminator units may well differ in properties such as labilities or ionic requirements for function, as well as in specificities with regard to their stimulating hormone, which may lead to an apparent separation of different adenyl cyclases. The situation in liver may well be analogous to that in the adipose tissue (see section B. II) where several of the functional membrane constituents can interact with each other and with adenyl cyclase to modify each other's activity. Little is known about this aspect of membrane structure and function at present. Such an interaction of neighbouring membrane constituents may be responsible for the action of insulin on liver adenyl cyclase because although insulin can reduce the cAMP content of perfused liver under a variety of conditions (JEFFERSON et al., 1968; EXTON and PARK, 1968a), probably by restraining adenyl cyclase activity, no *direct* effect of insulin on liver adenyl cyclase has yet been observed (WICKS, 1969).

Adenyl cyclase is present and sensitive to both adrenaline and to glucagon in foetal rat liver (WICKS, 1969; BITENSKY et al., 1970); that the enzyme may develop only at a late stage of gestation is suggested by studies of the synthesis of tyrosine transaminase. The synthesis of this enzyme is increased in response to either glucagon or adrenaline three days before birth; but an increased synthesis in response to cAMP itself occurs already 2 days earlier (GREENGARD, 1969). This observation suggests that the synthesis of cell membrane can occur without the synthesis of adenyl cyclase and/or the receptors associated with it. An attempt to demonstrate synthesis of new liver cell membrane without adenyl cyclase in adult rats has been unsuccessful; the adenyl cyclase of regenerating rat liver had the same specific activity and hormonal sensitivity at all stages of regeneration studied (BECKER and BITENSKY, 1969). However, the development of a hepatoma cell line in tissue culture that possesses no adenyl cyclase (GRANNER et al., 1968) also indicates that synthesis of functional adenyl cyclase does not necessarily accompany the assembly of the hepatic cell membrane.

The response of hepatic adenyl cyclase to hormones appears to decrease with age, particularly in male rats (BITENSKY et al., 1970). That this may be attributable to changes in the amount of sex hormones in the animal is suggested by the ability of injected testosterone to reduce adenyl cyclase activity (measured in the presence of adrenaline) in both male and female weanling rats.

Adrenocorticosteroids influence the sensitivity of liver adenyl cyclase to adrenaline, but are without effect on its response to glucagon. A marked increase in the response of both homogenate and washed particle adenyl cyclase to adrenaline occurs in adrenalectomized rats, whereas there is no change in the response to glucagon (BITENSKY et al., 1970). Adrenalectomy does not alter the rise in cAMP content of perfused liver that occurs with glucagon (FRIEDMANN et al., 1967). The increased responsiveness of adenyl cyclase to adrenaline is suppressed by treatment of the adrenalectomized rats with the glucocorticoid, prednisolone. This behaviour of the liver adenyl cyclase may seem paradoxical in view of the well known defect in several metabolic responses to catecholamines and to glucagon in the absence of glucocorticoids. However, it is now becoming clear that the glucocorticoids act at sites other than the initial site of interaction of adrenaline with its receptor and other than the adenyl cyclase system itself when they exert their "permissive" effects.

b) cAMP-dependent Protein Kinases

A cAMP-dependent protein kinase has been demonstrated to be present in liver (KUO and GREENGARD, 1969a). The activity of this enzyme towards endogenous substrates is increased by injection into rats of cAMP, dBcAMP or glucagon (LANGAN, 1969a and b). Insulin also has the same effect (LANGAN, 1969b) but it is possible that the major effect of insulin in the intact animal is to increase secretion of catecholamines or glucagon and that these secondarily activate liver adenyl cyclase and therefore cAMP-dependent protein kinase.

Although it has been postulated that all metabolic effects mediated by cAMP are in turn mediated by activation of one or more specific protein kinases (KUO and GREENGARD, 1969a and b), too little is known at present about the nature of the protein kinases and their natural substrates to permit a description of the metabolic effects of the catecholamines in these terms.

c) Glycogen Cycle

Early studies of the regulation by catecholamines of glycogen storage and mobilization in liver emphasized the activation of glycogen phosphorylase (see SUTHERLAND and RALL, 1960) whereas more recent studies have taken into consideration the regulation of the subsequently discovered glycogen synthetase (see LARNER, 1966). It now appears that, of the two enzymes involved in glycogen synthesis and glycogen breakdown, the synthetase is by far the more sensitive to regulation by cAMP (DEWULF and HERS, 1968b). Both enzymes exist in "active" (phosphorylase *a* and glycogen synthetase *a* or I) and "inactive" (phosphorylase *b* and synthetase *b* or D) forms. The transformation of the *b* form to the *a* form of glycogen phosphorylase is catalyzed by a kinase (RALL et al., 1956; SHIMAZU and AMAKAWA, 1968a) and the reverse reaction is catalyzed by a phosphatase (WOSILAIT and SUTHERLAND, 1956); cAMP accelerates the kinase reaction. Unlike muscle phosphorylase, liver phosphorylase *b* is inactive in the presence of AMP and total phosphorylase (*a* plus *b*) in liver can only be assayed after activation with the kinase (SHIMAZU and AMAKAWA, 1968a). The transformation *b* to *a* for glycogen synthetase is catalyzed by a phosphatase whereas the reverse reaction is catalyzed by a kinase which is activated by cAMP (see DEWULF and HERS, 1968a; LARNER, 1966), and also by other cyclic nucleotides (GLINSMANN and HERN, 1969). Thus cAMP stimulates one or more specific protein kinases which transfer phosphate from ATP to phosphorylase *b* and to synthetase *a*; this results in activation of the former and inactivation of the latter, which together bring about an acceleration of glycogen breakdown and a reduction of glycogen synthesis. Liver glycogen synthetase (both *a* and *b* forms) is stimulated by glucose-6-phosphate and phosphate (MERSMANN and SEGAL, 1967) and is inhibited by ATP and ADP (GOLD, 1970).

This reciprocal activation and inactivation of the enzymes of the glycogen cycle appears to be the principal basis for the glycogenolytic effect of the catecholamines and of glucagon; it also appears to be the basis of the action of insulin to increase the synthesis of glycogen (BISHOP and LARNER, 1967), since insulin lowers the concentration of cAMP in perfused rat liver (JEFFERSON et al., 1968; EXTON and PARK, 1968a). In intact dogs insulin activates glycogen synthetase and inactivates glycogen phosphorylase, both effects being antagonized by glucagon and assumed to be mediated by reduced cAMP levels (BISHOP and LARNER, 1967).

Other factors also regulate the operation of the glycogen cycle in liver in addition to the influence of cAMP on the relative amounts of the phosphorylase and synthetase in the active and inactive forms. For example, glycogen inhibits the conversion by the phosphatase of synthetase *b* to *a* (DEWULF and HERS, 1968a) and can thus impose a limit upon the amount of glycogen that can be stored. In addition to this special kind of feedback inhibition there is also a feed-forward stimulation by glucose itself. Injection of glucose into mice results in a very rapid activation of glycogen synthetase (DEWULF and HERS, 1967a and b), even in adrenalectomized animals (DEWULF and HERS, 1967a). Glucose has a similar action in the perfused liver: a high concentration of glucose causes activation of glycogen synthetase, inactivation of glycogen phosphorylase and a net increase in glycogen synthesis; glucose can, moreover, antagonize the opposite effect of glucagon without changing the concentration of cAMP (BUSCHIAZZO et al., 1970); the mechanism of this effect of glucose is not understood.

The glucocorticoids appear to increase the synthesis of glycogen in the liver by influencing the activation of synthetase *b* (DEWULF et al., 1968; DEWULF and HERS, 1968b); that this is most probably an influence on the synthesis of the activating enzyme (glycogen synthetase *b* phosphatase) is indicated by the lag period for activation after injection of prednisolone (DEWULF and HERS, 1968b; MERSMANN and SEGAL, 1969) and by the absence of the activating enzyme in adrenalectomized rats (MERSMANN and SEGAL, 1969). The preponderance of glycogen synthetase in the *b* form may provide a partial explanation for the reduced capacity for glycogen storage in the livers of adrenalectomized rats (FRIEDMAN et al., 1967). There appears to be no information available about the possible glucocorticoid-dependence of the phosphorylase *a* phosphatase. That this enzyme may also be glucocorticoid-dependent is suggested by two observations: 1, treatment of rabbits with cortisone causes inactivation of liver phosphorylase, an action that does not prevent the subsequent activation by injected adrenaline (KERRPOLA, 1952) and, 2, a preponderance of the *a* form is found in adrenalectomized rats (SCHAEFFER et al., 1969a).

The increase in glucose output from the perfused liver in response to catecholamines or to cAMP is due to both increased net breakdown of glycogen, brought about by changes in the activities of the enzymes of the glycogen cycle described here, and also to increased gluconeogenesis (see next section). The extent to which each process contributes to the increase in glucose output depends on the amount of glycogen present in the liver. Adrenaline and cAMP do cause disappearance of glycogen (LEVINE, 1965), activation of glycogen phosphorylase (LEVINE, 1965; GLINSMANN et al., 1969; NORTHROP and PARKS, 1964) and inactivation of glycogen synthetase (GLINSMANN et al., 1969; GLINSMANN and HERN, 1969); at the same time they cause increased glucose output by perfused liver from fed rats.

A physiological role for catecholamines in the regulation of the glycogen cycle of liver has been questioned by SOKAL, SARCIONE and HENDERSON (1964) because of the relatively large amounts of catecholamines needed to exert an effect. However, it is clear that stimulation of the sympathetic nerves to the liver can result in very rapid activation of glycogen phosphorylase (SHIMAZU and AMAKAWA, 1968a and b) and inactivation of glycogen synthetase (SHIMAZU, 1967) so that a physiological role for at least the noradrenaline liberated from nerve endings in the liver appears highly likely. It is of great interest that both effects of sympathetic stimulation can be opposed by stimulation of the parasympathetic nervous system (SHIMAZU and AMAKAWA, 1968a; SHIMAZU, 1967). No effect of parasympathomimetic agents on liver adenyl cyclase has been found (MURAD et al., 1962) although these agents do depress the activity of heart adenyl cyclase. However, it is possible that parasympathomimetic agents might only depress the stimulation of hepatic adenyl cyclase by, for example, the catecholamines, an action that might have been missed in the *in vitro* assay. No information appears to be available about the actions of parasympathomimetic agents on hepatic metabolism. It is obvious that an understanding of this aspect of the regulation of hepatic metabolism will be necessary for the complete understanding of the regulatory effects of the catecholamines.

d) Gluconeogenesis

Until relatively recently it was generally assumed that the hyperglycemic effect of the catecholamines was due principally to their action to promote liver glycogenolysis (see SUTHERLAND and ROBISON, 1966). It is now realized that not only is inhibition of insulin secretion also important in the production of the hyperglycemia but also a direct action on the liver to promote gluconeogenesis (see HIMMS-HAGEN, 1967 for review).

Adrenaline and noradrenaline increase gluconeogenesis from lactate in perfused liver (EXTON and PARK, 1968b) as also do glucagon and cAMP (EXTON et al., 1966). The exact mechanism by which gluconeogenesis from lactate is accelerated is still in doubt. Crossover analysis indicates that one major control point lies between pyruvate and phosphoenolpyruvate (WILLIAMSON et al., 1966b; EXTON et al., 1966). However, it is not yet known which enzymic reaction is involved. WILLIAMSON et al. (1966a) suggest that the increased concentration of acetyl CoA (produced as a result of the lipolytic effect of the hormones and of cAMP; see next section) activates pyruvate carboxylase. There is indeed considerable evidence that a raised concentration of fatty acid in liver, produced for example by infusion of oleate, does increase gluconeogenesis in this way (WILLIAMSON et al., 1969a and b) and some authors consider that the gluconeogenic effect of catecholamines and of glucagon is secondary to their lipolytic effect on liver. Exton and Park (1966) pointed out that among the many steps which intervene between pyruvate and phosphoenolpyruvate, is included transport across membranes, and recently Adam and Haynes (1969) have provided evidence that the transport of pyruvate into liver mitochondria is increased in rats treated with adrenaline or glucagon. Another possible mode of regulation which should not be overlooked is the transport of inhibitory cations from one cellular compartment to another (Bygrave, 1967; Rasmussen and Tenenhouse, 1968; Gevers and Krebs, 1966). The observation that pyruvate carboxylase, a key enzyme of gluconeogenesis that lies between pyruvate and phosphoenolpyruvate, is strongly inhibited by calcium ions has led Kimmich and Rasmussen (1969) to propose the hypothesis that acceleration by gluconeogenic stimuli of the transport of calcium out of mitochondria would have the effect of stimulating pyruvate carboxylase (by reducing the concentration of the inhibitory cation) and of inhibiting the pyruvate kinase in the cytosol (by the increase in the concentration of the inhibitory cation); there would thus be simultaneous stimulation of a gluconeogenic enzyme and inhibition of a glycolytic enzyme. The concentration of calcium in the different parts of the liver cell under these different conditions is unknown. However, it is known that noradrenaline, glucagon and also cAMP cause a large and rapid but transient loss of calcium from perfused liver: the amount lost may be as large as 20% of the total liver calcium (Friedmann and Park, 1968). Thus, it is likely that a reduction in the concentration of calcium may have a role in stimulating gluconeogenesis.

Not only gluconeogenesis from lactate but also gluconeogenesis and urea production from endogenous amino acids is increased by catecholamines (Exton and Park, 1968a; Malette et al., 1969), by glucagon (Exton and Park, 1968a; Garcia et al., 1966; Malette et al., 1969; Miller, 1965) and by cAMP (Menahan and Wieland, 1967; Malette et al., 1969). Insulin has the opposite effect (reduces gluconeogenesis and urea production) and inhibits competitively the effects of glucagon and of cAMP (Glinsmann and Mortimore, 1968). The amount of glucose produced is roughly equivalent to the amount of urea formed when the liver is stimulated by either dBcAMP (Menahan and Wieland, 1967) or glucagon (Garcia et al., 1966). That the regulation by cAMP involves the breakdown of the liver proteins is indicated by the increased release of amino acids from the perfused liver caused by both adrenaline and glucagon (Miller, 1965). Uptake of amino acids by liver is not altered by adrenaline (Chambers et al., 1968). Insulin reduces the release of amino acids and urea by perfused liver (Mondon and Mortimore, 1967) and livers from alloxan diabetic rats have a markedly enhanced release of amino acids and urea which is reduced by treating the rats with insulin (Wilcox et al., 1968). An effect of glucagon to promote proteolysis has been suggested by Garcia and co-workers (1966) and an effect of insulin to inhibit proteolysis has been suggested (Mondon and Mortimore, 1967; Mortimore and Mondon, 1970). Glucagon has in fact been observed to cause a three-fold increase in the number of lysosomes in rat liver perfused for only 4 hours (Ashford and Porter, 1962): the presence in these lysosomes of fragmented mitochondria and other cell constituents suggests a general increase in breakdown of cellular proteins under the influence of glucagon.

The delivery of more amino acids to the gluconeogenic pathway will by itself accelerate gluconeogenesis since this pathway is not operating at maximum capacity at physiological concentrations of its major substrates (Exton and Park, 1967; Malette et al., 1969). Moreover, a rate-limiting step between pyruvate and phosphoenolpyruvate (suggested above as one of the sites of alteration produced by the hormones and cAMP) would not be expected to influence the rate of gluconeogenesis from the bulk of the amino acids that are catabolized by the liver because most amino acids do not give rise to pyruvate in the course of their metabolism.

Whether the observed inhibition by adrenaline, glucagon (PRYOR and BERTHET, 1959) and cAMP (PRYOR and BERTHET, 1960) of amino acid incorporation into protein of liver slices is an expression of the accelerated proteolysis rather than of inhibition of protein synthesis is uncertain. Insulin does not alter amino acid incorporation into protein by perfused liver when it reduces the liberation of amino acids by the liver (MONDON and MORTIMORE, 1967).

Stimulation of gluconeogenesis by glucagon or by cAMP does not occur in perfused livers from adrenalectomized rats (FRIEDMANN et al., 1967; EISENSTEIN and STRACK, 1968). The reason for this is unknown. Neither the increase in cAMP content nor the movements of potassium and calcium produced by glucagon are prevented by lack of adrenal cortical hormones (FRIEDMANN et al., 1967).

e) Lipid Metabolism

In an intact animal one of the major influences of catecholamines on lipid metabolism in the liver is undoubtedly the large increase in the delivery of lipid substrate (FFA) to this organ, brought about principally by their action on the white adipose tissue. The first part of this discussion must, therefore, deal with the known effects of FFA on liver metabolism.

The liver takes up FFA in proportion to their concentration in plasma or in perfusion fluid, both *in vivo* (SPITZER and MCELROY, 1960; FINE and WILLIAMS, 1960) and *in vitro* (VAN HARKEN et al., 1969; HEIMBERG et al., 1969). The effects of an elevated FFA concentration include accelerated ketogenesis (EXTON et al., 1969; HEIMBERG et al., 1969; VAN HARKEN et al., 1969; STRUCK et al., 1965; EXTON and PARK, 1967) and accelerated gluconeogenesis from added substrate (STRUCK et al., 1965; WILLIAMSON et al., 1966, 1969a, b and c). Although increased ketogenesis occurs at fairly low concentrations of added FFA, accelerated gluconeogenesis is only seen when the concentration is high (VAN HARKEN et al., 1969; EXTON et al., 1969; WILLIAMSON et al., 1969b). The increased metabolism of FFA is accompanied by increases in the concentration of acetyl CoA, acyl CoA and citrate (WILLIAMSON et al., 1969b and c) and by a decrease in the concentration of free CoA. No change in the concentration of cAMP occurs (EXTON et al., 1969). The oxygen uptake of the liver increases (WILLIAMSON et al., 1969a), the output of triglyceride from the liver also increases (HEIMBERG et al., 1969) and the triglyceride content of the liver increases in proportion to the concentration of FFA (VAN HARKEN et al., 1969). A high concentration of FFA does not increase gluconeogenesis from endogenous amino acids, since there is no change in urea production (WILLIAMSON et al., 1969b and c) and since this effect is not seen in the absence of added substrate (WILLIAMSON et al., 1969a). However, it can accelerate gluconeogenesis from added amino acids (WILLIAMSON et al., 1969a). That fatty acid oxidation by the liver is a prerequisite for many of these effects is indicated by the fact that the acceleration by oleate of gluconeogenesis and ketogenesis is inhibited by (+)decanoylcarnitine, a compound which inhibits the transport of activated fatty acids to their site of oxidation (WILLIAMSON et al., 1969c). Similar increases in acetyl CoA and acyl CoA content, in ketone body content, in citrate content and in gluconeogenesis and ketogenesis occur in association with a high concentration of FFA in the blood in the livers of fed rats injected with glucagon (WILLIAMSON et al., 1966c; WILLIAMSON, 1967), with anti-insulin serum (WILLIAMSON, 1967; WILLIAMSON et al., 1966a) or with cortisol (SEUBERT et al., 1968).

Similar changes occur in the livers of starved rats and in these animals glucagon causes no further increase (WILLIAMSON et al., 1966c).

Although the principal way in which catecholamines modify lipid metabolism in the liver of intact animals is by causing an increase in the delivery of FFA to the liver, the catecholamines have, in addition, a direct action: they modify lipid and glucose metabolism of the liver in a way that resembles in many respects the change induced by a high concentration of FFA. Glucagon, dBcAMP and theophylline increase the concentration of acetyl CoA and acyl CoA and decrease the concentration of free CoA in liver slices (CLAYCOMB and KILSHEIMER, 1969). Glucagon and dBcAMP also increase ketogenesis (BEWSHER and ASHMORE, 1966; HEIMBERG et al., 1969; MENAHAN and WIELAND, 1967; STRUCK et al., 1965; VAN HARKEN et al., 1969; PENHOS et al., 1966; REGEN and TERRELL, 1968) as well as gluconeogenesis (see previous section). This similarity between the effects of glucagon and cAMP on the one hand and of FFA on the other has led to the hypothesis that the gluconeogenic and ketogenic actions of glucagon and of cAMP that mediate these effects are secondary to a rise in intracellular FFA concentration brought about by stimulation of a hepatic triglyceride lipase. This hypothesis was proposed by STRUCK, ASHMORE and WIELAND (1965) and received some support from the finding of an increased lipolytic activity in liver homogenates from rats injected with glucagon (BEWSHER and ASHMORE, 1966) and in liver slices incubated with glucagon or dBcAMP (CLAYCOMB and KILSHEIMER, 1969). Further indirect support for this hypothesis has been put forward by WILLIAMSON and co-workers (WILLIAMSON et al., 1966a and b; 1969a, b and c and WILLIAMSON, 1967). However, other workers have failed to find a lipolytic effect of glucagon in perfused liver (PENHOS et al., 1966). Although it is possible that part of the gluconeogenic and ketogenic effect of cAMP and of glucagon may be due to increased lipolysis, there exist several differences between the effects of glucagon or cAMP and those of FFA; these differences indicate that much of the gluconeogenic and ketogenic effect is not secondary to formation of FFA. The effects of glucagon and oleate on gluconeogenesis are additive (ROSS et al., 1967). Glucagon and cAMP increase urea production by an amount roughly equivalent to the amount of glucose formed in gluconeogenesis (MENAHAN and WIELAND, 1967 GARCIA et al., 1966) and are effective in the absence of added substrate whereas FFA have little or no effect on urea formation by perfused liver (WILLIAMSON et al., 1969b and c) and are ineffective in the absence of added substrate. Although both glucagon and cAMP can accelerate ketogenesis, as noted above, their effect is much smaller than that of added fatty acid (EXTON et al., 1969; WILLIAMSON et al., 1969c) and much more variable (EXTON et al., 1966). Indeed, some authors report that a supply of exogenous FFA is necessary for the ketogenic effect of glucagon (VAN HARKEN et al., 1969) while others report a greater ketogenic effect in livers from fasting animals than in livers from fed animals (PENHOS et al., 1966). Further evidence that the gluconeogenic and ketogenic effects of glucagon are not due to accelerated FFA production is provided by the failure of (+)decanoylcarnitine to inhibit the ketogenic, gluconeogenic and ureogenic effects of glucagon (WILLIAMSON et al., 1969c), although it inhibits the ketogenic and gluconeogenic effects of added FFA. Although WILLIAMSON and co-workers (1969c) interpret this finding as due to the utilization of endogenously produced fatty acids by carnitine-independent pathways, it might also be taken as providing some support for the idea that it is endogenous amino acids which are the substrates for the accelerated ketogenesis induced by glucagon. That some of the ketogenic amino acids, available as a consequence of the accelerated protein breakdown (see previous section), might be used to form ketone bodies does not seem to have been considered as a possible explanation for the ketogenic effects of glucagon and of cAMP.

Although the existence of a direct lipolytic effect of glucagon, catecholamines and cAMP on liver must remain in doubt there is no doubt that these compounds can modify the subsequent metabolism of FFA. The uptake of FFA by the liver is not altered by glucagon or dBcAMP (HEIMBERG et al., 1969) and is only slightly reduced by noradrenaline (HEIMBERG and FIZETTE, 1963); the latter effect was observed in the presence of phenoxybenzamine which may have modified somewhat the metabolic effect of the noradrenaline. In contrast to the lack of effect on uptake, noradrenaline (HEIMBERG and FIZETTE, 1963), glucagon (HEIMBERG et al., 1969; PENHOS et al., 1966) and dBcAMP (HEIMBERG et al., 1969) markedly inhibit the secretion of triglyceride by the liver. The biochemical basis for this inhibition of lipid secretion is not understood.

f) Protein Synthesis

In addition to promoting a general proteolysis in liver (MILLER, 1965; GARCIA et al., 1966) and possibly inhibiting general protein synthesis (PRYOR and BERTHET, 1959, 1960) catecholamines, glucagon and cAMP can increase the synthesis of certain specific enzyme proteins. Only three such proteins have been studied and of these three only one in any detail from this viewpoint. The extent to which synthesis of other enzyme proteins can be altered by cAMP and the physiological significance of such changes is not understood. The increase in amount of enzyme that occurs is generally referred to as due to enzyme induction: this term will be used here in this sense only and is not intended to imply any mechanism of action.

In normal liver cells in culture a variety of compounds can induce tyrosine transaminase: these include cAMP, dBcAMP, adrenaline, isopropylnoradrenaline and glucagon (WICKS, 1968, 1969). A similar induction due to glucagon has been observed in perfused liver from adrenalectomized rats (HAGER and KENNEY, 1968), and cAMP causes induction in perfused liver from normal rats (GLINSMANN et al., 1969). Similar effects are seen when cAMP, adrenaline or glucagon is administered to foetal or newborn rats (GREENGARD, 1969; HOLT and OLIVER, 1969). The response disappears in adult rats (GREENGARD, 1969) but does occur in adrenalectomized adult rats (GREENGARD, 1969; WICKS et al., 1969; CSANYI et al., 1967). In cultured liver cells derived from a Morris hepatoma this response to glucagon and also to dBcAMP or theophylline is lost, even though the ability to make this enzyme in response to glucocorticoids is retained (GRANNER et al., 1968; see also TOMKINS et al., 1969). In their lack of response to cAMP these cells resemble foetal liver at a very early stage of development (GREENGARD, 1969) but their response to glucocorticoids resembles that of adult liver.

The report that parasympathomimetic agents, too, can induce liver tyrosine transaminase in adrenalectomized rats (BLACK, 1970) may possibly be explained by stimulation of insulin secretion by these agents (see section B. VII).

Another enzyme that is induced by cAMP, dBcAMP, catecholamines or glucagon is phosphoenolpyruvate carboxykinase (YEUNG and OLIVER, 1968a and b; WICKS, 1969; WICKS et al., 1969). This enzyme, unlike the tyrosine transaminase, is not induced by hydrocortisone or by insulin; rather insulin inhibits the inducing effects of glucagon and of isopropylnoradrenaline (WICKS, 1969). Serine dehydratase is induced in intact or adrenalectomized rats by dBcAMP, cAMP and glucagon but not by hydrocortisone (WICKS et al., 1969; JOST et al., 1970). A number of other soluble enzymes of gluconeogenesis are not altered by any of these compounds (WICKS, 1969; YEUNG and OLIVER, 1968b).

The mechanism by which cAMP stimulates the synthesis of a specific protein such as tyrosine transaminase is unknown. Other hormones can exert a similar effect that is not mediated by cAMP; for example, the glucocorticoids, and also insulin (Wicks, 1969; Holten and Kenney, 1967; Hager and Kenney, 1968) despite the presumed decrease in cAMP that it produces.

There is at present no information concerning the mechanism by which any of these compounds can alter the synthesis of specific proteins. Wicks (1969) has noted that at least three separate mechanisms are involved for cAMP, insulin and hydrocortisone respectively. No physiological significance can be ascribed to these effects, except perhaps to the changes in phosphoenolpyruvate carboxykinase, which appear to occur in association with changes in rates of gluconeogenesis (Yeung and Oliver, 1968b). Wicks (1969) has proposed the interesting hypothesis that induction of tyrosine transaminase by adrenaline represents a feedback inhibition of the synthesis of adrenaline by accelerating the removal of the initial substrate for this pathway. This seems unlikely because the signal (concentration of adrenaline in the blood) does not indicate that there is no further need for adrenaline synthesis but rather that adrenaline has been secreted from the stores in the adrenal medulla. For the adrenal medulla to replenish its stores more tyrosine would be needed rather than less. It seems more likely that the increase in tyrosine transaminase in response to cAMP, adrenaline or glucagon represents, like the increase in serine dehydratase, an adaptation to accelerated gluconeogenesis from amino acids.

g) Ion Movements

It has been realized for many years, the evidence coming mainly from experiments with intact animals, that the catecholamines alter the movement of ions into and out of the liver (see Ellis, 1956; Ellis et al., 1967; Hornbrook, 1970 for reviews). The physiological significance of these ion movements has been largely ignored and is still not clear. However, since it is now apparent that metabolic processes can be markedly altered by rather small changes in the concentration of certain ions, it is necessary to consider the alterations in ion movements caused by the catecholamines together with their metabolic effects in order to see how far the metabolic effects can be ascribed to changes in ion concentration.

Adrenaline and noradrenaline cause a transient influx of potassium into perfused liver followed by a more prolonged and larger efflux (Craig, 1965; Friedmann and Park, 1968; Northrop, 1968; Exton and Park, 1968a): glucagon and cAMP have a similar effect, although with cAMP the initial small influx is sometimes not seen (Friedmann and Park, 1968; Northrop, 1968; Glinsmann and Mortimore, 1968; Exton and Park, 1968a; Burton et al., 1967). The changes in potassium movement appear to occur independently of the changes in glucose metabolism (Burton et al., 1967; Exton and Park, 1968a). They were originally ascribed to stimulation by the catecholamines of α-receptors (see Ellis, 1956; Ellis et al., 1967), receptors different from those for the other metabolic effects. However, since it is now apparent that the α-receptor blocking agents which inhibit the effects of catecholamines on ion movements also block the effect of cAMP on ion movements (Northrop, 1968) it seems more likely that the receptor responsible for changes in ion movement is identical with the receptor for stimulation of hepatic adenyl cyclase by adrenaline.

Metabolic consequences of the loss of potassium from the liver have not been clearly delineated. There is actually a depletion of potassium, both from the mitochondria and from the cytosol of the liver of adrenaline-treated animals (Auditore and Holland, 1956). Bygrave (1967) has pointed out that some enzymes of glycolysis (e.g. pyruvate kinase, phosphofructokinase) require potassium: thus a decrease in potassium concentration in the cytosol of the liver could conceivably lead to a reduction in the rate of glycolysis. A recent report that depletion of potassium inhibits the secretion of lipoproteins by the liver (JUDAH and NICHOLLS, 1970) suggests that the similar metabolic effect of the catecholamines might be secondary to the potassium depletion.

cAMP, and also noradrenaline and glucagon, cause a transient loss of calcium from the perfused liver (FRIEDMANN and PARK, 1968). As much as 20% of the total liver calcium may be lost in this way. However, the relative changes in calcium concentration in different cellular compartments are unknown. This loss of calcium is not a consequence of the other metabolic changes since it occurs equally well in livers from adrenalectomized rats in which the metabolic changes do not occur (FRIEDMANN and PARK, 1968). One possible metabolic consequence of a reduction in calcium concentration brought about by catecholamines and by glucagon would be a de-inhibition of mitochondrial pyruvate carboxylase leading to increased gluconeogenesis from pyruvate and lactate (see GEVERS and KREBS, 1966; KIMMICH and RASMUSSEN, 1969). This hypothesis assumes that the concentration of calcium inside the mitochondria is decreased under these conditions. One observation that is in keeping with this suggestion is the finding of ADAM and HAYNES (1969) of an increased capacity of mitochondria from livers of adrenaline-treated rats to fix CO_2 despite an apparently unchanged pyruvate carboxylase content. It has been postulated that an increased concentration of calcium in the cytosol inhibits glycolysis at the same time as mitochondrial pyruvate carboxylase is activated by a decreased concentration of calcium (GEVERS and KREBS, 1966; KIMMICH and RASMUSSEN, 1969; BYGRAVE, 1967). Another enzyme of liver that is influenced by calcium is adenyl cyclase itself which actually requires calcium (MARINETTI et al., 1969).

The mechanism by which cAMP increases calcium efflux is unknown. In heart muscle cAMP can increase the ATP-dependent uptake of calcium into isolated sarcoplasmic reticulum (ENTMAN et al., 1969b). Whether a similar cAMP-sensitive calcium transport exists in liver is unknown.

h) Summary: Effects of Catecholamines on Liver

There are numerous facets to the metabolic effects of catecholamines on liver which are difficult to fit together to provide an overall view of regulation of metabolism and function in the liver in the presence of the catecholamines. As far as can be ascertained at present all effects of the catecholamines on liver are mediated by stimulation of adenyl cyclase and increased formation of cAMP: cAMP phosphodiesterase appears to be regulated primarily by the availability of its substrate. Consequences of the rise in cAMP concentrations are listed in Table 1 and illustrated in Fig. 1. Some can be attributed to stimulation of specific enzymes by cAMP (all protein kinases); some may be due to reduced concentrations of cations in specific regions of the cell; some may be due to changed concentration of substrate (e.g., amino acids for gluconeogenesis); others are not explainable at present in these terms. Specific induction of enzyme synthesis appears to be yet another consequence of cAMP accumulation.

In an intact animal, in addition to these complex changes in regulatory processes caused by a direct action of adrenaline on the liver, changes will occur in response to altered concentrations in the blood of other compounds, caused by actions of adrenaline on other tissues. For example, increases in the concentrations of lactate and FFA will influence gluconeogenesis, fatty acid oxidation, triglyceride synthesis, ketogenesis; inhibition of insulin secretion will influence liver metabolism and a rise in glucose concentration should counteract some of the effects of cAMP on glycogen metabolism.

Thus, although the major consequence of the action of the catecholamines on liver can still be described as an increase in the output of glucose that contributes to the hyperglycemic effect in the intact animal, the mechanism of this action of

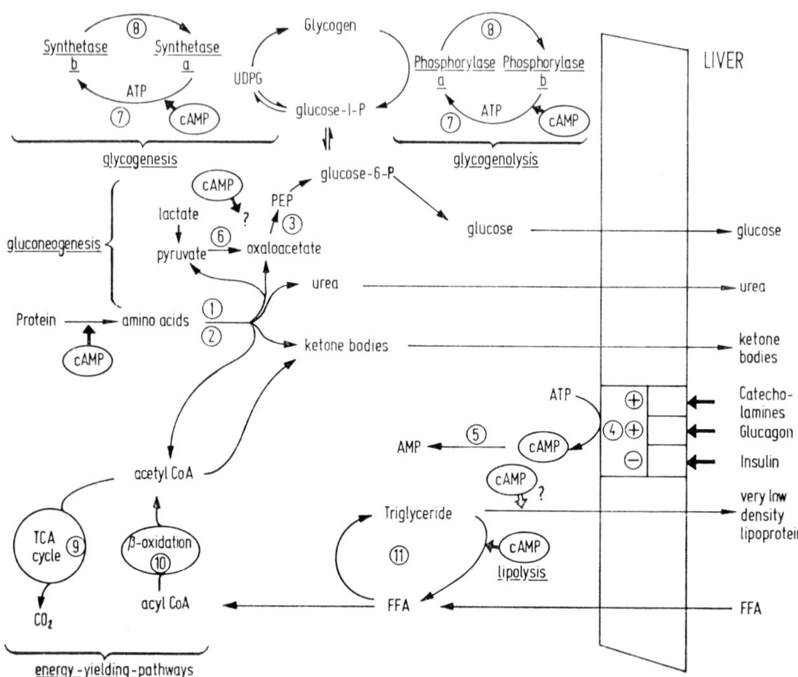

Fig. 1. *Summary of those aspects of liver metabolism known to be influenced by catecholamines.* Pathways are shown only in outline and most intermediates are omitted. The sites of *stimulation* by cAMP are shown by the solid arrows and sites of *inhibition* by cAMP are shown by open arrows. The approximate location of three enzymes of which the synthesis is increased by cAMP are shown by numbers: (1) tyrosine transaminase; (2) serine dehydratase; (3) phosphoenolpyruvate carboxykinase. Adenyl cyclase (indicated by (4)) is shown as being part of the plasma membrane and in contact with two stimulatory discriminator units and one inhibitory discriminator unit: (5) denotes cAMP phosphodiesterase. Pyruvate carboxylase is denoted by (6); note that this enzyme is involved in gluconeogenesis from lactate and from only some of the amino acids (those that give rise to pyruvate in the course of their metabolism). Ketone bodies are shown as arising from the metabolism of some amino acids and also from the metabolism of fatty acids. (7) denotes the cAMP-dependent protein kinase(s) responsible for the activation of phosphorylase *b* and for the inactivation of glycogen syntetase *a*. (8) denotes the phosphoprotein phophatase(s) responsible for the inactivation of phosphorylase *a* and for the activation of glycogen synthetase *b*; the synthesis of this phosphatase (or these phosphatases) is glucocorticoid-dependent. The major energy-yielding pathways of the liver, tricarboxylic acid cycle and β-oxidation cycle of fatty acid oxidation are shown by (9) and (10). The triglyceride cycle is shown by (11); utilization of plasma FFA for the synthesis of very low density lipoproteins must also be accompanied by the synthesis and incorporation into these lipoproteins of a specific protein, phospholipid and cholesterol. For further discussion of the actions of catecholamines and of insulin see the appropriate sections of the text (adenyl cyclase, Ia; glycogen cycle, Ic; gluconeogenesis (including protein brekdown), Id; lipid metabolism (including the role of FFA in promoting gluconeogenesis), Ie; enzyme induction, If). The intracellular location of ion movements and their alteration by catecholamines (section Ig) is not included in the diagram because insufficient information is available

the catecholamines is now realized to be considerably more complex than was once believed and can not at present be described in detail.

The "permissive" effects of glucocorticoids on certain of the metabolic effects of the catecholamines, especially those involving the liver, have been known for many years (see ELLIS, 1956 for review). However, it is now realized that the glucocorticoids are required only for some of the later consequences of the action of catecholamines on the liver and are not required for the initial events. The effects of the glucocorticoids can be seen to be in one sense *antagonistic* to the effects of the cAMP-producing hormones in that they shift the balance between active and inactive forms of the enzymes of the glycogen cycle towards synthesis whereas cAMP shifts them towards breakdown. In another sense, the glucocorticoids can be seen to have a *permissive* effect because the enzymes must first be in the forms that promote synthesis before they can be shifted by cAMP to the forms that promote breakdown.

II. White Adipose Tissue

The principal metabolic consequence of the action of catecholamines on white adipose tissue is an acceleration of the breakdown of triglyceride into free fatty acids and glycerol, the process of *lipolysis*. Since the functions of the white adipose tissue are the synthesis and storage of triglyceride and their mobilization as FFA when appropriate, the effect of the catecholamines is to elicit one of these functions, namely, the mobilization of triglyceride stores. The acceleration of lipolysis, which is a consequence of stimulation of the adenyl cyclase of white adipose tissue by the catecholamines, may be influenced by a variety of different metabolic processes and hormones, and has itself a profound influence on other metabolic processes in the adipose tissue. An abbreviated outline of the principal metabolic pathways of white adipose tissue is given in Fig. 2 as an aid in this discussion of their regulation. An extensive review of white adipose tissue metabolism has recently been made by JEANRENAUD (1968).

The introduction by RODBELL, first of a technique for the preparation of isolated white adipose tissue cells (RODBELL, 1964, 1965b) and later of a technique for the preparation of fat cell ghosts (RODBELL, 1967a and b) has made possible considerable advances in knowledge of the interaction of catecholamines and other hormones with the cell membrane of white adipose tissue and of the relation of adenyl cyclase to other functional components of the cell membrane. It seems likely that white adipose tissue may be the first tissue for which the nature of an adrenergic receptor will be identified: for this reason the evidence concerning the nature and properties of its cell membrane will be discussed in some detail here.

An earlier simple model for the mechanism of the lipolytic effect of catecholamines on white adipose tissue involved: (i) stimulation of adenyl cyclase, (ii) accumulation of its product, cAMP, and (iii) activation of the triglyceride lipase (see HIMMS-HAGEN, 1967 for earlier references). The adenyl cyclase was believed to be rather "nonspecific" in its responsiveness because it was also stimulated by a wide variety of other hormones (ACTH, TSH, glucagon). The rate of lipolysis was considered to depend on the concentration of cAMP, which in turn depended on the rate of production of this compound and the rate of its degradation. Methylxanthines such as theophylline or caffeine were found to inhibit the phosphodiesterase which degraded the cAMP; the accumulation of cAMP and the potentiation of the lipolytic effect of the catecholamines produced by the methylxanthines were therefore attributed to inhibition of this enzyme. Since a variety of adrenergic blocking agents, both α-adrenergic and β-adrenergic, were found to

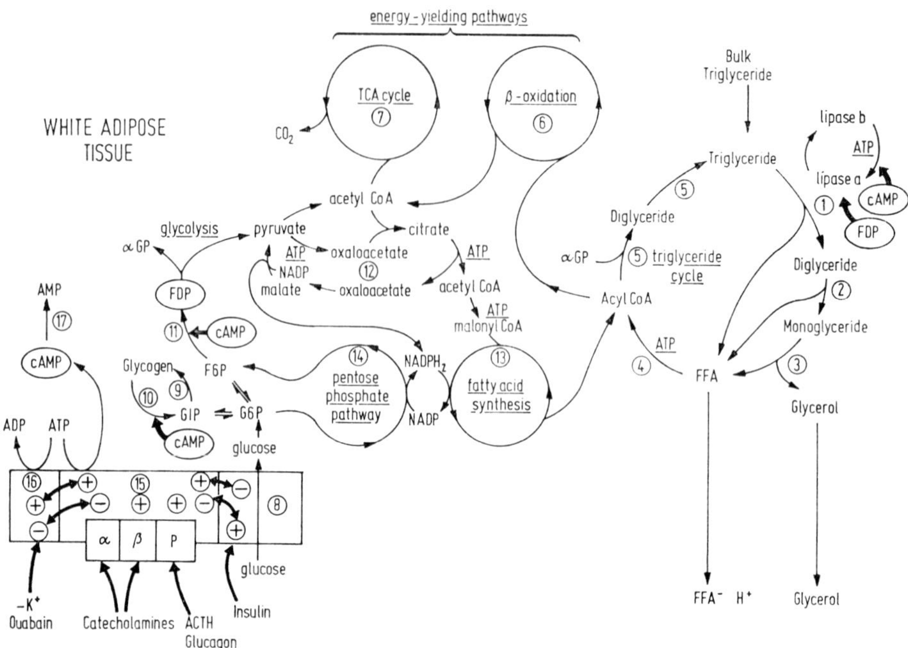

Fig. 2. *Summary of those aspects of the metabolism of white adipose tissue known to be influenced by catecholamines.* Pathways are shown only in outline and most intermediates are omitted. Sites of stimulation by cAMP and by FDP (fructose 1,6-diphosphate) are indicated by the appropriately labeled solid arrows. *Enzymes of lipolysis* are: (1) triglyceride lipase; (2) diglyceride lipase; (3) monoglyceride lipase. Enzymes of re-esterification of fatty acids are: (4) fatty acid activating enzyme (requires coenzyme A and splits ATP to AMP and pyrophosphate); (5) several acyltransferases and phosphatidic acid phosphatases. *Major energy-yielding pathways* are: (6) β-oxidation of fatty acids; (7) tricarboxylic acid cycle. *Enzymes of glucose disposal* are: (8) glucose transport component of the plasma membrane; (9) glycogen synthetase; (10) glycogen phosphorylase; (11) phosphofructokinase; (12) pyruvate cycle for the transport of acetyl groups from the mitochondrion to the cytosol; this includes the following enzymes and processes: pyruvate carboxylase (utilizes ATP), citrate synthase, transfer of citrate from mitochondrion to cytosol, citrate cleavage enzyme (utilizes ATP), malate dehydrogenase, malic enzyme, tranfer of pyruvate from cytosol to mitochondrion. The operation of malate dehydrogenase and malic enzyme results in the transfer of hydrogen from $NADH_2$ (derived for example from the glyceraldehyde 3-phosphate dehydrogenase reaction of glycolysis) to $NADPH_2$ and provides some of the reducing power needed for fatty acid synthesis. (13) fatty acid synthetase and the preceding step, acetyl CoA carboxylase (utilizes ATP), convert acetyl groups derived principally from glucose to fatty acids for subsequent storage as triglyceride. (14) pentose phosphate pathway; this provides the remainder of the $NADPH_2$ required for the synthesis of fatty acids. *Membrane components involved in the response to hormones are:* (15) adenyl cyclase; (16) Na^+-K^+-ATPase; (8) glucose transport. The other component of the adenyl cyclase system, cAMP phosphodiesterase, is denoted by (17). Adenyl cyclase is shown as being associated with three "receptors", one for peptide hormones (*P*), one for α-receptor actions of catecholamines and one for β-receptor actions of catecholamines. The effect of these receptors on the adenyl cyclase is indicated by (+) (stimulation) or by (—) (inhibition). The reciprocal relationship between adenyl cyclase and the neighbouring components of the membrane are indicated by the double-headed arrows. Inhibition of adenyl cyclase is associated with stimulation of glucose transport and vice versa; stimulation of adenyl cyclase is associated with inhibition of glucose transport. Inhibition of adenyl cyclase is associated with inhibition of Na^+-K^+-ATPase and vice versa; stimulation of Na^+-K^+-ATPase is associated with stimulation of adenyl cyclase. There appears also to be a reciprocal relationship between Na^+-K^+-ATPase and glucose transport; inhibition of Na^+-K^+-ATPase stimulates glucose transport. For further discussion see the text (B. II. 1)

inhibit the lipolytic effect of the catecholamines the suggestion was made that the receptor might be of a new type, neither α nor β. However, the subsequent recognition of a greater sensitivity to and greater specificity of inhibition by the β-receptor blocking agents (competitive inhibition) than of inhibition by the α-receptor blocking agents (noncompetitive inhibition) led to some acceptance of the idea that the receptor was more probably a β-receptor (STOCK and WESTERMANN, 1966a and b).

It is now apparent that this simple model cannot serve in discussion of the many observations of the regulation of adipose tissue lipolysis by catecholamines and other hormones. Three examples of such observations will be given here. Firstly, the concentration of cAMP is not always related to the rate of lipolysis. Thus, deoxyfrenolicin potentiates the actions of noradrenaline, of ACTH or of theophylline to increase cAMP concentration in fat cells, yet it inhibits their lipolytic actions (KUO, 1969). Cyclic GMP has been reported to raise cAMP concentration in fat cells and yet to inhibit lipolysis (MURAD et al., 1969b). It is known that the concentration of cAMP required for maximum activation of lipolysis is fairly low and that a higher concentration can be achieved without causing any further increase in lipolysis (BUTCHER et al., 1968; BUTCHER et al., 1965) but the situation described above in which raised cAMP concentration is associated with inhibition of lipolysis obviously requires a modification of the simple model. Secondly, it is possible for cAMP itself, and also dBcAMP, added to intact adipose tissue or cells, to have no effect, a lipolytic effect, or an antilipolytic effect depending on the incubation conditions or the pretreatment of the tissue (MOSINGER and VAUGHAN, 1967a and b; SWISLOCKI, 1970). Thirdly, the potentiation by insulin, under certain conditions, of the lipolytic effect of the catecholamines (JUNGAS and BALL, 1963; BURNS and LANGLEY, 1968; CHLOUVERAKIS, 1967) does not readily fit the simple model, in view of its well-documented action to inhibit catecholamine-induced increases in lipolysis (JUNGAS and BALL, 1964; FROESCH, 1967; BURNS and LANGLEY, 1968) in cAMP concentration (KUO and DE RENZO, 1969; BUTCHER et al., 1968) and in adenyl cyclase activity (JUNGAS, 1966).

In this review the simple and earlier model will therefore be modified in order to provide for the multitude of factors that have recently been shown to influence the lipolytic effect of the catecholamines. The discussion is divided into two main parts: those effects that can be localized to the cell membrane, and those effects which can be explained in terms of intracellular regulatory processes.

1. Events at the Cell Membrane

a) Functional Components of the Cell Membrane

The studies with fat cell ghosts (RODBELL, 1967a and b; BIRNBAUMER and RODBELL, 1969; BIRNBAUMER et al., 1969) in which events occurring at the cell membrane can be studied in the absence of any secondary regulation imposed by accelerated lipolysis (due to the catecholamines and other lipolytic hormones) or by accelerated lipogenesis (duc to insulin) among other processes, have led to the identification in the cell membrane of several hormone-sensitive processes; these have also been studied to some extent in particulate preparations of fat cells (VAUGHAN and MURAD, 1969). Such processes include: adenyl cyclase activity, cation transport, particularly the Na^{+}-K^{+}-stimulated ATPase or sodium pump ATPase, glucose transport and amino acid transport. There is, however, considerable interaction between the different processes in the membrane such that alteration in the activity of any one may lead to alterations in the activities of one or more of the others. The principal properties of each membrane component will be discussed in turn and possible interactions between individual components will be indicated.

The activity of adenyl cyclase is stimulated by the presence of catecholamines and of a number of peptide hormones (VAUGHAN and MURAD, 1969; BÄR and HECHTER, 1969; BIRNBAUMER and RODBELL, 1969; RODBELL, 1967a). Removal of calcium potentiates the stimulatory effects of adrenaline and of glucagon but inhibits the stimulatory effect of ACTH (BIRNBAUMER and RODBELL, 1969; BIRNBAUMER et al., 1969; BÄR and HECHTER, 1969); calcium inhibits the stimulatory effects of isopropylnoradrenaline (WILLIAMS et al., 1968a) and of fluoride (BIRNBAUMER et al., 1969). In this lack of requirement for calcium the adipose tissue adenyl cyclase resembles that of heart (DRUMMOND and DUNCAN, 1970) and differs from that of liver (MARINETTI et al., 1969) and brain (BRADHAM et al., 1970) both of which require calcium. Stimulation of adenyl cyclase activity by catecholamines may be observed in cells, ghosts and isolated particulate fractions. However, it has not been possible to identify in ghosts or particles certain actions of hormones on adenyl cyclase activity that are undoubtedly exerted at the plasma membrane. For example, the antilipolytic effect of insulin is demonstrable in isolated fat cells (KONO, 1969a and b; RODBELL and JONES, 1966) and is associated with diminished cAMP formation (KUO and DE RENZO, 1969; BUTCHER et al., 1968); it is generally presumed to be due to inhibition of adenyl cyclase activity. However, no measurable effect of insulin on adenyl cyclase of ghosts (RODBELL et al., 1968; CRYER et al., 1969) or of isolated subcellular particles (VAUGHAN and MURAD, 1969) or of isolated cells under most conditions (WILLIAMS et al., 1968a and b) has been found; the only report of a decrease in adenyl cyclase activity due to insulin involved the preincubation of intact tissue with insulin and no decrease could be seen when insulin was added after the cells were broken (JUNGAS, 1966). Insulin does not stimulate the phosphodiesterase responsible for the hydrolysis of cAMP (BLECHER et al., 1968; HEPP et al., 1969a). These characteristics of the effect of insulin are similar to the those of the effect of ouabain, an inhibitor of the Na^+-K^+-ATPase of fat cell membranes (LETARTE et al., 1969; MODOLELL and MOORE, 1967). Ouabain, like insulin, has an antilipolytic effect in fat cells (HO et al., 1966, 1967; MOSINGER and VAUGHAN, 1967a; FAIN, 1968), does not stimulate cAMP phosphodiesterase (HO et al., 1967) and may be presumed to inhibit adenyl cyclase activity and reduce the concentration of cAMP in the course of its action. Ouabain also has no direct effect upon adenyl cyclase although the adenyl cyclase activity of preparations from cells that have been preincubated with ouabain is reduced (HO et al., 1967). Thus, although the effects of insulin and of ouabain are associated with reduced adenyl cyclase activity, they do not appear to be exerted via direct inhibition of this enzyme. Thus stimulation of glucose transport by insulin and inhibition of the Na^+-K^+-ATPase by ouabain are both associated with inhibition of adenyl cyclase activity.

The ouabain-sensitive Na^+-K^+-ATPase of white adipose tissue (LETARTE et al., 1969; MODOLELL and MOORE, 1967) is presumably associated with the normal fluxes of sodium and potassium seen in this tissue (PERRY and HALES, 1969) and the sodium-dependent, ouabain-sensitive accumulation of potassium by fat cells (CLAUSEN et al., 1969). The activities of the other membrane components are dependent on the activity of this membrane ATPase. The lipolytic effect of the catecholamines is potassium dependent and is inhibited by ouabain (MOSINGER and KUJALOVA, 1966; KYPSON et al., 1968; HO et al., 1966; MOSINGER and VAUGHAN, 1967a; HO et al., 1967). The lipolytic effects of ACTH and glucagon are similarly inhibited (HO et al., 1966, 1967). The lipolytic agents whose action does not involve the stimulation of adenyl cyclase (theophylline, cAMP) still stimulate lipolysis in the absence of potassium and in the presence of ouabain (KYPSON et al., 1968; FAIN, 1968; HO et al., 1967). A reduction in adenyl cyclase activity has been demonstrated in cells preincubated with ouabain or in the absence of potassium (HO et al., 1967) and the absence of potassium reduces the effect of noradrenaline to increase cAMP formation in fat cells (KUO and DE RENZO, 1969); however, the effect of insulin to reduce cAMP formation by fat cells stimulated by noradrenaline plus theophylline is still seen in the absence of potassium (KUO and DE RENZO, 1969). Thus, the activity and hormonal sensitivity of the adenyl cyclase system is dependent on the normal functioning of the neighbouring ATPase.

A further instance of the interlocking of apparently different functional units in the membrane is provided by the observation that glucose transport in the membrane is influenced by the activity of the Na-K-ATPase. Glucose transport into fat cells is accelerated when the ATPase is inhibited by ouabain (HO and JEANRENAUD, 1967; CLAUSEN, 1969; MOSINGER and VAUGHAN, 1967a), by the absence of potassium (CLAUSEN, 1969; MOSINGER and VAUGHAN, 1967a; RODBELL, 1967b; LETARTE and RENOLD, 1969) or by the absence of sodium (LETARTE and RENOLD, 1969).

Since the functional state of the Na^+-K^+-ATPase appears to influence the activities of both the adenyl cyclase and the glucose transport components, the question arises as to whether this is a reciprocal arrangement, i.e., do changes in the activities of adenyl cyclase and glucose transport components influence the activity of the Na^+-K^+-ATPase? The existence of a reciprocal relationship between adenyl cyclase and the Na^+-K^+-ATPase is supported by the observation that adrenaline stimulates loss of potassium from fat cells by an action on α-receptors (PERRY and HALES, 1970), now known to be associated with inhibition of adenyl cyclase activity (see next section). However, insulin has little or no effect on potassium loss from fat pads (GOURLEY and BETHEA, 1964) or from fat cells (LETARTE et al., 1969).

The relationship between the adenyl cyclase and the glucose transport system is also a reciprocal one. Activation of glucose transport by insulin or (presumably indirectly) by ouabain is associated with reduced activity of the adenyl cyclase system (JUNGAS, 1966; HO et al., 1967). Activation of the adenyl cyclase system in fat cell ghosts by adrenaline, ACTH or glucagon reduces glucose transport (RODBELL, 1967b). This effect is not seen in cells where glucose transport is accelerated by these hormones because of the acceleration of lipolysis.

Another functional activity of the white adipose cell membrane, the transport of amino acids, is also related to the activity of the Na^+-K^+-ATPase but is not as directly linked as are the adenyl cyclase system and the glucose transport system. Although the transport of α-aminoisobutyric acid is inhibited by ouabain and is sodium- and potassium-dependent (TOUABI and JEANRENAUD, 1969; CLAUSEN and RODBELL, 1969), its rate of transport appears to depend on the intracellular potassium concentration or on the gradient of potassium concentration across the cell membrane rather than on the state of the ATPase itself and it is not altered by hormones that influence other membrane processes (insulin, adrenaline, ACTH) in ghosts (CLAUSEN and RODBELL, 1969). The transport of α-aminoisobutyric acid into fat cells is inhibited by adrenaline, ACTH and by caffeine (TOUABI and JEANRENAUD, 1969); this inhibition is most probably secondary to the accelerated lipolysis in these cells since it does not occur in the ghosts.

One very important property of the fat cell membrane which has only recently become apparent is that certain of its components can turn over rather rapidly.

The destruction by a low concentration of trypsin of that part of the membrane responsible for the action of insulin to increase glucose transport and to inhibit lipolysis (Kono, 1969a and b; Fain and Loken, 1969) is followed by a restoration of that component by a process that involves protein synthesis, since it is inhibited by both cycloheximide and by puromycin (Kono, 1969b). Since the restoration of this action of insulin is not inhibited by actinomycin it may be assumed that the mRNA preexists in the cell (Kono, 1969b). The "receptor" for insulin responsible for accelerated glucose transport is lost during isolation of a membrane fraction which still retains glucose transport activity: this fraction retains a stimulation by insulin when the cells from which it is prepared are preincubated with insulin but cannot itself respond directly to insulin (Martin and Carter, 1970). These findings may provide one possible explanation for the lack of insulin effect on adenyl cyclase in ghosts and particles: the appropriate "receptor" cannot be continually renewed in these preparations and the response, therefore, is missing.

Thus, the activity of the adenyl cyclase in the white adipose tissue membrane is influenced not only by the presence of the lipolytic hormones but also by the activity of the neighbouring glucose transport component of the membrane (sensitive to insulin) and by the activity of the neighbouring Na^+-K^+-ATPase of the membrane (sensitive to cation concentration and to ouabain). The relationship between adenyl cyclase and glucose transport and also that between glucose transport and the Na^+-K^+-ATPase are reciprocal. Each component influences the activity of the others. Thus any model for the adrenergic receptor in white adipose tissue (to be discussed in the next section) must take into account this interdependence of the membrane components. It is clear that when adenyl cyclase forms part of the intact plasma membrane certain of its properties differ from those of the adenyl cyclase of fragmented membrane: the organization of the structure of the membrane appropriate for the regulatory interactions between its component parts have been lost during the fragmentation and isolation. Adenyl cyclase would seem to be an excellent example of an *allotopic* enzyme, that is, an enzyme whose properties vary according to its state of attachment to a membrane (Racker, 1967). Similar thoughts about the embedding of adenyl cyclase in the macromolecular structure of the membrane with a configuration, and hence activity, determined by its surroundings have been expressed by several authors (Birnbaumer et al., 1969; Rodbell et al., 1968; Vaughan and Murad, 1969; Bär and Hechter, 1969: see Himms-Hagen, 1970a for a more detailed discussion of this problem).

b) The Nature of the Adrenergic Receptor

The elucidation of the nature of the adrenergic receptor in the white fat cell has been complicated by two factors: (i) the large number of different hormones that have a lipolytic action similar to that of the catecholamines, and (ii) the exceedingly large number and variety of compounds that can inhibit the lipolytic effect of the catecholamines. Figure 3 contains lists of compounds known to inhibit the lipolytic effect of catecholamines and indicates their site of action where this is known: the list of compounds which can be added to these is continually growing.

The existence of a single type of adenyl cyclase in the membrane is indicated by failure of the separate effects of the hormones which stimulate adenyl cyclase activity to summate (Bär and Hechter, 1969; Birnbaumer and Rodbell, 1969; Vaughan and Murad, 1969). However, there is good evidence for the interaction of the different lipolytic and antilipolytic hormones with different sites on the membrane. Thus the lipolytic effect of glucagon is abolished by mild treatment of the isolated cells with trypsin, a treatment that also abolishes the antilipolytic effect of insulin but which leaves intact the lipolytic effects of adrenaline and ACTH (KONO, 1969a and b; RODBELL et al., 1970) and of theophylline (FAIN

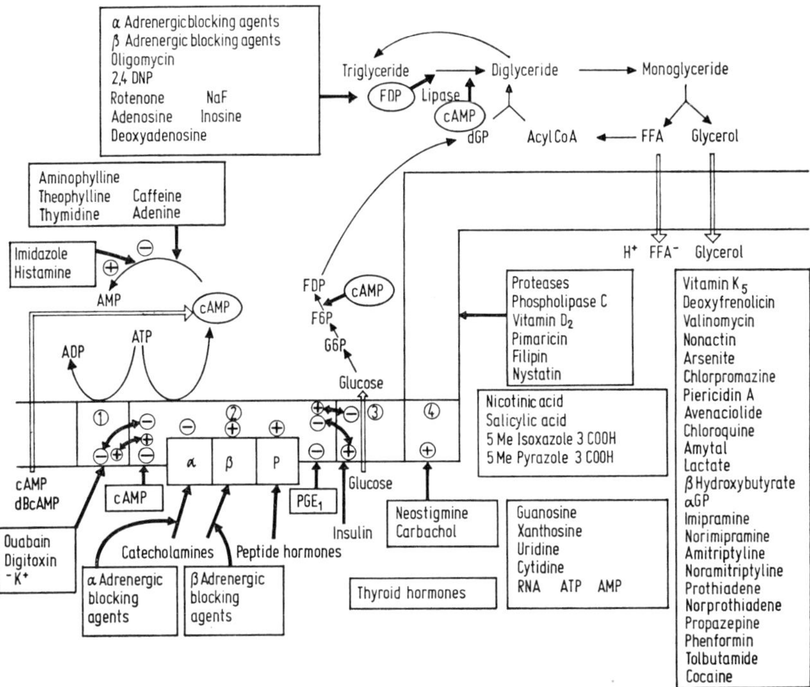

Fig. 3. *Compounds which inhibit the lipolytic effect of catecholamines on white adipose tissue.* Approximate sites of action of these compounds are shown when possible. Some compounds act at more than one site, for example, both the α-receptor blocking agents and the β-receptor blocking agents inhibit the lipase when they are present at high concentrations; at low concentrations only their effects on the actions of catecholamines are seen (an α-receptor blocking agent, phentolamine, potentiates the stimulation of lipolysis by the catecholamines whereas a β-receptor blocking agent, propranolol, reverses the stimulation by catecholamines to an inhibition of lipolysis). Abbreviations used are: PGE_1, prostaglandin E_1; *5 Me Isoxazole 3 COOH*, 5-methylisoxazole 3-carboxylic acid; *5 Me Pyrazole 3 COOH*, 5-methylpyrazole 3-carboxylic acid; $-K^+$ means no potassium in the incubation medium. Most references for the inhibitory actions of the compounds listed in this Figure will be found in a recent review (HIMMS-HAGEN, 1970a). Additional references are: histamine, GOODMAN (1968); cocaine, NAKANO et al. (1969); phenformin and tolbutamide, BROWN and STONE (1967); vitamin K_5 and deoxyfrenolicin, KUO (1969). Antimalarial drugs which have antilipolytic actions like chloroquine are quinine, quinidine, quinacrine, primaquine, hydroxychloroquine, (MARKUS and BALL, 1969). A variety of thiol containing compounds or compounds that react with thiol groups have antilipolytic actions; these include p-chloromercuribenzoate (MINEMURA and CROFFORD, 1969; CALVERT and LECH, 1970): N-ethylmaleimide (CALVERT and LECH, 1970); cysteine, glutathione, 2-mercaptoethanol, dithiothreitol (LAVIS and WILLIAMS, 1970). The four components of the membrane designated by numbers are: (1) Na^+-K^+-ATPase (inhibited by ouabain, digitoxin or lack of potassium); (2) adenyl cyclase with associated "receptors" for peptide hormones and catecholamines; (3) glucose transport component; (4) cholinergic component. (+) denotes an increase in activity; (—) denotes a decrease in activity. Where double-headed arrows connect these symbols a reciprocal relationship between the two changes exists, the one producing the other. Wide black arrows denote the approximate site of action of the compounds indicated. Narrow black arrows denote enzyme-catalyzed reactions or metabolic pathways. Open wide arrows denote transport of compounds across membranes

and LOKEN, 1969). The lipolytic response to glucagon is not restored by incubating the cells, unlike the antilipolytic response to insulin which can be restored in this way (KONO, 1969b). Further evidence for the existence of different receptors for the stimulation of lipolysis by the catecholamines and by the peptide hormones comes from the use of inhibitors (STOCK and WESTERMANN, 1966a and b). Propranolol (BIRNBAUMER and RODBELL, 1969) and Kö-592 (BÄR and HECHTER, 1969) inhibit the stimulating effect of adrenaline on adenyl cyclase in fat cell ghosts and pronethalol inhibits the increase in cAMP concentration of intact tissue induced by adrenaline (BUTCHER et al., 1968) but these β-adrenergic blocking agents do not influence the similar effects of ACTH or glucagon on these processes. The calcium-chelating compound, EGTA, specifically inhibits the stimulation of adenyl cyclase by ACTH in fat cell ghosts but actually potentiates the effect of adrenaline or of glucagon (BIRNBAUMER and RODBELL, 1969; BÄR and HECHTER, 1969). Whether the distinct sites of action of these four hormones (adrenaline, glucagon, ACTH, insulin) are on four different protein molecules which are part of the organized membrane structure or whether they involve more or fewer protein molecules is not yet known. These hormone-sensitive sites, termed discriminator units by BÄR and HECHTER (1969), may indeed influence not only the adenyl cyclase of the membrane but also the other membrane components. The complex network of regulatory connections between components of a hormone-sensitive and multifunctional membrane, such as that of the fat cell membrane, remains a problem for the future.

There is now evidence that both α-receptors and β-receptors are present in the white adipose tissue membrane, stimulation of the latter resulting in stimulation of adenyl cyclase and stimulation of the former resulting in inhibition of adenyl cyclase. The existence in this tissue of the β-receptor has been known for several years. However, the existence of the α-receptor was realized only recently: the evidence for this is: (i) adrenaline decreases the concentration of cAMP in white fat cells when its stimulatory effect is blocked by propanolol (TURTLE and KIPNIS, 1967); (ii) propranolol reverses the stimulation of lipolysis by the catecholamines to an inhibition of lipolysis (HIMMS-HAGEN, 1970a); this is best seen in fat cells from rats that have been fasting and re-fed, because the basal rate of lipolysis is high under these conditions and a decrease can readily be seen; a similar reversal by propranolol of the stimulation by adrenaline has been reported in human fat cells in which the basal rate of lipolysis is already high (BURNS and LANGLEY, 1969); (iii) phentolamine at low concentrations potentiates the lipolytic effects of the catecholamines on rat fat cells (HIMMS-HAGEN, 1970a); a similar observation has been reported for human adipose tissue (BURNS and LANGLEY, 1969; ÖSTMAN et al., 1969); (iv) phentolamine has been reported sometimes to enhance the effect of catecholamines to increase cAMP concentration (BUTCHER and SUTHERLAND, 1967). Although catecholamines have not been observed to inhibit directly the adenyl cyclase of particles or ghosts, either alone or in the presence of propranolol (BIRNBAUMER and RODBELL, 1969), pronethalol or DCI (VAUGHAN and MURAD, 1969) and phentolamine does not potentiate the stimulation of adenyl cyclase of ghosts by adrenaline (BIRNBAUMER and RODBELL, 1969), the results of experiments on which the above conclusions are based must be accepted with some caution since it is possible that appropriate concentrations of catecholamines or blocking agents have not always been used; indeed it is difficult to find suitable concentrations that will permit the reversal and potentiation of lipolysis described above (HIMMS-HAGEN, 1970a). However, it is also possible that part of the membrane that responds in the way attributed here to an α-receptor is missing in the modified preparations of fat cells studied in such experiments.

It is, therefore, apparent that the catecholamines are capable of both stimulating adenyl cyclase and thereby stimulating lipolysis, and of presumably inhibiting adenyl cyclase and thereby reducing lipolysis. The existence of two types of receptor may well be the explanation for the biphasic nature of the dose-response curve for the lipolytic effects of the catecholamines that is sometimes seen (ALLEN et al., 1969). Moreover, the existence of these two types of receptor, one inhibitory and the other stimulatory, and the observed biphasic nature of the dose-response curve prohibit the mathematical treatment of the slopes of such dose-response curves and their interpretation in terms of occupation of receptors (see for example LINCOVA et al., 1967 and WENKE, 1966).

If the α-receptor for the inhibition of lipolysis by the catecholamines is normally involved in restraining the lipolytic effects of the amines the question arises as to its physiological significance. The best evidence for the functioning of such a receptor in an intact animal comes from studies with the subcutaneous adipose tissue of the dog perfused *in situ*. Low-frequency stimulation of the nerves to this tissue causes liberation of FFA into the blood during the stimulation (ROSELL, 1966) whereas more rapid stimulation causes no release of FFA during the stimulation but only after the stimulation is stopped (ORÖ et al., 1965). This effect is not due to greater vasoconstriction produced by the more rapid stimulation (ROSELL, 1966). Recent evidence suggests that inhibitory α-receptors are involved. Both dihydroergotamine and phentolamine cause a marked potentiation of the effect of both slow and rapid stimulation of the nerves to cause release of FFA and of glycerol (FREDHOLM and ROSELL, 1968); this stimulation in the presence of dihydroergotamine can be inhibited by the β-receptor blocking agents, propranolol, pronethanol and INPEA (N-isopropyl-*p*-nitrophenylethanolamine) (FREDHOLM and ROSELL, 1968).

The greater part of the work quoted so far in this discussion of adipose tissue metabolism has been done with epididymal white adipose tissue of the rat. There are marked species differences in the response of white adipose tissue to catecholamines and there is also marked variability in response as evidenced by contradictory reports of the presence or absence of lipolytic effects of catecholamines in species other than the rat. For example, rabbit adipose tissue may (FAIN, 1970; HIMMS-HAGEN, 1967) or may not (RUDMAN and DEL RIO, 1969; LEWIS and MATTHEWS, 1968) respond to catecholamines by an increase in the rate of lipolysis. The same is true of guinea pig adipose tissue (ARNOLD and MCAULIFF, 1968a; RUDMAN, 1965). The effect of noradrenaline on human adipose tissue (ÖSTMAN et al., 1969; CARLSON et al., 1969) appears also to be rather variable. The response of adipose tissue in different regions of the dog to catecholamines is quite variable (BALLARD and ROSELL, 1969). An explanation for some of these species and regional differences may reside in differences in the relative proportions in the cell membranes of these tissues of structures which react with the catecholamines in a way described above as characteristic of α-receptor and β-receptors. The problem of the nature and significance of these so-called α-receptors in adipose tissue appears to be important for the study of this tissue in species other than the rat. The rat is not a suitable species for this study because of the predominance of the β-receptor stimulatory effect in this species.

2. Events Occurring Intracellularly

a) Known Effects of cAMP in White Adipose Tissue

α) Triglyceride Lipase. The rate-limiting step in the breakdown of triglycerides in the adipose tissue is believed to be the triglyceride lipase. The amount and activity of this enzyme are, therefore, of the greatest importance in determining the rate of lipolysis. Triglyceride lipase appears to exist in two forms, one more active than the other (HOLLETT and AUDITORE, 1967; GORIN and SHAFRIR, 1967; RIZACK, 1964; VAUGHAN et al., 1965) but this enzyme has not been very well characterized. *In vitro* the lipase is saturated at a substrate concentration of between 1 and 10 mM (HOLLETT and AUDITORE, 1967; RIZACK, 1961). However, this value clearly depends on the state of emulsification of the substrate and nothing is known about the physical state of the substrate attacked by this enzyme within the cell or whether substrate concentration in the cell can ever be the rate limiting factor in lipolysis. Although the activation of the lipase, demonstrable only in aged preparations of adipose tissue (HOLLETT and AUDITORE, 1967; VAUGHAN et al., 1965; GORIN and SHAFRIR, 1967), requires ATP (RIZACK, 1964) and is stimulated by cAMP, the lipase itself can be inhibited by ATP and by cAMP (RIZACK, 1965; WADE and HALES, 1969) and is activated only by a fairly narrow range of concentrations of these compounds. Fructose diphosphate can also stimulate the triglyceride lipase, an effect that appears to be unique to this hexose phosphate among the intermediates of glycolysis (CHLOUVERAKIS, 1968). The other two enzymes of lipolysis, diglyceride lipase and monoglyceride lipase, do not appear to be rate-limiting; diglycerides and monoglycerides do not normally accumulate in adipose tissue, even during very rapid lipolysis.

β) Phosphofructokinase. The activity of phosphofructokinase is a key factor in the regulation of glycolysis in adipose tissue (DENTON et al., 1966; HALPERIN and DENTON, 1969). This enzyme is inhibited by ATP and by citrate and is very sensitive to stimulation by cAMP (DENTON and RANDLE, 1966). Flux through the reaction catalyzed by this enzyme can be demonstrated to be increased when adipose tissue is stimulated by adrenaline (DENTON et al., 1966; HALPERIN and DENTON, 1969). The product of this reaction, fructose diphosphate, is not only a necessary substrate for the formation of α-glycerophosphate, but is also a stimulator of the triglyceride lipase, as noted above (CHLOUVERAKIS, 1968), and is also a stimulator and apparently an activator of pyruvate kinase (POGSON, 1968). The concentration of fructose diphosphate in adipose tissue is increased by adrenaline (HALPERIN and DENTON, 1969).

γ) Enzymes of the Glycogen Cycle. Glycogen phosphorylase of adipose tissue is activated by adrenaline (FRERICHS and BALL, 1962; VAUGHAN, 1960) and inactivated by insulin (JUNGAS, 1966) and appears to exist in AMP-stimulated and AMP-insensitive forms (JUNGAS, 1966). Glycogen synthetase appears to exist in two forms, stimulated by and independent of glucose-6-phosphate respectively, as in other tissues (JUNGAS, 1966); it is activated by insulin (JUNGAS, 1966) and presumably would be inactivated by adrenaline but no direct measurements of this appear to have been made. A report that adrenaline increases phosphorylase activity without altering glycogen synthetase activity in incubated adipose tissue is difficult to interpret because measurements were made in the presence of AMP (phosphorylase) and glucose-6-phosphate (synthetase) and represent only the sum of the active and inactive forms (GUTMAN and SHAFRIR, 1964). White adipose tissue normally stores very little glycogen and the activation of phosphorylase by adrenaline is of little significance in the overall metabolism of the tissue. Only in fasted and refed animals is there an appreciable quantity of glycogen in the adipose tissue and in this circumstance a major consequence of the action of adrenaline is accelerated glycogenolysis (FRERICHS and BALL, 1962).

δ) Protein Kinases. White adipose tissue contains a cAMP-dependent protein kinase (CORBIN and KREBS, 1969). The physiological substrate(s) for this enzyme is(are) as yet unknown.

b) Metabolic Consequences of the Action of Catecholamines on White Adipose Tissue

Major metabolic processes that are accelerated as a consequence of the action of catecholamines on adipose tissue are lipolysis (and the consequent release of FFA and glycerol), reesterification of fatty acids (and the consequent increase in ATP utilization), lipogenesis from glucose (only in the presence of insulin), glycogenolysis, glycolysis, tricarboxylic acid cycle activity (and oxygen uptake), glucose uptake and fatty acid oxidation; protein synthesis appears to be decreased. Some of these changes can be attributed directly to the rise in cAMP concentration caused by the catecholamines but many of them probably represent adjustments in rates of metabolic pathways secondary to the availability of one or another substrate. The complex relationships between different metabolic pathways of cytosol and mitochondria of adipose tissue have been studied in considerable detail in recent years (see FLATT, 1970; KATZ et al., 1966; KATZ and ROGNSTAD, 1969; ROGNSTAD and KATZ, 1969; JEANRENAUD, 1968) and the reader is referred to these studies for further discussion of this aspect of adipose tissue metabolism.

The extent of stimulation of lipolysis and the release of FFA and glycerol by the catecholamines can be modified by a number of factors. These include the FFA concentration within the cell and the availability of FFA acceptor (albumin) outside the cell: the stimulation of lipolysis does not occur in fat cells when no albumin is present in the incubation medium and lipolysis is inhibited by FFA (RODBELL, 1965a). The concentration of FFA within the cell during accelerated lipolysis depends upon their rate of production, their rate of release from the cell and also upon the rate at which they are re-esterified to form triglycerides again. This latter depends in turn upon the availablity of glucose as a source of α-glycerophosphate. The availability of glucose also determines how much fructose diphosphate, another stimulator of the triglyceride lipase, will be formed (CHLOUVERAKIS, 1968). Adrenaline does increase the concentration of fructose diphosphate in adipose tissue: however, this alone cannot be a sufficient stimulus for lipolysis because insulin also has this effect and in the presence of insulin adrenaline causes no further increase in fructose diphosphate concentration (HALPERIN and DENTON, 1969). The stimulation of lipolysis by the catecholamines is pH-dependent, whereas the mimicking effect of dBcAMP is not (POYART et al., 1967; POYART and NAHAS, 1968); this is most probably because of the pH dependence of adenyl cyclase. The extent to which inhibition by ATP plays a role in regulation of lipase activity is uncertain (RIZACK, 1965; GORIN and SHAFRIR, 1967; WADE and HALES, 1969). This inhibition has been reported to be reversed by low concentrations of cAMP (WADE and HALES, 1969). It could also perhaps be expected to be reversed in the cell stimulated by adrenaline by the reduction in ATP content of the tissue (DENTON and HALPERIN, 1968; HEPP et al., 1969b).

The increased re-esterification of fatty acids caused by the catecholamines appears to be due only to the rise in their concentration as a consequence of the acceleration of lipolysis. This is an ATP-consuming process and is probably the major cause of the fall in ATP concentration and the increase in oxygen uptake caused by adrenaline.

Depending on the circumstances, adrenaline can inhibit, leave unchanged, or accelerate the rate of lipogenesis from glucose; which effect is seen depends upon the incubation conditions. The mechanism of regulation of fatty acid synthesis in adipose tissue has been a puzzle for many years because, although several regulatory influences could be identified, none could be shown to be responsible for the observed changes in the rates of lipogenesis in the presence of hormones (see

Denton and Halperin, 1968). The recent proposal by Flatt (1970) of a hypothesis which attributes these difficulties to the failure to realize that lipogenesis is an energy-yielding process (ATP-yielding) has permitted the identification of the rate-limiting process in lipogenesis under most conditions. The rate of lipogenesis is limited by the rate at which ADP is regenerated from ATP. Flatt (1970) proposes that adrenaline accelerates lipogenesis by virtue of its effect on ATP utilization, principally for re-esterification of fatty acids: that adrenaline is sometimes observed to inhibit lipogenesis from glucose is explained by the ATP-requirement of some of the reactions of lipogenesis, which may not be met in the face of excessive ATP breakdown caused by adrenaline. A similar inhibition of lipogenesis also occurs with uncoupling agents such as DNP (see Flatt, 1970; Rognstad and Katz, 1969).

The significance of the decreased incorporation of amino acids into protein caused by adrenaline (Renold et al., 1960), by dBcAMP and by theophylline (Swislocki, 1970) is not clear. Although adrenaline does inhibit amino acid transport into fat cells (Touabi and Jeanrenaud, 1969) this does not appear to be due to a direct action of adrenaline on the cell membrane amino acid transport process (Clausen and Rodbell, 1969) but rather a consequence of the acceleration of lipolysis and is probably due to a reduction in the availability of the ATP necessary for the amino acid transport and the protein synthesis itself. The report that adrenaline, and also dBcAMP and caffeine, can inhibit the synthesis of lipoprotein lipase that occurs when fat pads are incubated (for 12 hours) in a medium containing insulin and glucose, may in part be attributable to lack of ATP (Wing et al., 1966; Wing and Robinson, 1968; Salaman and Robinson, 1966). A specific inhibitory effect of cAMP on the synthesis of this enzyme cannot, however, be excluded. Added FFA do not mimic the inhibition suggesting that it is not merely secondary to accelerated lipolysis.

An inhibitor of effects of cAMP on phosphorylase activation in preparations from liver and heart has been isolated from adipose tissue (Murad et al., 1969a); although so far unidentified this inhibitor appears to be very similar to cAMP and to be formed under conditions when cAMP is also formed, but it differs from cAMP in that its formation is inhibited by dBcAMP. Such an inhibitor may be involved in the reported accumulation of cAMP but inhibition of lipolysis caused by cGMP in adipose tissue (Murad et al., 1969b).

Since both α-receptors and β-receptors appear to exist in white adipose tissue (see II. I. b) and the former can be demonstrated to exert an inhibitory effect upon lipolysis, it is logical to look for other consequences of α-receptor stimulation. The only other metabolic effect so far attributable to such stimulation is increased uptake and oxidation of glucose (Blecher et al., 1969; Bray, 1967; Goodman and Bray, 1966; Bray and Goodman, 1968), an effect that appears to be a consequence only of accelerated transport of glucose into the cell due to an action of adrenaline at the cell membrane (see Himms-Hagen, 1970a). The physiological significance of this action is not known.

III. Cardiac Muscle

The rate of operation of the following metabolic processes in the heart is influenced by the catecholamines: glycogenolysis, glycogenesis, glycolysis, tricarboxylic acid cycle, fatty acid oxidation. However, because of the marked changes in the mechanical activity of the heart in the presence of catecholamines (positive inotropic and chronotropic responses), changes that impose an increased demand for substrate utilization, it is necessary to distinguish between primary and secondary consequences of the actions of catecholamines on the heart.

The observation, some 13 years ago, of an apparent correlation between activation of glycogen phosphorylase and the inotropic response to adrenaline or

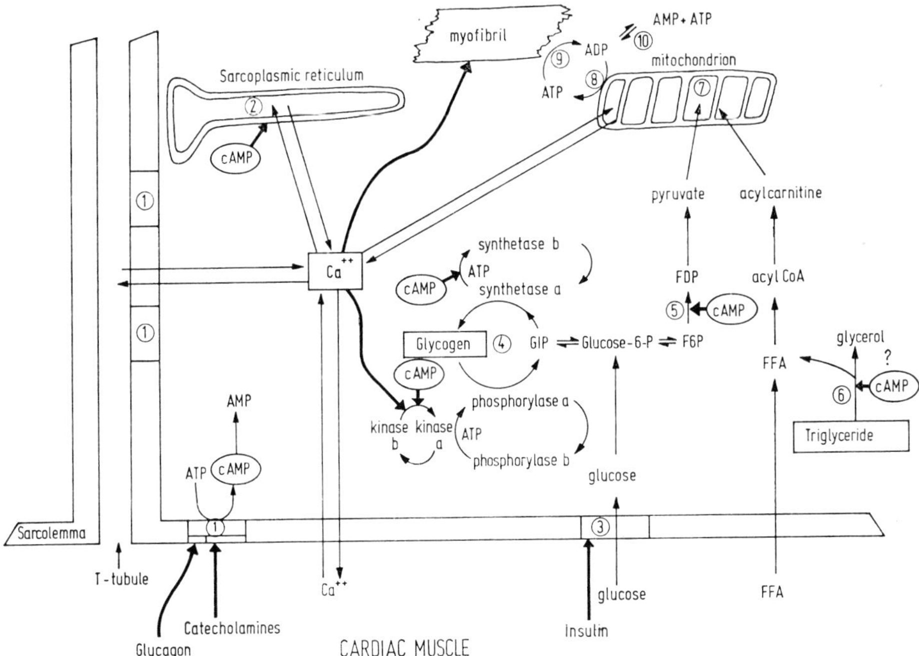

Fig. 4. *Summary of metabolic and other processes in heart which are influenced by catecholamines. Processes associated with sarcolemma and sarcoplasmic reticulum:* (1) is the adenyl cyclase of the sarcolemma, shown here as extending into the T-tubules (see text for discussion); the adenyl cyclase is associated with "receptors" for catecholamines and for glucagon. (2) is the sarcoplasmic reticulum, shown here to contain a cAMP-dependent (or cAMP-stimulated) calcium pump (ATPase). *Carbohydrate metabolism:* (3) is the insulin-sensitive glucose transport component; (4) is the glycogen cycle (the cAMP-stimulated enzymes are phosphorylase *b* kinase *b* kinase and glycogen synthetase *a* kinase); (5) is phosphofructokinase. *Lipid metabolism:* (6) is triglyceride lipase. *Major energy-yielding pathways* are denoted by (7) (which includes pyruvate dehydrogenase, β-oxidation of fatty acids and tricarboxylic acid cycle plus associated electron transport and oxidative phosphorylation (8)). *The major energy-using reaction* of muscle is contraction (9). When oxidative phosphorylation does not keep pace with the utilization of ATP for contraction the equilibrium concentrations of the reactants in the myokinase reaction (10) change and the concentration of AMP rises. *Calcium ion movements:* calcium moves in both directions across external membranes, sarcoplasmic reticulum membranes and mitochondrial membranes (see text for discussion). Two of the principal actions of calcium are illustrated: stimulation of contraction and stimulation of the activation of phosphorylase

to aminophylline by the perfused rat heart (Hess and Haugaard, 1958) led to a considerable amount of work (see Haugaard and Hess, 1965 for review). When subsequent studies showed that there could not be a cause-and-effect relationship between phosphorylase activation and the inotropic response the emphasis of such studies changed. Although attempts are still being made to establish a unitary hypothesis to explain all actions of catecholamines on the heart, the current studies are concerned with the actions of cyclic AMP, generated intracellularly in response to catecholamines acting at the cell membrane, on all aspects of cardiac function including movements of calcium ions and the role of these movements in regulating contractility, as well as on the activities of specific enzymes involved in the metabolic processes already mentioned.

In Fig. 4 is presented a diagram that illustrates in outline current knowledge of the consequences of the action of adrenaline on the heart. Evidence for individual statements in this diagram will be discussed in more detail below. However, it should be noted that the distribution of calcium ions into the four compartments implied in this diagram (in external medium, cytosol, sarcoplasmic reticulum and mitochondria) represents an oversimplification of the complex models proposed by muscle physiologists for calcium ion movements and for the role of calcium in the mechanism of excitation-contraction coupling (see for example BIANCHI, 1969). It is indeed difficult to integrate into a coherent whole the vast body of knowledge from such physiological studies with the similarly vast body of knowledge from biochemical studies. Not the least of the difficulties is the entirely different language used by the two groups. For a full understanding of the actions of catecholamines on the metabolism and function of the heart such an integration is essential.

a) Adenyl Cyclase

Stimulation of cardiac adenyl cyclase by catecholamines was first observed by MURAD et al. (1962) using washed particles prepared from dog heart. That stimulation occurs also in the intact heart is shown by the rapid and large increase in its cAMP content after contact with catecholamines (ROBISON et al., 1965; WILLIAMSON, 1966a; CHEUNG and WILLIAMSON, 1965; DRUMMOND et al., 1966; NAMM and MAYER, 1968; SHANFELD et al., 1969). ROBISON, BUTCHER and SUTHERLAND (1967) proposed a close relationship between the β-adrenergic receptor and adenyl cyclase. This proposal has led to several attempts to find changes in either the amount or the properties of adenyl cyclase in hearts which for various reasons have altered sensitivity to catecholamines. However, adenyl cyclase activity (basal, fluoride-stimulated and catecholamine-stimulated) is the same in denervated hearts (SOBEL et al., 1968), and in hearts from hyperthyroid cats (SOBEL et al., 1969; LEVEY et al., 1969b) as in normal hearts. Denervated hearts which are supersensitive to noradrenaline (DEMPSEY and COOPER, 1968) and depleted of their noradrenaline (COLEMAN et al., 1970) possess the normal amount of adenyl cyclase. In hyperthyroid hearts both adenyl cyclase and the inotropic response to noradrenaline are normal (LEVEY et al., 1969b). Although thyroid hormones have been reported to activate heart adenyl cyclase *in vitro* (LEVEY and EPSTEIN, 1969a) the physiological significance of such activation is doubtful because analogues of thyroid hormones which do not possess appreciable calorigenic activity *in vivo* also activate heart adenyl cyclase *in vitro*. The total amount of adenyl cyclase in the hearts of hypothyroid cats is less than in normal hearts. However, the sensitivity of the enzyme to noradrenaline and to fluoride is normal (LEVEY et al., 1969a). That such hearts do not have an impaired contractile response to noradrenaline indicates that, if adenyl cyclase is indeed to be equated with the β-adrenergic receptor, the capacity of the initial receptor system to respond to the external stimulus exceeds that of the contractile system to respond to receptor stimulation. This point will be considered further when the relation of the inotropic response to the adenyl cyclase system is discussed.

Another interesting property of the cardiac adenyl cyclase is its response to glucagon in washed particle preparations (MURAD and VAUGHAN, 1969; BROWN et al., 1968; LEVEY and EPSTEIN, 1969b). The stimulation by glucagon and that by the catecholamines are additive and, unlike the effect of the catecholamines, the stimulation by glucagon is not blocked by β-adrenergic blocking agents (MURAD and VAUGHAN, 1969; LEVEY and EPSTEIN, 1969b). Thus there must be separate binding sites for catecholamines and for glucagon. The loss of sensitivity to both catecholamines and glucagon by a solubilized preparation of adenyl cyclase (solubilized with Lubrol) and the retention by this preparation of basal and fluoride-stimulated activities (LEVEY, 1970) suggests that the binding sites for catecholamines and glucagon are either readily destroyed or that they are actually on separate protein molecules, distinct from adenyl cyclase.

Adenyl cyclase has usually been assumed to be present in the sarcolemma of cardiac muscle. However, a recent report suggests that adenyl cyclase may also be located in the sarcoplasmic reticulum (ENTMAN et al., 1969a). This interpretation of the existence of adenyl cyclase in a subcellular fraction sedimenting between 13,000 g and 100,000 g should be accepted only with caution because of the possibility that parts of fragmented transverse tubular system are isolated together with the fragmented sarcoplasmic reticulum; the former might reasonably be expected to contain adenyl cyclase since it is an extension of the sarcolemma. If adenyl cyclase should indeed be present in the sarcoplasmic reticulum then several problems arise concerning the polarity of the enzyme on the reticulum and the penetration of either catecholamine or ATP to the inside of the sarcoplasmic reticulum.

b) Effects of cAMP on Cardiac Muscle Enzymes

α) Enzymes of the Glycogen Cycle. The enzymes of the glycogen cycle directly activated by cyclic AMP are glycogen synthetase *a* kinase, the enzyme that "inactivates" glycogen synthetase (HUIJING and LARNER, 1966a and b), and the enzyme that converts phosphorylase *b* kinase to its active form, presumably phosphorylase *b* kinase (DRUMMOND et al., 1965; OZAWA and EBASHI, 1967). The consequences of the interaction of cAMP with these two enzymes in the cell would, therefore, be expected to be a conversion of glycogen phosphorylase to the *a* form, and consequently an increase in the rate of glycogenolysis, and a conversion of glycogen synthetase to the *b* form, and consequently a reduced rate of glycogenesis. These consequences do not necessarily arise in the beating heart when the concentration of cAMP is raised by adrenaline. The initial effect of adrenaline on the proportion of glycogen synthetase in the *a* form is to increase it (WILLIAMS and MAYER, 1966; WILLIAMSON, 1966a; BELFORD and CUNNINGHAM, 1968) and only subsequently to cause a decrease (WILLIAMS and MAYER, 1966; MAYER, 1967). The reason for the initial increase in synthetase *a* is not understood. It has been proposed that a local reduction in glycogen concentration brought about by the catecholamines results in reduced inhibition by glycogen of the synthetase *b* phosphatase, the enzyme that "activates" glycogen synthetase (MAYER, 1967). However, in the isolated perfused heart this effect is seen only in the presence of glucose (WILLIAMSON, 1966a) and thus appears to be a consequence of the accelerated glucose utilization. A similar effect of glucose on the glycogen synthetase of liver has been shown to be independent of changes in cAMP concentration (BUSCHIAZZO et al., 1970). There is clearly some additional glucose-initiated regulatory mechanism involved in the glycogen cycle that is not yet understood.

The usual effect of catecholamines on the phosphorylase system of enzymes is, as would be expected, an initial increase in the proportion of phosphorylase *b* kinase in the active form (DRUMMOND et al., 1966; NAMM et al., 1968); this coincides with the increase in cAMP concentration and is followed by an increase in the proportion of phosphorylase in the *a* form (ROBISON et al., 1965; WILLIAM-

SON, 1966a and b; ØYE, 1965; NAMM et al., 1968). The increase in phosphorylase *a* activity does not follow the increase in cAMP concentration and phosphorylase *b* kinase activity if calcium is lacking (NAMM et al., 1968). The explanation for this appears to be the requirement of the active form of phosphorylase *b* kinase for calcium (OZAWA and EBASHI, 1967). Indeed, calcium alone can increase the proportion of phosphorylase *a* (NAMM et al., 1968; FRIESEN et al., 1967 and 1969; KUKOVETZ and PÖCH, 1967) without any prior change in cAMP concentration or in phosphorylase *b* kinase *a* activity (NAMM et al., 1968). Although two possible explanations for this action of calcium exist, namely, the stimulation of phosphorylase *b* kinase activity by calcium (mentioned above) and the conversion of kinase *b* to kinase *a* by a calcium-dependent enzyme distinct from the cAMP-dependent enzyme (DRUMMOND et al., 1965) it seems likely that the former effect of calcium predominates in the intact heart because of the failure to find any increase in the proportion of phosphorylase *b* kinase in the *a* form in the calcium-stimulated hearts (NAMM et al., 1968).

The conversion of phosphorylase *b* to phosphorylase *a* appears to require a certain threshold of activation of phosphorylase *b* kinase; it is possible to produce an activation of phosphorylase *b* kinase without an increase in phosphorylase *a* by using low concentrations of adrenaline (NAMM and MAYER, 1968).

β) Enzymes of Glycolysis. Although phosphofructokinase of heart is stimulated by cAMP (MANSOUR, 1966) its activity is also regulated by the concentrations of a variety of other nucleotides and other compounds (ATP, ADP, AMP, orthophosphate, fructose-6-phosphate, citrate) and it is likely that the adrenaline-induced increase in the activity of the enzyme in the beating heart is largely secondary to the decrease in the concentration of ATP (as inhibitor) and the increase in the concentrations of AMP, ADP and orthophosphate (activators). Further control (reduction in activity) may be exerted by citrate (inhibitor) of which the concentration also rises (WILLIAMSON, 1966a and b). In heart the concentration of cAMP may play a rather minor role in the regulation of the action of this enzyme.

Activation of pyruvate dehydrogenase (from a *b* form to an *a* form) by a cAMP-dependent kinase has recently been reported by WIELAND and SIESS (1970): the role of this activation in regulation of pyruvate entry into the tricarboxylic acid cycle is not yet clear.

γ) Enzymes of Lipolysis. The evidence for activation of a lipase of heart by cAMP is that an increased release of glycerol occurs under the influence of adrenaline (WILLIAMSON, 1964; CHALLONER and STEINBERG, 1965; KREISBERG, 1966) or isopropylnoradrenaline (CHRISTIAN et al., 1969). The increase in glycerol release coincides with the increase in phosphorylase *a* activity and both these responses follow the initial increase in cAMP concentration and in contractile force caused by isopropylnoradrenaline; the dose-response curves for these two responses are also very similar (CHRISTIAN et al., 1969). The lipolytic response can also be produced by glucagon. Little is known, however, about the nature of the lipolytic system of enzymes or of the effects of cAMP upon it; the mediation of this lipolytic effect by cAMP cannot yet be regarded as proved.

δ) Protein Kinases. The extent to which the responses to cAMP are mediated by cAMP-dependent protein kinases, which do exist in the heart (rabbit and bovine heart with histone as substrate (KUO and GREENGARD, 1969a)) is uncertain. It seems probable that a cAMP-dependent protein kinase brings about the activation of phosphorylase *b* kinase *b* and the inactivation of glycogen synthetase *a*, but the role of similar enzymes in the acceleration of lipolysis and in the acceleration of calcium uptake is unknown.

c) Relation of the Inotropic Response to Cyclic cAMP Formation

The early correlations between activation of phosphorylase and the inotropic response (see HAUGAARD and HESS, 1965 and HIMMS-HAGEN, 1967 for reviews) have been succeeded by attempts to correlate activation of phosphorylase *b* kinase (DRUMMOND et al., 1966) and activation of adenyl cyclase with this response. With improved techniques for freezing and for enzyme assay now available it is fairly simple to demonstrate that the increase in activity of phosphorylase *a* occurs well after the initial increase in cAMP concentration and after the inotropic response (see for example ROBISON et al., 1965; WILLIAMSON, 1966a; SHANFELD et al., 1969; ØYE, 1965; NAMM et al., 1968) as also does the increase in lipolytic activity (CHRISTIAN et al., 1969). The increase in cAMP concentration occurs either simultaneously with the inotropic response (WILLIAMSON, 1966a; CHEUNG and WILLIAMSON, 1965; CHRISTIAN et al., 1969) or shortly before it (ROBISON et al., 1965; DRUMMOND et al., 1966; SHANFELD et al., 1969; NAMM et al., 1968). The increase in phosphorylase kinase activity accompanies that in cAMP concentration and both may precede the inotropic response (NAMM et al., 1968; DRUMMOND et al., 1966). Glucagon, like adrenaline, stimulates heart adenyl cyclase (MURAD and VAUGHAN, 1969) raises the concentration of cAMP in the heart (MAYER et al., 1970) and produces an inotropic response (LARAIA et al., 1968; MAYER et al., 1970) that coincides with the rise in cAMP and precedes the increase in phosphorylase *a* (MAYER et al., 1970). Current interest is, therefore, in the possible relationship between adenyl cyclase activation (and/or changes in cAMP concentration) and the inotropic response to catecholamines and to glucagon (see SUTHERLAND et al., 1968).

Several objections can be raised to a postulated role of cAMP in mediating the inotropic response to the catecholamines and these will be discussed before the evidence in favour of this role is mentioned. The first, and most important, objection is that cAMP, or dBcAMP, added to the perfused heart does not usually itself produce an inotropic response (ROBISON et al., 1965; see also SUTHERLAND and ROBISON, 1966; SUTHERLAND et al., 1968). This objection has now satisfactorily been answered by the finding of inotropic responses to dBcAMP by cardiac muscle of a number of species (SKELTON et al., 1970; KUKOVETZ and PÖCH, 1970).

Several experimental situations have been found in which the inotropic response can apparently be dissociated from the stimulation of adenyl cyclase. For example, hearts that possess less than the normal amount of adenyl cyclase (from hypothyroid cats) have a normal inotropic response to noradrenaline (LEVEY et al., 1969a). The effects of adrenaline and glucagon on the cAMP content of heart summate, whereas their effects on the contractile force do not (MAYER et al., 1970). Sometimes it is possible to obtain an inotropic response without any detectable change in cAMP concentration (MAYER et al., 1970; LARAIA et al., 1968; NAMM and MAYER, 1968; SHANFELD et al., 1969). This may be in part due to the technique used to freeze the heart, the rather small increases not appearing if the technique of freezing is inadequate (NAMM and MAYER, 1968), and in part because the assay methods fail to recognize very small changes in total cAMP concentration. The lack of a direct correlation between cAMP content and contractile force has also been used as an argument against a direct relationship between the two (WILLIAMSON, 1966a; CHEUNG and WILLIAMSON, 1965).

These findings can be explained if the following three assumptions are made: (1) the action of cAMP that has as its consequence the inotropic response reaches a maximum at very low concentrations (it may be assumed that the cAMP which exerts this effect exists in a distinct cellular compartment so that "low" here means a small change in the total cAMP but possibly a large change in a small compartment) (2) phosphorylase *b* kinase *b* kinase is much less sensitive to cAMP than the inotropic response mechanism, and a higher concentration of cAMP is needed to activate it (it should also be assumed that a certain minimum kinase *a* activity is necessary for phosphorylase *b* conversion to the *a* form) (3) the capacity of adenyl cyclase to respond to catecholamines (or to glucagon) by raising the intracellular concentration of cAMP considerably exceeds the sensitivity of the two responsive systems.

Thus the temporal separation between the different responses of the heart to catecholamines can be seen as a sequential switching on of several regulatory mechanisms by the rising concentration of cAMP and it is apparent that no direct correlation between the size of any of the responses and total cAMP concentration can be expected. In addition to the observation of a direct inotropic effect of dBcAMP (SKELTON et al., 1970; KUKOVETZ and PÖCH, 1970) considerable other evidence is in favour of a mediation by cAMP of the inotropic response to catecholamines. The relative effectiveness of adrenaline, noradrenaline and isopropylnoradrenaline to stimulate heart adenyl cyclase activity (MURAD et al., 1962) is the same as their relative effectiveness in producing the inotropic response. The pH optimum for the inotropic response is similar to that for activation of adenyl cyclase (DRUMMOND and DUNCAN, 1970). β-Adrenergic blocking agents, that inhibit the stimulation of adenyl cyclase by catecholamines (DCI: MURAD et al., 1962; propranolol: LEVEY and EPSTEIN, 1969a) and the rise in cAMP content of hearts treated with catecholamines (pronethalol: ROBISON et al., 1965; NAMM and MAYER, 1968), also inhibit the inotropic response.

Some of the links between cAMP and the other responses can be broken. For example, removal of calcium breaks the link between cAMP and the inotropic response and the link between phosphorylase *b* kinase activation and phosphorylase *b* activation (NAMM et al., 1968). The proposal that the link between a rise in cAMP concentration and the inotropic response involves calcium has been formulated in a variety of ways over the last few years (see for example, CHEUNG and WILLIAMSON, 1965; WILLIAMSON, 1966; RASMUSSEN and TENENHOUSE, 1968; ROBISON et al., 1967; SUTHERLAND and ROBISON, 1966; SUTHERLAND et al., 1968); however, no firm evidence has been found for it, largely because of lack of biochemical information about the mechanisms involved in the regulation of cardiac contractility.

It is now known that both adrenaline (see MAYER, 1967) and glucagon (NAYLER et al., 1970) increase the uptake of ^{45}Ca by beating hearts. Recently cAMP has been found to stimulate the uptake of calcium by a subcellular preparation from cardiac muscle (ENTMAN et al., 1969b). Adrenaline and glucagon also share this effect but the slower onset of response to these hormones and the presence of adenyl cyclase that is stimulated by them in the same preparation makes it likely that they act via cAMP formation (ENTMAN et al., 1969b). That the concentrations of adrenaline and glucagon needed for maximum calcium accumulation are much lower than the concentrations needed for maximum stimulation of adenyl cyclase illustrates again the greater capacity of the adenyl cyclase system to produce cAMP than needed for the responses to the cAMP.

In order to consider the possible physiological significance of this observation it is necessary first to discuss briefly the structure of cardiac muscle. Cardiac muscle contains four structural elements whose function involves calcium (BIANCHI, 1969): these are; the surface membrane (or sarcolemma) plus the transverse tubules (T-tubules) derived from it; the sarcoplasmic reticulum; the mitochondria; the contractile proteins. The first three contain "calcium pumps" and function in movement of calcium whereas the contractile elements are stimulated to contract by calcium. The T-tubule system consists of numerous sarcolemma-bound tubules running for the most part transversely but occasionally longitudinally, their lumen being continuous with the exterior of the cells (FAWCETT and McNUTT, 1969; see also SONNENBLICK and STAM, 1969). The sarcoplasmic reticulum, on the other hand, is an intracellular tubular system of which the lumen is not continuous with the exterior of the cell but which contains terminal cisternae which are in very close contact with the T-tubules (FAWCETT and McNUTT, 1969).

The role of calcium in determining the contractile state of the heart has been reviewed in detail by LANGER (1968) and by KATZ (1970). The account that follows is based largely upon the recent review of activation and contraction of cardiac muscle by SONNENBLICK and STAM (1969). The function of the calcium pump in the sarcoplasmic reticulum appears to be the removal of calcium from the cytosol, a process which leads to relaxation of the muscle. The calcium that activates the contractile process is in turn released principally from the sarcoplasmic reticulum as a consequence of depolarization of the sarcolemma, the amount released depending on the amount stored and determining the strength of the contraction. Thus, the more calcium available in the sarcoplasmic reticulum, the greater the force of contraction. The function of the calcium pump in the mitochondria is uncertain although it has also been suggested as playing a role in removal of calcium from the cytosol and thus regulating the concentration of free calcium (LEHNINGER, 1964; HAUGAARD et al., 1969); the mechanism and regulation of calcium exit from the mitochondria are unknown.

If it is assumed that cAMP functions within the cell to promote the uptake of calcium by the sarcoplasmic reticulum, as indicated by the evidence described above, then a mechanism for the mediation of the inotropic response to catecholamines becomes apparent. The amount of calcium that can be stored between beats is increased by cAMP and, therefore, the amount that can be released per beat is also increased and so is the force of contraction. This postulate is a present no more than a working hypothesis. The various lines of evidence that can be adduced to support it can be interpreted in different ways. A major problem is the purported presence of adenyl cyclase actually in the sarcoplasmic reticulum (ENTMAN et al., 1969a and b). The existence in the cardiac cell of two distinct tubular systems makes the interpretation of the nature of subcellular fractions very difficult. The isolated membrane-bound vesicles from dog heart have been reported to be 0.5—1.5 μ in diameter (ENTMAN et al., 1969a); however, within the cells of the heart (cat) the T-tubules have a diameter of approximately 0.2 μ and the diameter of the sarcoplasmic reticulum ranges from 0.1—1.0 μ, depending on its location (FAWCETT and McNUTT, 1969). Whether, as claimed by some workers, the isolated vesicle preparation is derived solely from the sarcoplasmic reticulum or whether both tubular systems (sarcoplasmic reticulum and T-tubules) are fragmented to form the vesicles that are isolated is impossible to say. The presence of adenyl cyclase, a typical cell membrane enzyme in all other mammalian cells studied (except perhaps skeletal muscle which resembles heart) should lead one to suspect in the so-called isolated sarcoplasmic reticulum preparation the presence of elements of sarcolemma, probably vesicles derived from the breakdown of the sarcolemma-derived T-tubules. In keeping with this interpretation is the observation that the specific activity and response to noradrenaline of the adenyl cyclase of the preparation of so-called "sarcoplasmic reticulum" (ENTMAN et al., 1969a and b) are less than that of the crude washed particulate preparation, sedimenting at fairly high speed (given as 10,000 rpm) and described as "sarcolemma" (LEVEY and EPSTEIN, 1969a; LEVEY et al., 1969a and b). This would be expected if the so-called "sarcoplasmic reticulum" fraction were contaminated with a small amount of sarcolemma with highly active adenyl cyclase. The variability of responses of isolated "sarcoplasmic reticulum" to catecholamines apparent in other reports may be due to different degrees of contamination with adenyl cyclase (see BAIRD and BINNION, 1969; HESS et al., 1968; SHINEBOURNE et al., 1969).

Other compounds in addition to cAMP and catecholamines can influence the uptake of calcium by sarcoplasmic reticulum. Fairly low concentrations of FFA inhibit calcium uptake (SCALES and MCINTOSH, 1968a): this action may underly their effect to reduce contractility in isolated hypoxic hearts (HENDERSON et al., 1969). Some β-adrenergic blocking agents may have another action on the heart in addition to and independent of their action to inhibit the effects of catecholamines on adenyl cyclase. For example, (+)-propranolol has the same inhibitory effect as (—)-propranolol on calcium uptake by isolated sarcoplasmic reticulum of heart and on the contractility of the heart (SCALES and MCINTOSH, 1968b) yet it is not a β-adrenergic blocking agent. Ouabain has a stimulatory effect on calcium uptake and the suggestion has been made that this is the basis of its positive inotropic action (ENTMAN et al., 1969c).

If it is true that catecholamines alter the movements of calcium as described above, then other metabolic consequences of changes in calcium concentration must be considered. That local changes in concentrations of ions have a significant role in influencing metabolic processes *in vivo* is a fairly recent concept (see BYGRAVE, 1967). The known roles of calcium in the heart are the activation of myosin ATPase, an effect not shared by cAMP (MCCARL et al., 1969) and a function as a cofactor for phosphorylase *b* kinase *a* (NAMM et al., 1968). The significance of its other effects, such as activation of an enzyme that converts kinase *b* to kinase *a* (DRUMMOND et al., 1965) and inhibition of adenyl cyclase (DRUMMOND and DUNCAN, 1970) is uncertain. The observation that hearts in a calcium-free medium have a higher cAMP content than hearts in a calcium-containing medium (NAMM et al., 1968) suggests that calcium may have a role in the regulation of adenyl cyclase in the intact heart. That increased cAMP content is not essential for an inotropic response to calcium itself is shown by the inotropic response to calcium which is accompanied by a decrease in cAMP concentration (FRIESEN et al., 1967 and 1969; NAMM et al., 1968). The concentration of calcium also influences the action of adrenaline on the movement of other ions. Adrenaline and isopropylnoradrenaline normally increase the uptake of potassium by beating heart muscle; however, as the concentration of calcium is lowered they either have no effect or actually cause a loss of potassium (STAFFORD, 1969).

In the heart, as in other tissues, cyclic AMP can be regarded as a second messenger bringing information into the cell about external events. Its function in the contractile mechanisms, as in the metabolic machinery, is to superimpose an external regulatory influence upon what is already a closely regulated system. The heart has mechanisms for increasing its force of contraction that do not involve cAMP (ØYE, 1967a and b; DHALLA and MCLAIN, 1967) just as it also has mechanisms for accelerating the breakdown of glycogen independently of cAMP (ØYE, 1967a and b; MAYER, 1967). The existence of such alternate mechanisms does not imply that cAMP is not important but illustrates again the remarkable adaptibility of mammalian cellular metabolism.

d) Summary: Metabolic Consequences of the Action of Catecholamines on the Heart

The functions of the metabolic and other effects of catecholamines on the heart should be discussed in the context of the function of such effects in the intact animal. Stimulation of the heart by catecholamines, whether noradrenaline from the nerve endings or adrenaline from the adrenal medulla, has as its primary function the acceleration of the transport in the blood of those substrates needed for energy production by other tissues (oxygen, glucose, FFA) and also by itself. Thus, the increased force of contraction and the simultaneous mobilization of endogenous stored substrates occur in response to a common stimulus; the subsequent utilization of these substrates by the heart is controlled largely by intracellular regulatory mechanisms as also is the utilization of the other substrates presented to the heart in the blood.

As might be expected, the action of the catecholamines on the heart is antagonized by acetylcholine. Cardiac adenyl cyclase is inhibited by acetylcholine (MURAD et al., 1962) and the proportion of phosphorylase in the *a* form is reduced by vagal stimulation (HESS et al., 1962; FRAZER and HESS, 1969) in the intact animal subjected to sympathetic stimulation. *In vitro* acetylcholine inhibits the activation of phosphorylase by adrenaline (BLUKOO-ALLOTEY et al., 1969). The inotropic response to adrenaline may not be inhibited by acetylcholine even although the activation of phosphorylase is inhibited completely (BLUKOO-ALLOTEY et al., 1969); under different conditions the inotropic response can be completely inhibited by acetylcholine as also can the inotropic response to theophylline although that to calcium cannot (MEESTER and HARDMAN, 1967). Although no measurement of cAMP content of the hearts appears to have been made, in the absence of contrary information it is probably justifiable to surmise that it would be reduced by the acetylcholine.

Insulin does not appear to be a physiological antagonist of the effect of catecholamines on adenyl cyclase of heart as it is in tissues such as liver or white adipose tissue. Insulin does however alter glucose transport in the heart (WILLIAMSON, 1964, 1966b). From a teleological viewpoint the lack of action of insulin on cardiac adenyl cyclase is understandable. Inhibition of adenyl cyclase by insulin occurs in those tissues whose storage material is principally for export (liver and adipose tissue) and in which both the storage of excess blood-borne substrate and the mobilization of stored material into the blood is regulated by the adenyl cyclase system. The storage material (both glycogen and triglyceride) of heart (and also skeletal muscle) is entirely for internal consumption and its metabolism is normally regulated by the energy needs of the tissue. Indeed, the stimulation by catecholamines is the only way in which the heart receives information about needs of other tissues. Its own needs can be met by a different kind of regulation. For example, anoxia can increase the rate of glycogenolysis in the heart much more than would be expected from the extent of activation of phosphorylase. This appears to be due to stimulation of the catalytic activity of both phosphorylase *a* and phosphorylase *b* by the relative concentrations of ATP (inhibitor), 5′-AMP (activator) and phosphate (substrate) (MORGAN and PARMEGGIANI, 1964). Nevertheless, an adrenergic component may also be involved in anoxia-induced glycogenolysis as evidenced by the rapid and transient rise in cAMP concentration (WOLLENBERGER et al., 1969), the rise in phosphorylase *b* kinase *a* activity (KRAUSE and WOLLENBERGER, 1967), the rise in phosphorylase *a* activity (WOLLENBERGER et al., 1969; MAYER et al., 1967; MAYER, 1967; ØYE, 1967a and b) and the release of endogenous noradrenaline (SHAHAB et al., 1969). Moreover, most of these metabolic effects of anoxia can be at least partially blocked by β-adrenergic blocking agents. Pronethalol partly blocks the rise in cAMP content (WOLLENBERGER et al., 1969) and the rise in the proportion of phosphorylase *a* (WOLLENBERGER et al., 1969; MAYER, 1967), although it does not prevent the disappearance of glycogen (MAYER, 1967; MAYER et al., 1967).

IV. Skeletal Muscle

Metabolic processes in skeletal muscle, like those in heart, are largely governed by intracellular regulatory mechanisms geared to the energy needs of the muscle itself. The major source of substrate for skeletal muscle, whether exercising or at rest, is the circulating plasma (glucose and FFA). Effects of catecholamines are superimposed on these endogenous regulatory mechanisms. The principal consequences of the action of the catecholamines on skeletal muscle are accelerated breakdown of its two main storage materials, glycogen and triglyceride (Fig. 5). The metabolic processes involved in the accelerated breakdown of glycogen are understood in some detail. However, by comparison practically nothing is known about the regulation of lipolysis in skeletal muscle and there is indeed considerable controversy at present regarding the role of muscle triglyceride stores in

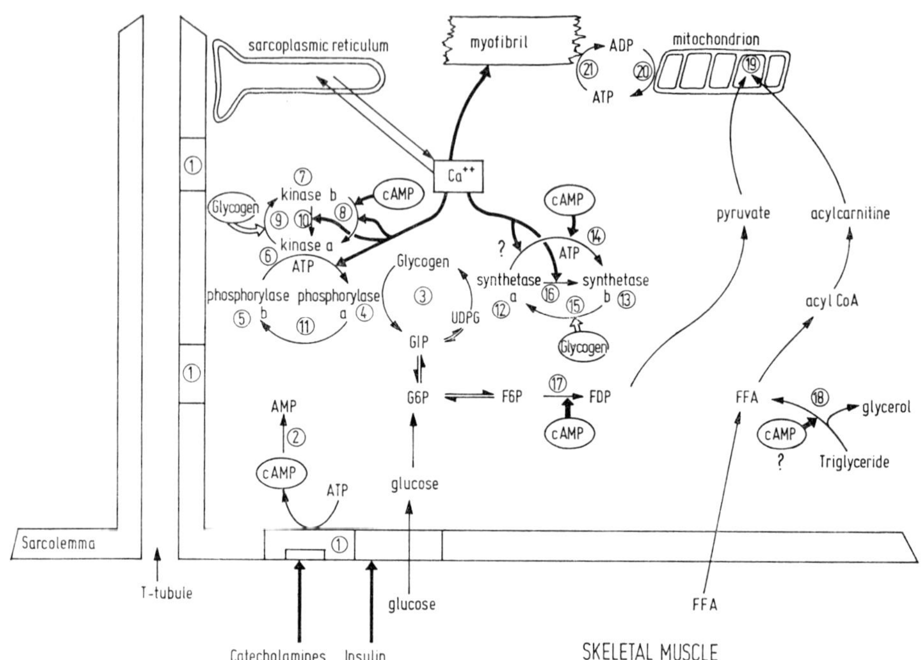

Fig. 5. *Summary of metabolic processes in skeletal muscle known to be influenced by catecholamines.* Adenyl cyclase (1) is shown as being present in sarcolemma and T-tubules and having associated with it a "receptor" for catecholamines. (2) denotes cAMP phosphodiesterase. Enzymes involved in the glycogen cycle (3) are shown in all the forms known to exist. These are: (4) glycogen phosphorylase *a*; (5) glycogen phophorylase *b*; (6) phosphorylase *b* kinase *a*; (7) phosphorylase *b* kinase *b*; (8) phosphorylase *b* kinase *b* kinase (or kinase kinase); (9) phosphorylase *b* kinase *a* phosphatase; (10) calcium-stimulated proteolytic activating enzyme(s); (11) phosphorylase *a* phosphatase; (12) glycogen synthetase *a*; (13) glycogen synthetase *b*; (14) glycogen synthetase *a* kinase; (15) glycogen synthetase *b* phosphatase; (16) calcium-stimulated proteolytic inactivating enzyme(s). Sites of stimulation by cAMP are shown by the labeled solid black arrows; sites of inhibition by glycogen are shown by the labeled open arrows. Two other cAMP-stimulated enzymes are phosphofructokinase (17) and triglyceride lipase (18). (19) denotes the major energy-yielding pathways of skeletal muscle: included here are pyruvate dehydrogenase, β-oxidation of fatty acids and tricarboxylic acid cycle plus associated electron transport and oxidative phosphorylation (20). The major energy-using reaction of skeletal muscle, contraction, is denoted by (21)

providing a source of substrate during exercise. In addition to their direct effect on skeletal muscle to alter its metabolism, the catecholamines also alter the contractile functioning of the muscle and may thus secondarily alter its metabolism in this way. Firstly, catecholamines appear to potentiate neuromuscular transmission and thus enhance the contractile response of muscle to a given stimulation of its motor nerve (BRECKENRIDGE et al., 1967; GOLDBERG and SINGER, 1969). Catecholamines can also enhance the force of contraction of skeletal muscle by a more direct effect on the muscle (see BOWMAN and RAPER, 1967; BOWMAN and RAPER, 1964) but the mechanism of this effect is very poorly understood.

a) Adenyl Cyclase

Adenyl cyclase is known to be present in muscle (SUTHERLAND et al., 1962). It can be stimulated by catecholamines both *in vitro* (KLAINER et al., 1962) and *in vivo* (POSNER et al., 1965; DRUMMOND et al., 1969). Adenyl cyclase is located in a membrane fraction which can be prepared from homogenates; the identity of these membranes has not been definitely established. Upon differential centrifugation of dog muscle homogenates adenyl cyclase activity (fluoride-stimulated) sediments in both the mitochondrial and microsomal fractions, the former having a considerably higher specific activity than the latter (RABINOWITZ et al., 1965). RABINOWITZ and co-workers (1965) identified the membranes as sarcoplasmic reticulum. However, a sarcolemma-derived tubule system is present in skeletal muscle, just as in the heart (see B. III. c). It is, therefore, possible that adenyl cyclase of these sarcolemma-derived tubules may be found in several subcellular fractions; the presence of adenyl cyclase in sarcolemma cannot be excluded on the basis of differential centrifugation studies alone.

b) Effect of cAMP on Skeletal Muscle Enzymes

α) Enzymes of the Glycogen Cycle. Like most other tissues, skeletal muscle contains cAMP-dependent protein kinases (KUO and GREENGARD, 1969a). The identity of the substrates for at least one of these kinases appears to be established. Activation of muscle phosphorylase *b* kinase *b* kinase is cAMP-dependent (WALSH et al., 1968; DRUMMOND and POWELL, 1970) and is accompanied by phosphorylation of the enzyme (DELANGE et al., 1968). Inactivation of glycogen synthetase *a* by synthetase *a* kinase is likewise stimulated by cAMP (ROSELL-PEREZ and LARNER, 1964; APPLEMAN et al., 1966) and associated with phosphorylation of the enzyme (LARNER and SANGER, 1965). A recent report suggests that these two phosphorylation reactions are catalyzed by a single kinase (SCHLENDER et al., 1969).

As would be expected from these known effects of cAMP the consequences of the action of adrenaline upon skeletal muscle are: an activation of phosphorylase *b* kinase (DRUMMOND et al., 1969; POSNER et al., 1965) an activation of phosphorylase (DANFORTH and HELMREICH, 1964; CRAIG et al., 1969; DRUMMOND et al., 1969; POSNER et al., 1965; WILLIAMS and MAYER, 1966), and a conversion of glycogen synthetase *a* to the *b* form (DANFORTH, 1965; CRAIG et al., 1969; WILLIAMS and MAYER, 1966). These changes may lead to a disappearance of glycogen from the muscle (WILLIAMS and MAYER, 1966). However, the influence of adrenaline on glycogen content is to decrease it when the glycogen content of the muscle is high and to decrease the accumulation of glycogen when the initial glycogen content is low (see HIMMS-HAGEN, 1967 for further review). A detailed review of regulation of glycogen metabolism has recently been made by HELMREICH (1969).

β) Enzymes of Glycolysis. Although phosphofructokinase of skeletal muscle is stimulated by cAMP (Passoneau and Lowry, 1962) the phosphofructokinase reaction appears to be regulated principally by the relative concentrations of ATP (inhibitor as well as substrate), ADP and AMP (stimulators), and it seems unlikely (for reasons that will be discussed later) that a stimulation of flow of glucose carbon through the phosphofructokinase reaction is an important consequence of the accumulation of cAMP that follows stimulation by adrenaline.

γ) Enzymes of Lipolysis. Although adrenaline can accelerate the breakdown of triglycerides in skeletal muscle, as judged by the increased production of FFA (Garland and Randle, 1963) and of glycerol (Randle et al., 1963) seen *in vitro* on the addition of adrenaline, nothing is known about the nature of the lipase(s) involved, about the possible role of cAMP or about the physiological significance of this effect.

c) Relation of Effect of Catecholamines on Contraction of Skeletal Muscle to cAMP Formation

Adrenaline has two distinct effects on contractile processes in skeletal muscle: firstly, it influences neuromuscular transmission and secondly, it exerts a more direct effect upon the muscle cells themselves to alter the tension developed during stimulation (see Bowman and Raper, 1967). The effect on neuromuscular transmission is considered to involve cAMP because it is potentiated by theophylline (Breckenridge et al., 1967; Goldberg and Singer, 1969) and is mimicked by dBcAMP (Goldberg and Singer, 1969). The increased frequency of single cell end plate potentials and the increased height of the compound end plate potential caused by adrenaline and by dBcAMP indicate that these compounds accelerate the release of packets of acetylcholine from the motor neurone (Goldberg and Singer, 1969).

The nature of the more direct effect of adrenaline on contraction depends upon the type of muscle involved. Fast-contracting muscles show an increase in twitch tension and a decreased rate of relaxation, whereas slow-contracting muscles show a decrease in twitch tension and an increased rate of relaxation (Bowman and Raper, 1967). Although it is tempting to interpret these effects in skeletal muscle in the same way as the rather similar effects in heart (see section 3 c), i.e., as a consequence of a change in the rate of movement of calcium ions into the sarcoplasmic reticulum caused by cAMP, there is at present no evidence for the participation of cAMP or of calcium ions in this effect.

d) Regulation of Metabolic Processes in Skeletal Muscle

Metabolic processes in skeletal muscle are regulated in such a way as to provide energy for muscular contraction; the substrates used come partly from the blood and partly from the endogenous stores, and if the endogenous stores are depleted during contraction they are replenished during rest. Regulation by catecholamines is superimposed upon a system that already possesses the capacity to regulate the breakdown of its endogenous stores in accordance with the need for them, at least in the case of carbohydrate.

Electrical stimulation of the motor nerve to skeletal muscle results in an exceedingly rapid conversion of phosphorylase *b* to phosphorylase *a* (Danforth et al., 1962; Posner et al., 1965; Drummond et al., 1969; Piras and Staneloni, 1969). This conversion is not accompanied by changes in cAMP concentration or by consistent changes in phosphorylase *b* kinase *a* activity (Posner et al., 1965; Drummond et al., 1969). This activation of phosphorylase by electrical stimulation differs from that caused by adrenaline in the speed at which it occurs (about 5 sec compared with several minutes) and in its mechanism. Conversion back to the *b* form during rest is also much more rapid than that occurring after adrenaline-induced stimulation (DANFORTH et al., 1962; PIRAS and STANELONI, 1969).

Glycogen synthetase *a* activity is reduced rapidly during electrical stimulation (also in about 5 sec) but only when it already constitutes a fairly large part of the total (PIRAS and STANELONI, 1969; STANELONI and PIRAS, 1969); however, its activity increases slowly during the resting period following electrical stimulation (DANFORTH, 1965; PIRAS and STANELONI, 1969). A 10 sec period of tetanic stimulation is accompanied, therefore, by a disappearance of glycogen, due largely to the rapid conversion of phosphorylase *b* to phosphorylase *a*; the concentrations of ATP and AMP do not change under these conditions and these metabolites presumably play little or no part in the acceleration of glycogenolysis (PIRAS and STANELONI, 1969). During the 10 min after stimulation the glycogen content is restored almost to its initial level; this is due in part to the conversion of glycogen synthetase *b* to the *a* form during this period and in part to the elevated concentration of glucose-6-phosphate (stimulator) compared to the unchanged concentrations of inhibitory metabolites (ATP, ADP, AMP, creatine phosphate) (PIRAS and STANELONI, 1969). The mechanism by which the two forms of phosphorylase and glycogen synthetase are interconverted under these conditions is poorly understood. As noted above, cAMP does not appear to be involved. The existence of calcium-stimulated enzymes that can convert phosphorylase *b* kinase *b* to phosphorylase *b* kinase *a* (HUSTON and KREBS, 1968) and convert glycogen synthetase *a* to glycogen synthetase *b* (BELOCOPITOW et al., 1965 and 1967) suggests one possible mechanism. However, these calcium-stimulated enzymes are proteases and their activating effects are irreversible (HUSTON and KREBS, 1968; BELOCOPITOW et al., 1965 and 1967). That they are not involved in the changes due to nerve stimulation is shown by the observation of STANELONI and PIRAS (1969) that four successive periods of tetanic stimulation followed by rest are each accompanied by similar and reciprocal changes in the proportion of phosphorylase *a* and of synthetase *a*. Thus, the processes of activation (and of inactivation) of each must be readily reversible.

However, the exclusion of calcium-dependent proteolytic activation mechanisms as an explanation of the activation of phosphorylase during contraction does not imply that calcium has no role in the activation of phosphorylase. Very low concentrations of calcium can stimulate the activity of phosphorylase *b* kinase (OZAWA et al., 1967) and can also stimulate the activity of phosphorylase *b* kinase *b* kinase (OZAWA and EBASHI, 1967); the many other similarities between synthetase *a* kinase and phosphorylase *b* kinase *b* kinase suggests that the synthetase *a* kinase too may be similarly stimulated by calcium. The reason for the large amount of phosphorylase *b* kinase in skeletal muscle (DELANGE et al., 1968) would then be apparent. The enzyme usually exerts its catalytic effect only for the few seconds that calcium is available to it: the large amount of the enzyme is necessary for the very rapid conversion of phosphorylase *b* to *a* and is normally inactive in the absence of calcium. Reconversion of phosphorylase *a* to the *b* form during rest involves the cessation of the action of the kinases and, therefore, the predominance of the actions of phosphorylase *a* phosphatase and of glycogen synthetase *b* phosphatase. If the above explanation were correct then restoration of phosphorylase *a* to *b* and of synthetase *b* to *a* during rest should proced at much the same rate; however, the phosphorylase *a* to *b* conversion requires only a few seconds whereas the synthetase *b* to *a* conversion takes minutes. The only plausible explanation for this difference at the moment is the inhibition of the activity of the synthetase *b* phosphatase by glycogen (Larner et al., 1968); in the phosphorylase enzyme system glycogen inhibits only the phosphorylase *b* kinase *a* phosphatase (Riley et al., 1968), an effect which would not restrict the conversion of phosphorylase *a* to *b*. There is known to be an inverse relationship between the proportion of glycogen synthetase in the *a* form and the concentration of glycogen in intact muscle under a variety of conditions (Danforth, 1965).

Skeletal muscle contains approximately equivalent stores of calories in the form of glycogen and of triglyceride (glycogen: 0.9 grams per 100 grams of muscle or 3690 calories per 100 grams (Piras and Staneloni, 1969); triglyceride, 0.34 grams per 100 grams of muscle or 3160 calories per 100 grams (Masoro et al., 1966a). However, it is not known whether lipid breakdown can be altered as a consequence of muscle contraction. The finding of an unchanged triglyceride content and turnover in monkey gastrocnemius muscle during 5 hours of stimulation of its motor nerve (*in vivo* in anaesthetized monkeys) suggests that no activation of lipolysis occurs under these conditions (Masoro et al., 1966b). However, when activation of the sympathetic nervous system accompanies contraction of skeletal muscle, as happens during exercise (see Himms-Hagen, 1967) the endogenous triglycerides of muscle do appear to serve as an energy source. The evidence for this is indirect and is based upon the oxidation by exercising muscle of more FFA than are taken up by it from the blood (see Havel et al., 1963, 1967; Issekutz et al., 1966).

Insulin can antagonize the effects of adrenaline on glycogen metabolism in skeletal muscle to some extent (Torres et al., 1968). However, it does not appear to exert this effect via the adenyl cyclase system as it does in liver and white adipose tissue. Insulin does not alter the concentration of cAMP in muscle, whether this has been raised by adrenaline or not (Craig et al., 1969; Larner et al., 1968; Goldberg et al., 1967); however, it does increase the proportion of glycogen synthetase in the *a* form without altering the proportion of phosphorylase in the *a* form (Larner et al., 1968; Craig et al., 1969). An effect of insulin to promote the conversion of synthetase *a* kinase to a cAMP-dependent form has been suggested as the means by which insulin normally increases the amount of glycogen synthetase *a* (Larner et al., 1968; Villar-Palasi, 1968) but the mechanism of this effect is unknown.

It is probably too soon to conclude that cAMP is not involved at all in the action of insulin on skeletal muscle. After preincubation with insulin, rat diaphragm does show a smaller initial increase in cAMP concentration with adrenaline (Craig et al., 1969); moreover, the proportion of synthetase *a* is increased by insulin in the presence of adrenaline, an effect that would not be expected if its only action were to convert the synthetase *a* kinase to a cAMP-dependent form. The lack of correlation between the measured cAMP content and synthetase *a* activity and between cAMP content and phosphorylase *a* activity suggests that only a small portion of the total cAMP participates in the activation or inactivation of these enzymes.

The existence of endogenous inhibitors of activation of enzymes by cAMP suggests that yet another regulatory mechanism may be important in muscle. Muscle and other tissues contain a protein inhibitor that is heat stable and that inhibits cAMP-dependent protein kinases in general (Brostrom, 1970) as well as cAMP stimulation of phosphorylase *b* kinase *b* kinase (Posner et al., 1964) and cAMP stimulated glycogen synthetase *a* kinase (Appleman et al., 1966). The physiological function of this inhibitor is unknown. Another inhibitor, which resembles cAMP very closely in its properties but is as yet unidentified, inhibits cAMP stimulation of phosphorylase activation (Murad et al., 1969a). This inhibitor is usually formed under conditions where cAMP itself is formed and its formation is enhanced by cAMP but inhibited by dBcAMP. MURAD, RALL and VAUGHAN (1969a) suggest that the existence of this inhibitor may explain the frequently observed lack of correlation between cAMP content of tissues and effect of stimulation and may also help to explain the greater effectiveness of dBcAMP in mimicking the effects of hormones. A complete understanding of the intricate regulation of the enzyme systems that respond to cAMP and to hormones will require an understanding of the nature and physiological functioning of these inhibitors.

Adrenal cortical hormones can influence the glycogenolytic response of skeletal muscle to catecholamines. Neither adrenaline nor cAMP stimulates muscle phosphorylase in adrenalectomized rats; the response is restored by treatment with hydrocortisone (SCHAEFFER et al., 1969b). This resembles the situation in liver. The nature of the defect in muscle produced by lack of adrenal cortical hormones is not known.

What is the physiological function of the action of catecholamines on skeletal muscle? The metabolic effects would appear to be superfluous since the muscle can bring about exactly the same changes, at least in glycogen metabolism, within a few seconds by means of its own intracellular regulatory mechanisms. It is possible that the effects of adrenaline may be of greater significance in fatigued muscle. Fatigued muscle loses its ability to maintain phosphorylase in the *a* form (DANFORTH and HELMREICH, 1964; PIRAS and STANELONI, 1969) but retains it to a much greater degree in the presence of adrenaline (DANFORTH and HELMREICH, 1964). The extent to which this effect of adrenaline is due to raised cAMP production or to acceleration of calcium accumulation is unknown. However, the combined effects of adrenaline on neuromuscular transmission, force of contraction and mobilization of endogenous glycogen and triglyceride presumably all enhance muscle function during severe exercise; these effects are of course supplemented by the increased supply of glucose and FFA to the muscle brought about the concomitant sympathetic stimulation of other tissues (liver, pancreatic islet β-cells, white adipose tissue).

V. Smooth Muscle

As far as they have been studied the metabolic actions of catecholamines on smooth muscle are similar to those on skeletal muscle.

a) Adenyl Cyclase

Although uterus is the only smooth muscle from which adenyl cyclase has been isolated and studied and its stimulation by catecholamines observed (TRINER et al., 1970; DOUSA and RYCHLIK, 1968) observations on cAMP accumulation in other smooth muscles (BUEDING et al., 1966; see also ROBISON et al., 1968) leave little doubt about the presence of the enzyme.

b) Effect of cAMP on Smooth Muscle Enzymes

The only metabolic consequence of catecholamine stimulation that has been studied in considerable detail for smooth muscle is the activation of phosphorylase. The properties of the phosphorylase enzyme system of smooth muscle are similar to those of the skeletal muscle enzyme system (MOHME-LUNDHOLM, 1963). Despite these similarities the smooth muscle phosphorylase is immunologically distinct from the skeletal muscle enzyme (BUEDING et al., 1964). It is, moreover, present in much smaller quantities and operates at lower substrate and activator concentrations (BUEDING et al., 1964). No information appears to be available about either the nature of the glycogen synthetase enzyme system of smooth muscle or about the significance of lipid metabolism in this tissue.

c) Relation of Effects of Catecholamines on Contraction and Relaxation of Smooth Muscle to cAMP Formation

Interest in the metabolic effects of catecholamines on smooth muscle has arisen in the course of studies of their effects on contraction and relaxation and on the relation of these effects to metabolic processes. The effects of catecholamines on contraction and relaxation of smooth muscle are difficult to fit into any unified scheme. There appear to be both α-receptors and β-receptors in most smooth muscles. α-Receptor stimulation usually results in contraction (uterus, vas deferens, vascular smooth muscle) and β-receptor stimulation usually results in relaxation (uterus, vascular smooth muscle, tracheal smooth muscle, intestinal smooth muscle). In some tissues it is also possible for α-receptor stimulation to cause relaxation and for β-receptor stimulation also to cause relaxation (intestinal smooth muscle). Thus, most tissues contain a mixture of α- and β-receptors whose stimulation usually has opposite effects but sometimes has the same effect. The actual mixture varies from one tissue to another, from one species to another, and even within a single tissue at different times.

There seems to be fairly general agreement that relaxation of smooth muscle caused by stimulation of β-receptors is associated with adenyl cyclase activation, cAMP accumulation and activation of phosphorylase (see ROBISON et al., 1967). That the relaxation is actually secondary to the rise in cAMP content is suggested by the similar effects of cAMP or dBcAMP (guinea pig tracheal chain: MOORE et al., 1968; rat ileum: KAWASAKI et al., 1969; rabbit ileum: KIM et al., 1968; rat uterus: DOBBS and ROBISON, 1968; TRINER et al., 1970), and by the similar or potentiating effects of theophylline or caffeine (rabbit ileum: WILKENFELD and LEVY, 1969; guinea pig tracheal chain: MOORE et al., 1968; rat ileum: KAWASAKI et al., 1969; rat uterus: DOBBS and ROBISON, 1968). A role for calcium in the relaxing effects of catecholamines on smooth muscle has frequently been suggested but no firm evidence has been forthcoming (see DANIEL et al., 1970). Cyclic AMP will inhibit calcium-induced contractions in the rat uterus (MITZNEGG et al., 1970) and cAMP or dBcAMP and also adrenaline will inhibit the calcium-dependent oxytocin induced contractions of uterus (TRINER et al., 1970; MITZNEGG et al., 1970). Moreover, calcium is required for the relaxant effect of isopropylnoradrenaline (DANIEL et al., 1970). There is, therefore, suggestive evidence that cAMP may have a role in transport of calcium from the cytosol of smooth muscle, as proposed for heart muscle, but more evidence for this is needed.

At one time, the role of phosphorylase activation in the effects of catecholamines on smooth muscle received considerable attention, just as it did also in the early studies on heart (see HIMMS-HAGEN, 1967 and BRODY and MCNEILL, 1970). Recent studies have clarified some of the early problems. For example, guinea pig taenia coli is now known to contain both α- and β-adrenergic receptors, both promoting relaxation (BRODY and DIAMOND, 1967); initial relaxation due to α-receptor stimulation precedes the relaxation due to β-receptor stimulation and can be separated from it by the use of α-adrenergic blocking agents. The increase in cAMP content (BUEDING et al., 1966) and the rise in phosphorylase *a* activity are associated with the β-receptor-induced relaxation that occurs at the later stage of the response. The fast α-receptor component of relaxation does not occur when isopropylnoradrenaline is used (BRODY and DIAMOND, 1967) except at high concentrations (ANDERSON and MOHME-LUNDHOLM, 1968).

In the uterine muscle phosphorylase is activated both when the uterus is relaxed by the stimulatory actions of catecholamines on β-receptors and when the uterus is made to contract, whether because of the stimulatory effects of catecholamines on α-receptors (DIAMOND and BRODY, 1966a), or because of the presence of other stimulatory agents such as oxytocin or serotonin, or because of spontaneous contractions (DIAMOND and BRODY, 1966b). Phosphorylase activation follows the contraction (DIAMOND and BRODY, 1966b) and, although there is so far no evidence for this, is presumably brought about in a fashion similar to the phosphorylase activation that accompanies contraction in skeletal muscle (see B. IV. d). The rise in phosphorylase *a* activity that occurs during relaxation due to β-receptor stimulation by isopropylnoradrenaline is associated with an increase in cAMP content of the uterus (DOBBS and ROBISON, 1968); the relaxation, the rise in cAMP content and the phosphorylase activation are all blocked by propranolol (DIAMOND and BRODY, 1966a; DOBBS and ROBISON, 1968).

The metabolic alterations that underly and/or accompany those effects of catecholamines on smooth muscle that are considered to be exerted by stimulation of α-receptors are entirely unknown. For those tissues where this effect is the opposite of the effect of β-receptor stimulation it is tempting to suppose that inhibition of adenyl cyclase may be involved, as originally suggested by ROBISON, BUTCHER and SUTHERLAND (1967). There is still no evidence that this can occur in smooth muscle. For those tissues, such as intestinal smooth muscle, where α-receptor stimulation has the same final effect as β-receptor stimulation, in this case relaxation, such a theory would not be applicable. No other hypothesis is available at present, except perhaps in terms of ion movements across the cell membrane (see DANIEL et al., 1970).

In summary, current knowledge of the metabolism of smooth muscle is very limited. Little is known of the mechanisms of contraction and relaxation and of the relationship between these aspects of smooth muscle function and the metabolic processes and their possible regulation by the catecholamines.

VI. Brown Adipose Tissue

The principal known metabolic function of brown adipose tissue is the production of heat: this function is under the control of the sympathetic nervous system and represents, therefore, a metabolic effect of the catecholamines. The brown adipose tissue stores triglyceride and, when stimulated to do so by catecholamines, either liberated from sympathetic nerve terminals in the tissue or borne by the blood from the adrenal medulla, breaks it down to provide an oxidizable substrate needed to support its calorigenic function. The calorigenic function is actually initiated by the products of lipolysis, the FFA set free as a consequence of the action of the catecholamines. Such a breakdown of storage material to support the function of the tissue itself is analogous to the breakdown of glycogen in heart to support the increased activity of the heart rather than to the breakdown of triglycerides in white adipose tissue to provide FFA for other organs. For this reason it is unfortunate that the term adipose tissue is included in its name because this implies a similarity to white adipose tissue and has led to many attempts to liken the functions the two tissues. Such attempts are no more useful than calling liver and skeletal muscle by two names including the term "glycogen-storing tissues" and then comparing their metabolism without taking into account their markedly different functions. Just as liver and skeletal muscle, although both subject to stimulation of glycogenolysis by the catecholamines, regulate their glycogen metabolism in entirely different ways, and in accordance with their respective functions of providing glucose for other tissues and of providing glucose as an internal energy source, so do white adipose tissue and brown adipose tissue, both subject to stimulation of lipolysis by catecholamines, regulate their triglyceride metabolism in different ways in accordance with their respective functions of providing in the one case FFA for other tissues and in the other case FFA as an internal energy source and promoter of calorigenesis.

Brown adipose tissue occurs in appreciable quantities only in certain newborn mammals, in hibernators and in cold acclimated animals: it is also present, but usually in lesser amounts, in the same species when they are adult, when they are not actually hibernating and when they are not adapted to cold. A comprehensive review of the distribution, structure and metabolism of brown adipose tissue and of the evidence for its function as a heat producing tissue can be found in a recent review by SMITH and HORWITZ (1969). The current live interest in this tissue has arisen for two reasons: (i) the regulation of its metabolism, and particularly of its mitochondrial oxidative metabolism, appears to be quite different from that of other tissues and it seems likely that elucidation of the mechanisms of these regulatory processes may bring light new concepts of mitochondrial function; (ii) the search for the elusive mechanism underlying nonshivering thermogenesis, the process of heat production that is switched on by noradrenaline in animals possessing the necessary adaptation, such as certain newborn mammals, hibernators and cold acclimated animals, has recently concentrated upon mechanisms of heat production in the brown adipose tissue; in addition, efforts to establish the relative contribution of this fairly small tissue to total heat production in animals that are producing heat by nonshivering thermogenesis have led to the disclosure of another function of this tissue, namely as an endocrine organ whose secretory product influences the capacity of other tissues to respond calorigenically to noradrenaline (HIMMS-HAGEN, 1969b, 1970b).

The brown adipose tissue is therefore unique in that both its metabolism and its calorigenic function are controlled directly by the sympathetic nervous system; it seems likely that its postulated endocrine function is similarly controlled, but evidence for this is not yet available. The growth of this tissue is also influenced by the sympathetic nervous system: the tissue actually grows when subjected to excessive stimulation (CAMERON and SMITH, 1964; SMITH and HORWITZ, 1969). The rich sympathetic innervation of this tissue is also unique in that it has a dual nature: cells and blood vessels are innervated by noradrenaline-containing nerves from different parts of the sympathetic nervous system (DERRY et al., 1969; DERRY and DANIEL, 1970; DANIEL and DERRY, 1969). Its vascularity is likewise very rich and the blood flow is increased by catecholamines (JANSKY and HART, 1968; HEIM and HULL, 1966; KUROSHIMA et al., 1967).

As might the be expected the metabolic changes that occur in the brown adipose tissue as a consequence of stimulation by catecholamines are very widespread and reach into every aspect of its metabolism. They will be discussed here under three headings: a) events at the cell membrane (including stimulation of adenyl cyclase); b) changes in lipid and carbohydrate metabolism; c) respiratory processes. These will be followed by brief discussions of: d) ultrastructural changes and growth; e) role of brown adipose tissue in nonshivering thermogenesis and f) function of brown adipose tissue: a summary.

a) Events at the Cell Membrane

An adenyl cyclase which is stimulated by noradrenaline and by fluoride is present in brown adipose tissue (MUIRHEAD and HIMMS-HAGEN, 1971). The cAMP content of brown adipose tissue slices is increased by noradrenaline

(BEVIZ et al., 1968) while dBcAMP and theophylline mimic the stimulatory effect of noradrenaline on oxygen uptake and lipolysis (REED and FAIN, 1968a and b; FAIN, 1970). Thus, as in other tissues, the initial effect of catecholamines on brown adipose tissue appears to be stimulation of adenyl cyclase activity.

The membranes of brown adipose tissue cells are depolarized by noradrenaline and by sympathetic nerve stimulation (GIRARDIER et al., 1968; HORWITZ et al., 1969), an effect of noradrenaline that is not mimicked by theophylline or by dBcAMP (HORWITZ et al., 1969). Propranolol blocks the noradrenaline-induced depolarization (HORWITZ et al., 1969) and also blocks other consequences of the interaction of noradrenaline with the membrane, such as accelerated lipolysis (FAIN, 1970) and increased oxygen uptake (LINDBERG et al., 1970; PRUSINER et al., 1968a); propranolol does not inhibit the stimulation of lipolysis by theophylline or by dBcAMP (FAIN, 1970). Phentolamine also inhibits the depolarization of brown adipose tissue cells by nerve stimulation (HORWITZ et al., 1969). This suggests that α-receptors may also be present; no other effect of phentolamine or of α-receptor stimulation is yet apparent.

b) Changes in Lipid and Carbohydrate Metabolism (Fig. 6)

Catecholamines stimulate lipolysis in brown adipose tissue (JOEL, 1965; JOEL, 1966; FAIN et al., 1967). This effect is mimicked by dBcAMP (REED and FAIN, 1968a) and is usually assumed to be due to stimulation or activation of a specific triglyceride lipase, although such an enzyme has not yet been identified in this tissue. Even though the brown adipose tissue itself uses the products of lipolysis, some FFA and glycerol can also be liberated from the tissue. In the brown adipose tissue FFA are first activated and then re-esterified or oxidized; the glycerol may be phosphorylated to form α-glycerophosphate. Fatty acid oxidation is increased by noradrenaline and, as will be discussed further under c), this increased oxidation supports the calorigenic effect.

Although there is a considerable utilization of glucose for re-esterification of fatty acids in brown adipose tissue of intact animals subjected to sympathetic stimulation (cold) (STEINER and CAHILL, 1964; HIMMS-HAGEN, 1965, 1969a; STEINER et al., 1970), this does not occur in response to noradrenaline *in vitro* (STEINER et al., 1969, 1970; KORNACKER and BALL, 1968; STEINER and CAHILL, 1966; FAIN et al., 1967). WILLIAMSON suggests that α-glycerophosphate is so rapidly removed that extensive re-esterification of fatty acids does not occur when lipolysis is stimulated *in vitro* (WILLIAMSON et al., 1970). Indeed, the high activities of cytoplasmic and mitochondrial α-glycerophosphate dehydrogenases suggests an important role for the α-glycerophosphate shuttle, possibly for utilization of the α-glycerophosphate formed from the glycerol liberated during lipolysis. The way in which the α-glycerophosphate shuttle is regulated so as to permit extensive re-esterification under conditions of lipolysis *in vivo* but not *in vitro* and to permit triglyceride synthesis to replenish the triglyceride stores *in vivo* is unknown although some regulation at this level would appear to be essential.

c) Respiratory Processes

Oxygen uptake of a cell represents the sum total of the organized complex of reactions occurring in the cell; it is extremely difficult to study a stimulation of oxygen uptake in any preparation except one which contains intact cells because the level or organization in subcellular preparations, such as homogenates or mitochondria, is not sufficient to permit an integrated change in cellular metabolism. Two criteria must be met in attempts to identify the process occurring *in vitro* that is responsible for the heat-producing function of the brown adipose tissue *in vivo* (HIMMS-HAGEN, 1970b): (i) the capacity of the process measured

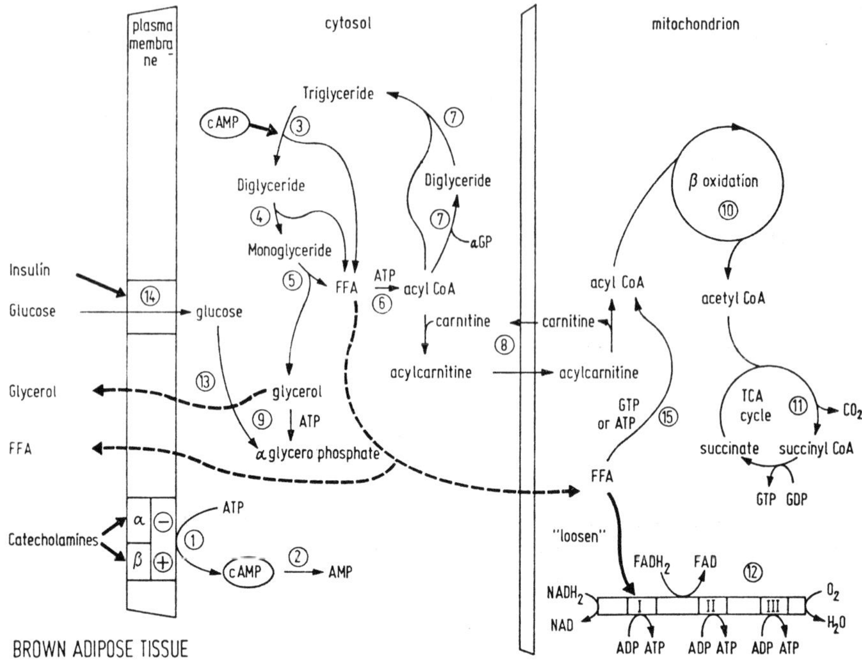

Fig. 6. *Summary of those aspects of brown adipose tissue metabolism known to be infleunced by catecholamines.* The cell membrane contains adenyl cyclase (1) plus associated "receptors" (the existence of the α-receptor is uncertain; see text for discussion). cAMP phosphodiesterase is denoted by (2). Enzymes of triglyceride breakdown are: (3) triglyceride lipase (cAMP-stimulated); (4) diglyceride lipase; (5) monoglyceride lipase. The FFA can be released from the cell, or they can enter the mitochondrion (see below) or they can be activated. (6) is the fatty acid activating enzyme of the cytosol and (7) represents the several enzymes involved in re-esterification of fatty acids. Activated fatty acids are transported into the mitochondrion via the carnitine transport cycle (8). The glycerol produced in lipolysis can be released from the cell or can be phosphorylated by glycerokinase (9). The α-glycerophosphate formed (αGP) can be used for re-esterification of fatty acids (7) or it can take part in the α-glycerophosphate shuttle for oxidation of $NADH_2$ produced in the cytosol (not shown). The major energy-yielding pathways in this tissue are β-oxidation of fatty acids (10) and tricarboxylic acid cycle (11). Glucose can also be used (13) and glucose entry is insulin-dependent (14). The heat-producing function of this tissue is determined largely by the rate of reoxidation of the reduced coenzymes in the electron transport chain (12); this is normally controlled by the rate of oxidative phosphorylation but can be "loosened" from it by FFA (see also Fig. 7). FFA in the mitochondria may be activated (15) or they may be transported from one compartment to another by a carnitine- and ATP-dependent process (not shown; see text for discussion)

in vitro should correspond to the capacity of the tissue in the intact animal; (ii) the operation of the putative calorigenic process should not be a permanent property of the tissue preparation in which it is studied but should be subject to switching on and off, i.e., the process must be a facultative one.

Data for meeting the first criterion can be obtained from measurements of oxygen uptake of stimulated slices or cells and from maximum activities of respiratory enzymes: this information sheds no light on the regulated operation of the calorigenic process. Data for meeting the second criterion come at present only from studies with intact tissue, slices or cells. Until it is possible to mimic in homogenates or isolated mitochondria the complex series of cytoplasmic events that occur in a catecholamine-stimulated tissue and culminate in the rise in mitochondrial respiration rate, it will probably not be possible to make meaningful studies of catecholamine-stimulated thermogenesis in such subcellular preparations. Evidence applicable to these two criteria will be discussed under two headings: firstly, that concerning *capacity*, and secondly, that concerning *operation*.

The observed capacity of brown adipose tissue to utilize oxygen in intact animals, either stimulated by infused noradrenaline or stimulated by exposure to cold, is fairly high. Values have been reported of 6.4 μatoms of oxygen per mg protein nitrogen per minute for newborn rabbits during infusion of noradrenaline (HEIM and HULL, 1966). (All quoted values of oxygen uptake have been converted to these same units for comparison; a nitrogen content of 15.4 mg per gram of wet tissue is used (SMITH and ROBERTS, 1964) if no other value is given by the authors.) For cold-acclimated rats values of about 2.5 μatoms of oxygen per minute per mg protein N can be calculated from the measured blood flow (JANSKY and HART, 1968; KUROSHIMA et al., 1967). These values for the rabbit and rat represent the minimum expected for the stimulated calorigenic process *in vitro*; they are described as the minimum values because it is possible for a tissue actually to possess a greater capacity for oxygen uptake than it is capable of using *in vivo* (JANSKY, 1963).

Noradrenaline-stimulated cells or slices from brown adipose tissue can achieve a rate of oxygen uptake as great or even greater than the minimum expected value (JOEL, 1965, 1966; REED and FAIN, 1968a and b; HAYWARD and BALL, 1966) although in many studies the rate of oxygen uptake has been very much lower (see HIMMS-HAGEN, 1970b) or cannot be calculated in this way because the protein content of the cells studied has not been measured.

The oxygen uptake of homogenates can also be very high when suitable substrates and co-factors are added, but there is no stimulation by catecholamines. Supplementation with ATP, carnitine, CoA and fumarate permits a rate of oxygen uptake of about 3.4 μatoms per minute per mg protein N (KORNACKER and BALL, 1968). Measurement of the cytochrome oxidase activity of brown adipose tissue homogenates indicates a capacity of 4.6 μatoms oxygen per minute per mg protein N at 25° (BARNARD et al., 1970) which would permit twice this rate at 37°.

Because in this tissue mitochondrial protein represents about 32—40% of the protein (THOMSON et al., 1968; ROBERTS and SMITH, 1967; SKALA et al., 1970) one would expect a rate of oxygen uptake of isolated mitochondria of approximately three times the minimum rate predicted; thus, for the rat a value of at least 7.8 μatoms oxygen per mg mitochondrial protein N per minute would be expected. Cytochrome oxidase activity of isolated mitochondria is high enough to meet this expected value: an activity of 8.2 μatoms oxygen per minute per mg protein N (measured at 23°) has been reported (SKALA et al., 1970). However, out of the more than twenty five reported rates of oxygen uptake of brown adipose tissue mitochondria only in one instance does the observed oxygen uptake reach that expected. This is the report by ALDRIDGE and STREET (1968); these authors studied a variety of procedures for the preparation and incubation of mitochondria, of which only one gave a high oxygen uptake (of 11.1 μatoms per minute per mg N). Other reported rates of oxygen uptake range mostly from 5—25% of the minimum expected (see HIMMS-HAGEN, 1970b).

Thus the respiration of isolated mitochondria is usually inhibited to a considerable extent. This is probably because they come into contact during their isolation with considerable quantities of fatty acids. Isolated mitochondria usually contain between 0.1 and 0.23 μmoles FFA per mg of protein (KORNACKER and BALL, 1968; DRAHOTA et al., 1968; HITTELMAN et al., 1969), which is considerably higher than the critical ratio for the uncoupling of oxidative phosphorylation by most fatty acids. The principal substrate for these mitochondria is the fatty acid they contain; these fatty acids cannot be activated to form the coenzyme A derivatives in the ATP-dependent activation reaction if the mitochondria are uncoupled and are unable to make ATP. If the isolated mitochondria are provided with co-factors that enable them to remove at least some of the damaging fatty acids (ATP or GTP (HOHORST and RAFAEL, 1968; RAFAEL et al., 1969); ADP plus α-ketoglutarate (RAFAEL et al., 1968); carnitine (HERD and HORWITZ, 1969); ATP plus carnitine (HERD and HORWITZ, 1969; DRAHOTA et al., 1968; HITTELMAN et al., 1969), they show reasonably normal coupled respiration. Brown adipose tissue mitochondria are more sensitive than are liver mitochondria to the inhibitory effects of fatty acids contacted during their isolation (THOMSON et al., 1968; LINDBERG et al., 1968) or added *in vitro* (RAFAEL et al., 1969).

In the light of these recent findings, the existence of the earlier variable reports of isolation of uncoupled, loosely, partially or fully coupled mitochondria from brown adipose tissue is understandable. Most of these reports can be found in a review by HIMMS-HAGEN (1970b). ALDRIDGE and STREET (1968) achieved a very high rate of oxygen uptake by use of an amount of albumin in the isolation, washing and incubation media that presumably permitted a concentration of FFA that was sufficient to stimulate respiration but not sufficient to inhibit it. Higher concentrations of albumin reduced the high rate of respiration, both in isolated mitochondria (ALDRIDGE and STREET, 1968) and in homogenates (KORNACKER and BALL, 1968) presumably because the albumin bound some of the fatty acids needed as substrates and/or stimulators. The role of uncoupling by fatty acids and of re-coupling by translocation or by oxidative removal of the fatty acids in heat production by brown adipose tissue (RAFAEL et al., 1969; HITTELMAN et al., 1969) will be discussed further below.

Thus the *capacity* to consume oxygen, at least of cells and slices, can correspond to that expected for the heat-producing function of this tissue (see criterion (i) above). In these brown adipose tissue preparations the *operation* also behaves as expected (see criterion (ii) above). Thus, basal respiration is low and is stimulated by noradrenaline, an effect mimicked by dBcAMP and by theophylline (see WILLIAMSON et al., 1970; BALL, 1970; FAIN and REED, 1970). This calorigenic effect of noradrenaline is also mimicked by fatty acids over a certain concentration range (see WILLIAMSON et al., 1970; FAIN and REED, 1970; PRUSINER et al., 1968a). The effect of noradrenaline, but not that of added fatty acid, is inhibited by propranolol (LINDBERG et al., 1970). These observations have led to the concept that the calorigenic effect of noradrenaline in this tissue is actually mediated by the rise in fatty acid concentration caused by the accelerated lipolysis.

Although the mechanism underlying the rise in oxygen uptake of brown adipose tissue caused by catecholamines is unknown several explanations have been proposed. In order to discuss such possible mechanisms it is advisable to consider first what is the usual mechanism for the regulation of the oxygen uptake. In most cells most of the time the primary factor influencing the rate of electron transport, and therefore oxygen uptake, is the availability of ADP, one of the substrates for oxidative phosphorylation. A rise in oxygen uptake occurs for two basic reasons: (1) An increase in the availability of ADP. Since ADP is derived from ATP an increase in the supply of ADP can only occur by means of an increased utilization of ATP for energy-consuming reactions. (2) An increased degree of independence of the concentration of ADP. This can take several forms: (a) a complete uncoupling of oxidative phosphorylation by such compounds as DNP, which results in complete lack of phosphorylation; (b) a "loosening" of coupling so that phosphorylation proceeds but relatively independently of electron transport; (c) a utilization of high-energy intermediates of the electron transport system for an energy-consuming reaction such as ion translocation; this differs from the increased utilization of ATP noted in (1) above only in the nature of the high-energy compound used. Of these alternative forms, (b) and (c) most probably represent two aspects of the same process. An increased utilization of some of the high-energy intermediates for a purpose other than phosphorylation of ADP would result in an apparent loosening of coupling.

Several metabolic pathways have been suggested as candidates for a process that results in increased ATP utilization. For example, accelerated operation of the triglyceride cycle, i.e., accelerated lipolysis together with accelerated re-esterification of the fatty acids produced, would have an ATPase-like effect. However, no evidence has been obtained for the occurrence of such an acceleration in brown adipose tissue *in vitro* (see B. VI. b). Similarly, there is no evidence for accelerated operation of other metabolic pathways that might also be considered. Although stimulation by noradrenaline does result in a marked lowering of the ATP/ADP ratio (WILLIAMSON, 1970) and also of the GTP/GDP ratio (PRUSINER et al., 1968b) the time-course of this reduction does not correspond to that of the rise in oxygen uptake. Moreover, noradrenaline can actually raise the ATP content of the cells under conditions where oxidative phosphorylation has been either uncoupled or inhibited, an observation that does not at all support the existence of a postulated ATPase-like pathway. Further evidence against the possibility of stimulation by noradrenaline of a cytoplasmic metabolic pathway with an ATPase-like effect is the observation that atractyloside does not inhibit the effect of noradrenaline to raise oxygen uptake: atractyloside inhibits the translocation of ADP and ATP in and out of the mitochondria and would be expected to inhibit the regeneration of ATP in the mitochondrion from ADP produced in the cytoplasm (WILLIAMSON, 1970; WILLIAMSON et al., 1970).

There seems to be fairly general agreement that the effect of noradrenaline and of the fatty acids to stimulate oxygen uptake falls into the category of (2) (b) or (2) (c), i.e., a form of loosening of the dependence of electron transport on ADP supply without complete ihibition of ATP formation. The suggestion that respiration is primarily controlled by concentration of substrate (see HORWITZ et al., 1970) is unlikely in view of the finding of an increased state of oxidation of respiratory chain components in noradrenaline-stimulated tissue both *in vivo* (PRUSINER et al., 1968c) and *in vitro* (PRUSINER, 1970; WILLIAMSON et al., 1970). The evidence for placing the mechanism in one of these categories rather than in (2) (a) (complete uncoupling) comes mainly from observations of the effects of a variety of inhibitors. Antimycin A inhibits respiration completely and also inhibits any stimulation by noradrenaline or oleate (WILLIAMSON, 1970; LINDBERG et al., 1970); rotenone also inhibits the effects of noradrenaline and of fatty acids (PRUSINER et al., 1968a; LINDBERG et al., 1970). These observations show that a normal respiratory chain is involved and that an NAD-linked substrate is being used. Uncoupling agents such as FCCP (carbonyl cyanide p-trifluoromethoxyphenylhydrazone) and related compounds themselves stimulate the basal respiration of brown adipose tissue cells (WILLIAMSON, 1970; LINDBERG et al., 1970). Such uncoupling agents appear to inhibit noradrenaline-induced stimulation of respiration only when their uncoupling effect is fairly complete. WILLIAMSON has measured the ATP content of cells in the presence of FCCP and found that 40% of the normal ATP content is still present, that the effect of noradrenaline is not completely inhibited under these conditions and that noradrenaline can actually induce an increase in ATP content (WILLIAMSON, 1970; WILLIAMSON et al., 1970). Thus, the basal respiration of these cells appears to be coupled in the usual way, and noradrenaline does not mimic the effect of an uncoupling agent.

Oligomycin inhibits the stimulatory effect of noradrenaline and of fatty acids in brown adipose tissue cells (WILLIAMSON, 1970; PRUSINER, 1970; FAIN and REED, 1970). This effect is interpreted to mean that at least the phosphate uptake step of normal oxidative phosphorylation occurs when the oxygen uptake is stimulated by noradrenaline. However, the inhibition of the noradrenaline response by oligomycin is not relieved by uncoupling, unlike the inhibition of respiration usually induced by oligomycin in other tissues (WILLIAMSON, 1970).

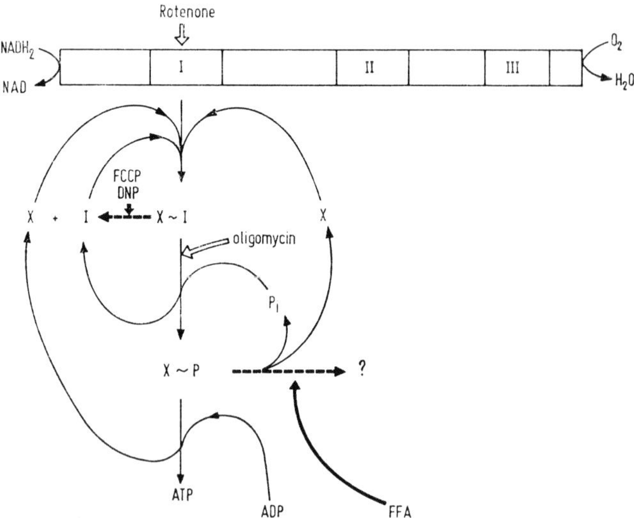

Fig. 7. Suggested mechanism for the action of FFA to "loosen" oxidative phosphorylation from electron transport in mitochondria of brown adipose tissue. See text, section VI.c for discussion

That the substrate-level phosphorylation (of GDP) associated with the tricarboxylic acid cycle is of considerable importance in the calorigenic effect of noradrenaline is suggested by the increase in ATP content produced by noradrenaline in partially uncoupled cells and by the inhibition of this increase caused by arsenite (WILLIAMSON, 1970). Oligomycin and arsenite together cause a very marked decrease of ATP in the cells.

These observations taken together suggest that the fatty acids produced by the increased lipolysis occurring in these cells in response to noradrenaline stimulate the utilization of a high-energy intermediate of oxidative phosphorylation for some unknown purpose. Energy-requiring transport of potassium (FAIN and REED, 1970; REED and FAIN, 1968b) and of calcium (HITTELMAN et al., 1967) have both been suggested as such energy-wasting processes. Figure 7 illustrates a conventional scheme of oxidative phosphorylation with hypothetical phosphorylated intermediates and suggests one possible site of action of the FFA, namely the stimulation of the utilization for some unknown purpose of the intermediate X$\sim$P. This suggestion is compatible with the inhibition by oligomycin, the failure of uncoupling agents to relieve this inhibition and the apparent "looseness" of the coupling. Also in keeping is the observation that phosphate (5 mM) can, under certain conditions, stimulate the respiration of mitochondria isolated from brown adipose tissue (GRAV et al., 1970). A higher concentration of phosphate (16.7 mM) such as that found in Krebs' Ringer phosphate solution, can partially inhibit the effect of noradrenaline (PRUSINER et al., 1968c; WILLIAMSON, 1970); this has been attributed to inhibition by phosphate of the GTP-dependent fatty acid activation (WILLIAMSON, 1970). The lack of inhibition of the stimulation by noradrenaline by atractyloside or by (+)-decanoylcarnitine (WILLIAMSON, 1970; WILLIAMSON et al., 1970) indicates a lack of dependence on either translocation of adenine nucleotides or of activated fatty acids: the means by which fatty acids arrive at the site appropriate for their action is not clear.

That free fatty acids can uncouple oxidative phosphorylation and completely inhibit respiration has been known for many years from studies with liver mitochondria. Mitochondria of brown adipose tissue behave similarly but are considerably more sensitive to low concentrations of fatty acid (RAFAEL et al., 1969). The concentration of fatty acids inside the mitochondrion must be very closely regulated in order to achieve the observed stimulation of respiration and to prevent the swelling, uncoupling and inhibition that would occur with higher concentrations of fatty acid. WILLIAMSON has been unable to detect any changes in intracellular FFA concentration during the stimulation of respiration by noradrenaline (WILLIAMSON, 1970). The compartmentation and activation of fatty acids in liver mitochondria is exceedingly complex and not well understood; however, there appear to be several different compartments, each with its own activating enzyme (see GARLAND et al., 1969; VAN DEN BERGH et al., 1969). Little is known about the detailed mechanism of fatty acid activation and oxidation in mitochondria of brown adipose tissue. However, the recent observation of an apparent intramitochondrial transport of fatty acids which was dependent on ATP and carnitine (HITTELMAN et al., 1969) suggests that the movements of fatty acids between different mitochondrial compartments may play an important role in the regulation of their concentration at the site where they initiate the loosening of the coupling process. In these experiments the apparent translocation of the fatty acids resulted in recoupling of oxidative phosphorylation in mitochondria that otherwise had a P/O ratio of zero (HITTELMAN et al., 1969).

In summary, the calorigenic effect of noradrenaline on brown adipose tissue appears to be due to a carefully controlled "loosening" of oxidative phosphorylation by fatty acids (or possibly by a specific fatty acid) released as a result of its lipolytic action. The mechanism of this "loosening" is not clear but studies with a variety of inhibitors suggest that it is *not* simply an uncoupling of oxidative phosphorylation but rather a utilization of a high-energy intermediate formed subsequent to the oligomycin-sensitive phosphate uptake reaction. Brown adipose tissue mitochondria differ from the mitochondria of other tissues in possessing the capacity to respond to fatty acids in this way. The use, if any, made of the energy liberated is unknown although ion transport is a possibility. Mechanisms of control of fatty acid concentration, by conversion to coenzyme A derivatives and/or translocation between different mitochondrial compartments, are not understood and are only just beginning to be studied. It is clear that an understanding of the mechanism of the calorigenic effect of noradrenaline in this tissue will depend upon an understanding not only of the control of fatty acid transport and metabolism within the cell and within the mitochondria, but also of the mechanism of oxidative phosphorylation and of how this process differs in brown adipose tissue from that in other tissues. Any depth of understanding of this latter appears to be still some distance away.

d) Ultrastructural Changes and Growth

The ultrastructure of the brown adipose tissue is characterized by the abundance of capillaries between the cells and of nerve endings on the cells (Bargmann et al., 1968) and the large number of mitochondria and lipid droplets closely packed into the cells. The appearance of these last two varies according to the functional state of the tissue and it seems likely that noradrenaline, liberated from the nerve endings, plays a role in the induction of these changes in structure. For example, one of the most remarkable features of newborn and fetal rat brown adipose tissue is the presence of dense inclusion bodies in the mitochondria (Suter, 1969a, c and d; Barnard, 1969; Barnard and Lindberg, 1969). These granules appear to be precursors of at least part of the cristae of the mitochondria: their disappearance is associated with the appearance of more closely packed cristae in the mitochondria (Barnard and Lindberg, 1969; Suter and Stäubli, 1970) and a rise in the specific activity of enzymes of the cristae (Skala et al., 1970). These dense granules disappear in 1—2 days in the normal newborn rat but their disappearance is hastened by exposure of the rat to a low temperature (20—22°) and prevented by maintenance of the rat at 37° (Suter, 1969a, c and d). Since the disappearance of the granules is also hastened by injection of noradrenaline or of theophylline or by incubation of isolated tissue with these agents, and since a β-receptor blocking drug (Trasicor) inhibits the disappearance in the cold *in vivo* and in the presence of noradrenaline *in vitro*, it has been suggested that noradrenaline provides the stimulus for the disappearance of the dense granules that occurs shortly after birth (Suter, 1969a and d; Barnard and Lindberg, 1969). However, during the first two days of life newborn rats do not have a functioning nerve supply to either the brown adipose tissue cells or to the blood vessels surrounding them (Derry and Daniel, 1970); they also do not have a functioning adrenal medulla (see Comline and Silver, 1966). It is, therefore, not possible to identify the physiological stimulus to granule disappearance as noradrenaline.

Exposure of older rats to cold for periods sufficiently long for them to become cold acclimated similarly causes the appearance of mitochondria containing tightly packed cristae (Suter, 1969b) together with high specific activities of enzymes of the cristae (Skala et al., 1970), changes which regress slowly when the acclimated rats are returned to the warm (Suter, 1969b). Noradrenaline liberated from nerve endings seems a likely candidate for the stimulus that produces these changes.

Exposure of a rat to cold actually stimulates the growth of the tissue. The new cells are derived from endothelial cells (Cameron and Smith, 1964; see also Smith and Horwitz, 1969), just as the normal brown adipose tissue cells are during differentiation before birth (Barnard, 1969). Thus during adaptation to cold the heat-producing capacity of this tissue can be surmised to become greater because it has more cells, because the cells contain more mitochondria (Skala et al., 1970) and because the mitochondria contain more cristae and respiratory enzymes (Skala et al., 1970).

e) Contribution of the Brown Adipose Tissue to Heat Production in Intact Animals

Although the heat-producing capacity of the brown adipose tissue increases during adaptation to cold the enlarged tissue still comprises less than 1% of the body weight. There are two questions that must be asked: first, what is the contribution of such a small heat-producing tissue to total heat production of the animal?; second, can the very small increase in size of the brown adipose tissue, relative to the size of the animal, account for the very large difference in capacity of cold acclimated animals to respond calorigenically to infusion of noradrenaline? In other words, is the increase in size of the brown adipose tissue an important part of the adaptation for nonshivering thermogenesis?

Several estimates of the contribution of brown adipose tissue to total oxygen uptake in an adapted animal during infusion of noradrenaline or during exposure to cold give values of between 6 and 12% of the total oxygen uptake (HIMMS-HAGEN, 1969b; SMITH et al., 1968; IMAI et al., 1968; HAYWARD and BALL, 1966; JANSKY and HART, 1968; HORWITZ et al., 1968). The total cytochrome oxidase activity in the interscapular brown adipose tissue of a cold acclimated rat (BARNARD et al., 1970) (the value is multiplied by two to correct for measurement at 23°) allows an estimate of a maximum possible contribution of approximately 13% of the total oxygen uptake of such a rat during infusion of noradrenaline (HIMMS-HAGEN, 1969b).

Newborn rabbits have a much larger amount of brown adipose tissue relative to their body weight (about 5%) and this amount can contribute to about 80% of the total heat production during either exposure to cold or during infusion of noradrenaline (HULL and SEGALL, 1965).

In a warm acclimated rat, in which the adaptation for non-shivering thermogenesis is not present to any appreciable extent, and the maximum oxygen uptake induced by infusion of noradrenaline is much smaller, the interscapular brown adipose tissue alone could account for a much larger proportion of the oxygen uptake during infusion of noradrenaline (36%) (HIMMS-HAGEN, 1969b). This is in keeping with the finding of large and rapid changes in oxygen tension of brown adipose tissue of warm acclimated animals when they are exposed to cold (SZELENYI, 1968; DONHOFFER and SZELENYI, 1968). These observations lead to the paradoxical conclusion that the heat-producing capacity of the brown adipose tissue is of greater *quantitative* significance in the warm acclimated animal, which does not possess the adaptation for nonshivering thermogenesis, than it is in the cold acclimated animal which does possess this adaptation. Only in the newborn rabbit is the brown adipose tissue the major heat-producing organ.

However, in the course of experiments designed to estimate the quantitative contribution of the brown adipose tissue to total thermogenic capacity in cold acclimated rats another function of this tissue has become apparent. Immediately after surgical removal of the interscapular brown adipose tissue the total oxygen uptake during infusion of noradrenaline is reduced by no more than 12% (HIMMS-HAGEN, 1969b). Further, within 1—4 days the total oxygen uptake during infusion of noradrenaline is reduced by 40% or more (HIMMS-HAGEN, 1969b; LEDUC and RIVEST, 1969). This slow and progressive loss of noradrenaline-sensitive thermogenic capacity, brought about by removal of a major part of the total brown adipose tissue, has led to the hypothesis that the tissue secretes a factor that alters the properties of other tissues to respond calorigenically to noradrenaline (HIMMS-HAGEN, 1969b). In support of this hypothesis is the finding that implantation of brown adipose tissue in the peritoneal cavity can partially prevent this initial loss (HIMMS-HAGEN, 1970b). It is, unfortunately, impossible to remove brown adipose tissue completely because of its diffuse location. Removal of the interscapular brown adipose tissue prior to exposure of rats to cold delays, but does not abolish, the development of the enhanced calorigenic response to noradrenaline that is characteristic of cold adapted animals:

however, the remaining brown adipose tissue elsewhere in the body (approximately 70% of the total) appears to grow even more than usual in these operated animals and presumably assumes, at least in part, the function of the interscapular brown adipose tissue under these conditions (BONIN and HIMMS-HAGEN, unpublished observations).

f) Summary: Thermogenic and Endocrine Functions of the Brown Adipose Tissue

Brown adipose tissue possesses a remarkable capacity for production of heat. This can be elicited by catecholamines, via stimulation of adenyl cyclase and acceleration of lipolysis. The fatty acids liberated as a consequence of accelerated lipolysis appear to provide both the stimulus for the increased heat production and the fuel to support it. The exact mechanism by which fatty acids can accelerate the rate of respiration is still uncertain but seems to involve a "loosening" of oxidative phosphorylation from electron transport. The mitochondria of brown adipose tissue appear to be unique in their capacity reversibly to "loosen" their oxidative phosphorylation in this way.

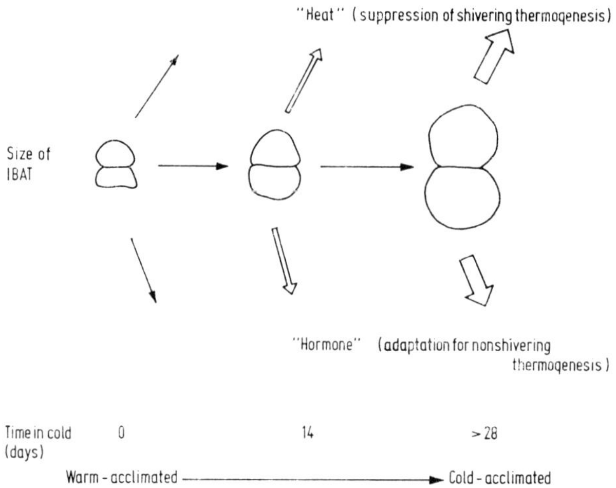

Fig. 8. Diagrammatic representation of the proposed progressive increase in heat-producing and hormone-producing capacities of the interscapular brown adipose tissue (IBAT) of the rat during acclimation to cold. After 4 weeks in the cold shivering is completely suppressed and the adaptation for nonshivering thermogenesis is at its maximum

The heat-producing capacity of this tissue, elicited by sympathetic nerve stimulation during exposure to cold, is particularly important in the maintenance of body temperature in newborn animals, In cold acclimated animals, in which the tissue is in the same adaptive state as in the newborn animals (cells packed with mitochondria, mitochondria packed with cristae, large size of tissue) the contribution of this tissue to total heat production is relatively small: this contribution is, however, important because of the distribution of the heat produced (SMITH and HORWITZ, 1969) and it seems likely that the principal use of the heat "secreted" by the brown adipose tissue is the suppression of shivering by means of the local warming of centres in the spinal cord (WÜNNENBERG and BRÜCK, 1968). In addition to the one secretion product, heat, another appears to be elaborated by brown adipose tissue. The function of this latter is to alter metabolic processes in other tissues so that they too can respond calorigenically to noradrenaline. The nature of this product is unknown but it is tempting to speculate that the unique property of brown adipose tissue mitochondria that allows them to "loosen" their oxidative phosphorylation from electron transport in a highly controlled manner, is somehow conveyed to other tissues so that their metabolism can be modified in a similar way. This idea is illustrated in Fig. 8 which shows in diagrammatic form the growth of brown adipose tissue during adaptation to cold and the progressive increase in "secretion" of heat (having as a consequence the progressive inhibition of shivering) and in secretion of the postulated factor (having as a consequence a progressive increase in the capacity of other tissues to respond to noradrenaline, i.e., the progressive development of nonshivering thermogenesis): all these changes are shown as occurring as a consequence of the excessive and prolonged stimulation of this tissue by noradrenaline.

VII. ß-Cells of Pancreatic Islets

In mammals catecholamines have a direct action on the β-cells of the pancreatic islets to inhibit the secretion of insulin. In view of the well known consequences of the lack of insulin in the intact animal it can be readily seen that this action of catecholamines can have pronounced effects on metabolic processes in most tissues, if for no other reason than because of the marked rises in blood glucose and FFA concentrations which result. Both reinforce the hyperglycemia due to the action of catecholamines on the liver and the rise in FFA concentration due to the action of catecholamines on adipose tissue.

Although an action of adrenaline to inhibit the secretion of insulin was suggested over 40 years ago (COLWELL and BRIGHT, 1930) it was only when modern techniques for accurately measuring insulin concentrations in plasma became available that this could be established (PORTE et al., 1965). The problem of the mechanism of regulation of insulin secretion is an old one, which is again receiving considerable attention in the light of present interest in the role of the catecholamines and of the adenyl cyclase system in this regulation. It is still not understood in detail and is obviously far more complex than originally supposed (for recent reviews see RENOLD, 1970; MAYHEW et al., 1969).

a) Adenyl Cyclase

No direct measurements of the activity of adenyl cyclase in normal islet tissue have been reported. However, adenyl cyclase has been measured in an insulin-producing islet cell adenoma (hamster) and found to be stimulated by glucagon (COHEN and BITENSKY, 1969). The cAMP content of incubated pancreatic islets is increased by theophylline and also by glucagon; however, adrenaline reduces the content of cAMP in the presence of theophylline (TURTLE and KIPNIS, 1967). In their response to catecholamines the pancreatic islets are, therefore, most unusual in that the predominant effect of adrenaline is an inhibition of adenyl cyclase. This inhibitory effect is prevented by α-adrenergic blockade (with phentolamine) but not by β-adrenergic blockade (with propranolol) (TURTLE and KIPNIS, 1967).

b) Effects of Changes in Adenyl Cyclase Activity on the Secretion of Insulin (Fig. 9)

Little or nothing is known about enzymes of the pancreatic islet β-cells that may be stimulated by cAMP although it is reasonable to suppose that such enzymes exist. The sole parameter of cAMP action that is readily accessible to observation is the secretion of insulin, the end-result of what must be a complex series of changes in intracellular regulation. The secretion of insulin by isolated islets can be increased by exogenous cAMP (Malaisse et al., 1967a); a similar effect of cAMP occurs in perfused pancreas (Sussmann and Vaughan, 1967).

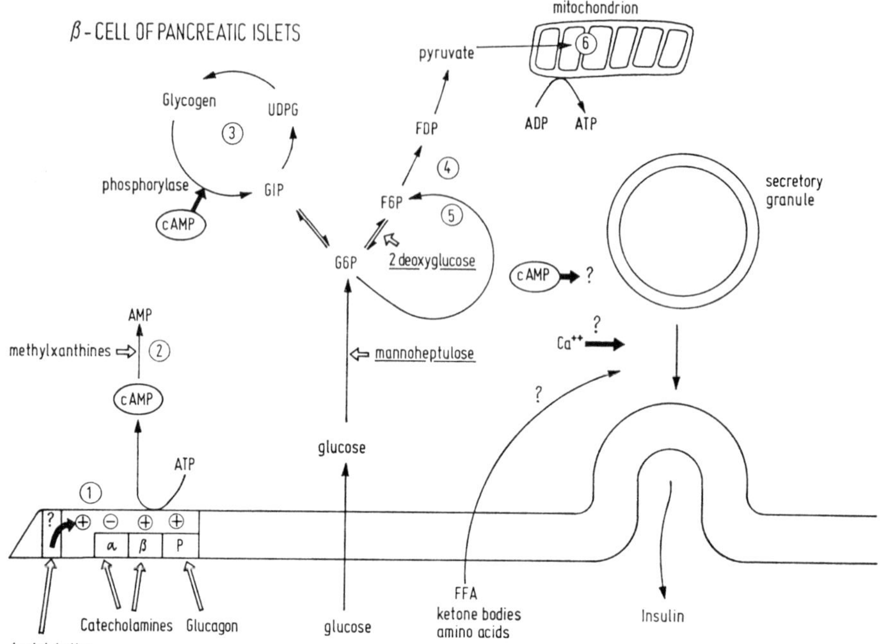

Fig. 9. *Summary of metabolic and other processes in β-cells of pancreatic islets known to be influenced by catecholamines.* Adenyl cyclase (1) is shown to be present in the cell membrane and associated with several "receptors". The four "receptors" shown are sensitive to peptide hormones (P), to an action of catecholamines that results in inhibition of adenyl cyclase (*α*), to an action of catecholamines that results in stimulation of adenyl cyclase (*β*) and possibly to an action of parasympathomimetic agents that results in stimulation of adenyl cyclase. (2) denotes cAMP phosphodiesterase. The glycogen cycle is present (3) but appreciable quantities of glycogen are not normally stored. Exogenous glucose is usually metabolized via glycolysis (4) and the pentose phosphate pathway (5). The sites of action of two commonly used inhibitors of glucose metabolism (mannoheptulose and 2-deoxyglucose) are shown. (6) represents oxidation of pyruvate to CO_2 in the mitochondrion. Insulin secretion occurs by the transfer of the contents of the secretory granules to the exterior of the cell, possibly by fusion of their membrane with the cell membrane (see Lacy et al., 1968b). The exact nature of the link between metabolic processes and secretion is uncertain. Both cAMP and calcium ions seem to be involved

However, for reasons that are not understood, this effect is not always seen (Lacy et al., 1968a). Other stimuli that are now known to raise the cAMP content of the islets also cause secretion of insulin. For example, theophylline (Turtle and Kipnis, 1967; Malaisse et al., 1967a; Wong et al., 1967) and caffeine (Lambert et al., 1967) stimute insulin secretion although, again for unknown reasons, not under all conditions (Sussmann and Vaughan, 1967; Lacy et al., 1968a). Glucagon also raises cAMP concentration (Turtle and Kipnis, 1967) and stimulates the secretion of insulin (Turtle and Kipnis, 1967; Malaisse et al., 1967a; Devrim and Recant, 1966; Lambert et al., 1967; Sussmann and Vaughan, 1967; Lacy et al., 1968a; Grodsky et al., 1967). Adrenaline reduces cAMP content (Turtle and Kipnis, 1967) and inhibits insulin secretion (Turtle and

Kipnis, 1967; Coore and Randle, 1964; Malaisse et al., 1967a and b; Wong et al., 1967; Edgar et al., 1969) as also does noradrenaline (Wong et al.,1967; Malaisse et al., 1967b). Like the effect on cAMP content, this effect of adrenaline to inhibit insulin secretion is prevented by α-receptor blocking agents (phentolamine: Turtle and Kipnis, 1967; Malaisse et al., 1967b; phenoxybenzamine: Malaisse et al., 1967b). However, although the predominant effect of adrenaline is an inhibitory one, a stimulatory effect can be uncovered by the use of blocking agents. In the presence of phentolamine, adrenaline (with theophylline) stimulates insulin secretion (Turtle and Kipnis, 1967). Isopropylnoradrenaline alone may stimulate insulin secretion at low concentrations of glucose (Gagliardino et al., 1968) while its inhibitory effect at higher concentrations of glucose can be reversed to a stimulation of insulin secretion by phenoxybenzamine (Malaisse et al., 1967a). The inhibition of insulin secretion by adrenaline is actually potentiated by β-receptor blocking agents (propranolol: Turtle and Kipnis, 1967).

A variety of other compounds can stimulate the secretion of insulin *in vitro*, in addition to glucose. These include fatty acids, ketone bodies, various amino acids, and other metabolites derived from these compounds (Malaisse and Malaisse-Lagae, 1968; Edgar et al., 1969; Renold, 1970). Moreover, the effects of these stimuli interact with the adenyl cyclase system as indicated by the enhancement by theophylline of the stimulatory effect of glucose (Malaisse et al., 1967a; Lambert et al., 1969a; Renold, 1970) and of amino acids (Malaisse and Malaisse-Lagae, 1968) and by the inhibition by adrenaline of the effects of glucose and arginine (Edgar et al., 1969).

The mechanism of insulin secretion is not understood. It appears to involve movement of storage granules to the surface of the cell where their contents are discharged (see Lacy et al., 1968b; Renold, 1970). This movement is initiated by metabolic changes within the cell, but the link between metabolism and secretion is unknown. Recently considerable interest has developed in the role of ions, particularly calcium, in providing this missing link (Rasmussen and Tenenhouse, 1968). Calcium is necessary for the stimulation of insulin secretion by glucose (Curry et al., 1968; Grodsky and Bennett, 1966) and by glucose plus caffeine (Lambert et al., 1969b) and when added to a calcium-depleted pancreas can actually stimulate the secretion of insulin (Curry et al., 1968). Recent observations of an effect of cAMP on calcium transport into sarcoplasmic reticulum of heart (see B. III. c) suggest a similar role for this compound in other tissues. No information is, however, at present available about calcium movements associated with secretion of insulin although a role for cAMP-induced movements of this cation in insulin secretion has been suggested (Lambert et al., 1969b). Adrenaline inhibits the uptake of calcium by pancreatic islets incubated in the presence of glucose (Malaisse-Lagae et al., 1969). This suggests that calcium entry into a specific cellular compartment may be involved in the initiation of insulin secretion and that adrenaline, *via* inhibition of adenyl cyclase, inhibits the entry of this cation. It is of interest in this connection that the secretion of insulin induced by dBcAMP (in mice *in vivo*) is blocked equally well by the β-adrenergic blocking agent (—)sotalol and by its isomer, (+)sotalol, which is not a β-receptor blocking agent (Bressler et al., 1969); likewise both (—) and (+) propranolol can block the effect of tolbutamide to stimulate secretion of insulin *in vivo*. These agents have antirrhytmic effects on the heart which are not associated with their β-adrenergic blocking activity but rather with inhibition of calcium uptake by sarcoplasmic reticulum (see section B. III. c and Scales and McIntosh, 1968a and b). It is tempting to suppose that they have a similar effect in pancreatic islets and that this is the basis for their inhibitory effect on insulin secretion.

c) Role of Catecholamines in the Regulation of Insulin Secretion in Intact Animals

A remarkably wide variety of compounds can influence the secretion of insulin in intact animals. Compounds which stimulate its secretion include glucose, FFA (SEYFFERT and MADISON, 1967; CRESPIN et al., 1969; GREENOUGH et al., 1967), ketone bodies, amino acids, intestinal hormones such as pancreozymin and secretin (ALLAN and TEPPERMAN, 1969; UNGER et al., 1967) and other hormones such as glucagon (CAMPBELL and RASTOGI, 1966; PORTE, 1967b; ALLAN and TEPPERMAN, 1969) and ACTH (LEBOVITZ and POOLER, 1967). That parasympathetic nerve stimulation also increases insulin secretion is indicated by the atropine-sensitive stimulatory effect of administered parasympathomimetic compounds *in vivo* (KAJINUMA et al., 1968) and *in vitro* (MALAISSE et al., 1967b) and by the increase in insulin secretion produced by vagal stimulation both *in vitro* (FINDLAY et al., 1969) and *in vivo* (KANETO et al., 1967; FROHMAN et al., 1967; DANIEL and HENDERSON, 1967). The sensitivity of pancreatic islets to these different stimuli varies according to the species. For example, the islet cells of ruminants are not very sensitive to glucose or to ketone bodies but are very sensitive to short chain fatty acids such as propionate and butyrate (HORINO et al., 1968). A raised FFA concentration can not only stimulate the secretion of insulin but can also inhibit the secretion of glucagon by the neighbouring α-cells of the islets (EDWARDS et al., 1969; LUYCKX and LEFEBVRE, 1970; MADISON et al., 1968).

A regulatory effect of endogenous adrenaline or noradrenaline must be considered against this background of the multiplicity of stimuli to insulin secretion. Activation of the sympathetic nervous system would be expected not only to produce an inhibition of insulin secretion but also to produce an increase in the concentration in blood of several compounds which stimulate insulin secretion (glucose, FFA, ketone bodies); indeed, the physiological function of the inhibition becomes apparent when considered as the prevention of the rise in insulin secretion that would normally occur in response to raised concentrations of these compounds. This inhibition by the catecholamines allows the pancreas to respond to the increased availability of substrate in the blood due to ingestion of a meal in the opposite way from the way it responds to the increased availability of substrate in the blood due to the sympathetic-mediated "fight or flight" reaction.

In order to consider the question of the existence of sympathetic tone in the basal regulation of insulin secretion, evidence for which comes mainly from the use of blocking agents, it is necessary first to consider briefly the effects of blocking agents on the secretion of insulin in the intact animal. Infusion of adrenaline or noradrenaline inhibits the rise in plasma insulin that would otherwise occur in response to hyperglycemia, produced either by the adrenaline itself or by administered glucose (PORTE et al., 1966; PORTE and WILLIAMS, 1966; KARAM et al., 1966; HERTELENDY et al., 1966; KRIS et al., 1966; CAMPBELL and RASTOGI, 1966). α-Adrenergic blockade with phentolamine prevents the inhibition and permits a rise in plasma insulin concentration (PORTE, 1967a; KANSAL and BUSE, 1967) whereas β-adrenergic blockade (with propranolol) potentiates the inhibition (PORTE, 1967a): stimulation of β-adrenergic receptors (with isopropylnoradrenaline) increases plasma insulin concentration (PORTE, 1967b).

Attempts to assess the extent to which catecholamines exert a tonic inhibitory effect on insulin secretion under basal conditions have employed the α-receptor blocking agent, phentolamine. Phentolamine does raise plasma insulin concentration (FROHMAN et al., 1967; SENFT et al., 1968c; WERRBACH et al., 1970;

BRESSLER et al., 1969) and potentiates the rise in insulin concentration produced by glucose (BUSE et al., 1970) or by theophylline (TURTLE et al., 1967). This can be interpreted as evidence for a continuous basal inhibition of insulin secretion by the catecholamines. However, it should be remembered that phentolamine also has other effects in intact animals. It raises plasma FFA concentration (BOSHART et al., 1965) and raises plasma lactate concentration by producing activation of muscle glycogenolysis (SALVADOR et al., 1968), both effects apparently due to increased catecholamine secretion, principally from the adrenal medulla (BOSHART et al., 1965; SALVADOR et al., 1968); it also raises plasma corticosterone concentration in rats (GOVIER et al., 1969). Thus, phentolamine may not only prevent the action of endogenous catecholamines to inhibit secretion of insulin but may at the same time cause the appearance in the blood of FFA which can stimulate insulin secretion. That a hypoglycemia ensues (SENFT et al., 1968c; SALVADOR et al., 1968) is probably due to the increased secretion of insulin. However, it is not clear to what extent the increased insulin secretion can really be attributed to reduction of sympathetic tone and to what extent it is due to stimulation of insulin secretion by the raised FFA concentration. Unfortunately, the use of β-receptor blocking agents to prevent the rise in plasma FFA concentration would not be helpful in resolving this question because these agents also block the rise in insulin secretion produced by a variety of other stimuli, including the administration of phentolamine (BRESSLER et al., 1969). It would be interesting to know what the effect of phentolamine on insulin secretion would be during the blockade of FFA release with an agent such as nicotinic acid.

Despite the above considerations there does appear to be little doubt that under a variety of conditions in which the sympathetic nervous system is activated inhibition of insulin secretion does occur as a consequence of the effect of adrenaline and/or noradrenaline on the pancreatic islets.

VIII. Salivary Glands

Salivary glands respond to the action of catecholamines by increasing their secretion of amylase. Zymogen granules move to the surface of the cell where their membrane fuses with the cell membrane: their contents are released and, as a consequence of the addition of zymogen granule membrane, the lumen becomes much larger (AMSTERDAM et al., 1969). This secretory process is accompanied and followed by resynthesis of the stored material. The rate of resynthesis itself is also stimulated by the catecholamines and is independent of their effect to stimulate secretion. The restoration of amylase content is associated with the uptake of lumen membrane into the cell.

If the stimulation by catecholamines is sufficiently great, sufficiently prolonged, or repeated often enough, an increase in size occurs due to a growth of the tissue. The salivary gland is not unique in its ability to grow in response to the chronic actions of catecholamines, since this ability is shared by the brown adipose tissue (see section B. VI. d). In neither case, however, is the biochemical basis of this response understood.

a) Adenyl Cyclase

Noradrenaline and isopropylnoradrenaline stimulate the adenyl cyclase of salivary glands *in vitro* (WOLFE et al., 1969): isopropylnoradrenaline has been observed to stimulate the adenyl cyclase of parotid glands of mice shortly after its injection (MALAMUD, 1969). Adrenaline increases the cAMP content of slices of rat parotid gland (RASMUSSEN and TENENHOUSE, 1968) and both dBcAMP and theophylline mimic the effects of the catecholamines to stimulate secretion of amylase; cAMP itself is ineffective in stimulating amylase secretion probably because of its failure to enter the cell (BDOLAH and SCHRAMM, 1965).

b) Metabolic Changes Associated with the Secretion and Resynthesis of Amylase

Stimulation of amylase secretion by adrenaline is clearly an energy-requiring process since it is inhibited when respiration and/or oxidative phosphorylation are blocked (with KCN, DNP or anaerobic conditions: BDOLAH et al., 1964; with oligomycin: BABAD et al., 1967). As in most tissues oxidative phosphorylation appears to be the major source of ATP in salivary glands and the contribution of glycolysis is of minor importance (FEINSTEIN and SCHRAMM, 1970). Glycolysis appears to provide very little of the energy for secretion, since the presence of glucose, with or without insulin, has no influence on the stimulation of secretion by adrenaline, and since iodoacetate does not inhibit the stimulation (BDOLAH et al., 1964). β-Hydroxybutyrate is the best substrate so far found for the support of the prolonged stimulation of amylase secretion *in vitro* (BABAD et al., 1967); however, the nature of the substrate used as the major source of energy by the gland *in vivo* in unknown. Adrenaline actually increases the rate of respiration of the salivary gland *in vitro* (BABAD et al., 1967; HAGEN, 1959). Since DNP also inhibits the stimulatory effects of both dBcAMP (BABAD et al., 1967) and theophylline (BDOLAH and SCHRAMM, 1965), ATP must be required not only for the activation by the catecholamines of adenyl cyclase, but also for the secretory process itself or for its activation by cAMP.

Calcium is necessary for stimulation by catecholamines of amylase secretion (RASMUSSEN and TENENHOUSE, 1968; DOUGLAS and POISNER, 1963). Since calcium is not required for the stimulation by adrenaline of cAMP formation the calcium probably has a role at a step between cAMP formation and the secretory process (RASMUSSEN and TENENHOUSE, 1968). The observed binding of cAMP to the smooth membranes of the salivary gland endoplasmic reticulum may also be related to this intermediate step (SALOMON and SCHRAMM, 1970). One report suggesting that calcium was not necessary for secretion (BDOLAH and SCHRAMM, 1964) may have an explanation in the exceedingly high calcium content of the gland (FEINSTEIN and SCHRAMM, 1970) which probably makes complete depletion of calcium difficult to achieve. Potassium is also necessary for the stimulation of amylase secretion by adrenaline (BDOLAH et al., 1964) and high concentrations of potassium mimic the effect of adrenaline on cAMP accumulation (RASMUSSEN and TENENHOUSE, 1968) and on amylase secretion (BDOLAH et al., 1964). There is some question as to whether the potassium acts directly or not on the adenyl cyclase since there is some evidence that this effect of potassium may be due, at least in part, to release of endogenous catecholamines (SCHRAMM, 1968).

The receptors for amylase secretion appear to be typical β-receptors since the stimulation by catecholamines is inhibited by the β-receptor blocking agents pronethalol and propranolol (SCHRAMM, 1968) but is not altered by the α-receptor blocking agents phentolamine (SCHRAMM, 1968) or dibenamine (HAGEN, 1959). Blocking agents do not alter the stimulatory effects of dBcAMP or theophylline (SCHRAMM, 1968).

Because a depletion of amylase occurs as a consequence of the stimulation of amylase secretion by the catecholamines, the restorative process is necessarily accompanied by an increased synthesis of amylase (BYRT, 1966; SIMSON, 1969). The amylase that is secreted in response to stimulation by catecholamines is that stored in the zymogen granules and not the newly synthesized amylase (BDOLAH et al., 1964; SCHRAMM and BDOLAH, 1964). However, adrenaline does have a direct stimulatory effect on the synthesis of amylase. This is demonstrable in slices and is mimicked by dBcAMP (GRAND and GROSS, 1969). Even when no further secretion of amylase can be produced by adrenaline because the glands are exhausted and have no further zymogen granules to secrete and one would expect the synthesis of amylase to be proceeding as rapidly as possible, adrenaline can still produce an acceleration of synthesis of new amylase. Thus the stimulation of amylase synthesis is not secondary to the secretory process itself. What is more, the increase in protein synthesis can occur in the absence of RNA synthesis, as indicated by the persistence of the stimulation of protein synthesis by adrenaline in slices in which RNA synthesis has been almost completely inhibited by actinomycin, either added to the incubation medium or injected into the animals 9 hours before. This suggests that cAMP stimulates protein synthesis at the translation level, i.e., it stimulates the reading of the mRNA, and that the mRNA template for synthesis of amylase in salivary gland is fairly stable (GRAND and GROSS, 1970).

Measurement of the stimulation of protein synthesis by adrenaline in salivary glands is complicated by the independent effect of this catecholamine to inhibit amino acid transport into the cells; this latter effect can be eliminated by washing off the adrenaline whereas the stimulation of amylase synthesis persists much longer. It seems likely that the inhibition of amino acid transport is due to a fairly direct interaction of adrenaline with the salivary gland cell membrane itself and is not due to cAMP accumulation (GRAND and GROSS, 1969; GRAND, 1969).

c) Metabolic Changes Associated with the Catecholamine-induced Growth of Salivary Glands

About 10 years ago the observation was first made that the administration of a large dose of isopropylnoradrenaline can lead to an enlargement of the salivary glands in rats (SELYE et al., 1961) and in mice (BROWN-GRANT, 1961). This observation has been repeatedly confirmed since that time. The increased size of the gland is due to both hypertrophy and hyperplasia (SELYE et al., 1961). An enlargement of salivary glands mediated by the sympathetic nervous system and occurring in response to tooth amputation had been observed previously (WELLS et al., 1959a and b; WELLS, 1962).

The administration of a large dose of isopropylnoradrenaline is followed approximately 24 hours later by an increase in the synthesis of DNA in salivary glands and somewhat later still by an increase in the rate of mitosis (BARKA, 1965a and b; BASERGA, 1966; BASERGA and HEFFLER, 1967; WHITLOCK et al., 1968). The time between injection and increased DNA synthesis shortens progressively when repeated injections of isopropylnoradrenaline are given (BARKA 1970; RADLEY, 1968) and even occurs in adrenalectomized rats (MALAMUD and BASERGA, 1967). The response of the salivary gland to isopropylnoradrenaline, is therefore suitable for the study of the mechanisms of stimulated DNA synthesis (SASAKI et al., 1969). However, the stimulatory effect of the catecholamines on the synthesis of amylase, which occurs whether or not accelerated mitosis occurs at a later stage, must accompany the early stage of the stimulation of DNA synthesis; this renders the search for an early stimulation of synthesis of a specific protein which precedes and is a prerequisite for stimulation of DNA synthesis (see SASAKI et al., 1969) rather difficult.

The synthesis of protein in salivary glands is increased shortly after the administration of isopropylnoradrenaline (MAYFIELD et al., 1968; SASAKI et al.,

1969). Administration of inhibitors of protein synthesis (puromycin, cycloheximide, Sasaki et al., 1969; 5-fluorophenylalanine, Baserga, 1966) shortly before or after the administration of isopropylnoradrenaline prevents the delayed increase in DNA synthesis; this suggests that in salivary glands, as is thought to be the case in other tissues, an early step in the stimulation of cell division is the formation of a specific protein. Temporary inhibition of protein synthesis with cycloheximide does not prevent the subsequent resynthesis of amylase but does prevent the changes responsible for the stimulation of DNA synthesis.

The increase in protein synthesis appears to occur predominantly on the free, rather than on the membrane-bound, ribosomes (Sasaki et al., 1969). However, the study of ribosomes isolated from stimulated glands (Sasaki et al., 1969; Robinovitch et al., 1969) may be complicated by the contamination of the preparation with ribonuclease, a component of the zymogen granules of the gland. Although increased numbers of polyribosomes and increased synthetic activity of the free ribosome fraction occur 1 and 8 hours after the administration of isopropylnoradrenaline (Sasaki et al., 1969) it is not clear to what extent these changes reflect decreased contamination of the preparation with ribonuclease (Robinovitch et al., 1969). Thus although there is no doubt that accelerated protein synthesis does occur as a direct response to stimulation by the catecholamines the extent to which this can be studied in cell-free preparations is uncertain.

Changes in enzyme activity in the catecholamine-stimulated gland include increases in thymidine kinase (Barka, 1965b; Whitlock et al., 1968), in DNA polymerase (Barka, 1965b), in peroxidase (Martin and Baserga, 1969) and in aspartate transcarbamylase, dihydroorotase, OMP pyrophosphorylase and OMP decarboxylase (Mayfield et al., 1968).

Another effect of the stimulation by isopropylnoradrenaline is an early increase in incorporation of ^{3}H-uridine into RNA of the salivary gland (Barka, 1966; Baserga and Heffler, 1967; Mayfield et al., 1968; Malamud and Baserga, 1969). Even though fluctuations in specific activity and pool size of the precursor (UTP) render the interpretation of such observations difficult (Baserga and Heffler, 1967; Malamud and Baserga, 1969), nevertheless the 8-fold increase in incorporation of uridine into nuclear RNA and lack of increase in microsomal RNA (Barka, 1966) do suggest a specific increase in nuclear RNA synthesis. Inhibition of RNA synthesis with actinomycin (Baserga and Heffler, 1967; Whitlock et al., 1968) also prevents the later increase in DNA synthesis.

Thus it may be concluded that the events set in train by the stimulation of the salivary gland by isopropylnoradrenaline which result in increased synthesis of DNA and mitosis include the synthesis of a specific protein, the synthesis of RNA and the synthesis of DNA, plus the synthesis of enzymes associated with the synthesis of these compounds. The exact sequence of events and the possible role of cAMP remain to be established. That theophylline potentiates the effect of small doses of isopropylnoradrenaline to increase DNA synthesis has been considered as evidence that cAMP is involved (Malamud, 1969) and this is supported by the observation that theophylline, administered repeatedly to rats, can also cause salivary gland enlargement (Wells, 1967). However, an attempt to dissociate stimulation of DNA synthesis from stimulation of amylase secretion by the use of a series of analogues of isopropylnoradrenaline was apparently successful (Kirby et al., 1969): amylase secretion could be stimulated without stimulation of DNA synthesis although the reverse could not be achieved. This might have been predicted from the known difficulty in producing salivary gland enlargement with noradrenaline (Campos and Parr, 1968) although this catecholamine does stimulate secretion of amylase. Stimulation of DNA synthesis may occur only as a result of excessive and prolonged stimulation of adenyl cyclase, achievable with isopropylnoradrenaline itself and with some of its analogues but not with others.

IX. Brain

Brain is a tissue in which the catecholamine-responsive adenyl cyclase system exists but the metabolic consequences of activation of this system by the catecholamines are poorly understood and the functional consequences are unknown. Brain contains adenyl cyclase and cAMP phosphodiesterase in fairly high concentrations (see RALL and KAKIUCHI, 1966). Moreover, adenyl cyclase activity is stimulated by a variety of compounds present in brain, including catecholamines, and is also stimulated by electrical impulses. However, because no parameter of brain function can be measured *in vitro* the significance of changes in the activity of the adenyl cyclase system is unknown. There are to be sure metabolic consequences of such changes but whether they are in themselves important physiologically or only incidental to some other function of the brain influenced by cAMP is unknown (see KAKIUCHI et al., 1969).

a) Adenyl Cyclase

Adenyl cyclase is present to a varying extent in different regions of the brain (WEISS and COSTA, 1968a) and is stimulated by catecholamines (KLAINER et al., 1962; SHIMIZU et al., 1969) and by histamine (SHIMIZU et al., 1969). For such stimulation the adenyl cyclase requires calcium but the enzyme is inhibited by excess calcium (BRADHAM et al., 1970).

The cAMP content of brain slices is increased by noradrenaline (KAKIUCHI and RALL, 1968a and b; KAKIUCHI et al., 1969) an effect that is potentiated by theophylline, inhibited by DCI and not altered by phenoxybenzamine (KAKIUCHI and RALL, 1968a). Electrical stimulation of slices likewise raises their cAMP content (KAKIUCHI et al., 1969). However, the effect of electrical stimulation differs from the effect of noradrenaline in that the rise in cAMP content is inhibited by theophylline (KAKIUCHI et al., 1969): the increase in cAMP caused by other depolarizing agents (batrachotoxin, veratridine, ouabain, potassium), like that caused by electrical stimulation, is also inhibited by theophylline (SHIMIZU et al., 1970a and b) but the mechanisms underlying this action of theophylline are not understood. Brain slices release adenosine in response to such depolarizing stimuli (SHIMIZU et al., 1970b) and the adenosine itself actually increases cAMP formation and potentiates the effect of noradrenaline (SHIMIZU et al., 1970b; SATTIN and RALL, 1970).

Brain contains a cAMP phosphodiesterase which differs from adenyl cyclase in its intracellular location. Adenyl cyclase is localized principally in a membranous fraction; cAMP phosphodiesterase is localized both in membranes and in a soluble fraction (DE ROBERTIS et al., 1967). The phosphodiesterase is fairly specific for cAMP and does not hydrolyze dBcAMP (DRUMMOND and POWELL, 1970). It is inhibited by a variety of nucleotides as well as by pyrophosphate, citrate and methylxanthines (CHEUNG, 1967). Adenosine is a rather weak inhibitor of this enzyme (SATTIN and RALL, 1970). Much of the phosphodiesterase of brain appears to be present in an inactive form but its activity can be unmasked by detergents (CHEUNG and SALGANICOFF, 1967), by snake venom (CHEUNG, 1969) or by an endogenous activator that appears to be a protein (CHEUNG, 1969, 1970).

b) Metabolic Consequences of the Formation of cAMP in Brain

cAMP stimulates a protein kinase in brain which is active at very low concentrations of cAMP (MIYAMOTO et al., 1969a and b; WELLER and RODNIGHT, 1970). The kinase studied by WELLER and RODNIGHT (1970) is of great interest because it is itself present in a membrane and phosphorylates seryl residues of a membrane-bound protein. At present however there is no physiological explanation for the presence of a cAMP-dependent phosphorylation of brain membranes.

Another cAMP-dependent protein kinase has also been isolated from brain in a highly purified form (MIYAMOTO et al., 1969a and b). One very interesting characteristic of this enzyme is worthy of mention, namely, that the stimulation of its activity by cAMP can be reduced by calcium, the inhibition being greater the lower the magnesium concentration: at low concentrations of magnesium cAMP actually inhibits the enzyme in the presence of calcium; ADP and adenosine also inhibit this enzyme (MIYAMOTO et al., 1969b).

In the present state of our knowledge it is difficult to attribute any metabolic consequences to the rise in cAMP concentration produced by catecholamines in the brain. Despite the large increase in cAMP content even phosphorylase is not activated as it is in other tissue slices stimulated by noradrenaline (KAKIUCHI and RALL, 1968b). Although phosphorylase is converted to the *a* form very rapidly in anoxic brains, maximum activation being apparent in only 5 sec, the concentration of cAMP at this time is low and may continue to rise for about 2 min (KAKIUCHI and RALL, 1968b; BRECKENRIDGE, 1964). Moreover, anoxia has exactly the opposite effect on glycogen synthetase from what would be expected if the changes in cAMP concentration were to influence the activation of this enzyme since the proportion in the *a* form is increased (GOLDBERG and O'TOOLE, 1969).

X. Pineal Gland

The pineal gland is of interest in the context of the present review because its function and, therefore, its metabolism, appear to be regulated principally by the sympathetic nervous system. The pineal has a rich sympathetic innervation in most species (KAPPERS, 1960; OWMAN, 1968) although not in man (OWMAN, 1968). Since the rat is the only species so far studied in any detail the discussion that follows should be taken as applying solely to the rat.

The pineal gland synthesizes melatonin; one activity of this hormone is to exert a control of the oestrous cycle and of the growth of the ovaries; the evidence for this hormonal function is largely indirect since melatonin itself has not been detected in the blood stream and variations in its secretion have not, therefore, been measured directly (see WURTMAN and AXELROD, 1968; AXELROD and WURTMAN, 1968). Environmental lighting is the principal factor influencing the activity of the pineal gland via its sympathetic innervation. However, in the past it has not been clear whether light exerts its influence by increasing or decreasing the discharge of noradrenaline from the sympathetic nerves to the pineal gland. Most authors are non-committal on this point, although implying an increased sympathetic discharge in light (see AXELROD and WURTMAN, 1968), whereas others suggest that there is a decreased sympathetic stimulation of the gland in the light (see WEISS, 1969b). Recently, direct measurements of electrical activity in postganglionic fibres in the pineal gland have been reported (TAYLOR and WILSON, 1970) that indicate that light depresses sympathetic stimulation of this organ; this effect of light is mediated by the retina and the superior cervical ganglion. In the discussion which follows it is asumed that sympathetic stimulation of the pineal gland occurs principally in the dark.

a) Adenyl Cyclase

Adenyl cyclase is present in particulate fractions derived from homogenates of rat pineal whereas cAMP phosphodiesterase is present in soluble fractions (WEISS and COSTA, 1968a). The adenyl cyclase is stimulated equally well by noradrenaline, adrenaline or isopropylnoradrenaline; the stimulation by noradrenaline is inhibited by propranolol and by DCI but not by phentolamine or by phenoxybenzamine (WEISS and COSTA, 1968b). Stimulation of this enzyme by fluoride is not blocked by any of these agents (WEISS, 1969a).

The pineal gland is one of the few tissues in which a modification of the amount of hormone-sensitive adenyl cyclase can be demonstrated. Continuous exposure of rats to light for nine days causes an increase in the amount of pineal adenyl cyclase measured either in the presence of noradrenaline or in the presence of fluoride (WEISS, 1969b). Denervation of the gland also causes a progressive rise in the amount of adenyl cyclase activity which reaches a maximum only in 4—6 weeks (WEISS, 1969b). A variation in the amount of adenyl cyclase during the oestrous cycle can be correlated with an effect of ovarian hormones to reduce the amount of adenyl cyclase (WEISS and CRAYTON, 1970). It should be noted that an increase in the amount of adenyl cyclase should not be equated with an increased functional activity of this enzyme in the intact animal. The amount of enzyme will determine the capacity of the gland to respond to noradrenaline by an increase in cAMP production whereas the catalytic activity actually expressed will depend upon the extent of stimulation by noradrenaline.

b) cAMP and Enzymes of the Pineal Gland

No direct and rapid effect of cAMP on any pineal enzyme has as yet been demonstrated. In particular it does not alter the activity of hydroxyindole-O-methyltransferase (HIOMT) (KLEIN et al., 1970a) or the activity of 5-hydroxytryptamine N-acetyltransferase (KLEIN et al., 1970b). A role for cAMP in pineal gland function is suggested only by the similarity between the slow effects of noradrenaline (described below) and the slow effects of dBcAMP on metabolic pathways in cultured pineal glands.

c) Effects of Noradrenaline and/or cAMP on Pathways of Indolalkylamine Metabolism in Pineal Gland

The synthesis of ^{14}C-melatonin from added ^{14}C-tryptophan in cultured pineal glands is increased by both noradrenaline (SHEIN and WURTMAN, 1969; AXELROD et al., 1969) and by dBcAMP (SHEIN and WURTMAN, 1969; KLEIN et al., 1970a). This effect is slow, being scarcely apparent after 4 hours of incubation and clearly evident only after 16 hours (SHEIN and WURTMAN, 1969). Conversion of ^{14}C-5-hydroxytryptamine to ^{14}C-melatonin is also increased by dBcAMP (KLEIN et al., 1970a); this suggests that the activity of one of the two enzymes involved in the conversion of 5-hydroxytryptamine to melatonin may be involved (Fig. 10). However, as noted above, no direct effect of dBcAMP on HIOMT activity or on N-acetyltransferase activity has been observed.

In earlier studies HIOMT was considered as the rate-limiting step in the pathway of melatonin synthesis (see WURTMAN and AXELROD, 1968) and emphasis was placed upon measurements of the activity of this enzyme under conditions where melatonin synthesis was accelerated. However, more recent studies have shown that under optimal assay conditions the activity of HIOMT is much higher than previously believed and that the HIOMT reaction is unlikely to be the rate-limiting step (WEISS, 1968; KLEIN et al., 1970a). Using appropriate assay conditions, KLEIN and co-workers (1970a) find no change in the enzymic activity in organ cultures of pineal gland during prolonged stimulation of melatonin synthesis by dBcAMP.

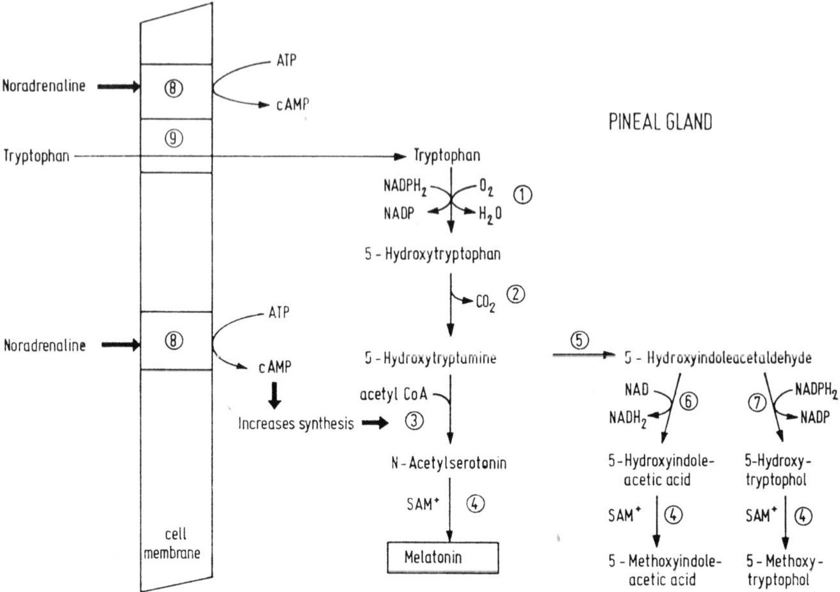

Fig. 10. *Pathways of metabolism in the pineal gland.* Enzymes indicated by number are: (1), tryptophan hydroxylase (in mitochondrion); (2), 5-hydroxytryptophan decarboxylase; (3), 5-hydroxytryptamine N-acetyltransferase; (4) 5-hydroxyindole-O-methyltransferase (HIOMT); (5), monoamine oxidase (in mitochondrion); (6) aldehyde dehydrogenase; (7) alcohol dehydrogenase; (8), adenyl cyclase; (9) tryptophan transport mechanism in the cell membrane. Synthesis of melatonin requires adequate amounts of enzymes (1) to (4) and of $NADPH_2$, SAM^+ (S-adenosylmethionine) and acetyl CoA. The rate-limiting step in the pathway of melatonin synthesis is enzyme (3), 5-hydroxytryptamine N-acetyltransferase

The obvious point of regulation of this branched pathway would be the N-acetyltransferase reaction which occurs immediately after the branch point. Recent reports (KLEIN et al., 1970b; KLEIN and WELLER, 1970) indicate that the activity of this enzyme is increased up to ten-fold by noradrenaline and by dBcAMP in cultured pineal glands. This increase appears to be due to increased protein synthesis because it is prevented by cycloheximide (KLEIN et al., 1970b).

Inspection of the pathway of melatonin synthesis and associated pathways reveals that the activities of other enzymes and the concentrations of other substrates may be important. Nothing is known, for example, about the intracellular supply of S-adenosylmethionine, of acetyl CoA in the cytosol or about the availability of $NADPH_2$. It is also conceivable that effects of noradrenaline and cAMP on metabolism of glucose or fatty acids by the pineal gland could alter the catalytic activity of several enzymes in the pathway by altering the availability of substrate.

Inhibition of monoamine oxidase can produce an increase in melatonin synthesis similar to that produced by noradrenaline (AXELROD et al., 1969; KLEIN and ROWE, 1970), presumably by diverting the 5-hydroxytryptamine in that direction; noradrenaline does not appear to act in this way (AXELROD et al., 1969). Melatonin itself can inhibit the activity of HIOMT (WEISS, 1968) but the physiological significance of such a possible feedback inhibition is unknown and perhaps doubtful in view of the observation that added melatonin does not alter the synthesis of ^{14}C-melatonin from ^{14}C-tryptophan in pineal cultures (AXELROD et al., 1969).

Noradrenaline has one effect on the pineal gland that is not shared by dBcAMP: this is an acceleration of tryptophan transport into the gland (WURTMAN et al., 1969).

In conclusion, noradrenaline, via activation of adenyl cyclase and cAMP production, appears to accelerate a rate-limiting step of melatonin synthesis. This is a slow effect and increased synthesis of new enzyme protein appears to be required. The rate-limiting enzyme is tentatively identified as 5-hydroxytryptamine N-acetyltransferase.

d) Relation of Metabolic Effects of Noradrenaline to Regulation of Pineal Gland Function

The secretion of melatonin by the pineal is influenced by environmental lighting in such a way that inhibition of secretion occurs in the light and stimulation of secretion occurs in the dark: the evidence for this comes from studies of effects of melatonin or effects of pinealectomy and of effects of light and dark on ovarian growth and function. That continuous light is to be equated with no secretion of melatonin should be borne in mind for the following discussion.

Table 3. *Changes in pineal gland causes by changes in environmental lighting conditions and by denervation*[a]

	Continuous dark	Continuous light	Denervation
Adenyl cyclase activity	*Low*	*Increases*	*Increases*
cAMP content	*Low*	*High*	
5-HTP decarboxylase activity	*Low*	*Increases*	*Increases*
5-hydroxytryptamine content	*Decreases*	*Increases*	*Increases*
N-acetyltransferase activity	*Increases*	*Decreases*	*?*
HIOMT activity	*Increases*	*Decreases*	*Decreases*
Synthesis of melatonin	*Increases*	*Decreases*	

[a] Information in this Table is based upon the following references: adenyl cyclase: WEISS, 1969b; cAMP content: EBADI et al., 1970; N-acetyltransferase activity: KLEIN and WELLER, 1970; all other changes: WURTMAN and AXELROD, 1968, AXELROD and WURTMAN, 1968, WURTMAN et al., 1964.

In Table 3 are listed the changes in enzyme activities and in 5-hydroxytryptamine and cAMP content that have been observed to occur in pineal glands of rats exposed to continuous light or to continuous dark. In attempting to correlate these changes in amounts of enzyme with concurrent changes in functional activity of the gland it must be remembered that the amount of enzyme determines only the maximum capacity of the cell to perform a particular reaction, a capacity that may never be expressed if, for example, the concentration of substrate or the concentration of activating agent should not be sufficient. In a metabolic pathway, such as that shown in Fig. 10, it is the flow through the slowest step in the pathway which determines the rate of formation of the final end-product, in this case melatonin. The changes may be summarized as follows:

in continuous light there is an apparent decrease in the capacity of the final part of the pathway of melatonin synthesis in keeping with the known reduction in melatonin secretion under these conditions; at the same time there is an apparent increase in the capacity of the first part of the pathway, as well as in the noradrenaline-responsive system itself (adenyl cyclase). In continuous dark all changes are in the opposite direction. There exists then a paradoxical situation in which the capacity to respond to noradrenaline by increasing cAMP formation and by forming 5-hydroxytryptamine in the first part of the synthetic pathway is increased at a time when the sympathetic stimulation of the gland and the capacity to synthesize melatonin from 5-hydroxytryptamine is actually decreased (i.e., continuous light or denervation) and vice versa. The significance of these reciprocal changes in the capacity of the two sections of the pathway is not clear. It may be connected with the need for dampened oscillations in the diurnal variation in melatonin secretion.

One observation which is not in keeping with the suggestion of increased sympathetic activity occurring in the dark and being responsible for the increases in the capacity of the final part of the synthetic pathway is the finding of a reduced amount of HIOMT activity in pineal glands of dark-adapted rats in which the sympathetic nerves to the gland had been directly stimulated (BROWNSTEIN and HELLER, 1968). The significance of the rather small and variable changes in HIOMT activity observed in these experiments remains to be established.

e) Summary: Regulation of Metabolic Processes in the Pineal Gland by Catecholamines

Noradrenaline stimulates adenyl cyclase of pineal gland. The principal metabolic consequence of this is accelerated synthesis of melatonin. This acceleration is secondary to cAMP formation, occurs slowly and appears to be due to increased synthesis of enzyme protein. The rate-limiting enzyme whose synthesis is increased by cAMP is tentatively identified as 5-hydroxytryptamine N-acetyltransferase.

There is a major problem in interpreting this effect of noradrenaline in terms of the regulation of pineal gland function by the sympathetic nervous system in the intact animal. This problem is whether light or dark is associated with increased sympathetic stimulation of the gland. It appears likely that increased sympathetic stimulation occurs when the animal is in the dark, but the evidence for this is largely indirect and more proof is needed before any sound hypothesis of regulation of pineal function and metabolism by the sympathetic nervous system can be formulated.

Changes in the pineal gland brought about by continuous exposure to light (equated here with lack of sympathetic stimulation) are an apparent *increase* in the capacity of the early part of the pathway of melatonin synthesis (including the noradrenaline-responsive system itself, adenyl cyclase) and a *decrease* in the last part of the pathway. Changes brought about by continuous exposure to dark are in the opposite direction. These reciprocal changes in capacity to interact with noradrenaline and capacity to synthesize product may serve to dampen the daily fluctuations in melatonin synthesis. This conclusion is based upon the assumption that these changes in enzyme activity represent similar changes in rate of operation: there is no evidence whatever for this assumption. This is another area in which more information is needed, in particular about rates of melatonin synthesis *in vivo* and how they are influenced by light and dark.

XI. Tissues which Contain Unusual Adenyl Cyclases

a) Red Blood Cells

Red blood cells of certain avian, mammalian and amphibian species contain a catecholamine-sensitive adenyl cyclase (ØYE and SUTHERLAND, 1966; DAVOREN and SUTHERLAND, 1963; SHEPPARD and BURGHARDT, 1969; ROSEN and ROSEN, 1968, 1969). The adenyl cyclase of frog erythrocytes is of great interest because it acquires its sensitivity to catecholamines only during metamorphosis (ROSEN and ROSEN, 1968). These frog erythrocytes provide a useful preparation for the study of the relation between catecholamine-sensitivity and adenyl cyclase activity. However, one difficulty with this type of study is that the enzyme readily loses its sensitivity to catecholamines in the course of its isolation from the cells (ROSEN and ROSEN, 1969).

b) Tumour Cells

Tumour cells may have unusual adenyl cyclases. A mouse mammary adenocarcinoma has been reported to have a very high catecholamine-stimulated adenyl cyclase activity (BROWN et al., 1969). In contrast, cultured liver cells derived from a Morris hepatoma have no adenyl cyclase (GRANNER et al., 1968).

c) Kidney Cortex and Medulla

The adenyl cyclase of kidney cortex and medulla differ in their hormonal sensitivities. The former is stimulated by parathyroid hormones (MELSON et al., 1970; NAGATA and RASMUSSEN, 1970) and but weakly by adrenaline and glucagon whereas the latter is stimulated by vasopressin and not by adrenaline or glucagon (MELSON et al., 1970; DOUSA et al., 1970).

The stimulation of kidney cortex adenyl cyclase by adrenaline is inhibited by propranolol but not by phentolamine (MELSON et al., 1970). The physiological significance, if any, of this response of the kidney cortex to catecholamines is not known. Adrenaline does not increase gluconeogenesis by perfused kidney although cAMP does have this effect (BOWMAN, 1970); the physiological stimulus for the cortex cyclase is uncertain but may be parathyroid hormone which does stimulate not only adenyl cyclase but also gluconeogenesis in this tissue (NAGATA and RASMUSSEN, 1970).

In the renal medulla the antidiuretic response to vasopressin is mediated by stimulating cAMP formation. The antidiuretic action of vasopressin in intact rats is inhibited by noradrenaline and this effect is prevented by an α-receptor blocking agent (phenoxybenzamine) but not by a β-receptor blocking agent (LIBERMAN et al., 1970). This suggests that an inhibitory effect of noradrenaline on the vasopressin-stimulated adenyl cyclase might occur. This has not been demonstrated in renal medulla but additional evidence from studies with two other rather similar tissues (toad bladder, frog skin) supports this concept (see B. XI. d and e).

d) Toad Bladder

The permeability of toad bladder to water is increased by vasopressin. That this effect is mediated by stimulation of adenyl cyclase is indicated by the rise in cAMP concentration (HANDLER et al., 1965), the mimicking action of cAMP (HANDLER et al., 1968; BOURGOIGNIE et al., 1969), and the similar effect of theophylline on both cAMP content (HANDLER et al., 1965; TURTLE and KIPNIS, 1967) and permeability (HANDLER et al., 1968). Catecholamines reduce the increase in cAMP content produced by theophylline (TURTLE and KIPNIS, 1967) and inhibit the effect of vasopressin on water permeability (HANDLER et al., 1968). α-Receptor blockade prevents these inhibitory effects of noradrenaline (TURTLE and KIPNIS, 1967; HANDLER et al., 1968). In fact, during blockade of α-receptors adrenaline increases the cAMP content of toad bladder in the presence of theophylline (TURTLE and KIPNIS, 1967) and isopropylnoradrenaline enhances the effect of vasopressin, an effect on β-receptors that is inhibited by propranolol (HANDLER et al., 1968).

Toad bladder may, therefore, be presumed to contain an adenyl cyclase that can be either inhibited or stimulated by the catecholamines. Inhibition of adenyl cyclase is mediated by α-receptors while stimulation is mediated by β-receptors.

e) Frog Skin

Frog skin also behaves as though it has α-receptors the stimulation of which inhibits adenyl cyclase activity and β-receptors the stimulation of which increases adenyl cyclase activity. Increased sodium flux occurs in response to noradrenaline, oxytocin, cAMP, theophylline (BASTIDE and JARD, 1968), adrenaline (WATLINGTON, 1968), isopropylnoradrenaline (WATLINGTON, 1968; MCAFEE, 1970) and other β-receptor stimulating agents (MCAFEE, 1970). This effect of catecholamines has therefore been attributed to stimulation of adenyl cyclase via stimulation of β-receptors. Stimulation of α-receptors with phenylephrine (WATLINGTON, 1969) or with adrenaline in the presence of pronethalol (WATLINGTON, 1968) reduces sodium flux and simultaneously antagonizes the stimulatory effect of vasopressin.

Interpretation of these changes in frog skin is complicated by the existence of mucous cells which also secrete sodium in response to β-receptor stimulation (WATLINGTON, 1968, 1969; MCAFEE, 1970). Moreover, frog skin contains another catecholamine-sensitive cell type, the melanophore. Thus measurements of cAMP content are not useful because of this heterogeneity of cell types in the frog skin.

The melanophores of both frog and lizard skin appear to respond to α-receptor stimulation by lightening of the skin and to β-receptor stimulation by darkening of the skin. Thus frog skin responds to catecholamines not only by changes in water and sodium transport and in mucus secretion but also by colour changes. Melanocyte-stimulating hormone causes darkening of the frog skin. Theophylline (ABE et al., 1969), cAMP and dBcAMP (NOVALES and DAVIS, 1967; HADLEY and GOLDMAN, 1969) mimic this effect. Stimulation of β-receptors by isopropylnoradrenaline or by salbutamol also causes darkening of the skin (GOLDMAN and HADLEY, 1969a and b). Stimulation of α-receptors by phenylephrine causes lightening of the skin (GOLDMAN and HADLEY, 1969b). Adrenaline or noradrenaline alone have rather variable effects (GOLDMAN and HADLEY, 1969b) but noradrenaline consistently lightens skin that has been darkened by melanocyte-stimulating hormone (ABE et al., 1969). In the presence of α-receptor blocking agents adrenaline and noradrenaline cause darkening of the skin (GOLDMAN and HADLEY, 1969b).

Thus frog and lizard skin melanophores appear to contain both α- and β-receptors, the one producing inhibition of adenyl cyclase and the other producing stimulation of adenyl cyclase. Measurements of cAMP content of frog skin in the presence of agents which lighten or darken the skin have shown that an increase in cAMP concentration is usually associated with darkening of the skin and a decrease in cAMP concentration is associated with lightening of the skin (ABE et al., 1969). It is likely that the cAMP measured in these skins is not only in the melanophores but also in epithelial cells and in mucous glands. However, since these three cell types appear to contain adenyl cyclases with similar responses to catecholamines there is nervertheless a correlation between overall cAMP content and physiological response.

C. Effects of Catecholamines on Metabolism of Intact Animals

The effects of catecholamines on the metabolism of intact animals may be divided into two classes: (1) the type of effect in which the actions of the catecholamines on individual tissues result in a rise in the concentration of a variety of compounds in the blood; this is referred to here as the mobilization of energy reserves, and (2) the type of effect in which the actions of catecholamines on individual tissues result in an increase in the overall metabolic rate of the animal, referred to here as the calorigenic effect. The first type of effect is usually assessed by measuring the changes either in the concentration of the appropriate compound in the blood or in the rate of its delivery into the blood; the second type of effect is assessed by measuring the oxygen uptake of the animal.

Neither type of measurement in itself can be considered to be a measure of any specific action of catecholamines on any one tissue. For this reason, attempts to quantitate, for example, the hyperglycemic effect, under a variety of conditions, or to identify, by the use of blocking agents, the receptors for the hyperglycemic effect, are unlikely to give meaningful results. To many workers the term "metabolic effects of catecholamines" is almost synonymous with the hyperglycemic, hyperketonemic, lacticacidemic, fatty acid-mobilizing and calorigenic effects of the catecholamines. However, this is an erroneous idea because both classes of effect are composite in nature; they both result from a variety of actions of the catecholamines on the metabolism of different tissues and both are but poor reflections of the precise nature of these different actions of the catecholamines.

I. Mobilization of Energy Reserves

From the foregoing discussion of the effects of catecholamines on individual tissues (sections B. I to B. XI) it is clear that not only liver and white adipose tissue break down their energy reserves (glycogen and triglyceride), largely for use by other tissues (in the form of glucose and FFA), but that skeletal, cardiac and smooth muscle and brown adipose tissue also break down their energy reserves (glycogen and triglyceride), largely for internal consumption, in response to stimulation by catecholamines. The liver uses not only its internal glycogen stores but also amino acids from a variety of sources to produce glucose when stimulated to do so by the catecholamines.

Measurements of the concentration of glucose or of FFA in the blood assess only the balance between the rate of their production and the rate of their utilization; of these processes either or both can be influenced by the catecholamines, not only by their direct actions to promote the release and utilization of these compounds but also by virtue of their actions to alter the secretion of other hormones which in turn influence these processes. The inhibition by the catecholamines of the secretion of insulin is of major importance in determining rates of production and utilization of glucose and also of FFA. Other hormones whose secretion may be influenced by catecholamines include ACTH and growth hormone, both of which influence carbohydrate and lipid metabolism. The secretion of ACTH is increased by the catecholamines (VERNIKOS-DANELLIS and MARKS, 1962); the increased secretion of glucocorticoids by the adrenal cortex which occurs as a consequence might be expected to promote gluconeogenesis. The effect of catecholamines on the secretion of growth hormone is predominantly an inhibitory one (PARRA et al., 1970; BLACKARD and HEIDINGSFELDER, 1968; IMURA et al., 1968); however, a stimulatory effect can be unmasked by the use of β-receptor blocking agents.

Table 4. *Processes involved in the hyperglycemic effect of catecholamines*

Tissue	Change in Metabolic Process	Change due to: (1) action of catecholamine on:	(2) lack of insulin	(3) raised FFA	(4) raised lactate	(5) raised gluco-corticoid
LIVER	increased glycogenolysis	liver	+			
	decreased glycogenesis	liver	+			
	increased gluconeogenesis	liver	+	+	+	+
	increased proteolysis	liver	+			
PANCREAS	decreased secretion of insulin - - - - (2)	β-cell				
MUSCLE	decreased uptake of glucose	β-cell	+	+		
	increased glycogenolysis - - - - (4)	muscle				
WHITE ADIPOSE TISSUE	increased lipolysis - - - - (3)	white adipose tissue	+			
	decreased uptake of glucose	β-cell	+			
ADRENAL CORTEX . . .	increased glucocorticoid secretion - - - - (5)	pituitary				

These agents potentiate and α-receptor blocking agents inhibit the rise in growth hormone secretion caused by hypoglycemia.

a) Hyperglycemic Effect

The rise in blood glucose concentration caused by catecholamines is attributed to both an increased production of glucose and a utilization of glucose that is smaller than would be expected from the concentration of glucose in the blood. At least five tissues participate in this effect: these tissues and the metabolic processes in them that are influenced by the catecholamines and that result in either increased production or decreased utilization of glucose are listed in Table 4.

The extent to which any one tissue contributes to the hyperglycemic effect depends on the nature of the stimulatory catecholamine and on the nutritional and hormonal status of the animal.

b) Fat-mobilizing Effect

The rise in blood FFA concentration (and also in glycerol concentration) caused by catecholamines is attributable to an increased liberation of these compounds from the white adipose tissue. This is due to a direct action of catecholamines on the white adipose tissue to accelerate lipolysis. Another factor involved is the inhibition by the catecholamines of insulin secretion by the β-cells of the pancreas (see Table 5). The mobilized FFA serve as the principal oxidizable substrate for those tissues (muscle and white adipose tissue) whose utilization of glucose is restricted by the relative lack of insulin.

Table 5. *Processes involved in the fat-mobilizing effect of catecholamines*

Tissue	Change in Metabolic Process	Change due to: (1) action of catecholamine on:	(2) lack of insulin
WHITE ADIPOSE TISSUE	increased lipolysis	white adipose tissue	+
	decreased uptake of glucose	β-cell	+
PANCREAS	decreased secretion of insulin - - - - - (2)	β-cell	

II. Calorigenic Effect

The calorigenic effect of the catecholamines is also a composite one. It is not possible to identify with any certainty the site or sites of this increased consumption of oxygen or the localization of the actions of the catecholamines that result in this increased oxygen uptake (see Himms-Hagen, 1967).

A number of metabolic processes whose operation involves utilization of ATP must contribute to this calorigenic effect. These include gluconeogenesis, urea synthesis and possibly also triglyceride breakdown plus re-esterification of the FFA. The return of the mobilized glucose and FFA to their stores following their liberation by the catecholamines is also an energy-consuming process that would necessitate an increase in oxygen uptake. These processes occur mainly in liver and the white adipose tissue. An increase in oxygen uptake of the brown adipose tissue due to a direct action of catecholamines on this tissue (see section B. VI) appears to be a major cause of the calorigenic effect of noradrenaline in warm acclimated rats.

In cold acclimated rats and in newborn animals the calorigenic effect of catecholamines is very much enhanced; it is much greater than in animals when not acclimated to cold or when adult. This is a reflection of an adaptation for non-shivering thermogenesis in these animals. The nature of the metabolic processes involved in this enhanced calorigenic effect of the catecholamines is not understood. Although the oxygen uptake of the brown adipose tissue is greatly enhanced it contributes relatively little, less than 12%, to the oxygen uptake of the whole animal under these conditions (see section B. VI).

D. Concluding Remarks

I. Metabolic Effects of Catecholamines

In almost all tissues that are sensitive to catecholamines the direct action of the catecholamines leads to an alteration in metabolic processes in the tissue as well as to a functional response of the tissue.

In some instances the change in function is a direct consequence of the alteration of metabolism (see Table 6, group 1). For example, the increased output of glucose by the isolated liver caused by the catecholamines is a direct consequence of the acceleration by the catecholamines of glycogenolysis and gluconeogenesis in this organ; the increased output of FFA by the white adipose tissue occurs as a consequence of the acceleration of lipolysis; the increased production of heat by the brown adipose tissue occurs as a consequence of the acceleration of lipolysis.

In other instances the change in function is not a direct consequence of the alteration in metabolism but appears rather to be supported by it (group 2, Table 6). For example, in isolated cardiac muscle the inotropic response caused by the catecholamines is not a consequence of the alterations in carbohydrate and lipid metabolism which occur at the same time, although these alterations undoubtedly lead to the provision of extra substrate at the time at which it is needed and thus support the alteration in function. Nevertheless, both the alteration in function and the alterations in metabolism in the heart appear to occur as a consequence of the initial stimulation by the catecholamines of adenyl cyclase activity. Insofar as increased utilization of ATP for formation of cAMP may be regarded as a "metabolic effect" of the catecholamines one may also regard the inotropic response as a consequence of this particular "metabolic effect" of the catecholamines.

Skeletal and smooth muscles fall into the same category as cardiac muscle in that the functions elicited by the catecholamines are not direct consequences of the alterations in carbohydrate and lipid metabolism but may nevertheless be consequences of adenyl cyclase stimulation (Table 6).

For those tissues in which the secretory function is altered by the catecholamines (group 3, Table 6), as a consequence of an alteration in adenyl cyclase activity, little information is available concerning alterations in metabolic processes that accompany this alteration in secretory function. The increased energy requirement for secretion and resynthesis of amylase in the salivary glands and for synthesis of melatonin in the pineal gland must be accompanied by alterations in other metabolic processes but it is not known whether these are altered simultaneously by the action of the catecholamines or whether they are altered only secondarily to the changes in demand for energy. The inhibition by catecholamines of insulin secretion as a consequence of inhibition of adenyl cyclase of the β-cells of the pancreatic islets, would not be expected to require significant alterations in energy-yielding metabolic processes.

Table 6. *Principal metabolic effects of catecholamines in several different tissues: the relation of these metabolic effects to the function of the tissue that is elicited by the catecholamines*

Tissue	Principal metabolic effect(s)	Section of this review	Relation to function elicited by the catecholamines: Function is a direct consequence of the metabolic effect	Function is not a direct consequence of the metabolic effect but is supported by it
1) LIVER	Increased glycogenolysis Increased gluconeogenesis	B. I	Increased output of glucose	
WHITE ADIPOSE TISSUE	Increased lipolysis	B. II	Increased output of FFA	
BROWN ADIPOSE TISSUE	Increased lipolysis	B. VI	Increased heat production	
2) CARDIAC MUSCLE . . .	Increased glycogenolysis Increased lipolysis	B. III		Increased force of contraction
SKELETAL MUSCLE . .	Increased glycogenolysis	B. IV		Increased force of contraction
SMOOTH MUSCLE . . .	Increased glycogenolysis	B. V		Relaxation
3) β-CELLS OF PANCREAS	?	B. VII		Inhibition of insulin secretion
SALIVARY GLANDS . .	?	B. VIII		Increased amylase secretion
PINEAL GLAND	?	B. X		Increased melatonin secretion
4) BRAIN	?	B. IX		?

The brain is listed (group 4, Table 6) in a class by itself because, although catecholamines do stimulate brain adenyl cyclase activity, the metabolic consequences of stimulation by catecholamines are poorly understood and the possible change in function that might result is entirely unknown.

In this review the actions of catecholamines on the metabolism of these individual tissues have been discussed and related as far as possible to the functional changes in the tissue also induced by the catecholamines.

The metabolic effects of catecholamines in intact animals may be divided into two classes: (1) the type of effect in which the actions of the catecholamines on individual tissues result in the rise in the concentration in the blood of a variety of compounds (glucose, FFA, lactic acid, ketone bodies, glycerol); this is referred to as the mobilization of energy reserves (see section C. I); (2) the type of effect in which the actions of the catecholamines on individual tissues result in an increase in the overall metabolic rate; this is referred to as the calorigenic effect (see section C. II). Neither of these types of effect, as measured by changes in concentration of metabolites in the blood or by changes in the oxygen consumption by the whole animal, can be considered to be a measure of a specific action of the catecholamines on any one tissue. Both represent the resultant of a variety of actions of the catecholamines on the metabolism of several individual tissues and both are poor reflections of these different actions.

II. Nature of Adrenergic Receptors for Metabolic Effects of Catecholamines

During the last few years there has been considerable interest in the nature of the receptors for metabolic responses to catecholamines as evidenced by the large number of reports on this subject and the devotion of an entire Symposium to this topic (see BRODY and MCNEILL, 1970; DANIEL et al., 1970; HIMMS-HAGEN, 1970a; HORNBROOK, 1970; MAYER, 1970). The problems involved in classifying these receptors have been discussed in some detail before (HIMMS-HAGEN, 1967). The main conclusions presented at that time were: (a) the metabolic responses to catecholamines in intact animals cannot be classified as α or β because of the composite nature of these responses; (b) even in isolated tissues where it may be possible by the usual techniques to classify the receptor as α or β, the acquisition of this knowledge does not actually give any information about the nature (structure, function) of the adrenergic receptor. The identification of a receptor in a given tissue as α or β is solely a matter of nomenclature: it cannot be taken as implying any knowledge of the nature of the receptor or of its relation to receptors with the same name in other types of cell (see also HIMMS-HAGEN, 1970b). These conclusions are still valid. The impossibility of identifying receptors for metabolic responses in intact animals will be reiterated here, with some selected examples, because of the current interest in attempts to achieve this type of classification. For example, the relative effectiveness of different catecholamines to raise blood glucose concentration cannot be related to their relative effectiveness in stimulating the "rat liver glycogenolytic receptor" (ARNOLD and MCAULIFF, 1968b) because this hyperglycemic response is dependent upon the actions of catecholamines on not only liver but also on pancreatic islets, on white adipose tissue on muscle and on the pituitary (see section C. I a). Likewise, the effects of blocking agents to alter effects of catecholamines on blood glucose and liver glycogen concentration cannot be equated with their effect to block actions of catecholamines on "rat liver receptors mediating glycogenolysis" (KENNEDY and ELLIS, 1969). Similar arguments can be used against attributing the rise in blood lactate produced by catecholamines to their actions on the muscle glycogenolytic receptor (ARNOLD and SELBERIS, 1968).

An important point about receptors for metabolic responses, which has only recently become apparent, is that what may be called α-receptors and β-receptors may both co-exist in a single tissue. This has been realized for many years for some of the "nonmetabolic" responses to catecholamines, although new examples of such tissues continue to appear as techniques for detecting the coexistence of both types of receptor become more sensitive. Only two examples are known so far for the coexistence in a single mammalian tissue of α- and β-receptors for metabolic responses. The pancreatic islet β-cells and white adipose tissue cells each contain both α- and β-receptors. In both instances the α-response appears to be associated with inhibition of adenyl cyclase and the β-response with stimulation of adenyl cyclase, as originally proposed by ROBISON, BUTCHER and SUTHERLAND (1967). Whether both kinds of receptor also co-exist in other tissues is not known.

It has not been possible to ascribe any physiological significance to the presence within a single cell of two kinds of receptors for catecholamines, one inhibitory and the other stimulatory. Normally one effect predominates. In pancreas the inhibitory effect predominates and in white adipose tissue the stimulatory effect predominates. Does the effect which is normally masked and revealed only by the use of blocking agents have any function? Does it serve to modulate the predominant opposing effect? Are there physiological conditions which unmask its activity? The only catecholamines that normally come into contact with these receptors are adrenaline and noradrenaline and they are both capable of stimulating both α- and β-receptors, at least to some extent. It seems likely that such a dual receptor system has a function, but its nature is not apparent at the moment. Perhaps when more is known about the detailed structure of cell membranes, about the functions of their different components and about the structural and functional interrelationships between these different components, the function of α-type receptors and β-type receptors within the framework of overall membrane function may become clearer.

References

ABE, K., BUTCHER, R.W., NICHOLSON, W.E., BAIRD, C.E., LIDDLE, R.A., LIDDLE, G.W.: Adenosine 3',5'-monophosphate (cyclic AMP) as the mediator of the actions of melanocyte stimulating hormone (MSH) and norepinephrine on the frog skin. Endocrinology **84**, 362—368 (1969).

ADAM, P.A.J., HAYNES, R.C., JR.: Control of hepatic mitochondrial CO_2 fixation by glucagon, epinephrine and cortisol. J. biol. Chem. **244**, 6444—6450 (1969).

ALDRIDGE, W.N., STREET, B.W.: Mitochondria from brown adipose tissue. Biochem. J. **107**, 315—317 (1968).

ALLAN, W., TEPPERMAN, H.M.: Stimulation of insulin secretion in the rat by glucagon, secretin and pancreozymin; effect of aminophylline. Life Sci. **8**, 307—317 (1969).

ALLEN, D.O., HILLMAN, C.C., ASHMORE, J.: Studies on a biphasic lipolytic response to catecholamines in isolated fat cells. Biochem. Pharmacol. **18**, 2233—2240 (1969).

AMSTERDAM, A., OHAD, I., SCHRAMM, M.: Dynamic changes in the ultrastructure of the acinar cell of the rat parotid gland during the secretory cycle. J. Cell Biol. **41**, 753—773 (1969).

ANDERSSON, R.G.G., MOHME-LUNDHOLM, E.: Metabolic actions associated with stimulation of α- and β-receptors for adrenaline in smooth muscle. Brit. J. Pharmacol. **34**, 204P—205P (1968).

APPLEMAN, M.M., BIRNBAUMER, L., TORRES, H.N.: Factors affecting the activity of muscle glycogen synthetase. III. The reaction with adenosine triphosphate, Mg^{++}, and cyclic 3',5'-adenosine monophosphate. Arch. Biochem. Biophys. **116**, 39—43 (1966).

ARNOLD, A., MCAULIFF, J.P.: Guinea pig adipose tissue responsiveness to catecholamines. Experientia (Basel) **24**, 436 (1968a).

— — Positive correlation of responsiveness to catecholamines of rat liver glycogenolytic receptor with other α-receptor responses. Experientia (Basel) **24**, 674—675 (1968b).

— SELBERIS, W.H.: Activities of catecholamines on the rat muscle glycogenolytic (β-2) receptor. Experientia (Basel) **24**, 1010—1011 (1968).

ASHFORD, T.P, PORTER, K.R.: Cytoplasmic components in hepatic cell lysosomes. J. Cell. Biol. **12**, 198—202 (1962).

AUDITORE, G.V., HOLLAND, W.C.: Further observations on the factors affecting the intracellular distribution of potassium in the kidney, liver, and brain of the rat, guinea pig and cat. J. Pharmacol. exp. Ther. **116**, 2 (1956).

AXELROD, J., SHEIN, H.M., WURTMAN, R.J.: Stimulation of ^{14}C-melatonin synthesis from ^{14}C-tryptophan by noradrenaline in rat pineal in organ culture. Proc. nat. Acad. Sci. (Wash.) **62**, 544—549 (1969).

— WURTMAN, R.J.: Photic and neural control of indoleamine metabolism in the rat pineal gland. Advanc. Pharmacol. **6A**, 157—166 (1968).

BABAD, H., BEN-ZVI, R., BDOLAH, A., SCHRAMM, M.: The mechanism of enzyme secretion by the cell. 4. Effects of inducers, substrates and inhibitors on amylase secretion by rat parotid slices. Europ. J. Biochem. **1**, 96—101 (1967).

BÄR, H.P., HECHTER, O.: Adenyl cyclase and hormone action: I. Effects of adrenocorticotropic hormone, glucagon, and epinephrine on the plasma membrane of rat fat cells. Proc. nat. Acad. Sci. (Wash.) **63**, 350—356 (1969).

BAIRD, T.J., BINNION, P.F.: Factors affecting the uptake of calcium by canine myocardial sarcoplasmic reticulum. Irish J. med. Sci. **2**, 585—593 (1969).

BALL, E.G.: Some aspects of fatty acid metabolism in brown adipose tissue. Lipids **5**, 220—223 (1970).

BALLARD, K., ROSELL, S.: The unresponsiveness of lipid metabolism in canine mesenteric adipose tissue to biogenic amines and to sympathetic nerve stimulation. Acta physiol. scand. **77**, 442—448 (1969).

BARGMANN, W., VON HEHN, G., LINDNER, E.: Über die Zellen des braunen Fettgewebes und ihre Innervation. Z. Zellforsch. **85**, 601—613 (1968).

BARKA, T.: Induced cell proliferation: the effect of isoproterenol. Exp. Cell Res. **37**, 662—679 (1965a).

— Stimulation of DNA synthesis by isoproterenol in the salivary gland. Exp. Cell Res. **39**, 355—364 (1965b).

— Stimulation of RNA synthesis in the salivary gland by isoproterenol. Exp. Cell Res. **41**, 573—579 (1966).

— Further studies on the stimulation of deoxyribonucleic acid synthesis in the submandibular gland by isoproterenol. Lab. Invest. **22**, 73—80 (1970).

BARNARD, T.: The ultrastructural differentiation of brown adipose tissue in the rat. J. Ultrastruct. Res. **29**, 311—332 (1969).

— LINDBERG, O.: Ultrastructural changes in the chondriome during perinatal development in brown adipose tissue of rats. J. Ultrastruct. Res. **29**, 293—310 (1969).

— SKÁLA, J., LINDBERG, O.: Changes in interscapular brown adipose tissue of the rat during perinatal and postnatal development and after cold acclimation. I. Activities of some respiratory enzymes in the tissue. Comp. Biochem. Physiol. **33**, 499—508 (1970).

BARRETT, A.M.: The role of plasma free fatty acids in the elevation of plasma cholesterol and phospholipids produced by adrenaline. J. Endocr. **36**, 301—316 (1966).

BASERGA, R.: Inhibition of stimulation of DNA synthesis by isoproterenol in submandibular glands of mice. Life Sci. **5**, 2033—2039 (1966).

— HEFFLER, S.: Stimulation of DNA synthesis by isoproterenol and its inhibition by actinomycin D. Exp. Cell Res. **46**, 571—580 (1967).

BASTIDE, F., JARD, S.: Actions de la noradrénaline et de l'oxytocine sur le transport actif de sodium et la perméabilité à l'eau de la peau de grenouille. Rôle du 3',5'-AMP cyclique. Biochim. biophys. Acta (Amst.) **150**, 113—123 (1968).

BDOLAH, A., BEN-ZVI, R., SCHRAMM, M.: The mechanism of enzyme secretion by the cell. II. Secretion of amylase and other proteins by slices of rat parotid gland. Arch. Biochem. Biophys. **104**, 58—66 (1964).

— SCHRAMM, M.: The function of 3',5' cyclic AMP in enzyme secretion. Biochem. biophys. Res. Commun. **18**, 452—454 (1965).

BECKER, F.F., BITENSKY, M.W.: Glucagon and epinephrine responsive adenyl cyclase activity of regenerating rat liver. Proc. Soc. exp. Biol. (N.Y.) **130**, 983—986 (1969).

BELFORD, J., CUNNINGHAM, M.A.: The effect of inotropic catecholamines, calcium and aminophylline on glycogen synthetase activity in the intact cat heart. J. Pharmacol. exp. Ther. **162**, 134—138 (1968).

BELOCOPITOW, E., APPLEMAN, M.M., TORRES, H.N.: Factors affecting the activity of muscle glycogen synthetase. II. The regulation by Ca^{++}. J. biol. Chem. **240**, 3473—3478 (1965).

— FERNANDEZ, M.C.G., BIRNBAUMER, L., TORRES, H.N.: Factors affecting muscle glycogen synthetase activity. IV. Comparative study of the different dependent forms of glycogen synthetase. J. biol. Chem. **242**, 1227—1231 (1967).

BEVIZ, A., LUNDHOLM, L., MOHME-LUNDHOLM, E.: Cyclic AMP as a mediator of hormonal metabolic effects in brown adipose tissue. Brit. J. Pharmacol. **34**, 198P—199P (1968).

BEWSHER, P.D., ASHMORE, J.: Ketogenic and lipolytic effects of glucagon on liver. Biochem. biophys. Res. Commun. **24**, 431—436 (1966).

BIANCHI, C.P.: Introduction: statement of the problem. (Symposium on Pharmacology of Excitation-Contraction Coupling in Muscle). Fed. Proc. **28**, 1624—1627 (1969).

BIRNBAUMER, L., POHL, S.L., RODBELL, M.: Adenyl cyclase in fat cells. I. Properties and the effects of adrenocorticotropin and fluoride. J. biol. Chem. **244**, 3468—3476 (1969).

— RODBELL, M.: Adenyl cyclase in fat cells. II. Hormone receptors. J. biol. Chem. **244**, 3477—3482 (1969).

BISHOP, J.S., LARNER, J.: Rapid activation-inactivation of liver uridine diphosphate glucose-glycogen transferase and phosphorylase by insulin and glucagon *in vivo*. J. biol. Chem. **242**, 1354—1356 (1967).

BITENSKY, M.W., RUSSELL, V., BLANCO, M.: Independent variation of glucagon and epinephrine responsive components of hepatic adenyl cyclase as a function of age, sex and steroid hormones. Endocrinology **86**, 154—159 (1970).

— — ROBERTSON, W.: Evidence for separate epinephrine and glucagon responsive adenyl cyclase systems in rat liver. Biochem. biophys. Res. Commun. **31**, 706—712 (1968).

BLACK, I.B.: Induction of hepatic tyrosine aminotransferase mediated by a cholinergic agent. Nature (Lond.) **225**, 648 (1970).

BLACKARD, W.G., HEIDINGSFELDER, S.A.: Adrenergic receptor control mechanism for growth hormone secretion. J. clin. Invest. **47**, 1407—1414 (1968).

BLECHER, M., MERLINO, N.S., RO'ANE, J.T.: Control of the metabolism and lipolytic effects of cyclic 3′,5′-adenosine monophosphate in adipose tissue by insulin, methylxanthines, and nicotinic acid. J. biol. Chem. **243**, 3973—3977 (1968).

— — — FLYNN, P.D.: Independence of the effects of epinephrine, glucagon, and adrenocorticotropin on glucose utilization from those on lipolysis in isolated rat adipose cells. J. biol. Chem. **244**, 3423—3429 (1969).

BLUKOO-ALLOTEY, J.A., VINCENT, N.H., ELLIS, S.: Interactions of acetylcholine and epinephrine on contractility, glycogen and phosphorylase activity of isolated mammalian hearts. J. Pharmacol. exp. Ther. **170**, 27—36 (1969).

BOSHART, C.R., WILL, L., PIRRÉ, A., RINGLER, I.: The effects of reserpine, guanethidine and other autonomic drugs on free fatty acid mobilization induced by phentolamine. J. Pharmacol. exp. Ther. **149**, 57—64 (1965).

BOURGOIGNIE, J., GUGGENHEIM, S., KIPNIS, D.M., KLAHR, S.: Cyclic guanosine monophosphate: effects on short-circuit current and water permeability. Science **165**, 1362—1363 (1969).

BOWMAN, R.H.: Gluconeogenesis in the isolated perfused rat kidney. J. biol. Chem. **245**, 1604—1612 (1970).

BOWMAN, W.C., RAPER, C.: The effects of adrenaline and other drugs affecting carbohydrate metabolism on contractions of the rat diaphragm. Brit. J. Pharmacol. **23**, 184—200 (1964).

— — Adrenotropic receptors in skeletal muscle. Ann. N.Y. Acad. Sci. **139**, 741—753 (1967).

BRADHAM, L.S., HOLT, D.A., SIMS, M.: The effect of Ca^{2+} on the adenyl cyclase of calf brain. Biochim. biophys. Acta (Amst.) **201**, 250—260 (1970).

BRAY, G.A.: Effects of epinephrine, corticotropin and thyrotropin on lipolysis and glucose oxidation in rat adipose tissue. J. Lipid Res. **8**, 300—307 (1967).

— GOODMAN, H.M.: Effects of epinephrine on glucose transport and metabolism in adipose tissue of normal and hypothyroid rats. J. Lipid Res. **9**, 714—719 (1968).

BRECKENRIDGE, B. McL.: The measurement of cyclic adenylate in tissues. Proc. nat. Acad. Sci. (Wash.) **52**, 1580—1586 (1964).

— BURN, J.H., MATSCHINSKY, F.M.: Theophylline, epinephrine and neostigmine facilitation of neuromuscular transmission. Proc. nat. Acad. Sci. (Wash.) **57**, 1893—1897 (1967).

BRESSLER, R., CORDON, M.V., BRENDEL, K.: Studies on the role of adenyl cyclase in insulin secretion. Arch. intern. Med. **123**, 248—251 (1969).

BRODY, T.M., DIAMOND, J.: Blockade of the biochemical correlates of contraction and relaxation in uterine and intestinal smooth muscle. Ann. N.Y. Acad. Sci. **139**, 772—780 (1967).

— McNEILL, J.H.: Adrenergic receptors for metabolic responses in skeletal and smooth muscles. Fed. Proc. **29**, 1375—1378 (1970).

BROSTROM, M.A., REIMANN, E.M., WALSH, D.A., KREBS, E.G.: A cyclic 3′,5′-AMP-stimulated protein kinase from cardiac muscle. Advances in Enzyme Regulation **8**, 191—203 (1970).

BROWN, H.D., CHATTOPADHYAY, S.K., MATTHEWS, W.S.: Glucagon stimulation of adenyl cyclase activity of cardiac muscle. Naturwissenschaften **55**, 181—182 (1968).

— — SPJUT, H.J., SPRATT, J.S., JR., PENNINGTON, S.N.: Adenyl cyclase activity in dimethylamino biphenyl-induced breast carcinoma. Biochim. biophys. Acta (Amst.) **192**, 372—375 (1969).

BROWN, J.D., STONE, D.B.: Antilipolytic effects of sulfonylurea drugs on induced lipolysis in isolated fat cells of the rat. Endocrinology **81**, 71—76 (1967).
BROWN-GRANT, K.: Enlargement of salivary gland in mice treated with isopropylnoradrenaline. Nature (Lond.) **191**, 1076—1078 (1961).
BROWNSTEIN, M.J., HELLER, A.: Hydroxyindole-O-methyltransferase activity: effect of sympathetic nerve stimulation. Science **162**, 367—368 (1968).
BUEDING, E., BUTCHER, R.W., HAWKINS, J., TIMMS, A.R., SUTHERLAND, E.W., JR.: Effect of epinephrine on cyclic adenosine 3′,5′-phosphate and hexose phosphates in intestinal smooth muscle. Biochim. biophys. Acta (Amst.) **115**, 173—178 (1966).
— KENT, N., FISHER, J.: Tissue specificity of glycogen phosphorylase b of intestinal smooth muscle. J. biol. Chem. **239**, 2099—2101 (1964).
BURNS, T.W., LANGLEY, P.: Observations on lipolysis with isolated adipose tissue cells. J. Lab. clin. Invest. **72**, 813—823 (1968).
— — The effect of α and β adrenergic blocking agents on basal and epinephrine stimulated lipolysis of human and rat isolated adipose tissue cells. Proc. Endocrine Soc. p. 32 (1969).
BURTON, S.D., MONDON, C.E., ISHIDA, T.: Dissociation of potassium and glucose efflux in isolated perfused rat liver. Amer. J. Physiol. **212**, 261—266 (1967).
BUSCHIAZZO, H., EXTON, J.H., PARK, C.R.: Effects of glucose on glycogen synthetase, phosphorylase and glycogen deposition in the perfused rat liver. Proc. nat. Acad. Sci. (Wash.) **65**, 383—387 (1970).
BUSE, M.G., JOHNSON, A.H., KUPERMINC, D., BUSE, J.: Effect of α-adrenergic blockade on insulin secretion in man. Metabolism **19**, 219—225 (1970).
BUTCHER, R.W., BAIRD, C.E., SUTHERLAND, E.W.: Effects of lipolytic and antilipolytic substances on adenosine 3′,5′-monophosphate levels in isolated fat cells. J. biol. Chem. **243**, 1705—1712 (1968).
— HO, R.J., MENG, H.C., SUTHERLAND, E.W.: Adenosine 3′,5′-monophosphate in biological materials. II. The measurement of adenosine 3′,5′-monophosphate in tissues and the role of the cyclic nucleotide in the lipolytic response of fat to epinephrine. J. biol. Chem. **240**, 4515—4523 (1965).
— SUTHERLAND, E.W.: The effects of catecholamines, adrenergic blocking agents, prostaglandin E_1 and insulin on cyclic AMP levels in the rat epididymal fat pad *in vitro*. Ann. N.Y. Acad. Sci. **139**, 849—859 (1967).
BYGRAVE, F.L.: The ionic enviroment and metabolic control. Nature (Lond.) **214**, 667—671 (1967).
BYRT, P.: Secretion and synthesis of amylase in the rat parotid gland after isoprenaline. Nature (Lond.) **212**, 1212—1215 (1966).
CALVERT, D.N., LECH, J.J.: Inhibition of lipolysis in isolated fat cells by sulfhydryl reagents. J. Pharmacol. exp. Ther. **171**, 135—140 (1970).
CAMERON, I.L., SMITH, R.E.: Cytological responses of brown fat tissue in cold-exposed rats. J. Cell Biol. **23**, 89—100 (1964).
CAMPBELL, J., RASTOGI, K.S.: Effects of glucagon and epinephrine on serum insulin and insulin secretion in dogs. Endocrinology **79**, 830—835 (1966).
CAMPOS, H.A., PARR, J.J.: Enlargement of the guinea pig salivary gland caused by catecholamines or tooth amputation. Europ. J. Pharmacol. **2**, 371—376 (1968).
CARLSON, L.A., HALLBERG, D., MICHELL, H.: Quantitative studies on the lipolytic response of human subcutaneous and omental adipose tissue to noradrenaline and theophylline. Acta med. scand. **185**, 465—469 (1969).
CHALLONER, D.R., STEINBERG, D.: Metabolic effect of epinephrine on the QO_2 of the arrested isolated perfused rat heart. Nature (Lond.) **205**, 602—603 (1965).
CHAMBERS, J.W., GEORG, R.H., BASS, A.D.: Effects of catecholamines and glucagon on amino acid transport in the liver. Endocrinology **83**, 1185—1192 (1968).
CHEUNG, W.Y.: Properties of cyclic 3′,5′-nucleotide phosphodiesterase from rat brain. Biochemistry **6**, 1079—1087 (1967).
— Cyclic 3′,5′-nucleotide phosphodiesterase: preparation of a partially inactive enzyme and its subsequent stimulation by snake venom. Biochim. biophys. Acta (Amst.) **191**, 303—315 (1969).
— Cyclic 3′,5′-nucleotide phosphodiesterase: demonstration of an activator. Biochem. biophys. Res. Commun. **38**, 533—538 (1970).
— SALGANICOFF, L.: Cyclic 3′,5′-nucleotide phosphodiesterase: localization and latent activity in rat brain. Nature (Lond.) **214**, 90—91 (1967).
— WILLIAMSON, J.R.: Kinetics of cyclic AMP changes in rat heart following epinephrine administration. Nature (Lond.) **207**, 979—981 (1965).
CHLOUVERAKIS, C.: Factors affecting the inhibitory action of insulin on lipolysis in a glucose-free medium. Endocrinology **81**, 521—526 (1967).
— The lipolytic action of fructose-1,6-diphosphate. Metabolism **17**, 708—716 (1968).
CHRISTIAN, D.R., KILSHEIMER, G.S., PETTETT, G., PARADISE, R., ASHMORE, J.: Advances in Enzyme Regulation **7**, 71—82 (1969).

CLAYCOMB, W.C., KILSHEIMER, G.S.: Effect of glucagon, adenosine-3',5'-monophosphate and theophylline on free fatty acid release by rat liver slices and on tissue levels of coenzyme A esters. Endocrinology **84**, 1179—1183 (1969).

CLAUSEN, T.: The relationship between the transport of glucose and cations across cell membranes in isolated tissues. V. Stimulating effect of ouabain, K^+-free medium and insulin on efflux of 3-O-methylglucose from epididymal adipose tissue. Biochim. biophys. Acta (Amst.) **183**, 625—634 (1969).

— RODBELL, M.: The metabolism of isolated fat cells. VIII. Amino acid transport in ghosts. J. biol. Chem. **244**, 1258—1262 (1969).

— — DUNAND, P.: The metabolism of isolated fat cells. VII. Sodium-linked, energy-dependent, and ouabain-sensitive potassium accumulation in ghosts. J. biol. Chem. **244**, 1252—1257 (1969).

COHEN, K.L., BITENSKY, M.W.: Inhibitory effects of alloxan on mammalian adenyl cyclase. J. Pharmacol. exp. Ther. **169**, 80—86 (1969).

COLEMAN, H.N., DEMPSEY, P.J., COOPER, T.: Myocardial oxygen consumption following chronic cardiac denervation. Amer. J. Physiol. **218**, 475—478 (1970).

COLWELL, A.R., BRIGHT, E.M.: The use of constant glucose injections for the study of induced variations in carbohydrate metabolism. Amer. J. Physiol. **92**, 555—567 (1930).

COMLINE, R.S., SILVER, M.: Development of activity in the adrenal medulla of the foetus and new-born animal. Brit. med. Bull. **22**, 16—20 (1966).

COORE, H.G., RANDLE, P.J.: Regulation of insulin secretion studied with pieces of rabbit pancreas incubated *in vitro*. Biochem. J. **93**, 66—78 (1964).

CORBIN, J.D., KREBS, E.G.: A cyclic AMP-stimulated protein kinase in adipose tissue. Biochem. biophys. Res. Commun. **36**, 328—336 (1969).

CRAIG, A.B., JR.: Vascular and metabolic effects of epinephrine in the isolated perfused rat liver. J. Pharmacol. exp. Ther. **149**, 346—350 (1965).

CRAIG, J.W., RALL, T.W., LARNER, J.: The influence of insulin and epinephrine on adenosine 3',5'-phosphate and glycogen transferase in muscle. Biochim. biophys. Acta (Amst.) **177**, 213—219 (1969).

CRESPIN, S.R., GREENOUGH, W.B., STEINBERG, D.: Stimulation of insulin secretion by infusion of free fatty acids. J. clin. Invest. **48**, 1934—1943 (1969).

CRYER, P.E., JARETT, L., KIPNIS, D.M.: Nucleotide inhibition of adenyl cyclase activity in fat cell membranes. Biochim. biophys. Acta (Amst.) **177**, 586—590 (1969).

CSÁNYI, V., GREENGARD, O., KNOX, W.E.: The induction of tyrosine aminotransferase by glucagon and hydrocortisone. J. biol. Chem. **242**, 2688—2692 (1967).

CURRY, D.L., BENNETT, L.L., GRODSKY, G.M.: Requirement for calcium ion in insulin secretion by the perfused rat pancreas. Amer. J. Physiol. **214**, 174—178 (1968).

DANFORTH, W.H.: Glycogen synthetase activity in skeletal muscle. Interconversion of two forms and control of glycogen synthesis. J. biol. Chem. **240**, 588—593 (1965).

— HELMREICH, E.: Regulation of glycolysis in muscle. I. The conversion of phosphorylase b to phosphorylase a in frog sartorius muscle. J. biol. Chem. **239**, 3133—3138 (1964).

— — CORI, C.F.: The effect of contraction and of epinephrine on the phosphorylase activity of frog sartorius muscle. Proc. nat. Acad. Sci. (Wash.) **48**, 1191—1199 (1962).

DANIEL, E.E., PATON, D.M., TAYLOR, G.S., HODGSON, B.J.: Adrenergic receptors for catecholamine effects on tissue electrolytes. Fed. Proc. **29**, 1410—1425 (1970).

DANIEL, H., DERRY, D.M.: Criteria for differentiation of brown and white fat in the rat. Canad. J. Physiol. Pharmacol. **47**, 941—945 (1969).

DANIEL, P.M., HENDERSON, J.R.: The effect of vagal stimulation on plasma insulin and glucose levels in the baboon. J. Physiol. (Lond.) **192**, 317—327 (1967).

DAVOREN, P.R., SUTHERLAND, E.W.: The effect of L-epinephrine and other agents on the synthesis and release of adenosine 3',5'-phosphate by whole pigeon erythrocytes. J. biol. Chem. **238**, 3009—3015 (1963).

DELANGE, R.J., KEMP, R.G., RILEY, W.D., COOPER, R.A., KREBS, E.G.: Activation of skeletal muscle phosphorylase kinase by adenosine triphosphate and adenosine 3',5'-monophosphate. J. biol. Chem. **243**, 2200—2208 (1968).

DEMPSEY, P.J., COOPER, T.: Supersensitivity of the chronically denervated feline heart. Amer. J. Physiol. **215**, 1245—1249 (1968).

DENTON, R.M., HALPERIN, M.L.: The control of fatty acid and triglyceride synthesis in rat epididymal adipose tissue. Roles of coenzyme A derivatives, citrate and L-glycerol 3-phosphate. Biochem. J. **110**, 27—38 (1968).

— RANDLE, P.J.: Citrate and the regulation of adipose tissue phosphofructokinase. Biochem. J. **100**, 420—423 (1966).

— YORKE, R.E., RANDLE, P.J.: Measurement of concentrations of metabolites in adipose tissue and effects of insulin, alloxan-diabetes and adrenaline. Biochem. J. **100**, 407—419 (1966).

De Robertis, E., Rodriguez de Lores Arnaiz, G., Alberici, M., Butcher, R. W., Sutherland, E. W.: Subcellular distribution of adenyl cyclase and cyclic phosphodiesterase in rat brain cortex. J. biol. Chem. **242**, 3487—3493 (1967).

Derry, D. M., Daniel, H.: Sympathetic nerve development in the brown adipose tissue of the rat. Canad. J. Physiol. Pharmacol. **48**, 160—168 (1970).

— Schönbaum, E., Steiner, G.: Two sympathetic nerve supplies to brown adipose tissue of the rat. Canad. J. Physiol. Pharmacol. **47**, 57—63 (1969).

Devrim, S., Recant, L.: Effect of glucagon on insulin release *in vitro*. Lancet (ii), 1227—1228 (1966).

De Wulf, H., Hers, H. G.: The stimulation of glycogen synthesis and of glycogen synthetase in the liver by the administration of glucose. Europ. J. Biochem. **2**, 50—56 (1967a).

— — The stimulation of glycogen synthesis and of glycogen synthetase in the liver by glucocorticoids. Europ. J. Biochem. **2**, 57—60 (1967b).

— — The interconversion of liver glycogen synthetase a and b *in vitro*. Europ. J. Biochem. **6**, 552—557 (1968a).

— — The role of glucose, glucagon and glucocorticoids in the regulation of liver glycogen synthesis. Europ. J. Biochem. **6**, 558—564 (1968b).

— Stalmans, W., Hers, H. G.: The influence of inorganic phosphate, adenosine triphosphate and glucose 6-phosphate on the activity of liver glycogen synthetase. Europ. J. Biochem. **6**, 545—551 (1968).

Dhalla, N. S., McLain, P. L.: Studies on the relationship between phosphorylase activation and increase in cardiac function. J. Pharmacol. exp. Ther. **155**, 389—396 (1967).

Diamond, J., Brody, T. M.: Effect of catecholamines on smooth muscle motility and phosphorylase activity. J. Pharmacol. exp. Ther. **152**, 202—211 (1966a).

— — Relationship between smooth muscle contraction and phosphorylase activation. J. Pharmacol. exp. Ther. **152**, 212—220 (1966b).

Dobbs, J. W., Robison, G. A.: Functional biochemistry of beta receptors in the uterus. Fed. Proc. **27**, 352 (1968).

Donhoffer, Sz., Szelényi, Z.: The role of brown adipose tissue in thermoregulatory heat production in the non-cold-adapted adult rat, guinea pig, ground squirrel and in the young rabbit. Acta physiol. Acad. Sci. hung. **28**, 349—361 (1965).

Douglas, W. W., Poisner, A. M.: The influence of calcium on the secretory response of the submaxillary gland to acetylcholine or to noradrenaline. J. Physiol. (Lond.) **165**, 528—541 (1963).

Douša, T., Hechter, O., Walter, R., Schwartz, I. L.: [8-Arginine]-vasopressinoic acid: an inhibitor of rabbit kidney adenyl cyclase. Science **167**, 1134—1135 (1970).

— Rychlik, I.: Adenyl cyclase and adenosine 3′,5′-cyclic phosphate phosphodiesterase in the receptor tissues of neurohypophysial hormones. Life Sci. **7**, part II, 1039—1044 (1968).

Drahota, Z., Honová, E., Hahn, P.: The effect of ATP and carnitine on the endogenous respiration of mitochondria from brown adipose tissue. Experientia (Basel) **24**, 431—432 (1968).

Drummond, G. I., Duncan, L.: Adenyl cyclase in cardiac tissue. J. biol. Chem. **245**, 976—983 (1970).

— — Friesen, A. J. D.: Some properties of cardiac phosphorylase b kinase. J. biol. Chem. **240**, 2778—2785 (1965).

— — Hertzman, E.: Effect of epinephrine on phosphorylase b kinase in perfused rat hearts. J. biol. Chem. **241**, 5899—5903 (1966).

— Harwood, J. P., Powell, C. A.: Studies on the activation of phosphorylase in skeletal muscle by contraction and by epinephrine. J. biol. Chem. **244**, 4235—4240 (1969).

— Powell, C. A.: Analogues of adenosine 3′,5′-cyclic phosphate as activators of phosphorylase *b* kinase and as substrates for cyclic 3′,5′-nucleotide phosphodiesterase. Molec. Pharmacol. **6**, 24—30 (1970).

Ebadi, M. S., Weiss, B., Costa, E.: Adenosine 3′,5′-monophosphate in rat pineal gland: increase induced by light. Science **170**, 188—190 (1970).

Edgar, P., Rabinowitz, D., Merimee, T. J.: Effects of amino acids on insulin release from excised rabbit pancreas. Endocrinology **84**, 835—843 (1969).

Edwards, J. C., Howell, S. L., Taylor, K. W.: Fatty acids as regulators of glucagon secretion. Nature (Lond.) **224**, 808—809 (1969).

Eisenstein, A. B., Strack, I.: Effects of glucagon on carbohydrate synthesis and enzyme activity in rat liver. Endocrinology **83**, 1337—1348 (1968).

Ellis, S.: The metabolic effects of epinephrine and related amines. Pharmacol. Rev. **8**, 485—562 (1956).

— Kennedy, B. L., Eusebi, A. J., Vincent, N. H.: Autonomic control of metabolism. Ann. N.Y. Acad. Sci. **139**, 826—832 (1967).

Entman, M. L., Cook, J. W., Jr., Bressler, R.: The influence of ouabain and alpha angelica lactone on calcium metabolism of dog cardiac "microsomes". J. clin. Invest. **48**, 229—234 (1969c).

ENTMAN, M. L., LEVEY, G. S., EPSTEIN, S. E.: Demonstration of adenyl cyclase activity in canine cardiac sarcoplasmic reticulum. Biochem. biophys. Res. Commun. **35**, 728—733 (1969a).

— — — Mechanism of action of epinephrine and glucagon on the canine heart. Evidence for increase in sarcotubular calcium stores mediated by cyclic 3′,5′-AMP. Circulat. Res. **25**, 429—438 (1969b).

EXTON, J. H., CORBIN, J. G., PARK, C. R.: Control of gluconeogenesis in liver. IV. Differential effects of fatty acids and glucagon on ketogenesis and gluconeogenesis in the perfused rat liver. J. biol. Chem. **244**, 4095—4102 (1969).

— JEFFERSON, L. S., JR., BUTCHER, R. W., PARK, C. R.: Gluconeogenesis in the perfused liver. The effects of fasting, alloxan diabetes, glucagon, epinephrine, adenosine 3′,5′-monophosphate and insulin. Amer. J. Med. **40**, 709—715 (1966).

— PARK, C. R.: Control of gluconeogenesis in liver. I. General features of gluconeogenesis in the perfused livers of rats. J. biol. Chem. **242**, 2622—2636 (1967).

— — The role of cyclic AMP in the control of liver metabolism. Adv. in Enzyme Regulation **6**, 391—407 (1968a).

— — Control of gluconeogenesis in liver. II. Effects of glucagon, catecholamines, and adenosine 3′,5′-monophosphate on gluconeogenesis in the perfused rat liver. J. biol. Chem. **243**, 4189—4196 (1968b).

FAIN, J. N.: Effect of K^+, valinomycin, tetraphenylborate and ouabain on lipolysis by white fat cells. Molec. Pharmacol. **4**, 349—357 (1968).

— Dihydroergotamine, propranolol and the β-adrenergic receptors of fat cells. Fed. Proc. **29**, 1402—1407 (1970).

— LOKEN, S. C.: Response of trypsin-treated brown and white fat cells to hormones. Preferential inhibition of insulin action. J. biol. Chem. **244**, 3500—3506 (1969).

— REED, N.: A mechanism for hormonal activation of lipolysis and respiration in free brown fat cells. Lipids **5**, 210—219 (1970).

— — SAPERSTEIN, R.: The isolation and metabolism of brown fat cells. J. biol. Chem. **242**, 1887—1894 (1967).

FAWCETT, D. W., MCNUTT, N. S.: The ultrastructure of the cat myocardium. I. Ventricular papillary muscle. J. Cell Biol. **42**, 1—45 (1969).

FEINSTEIN, H., SCHRAMM, M.: Energy production in rat parotid gland. Relation to enzyme secretion and effects of calcium. Europ. J. Biochem. **13**, 158—163 (1970).

FINDLAY, J. A., GILL, J. R., LEVER, J. D.: Increased insulin output following stimulation of the vagal supply to the perfused rabbit pancreas. J. Anat. (Lond.) **104**, 580 (1969).

FINE, M. B., WILLIAMS, R. H.: Effect of fasting, epinephrine and glucose and insulin on hepatic uptake of nonesterified fatty acids. Amer. J. Physiol. **199**, 403—406 (1960).

FLATT, J. P.: Conversion of carbohydrate to fat in adipose tissue: an energy-yielding and, therefore, self-limiting process J. Lipid Res. **11**, 131—143 (1970).

FRAZER, A., HESS, M. E.: Parasympathetic responses in hyperthyroid rats. J. Pharmacol. exp. Ther. **170**, 1—9 (1969).

FREDHOLM, B., ROSELL, S.: Effects of adrenergic blocking agents on lipid mobilization from canine subcutaneous adipose tissue after sympathetic nerve stimulation. J. Pharmacol. exp. Ther. **159**, 1—7 (1968).

FRERICHS, H., BALL, E. G.: Studies on the metabolism of adipose tissue. XI. Activation of phosphorylase by agents which stimulate lipolysis. Biochemistry **1**, 501—509 (1962).

FRIEDMAN, B., GOODMAN, E. H., JR., WEINHOUSE, S.: Effects of glucose feeding, cortisol, and insulin on liver glycogen synthesis in the rat. Endocrinology **81**, 486—496 (1967).

FRIEDMANN, N., EXTON, J. H., PARK, C. R.: Interaction of adrenal steroids and glucagon on gluconeogenesis in perfused rat liver. Biochem. biophys. Res. Commun. **29**, 113—119 (1967).

— PARK, C. R.: Early effects of 3′,5′-adenosine monophosphate on the fluxes of calcium and potassium in the perfused liver of normal and adrenalectomized rats. Proc. nat. Acad. Sci. (Wash.) **61**, 504—508 (1968).

FRIESEN, A. J. D., ALLEN, G., VALADARES, J. R. E.: Calcium-induced activation of phosphorylase in rat hearts. Science **155**, 1108—1109 (1967).

— OLIVER, N., ALLEN, G.: Activation of cardiac glycogen phosphorylase by calcium. Amer. J. Physiol. **217**, 445—450 (1969).

FROESCH, E. R.: The physiology and pharmacology of adipose tissue lipolysis: its inhibition and implications for the treatment of diabetes. Diabetologia **3**, 475—487 (1967).

FROHMAN, L. A., EZDINLI, E. Z., JAVID, R.: Effect of vagotomy and vagal stimulation on insulin secretion. Diabetes **16**, 443—448 (1967).

GAGLIARDINO, J. J., HERNANDEZ, R. E., RODRIGUEZ, R. R.: The β-receptors in the rat pancreas. Experientia (Basel) **24**, 1015 (1968).

GARCIA, A., WILLIAMSON, J. R., CAHILL, G. F., JR.: Studies on the perfused rat liver. II. Effect of glucagon on gluconeogenesis. Diabetes **15**, 188—193 (1966).

GARLAND, P.B., HADDOCK, B.A., YATES, D.W.: Components and compartments of mitochondrial fatty acid oxidation. FEBS Symposium **17**, 111—126 (1969). Ed. by L. ERNSTER and Z. DRAHOTA. London and New York: Academic Press 1969.

— RANDLE, P.J.: Effects of alloxan diabetes and adrenaline on concentrations of free fatty acids in rat heart and diaphragm muscles. Nature (Lond.) **199**, 381—382 (1963).

GEVERS, W., KREBS, H.A.: The effects of adenine nucleotides on carbohydrate metabolism in pigeon-liver homogenates. Biochem. J. **98**, 720—735 (1966).

GIRARDIER, L., SEYDOUX, J., CLAUSEN, T.: Membrane potential of brown adipose tissue. A suggested mechanism for the regulation of thermogenesis. J. gen. Physiol. **52**, 925—940 (1968).

GLINSMANN, W.H., HERN, E.P.: Inactivation of rat liver glycogen synthetase by 3′,5′-cyclic nucleotides. Biochem. biophys. Res. Commun. **36**, 931—936 (1969).

— — LINARELLI, L.G., FARESE, R.V.: Similarities between effects of adenosine 3′,5′-monophosphate and guanosine 3′,5′-monophosphate on liver and adrenal metabolism. Endocrinology **85**, 711—719 (1969).

— MORTIMORE, G.E.: Influence of glucagon and 3′,5′-AMP on insulin responsiveness of the perfused rat liver. Amer. J. Physiol. **215**, 553—559 (1968).

GOLD, A.H.: On the possibility of metabolite control of liver glycogen synthetase activity. Biochemistry **9**, 946—952 (1970).

GOLDBERG, A.L., SINGER, J.J.: Evidence for a role of cyclic AMP in neuromuscular transmission. Proc. nat. Acad. Sci. (Wash.) **64**, 134—141 (1969).

GOLDBERG, N.D., O'TOOLE, A.G.: The properties of glycogen synthetase and regulation of glycogen biosynthesis in rat brain. J. biol. Chem. **244**, 3053—3061 (1969).

— VILLAR-PALASI, C., SASKO, H., LARNER, J.: Effects of insulin treatment on muscle 3′,5′-cyclic adenylate levels *in vivo* and *in vitro*. Biochim. biophys. Acta (Amst.) **148**, 665—672 (1967).

GOLDMAN, J.M., HADLEY, M.E.: The effect of butoxamine, N-isopropylmethoxamine and salbutamol (AH-3365) on melanophore β-adrenergic receptors. J. Pharm. Pharmacol. **21**, 854—855 (1969a).

— — *In vitro* demonstration of adrenergic receptors controlling melanophore responses of the lizard, Anolis carolinensis. J. Pharmacol. exp. Ther. **166**, 1—7 (1969b).

GOODMAN, H.M.: Proposed mode of action of histamine. Nature (Lond.) **219**, 1053 (1968).

— BRAY, G.A.: Role of thyroid hormones in lipolysis. Amer. J. Physiol. **210**, 1053—1058 (1966).

GORIN, E., SHAFRIR, E.: Activation and inhibition of tri- and monoglyceride lipases in adipose tissue. Biochim. biophys. Acta (Amst.) **137**, 189—191 (1967).

GOURLEY, D.R.H., BETHEA, M.D.: Insulin effect on adipose tissue sodium and potassium. Proc. Soc. exp. Biol. (N.Y.) **115**, 821—823 (1964).

GOVIER, W.C., LOVENBERG, W., SJOERDSMA, A.: Studies on the role of catecholamines as regulators of tyrosine aminotransferase. Biochem. Pharmacol. **18**, 2661—2666 (1969).

GRAND, R.J.: Amino acid pools in rat parotid gland during epinephrine-stimulated protein synthesis. Biochim. biophys. Acta (Amst.) **195**, 252—254 (1969).

— GROSS, P.R.: Independent stimulation of secretion and protein synthesis in rat parotid gland. The influence of epinephrine and dibutyryl cyclic adenosine 3′,5′-monophosphate. J. biol. Chem. **244**, 5608—5615 (1969).

— — Translation-level control of amylase and protein synthesis by epinephrine. Proc. nat. Acad. Sci. (Wash.) **65**, 1081—1088 (1970).

GRANNER, D., CHASE, L.R., AURBACH, G.D., TOMKINS, G.M.: Tyrosine aminotransferase: enzyme induction independent of adenosine 3′,5′-monophosphate. Science **162**, 1018—1020 (1968).

GRAV, H.J., PEDERSEN, J.I., CHRISTIANSEN, E.N.: Conditions *in vitro* which affect respiratory control and capacity for respiration-linked phosphorylation in brown adipose tissue mitochondria. Europ. J. Biochem. **12**, 11—23 (1970).

GREENGARD, O.: The hormonal regulation of enzymes in prenatal and postnatal rat liver. Effects of adenosine 3′,5′-(cyclic)-monophosphate. Biochem. J. **115**, 19—24 (1969).

GREENOUGH, W.B., CRESPIN, S.R., STEINBERG, D.: Hypoglycaemia and hyperinsulinaemia in response to raised free-fatty-acid levels. Lancet (*ii*), 1334—1336 (1967).

GRODSKY, G.M., BENNETT, L.L.: Cation requirements for insulin secretion in the isolated perfused pancreas. Diabetes **15**, 910—913 (1966).

— — SMITH, D.F., SCHMID, F.G.: Effect of pulse administration of glucose or glucagon on insulin secretion *in vitro*. Metabolism **16**, 222—233 (1967).

GUTMAN, A., SHAFRIR, E.: Metabolic influences on enzymes of glycogen synthesis and breakdown in adipose tissue. Amer. J. Physiol. **207**, 1215—1220 (1964).

HADLEY, M.E., GOLDMAN, J.M.: Effect of cyclic 3′,5′-AMP and other adenine nucleotides on the melanophores of the lizard (Anolis carolinensis). Brit. J. Pharmacol. **37**, 650—658 (1969).

Hagen, J.M.: Stimulation of secretion and metabolism in mouse parotid glands *in vitro*. Biochem. Pharmacol. **2**, 206—214 (1959).
Hager, C.B., Kenney, F.T.: Regulation of tyrosine-α-ketoglutarate transaminase in rat liver. VII. Hormonal effects on synthesis in the isolated, perfused liver. J. biol. Chem. **243**, 3296—3300 (1968).
Halperin, M.L., Denton, R.M.: Regulation of glycolysis and L-glycerol 3-phosphate concentration in rat epididymal adipose tissue *in vitro*. Role of phosphofructokinase. Biochem. J. **113**, 207—214 (1969).
Handler, J.S., Bensinger, R., Orloff, J.: Effect of adrenergic agents on toad bladder response to ADH, 3′,5′-AMP, and theophylline. Amer. J. Physiol. **215**, 1024—1031 (1968).
— Butcher, R.W., Sutherland, E.W., Orloff, J.: The effect of vasopressin and of theophylline on the concentration of adenosine 3′,5′-phosphate in the urinary bladder of the toad. J. biol. Chem. **240**, 4524—4526 (1965).
Haugaard, N., Haugaard, E.S., Lee, N.H., Horn, R.S.: Possible role of mitochondria in regulation of cardiac contractility. Fed. Proc. **28**, 1657—1662 (1969).
— Hess, M.E.: Actions of autonomic drugs on cardiac phosphorylase activity and function. Pharmacol. Rev. **17**, 27—69 (1965).
Havel, R.J., Naimark, A., Borchgrevink, C.F.: Turnover rate and oxidation of free fatty acids of blood plasma in man during excercise: studies during continuous infusion of palmitate-1-C^{14}. J. clin. Invest. **42**, 1054—1063 (1963).
— Pernow, B., Jones, N.L.: Uptake and release of free fatty acids and other metabolites in legs of exercising men. J. appl. Physiol. **23**, 90—96 (1967).
Hayward, J.S., Ball, E.G.: Quantitative aspects of brown adipose tissue thermogenesis during arousal from hibernation. Biol. Bull. **131**, 94—103 (1966).
Heim, I., Hull, D.: The blood flow and oxygen consumption of brown adipose tissue in the new-born rabbit. J. Physiol. (Lond.) **186**, 42—55 (1966).
Heimberg, M., Fizette, N.B.: The action of norepinephrine on the transport of fatty acids and triglycerides by the isolated perfused rat liver. Biochem. Pharmacol. **12**, 392—394 (1963).
— Weinstein, I., Kohout, M.: The effects of glucagon, dibutyryl cyclic adenosine 3′,5′-monophosphate, and concentration of free fatty acid on hepatic lipid metabolism. J. biol. Chem. **244**, 5131—5139 (1969).
Helmreich, E.: Control of synthesis and breakdown of glycogen, starch and cellulose. In: M. Florkin and E.H. Stotz, Ed., Comprehensive Biochemistry, volume 17, Carbohydrate Metabolism, p. 17—92. Amsterdam: Elsevier 1969.
Henderson, A.H., Most, A.S., Sonnenblick, E.H.: Depression of contractility in rat heart muscle by free fatty acids during hypoxia. Lancet (*ii*), 825—826 (1969).
Hepp, D., Challoner, D.R., Williams, R.H.: Studies on the action of insulin in isolated adipose tissue cells. I. Stimulation of incorporation of 32P-labeled inorganic phosphate into mononucleotides in the absence of glucose. J. biol. Chem. **243**, 4020—4026 (1969b).
— Menahan, L.A., Wieland, O.: On the role of 3′,5′-cyclic AMP phosphodiesterase in insulin action on rat liver and adipose tissue. Hormone and Metabolic Res. **1**, 93—94 (1969a).
Herd, P.A., Horwitz, B.A.: Factors controlling brown mitochondrial respiration. Fed. Proc. **28**, 721 (1969).
Hertelendy, F., Machlin, L.J., Gordon, R.S., Horino, M., Kipnis, D.M.: Lipolytic activity and inhibition of insulin release by epinephrine in the pig. Proc. Soc. exp. Biol. (N.Y.) **121**, 675—677 (1966).
Hess, M.E., Haugaard, N.: The effect of epinephrine and aminophylline on the phosphorylase activity of perfused contracting heart muscle. J. Pharmacol. exp. Ther. **122**, 169—175 (1958).
— Shanfeld, J., Haugaard, N.: The role of the autonomic nervous system in the regulation of heart phosphorylase in the open-chest rat. J. Pharmacol. exp. Ther. **135**, 191—196 (1962).
Hess, M.L., Briggs, F.N., Shinebourne, E., Hamer, J.: Effect of adrenergic blocking agents on the calcium pump of the fragmented cardiac sarcoplasmic reticulum. Nature (Lond.) **220**, 79—80 (1968).
Himms-Hagen, J.: Lipid metabolism in warm-acclimated and cold-acclimated rats exposed to cold. Canad. J. Physiol. Pharmacol. **43**, 379—403 (1965).
— Sympathetic regulation of metabolism. Pharmacol. Rev. **19**, 367—461 (1967).
— The effect of age and cold-acclimation on the metabolism of brown adipose tissue in cold-exposed rats. Canad. J. Biochem. **47**, 251—256 (1969a).
— The role of brown adipose tissue in the calorigenic effect of adrenaline and noradrenaline in cold-acclimated rats. J. Physiol. (Lond.) **205**, 393—403 (1969b).
— Adrenergic receptors for metabolic responses in adipose tissue. Fed. Proc. **29**, 1388—1401 (1970a).
— Regulation of metabolic processes in brown adipose tissue in relation to nonshivering thermogenesis. Advanc. Enzyme Regulation **8**, 131—151 (1970b).

HITTELMAN, K.J., FAIRHURST, A.S., SMITH, R.E.: Calcium accumulation as a parameter of energy metabolism in mitochondria of brown adipose tissue. Proc. nat. Acad. Sci. (Wash.) **58**, 697—702 (1967).
— LINDBERG, O., CANNON, B.: Oxidative phosphorylation and compartmentation of fatty acid metabolism in brown fat mitochondria. Europ. J. Biochem. **11**, 183—192 (1969).
HO, R.J., JEANRENAUD, B.: Insulin-like action of ouabain. I. Effect on carbohydrate metabolism. Biochim. biophys. Acta (Amst.) **144**, 61—73 (1967).
— — POSTERNAK, TH., RENOLD, A.E.: Insulin-like action of ouabain. II. Primary antilipolytic effect through inhibition of adenyl cyclase. Biochim. biophys. Acta (Amst.) **144**, 74—82 (1967).
— — RENOLD, A.E.: Ouabain-sensitive fatty acid release from isolated fat cells. Experientia (Basel) **22**, 86—87 (1966).
HOHORST, H.-J., RAFAEL, J.: Oxydative Phosphorylierung durch Mitochondrien aus braunem Fettgewebe. Hoppe-Seylers Z. physiol. Chem. **349**, 268—270 (1968).
HOLLETT, C.R., AUDITORE, J.V.: Localization and characterization of a lipase in rat adipose tissue. Arch. Biochem. Biophys. **121**, 423—430 (1967).
HOLT, P.G., OLIVER, I.T.: Studies on the mechanism of induction of tyrosine aminotransferase in neonatal rat liver. Biochemistry **8**, 1429—1437 (1969).
HOLTEN, D., KENNEY, F.T.: Regulation of tyrosine α-ketoglutarate transaminase in rat liver. VI. Induction by pancreatic hormones. J. biol. Chem. **242**, 4372—4377 (1967).
HORINO, M., MACHLIN, L.J., HERTELENDY, F., KIPNIS, D.M.: Effect of short-chain fatty acids on plasma insulin in ruminant and nonruminant species. Endocrinology **83**, 118—128 (1968).
HORNBROOK, K.R.: Adrenergic receptors for metabolic responses in the liver. Fed. Proc. **29**, 1381—1385 (1970).
HORWITZ, B.A., HERD, P.A., SMITH, R.E.: Bioenergetics of brown adipose tissue. Lipids **5**, 30—34 (1970).
— HOROWITZ, J.M., JR., SMITH, R.: Norepinephrine-induced depolarization of brown fat cells. Proc. nat. Acad. Sci. (Wash.) **64**, 113—120 (1969).
— SMITH, R.E., PENGELLEY, E.T.: Estimated heat contribution of brown fat in arousing ground squirrels (Citellus lateralis). Amer. J. Physiol. **214**, 115—121 (1968).
HUIJING, F., LARNER, J.: On the effect of adenosine 3′,5′-cyclophosphate on the kinase of UDPG: α-1,4-glucan α-4-glucosyl transferase. Biochem. biophys. Res. Commun. **23**, 259—263 (1966a).
— — On the mechanism of action of adenosine 3′,5′-cyclophosphate. Proc. nat. Acat. Sci. (Wash.) **56**, 647—653 (1966b).
HULL, D., SEGALL, M.M.: The contribution of brown adipose tissue to heat production in the new-born rabbit. J. Physiol. (Lond.) **181**, 449—457 (1965).
HUSTON, R.B., KREBS, E.G.: Activation of skeletal muscle phosphorylase kinase by Ca^{2+}. II. Identification of the kinase activating factor as a proteolytic enzyme. Biochemistry **7**, 2116—2122 (1968).
IMAI, Y., HORWITZ, B.A., SMITH, R.E.: Calorigenesis of brown adipose tissue in cold-exposed rats. Proc. Soc. exp. Biol. (N.Y.) **127**, 717—719 (1968).
IMURA, H., KATO, Y., IKEDA, M., MORIMOTO, M., YAWATA, M., FUKASE, M.: Increased plasma levels of growth hormone during infusion of propranolol. J. clin. Endocr. **28**, 1079—1080 (1968).
ISSEKUTZ, B., JR., MILLER, H.I., RODAHL, K.: Lipid and carbohydrate metabolism during exercise. Fed. Proc. **25**, 1415—1420 (1966).
JANSKY, L.: Body organ cytochrome oxidase activity in cold- and warm-acclimated rats. Canad. J. Biochem. **41**, 1847—1854 (1963).
— HART, J.S.: Cardiac output and organ blood flow in warm- and cold-acclimated rats exposed to cold. Canad. J. Physiol. Pharmacol. **46**, 653—659 (1968).
JEANRENAUD, B.: Adipose tissue dynamics and regulation, revisited. Ergebn. Physiol. **60**, 57—140 (1968).
JEFFERSON, L.S., EXTON, J.H., BUTCHER, R.W., SUTHERLAND, E.W., PARK, C.R.: Role of adenosine 3′,5′-monophosphate in the effects of insulin and anti-insulin serum on liver metabolism. J. biol. Chem. **243**, 1031—1038 (1968).
JOEL, C.D.: The physiological role of brown adipose tissue. In: A.E. RENOLD and G.F. CAHILL, JR., Ed. Handbook of Physiology, section 5, pp. 59—85. American Physiological Society, 1965.
— Stimulation of metabolism of rat brown adipose tissue by addition of lipolytic hormones *in vitro*. J. biol. Chem. **241**, 814—821 (1966).
JOST, J.-P., HSIE, A., HUGHES, S.D., RYAN, L.: Role of cyclic adenosine 3′,5′-monophosphate in the induction of hepatic enzymes. I. Kinetics of the induction of rat liver serine dehydratase by cyclic adenosine 3′,5′-monophosphate. J. biol. Chem. **245**, 351—357 (1970).

JUDAH, J. D., NICHOLLS, M. R.: Role of liver-cell potassium ions in secretion of serum albumin and lipoproteins. Biochem. J. **116**, 663—669 (1970).
JUNGAS, R. L.: Role of cyclic-3',5'-AMP in the response of adipose tissue to insulin. Proc. nat. Acad. Sci. (Wash.) **56**, 757—763 (1966).
— BALL, E. G.: Studies on the metabolism of adipose tissue. XII. The effects of insulin and epinephrine on free fatty acid and glycerol production in the presence and absence of glucose. Biochemistry **2**, 383—388 (1963).
— — Studies on the metabolism of adipose tissue. XVII. *In vitro* effects of insulin upon the metabolism of the carbohydrate and triglyceride stores of adipose tissue from fasted-refed rats. Biochemistry **3**, 1696—1702 (1964).
KAJINUMA, H., KANETO, A., KUZUYA, T., NAKAO, K.: Effects of methacholine on insulin secretion in man. J. clin. Endocr. **28**, 1384—1388 (1968).
KAKIUCHI, S., RALL, T. W.: The influence of chemical agents on the accumulation of adenosine 3',5'-phosphate in slices of rabbit cerebellum. Molec. Pharmacol. **4**, 367—378 (1968a).
— — Studies on adenosine 3',5'-phosphate in rabbit cerebral cortex. Molec. Pharmacol. **4**, 379—388 (1968b).
— — McILWAIN, H.: The effect of electrical stimulation upon the accumulation of adenosine 3',5'-phosphate in isolated cerebral tissue. J. Neurochem. **16**, 485—491 (1969).
KANETO, A., KOSAKA, K., NAKAO, K.: Effects of stimulation of the vagus nerve on insulin secretion. Endocrinology **80**, 530—536 (1967).
KANSAL, P. C., BUSE, M. G.: The effect of adrenergic blocking agents on plasma insulin and blood glucose during urethan or epinephrine induced hyperglycemia. Metabolism **16**, 548—556 (1967).
KAPPERS, J. A.: The development, topographical relations and innervation of the epiphysis cerebri in the albino rat. Z. Zellforsch. **52**, 163—215 (1960).
KARAM, J. H., GRASSO, S. G., WEGIENKA, L. O., GRODSKY, G. M., FORSHAM, P. H.: Effects of selected hexoses, of epinephrine and of glucagon on insulin secretion in man. Diabetes **15**, 571—578 (1966).
KATZ, A. M.: Contractile proteins of the heart. Physiol. Rev. **50**, 63—158 (1970).
KATZ, J., LANDAU, B. R., BARTSCH, G. E.: The pentose cycle, triose phosphate isomerization, and lipogenesis in rat adipose tissue. J. biol. Chem. **241**, 727—740 (1966)
— ROGNSTAD, R.: The metabolism of glucose-2-T by adipose tissue. J. biol. Chem. **244**, 99—106 (1969).
KAWASAKI, A., KASHIMOTO, T., YOSHIDA, H.: Effects of 3',5'-cyclic adenosine monophosphate and its dibutyryl derivative on the motility of isolated rat ileum. Jap. J. Pharmacol. **19**, 494—501 (1969).
KENNEDY, B. L., ELLIS, S.: Interactions of catecholamines and adrenergic blocking agents at receptor sites mediating glycogenolysis in the rat. Arch. int. Pharmacodyn. **177**, 390—406 (1969).
KERRPOLA, W.: Inhibition of phosphorylase with cortisone and its activation with adrenaline in the rabbit. Endocrinology **51**, 192—202 (1952).
KIM, T. S., SHULMAN, J., LEVINE, R. A.: Relaxant effect of cyclic adenosine 3',5'-monophosphate on the isolated rabbit ileum. J. Pharmacol. exp. Ther. **163**, 36—42 (1968).
KIMMICH, G. A., RASMUSSEN, H.: Regulation of pyruvate carboxylase activity by calcium in intact rat liver mitochondria. J. biol. Chem. **244**, 190—199 (1969).
KIRBY, K. C., JR., SWERN, D., BASERGA, R.: The effect of structural modifications of the isoproterenol molecule on the stimulation of deoxyribonucleic acid synthesis in mouse salivary glands. Molec. Pharmacol. **5**, 572—579 (1969).
KLAINER, L. M., CHI, Y.-M., FREIDBERG, S. L., RALL, T. W., SUTHERLAND, E. W.: Adenyl cyclase. IV. The effects of neurohormones on the formation of adenosine 3',5'-phosphate by preparations from brain and other tissues. J. biol. Chem. **237**, 1239—1243 (1962).
KLEIN, D. C., BERG, G. R., WELLER, J.: Melatonin synthesis: adenosine 3',5'-monophosphate and norepinephrine stimulate N-acetyltransferase. Science **168**, 979—980 (1970b).
— — — GLINSMANN, W.: Pineal gland: dibutyryl cyclic adenosine monophosphate stimulation of labeled melatonin production. Science **167**, 1738—1740 (1970a).
— ROWE, J.: Pineal gland in organ culture. I. Inhibition by harmine of serotonin-^{14}C oxidation, accompanied by stimulation of melatonin-^{14}C production. Molec. Pharmacol. **6**, 164—171 (1970).
— WELLER, J. L.: Indole metabolism in the pineal gland: a circadian rhythm in N-acetyltransferase. Science **169**, 1093—1095 (1970).
KONO, T.: Destruction of insulin effector system of adipose tissue cells by proteolytic enzymes. J. biol. Chem. **244**, 1772—1778 (1969a).
— Destruction and restoration of the insulin effector system of isolated fat cells. J. biol. Chem. **244**, 5777—5784 (1969b).
KORNACKER, M. S., BALL, E. G.: Respiratory processes in brown adipose tissue. J. biol. Chem. **243**, 1638—1644 (1968).

KRAUSE, E.-G., WOLLENBERGER, A.: Über die Aktivierung der Phosphorylase b-Kinase im akut ischämischen Myokard. Acta biol. med. germ. **19**, 381—393 (1967).

KREISBERG, R. A.: Effect of epinephrine on myocardial triglyceride and free fatty acid utilization. Amer. J. Physiol. **210**, 385—389 (1966).

KRIS, A. O., MILLER, R. E., WHERRY, F. E., MASON, J. W.: Inhibition of insulin secretion by infused epinephrine in rhesus monkeys. Endocrinology **78**, 87—97 (1966).

KUKOVETZ, W. R., PÖCH, G.: The action of imidazole on the effects of methylxanthines and catecholamines on cardiac contraction and phosphorylase activity. J. Pharmacol. exp. Ther. **156**, 514—521 (1967).

— — Cardiostimulatory effects of cyclic 3',5'-adenosine monophosphate and its acylated derivatives. Naunyn-Schmiedeberg's Arch. Pharmak. exp. Path. **266**, 236—254 (1970).

KUO, J. F.: Effects of deoxyfrenolicin on isolated adipose cells. II. Lipolysis, adenosine 3',5'-monophosphate levels, and comparison with the effects of vitamin K_5. Biochem. Pharmacol. **18**, 757—766 (1969).

— DE RENZO, E. C.: A comparison of the effects of lipolytic and antilipolytic agents on adenosine 3',5'-monophosphate levels in adipose cells as determined by prior labeling with adenine-8-^{14}C. J. biol. Chem. **244**, 2252—2260 (1969).

— GREENGARD, P.: An adenosine 3',5'-monophosphate-dependent protein kinase from Escherichia coli. J. biol. Chem. **244**, 3417—3419 (1969b).

— — Cyclic nucleotide-dependent protein kinases. IV. Widespread occurrence of adenosine 3',5'-monophosphate-dependent protein kinase in various tissues and phyla of the animal kingdom. Proc. nat. Acad. Sci. (Wash.) **64**, 1349—1355 (1969a).

KUROSHIMA, A., KONNO, N., ITOH, S.: Increase in the blood flow through brown adipose tissue in response to cold exposure and norepinephrine in the rat. Jap. J. Physiol. **17**, 523—537 (1967).

KYPSON, J., TRINER, L., NAHAS, G. G.: Effects of ouabain and K^+-free medium on activated lipolysis and epinephrine-stimulated glycogenolysis. J. Pharmacol. exp. Ther. **159**, 8—17 (1968).

LACY, P. E., HOWELL, S. L., YOUNG, D. A., FINK, C. J.: New hypothesis of insulin secretion. Nature (Lond.) **219**, 1177—1179 (1968b).

— YOUNG, D. A., FINK, C. J.: Studies on insulin secretion *in vitro* from isolated islets of the rat pancreas. Endocrinology **83**, 1155—1161 (1968a).

LAMBERT, A. E., JEANRENAUD, B., RENOLD, A. E.: Enhancement by caffeine of glucagon-induced and tolbutamide-induced insulin release from isolated foetal pancreatic tissue. Lancet (*i*), 819—820 (1967).

— — JUNOD, A., RENOLD, A. E.: Organ culture of fetal rat pancreas. II. Insulin release induced by amino and organic acids, by hormonal peptides, by cationic alterations of the medium and by other agents. Biochim. biophys. Acta (Amst.) **184**, 540—553 (1969b).

— JUNOD, A., STAUFFACHER, W., JEANRENAUD, B., RENOLD, A. E.: Organ culture of fetal rat pancreas. I. Insulin release induced by caffeine and by sugars and some derivatives. Biochim. biophys. Acta. (Amst.) **184**, 529—539 (1969a).

LANGAN, T. A.: Action of adenosine 3',5'-monophosphate-dependent histone kinase *in vivo*. J. biol. Chem. **244**, 5763—5765 (1969a).

— Phosphorylation of liver histone following the administration of glucagon and insulin. Proc. nat. Acad. Sci. (Wash.) **64**, 1276—1283 (1969b).

LANGER, G. A.: Ion fluxes in cardiac excitation and contraction and their relation to myocardial contractility. Physiol. Rev. **48**, 708—757 (1968).

LARAIA, P. J., CRAIG, R. J., REDDY, W. J.: Glucagon: effect on adenosine 3',5'-monophosphate in the rat heart. Amer. J. Physiol. **215**, 968—970 (1968).

LARNER, J.: Hormonal and non-hormonal control of glycogen metabolism. Trans. N.Y. Acad. Sci. **29**, 192—209 (1966).

— SANGER, F.: The amino acid sequence of the phosphorylation site of muscle uridine diphosphoglucose α-1,4-glucan α-4-glucosyl transferase. J. molec. Biol. **11**, 491—500 (1965).

— VILLAR-PALASI, C., GOLDBERG, N. D., BISHOP, J. S., HUIJING, F., WENGER, J. I., SASKO, H., BROWN, N. B.: Hormonal and non-hormonal control of glycogen synthesis–control of transferase phosphatase and transferase I kinase. Advanc. Enzyme Regulation **6**, 409—423 (1968).

LAVIS, V. R., WILLIAMS, R. H.: Studies of the insulin-like actions of thiols upon isolated fat cells. J. biol. Chem. **245**, 23—31 (1970).

LEBOVITZ, H. E., POOLER, K.: ACTH-mediated insulin secretion: effect of aminophylline. Endocrinology **81**, 558—564 (1967).

LEDUC, J., RIVEST, P.: Effets de l'ablation de la graisse brune interscapulaire sur l'acclimatation au froid chez le rat. Rev. can. Biol. **28**, 49—66 (1969).

LEHNINGER, A. L.: The mitochondrion, molecular basis of structure and function. New York: W. A. Benjamin Inc. 1964.

LETARTE, J., JEANRENAUD, B., RENOLD, A.E.: Ionic effects on glucose transport and metabolism by isolated mouse fat cells incubated with or without insulin. II. Effect of replacement of K^+ and ouabain. Biochim. biophys. Acta (Amst.) **183**, 357—365 (1969).
— RENOLD, A.E.: Ionic effects on glucose transport and metabolism by isolated mouse fat cells incubated with or without insulin. I. Lack of effect of medium Ca^{+2} Mg^{+2}, or PO_4^{-3}. Biochim. biophys. Acta (Amst.) **183**, 350—356 (1969).
LEVEY, G.S.: Solubilization of myocardial adenyl cyclase. Biochem. biophys. Res. Commun. **38**, 86—92 (1970).
— EPSTEIN, S.E.: Myocardial adenyl cyclase; activation by thyroid hormones and evidence for two adenyl cyclase systems. J. clin. Invest. **48**, 1663—1669 (1969a).
— — Activation of adenyl cyclase by glucagon in cat and human heart. Circulat. Res. **24**, 151—156 (1969b).
— SKELTON, C.L., EPSTEIN, S.E.: Decreased myocardial adenyl cyclase activity in hypothyroidism. J. clin. Invest. **48**, 2244—2250 (1969a).
— — — Influence of hyperthyroidism on the effects of norepinephrine on myocardial adenyl cyclase activity and contractile state. Endocrinology **85**, 1004—1009 (1969b).
LEVINE, R.A.: Effects of glycogenolytic agents on phosphorylase activity of perfused liver. Amer. J. Physiol. **208**, 317—323 (1965).
LEWIS, G.P., MATTHEWS, J.: The mobilization of free fatty acids from rabbit adipose tissue in situ. Brit. J. Pharmacol. **34**, 564—578 (1968).
LIBERMAN, B., KLEIN, L.A., KLEEMAN, C.R.: Effect of adrenergic blocking agents on the vasopressin inhibiting action of norepinephrine. Proc. Soc. exp. Biol. (N.Y.) **133**, 131—134 (1970).
LINCOVÁ, D., ČERNOHORSKÝ, M., ČEPELÍK, J., MÜHLBACHOVÁ, E., WENKE, W.: Action of certain catechol and oxedrine sympathomimetics on lipid mobilization *in vitro*. Europ. J. Pharmacol. **2**, 53—58 (1967).
LINDBERG, O., DE PIERRE, J., RYLANDER, E., AFZELIUS, B.A.: Studies ofthe mitochondrial energy-transfer system of brown adipose tissue. J. Cell Biol. **34**, 293—310 (1968).
— PRUSINER, S.B., CANNON, B., CHING, T.M.: Metabolic control in isolated brown fat cells. Lipids **5**, 204—209 (1970).
LUNDHOLM, L., MOHME-LUNDHOLM, E., SVEDMYR, N.: Metabolic effects of catecholamines. In: E.E. BITTAR and N. BITTAR, Ed. The biological basis of medicine, volume 2 pp. 101—130. Academic Press, 1968.
LUYCKX, A.S., LEFEBVRE, P.J.: Arguments for a regulation of pancreatic glucagon secretion by circulating plasma free fatty acids. Proc. Soc. exp. Biol. (N.Y.) **133**, 524—528 (1970).
MADISON, L.L., SEYFFERT, W.A., JR., UNGER, R.H., BARKER, B.: Effect of plasma free fatty acids on plasma glucagon and serum insulin concentrations. Metabolism **17**, 301—304 (1968).
MAKMAN, M.H., SUTHERLAND, E.W.: Use of liver adenyl cyclase for assay of glucagon in human gastro-intestinal tract and pancreas. Endocrinology **75**, 127—134 (1964).
MALAISSE-LAGAE, F., MAHY, M., MALAISSE, W.J.: Effect of epinephrine upon ^{45}Ca uptake by isolated islets of Langerhans. Hormone and metabolic Res. **1**, 319—320 (1969).
MALAISSE, W.J., MALAISSE-LAGAE, F.: Stimulation of insulin secretion by noncarbohydrate metabolites. J. Lab. clin. Med. **72**, 438—448 (1968).
— — MAYHEW, D.: A possible role for the adenyl cyclase system in insulin secretion. J. clin. Invest. **46**, 1724—1734 (1967a).
— — WRIGHT, P.H., ASHMORE, J.: Effects of adrenergic and cholinergic agents upon insulin secretion *in vitro*. Endocrinology **80**, 975—978 (1967b).
MALAMUD, D.: Adenyl cyclase: relationship to stimulated DNA synthesis in parotid glands. Biochem. biophys. Res. Commun. **35**, 754—758 (1969).
— BASERGA, R.: On the mechanism of action of isoproterenol in stimulating DNA synthesis in salivary glands of rats and mice. Life Sci. **6**, 1765—1769 (1967).
— — Pool size and specific activity of UTP in isoproterenol-stimulated salivary glands. Biochim. biophys. Acta (Amst.) **195**, 258—261 (1969).
MALLETTE, L.E., EXTON, J.H., PARK, C.R.: Control of gluconeogenesis from amino acids in the perfused rat liver. J. biol. Chem. **244**, 5713—5723 (1969).
MANSOUR, T.E.: Factors influencing activation of phosphofructokinase. Pharmacol. Rev. **18**, 173—179 (1966).
MARINETTI, G.V., RAY, T.K., TOMASI, V.: Glucagon and epinephrine stimulation of adenyl cyclase in isolated rat liver plasma membranes. Biochem. biophys. Res. Commun. **36**, 185—193 (1969).
MARKUS, H.B., BALL, E.G.: Inhibition of lipolytic processes in rat adipose tissue by antimalarial drugs. Biochim. biophys. Acta (Amst.) **187**, 486—491 (1969).
MARTIN, A.P., BASERGA, R.: Changes in peroxidase activity in salivary gland after administration of isoproterenol. Proc. Soc. exp. Biol. (N.Y.) **131**, 1022—1025 (1969).

MARTIN, D.B., CARTER, J.R., JR.: Insulin-stimulated glucose uptake by subcellular particles from adipose tissue cells. Science **167**, 873—874 (1970).
MASORO, E.J., ROWELL, L.B., MCDONALD, R.M.: Intracellular muscle lipids as ernegy sources during muscular exercise and fasting. Fed. Proc. **25**, 1421—1424 (1966a).
— — — STEIERT, B.: Skeletal muscle lipids. II. Nonutilization of intracellular lipid esters as an energy source for contractile activity. J. biol. Chem. **241**, 2626—2634 (1966b).
MAYER, S.E.: Effect of epinephrine on carbohydrate metabolism in the heart. In: R.D. TANZ, F. KAVALER and J. ROBERTS, Ed. Factors influencing myocardial contractility, pp. 443—455. New York: Academic Press 1967.
— Adrenergic receptors for metabolic responses in the heart. Fed. Proc. (in press) (1970).
— NAMM, D.H., RICE, L.: Effect of glucagon on cyclic 3′,5′-AMP, phosphorylase activity and contractility of heart muscle of the rat. Circulat. Res. **26**, 225—233 (1970).
— WILLIAMS, B.J., SMITH, J.M.: Adrenergic mechanisms in cardiac glycogen metabolism. Ann. N.Y. Acad. Sci. **139**, 686—702 (1967).
MAYFIELD, E.D., JR., GHIDONI, J.J., BRESNICK, E., STANTON, H.C.: The effect of isoproterenol on pyrimidine biosynthesis in the salivary gland and heart of rats. Proc. Soc. exp. Biol. (N.Y.) **129**, 91—96 (1968).
MAYHEW, D.A., WRIGHT, P.H., ASHMORE, J.: Regulation of insulin secretion. Pharmacol. Rev. **21**, 183—212 (1969).
MCAFEE, R.D.: The action of β-adrenergic site stimulating catecholamines on isolated frog skin. Biochim. biophys. Acta (Amst.) **203**, 104—110 (1970).
MCCARL, R.L., MARGOSSIAN, S.S., JACKMAN, L.M., WEBB, R.L.: Characterization of rat heart myosin. II. Enzymatic properties. Biochemistry **8**, 3659—3664 (1969).
MEESTER, W.D., HARDMAN, H.F.: Blockade of the positive inotropic actions of epinephrine and theophylline by acetylcholine. J. Pharmacol. exp. Ther. **158**, 241—247 (1967).
MELSON, G.L., CHASE, L.R., AURBACH, G.D.: Parathyroid hormone-sensitive adenyl cyclase in isolated renal tubules. Endocrinology **86**, 511—518 (1970).
MENAHAN, L.A., WIELAND, O.: Glucagon-like action of N^6, 2′-O-dibutyryl cyclic 3′,5′-AMP on perfused rat liver. Biochem. biophys. Res. Commun. **29**, 880—885 (1967).
MERSMANN, H.J., SEGAL, H.L.: An on-off mechanism for liver glycogen synthetase activity.
— Proc. nat. Acad. Sci. (Wash.) **58**, 1688—1695 (1967).
— Glucocorticoid control of the liver glycogen synthetase-activating system. J. biol. Chem. **244**, 1701—1704 (1969).
MILLER, L.L.: Direct actions of insulin, glucagon and epinephrine on the isolated perfused rat liver. Fed. Proc. **24**, 737—744 (1965).
MINEMURA, T., CROFFORD, O.B.: Insulin-receptor interaction in isolated fat cells. I. The insulin-like properties of p-chloromercuribenzene sulfonic acid. J. biol. Chem. **244**, 5181 to 5188 (1969).
MITZNEGG, P., HEIM, F., MEYTHALER, B.: Influence of endogenous and exogenous cyclic 3′,5′-AMP on contractile responses induced by oxytocin and calcium in isolated rat uterus. Life Sci. **9**, part I, 121—128 (1970).
MIYAMOTO, E., KUO, J.F., GREENGARD, P.: Adenosine 3′,5′-monophosphate-dependent protein kinase from brain. Science **165**, 63—65 (1969a).
— — — Cyclic nucleotide-dependent protein kinases. III. Purification and properties of adenosine 3′,5′-monophosphate-dependent protein kinase from bovine brain. J. biol. Chem. **244**, 6395—6402 (1969b).
MODOLELL, J.B., MOORE, R.O.: ATPase activities of rat epididymal adipose tissue. Biochim. biophys. Acta (Amst.) **135**, 319—332 (1967).
MOHME-LUNDHOLM, E.: Smooth muscle phosphorylase and enzymes affecting its activity. Acta physiol. scand. **59**, 74—84 (1963).
MONDON, C.E., MORTIMORE, G.E.: Effects of insulin on amino acid release and urea formation in perfused rat liver. Amer. J. Physiol. **212**, 173—178 (1967).
MOORE, P.F., IORIO, L.C., MCMANUS, J.M.: Relaxation of the guinea pig tracheal chain preparation by N^6,2′-O-dibutyryl 3′,5′-cyclic adenosine monophosphate. J. Pharm. Pharmacol. **20**, 368—372 (1968).
MORGAN, H.E., PARMEGGIANI, A.: Regulation of glycogenolysis in muscle. II. Control of glycogen phosphorylase reaction in isolated perfused heart. J. biol. Chem. **239**, 2435—2439 (1964).
MORTIMORE, G.E., MONDON, C.E.: Inhibition by insulin on valine turnover in liver. Evidence for a general control of proteolysis. J. biol. Chem. **245**, 2375—2383 (1970).
MOSINGER, B., KUJALOVÁ, V.: Potassium-dependent lipomobilizing effect of adrenaline on incubated adipose tissue. Biochim. biophys. Acta (Amst.) **116**, 174—177 (1966).
— VAUGHAN, M.: Effects of electrolytes on epinephrine stimulated lipolysis in adipose tissue *in vitro*. Biochim. biophys. Acta (Amst.) **144**, 556—568 (1967a).
— — The action of cyclic 3′,5′-adenosine monophosphate on lipolysis in rat adipose tissue. Biochim. biophys. Acta (Amst.) **144**, 569—582 (1967b).

MUIRHEAD, M., HIMMS-HAGEN, J.: Changes in the amount and properties of adenyl cyclase in brown adipose tissue during acclimation of rats to cold. Canad. J. Biochem. **49**, 802—810 (1971).

MURAD, F., CHI, Y.-M., RALL, T.W., SUTHERLAND, E.W.: Adenyl cyclase. III. The effect of catecholamines and choline esters on the formation of adenosine 3′,5′-phosphate by preparations from cardiac muscle and liver. J. biol. Chem. **237**, 1233—1238 (1962).

— MANGANIELLO, V., VAUGHAN, M.: Effects of cyclic 3′,5′-GMP (cG) on the concentration of cyclic 3′,5′-AMP (cA) in fat cells. J. clin. Invest. **48**, 59a (1969b).

— RALL, T.W., VAUGHAN, M.: Conditions for the formation, partial purification and assay of an inhibitor of adenosine 3′,5′-monophosphate. Biochim. biophys. Acta (Amst.) **192**, 430—445 (1969a).

— VAUGHAN, M.: Effect of glucagon on rat heart adenyl cyclase. Biochem. Pharmacol. **18**, 1053—1059 (1969).

NAGATA, N., RASMUSSEN, H.: Parathyroid hormone, 3′,5′-AMP, Ca^{++}, and renal gluconeogenesis. Proc. nat. Acad. Sci. (Wash.) **65**, 368—374 (1970).

NAKANO, J., ISHII, T., PYRON, J.T., HOUSE, E.C.: Effect of cocaine on norepinephrine-induced lipolysis in anesthetized dogs and in isolated rat and dog fat cells. Arch. int. Pharmacodyn. **178**, 1—8 (1969).

NAMM, D.H., MAYER, S.E.: Effects of epinephrine on cardiac cyclic 3′,5′-AMP, phosphorylase kinase, and phosphorylase. Molec. Pharmacol. **4**, 61—69 (1968).

— — MALTBIE, M.: The role of potassium and calcium ions in the effect of epinephrine on cardiac cyclic adenosine 3′,5′-monophosphate, phosphorylase kinase, and phosphorylase. Molec. Pharmacol. **4**, 522—530 (1968).

NAYLER, W.G., McINNES, I., CHIPPERFIELD, D., CARSON, V., DAILE, P.: The effect of glucagon on calcium exchangeability, coronary blood flow, myocardial function and high energy phosphate stores. J. Pharmacol. exp. Ther. **171**, 265—275 (1970).

NORTHROP, G.: Effects of adrenergic blocking agents on epinephrine and 3′,5′-AMP-induced responses in the perfused rat liver. J. Pharmacol. exp. Ther. **159**, 22—28 (1968).

— PARKS, R.E., JR.: Studies on epinephrine and 3′,5′-AMP induced hyperglycemia employing the isolated perfused liver preparation. J. Pharmacol. exp. Ther. **145**, 135—141 (1964).

NOVALES, R.R., DAVIS, W.J.: Melanin-dispersing effect of adenosine 3′,5′-monophosphate on amphibian melanophores. Endocrinology **81**, 283—290 (1967).

ÖSTMAN, J., EFENDIĆ, S., ARNER, P.: Catecholamines and metabolism of human adipose tissue. Acta med. scand. **186**, 241—246 (1969).

ORÖ, L., WALLENBERG, L., ROSELL, S.: Ciculatory and metabolic processes in adipose tissue *in vivo*. Nature (Lond.) **205**, 178—179 (1965).

OWMAN, C.: On the significance of the 5-hydroxytryptamine stores in pineal gland. Advanc. Pharmacol. **6A**, 167—169 (1968).

ØYE, I.: The action of adrenaline in cardiac muscle. Dissociation between phosphorylase activation and inotropic response. Acta physiol. scand. **65**, 251—258 (1965).

— Glycogen phosphorylase: a specific secondary target system for adrenergic stimulation in the heart. Acta physiol. scand. **69**, 270—275 (1967b).

— The role of phosphorylase a and b for the control of glycogenolysis in the isolated working rat heart. Acta physiol. scand. **70**, 229—235 (1967a).

— SUTHERLAND, E.W.: The effect of epinephrine and other agents on adenyl cyclase in the cell membrane of avian erythrocytes. Biochim. biophys. Acta (Amst.) **127**, 347—354 (1966).

OZAWA, E., EBASHI, S.: Requirement of Ca ion for the stimulating effect of cyclic 3′,5′-AMP on muscle phosphorylase b kinase. J. Biochem. (Tokyo) **62**, 285—286 (1967).

— HOSOI, K., EBASHI, S.: Reversible stimulation of muscle phosphorylase b kinase by low concentrations of calcium ions. J. Biochem. (Tokyo) **61**, 531—533 (1967).

PARRA, A., SCHULTZ, R.B., FOLEY, T.P., JR., BLIZZARD, R.M.: Influence of epinephrine-propranolol infusion release on growth hormones in normal and hypopituitary subjects. J. clin. Endocr. **30**, 134—137 (1970).

PASSONEAU, J.V., LOWRY, O.H.: Phosphofructokinase and the Pasteur effect. Biochem. biophys. Res. Commun. **7**, 10—15 (1962).

PENHOS, J.C., WU, C.H., DAUNAS, J., REITMAN, M., LEVINE, R.: Effect of glucagon on the metabolism of lipids and on urea formation by the perfused rat liver. Diabetes **15**, 740—748 (1966).

PERRY, M.C., HALES, C.N.: Rates of efflux and intracellular concentrations of potassium, sodium and chloride ions in isolated fat-cells from the rat. Biochem. J. **115**, 865—871 (1969).

— — Factors affecting the permeability of isolated fat-cells from the rat to [42K] potassium and [36Cl] chloride ions. Biochem. J. **117**, 615—621 (1970).

PIRAS, R., STANELONI, R.: *In vivo* regulation of rat muscle glycogen synthetase activity. Biochemistry **8**, 2153—2160 (1969).

Pogson, C.I.: Adipose tissue pyruvate kinase. Properties and interconversion of two active forms. Biochem. J. **110**, 67—77 (1968).
Pohl, S.L., Birnbaumer, L., Rodbell, M.: Glucagon-sensitive adenyl cyclase in plasma membrane of hepatic parenchymal cells. Science **164**, 566—567 (1969).
Porte, D.: A receptor mechanism for the inhibition of insulin release by epinephrine in man. J. clin. Invest. **46**, 86—94 (1967a).
— Beta adrenergic stimulation of insulin release in man. Diabetes **16**, 150—155 (1967b).
— Sympathetic regulation of insulin secretion. Its relation to diabetes mellitus. Arch. intern. Med. **123**, 252—260 (1969).
— Graber, A., Kuzuya, T., Williams, R.H.: Epinephrine inhibition of insulin release. J. clin. Invest. **44**, 1087 (1965).
— — — — The effect of epinephrine on immunoreactive insulin levels in man. J. clin. Invest. **45**, 228—236 (1966).
— Williams, R.H.: Inhibition of insulin release by norepinephrine in man. Science **152**, 1248—1250 (1966).
Posner, J.B., Hammermeister, K.E., Bratvold, G.E., Krebs, E.G.: The assay of adenosine-3′,5′-phosphate in skeletal muscle. Biochemistry **3**, 1040—1044 (1964).
— Stern, R., Krebs, E.G.: Effects of electrical stimulation and epinephrine on muscle phosphorylase, phosphorylase b kinase and adenosine 3′,5′-phosphate. J. biol. Chem. **240**, 982—985 (1965).
Poyart, C.F., Nahas, G.G.: Inhibition of activated lipolysis by acidosis. Molec. Pharmacol. **4**, 389—401 (1968).
— Vulliemoz, Y., Nahas, G.G.: Regulation of activated lipolysis by albumin, glucose, and H^+. Proc. Soc. exp. Biol. (N.Y.) **125**, 863—868 (1967).
Prusiner, S.B.: Spectroscopic evidence for control of respiration prior to phosphorylation in hamster brown fat cells. J. biol. Chem. **245**, 382—389 (1970).
— Cannon, B., Lindberg, O.: Oxidative metabolism in cells isolated from brown adipose tissue. I. Catecholamine and fatty acid stimulation of respiration. Europ. J. Biochem. **6**, 15—22 (1968a).
— — Ching, T.M., Lindberg, O.: Oxidative metabolism in cells isolated from brown adipose tissue. 2. Catecholamine regulated respiratory control. Europ. J. Biochem. **7**, 51—57 (1968b).
— Williamson, J.R., Chance, B., Paddle, B.M.: Pyridine nucleotide changes during thermogenesis in brown fat tissue *in vivo*. Arch. Biochem. Biophys. **123**, 368—377 (1968c).
Pryor, J., Berthet, J.: Action du glucagon sur l'incorporation des acides aminés dans les protéines par le tissu hépatique. Arch. int. Physiol. Biochem. **68**, 227 (1959).
— — The action of adenosine 3′,5′-monophosphate on the incorporation of leucine into liver proteins. Biochim. biophys. Acta (Amst.) **43**, 556—557 (1960).
Rabinowitz, M., Desalles, L., Meisler, J., Lorand, L.: Distribution of adenyl-cyclase activity in rabbit skeletal muscle fractions. Biochim. biophys. Acta (Amst.) **97**, 29—36 (1965).
Racker, E.: Resolution and reconstitution of the inner mitochondrial membrane. Fed. Proc. **26**, 1335—1340 (1967).
Radley, J.M.: DNA synthesis in the rat submaxillary gland following injection of isoprenaline. Aust. J. exp. Biol. med. Sci. **46**, 795—797 (1968).
Rafael, J., Klaas, D., Hohorst, H.-J.: Mitochondrien aus braunem Fettgewebe: Enzyme und Atmungskettenphosphorylierung während der prä- und postnatalen Entwicklung des Interscapularen Fettkörpers des Meerschweinchens. Hoppe-Seylers Z. physiol. Chem. **349**, 1711—1724 (1968).
— Ludolph, H.-J., Hohorst, H.-J.: Mitochondrien aus braunem Fettgewebe: Entkopplung der Atmungskettenphosphorylierung durch langkettige Fettsäuren und Rekopplung durch Guanosintriphosphat. Hoppe-Seylers Z. physiol. Chem. **350**, 1121—1131 (1969).
Rall, T.W., Kakiuchi, S.: The influence of certain neurohormones and drugs on the accumulation of cyclic 3′,5′-AMP in brain tissue. In: O. Walaas, Ed. Molecular basis of some aspects of mental activity, pp. 417—427. London and New York: Academic Press 1966.
— Sutherland, E.W., Wosilait, W.D.: The relationship of epinephrine and glucagon to liver phosphorylase. III. Reactivation of liver phosphorylase in slices and in extracts. J. biol. Chem. **218**, 483—495 (1956).
Randle, P.J., Garland, P.B., Hales, C.N., Newsholme, E.A.: The glucose-fatty acid cycle; its role in insulin sensitivity and the metabolic disturbances of diabetes mellitus. Lancet (*i*), 785—789 (1963).
Rasmussen, H., Tenenhouse, A.: Cyclic adenosine monophosphate, Ca^{++}, and membranes. Proc. nat. Acad. Sci. (Wash.) **59**, 1364—1370 (1968).
Ray, T.K.: A modified method for the isolation of the plasma membrane from rat liver. Biochim. biophys. Acta (Amst.) **196**, 1—9 (1970).

REED, N., FAIN, J.N.: Stimulation of respiration in brown fat cells by epinephrine, dibutyryl-3′,5′-adenosine monophosphate, and m-chloro (carbonyl cyanide) phenylhydrazone. J. biol. Chem. **243**, 2843—2848 (1968a).

— — Potassium-dependent stimulation of respiration in brown fat cells by fatty acids and lipolytic agents. J. biol. Chem. **243**, 6077—6083 (1968b).

REGEN, D.M., TERRELL, E.B.: Effects of glucagon and fasting on acetate metabolism in perfused rat liver. Biochim. biophys. Acta (Amst.) **170**, 95—111 (1968).

REIK, L., PETZOLD, G.L., HIGGINS, J.A., GREENGARD, P., BARRNETT, R.J.: Hormone-sensitive adenyl cyclase: cytochemical localization in rat liver. Science **168**, 382—384 (1970).

RENOLD, A.E.: Insulin biosynthesis and secretion — a still unsettled topic. New Engl. J. Med. **282**, 173—182 (1970).

— CAHILL, G.F., JR., LEBOEUF, B., HERRERA, M.G.: Effect of adrenocortical hormones upon adipose tissue. In: CIBA foundation study group No. 5, Metabolic effects of adrenal hormones, pp. 68—79. Boston: Little, Brown and Co. 1960.

RILEY, W.D., DELANGE, R.J., BRATVOLD, G.E., KREBS, E.G.: Reversal of phosphorylase kinase activation. J. biol. Chem. **243**, 2209—2215 (1968).

RIZACK, M.A.: An epinephrine-sensitive lipolytic activity in adipose tissue. J. biol. Chem. **236**, 657—662 (1961).

— Activation of an epinephrine-sensitive lipolytic activity from adipose tissue by adenosine 3′,5′-phosphate. J. biol. Chem. **239**, 392—395 (1964).

— Hormone-sensitive lipolytic activity of adipose tissue. In: A.E. RENOLD and G.F. CAHILL. JR., Ed. Adipose Tissue, Handbook of Physiology, section 5, pp. 309—311. American Physiological Society, 1965.

ROBERTS, J.C., SMITH, R.E.: Time-dependent responses of brown fat in cold-exposed rats. Amer. J. Physiol. **212**, 519—525 (1967).

ROBINOVITCH, M.R., SMUCKLER, E.A.,SREEBNY, L.M.: Protein synthesis in a cell-free system, derived from the rat parotid gland. J. biol. Chem. **244**, 5361—5367 (1969).

ROBISON, G.A., BUTCHER, R.W., ØYE, I., MORGAN, H.E., SUTHERLAND, E.W.: The effect of epinephrine on adenosine 3′,5′-phosphate levels in the isolated perfused rat heart. Molec. Pharmacol. **1**, 168—177 (1965).

— — SUTHERLAND, E.W.: Adenyl cyclase as an adrenergic receptor. Ann. N. Y. Acad. Sci. **139**, 703—723 (1967).

— — — Cyclic AMP. Ann. Rev. Biochem. **37**, 149—174 (1968).

RODBELL, M.: Metabolism of isolated fat cells. I. Effects of hormones on glucose metabolism and lipolysis. J. biol. Chem. **239**, 375—380 (1964).

— Modulation of lipolysis in adipose tissue by fatty acid concentration in fat cell. Ann. N. Y. Acad. Sci. **131**, 302—314 (1965a).

— The metabolism of isolated fat cells. In: A.E. RENOLD and G.F. CAHILL, JR., Ed. Adipose tissue, Handbook of Physiology, section 5, pp. 471—482. American Physiological Society, 1965b.

— Metabolism of isolated fat cells. V. Preparation of "ghosts" and their properties; adenyl cyclase and other enzymes. J. biol. Chem. **242**, 5744—5750 (1967a).

— Metabolism of isolated fat cells. VI. The effects of insulin, lipolytic hormones, and theophylline on glucose transport and metabolism in "ghosts". J. biol. Chem. **242**, 5751—5756 (1967b).

— BIRNBAUMER, L., POHL, S.L.: Adenyl cyclase in fat cells. III. Stimulation by secretin and the effects of trypsin on the receptors for lipolytic hormones. J. biol. Chem. **245**, 718—722 (1970).

— JONES, A.B.: Metabolism of isolated fat cells. III. The similar inhibitory action of phospholipase C (Clostridium perfringens *a* toxin) and of insulin on lipolysis stimulated by lipolytic hormones and theophylline. J. biol. Chem. **241**, 140—142 (1966).

— — CHIAPPE DE CINGOLANI, G.E., BIRNBAUMER, L.: The actions of insulin and catabolic hormones on the plasma membrane of the fat cell. Recent Progr. Hormone Res. **24**, 215—247 (1968).

ROGNSTAD, R., KATZ, J.: The effect of 2,4-dinitrophenol on adipose-tissue metabolism. Biochem. J. **111**, 431—444 (1969).

ROSELL, S.: Release of free fatty acids from subcutaneous adipose tissue in dogs following sympathetic nerve stimulation. Acta physiol. scand. **67**, 343—351 (1966).

ROSELL-PEREZ, M., LARNER, J.: Studies on UDPG-*a*-glucan transglucosylase. V. Two forms of the enzyme in dog skeletal muscle and their interconversion. Biochemistry **3**, 81—88 (1964).

ROSEN, O.M., ROSEN, S.M.: The effect of catecholamines on the adenyl cyclase of frog and tadpole hemolysates. Biochem. biophys. Res. Commun. **31**, 82—91 (1968).

— — Properties of an adenyl cyclase partially purified from frog erythrocytes. Arch. Biochem. Biophys. **131**, 449—456 (1969).

Ross, B.D., Hems, R., Freedland, R.A., Krebs, H.A.: Carbohydrate metabolism of the perfused rat liver. Biochem. J. **105**, 869—875 (1967).

Rudman, D.: The mobilization of fatty acids from adipose tissue by pituitary peptides and catechol amines. Ann. N. Y. Acad. Sci. **131**, 102—112 (1965).

— Del Rio, A.E.: Responsiveness to lipolytic hormones, and inactivation of adrenocorticotropin, by adipose tissue slices and free fat cells from different mammalian species. Endocrinology **85**, 209—213 (1969).

Salaman, M.R., Robinson, D.S.: Clearing factor lipase in adipose tissue. A medium in which the enzyme activity of tissue from starved rats increases *in vitro*. Biochem. J. **99**, 640—647 (1966).

Salomon, Y., Schramm, M.: A specific binding site for 3′,5′-cyclic AMP in rat parotid microsomes. Biochem. biophys. Res. Commun. **38**, 106—111 (1970).

Salvador, R.A., April, S.A., Lemberger, L.: Phentolamine activation of glycogenolysis in rat skeletal muscle. Biochem. Pharmacol. **17**, 395—402 (1968).

Sasaki, T., Litwack, G., Baserga, R.: Protein synthesis in the early prereplicative phase of isoproterenol-stimulated synthesis of deoxyribonucleic acid. J. biol. Chem. **244**, 4831—4837 (1969).

Sattin, A., Rall, T.W.: The effect of adenosine and adenine nucleotides on the cyclic adenosine 3′,5′-phosphate content of guinea pig cerebral cortex slices. Molec. Pharmacol. **6**, 13—23 (1970).

Scales, B., McIntosh, D.A.D.: Studies on the radiocalcium uptake and the adenosine triphosphatases of skeletal and cardiac sarcoplasmic reticulum fractions. J. Pharmacol. exp. Ther. **160**, 249—260 (1968a).

— — Effects of propranolol and its optical isomers on the radiocalcium uptake and the adenosine triphosphatases of skeletal and cardiac sarcoplasmic reticulum fractions. J. Pharmacol. exp. Ther. **160**, 261—267 (1968b).

Schaeffer, L.D., Chenoweth, M., Dunn, A.: Adrenal corticosteroid involvement in the control of liver glycogen phosphorylase activity. Biochim. biophys. Acta (Amst.) **192**, 292—303 (1969a).

— — — Adrenal corticosteroid involvement in the control of phosphorylase in muscle. Biochim. biophys. Acta (Amst.) **192**, 304—309 (1969b).

Schlender, K.K., Wei, S.H., Villar-Palasi, C.: UDP-glucose: glycogen a-4-glucosyltransferase. I. Kinase activity of purified muscle protein kinase. Cyclic nucleotide specificity. Biochim. biophys. Acta (Amst.) **191**, 272—278 (1969).

Schramm, M.: Amylase secretion in rat parotid slices by apparent activation of endogenous catecholamine. Biochim. biophys. Acta (Amst.) **165**, 546—549 (1968).

— Bdolah, A.: The mechanism of enzyme secretion by the cell. III. Intermediate stages in amylase transport as revealed by pulse labeling of slices of parotid gland. Arch. Biochem. Biophys. **104**, 67—72 (1964).

Selye, H., Veilleux, R., Cantin, M.: Excessive stimulation of salivary gland growth by isoproterenol. Science **133**, 44—45 (1961).

Senft, G., Schultz, G., Munske, K., Hoffman, M.: Influence of insulin on cyclic 3′,5′-AMP phosphodiesterase activity in liver, skeletal muscle, adipose tissue, and kidney. Diabetologia **4**, 322—329 (1968a).

— — — — Effects of glucocorticoids and insulin on 3′,5′-AMP phosphodiesterase activity in adrenalectomized rats. Diabetologia **4**, 330—335 (1968b).

— Sitt, R., Losert, W., Schultz, G., Hoffmann, M.: Hemmung der Insulininkretion durch a-Receptoren stimulierende Substanzen. Naunyn-Schmiedeberg's Arch. Pharmak. exp. Path. **260**, 309—323 (1968c).

Seubert, W., Henning, H.V., Schoner, W., L'age, M.: Effects of cortisol on the levels of metabolites and enzymes controlling glucose production from pyruvate. Advanc. Enzyme Regulat. **6**, 153—180 (1968).

Seyffert, W.A., Jr., Madison, L.L.: Physiologic effects of metabolic fuels on carbohydrate metabolism. I. Acute effect of elevation of plasma free fatty acids on hepatic glucose output, peripheral glucose utilization, serum insulin, and plasma glucagon levels. Diabetes **16**, 765—776 (1967).

Shahab, L., Wollenberger, A., Haase, M., Schiller, U.: Noradrenalinabgabe aus dem Hundeherzen nach vorübergehender Okklusion einer Koronararterie. Acta biol. med. germ. **22**, 135—143 (1969).

Shanfeld, J., Frazer, A., Hess, M.E.: Dissociation of the increased formation of cardiac adenosine 3′,5′-monophosphate from the positive inotropic effect of norepinephrine. J. Pharmacol. exp. Ther. **169**, 315—320 (1969).

Shein, H.M., Wurtman, R.J.: Cyclic adenosine monophosphate stimulation of melatonin and serotonin synthesis in cultured rat pineals. Science **166**, 519—520 (1969).

SHEPPARD, H., BURGHARDT, C.: Adenylcyclase in non-nucleated erythrocytes of several mammalian species. Biochem. Pharmacol. **18**, 2576—2578 (1969).

SHIMAZU, T.: Glycogen synthetase activity in liver: regulation by the autonomic nerves. Science **156**, 1256—1257 (1967).

— AMAKAWA, A.: Regulation of glycogen metabolism in liver by the autonomic nervous system. II. Neural control of glycogenolytic enzymes. Biochim. biophys. Acta (Amst.) **165**, 335—348 (1968a).

— — Regulation of glycogen metabolism in liver by the autonomic nervous system. III. Differential effects of sympathetic nerve stimulation and of catecholamines on liver phosphorylase. Biochim. biophys. Acta (Amst.) **165**, 349—356 (1968b).

SHIMIZU, H., CREVELING, C.R., DALY, J.W.: Cyclic adenosine 3',5'-monophosphate formation in brain slices: stimulation by batrachotoxin, ouabain, veratridine, and potassium ions. Molec. Pharmacol. **6**, 184—188 (1970a).

— — — Stimulated formation of adenosine 3',5'-cyclic phosphate in cerebral cortex: synergism between electrical activity and biogenic amines. Proc. nat. Acad. Sci. (Wash.) **65**, 1033—1040 (1970b).

— DALY, J.W., CREVELING, C.R.: A radioisotopic method for measuring the formation of adenosine 3',5'-cyclic monophosphate in incubated slices of brain. J. Neurochem. **16**, 1609—1619 (1969).

SHINEBOURNE, E.A., HESS, M.L., WHITE, R.J., HAMER, J.: The effect of noradrenaline on the calcium uptake of the sarcoplasmic reticulum. Cardiovasc. Res. **3**, 113—117 (1969).

SIMSON, J.V.: Discharge and restitution of secretory material in the rat parotid gland in response to isoproterenol. Z. Zellforsch. **101**, 175—191 (1969).

SKÁLA, J., BARNARD, T., LINDBERG, O.: Changes in interscapular brown adipose tissue of the rat during perinatal and early postnatal development and after cold acclimation. II. Mitochondrial changes. Comp. Biochem. Physiol. **33**, 509—528 (1970).

SKELTON, C.L., LEVEY, G.S., EPSTEIN, S.E.: Positive inotropic effects of dibutyryl cyclic adenosine 3',5'-monophosphate. Circulat. Res. **26**, 35—43 (1970).

SMITH, R.E., HORWITZ, B.A.: Brown fat and thermogenesis. Physiol. Rev. **49**, 330—425 (1969).

— — IMAI, Y.: Quantitative thermogenesis of brown fat in hibernation and cold adaptation. In: Quantitative biology of metabolism, A. LOCKER, Ed. pp. 106—111. Springer-Verlag New York Inc., 1968.

— ROBERTS, J.C.: Thermogenesis of brown adipose tissue in cold-acclimated rats. Amer. J. Physiol. **206**, 143—148 (1964).

SOBEL, B.E., DEMPSEY, P.J., COOPER, T.: Adenyl cyclase activity in the chronically denervated cat heart. Biochem. biophys. Res. Commun. **33**, 758—762 (1968).

— — — Normal myocardial adenyl cyclase in hyperthyroid cats. Proc. Soc. exp. Biol. (N.Y.) **132**, 6—9 (1969).

SOKAL, J.E., SARCIONE, E.J., HENDERSON, A.M.: Relative potency of glucagon and epinephrine as hepatic glycogenolytic agents: studies with the isolated perfused rat liver. Endocrinology **74**, 930—938 (1964).

SONNENBLICK, E.H., STAM, A.C., JR.: Cardiac muscle: activation and contraction. Ann. Rev. Physiol. **31**, 647—674 (1969).

SPITZER, J.J., MCELROY, W.T., JR.: Some hormonal effects on uptake of free fatty acids by the liver. Amer. J. Physiol. **199**, 876—878 (1960).

STAFFORD, A.: Actions of adrenaline on the potassium balance of the isolated heart. Brit. J. Pharmacol. **36**, 571—581 (1969).

STANELONI, R., PIRAS, R.: Changes in glycogen synthetase and phosphorylase during muscular contraction. Biochem. biophys. Res. Commun. **36**, 1032—1038 (1969).

STEINER, G., CAHILL, G.F., JR.: Brown and white adipose tissue metabolism in cold-exposed rats. Amer. J. Physiol. **207**, 840—844 (1964).

— — Brown and white adipose tissue metabolism response to norepinephrine and insulin. Amer. J. Physiol. **211**, 1325—1328 (1966).

— JOHNSON, G.E., SELLERS, E.A., SCHÖNBAUM, E.: The nervous control of brown adipose tissue metabolism in normal and cold-acclimated rats. Fed. Proc. **28**, 1017—1021 (1969).

— LOVELAND, M., SCHÖNBAUM, E.: Effect of denervation on brown adipose tissue metabolism. Amer. J. Physiol. **218**, 566—570 (1970).

STOCK, K., WESTERMANN, E.: Hemmung der Lipolyse durch α- und β-Sympathicolytica, Nicotinsäure und Prostaglandin E_1. Naunyn-Schmiedeberg's Arch. Pharmak. exp. Path. **254**, 334—354 (1966a).

— — Competitive and non-competitive inhibition of lipolysis by α- and β-adrenergic blocking agents, methoxamine derivatives and prostaglandin E_1. Life Sci. **5**, 1667—1678 (1966b).

STRUCK, E., ASHMORE, J., WIELAND, O.: Stimulierung der Gluconeogenese durch langkettige Fettsäuren und Glucagon. Biochem. Z. **343**, 107—110 (1965).

SUSSMAN, K.E., VAUGHAN, G.D.: Insulin release after ACTH, glucagon and adenosine 3',5'-phosphate (cyclic AMP) in the perfused isolated rat pancreas. Diabetes **16**, 449—454 (1967).

SUTER, E.R.: The ultrastructure of brown adipose tissue in perinatal rats. Experientia (Basel) **25**, 286—287 (1969a).

— The fine structure of brown adipose tissue. I. Cold-induced changes in the rat. J. Ultrastruct. Res. **26**, 216—241 (1969b).

— The fine structure of brown adipose tissue. II. Perinatal development in the rat. Lab. Invest. **21**, 246—258 (1969c).

— The fine structure of brown adipose tissue. III. The effect of cold exposure and its mediation in newborn rats. Lab. Invest. **21**, 259—268 (1969d).

— STÄUBLI, W.: An ultrastructural histochemical study of brown adipose tissue from neonatal rats. J. Histochem. Cytochem. **18**, 100—106 (1970).

SUTHERLAND, E.W., ØYE, I., BUTCHER, R.W.: The action of epinephrine and the role of the adenyl cyclase system in hormone action. Recent Progr. Hormone Res. **21**, 623—646 (1965).

— RALL, T.W.: The relation of adenosine-3',5'-phosphate and phosphorylase to the actions of catecholamines and other hormones. Pharmacol. Rev. **12**, 265—299 (1960).

— — MENON, T.: Adenyl cyclase. I. Distribution, preparation and properties. J. biol. Chem. **237**, 1220—1227 (1962).

— ROBISON, G.A.: The role of cyclic-3',5'-AMP in responses to catecholamines and other hormones. Pharmacol. Rev. **18**, 145—161 (1966).

— — BUTCHER, R.W.: Some aspects of the biological role of adenosine 3',5'-monophosphate (cyclic AMP). Circulation **37**, 279—306 (1968).

SWISLOCKI, N.I.: Dissociation of lipolysis and protein anabolism by ACTH, bovine growth hormone and thyroid stimulating hormone in adipose tissue with dibutyryl cyclic AMP and theophylline. Biochim. biophys. Acta (Amst.) **201**, 242—249 (1970).

SZELÉNYI, Z.: Effect of cold exposure on oxygen tension in brown adipose tissue in the non-cold-adapted adult rat. Acta physiol. Acad. Sci. hung. **33**, 311—316 (1968).

TAYLOR, A.N., WILSON, R.W.: Electrophysiological evidence for the action of light on the pineal gland in the rat. Experientia (Basel) **26**, 267—269 (1970).

THOMSON, J.F., HABECK, D.A., NANCE, S.L., BEETHAM, K.L.: Ultrastructural and biochemical changes in brown fat in cold-exposed rats. J. Cell Biol. **41**, 312—334 (1969).

— SMITH, D.E., NANCE, S.L., HABECK, D.A.: Some metabolic characteristics of brown fat, with particular reference to the mitochondria. Comp. Biochem. Physiol. **25**, 783—804 (1968).

TOMKINS, G.M., GELEHRTER, T.D., GRANNER, D., MARTIN, D., JR., SAMUELS, H.H., THOMPSON, E.B.: Control of specific gene expression in higher organisms. Science **166**, 1474—1480 (1969).

TORRES, H.N., MARECHAL, L.R., BERNARD, E., BELOCOPITOW, E.: Control of muscle glycogen phosphorylase activity by insulin. Biochim. biophys. Acta (Amst.) **156**, 206—209 (1968).

TOUABI, M., JEANRENAUD, B.: α-Aminoisobutyric acid uptake in isolated mouse fat cells. Biochim. biophys. Acta (Amst.) **173**, 128—140 (1969).

TRINER, L., OVERWEG, N.I.A., NAHAS, G.G.: Cyclic 3',5'-AMP and uterine contractility. Nature (Lond.) **225**, 282—283 (1970).

TURTLE, J.R., KIPNIS, D.M.: An adrenergic receptor mechanism for the control of cyclic 3',5' adenosine monophosphate synthesis in tissues. Biochem. biophys. Res. Commun. **28**, 797—802 (1967).

— LITTLETON, G.K., KIPNIS, D.M.: Stimulation of insulin secretion by theophylline. Nature (Lond.) **213**, 727—728 (1967).

UNGER, R.H., KETTERER, H., DUPRÉ, J., EISENTRAUT, A.M.: The effects of secretin, pancreozymin, and gastrin on insulin and glucagon secretion in anesthetized dogs. J. clin. Invest. **46**, 630—645 (1967).

VAN DEN BERGH, S.G., MODDER, G.P., SOUVERIJN, J.H.M., PIERROT, H.C.J.M.: Some aspects of fatty acid oxidation by isolated mitochondria. In: L. ERNSTER and Z. DRAHOTA, Ed. Mitochondria: Structure and function, pp. 137—144. London and New York: Academic Press 1969.

VAN HARKEN, D.R., DIXON, C.W., HEIMBERG, M.: Hepatic lipid metabolism in experimental diabetes. V. The effect of concentration of oleate on metabolism of triglycerides and on ketogenesis. J. biol. Chem. **244**, 2278—2285 (1969).

VAUGHAN, M.: Effect of hormones on phosphorylase activity in adipose tissue. J. biol. Chem. **235**, 3049—3053 (1960).

— MURAD, F.: Adenyl cyclase activity in particles from fat cells. Biochemistry **8**, 3092—3099 (1969).

VAUGHAN, M., STEINBERG, D., LIEBERMAN, F., STANLEY, S.: Activation and inactivation of lipase in homogenates of adipose tissue. Life Sci. **4**, 1077—1083 (1965).

VERNIKOS-DANELLIS, J., MARKS, B.H.: Epinephrine-induced release of ACTH in normal human subjects: a test of pituitary function. Endocrinology **70**, 525—531 (1962).
VILLAR-PALASI, C.: The hormonal regulation of glycogen metabolism in muscle. Vitam. and Horm. **26**, 65—118 (1968).
WADE, D.R., HALES, C.N.: Activation of hormone-sensitive lipase by 3′,5′ cyclic AMP. Fed. Proc. **28**, 906 (1969).
WALSH, D.A., PERKINS, J.P., KREBS, E.G.: An adenosine 3′,5′-monophosphate-dependent protein kinase from rabbit skeletal muscle. J. biol. Chem. **243**, 3763—3765 (1968).
WATLINGTON, C.O.: Effect of catecholamines and adrenergic blockade on sodium transport of isolated frog skin. Amer. J. Physiol. **214**, 1001—1007 (1968).
— α-Adrenergic inhibition of Na^+-transport: the interaction of vasopressin and 3′,5′-AMP. Biochim. biophys. Acta (Amst.) **193**, 394—402 (1969).
WEISS, B.: Discussion of the formation, metabolism and physiologic effects of melatonin. Advanc. Pharmacol. **6**A, 152—155 (1968).
— Similarities and differences in the norepinephrine and sodium fluoride-sensitive adenyl cyclase system. J. Pharmacol. exp. Ther. **166**, 330—338 (1969a).
— Effects of environmental lighting and chronic denervation on the activation of adenyl cyclase of rat pineal gland by norepinephrine and sodium fluoride. J. Pharmacol. exp. Ther. **168**, 146—152 (1969b).
— COSTA, E.: Regional and subcellular distribution of adenyl cyclase and 3′,5′-cyclic nucleotide phosphodiesterase in brain and pineal gland. Biochem. Pharmacol. **17**, 2107—2116 (1968a).
— — Selective stimulation of adenyl cyclase of rat pineal gland by pharmacologically active catecholamines. J. Pharmacol. exp. Ther. **161**, 310—319 (1968b).
— CRAYTON, J.: Gonadal hormones as regulators of pineal adenyl cyclase activity. Endocrinology **87**, 527—533 (1970).
WELLER, M., RODNIGHT, R.: Stimulation by cyclic AMP of intrinsic protein kinase activity in ox brain membrane preparations. Nature (Lond.) **225**, 187—188 (1970).
WELLS, H.: Submandibular salivary gland weight increase by administration of isoproterenol to rat. Amer. J. Physiol. **202**, 425—428 (1962).
— Salivary gland enlargement in rats after administration of theophylline. Amer. J. Physiol. **212**, 1293—1296 (1967).
— HANDELMAN, C., MILGRAM, E.: Regulation by sympathetic nervous system of accelerated growth of salivary glands of rats. Amer. J. Physiol. **196**, 707—710 (1959a).
— ZACKIN, S.J., GOLDHABER, P., MUNSON, P.L.: Increase in weight of the submandibular salivary glands of rats following periodic amputation of the erupted portion of the incisor teeth. Amer. J. Physiol. **196**, 827—830 (1959b).
WENKE, M.: Effects of catecholamines on lipid mobilization. Advanc. Lipid Res. **4**, 69—105 (1966).
WERRBACH, J.H., GALE, C.C., GOODNER, C.J., CONWAY, M.J.: Effects of autonomic blocking agents on growth hormone, insulin and free fatty acids and glucose in baboons. Endocrinology **86**, 77—82 (1970).
WEST, E.S., TODD, W.R., MASON, H.S., VAN BRUGGEN, J.T.: Textbook of Biochemistry, 4th edition, p. 849. New York: MacMillan: and London: Collier-MacMillan 1966.
WHITLOCK, J.P., JR., KAUFMAN, R., BASERGA, R.: Changes in thymidine kinase and α-amylase activity during isoproterenol-stimulated DNA synthesis in mouse salivary gland. Cancer Res. **28**, 2211—2216 (1968).
WICKS, W.D.: Tyrosine-α-ketoglutarate transaminase: induction by epinephrine and adenosine-3′,5′-cyclic phosphate. Science **160**, 997—998 (1968).
— Induction of hepatic enzymes by adenosine 3′,5′-monophosphate in organ culture. J. biol. Chem. **244**, 3941—3950 (1969).
— KENNEY, F.T., LEE, K.-L.: Induction of hepatic enzyme synthesis in vivo by adenosine 3′,5′-monophosphate. J. biol. Chem. **244** 6008—6013 (1969).
WIELAND, O., SIESS, E.: Interconversion of phospho- and dephospho-forms of pig heart pyruvate dehydrogenase. Proc. nat. Acad. Sci. (Wash.) **65**, 947—954 (1970).
WILCOX, H.G., DISMON, G., HEIMBERG, M.: Hepatic lipid metabolism in experimental diabetes. IV. Incorporation of amino acid ^{14}C into lipoprotein-protein and triglyceride. J. biol. Chem. **243**, 666—675 (1968).
WILKENFELD, B.E., LEVY, B.: The effects of theophylline, diazoxide and imidazole on isoproterenol-induced inhibition of the rabbit ileum. J. Pharmacol. exp. Ther. **169**, 61—67 (1969).
WILLIAMS, B.J., MAYER, S.E.: Hormonal effects on glycogen metabolism in the rat heart *in situ*. Molec. Pharmacol. **2**, 454—464 (1966).
WILLIAMS, R.H., WALSH, S.A., ENSINCK, J.W.: Effect of metals upon the conversion of adenosine triphosphate to adenosine 3′,5′-monophosphate in lipocytes. Proc. Soc. exp. Biol. (N.Y.) **128**, 279—283 (1968a).

— — HEPP, D.K., ENSINCK, J.W.: Method for measuring hormonal effects on conversion of adenosine triphosphate to adenosine 3′,5′-monophosphate by isolated lipocytes. Metabolism XVII, 653—668 (1968b).

WILLIAMSON, J.R.: Metabolic effects of epinephrine in the isolated, perfused rat heart. I. Dissociation of the glycogenolytic from the metabolic stimulatory effect. J. biol. Chem. **239**, 2721—2729 (1964).

— Kinetic studies of epinephrine effects in the perfused rat heart. Pharmacol. Rev. **18**, 205—210 (1966a).

— Metabolic effects of epinephrine in the perfused rat heart. II. Control steps of glucose and glycogen metabolism. Molec. Pharmacol. **2**, 206—220 (1966b).

— Effects of fatty acids, glucagon and anti-insulin serum on the control of gluconeogenesis and ketogenesis in rat liver. Advanc. Enzyme Regulat. **5**, 229—255 (1967).

— Control of energy metabolism in hamster brown adipose tissue. J. biol. Chem. **245**, 2043—2050 (1970).

— BROWNING, E.T., SCHOLZ, R.: Control mechanisms of gluconeogenesis and ketogenesis. I. Effects of oleate on gluconeogenesis in perfused rat liver. J. biol. Chem. **244**, 4607 (1969a).

— — THURMAN, R.G., SCHOLZ, R.: Inhibition of glucagon effects in perfused rat liver by (+) decanoylcarnitine. J. biol. Chem. **244**, 5055—5064 (1969c).

— HERCZEG, B., COLES, H., DANISH, R.: Studies on the ketogenic effect of glucagon in intact rat liver. Biochem. biophys. Res. Commun. **24**, 437—442 (1966c).

— KREISBERG, R.A., FELTS, P.W.: Mechanism for the stimulation of gluconeogenesis by fatty acids in perfused rat liver. Proc. nat. Acad. Sci. (Wash.) **56**, 247—254 (1966b).

— PRUSINER, S., OLSON, M.S., FUKAMI, M.: Control of metabolism in brown adipose tissue. Lipids **5**, 1—14 (1970).

— SCHOLZ, R., BROWNING, E.T.: Control mechanisms of gluconeogenesis and ketogenesis. II. Interactions between fatty acid oxidation and the citric acid cycle in perfused rat liver. J. biol. Chem. **244**, 4617—4627 (1969b).

— WRIGHT, P.H., MALAISSE, W.J., ASHMORE, J.: Control of gluconeogenesis by acetyl CoA in rats treated with glucagon and anti-insulin serum. Biochem. biophys. Res. Commun. **24**, 765—770 (1966a).

WING, D.R., ROBINSON, D.S.: Clearing-factor lipase in adipose tissue. A possible role of adenosine 3′,5′-(cyclic)-monophosphate in the regulation of its activity. Biochem. J. **109**, 841—849 (1968).

— SALAMAN, M.R., ROBINSON, D.S.: Clearing-factor lipase in adipose tissue. Factor influencing the increase in enzyme activity produced on incubation of tissue from starved rats *in vitro*. Biochem. J. **99**, 648—656 (1966).

WOLFE, S.M., MUENZER, J., GORDON, R.S., JR.: Adenyl cyclase activity in salivary glands. Fed. Proc. **28**, 832 (1969).

WOLLENBERGER, A., KRAUSE, E.-G., HEIER, G.: Stimulation of 3′,5′-cyclic AMP formation in dog myocardium following arrest of blood flow. Biochem. biophys. Res. Commun. **36**, 664—670 (1969).

WONG, K.K., SYMCHOWICZ, S., STAUB, M.S., TABACHNICK, I.I.A.: The *in vitro* effect of catecholamines, diazoxide and theophylline on insulin release. Life Sci. **6**, 2285 (1967).

WOSILAIT, W.D., SUTHERLAND, E.W.: The relationship of epinephrine and glucagon to liver phosphorylase. II. Enzymatic inactivation of liver phosphorylase. J. biol. Chem. **218**, 469—481 (1956).

WÜNNENBERG, W., BRÜCK, K.: Zur Funktionsweise thermoreceptiver Strukturen im Cervicalmark des Meerschweinchens. Pflügers Arch. ges. Physiol. **299**, 1—10 (1968).

WURTMAN, R.J., AXELROD, J.: The formation, metabolism and physiologic effects of melatonin. Advanc. Pharmacol. **6A**, 141—151 (1968).

— — FISCHER, J.E.: Melatonin synthesis in the pineal gland. Effect of light mediated by the sympathetic nervous system. Science **143**, 1328—1330 (1964).

— SHEIN, H.M., AXELROD, J., LAREN, F.: Incorporation of ^{14}C-tryptophan into ^{14}C-protein by cultured rat pineals: stimulation by l-norepinephrine. Proc. nat. Acad. Sci. (Wash.) **62**, 749—755 (1969).

YEUNG, D., OLIVER, I.T.: Factors affecting the premature induction of phosphopyruvate carboxylase in neonatal rat liver. Biochem. J. **108**, 325—331 (1968a).

— — Induction of phosphopyruvate carboxylase in neonatal rat liver by adenosine 3′,5′-cyclic monophosphate. Biochemistry **7**, 3231—3239 (1968b).

Note added in proof: For recent literature on cyclic AMP see also

ROBISON, G.A., BUTCHER, R.W., SUTHERLAND, E.W.: Cyclic AMP. Academic Press, New York and London (1971).

GREENGARD, P., COSTA, E., editors: Role of cyclic AMP in cell function. Raven Press, New York (1970).

Chapter 12

Central Actions of Catecholamines

E. MARLEY and J.D. STEPHENSON

With 14 Figures

I. Introduction

The last twenty years have seen remarkable strides in understanding of the anatomy and function of the noradrenergic and dopaminergic components of the central nervous system. The discovery and mapping of noradrenaline in the brain (VOGT, 1954), apart from giving impetus to work in this field, also indicated what functions noradrenaline might serve by revealing its distribution. Dopamine is also present, mainly in the corpus striatum and median eminence. The distribution of amines was given meaning in terms of neuronal pathways by use of fluorescence microscopy (DAHLSTRÖM and FUXE, 1965; FUXE, 1965; HILLARP et al., 1966). Nigro-striatal and tubero-infundibular dopamine neurone systems were described as well as ascending and descending noradrenergic pathways. A further sophistication was development of substances which interfered with either the breakdown or synthesis of catecholamines, so increasing or depleting neuronal stores. That there were sites in the brain selectively responsive to catecholamines became evident from iontophoretic micro-electrode studies.

Almost as a chef-d'oeuvre, the effects of catecholamines could be witnessed in terms of changes in behaviour and electrical activity of large areas of the brain. Earlier work in which the amines were given intravenously was regarded with reserve, since the amines were unlikely to penetrate from the blood to the brain. FELDBERG and co-workers developed techniques which had important consequences; drugs were injected *via* a chronically implanted cannula so as to be distributed through the entire ventricular system or through a portion of it (see FELDBERG, 1963). Catecholamines so injected had central depressant effects quite the opposite of those obtained by intravenous injection. It is remarkable that even now the belief that catecholamines are exclusively central excitants has a considerable following. Catecholamines given by micro-infusion into selected areas of the brain, usually have depressant effects or effects compatible with a central depressant action as after intraventricular or intracisternal injection. Another method of acutely increasing the concentration of catecholamines in the brain is by administration of their amino-acid precursors. Although the effects are usually clear-cut, the interpretation is not easy since, apart from direct actions of their own, the amino acids are taken up into neurones, converted to the corresponding amines and released not only from noradrenergic or dopaminergic neurones but also from 5-hydroxytryptaminergic neurones.

This chapter deals with a few of these aspects. Wherever relevant, dose, route of injection and isomeric species of the particular drug are given.

II. Blood-Brain and Cerebrospinal Fluid-Brain Barriers

These aspects are considered since they are of utmost relevance to central actions of catecholamines.

1. Blood-Brain Barrier

The concept of a blood-brain barrier is currently under fire, partly because the original finding upon which it was fostered, i.e. that dyes injected parenterally failed to stain the brain although they coloured all other tissues — is based on fallacious premises and partly because the term covers such a heterogeneous collection of phenomena. "In some cases there is an almost complete mechanical barrier to entry, as with large molecules. With other substances considerable entry into the brain occurs, but the substance seems to be removed more rapidly than it arrives, so that the equilibrium position is one in which brain and cerebrospinal fluid concentrations are maintained far below those of the plasma. Again, entry of some material into brain may be actively facilitated, as with glucose, or completely unimpeded as in the case of water and the volatile anaesthetics. No anatomical structure, nor any single functional mechanism can account for all the blood-brain transport characteristics" (Dobbing, 1968).

The partition coefficient between fat (olive oil) and water relates to uptake of drugs into the brain (Meyer, 1899; Overton, 1901). The use of olive oil has been criticized in the light of subsequent knowledge that cell membrane constituents are composed chiefly of aliphatic alcohols and phospholipids (Albert, 1960). Oleyl alcohol has been suggested as a more satisfactory alternative. Partition coefficients between oleyl alcohol and an aqueous buffer were low for noradrenaline, α-methylnoradrenaline and adrenaline, i.e. 0.21, 0.26 and 0.26 respectively, in comparison to high values — 1.0 and 1.2 for phenethylamine and dexamphetamine respectively (Dewhurst and Marley, 1965a). This correlates with ready penetration of phenylethylamine and dexamphetamine to the brain, whereas catecholamines penetrate slowly or not at all. Thus in adult cats given tritium-labelled noradrenaline as a single intravenous dose or infused intravenously over 30 min, the hypothalamus was the only part of the brain, apart from the area postrema, where significant uptake of noradrenaline occurred; even there, uptake was slow compared with other tissues (Weil-Malherbe, 1960). Adrenaline infused intravenously into adult anaesthetized cats has been detected in the subarachnoid and ventricular spaces (Draškoci et al., 1960) but the dose used, 40 μg/kg/min, exceeds that likely to be achieved physiologically.

In immature brains the blood-brain barrier is said to be absent or not fully effective (Bakay, 1956; Lajtha, 1957). It was on this supposition that young chickens were used for testing the central effects of catecholamines (Key and Marley, 1961, 1962), inasmuch as the effects observed after systemic administration might be more valid than those in adults in which catecholamines would be excluded from the brain. Despite absence of the blood-brain barrier, the central nervous system was sufficiently mature for the chick to be behaviourally self-sufficient and for electrocortical activity to correlate highly with behavioural sleep or wakefulness (Key and Marley, 1962). Whereas intravenous catecholamines produced sleep in young chicks, they did not in the adult (Key and Marley, 1961, 1962). This accorded with the finding in adult animals of soporific effects when catecholamines were injected intraventricularly or intracisternally, by-passing the blood-brain barrier. For similar reasons, chicks were used for studying the central effects of 5-hydroxytryptamine (Hehman et al., 1961) and a variety of other drugs (Spooner and Winters, 1965).

Many substances penetrate more readily into immature than into adult brains. A higher exchange rate of chloride (LAJTHA, 1957; WAELSCH, 1955) and greater permeability of young than adult brains to glutamic acid (HIMWICH et al., 1957), lysine (LAJTHA, 1958), leucine (LAJTHA and TOTH, 1961), P^{32} (FRIES and CHAIKOFF, 1941), α-aminoisobutyric acid (KUTTNER et al., 1961) and thiocyanate (LAJTHA, 1957) were found. More recently, electron microscopists (CALEY, 1966) and physiologists (VERNADAKIS and WOODBURY, 1965) have demonstrated the large extracellular space in immature rat brains, amounting to a 40% space for inulin. Despite this large extracellular space, the blood-brain barrier was almost fully developed at birth since only a small amount of $(\pm)$-7-H^3-noradrenaline injected subcutaneously was taken up into the brain (GLOWINSKI et al., 1964). However, the presence of a large extracellular space could support the concept of blood-brain barrier immaturity, assuming that contraction of the space as the animal matures parallels development of the brain. Data along these lines were provided by SPOONER et al. (1966). Brain water content and extracellular space were determined in chickens and related to uptake of $(\pm)$-7-H^3-noradrenaline 2 min after its intravenous injection. The brain content of tritiated noradrenaline was: 93.0% of the plasma concentration at 1 day of age, 8.3% at 30 days, and 6.3% at 132 days. The maximum change in brain water content occurred during the first 30 days falling from 83% to 80.6%. The extracellular space decreased gradually from 31.5% at 1 day of age to 19.6% at 70 days. However, because a substance enters the brain in no way proves that it has an action there; such proof depends on being able to reproduce the effects by injecting the amine into sites of uptake.

The reduced entry of many biologically important substances into the brain may reflect cerebral metabolic requirements rather than blood-brain barrier function (BLASCHKO and CHRUŚCIEL, 1960). There may be better transport or metabolic mechanisms capable of restoring physiological concentration of the substance faster or to a greater degree in the adult than in the new-born brain (LAJTHA, 1962). Certainly, enzymes which inactivate sympathomimetic amines are present in low concentrations in immature animals (BIRKHÄUSER, 1940; EPPS, 1945) so that effects of these amines, should they penetrate to the brain, would persist longer. Enzymes such as DOPA decarboxylase and MAO are present in the vascular endothelium of the central nervous system (BERTLER et al., 1963) and constitute a proven barrier for DOPA and dopamine, one that is likely to apply for other catecholamines.

2. Cerebrospinal Fluid-Brain Barrier

Drugs may gain access to the brain not only through the blood-brain barrier but by secretion into the cerebrospinal fluid within the ventricles (ROTH et al., 1959). This brings another dimension into consideration, for while drug entry to the brain from the blood is largely governed by lipid solubility, entry from the cerebrospinal fluid to the brain is not (MAYER et al., 1959, 1960). Accordingly, effects of catecholamines given intraventricularly are of considerable interest since their relatively poor lipid solubility is no longer an impediment to absorption. The depth of penetration into the brain of substances injected into the ventricles differs greatly between various regions; substances may pass deeply into nuclear regions and even through the cerebral wall. The neuroglia appear to determine uptake of substances. The differences between uptake by grey and white matter and between different regions of grey matter would be due mainly to the fact that the distribution of the various glial cells varies between grey and white matter and, within the grey matter between different regions (FELDBERG, 1963). That uptake of substances from the cerebral ventricles is governed by neuroglial properties accords with electron microscopic findings (GERSCHENFELD et al., 1959; LUSE, 1959; LUSE and HARRIS, 1960), which indicate that neuroglial cells participate actively in movement of fluids within brain tissue.

There are two issues to consider. The first is the spread of an injectate within the ventricular system. For example, a radiopaque material (100 μl) given into the anterior horn of a cat lateral ventricle, was immediately distributed throughout the ventricular system including the lateral apertures of the 4th ventricle (McCARTHY and BORISON, 1966). The same volume of dye rapidly stained the brain's outer surfaces, indicating its swift transfer into subarachnoid spaces (CARR and MOORE, 1969). Large volumes of injectate may deform the ventricular system. Thus *30 μl* of ($\pm$)-H^3-noradrenaline injected intraventricularly in a *rat* dilated that ventricle (NOBLE et al., 1967) and 2 hr later, total tritium and H^3-noradrenaline contents were similar for injected and non-injected sides of the brain. In contrast, after administering only *10 μl* ($\pm$)-H^3-noradrenaline into a lateral ventricle of a *cat,* radioactivity was virtually confined to the ipsilateral and 3rd ventricles (CARR and MOORE, 1969); only a small amount was present in the contralateral ventricular lining. After injection into the 3rd ventricle, radioactivity was distributed caudal to the cannula, suggesting that the injectate moved with and not against flow of cerebrospinal fluid (CARR and MOORE, 1969).

The second point, that of the extent of uptake of drug from the ventricles into brain, can be most elegantly assessed by intraventricular injection of a radioactive isotope and subsequent determination of regional distribution of radioactivity. Although this has been done, the volume of material injected tends to be largish. GLOWINSKI and IVERSEN (1966a) injected radioactive noradrenaline or dopamine in a volume of 20—30 μl into a lateral ventricle of rats and killed the animals 1 and 24 hr later. Accumulation of H^3-noradrenaline in various brain portions correlated with regional distribution of endogenous noradrenaline, highest activity being present in the hypothalamus. Unexpectedly, there was considerable radioactivity in the striatum, a region with a high concentration of endogenous dopamine but little noradrenaline. Small amounts of activity were found in the hippocampus, cortex, cerebellum, midbrain and medulla oblongata. After intraventricular administration of H^3-dopamine there was rapid formation of H^3-noradrenaline in most brain regions except the striatum which had the largest activity of H^3-dopamine. REIVICH and GLOWINSKI (1967) re-examined this problem using autoradiography which permits more precise localization of radioactivity. Rats were injected intraventricularly with ($\pm$)-C^{14}-noradrenaline in a volume of 20—30 μl. In the diencephalon, the preoptic region and hypothalamus were intensely labelled. The reticular formation contained moderate amounts of radioactivity; in the medulla oblongata and pons, radioactivity was found in structures known to contain catecholamines either in nerve terminals such as the area grisea periventricularis, the inferior olivary complex and the raphe nuclei, or in cell bodies such as the locus coeruleus and the subependymal cells of the lateral part of the 4th ventricle. Overall and most striking was the uptake of amine into the limbic system. Similar findings were obtained by FUXE and UNGERSTEDT (1968a), whose approach differed in that they injected small doses (1—2 μg in 20 μl) of noradrenaline, dopamine or their α-methylated derivatives into a lateral ventricle of rats pretreated with reserpine or nialamide and assessed uptake by fluorescence microscopy. Uptake was confined to a limited zone, 300 μ wide, lining the ventricles and ventral part of the subarachnoid space. Uptake and accumulation of dopamine or noradrenaline did not occur unless monoamine oxidase had been inhibited, whereas the α-methylated compounds — which are resistant to monoamine oxidase, accumulated without inhibition of the enzyme. In a combined histochemical and autoradiographic study (FUXE et al., 1968), tritiated noradrenaline (15 μC in 20 μl or 30 μC in 40 μl) was injected into a lateral ventricle of rats. The above results were confirmed and good correlation noted between uptake of radioactive material and density of catecholamine neurones.

Tritiated noradrenaline given intracisternally in a 20 μl volume passes into the ventricular system of rats (SCHUBERT and LADISCH, 1969). There were two migration pathways into the brain for noradrenaline injected intracisternally, one from the subarachnoid space and one from the ventricular system, the amine penetrating 200—500 μ at these surfaces. Uptake was highest in regions rich in nerve cells, particularly those containing noradrenaline or dopamine in their terminals.

Finally, there is the possibility that substances injected into the brain enter the cerebrospinal fluid or blood, particularly if the volume of injectate is large. The rise in pressure produced by a large intracerebral injection (30 μl) in mice broke down the arachnoid villi with flow of injectate into the blood stream (CAIRNS, 1950; MIMS, 1960). Autoradiographic study indicated that a 20 μl injectate into the rabbit hypothalamus entered the brain stem, meninges and ventricular system (HARRISON, 1961). However, the technique is practical if adequate control is maintained over volume of injectate. At least 80% of radioactivity, 10 min after an intracerebral injection of 1.0 μl H^3-noradrenaline into the rat hypothalamus was recovered from brain tissue 2 mm laterally and rostrocaudally of the injection site (BOOTH, 1968). There was an average diffusion over an area of 1.9 mm diameter with injection of 1.0 μl of various dyes into the rat thalamus or hypothalamus (MYERS, 1966); a 1.0 μl droplet occupies a sphere, 1.1 mm in diameter (MYERS, 1964b). The validity of intracerebral injection techniques is discussed by RECH (1968).

III. Uptake, Storage and Release of Catecholamines and Catecholamine Precursors

Radioactive dopamine or noradrenaline, either formed endogenously from radioactive tyrosine or DOPA (BURACK and DRASKÓCZY, 1964; GOLDSTEIN and GERBER, 1963; GOLDSTEIN, 1964; UDENFRIEND and ZALTZMAN-NIRENBERG, 1963; IVERSEN and GLOWINSKI, 1966; NYBÄCK et al., 1968), or injected into the ventricles or cisterna magna (MILHAUD and GLOWINSKI, 1962, 1963; GOLDSTEIN and GERBER, 1963; GOLDSTEIN, 1964; MANNARINO et al., 1963; GLOWINSKI et al., 1965; GLOWINSKI et al., 1966a; GLOWINSKI et al., 1966c; SCHANBERG et al., 1967a; CARR and MOORE, 1969) mixes with endogenous catecholamines (GLOWINSKI and AXELROD, 1966; GLOWINSKI et al., 1966c; GLOWINSKI and IVERSEN, 1966b) and can be used as a tracer to monitor uptake, storage, turnover and metabolism of cerebral catecholamines. Estimation of noradrenaline turnover from the decline in endogenous noradrenaline concentration following α-methyltyrosine, an inhibitor of tyrosine hydroxylase, is limited by technical difficulties of measuring low concentrations of noradrenaline and by possible effects that these low concentrations have on turnover. Consequently, it is preferable to follow synthesis *in vivo* of radioactive catecholamines from radioactive tyrosine. Radioactive tyrosine, unlike radioactive DOPA or catecholamines, does not elevate endogenous catecholamine concentrations because conversion of tyrosine to DOPA is the step at which catecholamine synthesis is regulated.

Radioactivity was detected in a jugular vein, 2 min after intraventricular injection of C^{14}-noradrenaline (35 μg in 100 μl) in anaesthetized cats (MANNARINO et al., 1963). Some 50—60% of ($\pm$)-H^3-noradrenaline (20—30 μl) injected into a lateral ventricle or the cisterna magna of rats, appeared in the circulation within 6 min, after which there was no further loss of radioactivity from the brain until 1 hr (GLOWINSKI et al., 1965; SCHANBERG et al., 1967a). The immediate loss of radioactivity was probably due to the large volumes of injectate used, since in cats little radioactivity was detected in a jugular vein during the first hr after intraventricular injection of 10 μl ($\pm$)-H^3-noradrenaline (CARR and MOORE, 1969).

Four hours after intraventricular injection of ($\pm$)-H^3-noradrenaline, its subcellular distribution in various brain regions was similar to that of endogenous noradrenaline, although there was more exogenous than endogenous noradrenaline in the supernatant fraction (GLOWINSKI and IVERSEN, 1966b). However, specific activity of noradrenaline was higher in the particulate fraction of whole brain homogenates than in the supernatant (GLOWINSKI et al., 1966c). This discrepancy between results obtained in whole brain and in the cerebellum, cortex, medulla oblongata and hypothalamus may be related to differences in distribution of H^3-noradrenaline and endogenous noradrenaline among various brain regions e.g. caudate nucleus and hippocampus contain only low concentrations of endogenous noradrenaline, but accumulated large amounts of H^3-noradrenaline.

Radioactive noradrenaline, either taken up directly after intraventricular injection or synthesized *in vivo* from labelled precursors disappeared from the brain in several phases, as shown in Fig. 1 (UDENFRIEND and ZALTZMAN-NIRENBERG, 1963; BURACK and DRASKÓCZY, 1964; GLOWINSKI et al., 1965; IVERSEN and GLOWINSKI, 1966). There was a 45% decrease in H^3-noradrenaline between 1 and 2 hr corresponding to a half-life of about 70 min. From 2—12 hr (I in Fig. 1), the half-life of H^3-noradrenaline was about 3 hr, and from 12—48 hr (II in Fig. 1), the half-life was 17 hr (GLOWINSKI et al., 1965). In mice, half-lives of 3 hr (5 hr, NYBÄCK et al., 1968) and 17 hr were obtained for cerebral C^{14}-noradrenaline synthesized *in vivo* from DL-C^{14}-tyrosine or DL-C^{14}-DOPA (BURACK and DRASKÓCZY, 1964).

The rapid decline of radioactivity between 1 and 2 hr after administration of H^3-noradrenaline was probably due to incomplete mixing of accumulated H^3-noradrenaline with endogenous noradrenaline, with consequent preferential release of labelled catecholamine as occurs in the periphery (CHIDSEY and HARRISON, 1963; FISCHER and IVERSEN, quoted by IVERSEN, 1967). Thus, from 1—2 hr there was a rapid decline in H^3-noradrenaline of the supernatant fraction of whole brain (GLOWINSKI et al., 1966c).

At least two stores of noradrenaline have been postulated in peripheral sympathetic nervous tissue; a large storage pool in which noradrenaline is tightly bound and a small, functional pool with a more rapid turnover from which noradrenaline is readily released (TRENDELENBURG, 1961; STJÄRNE, 1961; STONE et al., 1962; CROUT et al., 1962; POTTER et al., 1962; POTTER and AXELROD, 1963). It seems likely that noradrenaline is stored in at least two pools in the brain, one with a rapid turnover — 3—4 hr, and the other with a slower turnover — 17—18 hr. Since a large proportion of accumulated H^3-noradrenaline disappeared in a single exponential decay within 8—12 hr of intraventricular injection, indicating a half-life of about 4 hr, regional turnover estimations were made during this time (IVERSEN and GLOWINSKI, 1966). An inverse relation between turnover and endogenous noradrenaline concentration was commonly found in the various brain regions. Thus, turnover of cerebellar noradrenaline (2 hr) was approximately twice that of hypothalamic noradrenaline (4 hr). Since total hypothalamic noradrenaline was approximately 10 times that of the cerebellum, the amount of noradrenaline synthesized in the hypothalamus per unit time was about 5 times greater (IVERSEN and GLOWINSKI, 1966; GLOWINSKI and BALDESSARINI, 1966).

It is probable that this relation between turnover and noradrenaline concentration is due to high concentrations of noradrenaline inhibiting synthesis of DOPA from tyrosine (section XI. 4., 6.). Disappearance of H^3-dopamine from rat brain after its intraventricular injection was similar to that of H^3-noradrenaline (IVERSEN and

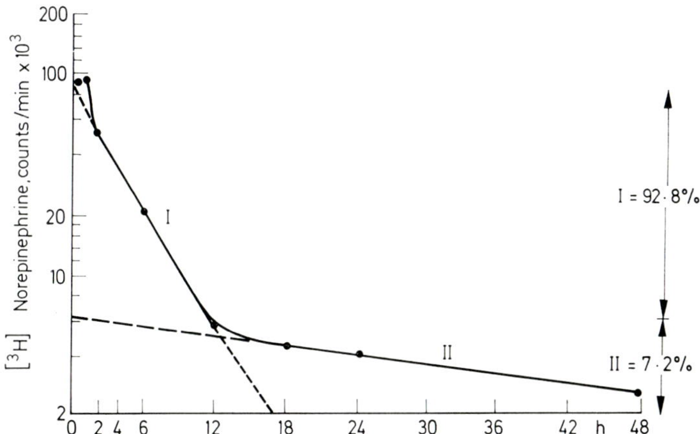

Fig. 1. Disappearance of H^3-noradrenaline from whole brain after intraventricular injection. H^3-Noradrenaline disappears in at least two phases: an initial rapid phase (I) accounts for the disappearance of the greater part of the catecholamine initially retained. (From IVERSEN, L.L. and GLOWINSKI, J., J. Neurochem. **13**, 671—682, 1966)

GLOWINSKI, 1966). However, its use is complicated by its possible synthesis to H^3-noradrenaline and its low endogenous concentration in most brain regions. In the caudate nucleus, turnover of H^3-dopamine was approximately 2 hr (IVERSEN and GLOWINSKI, 1966; UDENFRIEND and ZALTZMAN-NIRENBERG, 1963). However, after α-methyltyrosine half-life was increased to 4 hr; the reason for this increase is not known (IVERSEN and GLOWINSKI, 1966).

After intraventricular injection of H^3-noradrenaline, the major metabolite was H^3-normetanephrine in cats (MANNARINO et al., 1963; CARR and MOORE, 1969) and deaminated O-methylated catechols in rats, particularly 3-methoxy-4-hydroxy-phenylglycol (GOLDSTEIN and GERBER, 1963; GOLDSTEIN, 1964; GLOWINSKI et al., 1965). In rats, the ratio of H^3-normetanephrine to H^3-noradrenaline was higher after intraventricular injection of H^3-noradrenaline than after formation of H^3-noradrenaline *in vivo* from H^3-dopamine (GOLDSTEIN, 1964; GLOWINSKI et al., 1966b).

IV. Effect of Catecholamines on Innate Behaviour and Cerebral Electrical Activity

1. Catecholamines as Central Depressants

a) Intracisternal Injection

LEIMDORFER and METZNER (1949) observed that adrenaline (0.5—1.5 mg/kg) injected intracisternally in dogs produced brief excitement followed within 30 min first by sleep and then by anaesthesia lasting several hours; anaesthesia was sufficiently deep to permit laparotomy. No significant changes were noted in the electroencephalogram. In later experiments (LEIMDORFER, 1950), other catecholamines — noradrenaline, isoprenaline, butanephrine — given intracisternally evoked sleep and anaesthesia, whereas the phenolic amines, oxedrine or paredrine produced sleep but not anaesthesia. The lack of anaesthetic effect with the phenolic amines may have been due to insufficient dose. The volume of injectate is not mentioned in these papers, but the effects could be partly or wholly attributed to penetration of the amines into the ventricles and absorption from there into the brain.

It would be convenient to include in this section the effects in dogs of adrenaline (1.0 mg) injected into the arachnoid space overlying the cerebral cortex. Thirty min after injection the dog was drowsy and lying on its side (KOBAYASHI, 1965), the effect being maximal after 60 min with recovery at about 90 min. The mechanism of action is unknown since injection of a similar volume of dye indicated that the injectate would be confined to the upper half of the cerebral hemisphere without reaching the cisterna magna. BASS (1914) had observed sleep in dogs following injection of adrenaline under the dura or deeper into the brain.

b) Intraventricular Injection

The behavioural effects of adrenaline or noradrenaline injected intraventricularly in cats were the opposite of those seen after intravenous injection. It is worth recalling FELDBERG and SHERWOOD's (1954) description. "Within 10—20 min of an intraventricular injection of 20—80 μg of adrenaline into the cat, a state develops and subsequently deepens in which the animal appears to be under light anaesthesia. The condition is indistinguishable from that of sodium pentobarbitone anaesthesia. The cat lies in the cage, can be turned on its back, or lifted by its front or hind legs without struggling. The eyes are closed for most of the time the cat is left undisturbed, but when handled or disturbed, the cat stares with open apparently unseeing eyes interrupted by short periods in which the eyes fall shut. When pricked with a pin in the thighs, flank or head, it reacts very slowly if at all. When placed on the floor, the cat sags at once or can stand, and even jump, depending on the depth of the condition, but its gait is very slow and hesitant and consists of a few steps. The effect usually wears off within an hour and full recovery occurs within about 3 hr." Another interesting description is that of "catalepsy" induced in dogs by the intraventricular slow infusion of adrenaline or noradrenaline (6.25—12.5 μg/min) for 20 min (TRACZYK, 1964). To test for "catalepsy", wooden blocks were positioned under the dog's four paws. Untreated dogs usually stepped down within a few sec but after the infusion, "cataleptic" dogs stood on the blocks from 10—120 min. They no longer responded to auditory stimuli; muscular tonus was increased in the trunk and extremities. Transitory rigidity of forelegs and neck also occurs after adrenaline (0.5—1.0 mg/kg) injected intracisternally (LEIMDORFER and METZNER, 1949).

Central depressant effects have been elicited by intraventricular injection of adrenaline in mice (HALEY and McCORMICK, 1957; BRITTAIN and HANDLEY, 1967; CHAMBERS and ROBERTS, 1968; JONES and ROBERTS, 1968), rats (GRUNDEN, 1969), fowls (GRUNDEN and MARLEY, 1970), dogs (REITTER, 1957; GRUNDEN and KATZUNG, 1964), sheep (PALMER, 1959), monkeys (WADA, 1962) and man (LEIMDORFER et al., 1947; SHERWOOD, 1955). Catecholamines with similar effects include noradrenaline (FELDBERG and SHERWOOD, 1954; BRITTAIN and HANDLEY, 1967; GRUNDEN and MARLEY, 1970; PALMER, 1959), α-methylnoradrenaline (KADZIELAWA, 1967; GRUNDEN and MARLEY, 1970), isoprenaline (GRUNDEN, 1969; GRUNDEN and MARLEY, 1970), phenylephrine (GRUNDEN, 1969) and dopamine (SCHAIN, 1961; WADA et al., 1963; GRUNDEN and MARLEY, 1970).

The term central depressant as applied to catecholamines has been given loose connotation. Indeed, FELDBERG and SHERWOOD (1954) point out that the condition produced when adrenaline or noradrenaline was injected intraventricularly in cats was one of light general anaesthesia, but that previous workers had used the terms sleep and anaesthesia apparently interchangeably. It is valuable to specify the meaning since the effects seen in different species, although perhaps lying on the same phenomenal continuum, are not necessarily analogous. For example, the term central depressant has been construed to apply to decreased locomotor activity (FISCHER and AMALFARA, 1962; GRUNDEN and KATZUNG, 1964; GROSSMAN, 1968; GRUNDEN, 1969), sedation (BREGGIN, 1965; FINDLAY and ROBERTSHAW, 1967), stupor or partial anaesthesia (PALMER, 1959; BREGGIN, 1965), catalepsy (TRACZYK, 1964), analgesia (IVY et al., 1944), anaesthesia (LEIMDORFER and METZNER, 1949; FELDBERG and SHERWOOD, 1954; REITTER, 1957) and sleep (KEY and MARLEY, 1962; DEWHURST and MARLEY, 1965a, b; GRUNDEN and MARLEY, 1970; MARLEY and STEPHENSON, 1968a, 1969). We are indebted to Dr. L. R. GRUNDEN for the following comparison of the effects of catecholamines given intraventricularly in a number of species (GRUNDEN, 1967, 1969; GRUNDEN and KATZUNG, 1964; GRUNDEN and MARLEY, 1970). "The principal effect of intraventricular catecholamines in rats was a dose-dependent decrease in locomotor activity with less obvious "tranquillizing" or "soporific" phenomena. In dogs and cats, the effects of intraventricular adrenaline and related catecholamines strongly resembled those of chlorpromazine inasmuch as some animals appeared to be sleeping or drowsy, whereas others appeared fully awake but unconcerned about their surroundings. There was decreased locomotor activity, with ataxia usually being present in cats but not dogs. The effects were obtained with smaller doses if given into the 3rd rather than into the lateral ventricle. An anaesthesia-like state did not develop since the animals responded to painful stimuli and appeared to maintain consciousness. The "soporific" effects in these three species (rats, cats and dogs) were much less intense than those observed in young and adult chickens." Indeed, the soporific effects produced by intraventricular injection of catecholamines in the adult fowl are indistinguishable from normal sleep (Fig. 2). Thus postural reflexes are retained, the creature standing asleep, electrocortical activity is of the sleep pattern and electrocortical and behavioural arousal are elicited by sensory stimuli.

Intraventricularly applied, but not intravenously applied adrenaline (0.15 mg) caused vomiting in cats, an effect abolished by ablation of the emetic chemoreceptor trigger zone in the area postrema (BORISON, 1959). In cats, lip-licking, vocalisation, vomiting and defaecation were noted by KULKARNI (1967) and after larger doses of adrenaline (80 μg) by FELDBERG and SHERWOOD (1954). Intraventricular injection of adrenaline or noradrenaline in dogs caused salivation or vomiting (TRACZYK, 1964). Although vomiting may seem too gross a change to be considered in the context of behaviour, it is relevant when vomiting is also produced by amines injected parenterally in immature animals (MARLEY and KEY, 1963) or given by slow intravenous infusion in adult cats (SHARPLESS, 1959) for it suggests that the amines reached the vomiting centre in the medulla. Tachypnoea (respiratory rates up to 80/min) after intraventricular adrenaline has been seen in cats (LEIMDORFER et al., 1947; KULKARNI, 1967) and sheep (KULKARNI, 1967). In mice, intraventricular adrenaline has been reported to produce tachypnoea (HALEY and McCORMICK, 1957) or respiratory slowing (BRITTAIN and HANDLEY, 1967).

Just as there is gradation of behavioural change after catecholamines so is there variation in electrocortical response. In dogs (GRUNDEN and KATZUNG, 1964) and monkeys (WADA, 1962), "drowsiness" evoked by noradrenaline given into the lateral cerebral ventricle was accompanied by transition from alert electrocortical activity to the large amplitude slow frequency pattern associated with sleep. Electrocortical changes of sleep were noted by MATSUDA (1968) in rabbits after the intraventricular injection of adrenaline (200 μg) although in a number of animals this was preceded by electrocortical alerting. During the period of electro-

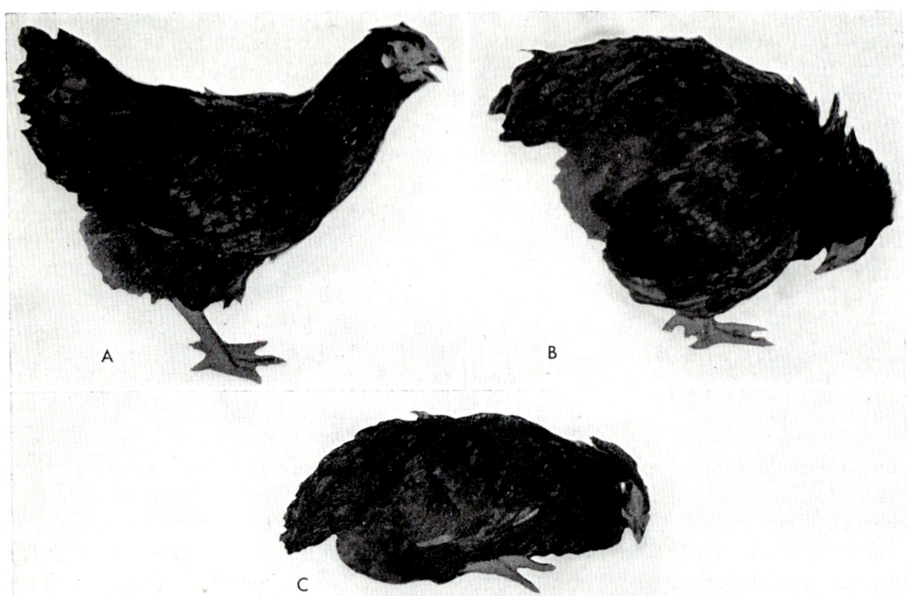

Fig. 2. Effects on posture of α-methylnoradrenaline (0.5 μmole, intraventricularly). A Normal alert adult chicken. B Chicken asleep 5 min after (—)-α-methylnoradrenaline, with head bowed, eyes closed and wings lowered. C The same chicken asleep in squatting position 30 min after administering the drug. (From GRUNDEN, L.R. and MARLEY, E., Neuropharmacology **9**, 119—128, 1970)

cortical synchrony, the arousal thresholds for reticular, hypothalamic or thalamic electrical stimulation were markedly elevated whereas the threshold for the recruiting response was unaltered. Electrocortical sleep patterns together with behavioural sleep were observed after injection of catecholamines into the third cerebral ventricle of adult fowls (GRUNDEN and MARLEY, 1970).

Discrepancies have been noted between the behavioural and electrocortical patterns produced by adrenaline injected intraventricularly in cats. Immediately after the injection, there was drowsy electrocortical activity but during the height of stupor electrocortical activation was conspicuous (ROTHBALLER, 1959). This dissociation between the behavioural and electrocortical response has been used to argue against the validity of the findings produced by intraventricular injection of catecholamines. However, this apparent electrocortical activation found at the height of stupor could well be that of "paradoxical sleep".

c) Injections into the Brain Substance

MYERS (1964a) defined a possible locus in cats for the soporific action of adrenaline injected intraventricularly. This he did by microinjecting the amine in 1 μl through a cannula into various parts of the brain. Adrenaline (5—10 μg) injected into the anterior, posterior, lateral or medial hypothalamic areas or into the cerebrospinal fluid, but not when injected into the dorsomedial thalamus, preoptic region or mesencephalon, induced a "drowsy" almost motionless state in which a prone position was adopted. Larger doses (25—50 μg) produced a "compulsive-like" sleep in which the cats awoke only briefly and frequently failed to respond to painful stimuli. That "drowsiness" was evoked by unilateral micro-

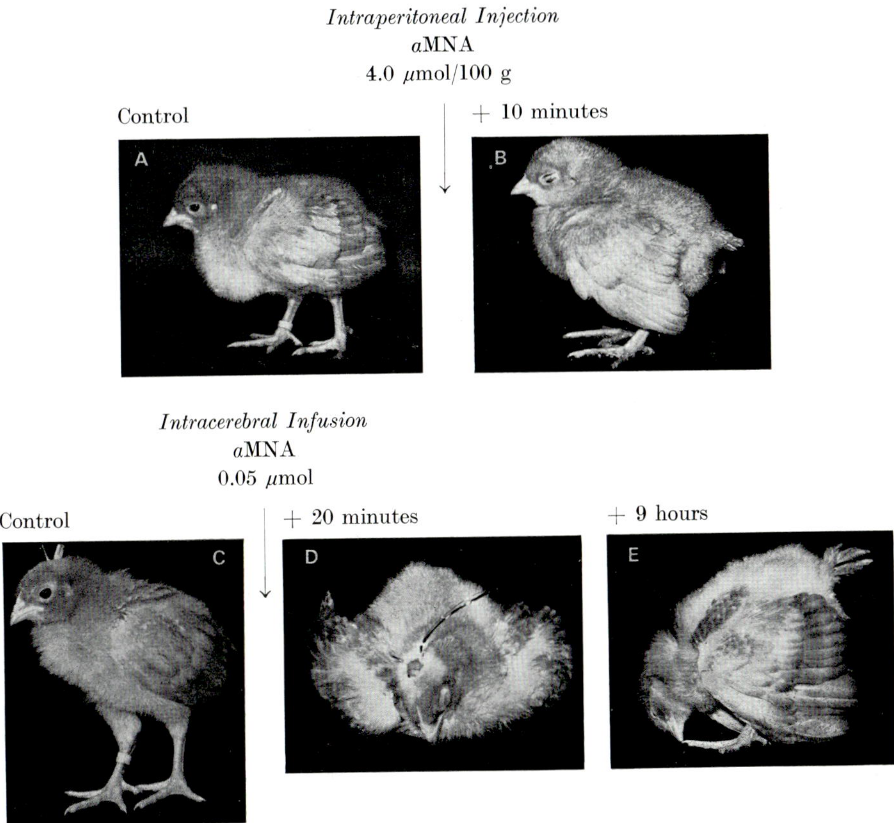

Fig. 3. Comparison of the behavioural effects of an intraperitoneal injection B of 4.0 μmole/100 g (—)-*a*-methylnoradrenaline (*a*MNA) with those of an infusion of 0.05 μmole *a*MNA into the posterior hypothalamic area (*D* and *E*). A and C, control alert behaviours. B Erect sleeping posture with wings lowered and applied closely to the trunk. Peak effect at 10 min with recovery in 30 min. D Prone sleeping posture assumed approx 8 min after infusion and lasting 4 hr. E Erect sleeping posture assumed 4 hr after infusion; recovery in 23 hr

injection of adrenaline into one hypothalamic nucleus is difficult to explain. The phenomenon is almost certainly not due to diffusion of the drug into other hypothalamic nuclei since 1.0 μl of dye diffused over an area approximately 1.9 mm in diameter (Myers 1966) while the feline hypothalamus is 6—7 mm long; nor is it likely that there was diffusion across the 3rd ventricle into contralateral hypothalamic nuclei.

(—)-Noradrenaline (2.0, 8.0 or 16 μg) in crystalline form or in 1 μl saline and positioned stereotactically into the midbrain reticular formation of rats reduced locomotor activity in an "open-field" test although drowsiness was not noted (Grossman, 1968). Startle reactions to sudden sounds, air-puffs or changes in cage illumination were also significantly reduced. Electrocortical activity contained significantly more slower frequencies and was of larger amplitude. In young chickens, (—)-adrenaline, (—)-noradrenaline, (—) and (±)-α-methylnoradrenaline (Fig. 3) and (—)-isoprenaline evoked profound behavioural sleep when microinfused in 0.5 μl into the ventral diencephalon or hypothalamus; dopamine had similar effects provided the chick had been pretreated with a monoamine oxidase inhibitor (Marley and Stephenson, 1968a, 1969, 1970). The effects, depending on dose and area of infusion, were maximal with infusions into or medial to the lateral hypothalamus. The response resulting from the application of 0.5 μl to the hypothalamus could not be ascribed to action on a particular nucleus since an injectate of this volume would encompass several ipsilateral and possibly contralateral hypothalamic nuclei in the diminutive chick brain. The electrocortical changes were less marked than those of behaviour. In some instances, electrocortical-behavioural dissociation occurred. The chick was asleep and prostrate, whilst the electrocorticogram displayed periods of characteristic drowsy activity alternating with bouts of small amplitude potentials; these were considerably longer lasting than the short epochs of paradoxical sleep activity during natural sleep.

d) Intravenous Injection in Immature Animals

The advantages of studying immature animals are twofold. The enzymes which inactivate sympathomimetic amines are present in low concentrations (Birkhäuser, 1940; Epps, 1945) so that central effects might be obtained with amines that are inactivated rapidly in adult brains. Secondly, the blood-brain barrier is absent or not fully effective (Bakay, 1956; Lajtha, 1957; Waelsch, 1955) and this should allow penetration of the brain by substances, e.g. catecholamines, which are excluded in adult animals. For these reasons the young of a number of species (cat, chicken, duck, guinea-pig) were examined and the chicken found the most useful (Key and Marley, 1961; Marley and Key, 1963; Marley, 1964, 1968a, b) inasmuch as catecholamines, administered systemically, evoked sleep in chicks up to the fourth or fifth weeks of life, a time the blood-brain barrier is said to become effective, whereas in adult fowls these amines were ineffective or elicited arousal.

The relevance of tests in young chickens is that similar effects were obtained with catecholamines given intravenously or by micro-infusion into the hypothalamus but no other part of the brain (Marley and Stephenson, 1968a, 1970), suggesting that intravenous catecholamines penetrate to and produce their effects by an action on the hypothalamus. In contrast, intravenous catecholamines have no effect on or elicit brief arousal in adult fowls (Key and Marley, 1962) but when given into the 3rd ventricle, by-passing the blood-brain barrier, they induce sleep as in young chicks (Grunden and Marley, 1970).

Catecholamines, [(—)-adrenaline, (—)-noradrenaline, their α-methyl derivatives and dopamine] of which adrenaline was the most potent, given intravenously to young chickens induced sleep accompanied by large amplitude (150—250 μV) slow frequency (1—4 Hz) electrocortical potentials associated with diminution of electromyographic activity (Fig. 4) and cessation of cheeping (Key and Marley, 1962; Dewhurst and Marley, 1964, 1965a, b). The sleep was physiological in nature, since the chick was roused by sensory stimuli and arousal was accompanied by electrocortical alerting. "Paradoxical sleep" electrocortical activity of low amplitude was also observed during deep sleep. The chicken normally sleeps standing or squatting with its head tucked under a wing, and identical postures were assumed during sleep elicited by catecholamines (Fig. 3B). Similar electrocortical patterns together with loss of electromyographic activity were induced by anaesthetics (KEY and MARLEY, 1962; MARLEY and STEPHENSON, 1968b). Response to the anaesthetics differed inasmuch as electrocortical arousal was not obtained with sensory stimuli; there was loss of postural reflexes and

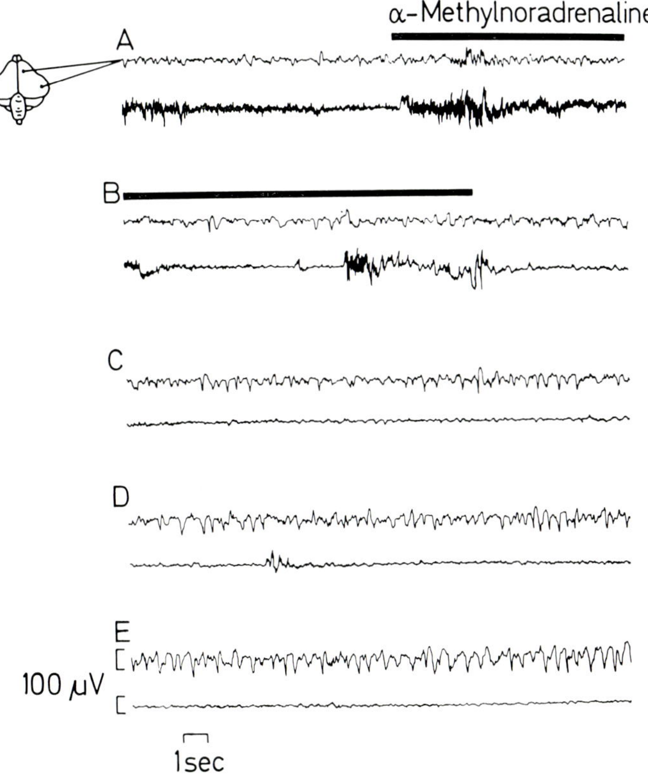

Fig. 4. Effect of (±)-α-methylnoradrenaline on electrocortical and electromyographic activity; recording from non-anaesthetized unrestrained 7-day chicken. A—E Consecutive records of electrocortical activity (upper trace) and electromyographic potentials (lower trace) over 100 sec. Slow intravenous injection of (±)-α-methylnoradrenaline, (10 μmole/kg i.v.) at bar (in A and B). Alert 25 μV electrocortical potentials and 40 μV electromyographic activity (A) change to 150 μV, 2 to 4 Hz electrocortical potentials and 10 μV electromyographic activity within 80 sec. E Chicken previously alert, now asleep. (From DEWHURST, W.G. and MARLEY, E., Brit. J. Pharmacol. **25**, 682—704, 1965)

during deep anaesthesia "suppression bursts" appeared in the electrocorticogram. Sleep produced by catecholamines but not that induced by anaesthetics was reversed by amphetamine-like amines.

Whereas adrenaline or noradrenaline produced behavioural and electrocortical arousal in adult cats, drowsiness and slow frequency large amplitude electrocortical activity were elicited in 3—4 week-old kittens (MARLEY and KEY, 1963). Parenteral injection of these amines produced retching and vomiting in the kittens, phenomena elicited in the adult cat by injecting the amines into the cerebral lateral ventricle, or by intravenous infusion of a large quantity of these amines. Interestingly, catecholamines elicited behavioural and electrocortical alerting in newborn as in adult guinea-pigs (MARLEY and KEY, 1963). The young guinea-pig is more mature than most species at birth (WINDLE, 1940); electrocortical activity (JASPER et al., 1937) and the blood-brain barrier (WAELSCH, 1955) are mature. This may account for the difference between the effects of catecholamines in young chickens and guinea-pigs.

2. Catecholamines as Central Excitants

Astonishingly few experiments have been made in unrestrained intact animals to study excitant effects of catecholamines, the majority of tests being confined to *encéphale isolé* preparations, with all the disadvantages that attach to the latter. Arousal usually follows intravenous injection of catecholamines into adult animals as opposed to soporific effects which occur after intraventricular injection of the amines or their administration into the brain.

a) Intact Animals

ROTHBALLER (1959) tested naturally sleeping cats that had a chronically implanted venous cannula and cortical recording electrodes and observed adrenaline (2—5 μg/kg i.v.) to elicit electrocortical and behavioural arousal. Arousal was also obtained with intravenous (—)-adrenaline, (—)-noradrenaline, (—)-isoprenaline or (±)-α-methylnoradrenaline given to 4 weeks or older kittens (MARLEY and KEY, 1963). Intravenous (—)-adrenaline or (—)-noradrenaline evoked behavioural and electrocortical alerting in guinea-pigs (MARLEY and KEY, 1963). In contrast, LONGO and SILVESTRINI (1957) found that adrenaline (20 μg) rarely elicited alerting when injected intravenously into intact rabbits.

Brief excitement sometimes precedes the central depressant effect of catecholamines. Thus there was a momentary increase of locomotor activity in rats (GRUNDEN, 1969); restlessness was noted also in cats (KULKARNI, 1967) and sheep (PALMER, 1959). Intraventricular α-methylnoradrenaline (50 μg) elicited behavioural activation in cats for 5—30 min followed by drowsiness lasting 4—5 hr (KADZIELAWA, 1967). Hyperexcitability was observed after intraventricular injection of adrenaline in mice (HALEY and MCCORMICK, 1957).

BENKERT (1969) studied the effect of noradrenaline given by microinjection (3 μl) via an implanted cannula into the hypothalamus of rats. With 45 μg, piloerection and tachypnoea developed and with 65 μg locomotor activity was markedly augmented; doses of 12—45 μg and 125—225 μg did not affect locomotor activity. CORDEAU et al. (1963) studied cats with chronically implanted cortical recording electrodes and a cannula in the brain-stem. Adrenaline (20 μg) injected through the cannula into the mesencephalic and rostral pontine reticular formation elicited behavioural and electrocortical arousal lasting 10—20 min. After 100 μg of adrenaline the cat paced and explored its cage for 30 min. Alerting was also obtained with adrenaline injected into the bulbar reticular formation, but was often complicated by retching, vomiting and salivation. The volume of these injections was 20 μl which may have intruded upon the effects of adrenaline since a volume exceeding 10 μl produces a lesion, the size of which is directly related to the volume of injectate, and which may simulate the effects of electrical stimulation of that area (RECH and DOMINO, 1959). Considering the site of injection, these doses of adrenaline are enormous, exceeding the amount of adrenaline in the cat's brain. Even so, alerting was evoked; the same dose given intraventricularly, intracisternally or intravenously produced drowsiness.

b) Encéphale Isolé Preparations and Curarized Animals

In feline *encéphale isolé* preparations, catecholamines evoke both electrocortical and behavioural arousal (BRADLEY, 1960), although the behavioural changes are necessarily restricted to the head and are brief. Long-lasting behavioural and electrocortical arousal were obtained with (±)-α-methylnoradrenaline (MARLEY and KEY, 1963). DELL (1960) argued that experiments in *encéphale isolé* preparations were inconclusive since with a blood pressure of only 60—80 mm Hg, the cortical activation evoked by adrenaline or noradrenaline might be a consequence of improved cerebral blood flow. Another objection is that the animal has recently recovered from anaesthesia. Many tests have been made in curarized animals (BONVALLET et al., 1954; CAPON, 1960; GOLDSTEIN and MUÑOZ, 1961; ROTHBALLER, 1956; SCHAEPPI, 1967) so the conclusions for adrenaline and noradrenaline apply only to *electrocortical* arousal. In the experiments of SCHAEPPI (1967), (—)-noradrenaline (10 μg) injected into the fourth ventricle of feline *encéphale isolé* preparations elicited transient electrocortical desynchronization, rise in blood pressure and retraction of the nictitating membranes.

Although electrocortical alerting is usually produced by intravenous injection of catecholamines the phenomenon is not consistent. In curarized rabbits and dogs, (—)-adrenaline (2—5 μg/kg) injected intravenously produced electrocortical alerting in only 20% of the animals (GOLDSTEIN and MUÑOZ, 1961). Alerting was not produced by (—)-adrenaline or (—)-noradrenaline (1—3 μg) when injected into the carotid or vertebral arteries of cats (MANTEGAZZINI et al., 1959), unless the dose was large enough (4—6 μg) for the amine to escape into the general circulation, when electrocortical alerting occurred 15—20 sec later. MANTEGAZZINI et al. (1959) suggested that this delayed arousal could be due to metabolites of adrenaline or noradrenaline. However, even large doses (150 μg/kg) or (±)-metanephrine, (±)-normetanephrine or 3-methoxy-4-hydroxymandelic acid given intravenously to intact cats did not affect electrocortical activity (MARLEY and KEY, 1963). The lack of effect of the intra-arterial injections of adrenaline or noradrenaline might also have been due to vasoconstriction of sufficient intensity in the brain to counteract the usual central effects.

It is uncertain whether the alerting produced by catecholamines is due to a direct action on the ascending reticular formation or is secondary to peripheral effects of the amines. BONVALLET et al. (1954) considered that hypertension was not responsible for the arousal; they showed discrepancies between the time-courses of hypertension and arousal, and arousal when blood pressure changes were negligible. This was confirmed by ROTHBALLER (1959); electrocortical activation occurred in cats with midbrain coagulation in which adrenaline was either ineffective on the blood pressure or produced a hypertension. In contrast, the results of BAUST et al. (1963) with cat *encéphale isolé* preparations supported the idea that arousal after catecholamines was due to the rise in blood pressure and was mediated through the reticular activating system. Electrocortical arousal after intravenous adrenaline either coincided with, or occurred 1—3 sec after, the rise in blood pressure. As also noted by CAPON (1960), electrocortical arousal was elicited with vasopressin injected intravenously, a substance which raises blood pressure without affecting adrenergic neurones. If blood pressure was kept constant during the intravenous injection of adrenaline, electrocortical arousal was delayed and briefer than if the pressure rose. When blood pressure was raised by rapidly injecting saline into the aorta, electrocortical arousal was elicited but disappeared before the pressure returned to normal. Again in rats lightly anaesthetized with tribromoethyl alcohol, intravenous injection of adrenaline produced electrocortical alerting (BRADLEY, P.B. and BURFORD, R. personal communication). When blood pressure was artificially maintained constant, electrocortical alerting did not usually occur with adrenaline (15 μg/kg i.v.) and if it did occur, it was significantly reduced (ALDRIDGE, J. and BRADLEY, P.B., personal communication); however, a larger dose (30 μg/kg) produced electrocortical arousal even with blood pressure stabilized. It was concluded that hypertension produced by adrenaline played an important role in the evocation of arousal but that the possibility of intrinsic excitatory effects of adrenaline on the brain was not excluded.

V. Effect of Catecholamines on Learnt Behaviour

The results with tests involving learnt behaviour were compatible with catecholamines having central depressant properties. Unfortunately, most of the tests depart from the ideal inasmuch as the animals were handled during the experiment or the drugs were given by routes which did not ensure they reached the brain. (—)-Adrenaline (0.25—1 mg/kg i.p.) prolonged climbing time in rats trained to climb a 5 ft rope under hunger drive. The effect began 10 min after the injection and was maximal at 50 min; it was dose-dependent (SMYTHIES and LEVY, 1960). More elaborate tests have been based on classical, instrumental and operant conditioning.

a) Classical Conditioning

Noradrenaline (15—50 μg/kg i.v.) suppressed conditioned motor, alimentary and salivary reflexes in dogs for up to 60 min after injection (FLORU et al., 1963). The physiological changes produced by catecholamines can also act as stimuli in the control of behaviour by virtue of their association with reinforcing environmental events. For example, they can become conditioned stimuli in avoidance conditioning (COOK and KELLEHER, 1961). In these experiments, beagles with an implanted intravenous cannula were injected with 10 μg/kg (—)-adrenaline or (—)-noradrenaline, the injections spaced sufficiently to allow autonomic responses to abate. On each conditioning trial and 30 sec after commencing the injection, electric shocks were given to a hind limb; flexion within the 30 sec prevented the shock. Before conditioning, neither amine produced leg flexion, but after training, the autonomic effects of adrenaline or noradrenaline became conditioned stimuli for the avoidance response.

b) Instrumental Conditioning

SHARPLESS (1959) infused (—)-adrenaline or (—)-noradrenaline into cats via a cannula implanted in a jugular vein and during performance of an instrumental hunger-motivated response. The cats had been conditioned to respond to a loud click (conditioning stimulus) by placing the head in a chamber to obtain food (conditioned response). Each animal received 24 trials daily, the first 12 being control trials during which a 5% dextrose-saline solution was infused intravenously. Adrenaline or noradrenaline was infused during the last 12 trials. Responding was markedly reduced after 6—12 min of the infusion of adrenaline at 4 or 6 μg/kg/min, but only after 30 min with noradrenaline infused at 6 μg/kg/min. The progressive reduction in responding was unlikely to be due to a rise in blood pressure, since with continued infusion of, or secretion of catecholamines, blood pressure returns gradually to its resting value (DRAŠKOCI et al., 1960; FELDBERG et al., 1934). The animals recovered within a few minutes of stopping the infusion. There were no excitatory effects even with infusion of small doses of the amines (0.5 or 1.0 μg/kg/min). Had small doses been excitatory, there would have been increased number of anticipatory errors, increased time spent in the reward chamber, or a decreased response latency.

The cat's behaviour during infusion of the larger doses resembled that elicited on injecting these amines into the lateral cerebral ventricle. The animal sometimes vomited; its respiration became rapid and continued so during the infusion. It gradually sank into stupor but remained capable of scratching, swallowing or retching. If such a cat was handled it could stand or walk more or less normally but, left to itself, it would lapse into stupor. During the infusion, the electrocorticogram displayed periods of spindling interspersed with apparently normal, low-voltage, waking activity.

These experiments by Sharpless emphasize again the central depressant effects of catecholamines and provide data for assessing whether sopor could be caused by secretion from the adrenal medulla, the largest and most easily mobilized source of catecholamines in the body. In cats, maximal secretion from one adrenal medulla on exciting *only* the major splanchnic nerve ranges from 1.5 to 5.0 μg/min (Duner, 1953; Folkow and Euler, 1954; Kaindl and Euler, 1951). It is clear from experiments of Sharpless that maximal secretion for 5—10 min would be required to elicit soporific effects. With stimuli to the splanchnic nerves providing complete spatial and temporal recruitment necessary for secretion of this magnitude (Marley and Prout, 1965), secretion declines rapidly as fatigue develops at the splanchnic-adrenal medullary junction (Marley and Paton, 1961). Even should sopor ensue, it would be terminated by this decline in secretion.

The effects of catecholamines have also been investigated in instrumental avoidance-escape situations. Adrenaline (6 mg/kg in oil) decreased the frequency of conditioned avoidance and escape by rats in a Skinner box (Kosman and Gerard, 1955). Smaller doses of adrenaline (0.3—0.9 mg/kg i.p.) did not facilitate avoidance learning (Moyer and Bunnell, 1958). Adrenaline (30—50 μg) or dopamine (200—400 μg) given intraventricularly to cats produced deterioration in avoidance responding (Wada et al., 1963). Adrenaline (0.5—40.0 mg) injected into the cerebral ventricles of dogs trained in a conditioned avoidance-escape situation, decreased or abolished the avoidance and escape responses (Grunden and Katzung, 1964). Similarly, (—)-noradrenaline positioned stereotactically into the midbrain reticular formation of rats reduced escape-avoidance responses to low intensity electric shocks (Grossman, 1968).

c) Operant Conditioning

Catecholamines diminish or suppress responding in operant experiments as shown for adrenaline in rats by Wentink (1938). Grossman (1968) tested the effects of (—)-noradrenaline (2.0, 4.0, 8.0 μg), positioned stereotactically into the midbrain reticular formation, on lever-pressing (Fixed Ratio 5) in rats with food or water as positive reinforcement; performance was significantly reduced. Wurtman et al. (1959) tested (—)-adrenaline and (—)-noradrenaline in relation to key-pecking in pigeons maintained either on Fixed Interval (FI) 15 min or Fixed Ratio (FR) 25 schedules with food reinforcement. Pecking was reduced in a dose-dependent fashion by both amines. A 50% reduction in pecking occurred with 30 μg (—)-adrenaline or with 100 μg (—)-noradrenaline given intramuscularly. Performance was not enhanced with any of the doses used (10, 30 and 100 μg adrenaline and 10, 30, 100 and 300 μg noradrenaline). Pecking during the FR 25 was much less affected than that on the FI 15 min, the reduction in pecking on the FI with 30 μg adrenaline exceeding that on the FR with 300 μg noradrenaline.

A number of possibilities besides a central action of the amines were considered for this reduction in pecking. One was that suppression of pecking was secondary to the pressor actions of the amines. In fowls, adrenaline has slightly greater pressor activity than noradrenaline (Harvey and Nickerson, 1951), a difference insufficient to account for the difference in potency in suppressing pecking. Adrenaline and noradrenaline reduce the tension developed in slow contracting muscles, e.g. the cat soleus (Bowman and Zaimis, 1958). An effect of this nature in the pigeon was considered unlikely because of the preservation of performance on the FR with a dose which abolished pecking on the FI. The FI generates a complex pattern of behaviour and is sensitive to drugs, whereas the FR generates a simpler pattern of responding more refractory to drugs (Morse and Herrnstein, 1956). A short FR is useful to include, since if it is affected it suggests that the drug doses used are too large and are producing incoordination.

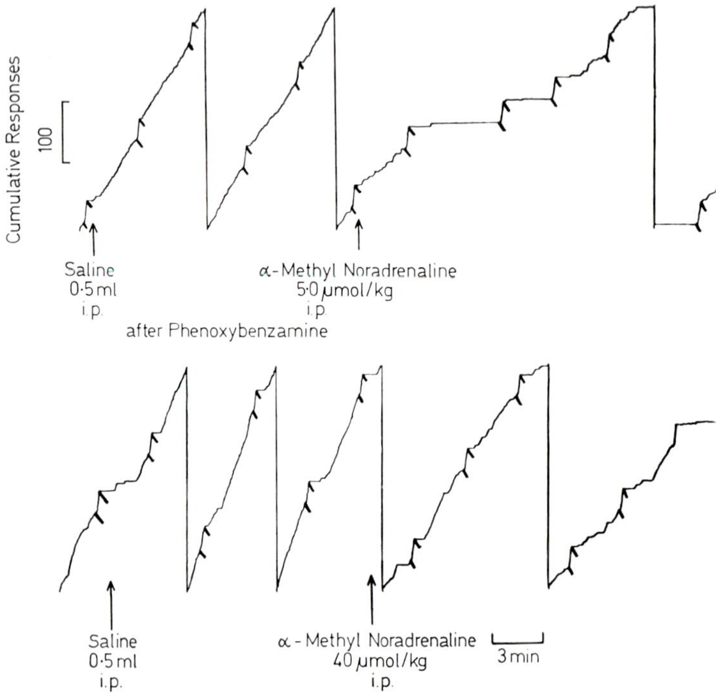

Fig. 5. Cumulative pecking records showing the effects of (±)-α-methylnoradrenaline on a multiple FR25, FI 3 min schedule. Ordinate: cumulative pecks. Abscissa: time. The fixed ratio (FR25) and fixed interval (FI 3) components alternated. The *short diagonal lines* on the records indicate presentations of the food reinforcer. Each record shows a portion of the performance by the same chicken in separate sessions following injections of saline and of α-methylnoradrenaline. Upper record; pecking was reduced in the FI but not the FR component by α-methylnoradrenaline (5.0 μmole/kg i.p.). Lower record; a 40 μmole/kg i.p. dose of α-methylnoradrenaline, after pretreating the chick with phenoxybenzamine (120 μmole/kg i.p. 3 days previously) was less effective than the 5 μmole/kg dose before phenoxybenzamine. (Adapted from Marley, E. and Morse, W.H., Brit. J. Pharmacol. **31**, 367—389, 1967)

Suppressant effects on key-pecking were also obtained with (±)-α-methylnoradrenaline (2.5—10 μmole/kg i.p.) in chickens (Fig. 5). Whereas α-methylnoradrenaline had a marked soporific action in young chickens but not in the adult, it suppressed pecking over the same dose range in young and adult chickens (Marley and Morse, 1967). In the operant situation, cheeping and pecking were reciprocally related so that when pecking was maximal cheeping was minimal, and *vice versa* (Marley and Morse, 1966). In a non-learnt situation, doses of α-methylnoradrenaline up to 1 mg/kg (4—5 μmole/kg) would have abolished cheeping. However in the operant situation pecking was reduced by this dose but cheeping increased, apparently as a consequence of the reduction in pecking; that is to say, the effect of α-methylnoradrenaline on a non-reinforced behaviour (cheeping) was at least partly dependent upon its effect on a reinforced behaviour (key-pecking). It was only with larger doses of α-methylnoradrenaline that cheeping as well as pecking were suppressed. This illustrates the fallibility of extrapolating drug effects from one situation to another let alone from one species to another.

VI. Effect of Catecholamines on Body Temperature

Since the effects on temperature in different species are considered separately, their possible mechanisms of action are discussed at the end of the section. In view of the importance of environmental temperature and injectate volume on the response, these are given whenever possible.

1. Mice

Intraventricular Injection

Noradrenaline or adrenaline (1—20 μg in 20 μl) injected into the 3rd cerebral ventricle produced dose-dependent falls in temperature with recovery in 3—4 hr (BRITTAIN, 1966; BRITTAIN and HANDLEY, 1967; COWELL and DAVEY, 1968). The hypothermic response to adrenaline was usually preceded by a brief rise in temperature (BRITTAIN and HANDLEY, 1967). Dopamine (10—80 μg) was much less potent than noradrenaline or adrenaline; recovery occurred within 40—60 min (BRITTAIN and HANDLEY, 1967). In contrast, isoprenaline (5—200 μg) evoked a dose-dependent rise in temperature lasting 60—90 min; after larger doses (200 μg), hyperthermia was followed by a fall in temperature. Straub tail phenomena, opisthotonus, hypotonia and reduced motor activity accompanied hyperthermia (BRITTAIN and HANDLEY, 1967).

2. Rats

Intracerebral or intraventricular injections of noradrenaline and adrenaline evoked hypo- or hyperthermia depending on dose (FELDBERG and LOTTI, 1967; MYERS and YAKSH, 1968; LOMAX et al., 1969) and ambient temperature (SCHMIDT, 1963).

a) Intraventricular and Intracisternal Administration

In *unrestrained* rats at an ambient temperature of 22°—24°C, whereas intraventricular injection of 20 μg noradrenaline increased temperature, 50 μg lowered it (Fig. 6); recovery occurred within 1—4 hr (MYERS and YAKSH, 1968). In *restrained* rats at the same ambient temperature, the dose-response slope for noradrenaline was shifted to the left. Thus 2—6 μg produced hyperthermia but larger doses (10—100 μg) induced hypothermia (FELDBERG and LOTTI, 1967). Paradoxically, after intracisternal injection, noradrenaline produced hypothermia with small doses but hyperthermia with large doses (BRUINVELS, 1970). For example, hypothermia was maximal following 4 μg noradrenaline; progressively larger doses had correspondingly smaller hypothermic effects until with 32 μg hyperthermia was obtained. Intraventricular injections of isoprenaline produced a dose-dependent rise in temperature (MYERS and YAKSH, 1968). Intraventricular injection of small doses of dopamine (10 μg) had little effect on body temperature but large doses (40 μg) often produced long lasting hyperthermia of slow onset (MYERS and YAKSH, 1968). Intracisternal injection of 4 μg dopamine lowered temperature, but the hypothermia was not increased by larger doses (BRUINVELS, 1970).

The effects of intraventricular (FELDBERG and LOTTI, 1967; MYERS and YAKSH, 1968) and intracerebral injections of adrenaline (vol 10 μl; SCHMIDT, 1963) were similar to those for noradrenaline.

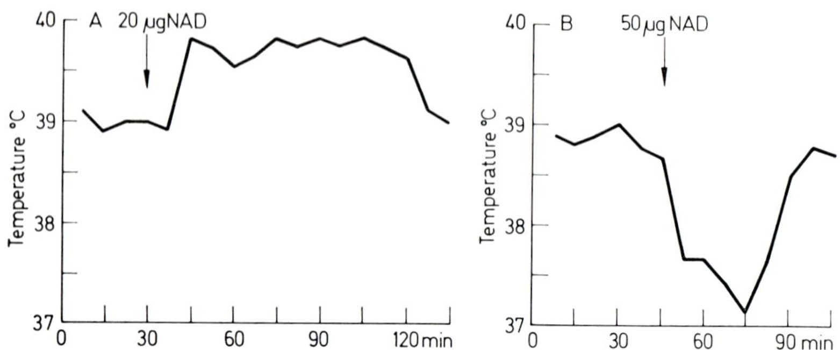

Fig. 6. Rise in body temperature (A) and fall in body temperature (B) in response to intraventricular injections of noradrenaline (*NAD*), 20 μg and 50 μg respectively in different rats. (From MYERS, R.D. and YAKSH, T.L., Physiol. and Behav. **3**, 917—928, 1968)

b) Intracerebral Injection

At thermoneutrality (22° C), intracerebral injections of noradrenaline (10 μg in 10 μl) lowered temperature 2° C. Below thermoneutrality (2° C) the fall was 4° C but at an elevated ambient temperature (32° C) rectal temperature increased 2° C (SCHMIDT, 1963); the locus of injection was not specified. (—)-Noradrenaline (0.5—5 μg in 1 μl) injected into the rostral hypothalamus raised temperature in some rats, lowered it in others or produced a fall followed by a prolonged rise; ambient temperature was 22 $\pm$ 0.5° C. To some extent the responses were dose-dependent, smaller doses being hyperthermic and larger doses hypothermic; 2.5 μg produced a consistent fall of 0.9 $\pm$ 0.15° C (LOMAX et al., 1969). An injection of noradrenaline (22 μg in 1 μl) into the lateral hypothalamus lowered temperature approximately 0.5° C (COONS, LEVAK, MILLER and WECHSLER — quoted by MILLER, 1965).

3. Rabbits

a) Intraventricular Administration

In a rabbit with fever produced as a result of widely opening a lateral ventricle, a drop of 1/10,000 adrenaline solution placed on the ventricular surface lowered body temperature (JACOBI and ROEMER, 1912). Hypothermia to adrenaline injected into the corpus striatum was also reported by BARBOUR and WING (1913) but hyperthermic responses to intraventricular injections of adrenaline were obtained by KONDO (1919) and EULER et al. (1943). Injections of (—)-noradrenaline (10 μg in 100 μl) into a lateral ventricle either raised rectal temperature 0.7°—1.3° C or were without effect (COOPER et al., 1965); ambient temperature was not specified. Noradrenaline lowered temperature in febrile rabbits (RUCKEBUSCH et al., 1965).

b) Intracerebral Administration

Of eight injections in six rabbits of (—)-noradrenaline (10 μg in 10 μl) into the anterior hypothalamus, four raised rectal temperature markedly, three were without effect and one produced a rise of 0.4° C (COOPER et al., 1965); ambient temperature was not specified. Injections of noradrenaline into either the medial preoptic area or the lateral ventricle did not produce significant or consistent changes in temperature (KALININA and REPIN, 1968); ambient temperature was not specified.

The inconsistencies in response to both intraventricular and intracerebral injection of catecholamines are probably due to differences in ambient temperature since at thermoneutrality (20° C), noradrenaline (20—75 μg in 50 μl) raised rectal temperature in a few rabbits only whereas above thermoneutrality (30 to 35° C), noradrenaline was markedly hyperthermic in all rabbits. In contrast, below thermoneutrality (5° C) noradrenaline lowered rectal temperature (BLIGH and COTTLE, 1969).

4. Cats

a) Intraventricular Administration

Intraventricular injections of noradrenaline or adrenaline (50—100 μg in 100 μl) consistently lowered rectal temperature 0.5° C—1.0° C and occasionally 1.3° C (FELDBERG and MYERS, 1964); ambient temperature was 20.5°—22.5° C. Temperature began to fall within a few min of injection, reaching a nadir within 60 min; after a further 30 min, temperature gradually returned to a level often somewhat higher than that prior to injection. Adrenaline was approximately twice as potent as noradrenaline. Slightly greater hypothermic responses to adrenaline were obtained by KULKARNI (1967) who observed falls of 3.2° C after adrenaline base (62.5 μg in 175 μl); ambient temperature was not specified.

b) Intracerebral Injection

Injections of adrenaline or noradrenaline into the anterior hypothalamus, but no other part of the brain, produced dose-dependent falls in rectal temperature whether it was normal, or elevated by either 5-hydroxytryptamine or typhoid vaccine (FELDBERG and MYERS, 1965); ambient temperature was 20.5—22.5° C. Typically, adrenaline (5 μg in 1 μl) lowered temperature approximately 1.6° C whereas the same dose of noradrenaline lowered temperature 0.6° C. Temperature began to fall less than 2 min after injection and reached a nadir within 30 min. With adrenaline, 2.5 μg, or noradrenaline, 5 μg, temperature returned to normal within 2 hr.

5. Dogs

Intraventricular Administration

Injections of noradrenaline or adrenaline (50—100 μg in 100 μl) into a lateral ventricle of anaesthetized dogs (FELDBERG et al., 1966) or third ventricle of unanaesthetized dogs (FELDBERG et al., 1967) lowered rectal temperature. Falls in body temperature have been observed after subdural, intracerebral or intracisternal administration of adrenaline (BASS, 1914; REITTER, 1957).

6. Sheep

Intraventricular Administration

Intraventricular injections of noradrenaline (100—250 μg in 200 μl) only significantly affected body temperature when shivering or panting were present (BLIGH and COTTLE, 1969). Thus above thermoneutrality (40° C), panting was depressed by noradrenaline in sheared and in non-sheared sheep and as a consequence rectal and para-carotid temperatures rose. At an ambient temperature of 10°—20° C, noradrenaline depressed shivering in sheared sheep and lowered body temperature, but in non-sheared sheep at an ambient temperature of 10° C shivering was absent and noradrenaline had only a slight hyperthermic effect. At an ambient temperature of 20°—30° C, noradrenaline consistently raised temperature in non-sheared sheep (also BLIGH, 1966) but lacked significant effects on sheared sheep at an ambient temperature of 30° C. Hyperthermia to intraventricular adrenaline was followed after about 2 hr by a prolonged fall in temperature (RUCKEBUSCH et al., 1966a); noradrenaline lowered temperature in febrile sheep (RUCKEBUSCH et al., 1965).

7. Goats

Intraventricular Administration

At thermoneutrality (18°—20° C) injections of noradrenaline or adrenaline (0.3—7 μg/kg) into the third ventricle had no significant effect on rectal temperature (ANDERSSON et al., 1966; BLIGH and COTTLE, 1969). Above thermoneutrality (30°—40° C), noradrenaline depressed panting and elevated temperature whereas below thermoneutrality (10° C), it diminished shivering and lowered body temperature (BLIGH and COTTLE, 1969).

8. Oxen

Intraventricular Administration

At an ambient temperature of 10°—20° C intraventricular injection of (—)-noradrenaline or adrenaline (3 mg in 3 ml) had no effect on rectal temperature, skin evaporative loss, respiratory rate, tidal volume or heat production. Ear temperature did not alter providing it was below 23° C. At an ambient temperature of 20° C, when ear temperature was between 30° and 34° C, noradrenaline or adrenaline lowered it 10°—14° C (FINDLAY and ROBERTSHAW, 1967).

9. Monkeys

a) Intraventricular Administration

Noradrenaline and adrenaline injected into the third ventricle of anaesthetized monkeys lowered rectal and ventricular temperatures (FELDBERG et al., 1967).

b) Intracerebral Administration

In an extensive study of the hypothalamic sites at which application of (—)-noradrenaline lowered temperature of unanaesthetized monkeys, responsive areas were located in the anterior, preoptic region ventral to the anterior commissure (MYERS and YAKSH, 1969). Thus, at an ambient temperature of 22°—25° C, (—)-noradrenaline (1.0—12.0 μg in 0.5—1.0 μl) produced a dose-dependent fall in temperature. The maximum fall elicited by dopamine, 12.0 μg was 0.3° C whereas the hypothermic effect of (—)-adrenaline was only slightly less than that of (—)-noradrenaline.

10. Chicks

a) Intravenous or Intraventricular Administration

Catecholamines given intravenously readily enter the central nervous system of young chicks (section II. A.). (—)-Adrenaline, (—)-noradrenaline and their α-methyl derivatives given intravenously lowered core and surface temperatures and reduced oxygen consumption (ALLEN and MARLEY, 1966, 1967; RUCKEBUSCH et al., 1966b). The effects of the α-methyl derivatives, compounds resistant to MAO (see BLASCHKO, 1952), were the most consistent and were dose-dependent

(ALLEN and MARLEY, 1967). This hypothermic action of noradrenaline in young chicks contrasts remarkably with that in other neonates in which noradrenaline acts on brown adipose tissue (HANNON et al., 1963; DAWKINS and HULL, 1964; STEINER and CAHILL, 1964) leading to hyperthermia and increased oxygen consumption (TAYLOR, 1960; MOORE and UNDERWOOD, 1963; SCOPES and TIZARD, 1963; DAWES and MESTYÁN, 1963); significantly, chicks do not possess brown adipose tissue (FREEMAN, 1967). In adult fowls, catecholamines given intravenously have little or no effect on behaviour, electrocortical activity or temperature (KEY and MARLEY, 1962; ALLEN and MARLEY, 1967), whereas after intraventricular injection they produced sopor and lowered temperature 1°—3°C (GRUNDEN and MARLEY, 1970).

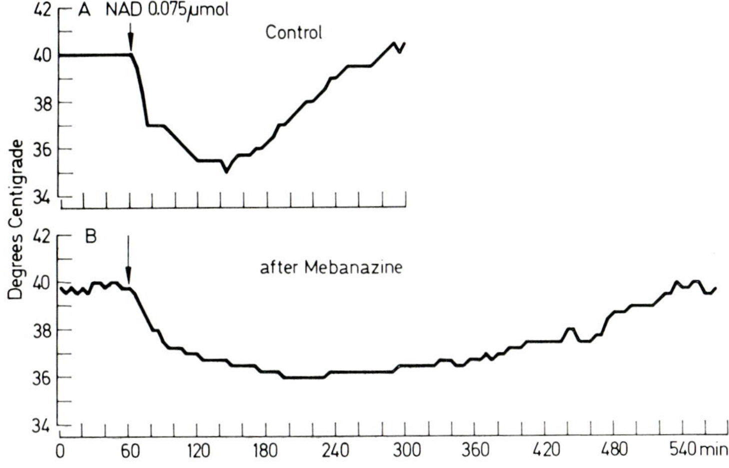

Fig. 7. Records of body temperature in a 16-day chicken. A Fall in temperature with recovery in 3.5 hr produced by an infusion of 0.075 μmole (—)-noradrenaline (NAd) into the hypothalamus. B Same chicken, 24 hr later, given mebanazine (10 μmole/100 g i.v. 18 hr and 1 hr previously) showing prolonged fall in temperature with recovery in 8 hr produced by a similar infusion of (—)-noradrenaline

b) Intracerebral Administration

Further evidence for a central action was the more profound and considerably longer-lasting effect of (—)-α-methylnoradrenaline or (—)-noradrenaline (0.5 μl) infused into the hypothalamus of young chicks over a 4 min period. Thus 0.01 to 0.2 μmole (2.2—44 μg) (—)-α-methylnoradrenaline or 0.05 μmole (8.5 μg) (—)-noradrenaline infused into the hypothalamus lowered temperature (Fig. 7) and oxygen consumption and produced behavioural sleep (Fig. 3D, E) (MARLEY and STEPHENSON, 1968a, 1969, 1970); ambient temperature was 29°—31°C. The duration of response was dependent on its intensity and varied between 3 and 4 hr for noradrenaline and between 7 and 12 hr for α-methylnoradrenaline; falls in temperature of up to 6°C were recorded. The onset of the effect was most rapid with infusions into the hypothalamic region but owing to the diminutive size of the chick brain the effect could not be localized to a specific hypothalamic nucleus or group of nuclei. The intensity was greatest with infusions close to the midline but rather than suggesting an action on medial nuclei, this may represent a bilateral distribution and action of the amine on hypothalamic nuclei. (—)-Isoprenaline 0.05—0.1 μmole (14—28 μg) infused into the same area produced effects similar to, but less intense, than those produced by (—)-noradrenaline. However, the duration of action was longer and falls in temperature of 1.75°—5°C persisted for 5—6 hr. Dopamine (0.15—0.3 μmole, 28—56 μg) was without significant effect on temperature.

11. Discussion

Since noradrenaline, adrenaline and 5-hydroxytryptamine are present in relatively high concentrations in the hypothalamus (VOGT, 1954; AMIN et al., 1954) it was suggested by BRODIE and SHORE (1957) and VON EULER (1961) that their presence might be related to temperature regulation. The possible importance of dopamine has been neglected probably because its effects after intracerebral injection are short, a consequence of rapid deamination. However, when released physiologically it is likely to be considerably more effective and may play a role in temperature regulation (BARNETT and TABER, 1968). Since rectal temperature of the cat was increased by intraventricular injections of 5-hydroxytryptamine but decreased by noradrenaline or adrenaline, FELDBERG and MYERS (1964) proposed body temperature to be regulated by release of amines in the hypothalamus by one of two mechanisms. Either amines were continuously liberated, normal temperature being the outcome of a fine balance between 5-hydroxytryptamine and catecholamine release with temperature changes a consequence of disturbing this balance, or normal temperature was maintained by other means, release of hypothalamic amines effecting changes in temperature.

MYERS and SHARPE (1968) postulated that in the monkey two anatomically distinct neurochemical pathways originated in the anterior preoptic region of the hypothalamus and projected to the posterior hypothalamus. One pathway was thought to control catecholamine release to cause heat loss, and the other by liberation of 5-hydroxytryptamine to lead to heat production. Later experiments undermined this theory for although 5-hydroxytryptamine activated a cholinergic heat-production pathway projecting from the anterior to posterior hypothalamus, a neurochemical pathway which activated heat loss could not be demonstrated (MYERS and YAKSH, 1969). A sustained liberation of 5-hydroxytryptamine within the anterior hypothalamus was therefore thought necessary for maintenance of heat production (Fig. 8). Release of noradrenaline could influence the 5-hydroxytryptamine-cholinergic heat production pathway in one of two ways. First, noradrenaline could antagonize the hypothalamic action of 5-hydroxytryptamine either by inhibiting its release or by competing for its post-synaptic receptor sites. Second, and as favoured by MYERS and YAKSH (1969), noradrenaline would inhibit the cholinergic heat production pathway, possibly at synapses.

The above hypothesis is not applicable to those species (i.e. sheep, goat, rabbit and ox) which react differently from cat and monkey to intraventricular injection of amines. Instead, a neuronal model with reciprocal inhibition between heat production and heat loss functions which allowed for reciprocal effects of amines at high and low ambient temperatures (Fig. 9) was proposed by BLIGH and COTTLE (1969). The effect of 5-hydroxytryptamine was to increase heat loss and reduce heat production. It was therefore most effective at low ambient temperatures when both these responses contributed to a fall in body temperature and was least effective at high ambient temperatures, when there could be little further increase in heat loss and little or no decrease in heat production. Noradrenaline was thought to cause inhibition of heat-loss and heat-production systems at synapses posterior to those for 5-hydroxytryptamine. Thus at low ambient temperatures when heat production was maximally activated and heat loss maximally inhibited, noradrenaline reduced heat production and lowered body temperature; at high ambient temperatures, when heat loss mechanisms were maximally activated and heat production mechanisms maximally inhibited, noradrenaline reduced heat loss and raised body temperature. In the sheep and goat, acetylcholine was proposed as a transmitter at synapse *b*, (Fig. 9) (BLIGH and MASKREY, 1969; BLIGH et al., 1971). The neuronal models of BLIGH and COTTLE (1969) and MYERS and YAKSH (1969) are similar in many respects and if the effects of intraventricular or intrahypothalamic injections of 5-hydroxytryptamine and catecholamines on body temperature of the cat, dog and monkey at *different* ambient temper-

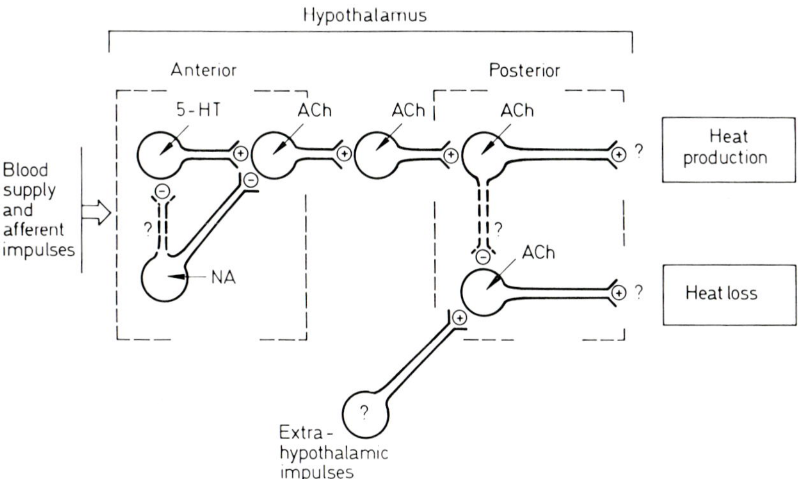

Fig. 8. A neuronal model of the hypothalamic system regulating body temperature. When the cells containing 5-hydroxytryptamine (5-HT) are stimulated by cooling or a pyrogen, a cholinergic heat-production pathway to the posterior hypothalamus is activated. When noradrenaline (NA) containing cells are stimulated by warming or antipyretics, the 5-hydroxytryptamine-cholinergic heat pathway is inhibited either by interference with the 5-hydroxytryptamine cell system or blockade of the acetylcholine cell system. The suppression of the heat-production pathway permits the second cholinergic system in the posterior hypothalamus to activate the efferent heat-loss pathway, which could also be influenced by extrahypothalamic structures. (From MYERS, R. D. and YAKSH, T. L., J. Physiol. (Lond.) **202**, 483—500, 1969)

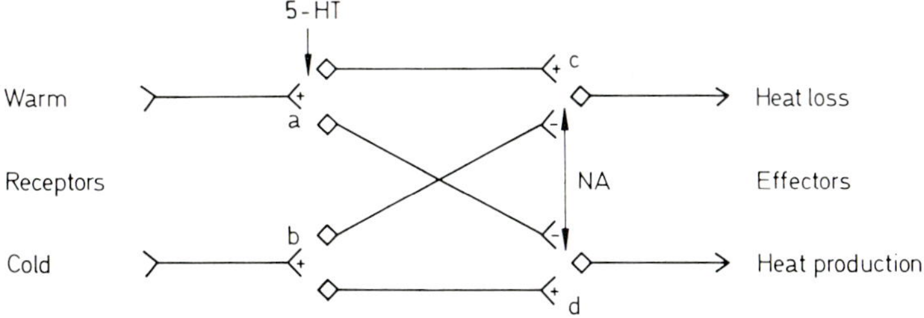

Fig. 9. A neuronal model with pathways for reciprocal inhibition between heat production and heat loss. Increase in heat loss (synapses a and c) and decrease in heat production (synapses a and d) in response to 5-hydroxytryptamine acting at synapse a is most effective in lowering body temperature at low ambient temperatures. Noradrenaline reduces heat production (synapse d), most effectively at high ambient temperatures or decreases heat loss (synapse c), most effectively at low ambient temperatures (+ = facilitates; — = inhibits). (From BLIGH, J. and COTTLE, W.H., Experientia (Basel) **25**, 608—609, 1966). Acetylcholine is a putative transmitter at synapse b (BLIGH, J. and MASKREY, M., J. Physiol. (Lond.) **203**, 55—57P, 1969; BLIGH, J., COTTLE, W.H. and MASKREY, M., J. Physiol. (Lond.) **212**, 377—392, 1971)

atures were known, then it might be possible to interpret their actions in terms of one model. The model of Bligh and Cottle (1969) explains hypo- and hyperthermia evoked in the rat at different ambient temperatures and variable effects obtained at thermoneutrality by intraventricular or intracerebral injection of noradrenaline (section VI. 2.).

Effects of monoamines on hypothalamic circulation may also influence body temperature. Since the hypothalamus is normally cooled by the blood flowing through it, vasoconstriction within the hypothalamus reduces blood flow and increases hypothalamic temperature (McCook et al., 1962); an increase in hypothalamic temperature leads to decreased heat production and increased heat loss and *vice versa* (Ström, 1960). Such explanations are not readily applied to chicks since infusions into the hypothalamus of noradrenaline and isoprenaline, which have opposite effects on peripheral vessels, lowered body temperature (Marley and Stephenson, 1969).

VII. Effect of Catecholamines on Food and Water Intake

Injection of solid crystalline salts of (—)-noradrenaline, (—)-adrenaline or dopamine (1—5 μg) into the lateral hypothalamus evoked a reproducible eating response in satiated rats (Grossman, 1960, 1962a). Eating, which commenced 5—10 min after injection, continued for 20—40 min after (—)-adrenaline and for longer after (—)-noradrenaline; food consumption averaged 3.0 g after (—)-adrenaline and 4.3 g after (—)-noradrenaline. Doses greater than 5 μg induced somnolence and hypoactivity, and so eating was reduced. Drinking sometimes occurred towards the end of the test period but this appeared to be prandial since it did not occur in rats with access to water but not food. Cholinergic agents injected into the same site produced drinking but not eating but the different effects of adrenergic and cholinergic agents were not mediated by different motor systems since noradrenaline or adrenaline (1 μl) injected into the lateral hypothalamus caused rats to drink liquid food of similar density to water, but not water (Fig. 10) whereas carbachol had the opposite effect (Miller et al., 1964). Feeding and drinking were mutually antagonistic activities since adrenergic substances elicited eating in satiated rats but inhibited drinking in thirsty rats, whereas cholinergic substances evoked drinking in satiated animals but inhibited eating in hungry animals (Grossman, 1962a; Grossman, 1964). The opposite effects were observed by Myers (1964b) and Cicero (1968), application of catecholamines to the lateral hypothalamic region of rats producing drinking more often than feeding. Miller (1965) and Fisher and Coury (1962) encountered this paradoxical effect in rats only rarely. (—)-Noradrenaline and (—)-adrenaline injected into the rat lateral hypothalamus evoked eating and a variable amount of drinking (Booth, 1968).

These discrepancies are clarified by findings of Hutchinson and Renfrew (1967). Injections of noradrenaline into the dorsomedial or lateral hypothalamic nuclei, increased bar pressing for food in both satiated and starved rats, confirming earlier findings of Wagner and de Groot (1963). However, in rats given injections into the anterior hypothalamus or preoptic area, the response was dependent on degree of deprivation. Thus in food-deprived rats, noradrenaline increased drinking and reduced eating whereas in water-deprived rats, it increased eating but decreased drinking. In non-deprived rats, noradrenaline decreased drinking but left eating unaffected. Therefore, the discrepancies could be explained by diffusion of noradrenaline from the lateral hypothalamus to the contiguous anterior hypothalamus or preoptic area together with variations in the state of food and water deprivation of the rats.

There are species differences in response, since in rabbits injections of carbachol into the lateral hypothalamus and preoptic area evoked eating and drinking whereas noradrenaline was without effect (SOMMER et al., 1967). Conversely, (—)-noradrenaline or dopamine (6—50 μg in 1 μl) injected into various diencephalic sites of satiated monkeys induced eating, prandial drinking and lowered

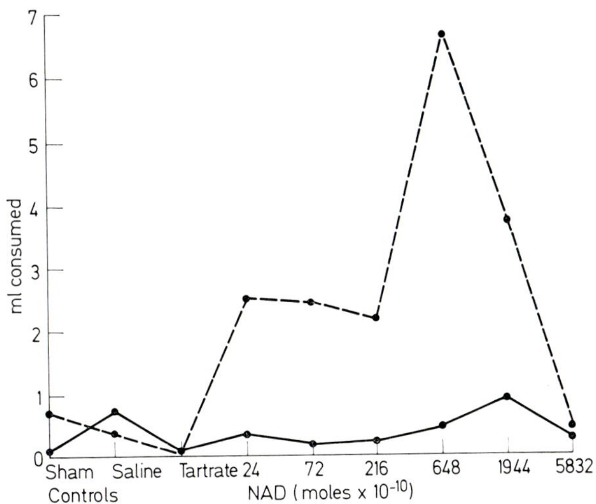

Fig. 10. Effects of different doses of noradrenaline (NAD) and of control ("*sham*", *saline*, *tartrate*) injections into the lateral hypothalamus on liquid food (broken line) and water intake (continuous line) of satiated rats. Noradrenaline selectively increased liquid food intake. (From MILLER, N.E., GOTTESMAN, K.S. and EMERY, N., Amer. J. Physiol. **206**, 1384—1388, 1964)

temperature (MYERS and SHARPE, 1968; SHARPE and MYERS, 1969).Cholinergic compounds inhibited both food and water intake in hungry, thirsty monkeys. Ingestive responses resulting from catecholamines have not been observed in cats (MYERS, 1964b; HERNANDEZ-PEÓN et al., 1963; BAXTER, 1967). In some chicks, injection of (—)-α-methylnoradrenaline into the preoptic area led to hyperphagia followed by sleep (MARLEY and STEPHENSON, unpublished data). In rats, evidence was obtained for separate motivational and consummatory ingestive pathways from injections of noradrenaline and carbachol into the lateral hypothalamus and perifornical area (MORGANE, 1961).

The concept of superimposed but independent feeding and drinking centres in the lateral hypothalamus with a satiety centre in the ventromedial hypothalamic nucleus exerting its effect by inhibiting the lateral hypothalamus (ANAND and BROBECK, 1951; ANAND and DUA, 1958; ANAND, 1961; WAGNER and DE GROOT, 1963; SMITH and MCCANN, 1961) is too simple to satisfy results from chemical (see above) and electrical stimulation studies (ROBINSON and MISHKIN, 1962, 1968; WYRWICKA and DOTY, 1966) and from lesion experiments (REYNOLDS, 1965; SKULTETY, 1966; PARKER and FELDMAN, 1967). Moreover, comparison of results from chemical and electrical stimulation poses certain problems. In rats, thresholds for eliciting feeding and drinking by electrical stimulation of the same hypothalamic site differed and since both decreased with repeated testing, response to a repeated stimulus changed (WISE, 1968). In monkeys, electrical stimulation evoked eating in less than 30% of cases (ROBINSON and MISHKIN, 1968) compared to over 75% following (—)-noradrenaline (SHARPE and MYERS,

1969). The greater efficacy of noradrenaline may be due to selective action on neurones whereas the response to electrical stimulation is usually that of the system with the lowest threshold. Response to catecholamines frequently depended on the catecholamine used. Thus, noradrenaline injected into the ventromedial nucleus inhibited intake of liquid food in food-deprived and in satiated rats, but adrenaline increased liquid food intake in both situations (WAGNER and DE GROOT, 1963). In contrast, isoprenaline injected into the lateral hypothalamus of rats did not elicit eating (BOOTH, 1968; MYERS and YAKSH, 1968; SLANGEN and MILLER, 1969; LEIBOWITZ, 1970). Antagonism between an α-adrenoceptive "hunger" system and a β-adrenoceptive "satiety" system has been described for the rat hypothalamus (LEIBOWITZ, 1970 and section XII., 4.).

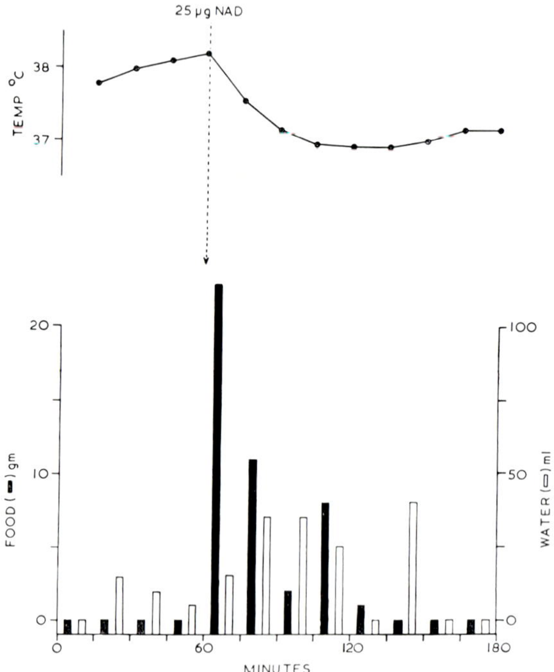

Fig. 11. Effects of an injection of noradrenaline (NAD), 25 μg (at arrow) into the periventricular grey region on temperature (top trace), food (solid bars) and water (open bars) intake of a satiated monkey. Food and water intake were recorded every 15 min. Noradrenaline lowered temperature and increased food and water intake (From SHARPE, L.G. and MYERS, R.D., Exp. Brain Res. 8, 295—310, 1969)

Relations of Temperature Regulation to Food and Water Intake

There is an intimate relationship between food and water intake and thermoregulation. Since the areas from which catecholamines evoke ingestive and thermoregulatory responses are contiguous or overlap it is not surprising to find that the two types of response are often associated (Fig. 11). In goats, heating the anterior hypothalamic preoptic area induced tachypnoea, peripheral vasodilatation, with consequent lowering of body temperature, and drinking; cooling the same area induced eating, peripheral vasoconstriction, with consequent increase in body temperature and, provided ambient temperature was below 18°C, shivering (ANDERSSON and LARSSON, 1961; ANDERSEN et al., 1962). Similarly, food intake of rats increased when core temperature was reduced as a consequence of heating the anterior hypothalamic preoptic area (SPECTOR et al., 1968). However, whereas noradrenaline injected into the lateral hypothalamus of rats lowered body temperature and induced eating, carbachol, injected into the same site lowered temperature further but induced drinking and not eating (MILLER, 1965). Also in rats, hyperphagia was evoked by intraventricular injection of noradrenaline in doses which produced either hypo- or hyperthermia (MYERS and YAKSH, 1968).

Thus it seems unlikely that ingestive responses are elicited primarily by effects of catecholamines on thermo-regulatory mechanisms but that their association is due to the close proximity of functionally specific systems traversing the area encompassed by the injectate which may or may not respond to the catecholamine.

VIII. Oxygen Consumption

Increase in metabolic rate produced by catecholamines is referred to as their calorigenic action and equated in terms of increased oxygen consumption. Adrenaline has greater calorigenic effect than noradrenaline in adult rats (HSIEH and CARLSON, 1957; TAYLOR, 1960), rabbits (COTTLE, 1963; LUNDHOLM, 1950), guinea-pigs (LUNDHOLM, 1949) and cats (MOORE and UNDERWOOD, 1963); in dogs (HAVEL, 1963), and man (HARRIS et al., 1965; HAVEL et al., 1964), adrenaline and noradrenaline have similar calorigenic properties; in adult fowls, adrenaline and noradrenaline neither raise nor lower temperature (RUCKEBUSCH et al., 1966b; ALLEN and MARLEY, 1966, 1967). By contrast, noradrenaline has greater calorigenic effects than adrenaline in neonatal guinea-pigs (DAWES and MESTYÁN, 1963), rabbits (DAWKINS and HULL, 1964) and cats (MOORE and UNDERWOOD, 1963). These effects, obtained with subcutaneous, intramuscular or intravenous administration in the various species, are discussed in an exemplary review by HIMMS-HAGEN (1967). For species in which catecholamines lower temperature when given intraventricularly, there is every likelihood that oxygen consumption would be simultaneously reduced. Surprisingly, this possibility seems not to have been examined. Heat production was measured in oxen by FINDLAY and ROBERTSHAW (1967), but was unaltered, as was temperature, by adrenaline or noradrenaline given intraventricularly.

In marked contrast to neonates of other species, catecholamines given intravenously (RUCKEBUSCH et al., 1966b; ALLEN and MARLEY, 1966, 1967; ALLEN et al., 1970) or by micro-infusion into the hypothalamus of young chicks (MARLEY and STEPHENSON, 1968a, 1969) lower oxygen consumption and temperature. The depressant effects of catecholamines on oxygen consumption were more marked after micro-infusion into the hypothalamus than after intravenous injection. Since, oxygen consumption increases two to three-fold in chicks tested below thermoneutrality (FREEMAN, 1964), the depressant effects of catecholamines on oxygen consumption were the more clearly observed. Figure 12 illustrates that the *increase* in oxygen consumption due to chilling was halved by intravenous injection of (—)-α-methylnoradrenaline. The significance of this is discussed in Section IX.

IX. Shivering, Tremor and Electromyographic Activity

Shivering, associated with a fall in temperature and evident by visual inspection, was induced in cats 30—150 min after injection of chlorpromazine intramuscularly or pentobarbitone intraperitoneally. As shown in Fig. 13 shivering induced by pentobarbitone was abolished by 0.5 μg of adrenaline or noradrenaline given into a lateral ventricle (Domer and Feldberg, 1960); isoprenaline, phenylephrine, ephedrine or amphetamine given intraventricularly in doses from 5—500 μg did not affect shivering.

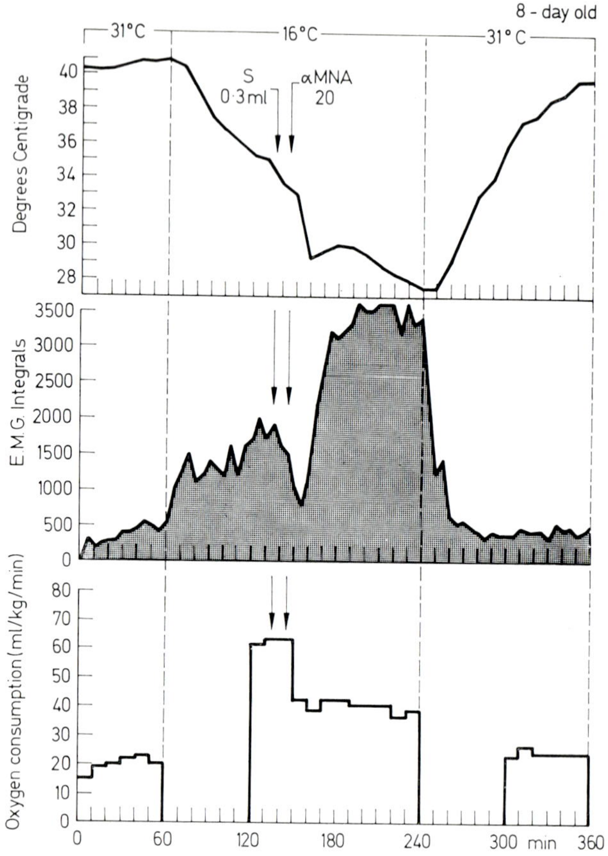

Fig. 12. From above downwards: graph of body temperature, integrated electromyographic activity and histograms of oxygen consumption in an 8-day chick at serial environmental temperatures of 31 °C, 16 °C and 31 °C. The breaks between histograms of oxygen consumption are periods allowed for thermal equilibrium to re-establish after transfer of the oxygen consumption chamber from 31° to 16 °C or *vice versa*. Note reduction in oxygen consumption by (—)-*a*-methylnoradrenaline (*a*MNA) 20 μmole/kg i.v., which persists throughout the period at 16 °C, with further decrease in temperature. In contrast, there is much briefer reduction in electromyographic activity. S, saline. (From Allen, D.J., Garg, K.N. and Marley, E., Brit. J. Pharmacol. **381**, 667—687, 1970)

In experiments of Bligh and Cottle (1969), shivering was recorded electromyographically in non-anaesthetized rabbits, goats and sheep at an environmental temperature of 10 °C. Noradrenaline (20—75 μg for rabbits, 100—250 μg for goats and sheared sheep) given into a lateral ventricle reduced shivering. Even at thermoneutrality, catecholamines substantially diminished the electromyogram in non-anaesthetized young chickens as shown for intravenous (±)-*a*-methylnoradrenaline in Fig. 4; the effects with this dose lasted up to 30 min. Below thermoneutrality (16 °C) however, shivering — measured electromyographically — was diminished but only evanescently (Fig. 12) by twice the dose of (—)-*a*-methylnoradrenaline used in the experiment from which tracings for Fig. 4 were obtained. Although electromygraphic activity returned to pre-injection values 15 min after α-methylnoradrenaline, as also shown in Fig. 12, the threefold increase in oxygen

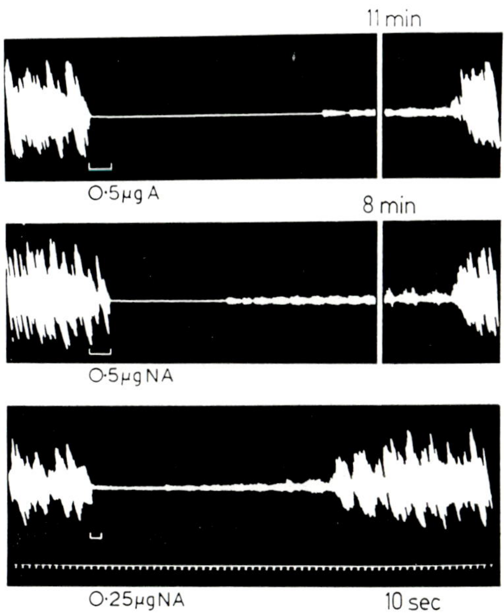

Fig. 13. Tremor recorded from left tibialis anterior muscle of a cat anaesthetized with pentobarbitone sodium. At the signals, perfusion was with adrenaline (A) or noradrenaline (NA) from lateral ventricle to aqueduct at a rate of 0.1 ml/min for 30 sec (0.5 μg) or for 15 sec (0.25 μg). In the upper two records the intervals between the two sections were 11 and 8 min respectively. Time signals in 10 sec. (From Domer, F.R. and Feldberg, W., Brit. J. Pharmacol. **15**, 578—587, 1960)

consumption due to chilling was halved for the subsequent 95 min before the chicken was restored to a thermoneutral environment. Presumably, the residual increase in oxygen consumption was associated with shivering which continued and increased despite temporary abatement after α-methylnoradrenaline. There was suggestive evidence that the halving of the increase in oxygen consumption was due to reduced fat metabolism (Allen et al., 1970).

Tremor elicited in cats by tubocurarine perfused from a lateral ventricle to the aqueduct was also abolished by intraventricular adrenaline or noradrenaline (Feldberg and Malcolm, 1959). Evidence locating this action of catecholamines to the diencephalon was obtained from anaesthetized cats in which tremor was recorded from the freed tendon of the anterior tibialis muscle. Both lateral ventricles were perfused, whereby perfusate from one lateral ventricle did not enter the other, the fluids meeting in the third ventricle. Tubocurarine was perfused through one lateral ventricle and artificial cerebrospinal fluid through the other until tremor developed. Adrenaline or noradrenaline then replaced the artificial cerebrospinal fluid and tremor stopped within 20 sec (Carmichael et al., 1962). Surprisingly after intracisternal injection, noradrenaline and adrenaline produced fasciculation of the trapezius and sternomastoid muscles of anaesthetized cats but this was attributed to an action on the lateral aspects of the upper cervical cord (Rocha e Silva and Sproull, 1966). Inhibition of shivering has been obtained by electrical stimulation of the hypothalamus (HEMINGWAY et al., 1954), particularly the ventromedial septal region and the anterior or ventrolateral posterior hypothalamus (STUART et al., 1961). Electrical stimulation of the preoptic area in the goat inhibited shivering and lowered temperature (ANDERSSON et al., 1956).

In animals other than the chick, intravenous injections of catecholamines produce effects opposite to those obtained by intraventricular injection. For example, in man, intravenous adrenaline enhances tremor (BARCROFT et al., 1952). Since finger tremor induced by intravenous adrenaline was abolished by interrupting arterial supply to the arm by an occlusive cuff above that elbow (OWEN and MARSDEN, 1965), tremor was likely to be due to a peripheral action. Intra-arterial infusion of adrenaline or isoprenaline into a brachial artery caused increased ipsilateral finger tremor in dose-dependent fashion (FOLEY et al., 1967).

X. Effect of Catecholamines on Central Control of Blood Pressure

(—)-Noradrenaline (0.05—0.5 mg) or DOPA (0.5—10 mg) given into a lateral ventricle of anaesthetized dogs, produced bradycardia, lowered blood pressure 26—28 mm Hg for about 1 hr and diminished pressor responses to carotid occlusion (McCUBBIN et al., 1960). Since the effects were opposed by intraventricular administration of vasodilator substances (sodium nitroprusside, histamine) and simulated by intraventricular injection of vasoconstrictor substances (angiotensin, vasopressin), the possibility was canvassed (KANEKO et al., 1960) that they were due to changes in blood supply of vasomotor centres. Adrenaline, given intraventricularly to lightly anaesthetized cats, lowered blood pressure (NASHOLD et al., 1962); (—)-noradrenaline (40 or 80 μg) given intraventricularly to anaesthetized cats elicited bradycardia, which when marked was accompanied by a small fall in blood pressure (SHARE and MELVILLE, 1963). Although these results are compatible with a central depressant action of noradrenaline, interpretation was complicated by the finding that when noradrenaline was injected intraventricularly to cats given intraventricular reserpine 18—22 hr previously, increases in blood pressure of 30—150 mm Hg ensued together with tachycardia. This suggested leakage of noradrenaline from the cerebrospinal fluid into the systemic circulation, despite significant reduction of these effects after section of the spinal cord at C2 (SHARE and MELVILLE, 1963). Another possibility, and one mooted by MELVILLE and JOHNSON (1970), was that the rise in blood pressure and tachycardia observed during perfusion of the ventricle with large concentrations of noradrenaline were due to an increased loss of brain potassium since there was marked increase of potassium in the perfusate.

That isoprenaline (1.5, 15 and 75 μg), given intraventricularly to anaesthetized cats, lowered blood pressure but induced *tachycardia* (GAGNON and MELVILLE, 1967) again suggests leakage into the systemic circulation, yet paradoxically these effects, also obtained after pretreatment with intraventricular reserpine, were abolished by spinal cord section. The effects of intraventricular (—)-adrenaline (10—200 μg), (—)-noradrenaline (50 μg) or (—)-isoprenaline (50—200 μg) on blood pressure and cardiac rate of anaesthetized rabbits (TODA et al., 1969) were the same as in anaesthetized cats. COWELL and DAVEY (1968) noted pressor responses of about 75 mm Hg lasting 15 min to (—)-noradrenaline (10 μg) given intraventricularly in anaesthetized mice. These effects were potentiated by doses of pempidine sufficient to abolish pressor effects of dimethylphenyl-piperazinium. The results again imply passage of noradrenaline from the brain into the general circulation, but then the technique of acute intraventricular injection in mice leaves much to be desired compared with that of injection via a chronically implanted intraventricular cannula as used by the other investigators.

Since anaesthesia vitiates the action of many drugs on the central nervous system and often lowers blood pressure, it is remarkable that such clear-cut effects were observed by McCubbin et al. (1960). The fall in blood pressure they noted was only just short of the mean fall of 35 mm Hg lasting some hours in non-anaesthetized young chicks given (—)-α-methylnoradrenaline (0.05 μmole in 0.5 μl) by micro-infusion into the hypothalamus (Marley and Stephenson, 1970). In unanaesthetized rabbits, intraventricular (—)-adrenaline (200 μg) evoked a rise followed by a substantial fall in blood pressure (Toda et al., 1969).

XI. Drugs Affecting Catecholamine Synthesis, Storage, Release and Metabolism

The effects of drugs which alter synthesis, storage, release or metabolism of catecholamines are discussed inasmuch as they affect behavioural responses of exogenous DOPA, dopamine or noradrenaline. Effects of these drugs on endogenous catecholamines are dealt with in the chapters 6, 7, 13 of this volume.

1. Monoamine Precursors and Inhibitors of DOPA Decarboxylase

a) Mechanism of Action

The amino acids, DOPA and 3,4-dihydroxyphenylserine, penetrate the blood-brain barrier after which they undergo decarboxylation in the brain by aromatic-L-amino acid decarboxylase (hereafter DOPA decarboxylase) to dopamine and noradrenaline respectively (Carlsson et al., 1957; Carlsson, 1964). Since dopamine is a precursor of noradrenaline, administration of DOPA leads to an increase in the brain concentrations of both dopamine and noradrenaline in chicks (Abuzzahab, 1966) and mammals (Bertler and Rosengren, 1959; McGeer et al., 1963) but the increase of noradrenaline is less than that of dopamine (Bertler and Rosengren, 1959; McGeer et al., 1963; Weil-Malherbe et al., 1961a; Dagirmanjian et al., 1963) possibly because of a slow rate of β-hydroxylation. Also conversion of dopamine to noradrenaline by dopamine β-hydroxylase *in vitro* is quantitatively less than conversion of dopamine to 3,4-dihydroxyphenylacetic acid, homovanillic acid and 3-O-methyltyramine by MAO and COMT (Rutledge and Jonason, 1967). *In vivo*, concentrations of 3,4-dihydroxyphenylacetic acid and homovanillic acid increase considerably in the caudate nucleus following administration of L-DOPA (Andén et al., 1963; Carlsson and Hillarp, 1962). However, in certain regions of the brain where dopamine β-hydroxylase activity is high, e.g. hypothalamus (Udenfriend and Creveling, 1959), rapid synthesis of noradrenaline from dopamine occurs (Glowinski and Iversen, 1966a). 3,4-Dihydroxyphenylserine is decarboxylated slowly so that concentrations of noradrenaline in the brain only rise significantly after its administration following pretreatment with an MAO inhibitor (Carlsson, 1964).

b) Behaviour, Temperature and Electrocortical Activity

The central actions of DOPA have been studied in many species, particularly after pretreatment with catecholamine-depleting agents or inhibitors of catecholamine synthesis and metabolism. In general, large doses of DOPA produce electroencephalographic arousal (see below), locomotor stimulation and hyperthermia accompanied by autonomic phenomena such as piloerection, salivation, pupillary dilatation etc; the effects of reserpine are also reversed (BERTLER and ROSENGREN, 1959; BLASCHKO and CHRUŚCIEL, 1960; CARLSSON et al., 1957; EVERETT and WIEGAND, 1962; HALPERN et al., 1963; KIKUCHI, 1962; GRIESEMER and GASNER, 1962; DEWHURST and MARLEY, 1965a; SPOONER and WINTERS, 1965; LAMMERS and VAN ROSSUM, 1968).

In contrast, some investigators obtained suppression of spontaneous motor activity or of operant behaviour after DL- or L-DOPA, with doses less than 500 mg/kg in rats and mice (BOFF and HEISE, 1963; BOISSIER and SIMON, 1966; EIDUSON, 1959; SCHECKEL et al., 1965; SMITH and DEWS, 1962; ESTLER and AMMON, 1970). Evidence that the suppression of activity following DOPA is due to a peripheral action of its catabolites was obtained by BUTCHER and ENGEL (1969a, b) using an inhibitor of DOPA decarboxylase that does not readily pass the blood-brain barrier, Ro 4-4602 (N-(DL-seryl)-N^1-(2,3,4-hydroxybenzyl)-hydrazine) and consequently selectively inhibits extracerebral DOPA decarboxylase (BARTHOLINI et al., 1967). After pretreatment with Ro 4-4602, DOPA concentration in the blood and dopamine concentrations in the brain were augmented, presumably due to an increased amount of DOPA entering the brain (BARTHOLINI and PLETSCHER, 1968; see BERTLER et al., 1963). L-DOPA (150 mg/kg i.p.) reduced operant avoidance responding and produced autonomic symptoms culminating in death; lower doses were ineffective (BUTCHER and ENGEL, 1969b). However, after pretreatment with Ro 4-4602 (50 mg/kg) which itself did not influence responding, L-DOPA (150 or 200 mg/kg) increased avoidance responses in the absence of autonomic phenomena. Conversion of DOPA to dopamine and noradrenaline in the periphery was inhibited by Ro 4-4602, suggesting that the autonomic effects and suppression of activity seen after DOPA alone, were due to a peripheral action of DOPA catabolites; suppression or reduction of operant responding occurs after peripheral administration of dopamine or noradrenaline (section V). DOPA is preferentially decarboxylated extracerebrally because of higher DOPA decarboxylase activity in the periphery (BLASCHKO and CHRUŚCIEL, 1960). Thus after injection of L-DOPA (400 mg/kg i.p.) in reserpinized mice, the dopamine concentration in the heart was approximately five times that in the brain (SEIDEN and CARLSSON, 1964). However, increased responding to DOPA after Ro 4-4602 was not easily related to any one change in brain monoamine concentrations since there was a 7—8 times increase in dopamine, an 80—84% reduction in 5-HT and a significant decrease in noradrenaline; doses of L-DOPA which did not influence responding after Ro 4-4602 still increased cerebral dopamine concentrations 3—5 times and significantly reduced 5-hydroxytryptamine and noradrenaline (BUTCHER and ENGEL, 1969b). The decrease in concentration of 5-hydroxytryptamine may have been due to its displacement by newly synthesized dopamine (BARTHOLINI et al., 1968; BUTCHER et al., 1970), competitive inhibition of DOPA decarboxylase by L-DOPA or competition between L-DOPA and 5-hydroxytryptophan for DOPA decarboxylase (BUTCHER and ENGEL, 1969b). Increased motor activity does not become apparent until brain dopamine concentration is increased 3—4 fold (EVERETT and WIEGAND, 1962).

Intravenous or intracarotid injections of DOPA (20—50 mg/kg i.v.; 8—20 mg i.a.) produced electrocortical desynchronization in cat or rabbit *cerveau isolé* preparations (MONNIER and TISSOT, 1958; MONNIER, 1960; MANTEGAZZINI and GLÄSSER, 1960) and selectively increased brain dopamine (DAGIRMANJIAN et al., 1963). In contrast intravenous or intracarotid injections of L-DOPA (5—20 mg/kg i.v.; 22 or 44 mg i.a.) or DL-DOPA (25—30 mg/kg i.v.) did not consistently evoke electrocortical desynchronization in curarized rabbits (COSTA et al., 1960a), gallamine-immobilized or *encéphale isolé* cat preparations (KADZIELAWA and

WIDY-TYSZKIEWICZ, 1970a). Presumably in intact or *encéphale isolé* preparations ascending influences from bulbar synchronizing centres, removed by more anterior transections, inhibited DOPA-induced desynchronization (KADZIELAWA and WIDY-TYSZKIEWICZ, 1970a). That desynchronization was prevented by Ro 4-4602 suggested that peripheral actions of dopamine and noradrenaline were responsible, not central actions as assumed by KADZIELAWA and WIDY-TYSZKIEWICZ (1970b) since Ro 4-4602 does not inhibit cerebral DOPA decarboxylase (BARTHOLINI et al., 1967). Bilateral injections of DOPA (0.1 mg) into various pontine nuclei of the rabbit evoked electrocortical desynchronization, diminished awareness and reduced electromyographic activity of neck muscles (LEDEBUR and TISSOT, 1966). After a short latent period, DL-3,4-dihydroxyphenylserine (200 mg i.v.) induced behavioural and electrocortical sleep in rats (HAVLÍČEK, 1967).

Many investigators consider DOPA to be pharmacologically inert (CARLSSON, 1966; HORNYKIEWICZ, 1966) but in 1—28 day chicks, L-DOPA produced behavioural and electrocortical alerting, whereas dopamine and noradrenaline induced behavioural and electrocortical sleep (DEWHURST and MARLEY, 1965a; SPOONER and WINTERS, 1965). L- and DL-DOPA applied by micro-pipettes excited feline cortical neurones, whereas dopamine and noradrenaline depressed cortical neuronal discharge initiated by synaptic activity or by the application of L-glutamate (KRNJEVIĆ and PHILLIS, 1963).

2. Inhibitors of Monoamine Storage

Two types of inhibitor markedly deplete monoamines, on the one hand, the DOPA analogues, α-methyl DOPA and α-MMT, and on the other, the Rauwolfia alkaloids (e.g. reserpine) and benzoquinolizines.

a) Mechanism of Action

The DOPA analogues rapidly reduce brain monoamine concentrations but whereas those of 5-hydroxytryptamine and dopamine return to normal within 24 hr, that of noradrenaline remains low for several days (HESS et al., 1961; PORTER et al., 1961; SOURKES et al., 1961; CARLSSON and LINDQVIST, 1962). Although these amino acids are competitive inhibitors of DOPA decarboxylase, inhibition of this enzyme does not contribute to their action since this enzyme is present in great excess and is not rate-limiting (HESS et al., 1961; UDENFRIEND et al., 1966). Furthermore, potent inhibitors of DOPA decarboxylase do not reduce monoamine concentrations (DRAIN et al., 1962; BRODIE et al., 1962). The prolonged depletion of noradrenaline by α-MMT and α-methyl DOPA is due to the formation of (—)-metaraminol and α-methylnoradrenaline, respectively (UDENFRIEND and ZALTZMAN-NIRENBERG, 1962; GESSA et al., 1962; CARLSSON and LINDQVIST, 1962) which displace noradrenaline stoichiometrically (ANDÉN, 1964; SHORE et al., 1964; PORTER et al., 1965; but see MUSCHOLL, 1966).

b) Behaviour and Electrocortical Activity

Reserpine depletes brain catecholamines and 5-hydroxytryptamine, producing characteristic sedation probably by preventing incorporation of monoamines into storage vesicles (GLOWINSKI and AXELROD, 1965; GLOWINSKI et al., 1966b). The connexion between depletion of brain amines and sedation was not immediately apparent since the time-course of behavioural recovery in acutely reserpinized animals was unrelated to restoration of brain catecholamines (BERTLER, 1961; COSTA et al., 1962; HÄGGENDAL and LINDQVIST, 1963; MCGEER et al., 1963). The existence of a small, functional storage pool (section III), restoration of which parallels behavioural recovery was revealed by chronic reserpine experiments (HÄGGENDAL and LINDQVIST, 1964). The importance of this pool has been confirmed by tests using H^3-noradrenaline (GLOWINSKI et al., 1966a).

The sedative effects of reserpine were reversed 15—30 min after injecting large doses of DOPA in mice (CARLSSON et al., 1957; CHRUŚCIEL, 1960; BLASCHKO and CHRUŚCIEL, 1960), monkeys (EVERETT and TOMAN, 1959), cats (McGEER et al., 1963) but not consistently in rats (CARLSSON, 1966). This time interval suggests that reversal was due to synthesis of either dopamine or noradrenaline. Dopamine was the more obvious candidate since in reserpinized cats, behavioural recovery was associated with a return to normal of dopamine concentration in the brain but only partial recovery of noradrenaline; 5-hydroxytryptamine was unaffected (McGEER et al., 1963). Further, in reserpinized mice, DL-threo-3,4-dihydroxyphenylserine, which is decarboxylated directly to noradrenaline, restored brain concentration of noradrenaline but did not reverse the behavioural effects (CREVELING et al., 1968) except after MAO inhibition (CARLSSON, 1966), thus confirming earlier findings of BLASCHKO and CHRUŚCIEL (1960). Reserpine inhibits synthesis of noradrenaline *in vitro* in peripheral sympathetic nerve tissue, adrenal medulla and heart probably as a consequence of blockade of the storage mechanism since dopamine β-hydroxylase is confined to storage vesicles (KIRSHNER, 1962; RUTLEDGE and WEINER, 1967; STJÄRNE, 1966; STJÄRNE and LISHAJKO, 1966; STJÄRNE et al., 1967; ROTH and STONE, 1968); inhibition of noradrenaline synthesis *in vivo* and in the brain is less certain (KRONEBERG and SCHÜMANN, 1958, 1960; ANDÉN et al., 1964; PHILIPPU and SCHÜMANN, 1967; KOPIN and WEISE, 1968; CARLSSON et al., 1968a). DL-DOPA reduced the threshold for EEG arousal, produced by electrical stimulation of the brain stem in rabbits pretreated with tetrabenazine (TAKAGI et al., 1968).

c) Conclusion

Great caution should be exercised when attempting to relate behaviour to concentrations of brain monoamines, particularly in view of the existence of the small but important functional pool. Reserpine lowers concentrations of noradrenaline, dopamine and 5-hydroxytryptamine about the same extent and time (SHORE, 1962; CARLSSON, 1966) and a causal relation between sedation and depletion of 5-hydroxytryptamine has been suggested (BRODIE et al., 1956). Absence of sedation after α-MMT, which has a lesser effect on 5-hydroxytryptamine concentration than reserpine, has been used as an argument in favour of this relation. In fact, α-MMT which itself produces locomotor stimulation (PORTER et al., 1961; VAN ROSSUM, 1963; CARLTON, 1963; SCHECKEL and BOFF, 1964; WEISSMAN and KOE, 1967), and α-methyl DOPA partly antagonize the effects of reserpine (CARLSSON, 1966; NEČINA, 1962). However, noradrenergic transmission is impaired by reserpine (BERTLER et al., 1956; BERTLER et al., 1958; MUSCHOLL and VOGT, 1958; GAFFNEY et al., 1963) but not by α-MMT (or (+)-adrenaline which also displaces noradrenaline stoichiometrically) even in doses which deplete 97% of noradrenaline in the brain, spleen and heart of cats and rats (ANDÉN and MAGNUSSON, 1963). Therefore an additional action of reserpine must be sought to explain impairment of transmission. This action is probably blockade of the uptake mechanism in storage vesicles leading to depletion of noradrenaline in the small functional pool essential for transmission. This pool can also be depleted of noradrenaline by inhibition of catecholamine synthesis. A complication attached to the use of α-methyl DOPA and α-MMT is that the catabolites, α-methylnoradrenaline and (—)-metaraminol are released by nervous activity and act as "false transmitters" (DAY and RAND, 1963) albeit with reduced efficacy compared to noradrenaline.

3. Inhibitors of Monoamine Uptake

Desmethylimipramine and imipramine significantly alter response of the central nervous system to injected monoamines without altering their endogenous concentration in the brain (SULSER et al., 1962, 1964; SCHWARTZ et al., 1963; NYBÄCK et al., 1968) or the fluorescence of central nerve terminals containing catecholamines (BARTONIČEK et al., 1964). In the following experiments imipramine and desmethylimipramine were given intraperitoneally or intravenously.

a) Mechanism of Action

Accumulation of H^3-noradrenaline in rat brain following its intraventricular or intracisternal injection was reduced by imipramine or desmethylimipramine (GLOWINSKI and AXELROD, 1964, 1966; SCHANBERG et al., 1967b; GLOWINSKI et al., 1966a; FUXE and UNGERSTEDT, 1968b). Desmethylimipramine, but not imipramine, reduced accumulation of C^{14}-noradrenaline in mouse brain, following intravenous injection of C^{14}-tyrosine (NYBÄCK et al., 1968; SCHUBERT et al., 1970). Since the effects of imipramine on noradrenaline uptake are due to its demethylated metabolite, desmethylimipramine (GILLETTE et al., 1961), it was inactive in species (rabbits, mice) in which demethylation was negligible (SULSER et al., 1964).

Accumulation of H^3-dopamine after intraventricular injection, or of C^{14}-dopamine following intravenous injection of C^{14}-tyrosine was unaffected by imipramine or desmethylimipramine (GLOWINSKI et al., 1966a; NYBÄCK et al., 1968; SCHUBERT et al., 1970). Desmethylimipramine prevented the reserpine-resistant accumulation of dopamine and noradrenaline, following their intraventricular injection, in noradrenaline neurones (FUXE and UNGERSTEDT, 1968b) but not in dopamine neurones (FUXE and HILLARP, 1964; FUXE et al., 1966, 1967; FUXE and UNGERSTEDT, 1968b). Similarly, after administration of L-DOPA to reserpinized animals, desmethylimipramine prevented accumulation of catecholamines in central noradrenaline neurones, but not in central dopamine neurones, *in vitro* and *in vivo* (CARLSSON et al., 1966a). Interestingly, anti-parkinsonian drugs are non-competitive inhibitors of dopamine uptake in the rat corpus striatum; this inhibition may account for their therapeutic action (COYLE and SNYDER, 1969).

Reduced accumulation of radioactive noradrenaline after imipramine or desmethylimipramine was associated with increase in brain normetanephrine (GLOWINSKI et al., 1966a; SCHANBERG et al., 1967b); this was not due to enhanced release of noradrenaline since the rate of disappearance of previously accumulated C^{14}-noradrenaline (synthesized from C^{14}-tyrosine) in mouse brain was unaltered by desmethylimipramine (NYBÄCK et al., 1968; SCHUBERT et al., 1970). In rats, imipramine and desmethylimipramine retarded disappearance of H^3-noradrenaline from the brain (GLOWINSKI and AXELROD, 1966; NOBLE et al., 1967; SCHANBERG et al., 1967b) but paradoxically increased disappearance of endogenous noradrenaline, but not dopamine, after inhibition of synthesis with α-methyltyrosine (NEFF and COSTA, 1966a). Desmethylimipramine and to a lesser extent, imipramine also slowed disappearance of noradrenaline from the brain following an amine-releasing compound, 4-α-dimethyl-meta-tyramine (CARLSSON et al., 1969a); desmethylimipramine reduced release of noradrenaline from electrically stimulated brain slices (BALDESSARINI and KOPIN, 1967).

Although large concentrations of imipramine inhibit dopamine β-hydroxylase *in vitro* (GOLDSTEIN and CONTRERA, 1961a), this would not account for reduced accumulation of H^3-noradrenaline following its intraventricular administration. Indeed, slowed accumulation of noradrenaline in the brain following desmethylimipramine is thought to be due to competitive inhibition of noradrenaline uptake at neuronal membranes (FUXE and UNGERSTEDT, 1968b) and at storage vesicle membranes (PHILIPPU et al., 1969), as occurs in the periphery (HAMBERGER, 1967; BERTI and SHORE, 1967). Since inhibition is competitive, impairment of uptake depends on the relative concentrations of desmethylimipramine and noradrenaline. Thus, after an intraperitoneal injection of desmethylimipramine, uptake of an intraventricular injection of noradrenaline was impaired most in the medulla oblongata, away from the injection site and where noradrenaline concentration was low, and least in the hippocampus where noradrenaline concentration was high (FUXE and UNGERSTEDT, 1968b; GLOWINSKI et al., 1966a). Sensitivity of the uptake mechanism to desmethylimipramine varied in different brain regions, being greatest in the cerebellum and least in the striatum, *in vitro* (SNYDER et al., 1968) and *in vivo* (GLOWINSKI et al., 1966a).

Actions of imipramine-like drugs on release and uptake of 5-hydroxytryptamine should not be ignored. Imipramine, but not desmethylimipramine, inhibited reserpine-resistant uptake of 5-hydroxytryptamine in rats (FUXE and UNGERSTEDT, 1967; CARLSSON et al., 1968b) and reduced the accumulation of H^3-5-hydroxytryptamine in mouse brain (SCHUBERT et al., 1970). Desmethylimipramine did not affect uptake of C^{14}-5-hydroxytryptamine from rat cerebral ventricles (PALAIČ et al., 1967). Unexpectedly, imipramine did not affect uptake of H^3-5-hydroxytryptamine by rat brain (SCHILDKRAUT et al., 1969; D. ECCLESTON quoted by SCHILDKRAUT et al., 1969). Imipramine but not desmethylimipramine retarded the release of H^3-5-hydroxytryptamine from rat brain (SCHILDKRAUT et al., 1969). Imipramine and amitriptyline but not desmethylimipramine and nortriptyline retarded disappearance of H^3-5-hydroxytryptamine from mouse brain (SCHUBERT et al., 1970) and of endogenous 5-hydroxytryptamine following an amine releasing compound, 4-methyl-α-ethyl-meta-tyramine (CARLSSON et al., 1969b) or a synthesis inhibitor (CORRODI and FUXE, 1968, 1969). Thus, dimethylated compounds affected predominantly brain 5-hydroxytryptamine whereas monomethylated compounds affected noradrenaline.

b) Behaviour, Temperature and Electrocortical Activity

The effects of noradrenaline are potentiated by desmethylimipramine presumably because inhibition of noradrenaline uptake increases the concentration of noradrenaline at postsynaptic sites (AXELROD et al., 1961a; HERTTING et al., 1961; GLOWINSKI and AXELROD, 1964; IVERSEN, 1965). Thus, prior administration of imipramine and desmethylimipramine prevented many behavioural effects of reserpine or benzoquinolizines, including sedation and reduced locomotor activity (DOMENJOZ and THEOBALD, 1959; COSTA et al., 1960b; GILLETTE et al., 1961; MAXWELL and PALMER, 1961; GARATTINI et al., 1962; SULSER et al., 1962; WILSON and TISLOW, 1962; ASKEW, 1963; HALLIWELL et al., 1964) but did not prevent depletion of cerebral monoamines by reserpine (GARATTINI et al., 1962) although the rate of depletion of noradrenaline was slowed (MANARA et al., 1966). Rapid depletion was essential for prevention of reserpine effects since these were not found in cats, because of slow monoamine release following reserpine, nor in rats following repeated administration of small doses of reserpine (SULSER et al., 1964). Because of negligible demethylation imipramine did not prevent reserpine sedation in mice, rabbits and dogs (SULSER et al., 1962, 1964) but surprisingly reserpine ptosis was reversed in rabbits (MAXWELL and PALMER, 1961). According to ROSS and RENYI (1967) desmethylimipramine prevented reserpine ptosis and hypothermia, in mice, but not sedation; it was acting centrally since its methiodide, which fails to penetrate the blood-brain barrier, did not prevent these phenomena. Potentiation by desmethylimipramine of the excitant effects in mice of DL- and L-DOPA (McGrath and Ketteler, 1963; Everett et al., 1964) is used as a screening test for possible antidepressant drugs (Everett, 1966).

The increase in body temperature produced by desmethylimipramine in reserpinized rats was attributed to extraneuronal accumulation of noradrenaline since it was prevented by pretreatment with α-methyltyrosine or diethyldithiocarbamate (Jori et al., 1966). Imipramine potentiated the hypothermic effects of noradrenaline injected intracisternally in rats (Bruinvels, 1970). Hyperthermia evoked by intravenous or subcutaneous injection of noradrenaline in rats and mice was potentiated by desmethylimipramine (Jori and Garattini, 1965; Cowell and Davey, 1968). Paradoxically, nortriptyline and imipramine antagonized the hypothermic effect of an intraventricular injection of noradrenaline in mice (Brittain, 1966; Cowell and Davey, 1968); this was attributed to potentiation of the hyperthermic effects of noradrenaline leaking into the systemic circulation (Cowell and Davey, 1968). However, in mice reduction in locomotor activity following intracisternal injection of noradrenaline or dopamine was partially prevented by oral pretreatment with amitriptyline (Broadley and Roberts, 1967) whereas imipramine completely reversed actions of L-DOPA on electrocortical activity of cat *cerveau isolé* preparations, intense synchronization resulting (Kadzielawa and Widy-Tyszkiewicz, 1970b).

Eating responses elicited by noradrenaline injected into the rat hypothalamus were antagonized when desmethylimipramine was given into the hypothalamus 5 min previously but potentiated when given 20 min previously, suggesting that neural uptake of noradrenaline was important in mediating the eating response, at least initially (Booth, 1968). Antagonism of the behavioural depressant effects of noradrenaline by imipramine in young chicks was attributed to a postsynaptic action (Mandell et al., 1969).

4. Inhibitors of Tyrosine Hydroxylase

a) Mechanism of Action

Tyrosine hydroxylase, the rate-limiting enzyme in the synthesis of noradrenaline (Udenfriend and Wijngaarden, 1956; Levitt et al., 1965; Udenfriend et al., 1965), has been isolated (Nagatsu et al., 1964). 5-HTP and several analogues of tyrosine and tryptophan were found to be potent inhibitors of this enzyme *in vitro* and *in vivo* (Udenfriend et al., 1966; Spector et al., 1965a: Zhelyaskov et al., 1968; Carlsson et al., 1963a). The most widely used inhibitor is α-methyltyrosine (Spector et al., 1965a), particularly in the form of the soluble methylester hydrochloride (Hanson, 1965; Corrodi and Hanson, 1966); this is slowly converted to α-methyl-DOPA and α-methylnoradrenaline (Maître, 1965) but these are unlikely to contribute to its action (Udenfriend et al., 1966). Other inhibitors include iodinated derivatives of tyrosine, some of which occur endogenously and are involved in thyroid hormone synthesis (Goldstein et al., 1965; Spector et al., 1965b).

The rate of noradrenaline and dopamine depletion after inhibition of tyrosine hydroxylase is dependent on rate of utilization and so is more rapid in tissues with a fast turnover e.g. brain (Udenfriend and Zaltzman-Nirenberg, 1963). In brain, minimum catecholamine concentrations were reached about 8 hr after a single injection of α-methyltyrosine but after repeated injections to maintain enzyme inhibition over a period of time sufficient for utilization of catecholamine stores, noradrenaline and dopamine were undetectable; 5-hydroxytryptamine was unaffected (Spector et al., 1965a). However, since there is only slow exchange between storage and functional pools (CROUT et al., 1962) and repletion of the functional pool by reuptake is probably less than that resulting from synthesis (KOPIN et al., 1965), disruption of function may be achieved without total catecholamine depletion. Prior depletion of the storage pool by a small dose of reserpine intensifies and hastens onset of depletion by α-methyltyrosine (HANSON, 1966; MENON et al., 1967; CARR and MOORE, 1968).

b) Behaviour

Following chronic treatment with α-methyltyrosine, guinea-pigs (80 mg/kg i.p. every 3 hr for 24 hr) and cats (80 mg/kg every 12 hr for 2 weeks) were less active, slightly sedated but easily roused (SPECTOR et al., 1965a). Single injections of the α-methyltyrosine methylester (150—200 mg/kg i.p. in cats and 125 or 250 mg/kg i.p. in rats) produced sedation of varying depth and duration and disrupted conditioned avoidance responses (cats — shuttle box; rats — Skinner box); the effects coincided with selective depletion of cerebral catecholamines (HANSON, 1965). α-Methyltyrosine-induced suppression of self-stimulation in rats was also associated with a decrease in brain noradrenaline concentrations (POSCHEL and NINTEMAN, 1966). WEISSMAN and KOE (1965) suggested that doses of α-methyltyrosine frequently used were toxic and that this contributed to its sedative effect; they were unable, whatever the dose, to disrupt a conditioned "jump-out" avoidance response in rats. However, single injections of non-toxic doses of α-methyltyrosine (80 mg/kg i.p.) reduced avoidance in the shuttle-box, whereas multiple injections (80 mg/kg i.p. every 6 hr for 4 doses) increased avoidance and diminished escape-responses (MOORE, 1966), suggesting that the "jump-out" procedure is less sensitive. Toxicity, due to kidney damage caused by deposition of insoluble α-methyltyrosine in the kidney tubules, can be diminished by water-loading, or procedures which reduce its blood concentration, such as oral administration, repeated small doses, or its incorporation in the diet (MOORE et al., 1967; JOHNSON et al., 1967; MOORE, 1968a, 1968b).

L-DOPA (100 mg/kg) reversed the effects of α-methyltyrosine on conditioned avoidance behaviour in cats, rats and mice and caused excitement, increased motor activity, piloerection, mydriasis and exophthalmos; dopamine concentration in the brain rose above and then decreased rapidly to normal after 30 min whereas noradrenaline concentration had risen to normal values by 60 min (HANSON, 1965; CORRODI and HANSON, 1966). HANSON (1965) did not detect significant changes in cerebral noradrenaline concentration after L-DOPA. The effects of L-DOPA after α-methyltyrosine were considerably longer-lasting than after reserpine. This could be attributed to intact intraneuronal storage mechanisms so that newly synthesized catecholamines were incorporated and protected from MAO (see below and CORRODI et al., 1966; CORRODI and FUXE, 1967). Extraneuronal dopamine, located in the pericytes, was partly responsible for the overshoot in dopamine concentration after L-DOPA (CORRODI et al., 1966).

Hyperactivity and stereotyped behaviour due to amphetamine were not seen in rats pretreated with α-methyltyrosine (100 mg/kg 9, 6 and 3 hr previously), but when L-DOPA (200 mg/kg) which by itself was without effect, was given at the same time as amphetamine, the typical amphetamine syndrome developed (RANDRUP and MUNKVAD, 1966). Similarly, (+)-amphetamine failed to restore a conditioned avoidance response in cats treated with reserpine (0.1 mg/kg) and α-methyltyrosine (100 mg/kg) but subsequently administered L-DOPA (12.5 or 25 mg/kg) caused prompt restoration (HANSON, 1967a). These results, which were confirmed using 3-α-dimethyltyrosine methylester (HANSON, 1967b), an inhibitor of tyrosine hydroxylase that is not converted to α-methyl DOPA and α-methylnoradrenaline which may act as "false transmitters", suggest that catecholamines are necessary for central actions of dexamphetamine. α-Methyltyrosine prevented the effects of amphetamine in doses that did not reduce cerebral catecholamine concentrations; probably the functional pool was selectively depleted of catecholamines because of its more rapid turnover (DOMINIC and MOORE, 1969).

Since intraneuronal storage mechanisms are intact in animals treated with α-methyltyrosine, but not reserpine (CORRODI et al., 1966; CORRODI and FUXE, 1967), restoration of cerebral catecholamine concentrations with L-DOPA presumably restores normal functioning of sympathetic neurones. It cannot be stated whether or not reversal of sedation and restoration of conditioned avoidance responses produced by DOPA is due to increase of dopamine or noradrenaline, since concentrations of catecholamines in whole brain do not necessarily reflect concentrations in the "functional pool" and dopamine may substitute for noradrenaline as a transmitter.

5. Inhibitors of Dopamine β-Hydroxylase

a) Mechanism of Action

Dopamine β-hydroxylase catalyzes conversion of dopamine to noradrenaline (LEVIN et al., 1960), once considered to be the rate-limiting step in synthesis of noradrenaline (GOLDSTEIN and CONTRERA, 1961b; COLLINS, 1965). The enzyme is inhibited by a variety of chelating agents *in vitro* (GOLDSTEIN et al., 1964a; GREENE, 1964). Among these, disulfiram (tetraethylthiuram disulphide) which is reduced *in vivo* to its active form, diethyldithiocarbamate, was sufficiently potent *in vivo* (GOLDSTEIN et al., 1964b; COLLINS, 1965; CARLSSON et al., 1966b; MUSACCHIO et al., 1964) for hydroxylation to be rate-limiting (MUSACCHIO et al., 1964, 1966; GOLDSTEIN et al., 1964b). More potent selective inhibitors have recently been introduced (SVENSSON and WALDECK, 1969; MAJ and VETULANI, 1969, 1970; JOHNSON et al., 1970). Reduction in cerebral noradrenaline concentration by inhibition of dopamine β-hydroxylase, in rats and mice was associated with a consistent but not significant ($p = 0.05$) increase in cerebral dopamine (GOLDSTEIN and NAKAJIMA, 1967; SEIDEN and PETERSON, 1968; CARLSSON et al., 1966b; LITTLETON, 1967; MAJ and VETULANI, 1969, 1970). Disulfiram did not reduce noradrenaline concentrations in guinea-pig brain (UDENFRIEND et al., 1966); possible explanations have been advanced for this discrepancy (GOLDSTEIN and NAKAJIMA, 1967).

Rate of depletion of cerebral noradrenaline after disulfiram was greater than after α-methyltyrosine (GOLDSTEIN and NAKAJIMA, 1967; PERSSON and WALDECK, 1970) possibly because some brain dopamine following tyrosine hydroxylase inhibition was available as a precursor for noradrenaline, whereas after disulfiram, noradrenaline synthesis ceased immediately. The problem may be more complex, however, since after simultaneous inhibition of tyrosine hydroxylase and dopamine β-hydroxylase, the rates of noradrenaline and dopamine depletion were slower than after selective inhibition of dopamine β-hydroxylase and tyrosine hydroxylase respectively (GOODCHILD, 1969; PERSSON and WALDECK, 1970). Cerebral dopamine concentrations following disulfiram were only slightly increased by pretreatment with nialamide (GOLDSTEIN and NAKAJIMA, 1967; CARLSSON et al., 1967). Since inhibition of β-hydroxylation interferes with binding of the amine in neuronal vesicles to the ATP-protein complex (MUSACCHIO et al., 1965), an increase of free dopamine in the cytoplasm would occur, further inhibiting its synthesis by a feed-back mechanism (CARLSSON et al., 1967). A similar mechanism would explain a fall in cerebral dopamine concentration occurring four hours after disulfiram (JOHNSON et al., 1970).

Interpretation of results after dopamine β-hydroxylase inhibition should allow for dopamine possibly replacing noradrenaline as a transmitter. Dopamine and noradrenaline were released by splenic nerve stimulation in cats pretreated with disulfiram (THOENEN et al., 1965, 1967).

b) Behaviour, Temperature and Electrocortical Activity

Diethyldithiocarbamate produced sedation in rats and mice (PFEIFER et al., 1966; RANDRUP and SCHEEL-KRÜGER, 1966; CARLSSON et al., 1966b; AIGNER et al., 1967; MOORE, 1968c). In mice pretreated with reserpine or α-methyltyrosine, restoration of motility by nialamide together with DOPA, appeared to depend on replenishment of brain noradrenaline, since it was prevented by disulfiram (MAJ et al., 1968). Similarly disulfiram, which itself disrupted conditioned avoidance responding (KRANTZ and SEIDEN, 1968) prevented reversal or reserpine-induced suppression of responding by L-DOPA (SEIDEN and PETERSON, 1968). Increase in locomotor activity by amphetamine was also prevented by disulfiram and diethyldithiocarbamate (MAJ and PRZEGALIŃSKI, 1967; PFEIFER et al., 1966) but not the effects of amphetamine on stereotyped behaviour (RANDRUP and SCHEEL-KRÜGER, 1966; MAJ and PRZEGALIŃSKI, 1967; MAJ and VETULANI, 1970). However, depression of spontaneous motor activity might not result exclusively from a depletion of brain noradrenaline (AIGNER et al., 1967; MOORE, 1968c; MAJ and VETULANI, 1970). The effects of nialamide on diethyldithiocarbamate-induced sedation in rats were inconclusive (CARLSSON et al., 1966b, 1967). Diethyldithiocarbamate also inhibited the hyperthermic response to DOPA in reserpinized rats (JORI et al., 1966). Diethyldithiocarbamate raised temperature in reserpinized mice but lowered it in normal mice (BARNETT and TABER, 1968). Electrocortical desynchronization to DOPA in cat *encéphale isolé* preparations was reduced by disulfiram (KADZIELAWA and WIDY-TYSZKIEWICZ, 1970b).

6. Inhibitors of Monoamine Oxidase

a) Mechanism of Action

Oxidative deamination by MAO and O-methylation by COMT are the major enzymatic pathways of catecholamine metabolism in the brain (MANNARINO et al., 1963; MATSUOKA, 1964; GLOWINSKI et al., 1965; AXELROD, 1966; GLOWINSKI and BALDESSARINI, 1966; PLETSCHER et al., 1966; GLOWINSKI et al., 1966b). Indirect evidence suggests that MAO, present in brain mitochondria (BOGDANSKI et al., 1957; WEIL-MALHERBE et al., 1961b; NUKADA et al., 1963) mainly at synaptic endings (RODRIGUEZ DE LORES ARNAIZ and DE ROBERTIS, 1962), functions intraneuronally whereas COMT, present in a soluble supernatant fraction (AXELROD and TOMCHICK, 1958) associated with synaptosomes (ALBERICI et al., 1965), functions extraneuronally. Thus, following intravenous injection of DOPA, dihydroxyphenylacetic acid appeared in brain before homovanillic acid suggesting that deamination occurred first, close to the site of dopamine formation (CARLSSON and HILLARP, 1962). Also, the ratio of H^3-normetanephrine to H^3-noradrenaline was higher after administration of H^3-noradrenaline than after formation of C^{14}-noradrenaline intraneuronally from C^{14}-tyrosine (GLOWINSKI et al., 1966b).

Pretreatment with a monoamine oxidase inhibitor increased brain concentrations of endogenous monoamines in rats (GREEN and ERICKSON, 1960; CROUT et al., 1961; PSCHEIDT et al., 1963), mice (CARLSSON et al., 1959; WIEGAND and

Perry, 1961; Pscheidt et al., 1963), rabbits (Spector et al., 1958; Bertler, 1961; Pscheidt et al., 1963), guinea-pigs (Pscheidt et al., 1963), monkeys (Pscheidt et al., 1963) and chickens (Pscheidt and Himwich, 1965). In cats and dogs, 5-hydroxytryptamine, but not noradrenaline was increased (Vogt, 1954, 1959; Spector et al., 1960; Pscheidt et al., 1963; Mannarino et al., 1963; Maling et al., 1962).

Where concentration of monoamines was raised, that of 5-hydroxytryptamine was usually increased more than that of catecholamines. Accumulation of H^3-noradrenaline, following its intraventricular administration, was enhanced by pretreatment with a MAO inhibitor in rats (Glowinski and Axelrod, 1965; Glowinski et al., 1966a) but not in cats (Mannarino et al., 1963). The increase of catecholamines following DOPA was enhanced by MAO inhibition (Carlsson et al., 1958; Weil-Malherbe et al., 1961a; Everett and Wiegand, 1962) that of dopamine being greater than that of noradrenaline; this may be due either to a slow rate of β-hydroxylation or, after hydrazine-MAO inhibitors, to inhibition of dopamine β-hydroxylase since benzylhydrazines are potent inhibitors of this enzyme *in vitro* and *in vivo* (Creveling et al., 1962; Kuntzman et al., 1962). Increase in cerebral concentration of dopamine and noradrenaline following MAO inhibition was associated with increase in their respective O-methylated catabolites, 3-methoxytyramine and normetanephrine (Carlsson and Waldeck, 1964; Axelrod, 1958; Glowinski et al., 1966a).

Interpretation of results after monoamine oxidase inhibition is not easy. Many MAO inhibitors, particularly those with a phenylisopropyl moiety (e.g. phenylisopropylhydrazine) produce amphetamine-like stimulation independent of their enzyme inhibiting activity (Eltherington and Horita, 1960; Pirch and Norton, 1965). Tranylcypromine releases noradrenaline in the brain (Carlsson et al., 1960); this may explain the similar hypothermic effects of intraventricular injections of tranylcypromine and noradrenaline in rats (Feldberg and Lotti, 1967). Phenylisopropylhydrazine reduced the rate of disappearance of H^3-noradrenaline from brain (Glowinski and Axelrod, 1965) suggesting that MAO inhibitors either reduce release of catecholamines from storage sites (Glowinski and Axelrod, 1965; Axelrod et al., 1961b) or increase the half-life of intracellular catecholamines by preventing their oxidative deamination (Carlsson, 1966). The turnover of endogenous brain noradrenaline is reduced by MAO inhibition, probably due to increased catecholamine concentration inhibiting tyrosine hydroxylation (Neff and Costa, 1966b); catecholamines are potent inhibitors of tyrosine hydroxylase (Udenfriend et al., 1965).

b) Behaviour, Temperature and Electrocortical Activity

The behavioural and autonomic effects of DOPA were intensified by pretreatment with an MAO inhibitor (Carlsson et al., 1958; Blaschko and Chruściel, 1960; Weil-Malherbe et al., 1961a; Everett and Wiegand, 1962; Spooner and Winters, 1965; Boissier and Simon, 1966). Behavioural effects of catecholamines injected intracerebrally were potentiated in species in which MAO inhibition elevates cerebral catecholamine concentration. Thus in mice, behavioural depression following intraventricular injection of noradrenaline (25—100 μg/100 g) was potentiated by pretreatment with iproniazid (Chambers and Roberts, 1968). In rats, intracerebral injection of noradrenaline (1×10^{-7} mole) lowered temperature 2.5°C after MAO inhibition with nialamide compared to a fall of 1°C before nialamide (Schmidt and Fähse, 1964). In chicks, injection of (—)-noradrenaline (0.05 μmole) into the hypothalamus lowered temperature the same extent before and after MAO inhibition, but the duration of response after mebanazine, a hydrazine MAO inhibitor, was increased from a control of between 3 and 4 hr to between 8 and 9 hr (Marley and Stephenson, 1970 and Fig. 7). Injection of dopamine (0.1 μmole) into the hypothalamus of chicks was without significant effect, but after mebanazine, dopamine lowered temperature and produced behavioural sleep (Marley and Stephenson, 1969, 1970). In contrast in cats, the behavioural effects of an intraventricular injection of noradrenaline or adrenaline were only slightly increased by pretreatment with phenylisopropylhydrazine (Schain, 1961).

The effects of reserpine, α-MMT or tetrabenazine after MAO inhibition were similar to, but more intense than those of DOPA suggesting that they were due to release of free monoamines instead of deaminated metabolites caused by block of monoamine storage and/or uptake (Carlsson, 1966; Pletscher et al., 1966; Graeff, 1966). Depletion of catecholamines by α-methyltyrosine was reduced by pretreatment with an MAO inhibitor (Moore and Rech, 1967). In rats, behavioural and electrocortical sleep produced by DL-3,4-dihydroxyphenylserine were potentiated by pretreatment with nialamide (Havlíček, 1967). Unilateral injections of dopamine (1—50 μg in 5 μl) into the rat striatum produced turning contralateral to the side of injection and an asymmetric posture which were potentiated by pretreatment with nialamide (Ungerstedt et al., 1969).

7. Inhibitors of Catechol-O-Methyl Transferase

a) Mechanism of Action

Whereas there are many selective potent inhibitors of MAO, there are none for COMT; consequently, study of its role in catecholamine metabolism has been retarded, A variety of compounds inhibit COMT *in vitro* including catechol, pyrogallol, 3,4-dihydroxyphenylacetamide, tropolone and their respective derivatives, L-DOPA and its amine derivatives and degradation products of adrenaline and noradrenaline, adnamine and noradnamine (Axelrod and Laroche, 1959; Bacq et al., 1959; Belleau and Burba, 1961; Crout, 1961; Carlsson et al., 1962; Ross and Haljasmaa, 1964a; Abbs et al., 1967) but few are effective *in vivo*; of these pyrogallol, 2,3,4-trihydroxyacetophenone and derivatives of 3,4-dihydroxyphenylacetamide are the most potent (Carlsson et al., 1963a; Carlsson, 1964; Ross and Haljasmaa, 1964b). With some compounds, e.g. tropolones, inhibition of peripheral COMT was greater than that of cerebral COMT (Ross and Haljasmaa, 1964b), possibly because of poor penetration to the brain. Side effects are common. Thus, some derivatives of 3,4-dihydroxyphenylacetamide inhibit catecholamine and 5-hydroxytryptamine synthesis (Carlsson et al., 1963a; Roos and Werdinius, 1963; Carlsson, 1964); tropolones inhibit dopamine β-hydroxylase *in vitro* (Goldstein et al., 1964a). Since pyrogallol is rapidly metabolized by COMT (Archer et al., 1960), repeated injections were necessary to maintain inhibition; these cause methaemoglobinaemia and paresis of hind limbs (Crout et al., 1961). In mice, pyrogallol and catechol produced convulsions unrelated to inhibition of COMT (Angel and Rogers, 1968). U-0521 (3,4-dihydroxy-2-methyl propiophenone), a competitive inhibitor of COMT (Giles and Miller, 1967a), produced drowsiness and sleep in rats and mice (Moffett et al., 1964). This was unlikely to be related to inhibition of COMT unless its methoxy derivatives, devoid of inhibitory activity *in vitro* but still producing sedation (Moffett et al., 1964), were demethylated *in vivo* (Giles and Miller, 1967b).

Brain catecholamines were not elevated in rats by repeated administration of pyrogallol, 50 mg/kg i.p., every 30 min for 18 hr (Crout et al., 1961) or daily for several weeks (MAÎTRE, 1966). Instead, catecholamines were slightly reduced (CROUT et al., 1961) due possibly to release or inhibition of synthesis. Surprisingly, pyrogallol (10 mg/kg) increased catecholamines in various regions of mouse and rat brain within 1 hr of intraperitoneal injection (IZQUIERDO et al., 1964). Cerebral catecholamines were decreased slightly in rabbits by intracarotid injection of pyrogallol, 50 mg/kg, but elevated by intracisternal injection of 20 mg/kg (MATSUOKA et al., 1962). Accumulation of cerebral dopamine and noradrenaline following intraperitoneal injection of DOPA or 3,4-dihydroxyphenylserine respectively, was increased after inhibition of COMT with α-ethoxydopacetamide or 2-(3,4-dihydroxyphenyl)-pentanoyl amide (CARLSSON, 1964). Tropolone, 40 mg/kg i.p. 2 hr and 30 min prior to intraperitoneal injection of C^{14}-DOPA enhanced accumulation of cerebral catecholamines (GOLDSTEIN, 1964). Tropolone-4-acetamide (25 mg/kg i.p.) markedly decreased formation of normetanephrine in rat brain without affecting cerebral noradrenaline (GLOWINSKI and AXELROD, 1965). Similarly, 2-(3,4-dihydroxyphenyl)-hexanoyl amide (500 mg/kg i.v.) reduced normetanephrine in rabbit brain to 10% of normal without affecting noradrenaline (HÄGGENDAL, 1963).

b) Behaviour

Pyrogallol and 3,4-dihydroxyphenylacetamide produced dose-dependent suppression of exploratory behaviour in mice (MERLO and IZQUIERDO, 1963); in rats, establishment of a conditioned reflex was slowed and its extinction enhanced (IZQUIERDO and MERLO, 1963; MERLO and IZQUIERDO, 1965). In rabbits, intracisternal injection of pyrogallol (20 mg/kg) produced hypotonia and ataxia and eventually abolished motor activity (MATSUOKA et al., 1962). α-Ethoxydopacetamide or 2-(3,4-dihydroxyphenyl)-pentanoyl amide potentiated locomotor activity following intraperitoneal injection of DOPA or 3,4-dihydroxyphenylserine in mice (CARLSSON, 1964). However, pyrogallol (100 mg/kg i.p.) did not affect response to intraventricular injection of noradrenaline in mice (CHAMBERS and ROBERTS, 1968).

XII. Antagonism

Experiments to determine whether central effects of catecholamines are reduced or abolished by selective antagonists active at peripheral α- or β-receptors for catecholamines provide a basis for ascertaining whether receptors mediating the central action of catecholamines are similar to those in the periphery. The pitfalls inherent in interpretation of such experiments are cogently assessed by NICKERSON and HOLLENBERG (1967).

1. Electrocortical Activity and Innate Behaviour

Central depressant effects in mice (reduced locomotor activity and muscle tone, slowed respiration) due to noradrenaline (2 μg intracisternally) were not obtained when phentolamine (2 μg intracisternally), an antagonist at α-receptors for catecholamines, was injected simultaneously with noradrenaline; antagonism was surmounted by larger doses of noradrenaline (BRITTAIN and HANDLEY, 1967). Propranolol, an antagonist at β-receptors for catecholamines, neither antagonized nor potentiated these central effects of catecholamines. Other evidence for central depressant effects of catecholamines being mediated via α-receptors for catecholamines derive from experiments with chickens (DEWHURST and MARLEY, 1965a, b). Thus behavioural and electrocortical sleep induced by intravenous ($\pm$)-α-methylnoradrenaline were prevented by prior treatment with large doses of phenoxybenzamine, but not propranolol, pronethalol, hyoscine or a histamine antagonist, chlorpheniramine; it proved difficult to antagonize the soporific effects of (—)-adrenaline or (—)-noradrenaline. However, the intense soporific effects of (—)-noradrenaline (0.05—0.075 μmole), (—)-isoprenaline (0.05—0.1 μmole) and (±)-α-methylnoradrenaline (0.01—0.2 μmole) given by micro-infusion (0.05 μl over 4 min) into the hypothalamus of young chickens were prevented or substantially reduced by the prior intravenous injection of phenoxybenzamine or by its micro-infusion into the hypothalamus (MARLEY and STEPHENSON, 1968a, 1969, 1970).

It is readily conceivable that in some species, the central depressant effects of catecholamines are mediated via β-receptors or by an action on both α- and β-receptors. That the issue is far from solved is clear from results of GRUNDEN (1969) who found that rank order potency of catecholamines given intraventricularly to rats suggested an action on β-receptors, in that (±)-isoprenaline was more active than (—)-adrenaline which in turn was more potent than (±)-noradrenaline. However, pretreatment with either phenoxybenzamine or propranolol *potentiated* the central actions of these amines.

GOLDSTEIN and MUÑOZ (1961) postulated, on the basis of the effect of catecholamines on electrocortical activity after administration of pharmacological antagonists, that there were separate receptors in the brain mediating their "excitant" and "depressant" actions. The reactivity of animals, in this case cats, would depend on the degree of "activation" of these receptors. Should receptors mediating the central depressant effects of the amines be activated, any activation of "excitant" receptors by these amines would be counteracted and no change in electrocortical patterns ensue. If receptors mediating central depressant effects of the amines were occupied, as after dichloroisoprenaline, no counteraction would be possible, and an excitant effect i.e. electrocortical alerting would be obtained. Conversely, when "excitant" receptors were occupied, activation of "depressant" receptors would lead to electrocortical sleep, as for example when isoprenaline or a large dose of adrenaline was given after phenoxybenzamine. This interpretation implies that catecholamines normally have dual actions on central receptors or actions on two types of receptors, but with a predominant effect on one or other group. It is also compatible with their actions in the periphery, where amines such as noradrenaline (KARIM, 1964) and many other sympathomimetic amines (BLACKWELL and MARLEY, 1967) previously thought to act entirely at α-receptors for catecholamines have been found to activate β-receptors, an action that becomes very conspicuous when α-receptors are blocked. There are objections to these interpretations of GOLDSTEIN and MUÑOZ, as they themselves recognized. Thus, electrocortical alerting was obtained with dichloroisoprenaline, and this could be interpreted as an activation of "excitant" receptors and not, as they assumed, a suppression of the action of hypothetical "depressant" receptors. Electrocortical alerting evoked by adrenaline in a cat in which it was previously ineffective, but in the meantime dichloroisoprenaline had been given, could be attributed to summation of the "excitant" actions of adrenaline and dichloroisoprenaline rather than to blockade of the "depressant" effects of adrenaline.

Support for GOLDSTEIN and MUÑOZ's ideas derive from work of MATSUDA (1968). The conclusions again apply solely to electrocortical activity since experiments were made within 2 hr of implantation of a cannula into the lateral ventricle of rabbits. MATSUDA noted that the large amplitude slow frequency electrocortical potentials, normally associated with sleep and evoked by intraventricular adrenaline (200 μg), were not obtained when noradrenaline was given 2 hr after phenoxybenzamine or phentolamine (2.0 mg intraventricularly); instead, electrocortical alerting occurred. In contrast, following the same dose of intraventricular adrenaline given 90 min after β-receptor antagonists, dichloroisoprenaline, propranolol or pronethalol (4.0 mg intraventricularly), the large amplitude slow frequency electrocortical potentials appeared unimpaired.

2. Learnt Behaviour

Suppressant effects of (—)-adrenaline on key-pecking in pigeons were almost completely annulled by pretreating the birds with phenoxybenzamine (1 mg daily for at least 3 days), doses which did not modify behaviour (WURTMAN et al., 1959). As much as 300 μg (—)-adrenaline, given intramuscularly, now caused less reduction in pecking than did 30 μg in the absence of phenoxybenzamine. The almost ten-fold shift in dose-response slope accords with GADDUM's (1961) notion that high values for the dose-ratio (ratio by which the dose is increased to reproduce the original effects) are seldom seen in experiments on the central nervous system. Phentolamine also antagonized suppressant effects of (—)-adrenaline on pecking (DEWS, 1962); in contrast, the effects of adrenaline were enhanced by dichloroisoprenaline. In chickens, and as shown in Fig. 5, suppressant effects of ($\pm$)-a-methylnoradrenaline on key-pecking were also antagonized by pretreatment with phenoxybenzamine and again there was a ten-fold shift in dose-response slope; antagonism was surmounted by increasing the dose of agonist (MARLEY and MORSE, 1967). The effects of ($\pm$)-a-methylnoradrenaline were unaffected or enhanced by chlorpromazine, by pronethalol and by a tryptamine antagonist, methysergide.

3. Body Temperature

One of the drawbacks of using catecholamine antagonists is that they often lower temperature. In the studies discussed below, these difficulties have been allowed for so far as possible. Noradrenaline (5 μg) injected into the cerebral ventricles of mice lowered oesophageal temperature almost 3°C with recovery after about 5 hr. The same dose of noradrenaline given together with phentolamine (2 μg) into the ventricles lowered temperature less than 1°C with recovery after about 3 hr (BRITTAIN and HANDLEY, 1967), a smaller effect on temperature than produced by phentolamine alone; the behavioural effects of noradrenaline were simultaneously antagonized. Antagonism was surmounted with larger doses of noradrenaline. Propranolol, in intraventricular doses which did not affect body temperature, neither antagonized nor potentiated the effects of intraventricular noradrenaline.

Given intravenously, (—)- or ($\pm$)-a-methylnoradrenaline and other catecholamines lowered temperature and oxygen consumption in chicks (ALLEN and MARLEY, 1967). For example, ($\pm$)-a-methylnoradrenaline (10 μmole/kg i.v.) lowered mediastinal temperature 3.9°C in a 13-day chick with recovery after about 3 hr; this dose produced deep sleep with loss of electromyographic activity from the neck muscles. Phenoxybenzamine (100 μmole/kg i.p.) was then given and the chick re-tested after 3 days. ($\pm$)-a-Methylnoradrenaline (10 μmole/kg i.v.) now elicited a fall of 1.0°C with recovery in 2 hr; a subsequent dose of 20 μmole/kg was ineffective. The soporific effects of a-methylnoradrenaline were also antagonized. The large dose of phenoxybenzamine used had been previously found necessary for antagonism of effects of catecholamines on innate and learnt behaviours. The actions of the β-halo-alkylamines may be atypical in fowls, for HARVEY and NICKERSON (1951) observed that surprisingly large doses of dibenamine were required to abolish the pressor action of noradrenaline.

Catecholamines micro-infused into the hypothalamus of young chicks at thermoneutral environments, apart from producing sleep, also lowered temperature (Marley and Stephenson, 1968a, 1969). For example, (—)-noradrenaline (0.05—0.75 μmole) lowered temperature 2.5°—6°C and reduced oxygen consumption by up to 24% with recovery after 3—4 hr; (±)-α-methylnoradrenaline (0.01—0.2 μmole) lowered temperature 1.1°—8.0°C with 21—52% diminution of oxygen consumption, recovery occurring after 3—8 hr; (—)-isoprenaline (0.5 to 0.1 μmole) lowered temperature 1.7°—5°C with recovery after 5—6 hr; dopamine (0.1 μmole), after pretreating chicks with mebanazine, lowered temperature 3°C for 5—6 hr. These effects together with those on behaviour were abolished or reduced by pretreatment with intravenous phenoxybenzamine, but not propranolol. Unexpectedly, propranolol as well as phenoxybenzamine micro-infused into the hypothalamus prevented the effects on temperature of noradrenaline given 2 hr later; in contrast, phenoxybenzamine, but not propranolol prevented the behavioural effects (Marley and Stephenson, 1970).

In cats, intraventricular adrenaline or noradrenaline (50 or 100 μg), which induced a fall in rectal temperature, no longer had this effect after intraventricular ergotamine (100 μg) (Banerjee et al., 1968). Instead, the catecholamines elicited shivering lasting 10—30 min which began almost immediately after the injection and was associated with an elevation in temperature of 0.1°—0.3°C. This short-lasting temperature "reversal" occurred only with the first injection of adrenaline or noradrenaline, subsequent doses having no effect. Although ergotamine — considered to be a classical α-receptor blocking agent in peripheral tissues — prevented the hypothermic effects of adrenaline and noradrenaline, it was construed that "the widely accepted concept of α- and β-receptors developed for the peripheral actions of catecholamines may not extend to the hypothalamus and possibly also not to other central sites on which catecholamines act".

4. Food and Water Intake

Solid noradrenaline bitartrate (1—5 μg) applied to the hypothalamic ventromedial nuclei via a stereotactically implanted cannula, induced vigorous and prolonged eating in food-satiated rats, as did adrenaline. These effects were reduced in a dose-dependent manner by ethoxybutamoxane (1.0, 2.5 and 5.0 mg/kg i.p.) given 1 hr prior to noradrenaline; drinking in water-satiated rats induced by carbachol positioned stereotactically into the hypothalamus was not significantly altered (Grossman, 1962b). Conversely, intraperitoneal doses of atropine that antagonized those of carbachol on drinking did not significantly alter the effects of noradrenaline on eating. Phenoxybenzamine (1 μg in 1 μl) and phentolamine (0.04 μmol in 1 μl) prevented the eating response to (—)-noradrenaline injected 1 hr later via the same hypothalamic cannula in rats with access to food and water, whereas propranolol (6.75 μg in 1 μl and 0.04—0.12 μmol in 1 μl) did not (Booth, 1968; Slangen and Miller, 1969). Injections of (—)-isoprenaline (0.15 μmol in 1 μl) and (—)-adrenaline (0.1 μmol in 1 μl) into the posterior part of the anterior hypothalamus of food-deprived rats reduced eating; (—)-noradrenaline (0.02 μmol in 1 μl) increased eating (Leibowitz, 1970). Propranolol (0.14 μmol in 1 μl) given via the same hypothalamic cannula 5 min previously, prevented this effect of isoprenaline and reversed that of adrenaline; phentolamine (0.07 μmol in 1 μl) potentiated the effects of isoprenaline and adrenaline. These results suggest the presence, in the rat hypothalamus, of an α-adrenoceptive "hunger" system which mediates eating and a β-adrenoceptive "satiety" system which suppresses eating (Leibowitz, 1970).

5. Blood Pressure

An action on α-receptors in the central nervous system was implied from the work of KANEKO et al., 1960, using anaesthetized dogs. Thus the lowered blood pressure, bradycardia and diminished pressor effects to carotid occlusion, induced by intraventricular noradrenaline (100 μg), were temporarily reversed by phentolamine (5 mg) injected intraventricularly. β-Receptors would also appear to be present (GAGNON and MELVILLE, 1967), since prior intraventricular injection of pronethalol (300 μg) or propranolol (30 μg) to anaesthetized cats, significantly diminished the hypotension and tachycardia evoked by intraventricular isoprenaline (15 μg); in contrast, phenoxybenzamine (2 mg) failed to attenuate the effects of isoprenaline. GAGNON and MELVILLE (1969) later investigated the effects of intraventricular phentolamine or pronethalol on cardiovascular effects of noradrenaline injected intraventricularly. Although they concluded there were α-and β-receptors for catecholamines in the central nervous system, unfortunately the cats had been pretreated with reserpine, imipramine or chlorpromazine which complicated interpretation as intraventricular noradrenaline now evoked a rise rather than a fall in blood pressure.

The balance of evidence then favours the presence of α-receptors in the nervous system, receptors mediating the central effects of catecholamines. The evidence is far from decisive. The position has been paraphrased by NICKERSON and HOLLENBERG (1967). "Although many "suggestive" observations have been reported, each must be assessed separately. The many apparently direct effects of α-adrenergic blocking agents on the central nervous system make it hazardous to lump these very diverse observations together under the "where there is smoke there must be fire" philosophy."

XIII. Structure-Activity Studies

There is a dearth of information in this field. Ideally, the drugs to be compared should be delivered directly to an aggregate of neurones which influence a single behavioural and/or physiological variable and to the extent that a change can be recorded and quantitated. Outside the context of iontophoretic application of drugs, this ideal has remotely been achieved. For the most part, catecholamines have been given by routes (intravenous, intraperitoneal) not necessarily ensuring entry to the brain, or should entry occur, do not guarantee equimolar distribution at receptor sites. The intraventricular route is more satisfactory but because of the vast populations of neurones affected, both excitatory and inhibitory mechanisms may be activated, so vitiating conclusions about drug structure and potency. Micro-infusion to some selected site in the brain is promising but also has disadvantages, not the least of which is neuronal damage by repeated infusions.

1. Innate Behaviour and Cerebral Electrical Activity

a) Intracisternal Injection

An observation never given the prominence it merits is that of LEIMDORFER (1950) who noted that whereas noradrenaline, isoprenaline, butanephrine and to a lesser extent oxedrine and paredrine injected intracisternally elicited sopor; by contrast amphetamine, phenylpropanolamine, ephedrine, phenylephrine and tuaminoheptane evoked excitement. Unfortunately, relative potencies of these amines were not indicated although the long persistence of catecholamines in cerebrospinal fluid was mentioned, and the different qualitative effects of the amines on the central nervous system stressed for the first time. Sympathomimetic amines have been divided into two main groups for their peripheral actions, those of the directly-acting catecholamines and those of the amphetamine-like amines which act indirectly through noradrenaline release (BURN and RAND, 1958). Of the amines tested by LEIMDORFER, adrenaline, noradrenaline, isoprenaline and butanephrine would fall into the predominantly directly-acting group, whereas amphetamine, phenylpropanolamine, ephedrine and tuaminoheptane would be classified as predominantly indirectly-acting. This division of the amines into two groups for their central effect no doubt reflects a fundamental difference in mode of action, although not necessarily the same as that underlying their peripheral effects.

b) Intraventricular and Intracerebral Injections

Given intraventricularly, adrenaline has been noted as more potent in eliciting sopor than noradrenaline (TRACZYK, 1964). (±)-Isoprenaline, (—)-adrenaline and (—)-phenylephrine, in descending order of potency, reduced locomotor activity when given into the 3rd cerebral ventricle of rats; phenylethylamine, lacking hydroxyl groups on the benzene ring and aliphatic side-chain, produced excitement (GRUNDEN, 1969). (—)-Adrenaline, (—)-noradrenaline, (—)-a-methylnoradrenaline or (—)-isoprenaline injected into the 3rd cerebral ventricle of adult fowls elicited behavioural and electrocortical sleep, their effects differing in duration rather than intensity. With equimolar doses (0.5 μmole), (—)-a-methylnoradrenaline had the longest (>6 hr) and (—)-noradrenaline the shortest (<2 hr) duration of effect; dexamphetamine elicited mild excitement (GRUNDEN and MARLEY, 1970). Again duration rather than intensity of effect was the distinguishing criterion for assessing action of catecholamines micro-infused into the hypothalamus of young chickens. Equimolar doses of (—)-a-methylnoradrenaline, (—)-isoprenaline and (—)-noradrenaline, in diminishing order for duration of effect, evoked behavioural and electrocortical sleep (MARLEY and STEPHENSON, 1970). Dopamine was normally inactivated too rapidly to have effect, for it was only when the chick had been pretreated with an amine oxidase inhibitor that it produced sleep. A number of catecholamines and congeners given by microinjection via an implanted cannula into the lateral hypothalamus were tested for their effects on eating in rats (BOOTH, 1968). There was stereospecificity, (—)-noradrenaline being ten times more active than the dextro-isomer. (—)-Adrenaline was equiactive with (—)-noradrenaline; the catecholamines, (±)-isoprenaline and dopamine were much less potent than (—)-noradrenaline; the phenolic amine (—)-phenylephrine and the (±)-isomers of the metabolites, metanephrine and normetanephrine had small or nil effects. These results in rats and fowls are conflicting and do not permit conclusions about structure-activity relations of catecholamines. They probably reflect rate of degradation of catecholamines by enzymes rather than activity at receptors, a fault probably of most *in vivo* systems.

c) Intravenous Injection

CLYMER and SEIFTER (1947) used young chicks for screening compounds with amphetamine-like properties since these evoked excitement and characteristic postural changes. The drugs were given subcutaneously in very large doses. Catecholamines were also tested and noted to induce drowsiness. A much larger series of compounds given intravenously was tested on innate behaviour, including cheeping, and electrocortical activity in young chickens (KEY and MARLEY, 1962; DEWHURST and MARLEY, 1965a, b). Insomuch as intravenous noradrenaline passes into the brain of chicks (SPOONER et al., 1966) and identical effects to those obtained on intravenous injection of catecholamines were elicited with 1/200th—1/100th the intravenous dose but by micro-infusion into the brain (MARLEY and STEPHENSON, 1968a, 1969), the results are relevant. The effect of chemical substitution of the phenylethylamine molecule was tested in terms of the drug's soporific potency. Since relative potencies of the amines given intravenously differed from those obtained by micro-infusion into the hypothalamus — presumably because of differences in uptake into the brain and in rate of enzymic degradation, the effects of substitution will be considered only in general terms. Paradoxically, interpretation was easier than when catecholamines were given intraventricularly or into the hypothalamus.

N-Methylation of noradrenaline to form adrenaline increased soporific potency, whereas a larger substituent, isopropyl as in isoprenaline, diminished activity. N-Methylation in the absence of the hydroxyl on the β-carbon atom had a reverse effect since dopamine was considerably more potent than epinine. Substituents on the α-carbon atom also reduced potency. For example, α-methylnoradrenaline was five times less active than noradrenaline in terms of threshold dose but its effect was more prolonged. α-Ethylnoradrenaline was 1/20th as active as noradrenaline and α-methylation of dopamine rendered it inactive. The importance of a β-hydroxyl was evident from the greater potency of adrenaline and noradrenaline compared to epinine and dopamine respectively; the latter two lack the β-hydroxyl. Thus (—)-adrenaline was 400 times more active than epinine on cheeping and the electrocorticogram. (—)-Noradrenaline was six times more potent than dopamine on cheeping and twenty times more active on the electrocorticogram. Stereospecificity was important, (—)-noradrenaline being much more active than its dextro-isomer. Similarly, racemic α-methylnoradrenaline (with respect to the β-carbon atom) was forty times as potent as the dextro-form. Absence of the side-chain, as in catechol or pyrogallol, deprived the molecule of soporific activity. Ring substitution or modification altered potency. Thus a phenolic amine, phenylephrine, which differs from adrenaline only by lack of a hydroxyl on the 4-position in the ring was considerably less potent; oxedrine which lacks the hydroxyl in the 3-position was less active than phenylephrine. Other phenolic amines with a hydroxyl group substituted in the 3- or 4-position on the ring (metatyramine and tyramine) were much less potent than dopamine with hydroxyl groups in the 3- and 4-positions. Amines with methoxy- (mescaline, metanephrine) or chloro- substituents (dichloroisoprenaline) on the ring had less central depressant activity than the parent catecholamine.

It would appear that the same alterations in chemical structure which influence potency of the amines on peripheral receptors in mammals, determined activity in the chick's central nervous system. For example, central depressant potency was reduced in molecules with alkyl substituents on the terminal nitrogen or on the α-carbon atom, or in the absence of the β-hydroxyl group. Similar findings for substitution on the terminal nitrogen atom or the α-carbon atom applied for central excitant amines (DEWHURST and MARLEY, 1965a, b). Since the same conclusions apply for excitant amines, which readily penetrate to the nervous system, this would mitigate against a primary peripheral and secondary central action to account for the effects of catecholamines. Optical activity also determined potency, the laevo- being more active than the dextro-isomer for central depressant activity whereas the reverse applied for excitant properties. The aliphatic side-chain was important for central depressant activity and molecules without the side-chain but possessing hydroxyls on the ring structure lacked this property. Excitant amines also had an aliphatic side-chain attached to one of a number of lipophilic radicals which were aromatic (phenyl, indolyl), alicyclic (cyclopentyl), mixed (tetrahydronaphthyl), or straight chain aliphatic (tuaminoheptane). It was tentatively concluded that these amines bond primarily at the cationic head and secondarily at the planar ring structure, presumably through VAN DER WAAL's forces. Since a hydroxyl on the β-carbon atom increased central depressant potency, hydrogen bonding may also occur through this substituent.

LEIMDORFER (1950) on the basis of findings with sympathomimetic amines injected intracisternally in dogs, suggested that with molecules of the phenylethylamine structure, the sedative effects were related to the catechol moiety, and the excitant effects to the aliphatic portion. This may be an oversimplification. Results with young chickens showed that both central depressants and excitants possessed an aliphatic component. Where a ring structure was present and had electronegative substituents (OH, CH_3O, Cl) so that electrostatic pairing was possible, then the compound was a central depressant; those having none, or electropositive substituents (CH_3) had excitant properties. The phenolic groups of sympathomimetic amines are ionized little, if at all, at physiological pH (LEWIS, 1954). However, the difference in effects between central depressants, α-methylnoradrenaline or α-methyladrenaline, and the central excitants, amphetamine or N-methylamphetamine, which are otherwise structurally identical but lack the phenolic hydroxyls, could be best accounted for by the hydroxyls on the ring structure modifying electronic properties of the molecule.

2. Learnt Behaviour

The literature is scanty and the experiments alluded to were not intended to elucidate structure-activity relations. Adrenaline was more potent than noradrenaline in suppressing respondent conditioning in cats (SHARPLESS, 1959) or operant conditioned key-pecking in pigeons (WURTMAN et al., 1959). In cats, there was greater suppression of conditioned avoidance responding with noradrenaline than with adrenaline and less still with dopamine (WADA et al., 1963).

3. Temperature

Temperature effects of catecholamines are difficult to assess in terms of chemical structure, partly because of the variation in response between species, partly because one dose of an amine may lower temperature whereas another of the same amine raises it and partly because of the marked influence of environmental temperature on response, a factor not allowed for in many experiments. For these reasons, consideration is not attempted.

XIV. Effects of Catecholamines on Spinal Cord Reflexes

The effects of drugs on spinal cord reflexes are not difficult to study but likewise are not easy to interpret. It is conceivable, for example, that the effects of a drug on blood flow to the spinal cord are sufficiently considerable to alter reflexes, yet the drug may have little or no direct action on spinal cord neurones. The drug may not directly affect a reflex arc but act on afferent neurones entering the spinal cord at a different level or even the brain, so modifying reflex activity. Since anaesthesia generally reduces spinal cord reflex activity and reduces or even abolishes effects of drugs on spinal cord reflexes, it is difficult to compare results in such animals with those in spinal cats, in which ipsilateral flexor reflexes are readily elicited, or those in decerebrate cats which allow easy evocation of contralateral extensor reflexes. These influences may explain some of the discrepancies between results detailed below.

1. Effects of Catecholamines

a) Extensor Reflexes

Large intravenous doses of adrenaline (>50 μg/kg) depressed amplitude of the patellar reflex (an ipsilateral monosynaptic reflex) independently of blood pressure changes in cats anaesthetized with chloralose, pentobarbitone or urethane (SCHWEITZER and WRIGHT, 1937; SIGG et al., 1955; TEN CATE et al., 1959; McLENNAN, 1961); depression was usually preceded by brief facilitation. Occasionally a "triphasic response" was seen, a short initial depression, then enhancement lasting several minutes followed by prolonged depression (SCHWEITZER and WRIGHT, 1937). Noradrenaline was less potent than adrenaline and dopamine was almost inactive; after topical administration to the spinal cord as opposed to intravenous injection, the order of potency was reversed (McLENNAN, 1961). In contrast, smaller doses of adrenaline (5—20 μg i.v.) increased amplitude of the patellar reflex in cats lightly anaesthetized with pentobarbitone (SIGG et al., 1955); deep anaesthesia or larger doses of adrenaline depressed the reflex. In vagotomized spinal cats, adrenaline (10—20 μg/kg i.v.) produced a "triphasic response" on the patellar reflex followed by a second period of facilitation superimposed on occasions by brief periods of tonic extension and clonus (KISSEL and DOMINO, 1959a); infrequently, adrenaline only depressed reflex amplitude. Surprisingly, in cats anaesthetized with pentobarbitone, adrenaline-induced facilitation of the patellar reflex was abolished by decerebration rostral to the tentorium or by spinal transection (SIGG et al., 1955). In chloralosed spinal dogs with separately perfused spinal cord and hind legs, adrenaline (1 mg i.v. or >100 μg i.a. to the spinal cord) increased amplitude of the patellar reflex (BÜLBRING and BURN, 1941). Intra-arterial injection of adrenaline to the spinal cord of acute and chronic spinal cats, consistently increased the amplitude of monosynaptic reflex potentials elicited by peripheral nerve stimulation (WILSON, 1956; BERNHARD and SKOGLUND, 1953).

The effects of catecholamines on a polysynaptic crossed extensor reflex varied. This reflex was enhanced by intravenous infusion of (—)-adrenaline (2 μg/kg/min) or (—)-noradrenaline (10 μg/kg/min) in chronic spinal dogs (MARTIN and EADES, 1967). In acute spinal cats, adrenaline (10—20 μg/kg i.v.) did not affect a crossed extensor reflex, elicited by electrical stimulation of the contralateral sciatic nerve, except when elicited during the second period of patellar reflex facilitation, when it increased (KISSEL and DOMINO, 1959a). (—)-Methylnoradrenaline (0.025 to 0.1 μmole i.v.) produced a dose-dependent reduction in amplitude of this reflex in acute spinal chicks (Fig. 14, MARLEY and STEPHENSON, unpublished observations); noradrenaline (2 μg i.v.) was ineffective in chloralosed spinal chicks (BOWMAN et al., 1964).

b) Flexor Reflexes

A polysynaptic ipsilateral flexor reflex was facilitated in chronic spinal dogs by intravenous infusion of (—)-adrenaline, 2 μg/kg/min or (—)-noradrenaline, 10 μg/kg/min (MARTIN and EADES, 1967). Close intra-arterial injections of adrenaline (5—40 μg/kg) to the spinal cord of acute and chronic spinal cats, produced variable effects on monosynaptic and polysynaptic spinal flexor reflexes (WILSON, 1956); increases, decreases, decreases preceded by transient increases and instances without obvious change, were noted. In acute spinal cats, adrenaline and noradrenaline (10—15 μg i.a.) frequently diminished reflex amplitude (BERNHARD and SKOGLUND, 1953); (—)-noradrenaline (5 μg/kg i.v.) was ineffective (MARLEY and VANE, 1967).

Reciprocal effects of adrenaline on extensor and flexor reflexes evoked by medullary stimulation in decerebrate cats were observed by BÜLBRING et al. (1948). Adrenaline, and its metabolites attenuated reciprocal inhibition of the

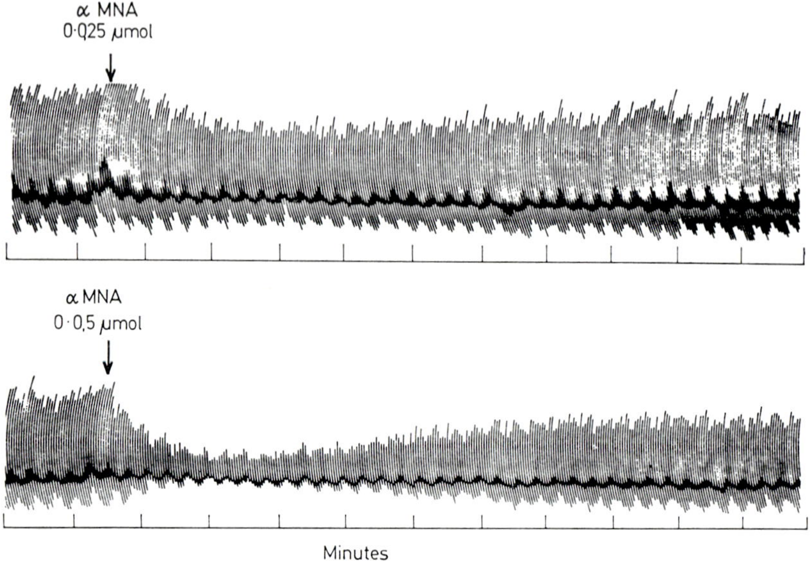

Fig. 14. Crossed extensor reflex in a spinal chick (90 g). (—)-a-Methylnoradrenaline (aMNA 0.025—0.05 μmole/100 g i.v.) produced a dose-dependent reduction of twitch height. Larger doses (not shown in Fig. 1) temporarily abolished the reflex. (MARLEY, E. and STEPHENSON, J.D., unpublished results)

patellar reflex and increased contralateral inhibition of the ipsilateral flexor reflex in anaesthetized cats (ARUSHANYAN and BELOZERTSER, 1964). Adrenaline increased the ipsilateral flexor withdrawal reflex and patellar reflex in chronic spinal monkeys (JACOBSEN and KENNARD, 1933).

In spinal cats anaesthetized with pentobarbitone, intra-arterial injections of adrenaline or noradrenaline (5—100 μg) to the spinal cord, lacked effect on amplitude of evoked monosynaptic reflex potentials or on spinal interneurones of the Renshaw type (CURTIS et al., 1957). In contrast, in decerebrate, curarized cats, intravenous or intra-arterial injections of noradrenaline (1—3 μg/kg) increased spontaneous firing rate of spinal interneurones and their response to single afferent volleys (SKOGLUND, 1961).

Effects of catecholamines on reflexes were thought not to be secondary to vascular changes for several reasons: a) effects of adrenaline on the patellar reflex were similar with and without blood pressure stabilization (KISSEL and DOMINO, 1957, 1959a), b) the patellar reflex was unaffected when blood pressure was raised artificially (KISSEL and DOMINO, 1959a) or reflexly by carotid occlusion (SCHWEITZER and WRIGHT, 1937), c) there was no consistent relation between pressor effects of catecholamines and their activity on reflexes, d) adrenaline decreased venous blood flow from the spinal cord of the dog despite an elevated blood pressure (BÜLBRING and BURN, 1941). In rabbits, the effects of intravenous infusions of adrenaline on spinal cord vasculature were dose-dependent, 1—2 μg/kg/min producing vasoconstriction and 10 μg/kg/min, vasodilatation (FIELD et al., 1951). After intra-arterial injection of adrenaline to the spinal cord, regional changes in blood flow within the spinal cord occurred without changes in systemic blood pressure (SKOGLUND, 1961). e) If vasoconstriction occurred then polysynaptic pathways should be affected before monosynaptic pathways since they are more susceptible to hypoxia (KISSEL and DOMINO, 1959b); monosynaptic pathways were more sensitive to adrenaline (KISSEL and DOMINO, 1959a). However, effects of noradrenaline on fusiform neurones in decerebrate cats were considered to be due to an increase in spinal cord blood flow, since effects were only occasionally observed when arterial blood pressure was above a critical level (VOORHOEVE, 1960).

2. Reserpine

Effects of reserpine were inconsistent. Reserpine (5 mg/kg i.v., dissolved in a mixture of benzyl alcohol, citric acid, propylene glycol and water) increased amplitudes of the patellar reflex and of evoked monosynaptic potentials in spinal cats (SCHNEIDER et al., 1955); the solvent produced some facilitation. In contrast, reserpine (10 mg/kg i.v.) lacked effect on amplitude of evoked monosynaptic and polysynaptic potentials in acute spinal cats, but reduced post-tetanic potentiation potentials (ESPLIN and HEATON, 1957). In chronic spinal dogs, whereas a single injection of reserpine (2 mg/kg i.v.) increased amplitude of the patellar reflex, it was decreased by chronic reserpine treatment (MARTIN and EADES, 1967). Reserpine prevented convulsive motor activity following decapitation of rats (HERMAN and BARNES, 1967).

3. Inhibitors of Monoamine Oxidase

Pretreatment with β-phenylethylhydrazine potentiated depressant actions on spinal cord reflexes of dopamine and adrenaline in cats anaesthetized with chloralose or urethane (MCLENNAN, 1961). Amplitude of monosynaptic potentials were increased in spinal decorticate cats by pargyline, nialamide, tranylcypromine and α-ethyltryptamine; polysynaptic potentials were unaffected (ANDERSON et al., 1967). Facilitation was probably related to the 70% increase in 5-hydroxytryptamine content of the spinal cord since it was prevented by methysergide (1 mg/kg i.v.) but not phenoxybenzamine (10 mg/kg i.v.).

4. Catecholamine Antagonists

Phenoxybenzamine (4—5 mg/kg i.v.) prevented facilitation of a polysynaptic flexor reflex in chronic spinal dogs by (—)-adrenaline (MARTIN and EADES, 1967) but not facilitation of the patellar reflex by noradrenaline or adrenaline in vagotomized spinal cats (KISSEL and DOMINO, 1957, 1959a). Phenoxybenzamine (15 mg/kg i.v.) but not dichloroisoprenaline (10 mg/kg i.v.) prevented depression of the amplitude of patellar reflex by an intravenous injection of adrenaline; dichloroisoprenaline, but not phenoxybenzamine, prevented depression of the reflex by dopamine applied directly to the cord (MCLENNAN, 1961). Phenoxybenzamine prevented convulsive motor activity in rats following decapitation (HERMAN and BARNES, 1967). Reflex inhibition of spinal cord reflexes produced by electrical stimulation of the reticular formation was prevented by intravenous infusion of phenoxybenzamine, 0.025 mg/min (CRAMMER et al., 1959) or by intravenous injection of dichloroisoprenaline (MCLENNAN, 1961); intravenous injection of phenoxybenzamine (20 mg/kg) was ineffective (MCLENNAN, 1961).

5. Monoamine Precursor

DOPA facilitated a flexor reflex evoked by pinching the skin of a spinal cat (CARLSSON et al., 1963b). L-DOPA (5—30 mg/kg i.v.) increased amplitude of monosynaptic potentials evoked by stimulation of a dorsal root or peripheral nerve and depressed polysynaptic activity in spinal decorticate cats (Baker and Anderson, 1965, 1970a); larger doses (67—100 mg/kg i.v.) increased polysynaptic activity (Andén et al., 1966a). These effects were assumed to be due to the formation from DOPA of noradrenaline (Andén et al., 1966b) and/or dopamine (Baker and Anderson, 1970a) and were prevented by α-adrenoceptor blockade (Andén et al., 1966b; Baker and Anderson, 1970b). The mode of action of large doses of DOPA has been extensively studied using electrophysiological techniques (Andén et al., 1966a, 1966b, 1966c; Jankowska et al., 1966, 1967a, 1967b).

XV. Conclusions

The future for research into catecholamines and the central nervous system is rosy, if indeed not more colourful. A plea ought to be entertained that alongside anticipated leaps forward some of the ground already examined would repay re-scrutiny. This is particularly necessary in the realms of behaviour and temperature regulation, where, in the one, there is ambiguity in descriptive terms and in the other there is late realization of the considerable influence of environmental temperature. With species where catecholamines have biphasic effects on temperature, in addition to excluding environmental factors as causal, the use of antagonists at α- or β-receptors could clarify whether these effects depend on actions mediated via α- or β-receptors or both. Structure activity relations deduced from systematically administered amines seem doomed to constitute heresay evidence, in contrast to true testimony derived from iontophoretic studies. Perhaps the most promising candidate for investment resides in investigations linking catecholamine effects with their metabolic turnover in the brain. In conclusion, the theme "Catecholamines and the Central Nervous System", so long a simulacrum, has been at least partly divested of its mystery.

Acknowledgements: We should like to acknowledge indebtedness to authors, journals and publishers for kind permission to reproduce Figs. 1, 2, 4—6, 8—13.

The manuscript was prepared under the auspices of grants from the Bethlem Royal and Maudsley Hospitals Research Fund and the Medical Research Council.

References

Abbs, E.T., Broadley, K.J., Roberts, D.J.: Inhibition of catechol-O-methyl transferase by some acid degradation products of adrenaline and noradrenaline. Biochem. Pharmacol. **16**, 279—282 (1967).

Abuzzahab, F.S.: Dopa induced changes in brain norepinephrine in the newly hatched chick. Fed. Proc. **25**, 451 (1966).

Aigner, A., Hornykiewicz, O., Lisch, H.-J., Springer, A.: Beeinflussung der Gehirn-Katecholamine, der Spontanaktivität und der L-DOPA-Hyperactivität durch Diäthyldithiocarbamat. Med. Pharmacol. exp. **17**, 576—585 (1967).

Alberici, M., Rodriguez de Lores Arnaiz, G., de Robertis, E.: Catechol-O-methyltransferase in nerve endings of rat brain. Life Sci. **4**, 1951—1960 (1965).

Albert, A.: *Selective Toxicity*, 2nd. ed. p. 196. London: Methuen 1960.

Allen, D.J., Garg, K.N., Marley, E.: Mode of action of α-methylnoradrenaline on temperature and oxygen consumption in young chickens. Brit. J. Pharmacol. **38**, 667—687 (1970).

— Marley, E.: Actions of amines on temperature in the chicken. J. Physiol. (Lond.) **183**, 61—62P (1966).

— — Effect of sympathomimetic and allied amines on temperature and oxygen consumption. Brit. J. Pharmacol. **31**, 290—312 (1967).

Amin, A.N., Crawford, T.B.B., Gaddum, J.H.: The distribution of substance P and 5-hydroxytryptamine in the central nervous system of the dog. J. Physiol. (Lond.) **126**, 598—618 (1954).

Anand, B.K.: Nervous regulation of food intake. Physiol. Rev. **41**, 677—708 (1961).

ANAND, B.K., BROBECK, J.R.: Localization of a "feeding centre" in the hypothalamus of the rat. Proc. Soc. exp. Biol. (N.Y.) **77**, 323—324 (1951).

— DUA, S.: Hypothalamic control over water consumption in the rat. Indian J. med. Res. **46**, 426—430 (1958).

ANDÉN, N.-E.: On the mechanism of noradrenaline depletion by α-methyl metatyrosine and metaraminol. Acta pharmacol. (Kbh.) **21**, 260—271 (1964).

— JUKES, M.G.M., LUNDBERG, A.: The effect of DOPA on the spinal cord. 2. A pharmacological analysis. Acta physiol. scand. **67**, 387—397 (1966b).

— — — VYKLICKÝ, L.: The effect of DOPA on the spinal cord. 1. Influence on transmission from primary afferents. Acta physiol. scand. **67**, 373—386 (1966a).

— — — — The effect of DOPA on the spinal cord. 3. Depolarization evoked in the central terminals of ipsilateral Ia afferents by volleys in the flexor reflex afferents. Acta physiol. scand. **68**, 322—336 (1966c).

— MAGNUSSON, T.: Functional significance of noradrenaline depletion by α-methyl metatyrosine, metaraminol and dextro-adrenaline. In: "Proceedings of the 2nd International Pharmacological Meeting", vol. 3. Pharmacology of cholinergic and adrenergic transmission, pp. 319—328. Eds. G.B. KOELLE, W.W. DOUGLAS and A. CARLSSON. Oxford: Pergamon Press; Praha, Czechoslovak Medical Press 1963.

— ROOS, B.E., WERDINIUS, B.: On the occurrence of homovanillic acid in brain and cerebrospinal fluid and its determination by a fluorimetric method. Life Sci. **2**, 448—458 (1963).

— — — Effects of chlorpromazine, haloperidol and reserpine on the levels of phenolic acids in rabbit corpus striatum. Life Sci. **3**, 149—158 (1964).

ANDERSEN, H.T., ANDERSSON, B., GALE, C.: Central control of cold defence mechanisms and the release of "endopyrogen" in the goat. Acta physiol. scand. **54**, 159—174 (1962).

ANDERSON, E.G., BAKER, R.G., BANNA, N.R.: The effects of monoamine oxidase inhibitors on spinal synaptic activity. J. Pharmacol. exp. Ther. **158**, 405—415 (1967).

ANDERSSON, B., GRANT, R., LARSSON, S.: Central control of heat loss mechanisms in the goat. Acta physiol. scand. **37**, 261—280 (1956).

— JOBIN, M., OLSSON, K.: Serotonine and temperature control. Acta physiol. scand. **67**, 50 to 56 (1966).

— LARSSON, B.: Influence of local temperature changes in the pre-optic area and rostral hypothalamus on the regulation of food and water intake. Acta physiol. scand. **52**, 75—89 (1961).

ANGEL, A., ROGERS, K.J.: Convulsant activity of polyphenols. Nature (Lond.) **217**, 84—85 (1968).

ARCHER, S., ARNOLD, A., KULLNIG, R.K., WYLIE, D.W.: The enzymic methylation of pyrogallol. Arch. Biochim. Biophys. **87**, 153—154 (1960).

ARUSHANYAN, E.B., BELOZERTSER, YU. A.: [The influence of adrenaline and chlorpromazine on the inhibition of spinal reflexes] — Russian. Fiziol. Zh. Sechenov. **50**, 580—586 (1964).

ASKEW, B.M.: A simple screening procedure for imipramine-like antidepressant agents. Life Sci. **2**, 725—730 (1963).

AXELROD, J.: Presence ,formation and metabolism of normetanephrine in the brain. Science **127**, 754—755 (1958).

— Methylation reactions in the formation and metabolism of catecholamines and other biogenic amines. Pharmacol. Rev. **18**, 95—113 (1966).

— HERTTING, G., PATRICK, R.W.: Inhibition of H^3-norepinephrine release by monoamine oxidase inhibitors. J. Pharmacol. exp. Ther. **134**, 325—328 (1961b).

— LAROCHE, M.J.: Inhibitors of O-methylation of epinephrine and norepinephrine *in vivo* and *in vitro*. Science **130**, 800 (1959).

— TOMCHICK, R.: Enzymatic O-methylation of epinephrine and other catechols. J. biol. Chem. **233**, 702—705 (1958).

— WHITBY, L.G., HERTTING, G.: Effect of psychotropic drugs on the uptake of H^3-norepinephrine by tissues. Science **133**, 383—384 (1961a).

BACQ, Z.M., GOSSELIN, L., DRESSE, A., RENSON, J.: Inhibition of O-methyltransferase by catechol and sensitization to epinephrine. Science **130**, 453 (1959).

BAKAY, L.: *The Blood-Brain Barrier*. Springfield, Ill.: Thomas 1956.

BAKER, R.G., ANDERSON, E.G.: The effect of L-3,4-dihydroxyphenylalanine on spinal synaptic activity. Pharmacologist **7**, 142 (1965).

— — The effects of L-3,4-dihydroxyphenylalanine on spinal reflex activity. J. Pharmacol. exp. Ther. **173**, 212—223 (1970a).

— — The antagonism of the effects of L-3,4-dihydroxyphenylalanine on spinal reflexes by adrenergic blocking agents. J. Pharmacol. exp. Ther. **173**, 224—231 (1970b).

BALDESSARINI, R.J., KOPIN, I.J.: The effect of drugs on the release of norepinephrine-H^3 from central nervous system tissues by electrical stimulation *in vitro*. J. Pharmacol. exp. Ther. **156**, 31—38 (1967).

BANERJEE, U., FELDBERG, W., LOTTI, V. J.: Effect on body temperature of morphine and ergotamine injected into the cerebral ventricle of cats. Brit. J. Pharmacol. **32**, 523—538 (1968).

BARBOUR, H.G., WING, E.S.: The direct application of drugs to the temperature centres. J. Pharmacol. exp. Ther. **5**, 105—147 (1913).

BARCROFT, H., PETERSON, E., SCHWAB, R.S.: Action of adrenaline and noradrenaline on the tremor in Parkinson's disease. Neurology **26**, 600—601 (1952).

BARNETT, A., TABER, R.I.: The effects of diethyldithiocarbamate and L-DOPA on body temperature in mice. J. Pharm. Pharmacol. **20**, 600—604 (1968).

BARTHOLINI, G., BURKARD, W.P., PLETSCHER, A., BATES, H.M.: Increase of cerebral catecholamines caused by 3,4-dihydroxyphenylalanine after inhibition of peripheral decarboxylase. Nature (Lond.) **215**, 852—853 (1967).

— DA PRADA, M., PLETSCHER, A.: Decrease of cerebral 5-hydroxytryptamine by 3,4-dihydroxyphenylalanine after inhibition of extracerebral decarboxylase. J. Pharm. Pharmacol. **20**, 228—229 (1968).

— PLETSCHER, A.: Cerebral accumulation and metabolism of C^{14}-dopa after selective inhibition of peripheral decarboxylase. J. Pharmacol. exp. Ther. **161**, 14—20 (1968).

BARTONIČEK, V., DAHLSTRÖM, A., FUXE, K.: Effects of certain psychopharmaca on the intraneuronal levels of 5-HT and catecholamines in the specific monoamine neurons of the rat brain. Experientia (Basel) **20**, 690 (1964).

BASS, A.: Über eine Wirkung des Adrenalins auf das Gehirn. Z. ges. Neurol. Psychiat. **26**, 600—601 (1914).

BAUST, W., NIEMCYZYK, H., VIETH, J.: The action of blood pressure on the ascending reticular activating system with special reference to adrenaline-induced EEG arousal. Electroenceph. clin. Neurophysiol. **15**, 63—72 (1963).

BAXTER, B.L.: Comparison of the behavioural effects of electrical or chemical stimulation applied at the same brain loci. Exp. Neurol. **19**, 412—432 (1967).

BELLEAU, B., BURBA, J.: Tropolones: unique class of potent noncompetitive inhibitors of S-adenosylmethionine-catecholmethyltransferase Biochim. biophys. Acta (Amst.) **54**, 195—196 (1961).

BENKERT, O.: Measurement of hyperactivity in rats in a dose-response-curve after intrahypothalamic norepinephrine injection. Life Sci. **8**, 943—946 (1969).

BERNHARD, C.G., SKOGLUND, C.R.: Potential changes in spinal cord following intra-arterial administration of adrenaline and noradrenaline as compared with acetylcholine effects. Acta physiol. scand. **29**, Suppl. 106, 435—454 (1953).

BERTI, F., SHORE, P.A.: A kinetic analysis of drugs that inhibit the adrenergic neuronal membrane amine pump. Biochem. Pharmacol. **16**, 2091—2094 (1967).

BERTLER, Å.: Effect of reserpine on the storage of catecholamines in brain and other tissues. Acta physiol. scand. **51**, 75—83 (1961).

— CARLSSON, A., LINDQVIST, M., MAGNUSSON, T.: On the catechol amine levels in blood plasma after stimulation of the sympatho-adrenal system. Experientia (Basel) **14**, 184 (1958).

— — ROSENGREN, E.: Release by reserpine of catecholamines from rabbits' hearts. Naturwissenschaften **22**, 521 (1956).

— FALCK, B., ROSENGREN, E.: The direct demonstration of a barrier mechanism in the brain capillaries. Acta pharmacol. (Kbh.) **20**, 317—321 (1963).

— ROSENGREN, E.: On the distribution in brain of monoamines and of enzymes responsible for their formation. Experientia (Basel) **15**, 382—384 (1959).

BIRKHÄUSER, H.: Fermente im Gehirn geistig normaler Menschen. Helv. chir. Acta **23**, 1071—1086 (1940).

BLACKWELL, B., MARLEY, E.: Depressor effects with sympathomimetic amines after blockade of cardiovascular α-receptors. Nature (Lond.) **213**, 840 (1967).

BLASCHKO, H.: Amine oxidase and amine metabolism. Pharmacol. Rev. **4**, 415—458 (1952).

— CHRUŚCIEL, T.L.: The decarboxylation of amino acids related to tyrosine and their awakening action in mice. J. Physiol. (Lond). **151**, 272—284 (1960).

BLIGH, J.: Effects on temperature of monoamines injected into the lateral ventricle ofsheep. J. Physiol. (Lond.) **185**, 46P (1966).

— COTTLE, W.H.: The influence of ambient temperature on thermoregulatory responses to intraventricularly injected monoamines in sheep, goats and rabbits. Experientia (Basel) **25**, 608—609 (1969).

— — MASKREY, M.: Influence of ambient temperature on the thermoregulatory responses to 5-hydroxytryptamine, noradrenaline and acetylcholine injected into the lateral cerebral ventricles of sheep, goats and rabbits. J. Physiol. (Lond.) **212**, 377—392 (1971).

— MASKREY, M.: A possible role of acetylcholine in the central control of body temperature in sheep. J. Physiol. (Lond.) **203**, 55—57P (1969).

BOFF, E., HEISE, G.A.: Attenuation of tetrabenazine "reversal" by chlordiazepoxide hydrochloride. Fed. Proc. **22**, 510 (1963).

BOGDANSKI, D.F., WEISSBACH, H., UDENFRIEND, S.: The distribution of serotonin, 5-hydroxytryptophan decarboxylase and monoamine oxidase in brain. J. Neurochem. **1**, 272—278 (1957).

BOISSIER, J.R., SIMON, P.: De la potentialisation des effects de la DOPA par les inhibiteurs de la monoamineoxydase. Psychopharmacologia (Berl.) **8**, 428—436 (1966).

BONVALLET, M., DELL, P., HIEBEL, G.: Tonus sympathique et activité électrique cortical. Electroenceph. clin. Neurophysiol. **6**, 119—144 (1954).

BOOTH, D.A.: Mechanism of action of norepinephrine in eliciting an eating response on injection into the rat hypothalamus. J. Pharmacol. exp. Ther. **160**, 336—348 (1968).

BORISON, H.L.: Effect of ablation of medullary emetic chemoreceptor trigger zone on vomiting responses to cerebral intraventricular injection of adrenaline, apomorphine and pilocarpine in the cat. J. Physiol. (Lond.) **147**, 172—177 (1959).

BOWMAN, W.C., CALLINGHAM, B.A., OSUIDE, G.: Effects of tyramine on a spinal reflex in the anaesthetized chick. J. Pharm. Pharmacol. **16**, 505—515 (1964).

— ZAIMIS, E.: The effects of adrenaline, noradrenaline and isoprenaline on skeletal muscle contractions in the cat. J. Physiol. (Lond.) **144**, 92—107 (1958).

BRADLEY, P.B.: Electrophysiological evidence relating to the role of adrenaline in the central nervous system. In: "Adrenergic Mechanisms", pp. 410—420. Eds. J. R. VANE, G.E.W. WOLSTENHOLME and M. O'CONNOR. London: Churchill 1960.

BREGGIN, P.R.: Sedative-like effect of epinephrine. Arch. gen. Psychiat. **12**, 255—259 (1965).

BRITTAIN, R.T.: The intracerebral effects of noradrenaline and its modification by drugs in the mouse. J. Pharm. Pharmacol. **18**, 621—623 (1966).

— HANDLEY, S.L.: Temperature changes produced by the injection of catecholamines and 5-hydroxytryptamine into the cerebral ventricles of the conscious mouse. J. Physiol. (Lond.) **192**, 805—813 (1967).

BROADLEY, K.J., ROBERTS, D.J.: The influence of antidepressant drugs on akinesia produced in mice by intracisternally administered noradrenaline, dopamine and noradnamine. Experientia (Basel) **23**, 807—808 (1967).

BRODIE, B.B., KUNTZMAN, R., HIRSCH, C.W., COSTA, E.: Effects of decarboxylase inhibition on the biosynthesis of brain monoamines. Life Sci. **3**, 81—84 (1962).

— SHORE, P.A.: A concept of the role of serotonin and norepinephrine as chemical mediators in the brain. Ann. N. Y. Acad. Sci. **66**, 631—642 (1957).

— — PLETSCHER, A.: Serotonin-releasing activity limited to Rauwolfia alkaloids with tranquilizing action. Science **123**, 992—993 (1956).

BRUINVELS, J.: Effect of noradrenaline, dopamine and 5-hydroxytryptamine on body temperature in the rat after intracisternal administration. Neuropharmacology **9**, 277—282 (1970).

BÜLBRING, E., BURN, J.H.: Observations bearing on synaptic transmission by acetylcholine in the spinal cord. J. Physiol. (Lond.) **100**, 337—368 (1941).

— — SKOGLUND, C.R.: The action of acetylcholine and adrenaline on flexor and extensor movements evoked by stimulation of the descending motor tracts. J. Physiol. (Lond.) **107**, 289—299 (1948).

BURACK, W.R., DRASKÓCZY, P.R.: The turnover of endogenously labelled catecholamine in several regions of the sympathetic nervous system. J. Pharmacol. exp. Ther. **144**, 66—75 (1964).

BURN, J.H., RAND, M.J.: The action of sympathomimetic amines in animals treated with reserpine. J. Physiol. (Lond.) **144**, 314—336 (1958).

BUTCHER, L.L., ENGEL, J.: Peripheral factors in the mediation of the effects of L-dopa on locomotor activity. J. Pharm. Pharmacol. **21**, 614—616 (1969a).

— — Behavioural and biochemical effects of L-dopa after peripheral decarboxylase inhibition. Brain Res. **15**, 233—242 (1969b).

— — FUXE, K.: L-DOPA induced changes in central monoamine neurones after peripheral decarboxylase inhibition. J. Pharm. Pharmacol. **22**, 313—316 (1970).

CAIRNS, H.J.F.: Intracerebral inoculation of mice: fate of the inoculum. Nature (Lond.) **166**, 910—911 (1950).

CALEY, D.W.: Light and electron microscope study of the developing rat cerebral cortex. Anat. Rec. **154**, 325—326 (1966).

CAPON, A.: Analyse de l'effet d'éveil exercé par l'adrénaline et d'autres amines sympathicomimétiques sur l'électrocorticogramme du lapin non narcotisé. Arch. int. Pharmacodyn. **127**, 141—162 (1960).

CARLSSON, A.: Functional significance of drug-induced changes in brain monoamine levels. pp. 9—27. In: "Progress in Brain Research, Vol. 8. Biogenic Amines", Ed. H.E. HIMWICH and W.A. HIMWICH. Amsterdam: Elsevier Publishing Co. 1964.

Carlsson, A.: Drugs which block the storage of 5-hydroxytryptamine and related amines. In: "Handbuch der Experimentellen Pharmakologie, Vol. 19. 5-Hydroxytryptamine and related indolealkylamines", pp. 529—592. Ed. V. Erspamer. Berlin-Heidelberg-New York: Springer 1966.
— Corrodi, H., Fuxe, K., Hökfelt, T.: Effect of some antidepressant drugs on the depletion of intraneuronal brain catecholamine stores caused by 4,α-dimethyl-meta-tyramine. Europ. J. Pharmacol. **5**, 367—373 (1969a).
— — — — Effect of antidepressant drugs on the depletion of intraneuronal brain 5-hydroxytryptamine stores caused by 4-methyl-α-ethyl-meta-tyramine. Europ. J. Pharmacol. **5**, 357—366 (1969b).
— — Waldeck, B.: α-Substituierte Dopacetamide als Hemmer der Catechol-O-methyltransferase und der enzymatischen Hydroxylierung aromatischer Aminosäuren. In den Catecholamin-Metabolismus eingreifende Substanzen. Helv. chim. Acta. **46**, 2271—2285 (1963a).
— Fuxe, K., Hamberger, B., Lindqvist, M.: Biochemical and histochemical studies on the effects of imipramine-like drugs and (+)-amphetamine on central and peripheral catecholamine neurones. Acta physiol. scand. **67**, 481—497 (1966a).
— — Hökfelt, T.: Failure of dopamine to accumulate in central noradrenaline neurones after depletion with diethyldithiocarbamate. J. Pharm. Pharmacol. **19**, 481—483 (1967).
— — Ungerstedt, U.: The effect of imipramine on central 5-hydroxytryptamine neurones. J. Pharm. Pharmacol. **20**, 150—151 (1968b).
— Hillarp, N.-Å.: Formation of phenolic acids in brain after administration of 3,4-dihydroxyphenylalanine. Acta physiol. scand. **55**, 95—100 (1962).
— Lindqvist, M.: *In vivo* decarboxylation of α-methyl DOPA and α-methyl metatyrosine. Acta physiol. scand. **54**, 87—94 (1962).
— — Fila-Hromadko, S., Corrodi, H.: Synthese von Catechol-O-methyl-transferasehemmenden Verbindungen. In den Catecholaminmetabolismus eingreifende Substanzen 1. Mitteilung. Helv. chim. Acta **45**, 270—276 (1962).
— — Fuxe, K., Hökfelt, T.: Histochemical and biochemical effects of diethyldithiocarbamate on tissue catecholamines. J. Pharm. Pharmacol. **18**, 60—62 (1966b).
— — Magnusson, T.: 3,4-dihydroxyphenylalanine and 5-hydroxytryptophan as reserpine antagonists. Nature (Lond.) **180**, 1200 (1957).
— — — The effect of monoamine oxidase inhibitors on the metabolism of the brain catecholamines. J. Soc. Ciénc. méd. Lisboa. **123**, Suppl. 96 (1959).
— — — "On the biochemistry and possible functions of dopamine and noradrenaline in brain". In: "Ciba Symposium on Adrenergic Mechanisms", pp. 434—439. Eds. J.R. Vane, G.E.W. Wolstenholme and M. O'Connor. London: Churchill 1960.
— — — Waldeck, B.: On the presence of 3-hydroxytyramine in brain. Science **127**, 471 (1958).
— Magnusson, T., Rosengren, E.: 5-hydroxytryptamine of the spinal cord, normally and after transection. Experientia (Basel) **19**, 359—360 (1963b).
— Meisch, J.-J., Waldeck, B.: On the β-hydroxylation of ($\pm$)-α-methyldopamine *in vivo*. Europ. J. Pharmacol. **5**, 85—92 (1968a).
— Waldeck, B.: A method for the fluorimetric determination of 3-methoxytyramine in tissues and the occurrence of this amine in brain. Scand. J. clin. Lab. Invest. **16**, 133—138 (1964).
Carlton, P.L.: Behavioural stimulation due to α-methyl-meta-tyrosine. Nature (Lond.) **200**, 586—587 (1963).
Carmichael, E.A., Feldberg, W., Fleischhauer, K.: The site of origin of the tremor produced by tubocurarine acting from the cerebral ventricles. J. Physiol. (Lond.) **162**, 539—554 (1962).
Carr, L.A., Moore, K.E.: Effects of reserpine and α-methyl-tyrosine on brain catecholamines and the pituitary adrenal response to stress. Neuroendocrinology, **3**, 285—302 (1968).
— — Distribution and metabolism of norepinephrine after its administration into the cerebroventricular system of the cat. Biochem. Pharmacol. **18**, 1907—1918 (1969).
Cate, J. ten., Boeles, J.T.F., Biersteker, P.A.: The action of adrenaline and noradrenaline on the knee-jerk. Arch. int. Physiol. **67**, 468—488 (1959).
Chambers, D.M., Roberts, D.J.: Some pharmacological effects of noradrenaline and its metabolites injected into the cerebral ventricles in mice. Brit. J. Pharmacol. **34**, 223—224P (1968).
Chidsey, C.A., Harrison, D.C.: Studies on the distribution of exogenous norepinephrine in the sympathetic neurotransmitter stores. J. Pharmacol. exp. Ther. **140**, 217—223 (1963).
Chruściel, T.L.: Awakening actions of derivatives of phenylalanine. In: "Adrenergic Mechanisms". Ciba Foundation Symposium, pp. 440—443. Eds. J.R. Vane, G.E.W. Wolstenholme and M. O'Connor. London: Churchill 1960.

Cicero, T.J.: Self-selection of ethanol in rats: behavioural, physiological and neurochemical mechanisms. Doctoral Dissertation, Purdue University (1968).

Clymer, N.V., Seifter, J.: A method of screening sympathomimetic amines for stimulant action on the cerebrum. J. Pharmacol. exp. Ther. **89**, 149—152 (1947).

Collins, G.G.S.: Inhibition of dopamine β-oxidase by diethyldithiocarbamate. J. Pharm. Pharmacol. **17**, 526—527 (1965).

Cook, L., Kelleher, R.T.: The interaction of drugs and behaviour. In: "Neuropharmacology", vol. 2, pp. 77—92. Ed. E. Rothlin. Amsterdam: Elsevier 1961.

Cooper, K.E., Cranston, W.I., Honour, A.J.: Effects of intraventricular and intrahypothalamic injection of noradrenaline and 5-HT on body temperature in conscious rabbits. J. Physiol. (Lond.) **181**, 852—864 (1965).

Cordeau, J.P., Moreau, A., Beaulnes, A., Laurin, C.: EEG and behavioural changes following microinjection of acetylcholine and adrenaline in the brain stem of cats. Arch. ital. Biol. **101**, 30—47 (1963).

Corrodi, H., Fuxe, K.: The effect of catecholamine precursors and monoamine oxidase inhibition on the amine levels of central catecholamine neurones after reserpine treatment or tyrosine hydroxylase inhibition. Life Sci. **6**, 1345—1350 (1967).

— — The effect of imipramine on central monoamine neurones. J. Pharm. Pharmacol. **20**, 230—231 (1968).

— — Decreased turnover in central 5-HT nerve terminals induced by antidepressant drugs of the imipramine type. Europ. J. Pharmacol. **7**, 56—59 (1969).

— — Hökfelt, T.: Refillment of the catecholamine stores with 3,4-dihydroxyphenylalanine after depletion induced by inhibition of tyrosine hydroxylase. Life Sci. **5**, 605—611 (1966).

— Hanson, L.C.F.: Central effects of an inhibitor of tyrosine hydroxylation. Psychopharmacologia (Berl.) **10**, 116—125 (1966).

Costa, E., Garattini, S., Valzelli, L.: Interactions between reserpine, chlorpromazine and imipramine. Experientia (Basel) **16**, 461—463 (1960b).

— Gessa, G.L., Kuntzman, R., Brodie, B.B.: The effect of drugs on storage and release of serotonin and catecholamines in brain. In: "Proceedings of the 1st International Pharmacological Meeting, Vol. 8. Pharmacological Analysis of central nervous action", pp. 43—71. Ed. W.D.M. Paton and P. Lindgren. Oxford: Pergamon Press 1962.

— Pscheidt, G.R., van Meter, W.G., Himwich, H.E.: Brain concentrations of biogenic amines and EEG patterns of rabbits. J. Pharmacol. exp. Ther. **130**, 81—88 (1960a).

Cottle, W.H.: Calorigenic response of cold-adapted rabbits to adrenaline and to noradrenaline. Canad. J. Biochem. Physiol. **41**, 1334—1337 (1963).

Cowell, P., Davey, M.J.: The reversal of the central effects of noradrenaline by antidepressant drugs in mice. Brit. J. Pharmacol. **34**, 159—168 (1968).

Coyle, J.T., Snyder, S.H.: Antoparkinsonian drugs: Inhibition of dopamine uptake in the corpus striatum as a possible mechanism of action. Science **166**, 899—901 (1969).

Crammer, J.I., Brann, A.W., Bach, L.M.N.: An adrenergic basis for bulbar inhibition. Amer. J. Physiol. **197**, 835—838 (1959).

Creveling, C.R., Daly, J., Tokuyama, T., Witkop, B.: The combined use of α-methyltyrosine and threo-dihydroxyphenylserine — selective reduction of dopamine levels in the central nervous system. Biochem. Pharmacol. **17**, 65—70 (1968).

— Van der Schoot, J.B., Udenfriend, S.: Phenethylamine isosteres as inhibitors of dopamine β-oxidase. Biochem. biophys. Res. Commun. **8**, 215—219 (1962).

Crout, J.R.: Inhibition of catechol-O-methyl transferase by pyrogallol in the rat. Biochem. Pharmacol. **6**, 47—54 (1961).

— Creveling, C.R., Udenfriend, S.: Norepinephrine metabolism in rat brain and heart. J. Pharmacol. exp. Ther. **132**, 269—277 (1961).

— Muskus, A.J., Trendelenburg, U.: Effect of tyramine on isolated guinea-pig atria in relation to their noradrenaline stores. Brit. J. Pharmacol. **18**, 600—611 (1962).

Curtis, D.R., Eccles, J.C., Eccles, R.M.: Pharmacological studies on spinal reflexes. J. Physiol. (Lond.) **136**, 420—434 (1957).

Dagirmanjian, R., Laverty, R., Mantegazzini, P., Sharman, D.F., Vogt, M.: Chemical and physiological changes produced by arterial infusion of dihydroxyphenylanine into one cerebral hemisphere of the cat. J. Neurochem. **10**, 177—182 (1963).

Dahlström, A., Fuxe, K.: Evidence for the existence of monoamine neurones in the central nervous system. II. Experimentally induced changes in the intraneuronal amine levels of bulbospinal neuron systems. Acta physiol. scand. **64**, Suppl. 247, 7—36 (1965).

Dawes, G.S., Mestyán, G.: Changes in the oxygen consumption of new-born guinea-pigs and rabbits on exposure to cold. J. Physiol. (Lond.) **168**, 22—42 (1963).

Dawkins, M.J.R., Hull, D.: Brown adipose tissue and the response of new-born rabbits to cold. J. Physiol. (Lond.) **172**, 216—238 (1964).

Day, M., Rand, M.J.: A hypothesis for the mode of action of α-methyldopa in relieving hypertension. J. Pharm. Pharmacol. **15**, 221—224 (1963).
Dell, P.: Intervention of an adrenergic mechanism during brain-stem reticular activation. In: "Adrenergic Mechanisms" Ciba Foundation Symposium, pp. 393—409. Eds. J.R. Vane, G.E.W. Wolstenholme and M. O'Connor. London: Churchill 1960.
Dewhurst, W.G., Marley, E.: Differential effect of sympathomimetic amines on the central nervous system. In: "Animal Behaviour and Drug Action". Ciba Foundation Symposium, pp. 175—188. Eds. H. Steinberg, A.V.S. de Reuck and J. Knight. London: Churchill 1964.
— — Action of sympathomimetic and allied amines on the central nervous system of the chicken. Brit. J. Pharmacol. **25**, 705—727 (1965a).
— — The effects of α-methyl derivatives of noradrenaline, phenethylamine and tryptamine on the central nervous system of the chicken. Brit. J. Pharmacol. **25**, 682—704 (1965b).
Dews, P.B.: Monoamines and conditioned behaviour. In: "Monoamines et Systeme Nerveux-Central", pp. 143—151. Ed. J. Ajuriaguerra. Geneva: Georg 1962.
Dobbing, J.: The blood-brain barrier. In: "Applied Neurochemistry", pp. 317—331. Eds. A.N. Davison and J. Dobbing. Oxford: Blackwell 1968.
Domenjoz, R., Theobald, W.: Zur Pharmakologie des Tofranil (N-3(3-Dimethylaminopropyl)-iminodibenzyl-Hydrochlorid). Arch. int. Pharmacodyn. **120**, 450—489 (1959).
Domer, F.R., Feldberg, W.: Tremor in cats: the effect of administration of drugs into the cerebral ventricles. Brit. J. Pharmacol. **15**, 578—587 (1960).
Dominic, J.A., Moore, K.E.: Acute effects of α-methyltyrosine on brain catecholamine levels and on spontaneous and amphetamine-stimulated motor activity in mice. Arch. int. Pharmacodyn. **178**, 166—176 (1969).
Drain, D.J., Horlington, M., Lazare, R., Poulter, G.A.: The effect of α-methyl DOPA and some other decarboxylase inhibitors on brain 5-hydroxytryptamine. Life Sci. **3**, 93—97 (1962).
Draškoci, M., Feldberg, W., Haranath, P.S.R.: Passage of circulating adrenaline into perfused cerebral ventricles and subarachnoidal space. J. Physiol. (Lond.) **150**, 34—49 (1960).
Duner, H.: The influence of the blood glucose on the secretion of adrenaline and noradrenaline from the suprarenal. Acta physiol. scand. **28**, Suppl. 102, 3—77 (1953).
Eiduson, S.: Effects of DOPA, 5-HTP and iproniazid on self-stimulation of the brain. Fed. Proc. **18**, 221 (1959).
Eltherington, L.G., Horita, A.: Some pharmacological actions of β-phenylisopropylhydrazine. J. Pharmacol. exp. Ther. **128**, 7—14 (1960).
Epps, H.M.R.: The development of amine oxidase activity by human tissues after birth. Biochem. J. **39**, 37—42 (1945).
Esplin, D.W., Heaton, D.G.: Effects of reserpine on spinal cord synaptic transmission. J. Pharmacol. exp. Ther. **121**, 267—271 (1957).
Estler, C.J., Ammon, H.P.T.: Antagonistic effects of dopa and propranolol on brain glycogen. J. Pharm. Pharmacol. **22**, 146—147 (1970).
Euler, C. von: Physiology and pharmacology of temperature regulation. Pharmacol. Rev. **13**, 361—398 (1961).
Euler, U.S. von, Lindner, E., Myrin, S.-O.: Über die fiebererregende Wirkung des Adrenalins. Acta physiol. scand. **5**, 85—96 (1943).
Everett, G.M.: The dopa response potentiation test and its use in screening for antidepressant drugs. In: "Antidepressant Drugs" Proceedings of the 1st International Symposium, pp. 164—167. Eds. S. Garattini and M.N.G. Dukes. Amsterdam: Excerpta Medica Foundation 1966.
— Toman, J.E.P.: Mode of action of Rauwolfia alkaloids and motor activity. Biol. Psychiat. **2**, 75—81 (1959).
— Wiegand, R.G.: Central amines and behavioural states: a critique and new data. In: "Proceedings of the 1st International Pharmacological Meeting, vol. 8. Pharmacological analysis of central nervous action", pp. 85—92. Eds. W.D.M. Paton and P. Lindgren. Oxford: Pergamon Press 1962.
— Will, F., Evans, A.: The search for new antidepressant drugs. Fed. Proc. **23**, 198 (1964).
Feldberg, W.: A pharmacological approach to the brain from its inner and outer surface. London: Arnold 1963.
— Hellon, R.F., Lotti, V.J.: Temperature effects produced in dogs and monkeys by injections of monoamines and related substances into the third ventricle. J. Physiol. (Lond.) **191**, 501—515 (1967).
— — Myers, R.D.: Effects on temperature of monoamines injected into the cerebral ventricles of anaesthetized dogs. J. Physiol. (Lond.) **186**, 416—423 (1966).
— Lotti, V.J.: Temperature responses to monoamines and an inhibitor of MAO injected into the cerebral ventricles of rats. Brit. J. Pharmacol. **31**, 152—161 (1967).

FELDBERG, W., MALCOLM, J.L.: Experiments on the site of action of tubocurarine when applied via the cerebral ventricles. J. Physiol. (Lond.) **149**, 58—77 (1959).
— MINZ, B., TSUDZIMURA, H.: The mechanism of the nervous discharge of adrenaline. J. Physiol. (Lond.) **81**, 286—304 (1934).
— MYERS, R.D.: Effects on temperature of amines injected into the cerebral ventricles. A new concept of temperature regulation. J. Physiol. (Lond.) **173**, 226—237 (1964).
— — Changes in temperature produced by microinjections of amines into the anterior hypothalamus of cats. J. Physiol. (Lond.) **177**, 239—245 (1965).
— SHERWOOD, S.L.: Injections of drugs into the lateral ventricles of the cat. J. Physiol. (Lond.) **123**, 148—167 (1954).
FIELD, E.J., GRAYSON, J., ROGERS, A.F.: Observations on the blood flow in the spinal cord of the rabbit. J. Physiol. (Lond.) **114**, 56—70 (1951).
FINDLAY, J.D., ROBERTSHAW, D.: The mechanism of body temperature changes induced by intraventricular injections of adrenaline, noradrenaline and 5-hydroxytryptamine in the ox (Bos Taurus). J. Physiol. (Lond.) **189**, 329—336 (1967).
FISCHER, E., AMALFARA, M.L.: Effect of catecholamines on the psychomotor activity of mice. Nature (Lond.) **193**, 590—591 (1962).
FISHER, A., COURY, J.: Cholinergic tracing of a central neural circuit underlying the thirst drive. Science **138**, 691—693 (1962).
FLORU, R., STERESCU-VOLANSCHI, M., NESTIANU, V.: Research on the psychopharmacology of norepinephrine. In: "Psychopharmacological Methods", pp. 209—218. Eds. Z. VOTAVA, M. HORVATH and O. VINAR. London: Pergamon Press 1963.
FOLEY, T.H., MARSDEN, C.D., OWEN, D.A.L.: Evidence for a direct peripheral effect of adrenaline on physiological tremor in man. J. Physiol. (Lond.) **189**, 65—66P (1967).
FOLKOW, B., EULER, U.S. VON: Selective activation of noradrenaline and adrenaline producing cells in the cat's adrenal gland by hypothalamic stimulation. Circulat. Res. **2**, 191—195 (1954).
FREEMAN, B.M.: The emergence of the homeothermic-metabolic response in the fowl (Gallus domesticus). Comp. Biochem. Physiol. **13**, 413—422 (1964).
— Some effects of cold on the metabolism of the fowl during the perinatal period. Comp. Biochem. Physiol. **20**, 179—193 (1967).
FRIES, B.A., CHAIKOFF, I.L.: Factors influencing recovery of injected labelled phosphorus in various organs of the rat. J. biol. Chem. **141**, 479—485 (1941).
FUXE, K.: The distribution of monoamine terminals in the central nervous system. Acta physiol. scand. **64**, Suppl. 247, 41—85 (1965).
— HAMBERGER, B., MALMFORS, T.: Inhibition of amine uptake in tubero-infundibular dopamine neurones and in catecholamine cell bodies of the area postrema. J. Pharm. Pharmacol. **18**, 543—544 (1966).
— — — The effect of drugs on accumulation of monoamines in tubero-infundibular dopamine neurones. Europ. J. Pharmacol. **1**, 334—341 (1967).
— HILLARP, N.-Å.: Uptake of L-dopa and noradrenaline by central catecholamine neurones. Life Sci. **3**, 1403—1406 (1964).
— HÖKFELT, T., RITZÉN, M., UNGERSTEDT, U.: Studies on uptake of intraventricularly administered tritiated noradrenaline and 5-hydroxytryptamine with combined fluorescence, histochemical and autoradiographic techniques. Histochemie **16**, 186—194 (1968).
— UNGERSTEDT, U.: Localization of 5-hydroxytryptamine uptake in rat brain after intraventricular injection. J. Pharm. Pharmacol. **19**, 335—336 (1967).
— — Histochemical studies on the distribution of catecholamines and 5-hydroxytryptamine after intraventricular injections. Histochemie **13**, 16—28 (1968a).
— — Histochemical studies on the effect of (+)-amphetamine, drugs of the imipramine group and tryptamine on central catecholamine and 5-hydroxytryptamine neurones after intraventricular injection of catecholamines and 5-hydroxytryptamine. Europ. J. Pharmacol. **4**, 135—144 (1968b).
GADDUM, J.H.: Antagonisms between drugs. In: "Neuro-Psychopharmacology", vol. 2, pp. 19—24. Ed. E. ROTHLIN. Amsterdam: Elsevier 1961.
GAFFNEY, T.E., CHIDSEY, C.A., BRAUNWALD, E.: Study of the relationship between the neurotransmitter store and adrenergic nerve block induced by reserpine and guanethidine. Circulat. Res. **12**, 264—268 (1963).
GAGNON, D.J., MELVILLE, K.I.: Centrally mediated cardiovascular responses to isoprenaline. Int. J. Neuropharmacol. **6**, 245—251 (1967).
— — Alteration of centrally mediated cardiovascular manifestations by intraventricular pronethalol and phentolamine. Int. J. Neuropharmacol. **8**, 587—592 (1969).
GARATTINI, S., GIACHETTI, A., JORI, A., PIERI, L., VALZELLI, L.: Effect of imipramine, amitriptyline and their monomethyl derivatives on reserpine activity. J. Pharm. Pharmacol. **14**, 509—514 (1962).

Gerschenfeld, H.M., Wald, F., Zadunaisky, J.A., de Robertis, E.P.D.: Function of astroglia in the water-ion metabolism of the central nervous system. Neurology **9**, 412 to 425 (1959).

Gessa, G.L., Costa, E., Kuntzman, R., Brodie, B.B.: Evidence that the loss of brain catecholamine stores due to blockade of storage does not cause sedation. Life Sci. **2**, 605—616 (1962).

Giles, R.E., Miller, J.W.: A comparison of certain properties of catechol-O-methyl transferase to those of adrenergic beta receptors. J. Pharmacol. exp. Ther. **156**, 201—206 (1967a).

— — The catechol-O-methyl transferase activity and endogenous catecholamine content of various tissues in the rat and the effect of administration of U-0521 (3-4-dihydroxy-2-methyl propiophenone). J. Pharmacol. exp. Ther. **158**, 189—194 (1967b).

Gillette, J.R., Dingell, J.V., Sulser, F., Kuntzman, R., Brodie, B.B.: Isolation from rat brain of a metabolic product, desmethylimipramine, that mediates the antidepressant activity of imipramine (Tofranil). Experientia (Basel) **17**, 417—418 (1961).

Glowinski, J., Axelrod, J.: Inhibition of uptake of tritiated noradrenaline in the intact rat brain by imipramine and related compounds. Nature (Lond.) **204**, 1318—1319 (1964).

— — Effect of drugs on the uptake, release and metabolism of H^3-norepinephrine in rat brain. J. Pharmacol. exp. Ther. **149**, 43—49 (1965).

— — Effect of drugs on the disposition of H^3-norepinephrine in the rat brain. Pharmacol. Rev. **18**, 775—786 (1966).

— — Iversen, L.: Regional studies of catecholamines in the rat brain. IV. Effects of drugs on the disposition and metabolism of H^3-norepinephrine and H^3-dopamine. J. Pharmacol. exp. Ther. **153**, 30—41 (1966a).

— — Kopin, I.J., Wurtman, R.J.: Physiological disposition of H^3-norepinephrine in the developing rat. J. Pharmacol. exp. Ther. **146**, 48—53 (1964).

— Baldessarini, R.J.: Metabolism of norepinephrine in the central nervous system. Pharmacol. Rev. **18**, 1201—1238 (1966).

— Iversen, L.L.: Regional studies of catecholamines in the rat brain — I: The disposition of (H^3)-norepinephrine, (H^3)-dopamine and (H^3)-dopa in various regions of the brain. J. Neurochem. **13**, 655—669 (1966a).

— — Regional studies of catecholamines in the rat brain — III: Subcellular distribution of endogenous and exogenous catecholamines in various brain regions. Biochem. Pharmacol. **15**, 977—987 (1966b).

— — Axelrod, J.: Storage and synthesis of norepinephrine in the reserpine-treated rat brain. J. Pharmacol. exp. Ther. **151**, 385—399 (1966b).

— Kopin, I.J., Axelrod, J.: Metabolism of H^3-norepinephrine in the rat brain. J. Neurochem. **12**, 25—30 (1965).

— Snyder, S.H., Axelrod, J.: Subcellular localization of H^3-norepinephrine in the rat brain and the effect of drugs. J. Pharmacol. exp. Ther. **152**, 282—292 (1966c).

Goldstein, L., Muñoz, C.: Influence of adrenergic stimulant and blocking drugs on cerebral electrical activity in curarized animals. J. Pharmacol. exp. Ther. **132**, 345—353 (1961).

Goldstein, M.: Cerebral metabolism of DOPA-C^{14} in rats. Int. J. Neuropharmacol. **3**, 37—43 (1964).

— Anagnoste, B., Lauber, E., McKereghan, M.R.: Inhibition of dopamine β-hydroxylase by disulfiram. Life Sci. **3**, 763—767 (1964b).

— — Nakajima, K.: Inhibition of endogenous catecholamine biosynthesis by 3-iodo-l-tyrosine. Biochem. Pharmacol. **14**, 1914—1916 (1965).

— Contrera, J.F.: Inhibition of dopamine β-oxidase by imipramine. Biochem. Pharmacol. **7**, 278—279 (1961a).

— — Studies on inhibition of 3,4-dihydroxyphenylethylamine (dopamine) β-oxidase *in vitro*. Experientia (Basel) **17**, 267 (1961b).

— Gerber, H.: Phenolic alcohols in the brain after administration of DOPA-C^{14} or dopamine-C^{14}. Life Sci. **2**, 97—100 (1963).

— Lauber, E., McKereghan, M.R.: The inhibition of dopamine β-hydroxylase by tropolone and other chelating agents. Biochem. Pharmacol. **13**, 1103—1106 (1964a).

— Nakajima, K.: The effect of disulfiram on catecholamine levels in the brain. J. Pharmacol. exp. Ther. **157**, 96—102 (1967).

Goodchild, M.A.: The effects of two inhibitors of catecholamine synthesis on the content of noradrenaline and dopamine of the rat brain. Brit. J. Pharmacol. **36**, 39—40P (1969).

Graeff, F.G.: The role of dopamine in motor excitation of mice induced by brain catecholamine releasers. J. Pharm. Pharmacol. **18**, 627—628 (1966).

Green, H., Erickson, B.W.: Effect of trans-2-phenylcyclopropylamine upon norepinephrine concentration and monoamine oxidase activity of rat brain. J. Pharmacol. exp. Ther. **129**, 237—242 (1960).

GREENE, A.L.: The inhibition of dopamine-β-oxidase by chelating agents. Biochim. biophys. Acta (Amst.) **81**, 394—397 (1964).

GRIESEMER, E.C., GASNER, L.T.: Altered DOPA antagonism of reserpine hypothermia by α-methyl DOPA. Fed. Proc. **2**, 333 (1962).

GROSSMAN, S.P.: Eating or drinking elicited by direct adrenergic or cholinergic stimulation of hypothalamus. Science **132**, 301—302 (1960).

— Direct adrenergic and cholinergic stimulation of hypothalamic mechanisms. Amer. J. Physiol. **202**, 872—882 (1962a).

— Effects of adrenergic and cholinergic blocking agents on hypothalamic mechanisms. Amer. J. Physiol. **202**, 1230—1236 (1962b).

— Behavioural effects of chemical stimulation of the ventral amygdala. J. comp. physiol. Psychol. **57**, 29—36 (1964).

— Behavioural and electroencephalographic effects of micro-injections of neurohumors into the midbrain reticular formation. Physiol. Behav. **3**, 777—786 (1968).

GRUNDEN, L.R.: Studies on the central action of epinephrine, Doctoral Dissertation. San Francisco: University of California 1967.

— Action of intracerebro-ventricular epinephrine on gross behavior, locomotor activity and hexobarbital sleeping times in rats. Int. J. Neuropharmacol. **8**, 573—586 (1969).

— KATZUNG, B.G.: Studies on the central action of large doses of epinephrine. Fed. Proc. **23**, 455 (1964).

— MARLEY, E.: Effects of sympathomimetic amines injected into the third ventricle in adult chickens. Neuropharmacology **9**, 119—128 (1970).

HÄGGENDAL, J.: The presence of 3-O-methylated noradrenaline (normetanephrine) in normal brain tissue. Acta physiol. scand. **59**, 261—268 (1963).

— LINDQVIST, M.: Behaviour and monoamine levels during long term administration of reserpine to rabbits. Acta physiol. scand. **57**, 431—436 (1963).

— — Disclosure of labile monoamine fractions in brain and their correlation to behaviour. Acta physiol. scand. **60**, 351—357 (1964).

HALEY, T.J., MCCORMICK, W.G.: Pharmacological effects produced by intracerebral injection of drugs in the conscious mouse. Brit. J. Pharmacol. **12**, 12—15 (1957).

HALLIWELL, G., QUINTON, R.M., WILLIAMS, F.E.: A comparison of imipramine, chlorpromazine and related drugs in various tests involving autonomic functions and antagonism of reserpine. Brit. J. Pharmacol. **23**, 330—350 (1964).

HALPERN, B.N., DRUDI-BARACCO, C., BESSIRARD, D.: dl-DOPA et compartement émotionnel élémentaire. C.R. Soc. Biol. (Paris) **157**, 85—90 (1963).

HAMBERGER, B.: Reserpine-resistant uptake of catecholamines in isolated tissues of the rat. Acta physiol. scand. **71**, Suppl. 295, 7—56 (1967).

HANNON, J.P., EVONUK, E., LARSON, A.M.: Some physiological and biochemical effects of norepinephrine in the cold-acclimatized rat. Fed. Proc. **22**, 783—788 (1963).

HANSON, L.C.F.: The disruption of conditioned avoidance response following selective depletion of brain catecholamines. Psychopharmacologia (Berl.) **6**, 100—110 (1965).

— Evidence that the central action of amphetamine is mediated via catecholamines. Psychopharmacologia (Berl.) **9**, 78—80 (1966).

— Evidence that the central action of (+)-amphetamine is mediated via catecholamines. Psychopharmacologia (Berl.) **10**, 289—297 (1967a).

— Biochemical and behavioural effects of tyrosine hydroxylase inhibition. Psychopharmacologia (Berl.) **11**, 8—17 (1967b).

HARRIS, W.S., SCHOENFELD, C.D., BROOKS, R.H., WEISSLER, A.M.: Receptor mechanisms for the metabolic and circulatory actions of epinephrine in man. J. clin. Invest. **44**, 1058 (1965).

HARRISON, T.S.: Some factors influencing thyrotropin release in the rabbit. Endocrinology **68**, 466—478 (1961).

HARVEY, S.C., NICKERSON, M.: Adrenergic mechanisms in the chicken. Fed. Proc. **10**, 307 (1951).

HAVEL, R.J.: Transport of fatty acids between adipose tissue and blood. Role of catecholamines and the sympathetic nervous system. In: "Effects of Drugs on Synthesis and Mobilization of Lipids", pp. 43—65: Ed. E.C. HORNING. London: Pergamon Press 1963.

— CARLSON, L.A., EKELUND, L.-G., HOLMGREN, A.: Studies on the relation between mobilization of free fatty acids and energy metabolism in man: effects of norepinephrine and nicotinic acid. Metabolism **13**, 1402—1412 (1964).

HAVLÍČEK, V.: The effect of dl-3,4-dihydroxyphenylserine (precursor of noradrenaline) on the ECoG of unrestrained rats. Int. J. Neuropharmacol. **6**, 83—88 (1967).

HEHMAN, K.N., VONDERAHE, A.R., PETERS, J.J.: Effect of serotonin on behavior, electrical activity of the brain, and seizure threshold of the newly hatched chick. Neurology **11**, 1011—1016 (1961).

Hemingway, A., Forgrave, P., Birzis, L.: Shivering suppression by hypothalamic stimulation. J. Neurophysiol. **17**, 375—386 (1954).

Herman, E.H., Barnes, C.D.: Observations of drug effects on a type of spinal motor activity. Arch. int. Pharmacodyn. **165**, 425—429 (1967).

Hernández-Peón, R., Chávez-Ibarra, G., Morgane, P.J., Timo-Iaria, C.: Limbic cholinergic pathways involved in sleep and emotional behaviour. Exp. Neurol. **8**, 93—111 (1963).

Hertting, G., Axelrod, J., Whitby, L.G.: Effect of drugs on the uptake and metabolism of H^3-norepinephrine. J. Pharmacol. exp. Ther. **134**, 146—153 (1961).

Hess, S.M., Connamacher, R.H., Ozaki, M., Udenfriend, S.: The effects of α-methyl-DOPA and α-methyl-*m*-tyrosine on the metabolism of norepinephrine and serotonin *in vivo*. J. Pharmacol. exp. Ther. **134**, 129—138 (1961).

Hillarp, N.-Å., Fuxe, K., Dahlström, A.: Demonstration and mapping of central neurons containing dopamine, noradrenaline and 5-hydroxytryptamine and their reactions to psychopharmaca. Pharmacol. Rev. **18**, 727—741 (1966).

Himms-Hagen, J.: Sympathetic regulation of metabolism. Pharmacol. Rev. **19**, 367—461 (1967).

Himwich, W.A., Petersen, J.C., Allen, M.L.: Hematoencephalic exchange as a function of age. Neurology **7**, 705—710 (1957).

Hornykiewicz, O.: Dopamine (3-hydroxytyramine) and brain function. Pharmacol. Rev. **18**, 925—964 (1966).

Hsieh, A.C.L., Carlson, L.D.: Role of adrenaline and noradrenaline in chemical regulation of heat production. Amer. J. Physiol. **190**, 243—246 (1957).

Hutchinson, R.R., Renfrew, J.W.: Modification of eating and drinking: Interactions between chemical agent, deprivation state, and site of stimulation. J. comp. physiol. Psychol. **63**, 408—416 (1967).

Iversen, L.L.: Inhibition of noradrenaline uptake by drugs. J. Pharm. Pharmacol. **17**, 62—64 (1965).

— The uptake and storage of noradrenaline in sympathetic nerves. Cambridge: University Press 1967.

— Glowinski, J.: Regional studies of catecholamines in the rat brain. II. Rate of turnover of catecholamines in various brain regions. J. Neurochem. **13**, 671—682 (1966).

Ivy, A.C., Goetzl, F.R., Harris, S.C., Burrill, D.Y.: The analgesic effect of intracarotid and intravenous injection of epinephrine in dogs and of subcutaneous injection in man. Quart. Bull. Northw. Univ. med. Sch. **18**, 298—306 (1944).

Izquierdo, J.A., Jofre, I.J., Dezza, M.: Effect of pyrogallol on the catecholamine content of cortex, diencephalon, mesencephalon and cerebellum of mouse and rat. Med. exp. (Basel) **10**, 45—55 (1964).

Izquierdo, I., Merlo, A.B.: Effect of pyrogallol on acute learning in rats. J. Pharm. Pharmacol. **15**, 154—155 (1963).

Jacobi, C., Roemer, C.: Beiträge zur Erklärung der Wärmestichhyperthermie. Naunyn-Schmiedebergs Arch. exp. Path. Pharmak. **70**, 149—182 (1912).

Jacobsen, C.F., Kennard, M.A.: The influence of ephedrine sulphate on the reflexes of the spinal monkey. J. Pharmacol. exp. Ther. **49**, 362—374 (1933).

Jankowska, E., Jukes, M.G.M., Lund, S., Lundberg, A.: The effect of DOPA on the spinal cord. 5. Reciprocal organization of pathways transmitting excitatory action to alpha motoneurones of flexors and extensors. Acta physiol. scand. **70**, 369—388 (1967a).

— — — — The effect of DOPA on the spinal cord. 6. Half-centre organization of interneurones transmitting effects from the flexor reflex afferents. Acta physiol. scand. **70**, 389—402 (1967b).

— Lund, S., Lundberg, A.: The effect of DOPA on the spinal cord. 4. Depolarization evoked in the central terminals of contralateral Ia afferent terminals by volleys in the flexor reflex afferents. Acta physiol. scand. **68**, 337—341 (1966).

Jasper, H.H., Bridgman, C.S., Carmichael, L.: An ontogenetic study of cerebral electrical potentials in the guinea-pig. J. exp. Psychol. **21**, 63—67 (1937).

Johnson, G.A., Boukma, S.J., Kim, E.G.: *In vivo* inhibition of dopamine β-hydroxylase by 1-phenyl-3-(2-thiazolyl)-2-thiourea (U-14, 624). J. Pharmacol. exp. Ther. **171**, 80—87 (1970).

— Kim, E.G., Veldkamp, W., Russel, R.: Difference in oral effectiveness of two tyrosine hydroxylase inhibitors. Biochem. Pharmacol. **16**, 401—403 (1967).

Jones, B.J., Roberts, D.J.: The effects of intracerebroventricularly administered noradnamine and other sympathomimetic amines upon leptozol convulsions in mice. Brit. J. Pharmacol. **34**, 27—31 (1968).

Jori, A., Carrara, M.C., Garattini, S.: Importance of noradrenaline synthesis for the interaction between desipramine and reserpine. J. Pharm. Pharmacol. **18**, 619—620 (1966).

— Garattini, S.: Interaction between imipramine-like agents and catecholamine-induced hyperthermia. J. Pharm. Pharmacol. **17**, 480—488 (1965).

KADZIELAWA, K.: Studies on the pharmacology of α-methyl-3,4-dihydroxyphenylalanine (α-methyl-dopa) and α-methylnorepinephrine. Int. J. Neuropharmacol. **6**, 453—462 (1967).
— WIDY-TYSZKIEWICZ, E.: Electroencephalographic analysis of the central action of dihydroxyphenylalanine. Electroenceph. clin. Neurophysiol. **28**, 259—265 (1970a).
— — The influence of various pharmacological agents on the desynchronization produced by DOPA in the *cerveau isolé* preparation. Electroenceph. clin. Neurophysiol. **28**, 266—272 (1970b).
KAINDL, F., EULER, U.S. VON: Liberation of noradrenaline and adrenaline from the suprarenals of the cat during carotid occlusion. Amer. J. Physiol. **166**, 284—288 (1951).
KALININA, N.A., REPIN, I.S.: [On the role of hypothalamic serotonin and noradrenaline in body temperature regulation] — Russian Fiziol. Zh. Sechenov. **54**, 1371—1377 (1968).
KANEKO, Y., MCCUBBIN, J.W., PAGE, I.H.: Mechanism by which serotonin, norepinephrine and reserpine cause central vasomotor inhibition. Circulat. Res. **8**, 1228—1234 (1960).
KARIM, S.M.M.: The mechanism of the depressor action of noradrenaline in the cat. Brit. J. Pharmacol. **23**, 592—599 (1964).
KEY, B.J., MARLEY, E.: The effect of some sympathomimetic amines on electrocortical activity and behaviour of young and adult animals. J. Physiol. (Lond.) **155**, 39—41P (1961).
— — The effect of the sympathomimetic amines on behaviour and electrocortical activity of the chicken. Electroenceph. clin. Neurophysiol. **14**, 90—105 (1962).
KIKUCHI, T.: Electroencephalographic studies on the action of reserpine, DOPA and 5-HTP in reference to the effects of pretreatment with β-phenylisopropylhydrazine. Jap. J. Pharmacol. **11**, 151—170 (1962).
KIRSHNER, N.: Uptake of catecholamines by a particulate fraction of the adrenal medulla. J. biol. Chem. **237**, 2311—2317 (1962).
KISSEL, J.W., DOMINO, E.F.: Effects of serotonin, adrenergic and adrenergic blocking agents on spinal cord reflexes before and after blood pressure stabilization. J. Pharmacol. exp. Ther. **119**, 157—158 (1957).
— — The effects of some possible neurohumoral agents on spinal cord reflexes. J. Pharmacol. exp. Ther. **125**, 168—177 (1959a).
— — Effects of controlled progressive hypotension on some spinal reflexes in the cat. Amer. J. Physiol. **196**, 59—64 (1959b).
KOBAYASHI, T.: Behavioural changes of dogs following injection of neurotropic drugs into the arachnoid space overlying the cerebral cortex. In: "Progress in Brain Research, vol. 16. Horizons in Neuropharmacology", pp. 106—120. Eds. W.A. HIMWICH and J.P. SCHADÉ. Amsterdam: Elsevier 1965.
KONDO, S.: Über die Wirkung des Adrenalins auf die Wärmeregulation. Acta Sch. med. Univ. Kioto **3**, 169—205 (1919).
KOPIN, I.J., GORDON, E.K., HORST, W.D.: Studies of uptake of l-norepinephrine-C^{14}. Biochem. Pharmacol. **14**, 753—759 (1965).
— WEISE, V.K.: Effect of reserpine and metaraminol on excretion of homovanillic acid and 3-methoxy-4-hydroxyphenolglycol in the rat. Biochem. Pharmacol. **17**, 1461—1464 (1968).
KOSMAN, M.E., GERARD, R.W.: The effect of adrenaline on a conditioned avoidance response. J. comp. physiol. Psychol. **48**, 506—508 (1955).
KRANTZ, K.D., SEIDEN, L.S.: Effects of diethyldithiocarbamate on the conditioned avoidance response of the rat. J. Pharm. Pharmacol. **20**, 166—167 (1968).
KRNJEVIĆ, K., PHILLIS, J.W.: Actions of certain amines on cerebral cortical neurones. Brit. J. Pharmacol. **20**, 471—490 (1963).
KRONEBERG, G., SCHÜMANN, H.J.: Adrenalinsekretion und Adrenalinverarmung der Kaninchennebennieren nach Reserpin. Naunyn-Schmiedebergs Arch. exp. Path. Pharmak. **234**, 133—146 (1958).
— — Der Einfluß von Iproniacid auf die durch Reserpin gesteigerte Sekretion des Kaninchennebennierenmarks. Naunyn-Schmiedebergs Arch. exp. Path. Pharmak. **239**, 29—34 (1960).
KULKARNI, A.S.: Effects on temperature of serotonin and epinephrine injected into the lateral cerebral ventricle of the cat. J. Pharmacol. exp. Ther. **157**, 541—545 (1967).
KUNTZMAN, R., COSTA, E., CREVELING, C.R., HIRSCH, C., BRODIE, B.B.: Inhibition of norepinephrine synthesis in mouse brain by blockade of dopamine β-oxidase. Life Sci. **1**, 85—92 (1962).
KUTTNER, R., SIMS, J.A., GORDON, W.: The uptake of a metabolically inert amino acid by brain and other organs. J. Neurochem. **6**, 311—317 (1961).
LAJTHA, A.: The development of the blood-brain barrier. J. Neurochem. **1**, 216—227 (1957).
— Amino acid and protein metabolism of the brain. II. The uptake of L-lysine by brain and other organs of the mouse at different ages. J. Neurochem. **2**, 209—215 (1958).
— In: "Neurochemistry", 2nd. ed., p. 399. Eds. K.A.C. ELLIOTT, I.H. PAGE and J.H. QUASTEL. Springfield, Ill.: Thomas 1962.

Lajtha, A., Toth, J.: The brain barrier system. II. Uptake and transport of amino acids by the brain. J. Neurochem. **8**, 216—225 (1961).
Lammers, A.J., van Rossum, J.M.: Bizzarre social behaviour in rats induced by a combination of a peripheral decarboxylase inhibitor and DOPA. Europ. J. Pharmacol. **5**, 103—106 (1968).
Ledebur, I.X., Tissot, R.: Modification de l'activité électrique cérébrale du lapin sous l'effet de microinjections de précurseures de monoamines dans les structures somnogènes bulbaire et pontiques. Electroenceph. clin. Neurophysiol. **20**, 370—381 (1966).
Leibowitz, S.F.: Hypothalamic β-adrenergic "satiety" system antagonizes an α-adrenergic "hunger" system in the rat. Nature (Lond.) **226**, 963—964 (1970).
Leimdorfer, A.: The action of sympathomimetic amines on the central nervous system and the blood sugar. Mechanism of action. J. Pharmacol. exp. Ther. **98**, 62—71 (1950).
— Arana, R., Hack, M.A.: Hyperglycemia induced by the action of adrenaline on the central nervous system. Amer. J. Physiol. **150**, 588—595 (1947).
— Metzner, W.R.T.: Analgesia and anaesthesia induced by epinephrine. Amer. J. Physiol. **157**, 116—121 (1949).
Levin, E.Y., Levenberg, B., Kaufman, S.: The enzymatic conversion of 3,4-dihydroxyphenylethylamine to norepinephrine. J. biol. Chem. **235**, 2080—2086 (1960).
Levitt, M., Spector, S., Sjoerdsma, A., Udenfriend, S.: Elucidation of the rate-limiting step in norepinephrine biosynthesis in the perfused guinea-pig heart. J. Pharmacol. exp. Ther. **148**, 1—8 (1965).
Lewis, G.P.: The importance of ionization in the activity of sympathomimetic amines. Brit. J. Pharmacol. **9**, 488—493 (1954).
Littleton, J.M.: The interaction of dexamphetamine with inhibitors of noradrenaline biosynthesis in rat brain *in vivo* J. Pharm. Pharmacol. **19**, 414—415 (1967).
Lomax, P., Foster, R.S., Kirkpatrick, W.E.: Cholinergic and adrenergic interactions in the thermoregulatory centres of the rat. Brain Res. **15**, 431—438 (1969).
Longo, V.G., Silvestrini, B.: Effects of adrenergic and cholinergic drugs injected by intracarotid route on electrical activity of brain. Proc. Soc. exp. Biol. (N.Y.) **95**, 43—47 (1957).
Lundholm, L.: The effect of *l*-noradrenaline and ergotamine on the oxygen consumption of guinea-pigs. Acta physiol. scand. **18**, 341—354 (1949).
— The effect of *l*-noradrenaline on the oxygen consumption and lactic acid content in the rabbit. Acta physiol. scand. **21**, 195—204 (1950).
Luse, S.A.: The fine structure of the morphogenesis of myelin. In: "Biology of Myelin", pp. 59—80. Ed. S.R. Korey. New York: Harper 1959.
— Harris, B.: Electron microscopy of the brain in experimental edema. J. Neurosurg. **17**, 439—446 (1960).
McCarthy, L.E., Borison, H.L.: Volumetric compartmentalization of the cranial cerebrospinal fluid system determined radiographically in the cat. Anat. Rec. **155**, 305—314 (1966).
McCook, R.D., Peiss, C.N., Randall, W.C.: Hypothalamic temperatures and blood flow. Proc. Soc. exp. Biol. (N.Y.) **109**, 518—521 (1962).
McCubbin, J.W., Kaneko, Y., Page, I.H.: Ability of serotonin and norepinephrine to mimic the central effects of reserpine on vasomotor activity. Circulat. Res. **8**, 849—858 (1960).
McGeer, P.L., McGeer, E.G., Wada, J.A.: Central aromatic amine levels and behaviour. II. Serotonin and catecholamine levels in various cat brain areas following administration of psychoactive drugs or amine precursors. Arch. Neurol. (Chic.) **9**, 81—89 (1963).
McGrath, W.R., Ketteler, H.J.: Potentiation of the antireserpine effects of dihydroxyphenylalanine by antidepressants and stimulants. Nature (Lond.) **199**, 917—918 (1963).
McLennan, H.: The effect of some catecholamines upon a monosynaptic reflex pathway in the spinal cord. J. Physiol. (Lond.) **158**, 411—425 (1961).
Maître, L.: Presence of α-methyl-dopa metabolites in heart and brain of guinea-pigs treated with α-methyl-tyrosine. Life Sci. **4**, 2249—2256 (1956).
— Effects of long term administration of pyrogallol on tissue catecholamine levels, monoamine oxidase and catechol-O-methyltransferase activities in the rat. Biochem. Pharmacol. **15**, 1935—1945 (1966).
Maj, J., Przegaliński, E.: Disulfiram and some effects of amphetamine in mice and rats. J. Pharm. Pharmacol. **19**, 341—342 (1967).
— — Wielosz, M.: Disulfiram and the drug-induced effects on motility. J. Pharm. Pharmacol. **20**, 247—248 (1968).
— Vetulani, J.: Effect of some N,N-disubstituted dithiocarbamates on catecholamine levels in rat brain. Biochem. Pharmacol. **18**, 2045—2047 (1969).
— — Some pharmacological properties of N,N-disubstituted dithiocarbamates and their effect on the brain catecholamine levels. Europ. J. Pharmacol. **9**, 183—189 (1970).
Maling, H.M., Highman, B., Spector, S.: Neurologic, neuropathologic and neurochemical effects of prolonged administration of phenylisopropyl-hydrazine (JB516), phenylisobutylhydrazine (JB835) and other MAO inhibitors. J. Pharmacol. exp. Ther. **137**, 334—343 (1962).

MANARA, L., ALGERI, S., SESTINI, M.G.: Some modifications of the adrenergic mechanism induced by DMI-reserpine interactions. In: "Antidepressant Drugs" Proceedings of the 1st International Symposium 1966, pp. 51—60. Eds. S. GARATTINI and M.N.G. DUKES. Amsterdam: Excerpta Medical Foundation 1966.

MANDELL, A.J., SPOONER, C.E., WINTERS, W.D., CRUIKSHANK, M., SABBOT, I.M.: Imipramine antagonism of the CNS effects of norepinephrine behavioural and biochemical correlates. Int. J. Neuropharmacol. **8**, 235—244 (1969).

MANNARINO, E., KIRSHNER, N., NASHOLD, B.S.: The metabolism of C^{14}-noradrenaline by cat brain *in vivo*. J. Neurochem. **10**, 373—379 (1963).

MANTEGAZZINI, P., GLÄSSER, A.: Action de la DL-3-4-dioxyphenilalanine (DOPA) et de la dopamine sur l'activité électrique du chat "*cerveau isolé*". Arch. ital. Biol. **98**, 367—374 (1960).

— POECK, K., SANTIBAÑEZ, H.G.: The action of adrenaline and noradrenaline on the cortical electrical activity of the "*encéphale isolé*" cat. Arch. ital. Biol. **97**, 222—242 (1959).

MARLEY, E.: The adrenergic system and sympathomimetic amines. In: "Advances in Pharmacology", vol. 3, pp. 167—266. Eds. S. GARATTINI and P.A. SHORE. New York: Academic Press (1964).

— Action of sympathomimetic and allied amines on the central nervous system. In: "The Scientific Basis of Medicine" Annual Reviews, pp. 359—382. London: Athlone Press 1968a.

— Pharmacological studies. In: "Studies in Psychiatry", pp. 253—288. Eds. M. SHEPHERD and D.L. DAVIES. Oxford: University Press 1968b.

— KEY, B.J.: Maturation of the electrocorticogram and behaviour in the kitten and guinea-pig and the effect of some sympathomimetic amines. Electroenceph. clin. Neurophysiol. **15**, 620—636 (1963).

— MORSE, W.H.: Operant conditioning in the newly hatched chick. J. exp. Anal. Behav. **9**, 95—103 (1966).

— — Effects of α-methyl derivatives of noradrenaline, phenethylamine and tryptamine on operant conditioning in chickens. Brit. J. Pharmacol. **31**, 367—389 (1967).

— PATON, W.D.M.: The output of sympathetic amines from the cat's adrenal gland in response to splanchnic nerve activity. J. Physiol. (Lond.) **155**, 1—27 (1961).

— PROUT, G.I.: Physiology and pharmacology of the splanchnic adrenal medullary junction. J. Physiol. (Lond.) **180**, 483—513 (1965).

— STEPHENSON, J.D.: Intracerebral microinfusions of amines in young chickens. J. Physiol. (Lond.) **196**, 116—117P (1968a).

— — Some pharmacological effects of halothane in fowls. Int. J. Neuropharmacol. **7**, 165 to 184 (1968b).

— — Effects of some catecholamines infused into the hypothalamus of young chickens. Brit. J. Pharmacol. **36**, 194P (1969).

— — Effects of catecholamines infused into the brain of young chickens. Brit. J. Pharmacol. **40**, 639—658 (1970).

— VANE, J.R.: Tryptamines and spinal cord reflexes in cats. Brit. J. Pharmacol. **31**, 447—465. (1967).

MARTIN, W.R., EADES, C.G.: Pharmacological studies of spinal cord adrenergic and cholinergic mechanisms and their relation to physical dependence on morphine. Psychopharmacologia (Berl.) **11**, 195—223 (1967).

MATSUDA, Y.: Effects of intraventricularly administered adrenaline on rabbits EEG and their modifications by adrenergic blocking agents. Jap. J. Pharmacol. **18**, 139—152 (1968).

MATSUOKA, M.: Function and metabolism of catecholamines in the brain. Jap. J. Pharmacol. **14**, 181—193 (1964).

— YOSHIDA, H., IMAIZUMI, R.: Effect of pyrogallol on the catecholamine content of the rabbit brain. Biochem. Pharmacol. **11**, 1109—1110 (1962).

MAXWELL, D.R., PALMER, H.T.: Demonstration of anti-depressant or stimulant properties of imipramine in experimental animals. Nature (Lond.) **191**, 84—85 (1961).

MAYER, S.E., MAICKEL, R.P., BRODIE, B.B.: Kinetics of penetration of drugs and other foreign compounds into cerebrospinal fluid and brain. J. Pharmacol. exp. Ther. **127**, 205—211 (1959).

— — — Disappearance of various drugs from the cerebrospinal fluid. J. Pharmacol. exp. Ther. **128**, 41—43 (1960).

MELVILLE, K.I., JOHNSON, M.C.: Cerebrospinal fluid electrolyte changes during lateral ventricular perfusion with noradrenaline and associated cardiovascular responses. Neuropharmacology **9**, 79—95 (1970).

MENON, M.K., DANDIYA, P.C., BAPNA, J.S.: Modification of the effects of tranquilizers in animals treated with α-methyl-l-tyrosine. J. Pharmacol. exp. Ther. **156**, 63—69 (1967).

MERLO, A.B., IZQUIERDO, I.: The action of inhibitors of catechol-O-methyl-transferase on the exploratory activity of mice. J. Pharm. Pharmacol. **15**, 629—630 (1963).

MERLO, A.B., IZQUIERDO, I: Effect of inhibitors of O-methyl-transferase and of adrenergic blocking agents on conditioning and extinction in rats. Med. exp. (Basel) **13**, 217—226 (1965).
MEYER, H.: Zur Theorie der Alkoholnarkose. Naunyn-Schmiedeberg's Arch. exp. Path. Pharmak. **42**, 109—118 (1899).
MILHAUD, G., GLOWINSKI, J.: Métabolisme de la dopamine-C^{14} dans le cerveau du rat. Etude de mode d'administration. C.R. Acad. Sci. (Paris) **255**, 203—205 (1962).
— — Métabolisme de la noradrenaline-C^{14} dans le cerveau du rat. C.R. Acad. Sci. (Paris) **256**, 1033—1035 (1963).
MILLER, N.E.: Chemical coding of behaviour in the brain. Science **148**, 328—338 (1965).
— GOTTESMAN, K.S., EMERY, N.: Dose response to carbachol and norepinephrine in rat hypothalamus. Amer. J. Physiol. **206**, 1384—1388 (1964).
MIMS, C.A.: Intracerebral injections and growth of viruses in the mouse brain. Brit. J. exp. Path. **41**, 52—59 (1960).
MOFFETT, R.B., HANZE, A.R., SEAY, P.H.: Central nervous system depressants. V. polyhydroxy and methoxyphenyl ketones, carbinols and their derivatives. J. Med. Chem. **7**, 178—186 (1964).
MONNIER, M.: Action électro-physiologiques des stimulants du système nerveux central. I. Systèmes adrénergiques, cholinergiques et neurohumeures sérotoniques. Arch. int. Pharmacodyn. **124**, 281—301 (1960).
— TISSOT, R.: Action de la réserpine et de ses médiateurs (5-hydroxytryptophan-sérotonine et Dopa-noradrénaline) sur le comportement et le cerveau du lapin. Helv. physiol. Acta **16**, 255—267 (1958).
MOORE, K.E.: Effects of α-methyltyrosine on brain catecholamines and conditioned behaviour in guinea-pigs. Life Sci. **5**, 55—65 (1966).
— Behavioural effects of α-methyltyrosine administered in the diets of mice pretreated with a monoamine oxidase inhibitor. J. Pharm. Pharmacol. **20**, 656—657 (1968a).
— Development of tolerance to the behavioural depressant effects of α-methyltyrosine. J. Pharm. Pharmacol. **20**, 805—807 (1968b).
— Behaviour and brain catecholamines after disulfiram (D.S.) and diethyldithiocarbamate (DDC). Fed. Proc. **27**, 274 (1968c).
— RECH, R.H.: Antagonism by monoamine oxidase inhibitors of α-methyltyrosine-induced catecholamine depletion and behavioural depression. J. Pharmacol. exp. Ther. **156**, 70—75 (1967).
— WRIGHT, P.F., BERT, J.K.: Toxicologic studies with α-methyltyrosine, an inhibitor of tyrosine hydroxylase. J. Pharmacol. exp. Ther. **155**, 506—515 (1967).
MOORE, R.E., UNDERWOOD, M.C.: The thermogenic effects of noradrenaline in new-born and infant kittens and other small animals. A possible hormonal mechanism in the control of heat production. J. Physiol. (Lond.) **168**, 290—317 (1963).
MORGANE, P.J.: Evidence of a "hunger motivational" system in the lateral hypothalamus of the rat. Nature (Lond.) **191**, 672—674 (1961).
MORSE, W.H., HERRNSTEIN, R.J.: Effects of drugs on characteristics of behavior maintained by complex schedules of intermittent positive reinforcement. Ann. N.Y. Acad. Sci. **65**, 303—317 (1956).
MOYER, K.E., BUNNELL, B.N.: Effect of injected adrenaline on an avoidance response in the rat. J. genet. Psychol. **92**, 247—251 (1958).
MUSACCHIO, J.M., GOLDSTEIN, M., ANAGNOSTE, B., PÖCH, G., KOPIN, I.J.: Inhibition of dopamine β-hydroxylase by disulfiram *in vivo*. J. Pharmacol. exp. Ther. **152**, 56—61 (1966).
— KOPIN, I.J., SNYDER, S.H.: Effects of disulfiram on tissue norepinephrine content and subcellular distribution of dopamine, tyramine and their β-hydroxylated metabolites. Life Sci. **3**, 769—775 (1964).
— — WEISE, V.K.: Subcellular distribution of some sympathomimetic amines and their β-hydroxylated derivatives in the rat heart. J. Pharmacol. exp. Ther. **148**, 22—28 (1965).
MUSCHOLL, E.: "Autonomic nervous system; newer mechanisms of adrenergic blockade". In: "Annual Review of Pharmacology", vol. 6, pp. 107—128. Ed. H.W. ELLIOTT. California: Annual Reviews, Inc. 1966.
— VOGT, M.: The action of reserpine on the peripheral sympathetic system. J. Physiol. (Lond.) **141**, 132—155 (1958).
MYERS, R.D.: Emotional and autonomic responses following hypothalamic chemical stimulation. Canadian J. Psychol. **18**, 6—14 (1964a).
— Modification of drinking patterns by chronic intracranial infusion. In: "Thirst in the Regulation of Body Water", pp. 533—551. Ed. M.J. WAYNER. Oxford: Pergamon Press 1964b.
— Injection of solutions into cerebral tissue: relation between volume and diffusion. Physiol. Behav. **1**, 171—174 (1966).
— SHARPE, L.G.: Chemical activation of ingestive and other hypothalamic regulatory mechanisms. Physiol. Behav. **3**, 987—995 (1968).

MYERS, R.D., YAKSH, T.L.: Feeding and temperature responses in the unrestrained rat after injections of cholinergic and aminergic substances into the cerebral ventricles. Physiol. Behav. **3**, 917—928 (1968).

— — Control of body temperature in the unanaesthetized monkey by cholinergic and aminergic systems in the hypothalamus. J. Physiol. (Lond.) **202**, 483—500 (1969).

NAGATSU, T., LEVITT, M., UDENFRIEND, S.: Tyrosine hydroxylase. The initial step in norepinephrine biosynthesis. J. biol. Chem. **239**, 2910—2917 (1964).

NASHOLD, B.S., MANNARINO, E., WUNDERLICH, M.: Pressor-depressor blood pressure responses in the cat after intraventricular injection of drugs. Nature (Lond.) **193**, 1297—1298 (1962).

NEČINA, J.: Antagonism between α-methyl DOPA and reserpine. Life Sci. **1**, 301—303 (1962).

NEFF, N.H., COSTA, E.: Effect of tricyclic antidepressants and chlorpromazine on brain catecholamine synthesis. In: "Antidepressant Drugs" Proceedings of the 1st International Symposium 1966, pp. 28—34. Eds. S. GARATTINI and M.N.G. DUKES. Amsterdam: Excerpta Medica Foundation 1966a.

— — The influence of monoamine oxidase inhibition on catecholamine synthesis. Life Sci. **5**, 951—959 (1966b).

NICKERSON, M., HOLLENBERG, N.K.: Blockade of α-adrenergic receptors. In: "Physiological Pharmacology", vol. IV, pp. 243—305. The Nervous System. Eds. W.S. ROOT and F.G. HOFMANN. New York: Academic Press 1967.

NOBLE, E.P., WURTMAN, R.J., AXELROD, J.: A simple and rapid method for injecting H^3-norepinephrine into the lateral ventricle of the rat brain. Life Sci. **6**, 281—291 (1967).

NUKADA, T., SAKURAI, T., IMAIZUMI, R.: Monoamine oxidase activity and mitochondrial structure of the brain. Jap. J. Pharmacol. **13**, 124 (1963).

NYBÄCK, H., BORZECKI, Z., SEDVALL, G.: Accumulation and disappearance of catecholamines formed from tyrosine-C^{14} in mouse brain; effect of some psychotropic drugs. Europ. J. Pharmacol. **4**, 395—403 (1968).

OVERTON, E.: Studien über die Narkose. Jena: Gustav Fischer 1901.

OWEN, D.A.L., MARSDEN, C.D.: Effect of adrenergic β-blockade of parkinsonian tremor. Lancet ii, 1259—1262 (1965).

PALAIČ, D., PAGE, I.H., KHAIRALLAH, P.A.: Uptake and metabolism of (^{14}C)-serotonin in rat brain. J. Neurochem. **14**, 63—69 (1967).

PALMER, A.C.: Injection of drugs into the cerebral ventricle of sheep. J. Physiol. (Lond.) **149**, 209—214 (1959).

PARKER, S.W., FELDMAN, S.M.: Effect of mesencephalic lesions on feeding behaviour in rats. Exp. Neurol. **17**, 313—326 (1967).

PERSSON, T., WALDECK, B.: Is there an interaction between dopamine and noradrenaline containing neurones in the brain? Acta physiol. scand. **78**, 142—144 (1970).

PFEIFER, A.K., GALAMBOS, E., GYÖRGY, L.: Some central nervous properties of diethyldithiocarbamate. J. Pharm. Pharmacol. **18**, 254 (1966).

PHILIPPU, A., BECKE, H., BURGER, A.: Effect of drugs on the uptake of noradrenaline by isolated hypothalamic vesicles. Europ. J. Pharmacol. **6**, 96—101 (1969).

— SCHÜMANN, H.J.: Bildung und Speicherung von α-Methylnoradrenalin. Naunyn-Schmiedebergs Arch. Pharmak. exp. Path. **256**, 183—195 (1967).

PIRCH, J.H., NORTON, S.: Beta-phenylisopropylhydrazine (JB-516) on septal hyperirritability and brain amine levels in the rat. J. Pharmacol. exp. Ther. **155**, 506—515 (1965).

PLETSCHER, A., GEY, K.F., BURKARD, W.P.: Inhibitors of monoamine oxidase and decarboxylase of aromatic amino acids. In: "Handbook of Experimental Pharmacology, vol. XIX, pp. 593—735. 5-hydroxytryptamine and related indolealkylamines". Ed. V. ERSPAMER. Heidelberg: Springer 1966.

PORTER, C.C., TOTARO, J.A., BURCIN, A.: The relationship between radioactivity and norepinephrine concentrations in the brains and hearts of mice following administration of labelled methyldopa or 6-hydroxydopamine. J. Pharmacol. exp. Ther. **150**, 17—22 (1965).

— — LEIBY, C.M.: Some biochemical effects of α-methyl-3,4-dihydroxyphenylalanine and related compounds in mice. J. Pharmacol. exp. Ther. **134**, 139—145 (1961).

POSCHEL, B.P.H., NINTEMAN, F.W.: Hypothalamic self-stimulation: its supression by blockade of norepinephrine biosynthesis and reinstatement by methamphetamine. Life Sci. **5**, 11—16 (1966).

POTTER, L.T., AXELROD, J.: Studies on the storage of norepinephrine and the effect of drugs. J. Pharmacol. exp. Ther. **140**, 199—206 (1963).

— — KOPIN, I.J.: Differential binding and release of norepinephrine and tachypylaxis. Biochem. Pharmacol. **11**, 254—256 (1962).

PSCHEIDT, G.R., HIMWICH, H.E.: Chicken brain amines: normal levels and effect of reserpine and monoamine oxidase inhibitors. In: "Progress in Brain Research, vol. 16, pp. 245—249. Horizons in Neuropsychopharmacology". Eds. W.A. HIMWICH and J.P. SCHADÉ. Amsterdam: Elsevier 1965.

Pscheidt, G.R., Morpurgo, C., Himwich, H.E.: Studies on norepinephrine and 5-hydroxytryptamine in various species. In: "Comparative Neurochemistry. 5th International Neurochemical Symposium", pp. 401—402. Ed. D. Richter. New York: Pergamon Press 1964.
Randrup, A., Munkvad, I.: Role of catecholamines in the amphetamine excitatory response. Nature (Lond.) **211**, 540 (1966).
— Scheel-Krüger, J.: Diethyldithiocarbamate and amphetamine stereotype behaviour. J. Pharm. Pharmacol. **18**, 752 (1966).
Rech, R.H.: The relevance of experiments involving injection of drugs into the brain. In: "Importance of fundamental principles in drug evaluation", pp. 325—360. Ed. D.H. Tedeschi and R.E. Tedeschi. New York: Raven Press 1968.
— Domino, E.F.: Observations on injections of drugs into the brain substance. Arch. int. Pharmacodyn. **121**, 429—442 (1959).
Reitter, H.: Narkoseeffekt durch intrazisternale Adrenalin injektion. Anaesthesist **6**, **131** to 135 (1957).
Reivich, M., Glowinski, J.: An autoradiographic study of the distribution of C^{14}-norepinephrine in the brain of the rat. Brain **90**, 633—646 (1967).
Reynolds, R.W.: An irritative hypothesis concerning the hypothalamic regulation of food intake. Psychol. Rev. **72**, 105—116 (1965).
Robinson, B.W., Mishkin, M.: Alimentary responses evoked from forebrain structures in Macaca mulatta. Science **136**, 260—261 (1962).
— — Alimentary responses to forebrain stimulation in monkeys. Exp. Brain Res. **4**, 330—366 (1968).
Rocha e Silva, M., Sproull, D.H.: An excitatory action of adrenaline, noradrenaline and 5-hydroxytryptamine on the spinal cord. J. Physiol. (Lond.) **185**, 445—454 (1966).
Rodriguez de Lores Arnaiz, G., de Robertis, E.: Cholinergic and non-cholinergic nerve endings in the rat brain. II. Subcellular localization of monoamine oxidase and succinate dehydrogenase. J. Neurochem. **9**, 503—508 (1962).
Roos, B.E., Werdinius, B.: The effect of α-methyl dopa on the metabolism of 5-hydroxytryptamine in brain. Life Sci. **2**, 92—96 (1963).
Ross, S.B., Haljasmaa, Ö.: Catechol-O-methyl transferase inhibitors. *In vitro* inhibition of the enzyme in mouse-brain extract. Acta pharmacol. (Kbh.) **21**, 205—214 (1964a).
— — Catechol-O-methyl transferase inhibitors. *In vivo* inhibition in mice. Acta pharmacol. (Kbh.) **21**, 215—225 (1964b).
— Renyi, A.L.: Inhibition of the uptake of tritiated catecholamines by antidepressant and related drugs. Europ. J. Pharmacol. **2**, 181—186 (1967).
Rossum, J.M. van: Mechanism of the central stimulant action of α-methyl-meta-tyrosine. Psychopharmacologia (Berl.) **4**, 271—280 (1963).
Roth, L.J., Schoolar, J.C., Barlow, C.F.: Sulfur-35 labeled acetazolamide in cat brain. J. Pharmacol. exp. Ther. **125**, 128—136 (1959).
Roth, R.H., Stone, E.A.: The action of reserpine on noradrenaline biosynthesis in sympathetic nerve tissue. Biochem. Pharmacol. **17**, 1581—1590 (1968).
Rothballer, A.B.: Studies on the adrenaline-sensitive component of the reticular activating system. Electroenceph. clin. Neurophysiol. **8**, 603—621 (1956).
— The effects of catecholamines on the central nervous system. Pharmacol. Rev. **11**, 494—547 (1959).
Ruckebusch, Y., Grivel, M.L., Laplace, J.P.: Variations interspécifiques des modifications de la température centrale liées à l'injection cérébro-ventriculaire de catécholamines et de 5-hydroxytryptamine. C.R. Soc. Biol. (Paris) **159**, 1748—1750 (1965).
— — — Effects comportementaux et électrographiques de l'injection cérébroventriculaire de catécholamines chez le mouton. Thérapie **21**, 483—491 (1966a).
— Laplace, J.P., Grivel, M.L.: Variations de l'activité médicamenteuse en fonction de l'âge: étude chez le poussin. Thérapie **21**, 1113—1120 (1966b).
Rutledge, C.O., Jonason, J.: Metabolic pathways of dopamine and norepinephrine in rabbit brain *in vitro*. J. Pharmacol. exp. Ther. **157**, 493—502 (1967).
— Weiner, N.: The effect of reserpine upon the synthesis of norepinephrine in the isolated rabbit heart. J. Pharmacol. exp. Ther. **157**, 290—302 (1967).
Schaeppi, U.: Drug injection into the cat's 4th ventricle: effects upon EEG and autonomic system. Arch. int. Pharmacodyn. **169**, 44—54 (1967).
Schain, R.J.: Some effects of a monoamine oxidase inhibitor upon changes produced by centrally administered amines. Brit. J. Pharmacol. **17**, 261—266 (1961).
Schanberg, S.M., Schildkraut, J.J., Kopin, I.J.: The effects of pentobarbital on the fate of intracisternally administered norepinephrine-H^3. J. Pharmacol. exp. Ther. **157**, 311—318 (1967a).
— — — The effects of psychoactive drugs on norepinephrine metabolism in brain. Biochem. Pharmacol. **16**, 393—399 (1967b).

SCHECKEL, C.L., BOFF, E.: Behavioural stimulation in rats associated with a selective release of brain norepinephrine. Arch. int. Pharmacodyn. **152**, 479—490 (1964).

— — PAZERY, L.M.: Behavioural and biochemical effects of interacting 3,4-dihydroxyphenylalanine (DOPA) and an inhibitor of aromatic acid decarboxylase (Ro 4-4602). Fed. Proc. **24**, 195 (1965).

SCHILDKRAUT, J.J., SCHANBERG, S.M., BREESE, G.R., KOPIN, I.J.: Effects of psychoactive drugs on the metabolism of intracisternally administered serotonin in rat brain. Biochem. Pharmacol. **18**, 1971—1978 (1969).

SCHMIDT, J.: Die Abhängigkeit der Temperaturbeeinflussung von Ratten durch biogene Amine von der Applikationsart und der Umgebungstemperatur. Acta biol. med. germ. **10**, 350 to 356 (1963).

— FÄHSE, C.: Die Wirkung von Hemmstoffen der Monoaminoxydase auf die Körpertemperatur von Ratten. Acta biol. med. germ. **13**, 607—614 (1964).

SCHNEIDER, J.A., PLUMMER, A.J., EARL, A.E., GAUNT, R.: Neuropharmacological aspects of reserpine. Ann. N.Y. Acad. Sci. **61**, 17—26 (1955).

SCHUBERT, J., NYBÄCK, H., SEDVALL, G.: Effect of antidepressant drugs on accumulation and disappearance of monoamines formed *in vivo* from labelled precursors in mouse brain. J. Pharm. Pharmacol. **22**, 136—138 (1970).

SCHUBERT, P., LADISCH, W.: Chronic administration of electroconvulsive shock and norepinephrine metabolism in the rat brain. Psychopharmacologia (Berl.) **15**, 289—295 (1969).

SCHWARTZ, D.E., BURKARD, W.P., ROTH, M., GEY, K.F., PLETSCHER, A.: Effect of chlorpromazine on the penetration of MAO inhibitors and monoamine releasers into rat brain. Arch. int. Pharmacodyn. **141**, 135—144 (1963).

SCHWEITZER, A., WRIGHT, S.: The action of adrenaline on the knee-jerk. J. Physiol. (Lond.) **88**, 476—491 (1937).

SCOPES, J.W., TIZARD, J.P.M.: The effect of intravenous noradrenaline on the oxygen consumption of new born mammals. J. Physiol. (Lond.) **156**, 305—326 (1963).

SEIDEN, L.S., CARLSSON, A.: Brain and heart catecholamine levels after L-DOPA administration in reserpine treated mice: Correlations with a conditioned avoidance response. Psychopharmacologia (Berl.) **5**, 178—181 (1964).

— PETERSON, D.D.: Blockade of L-dopa reversal of reserpine-induced conditioned avoidance response suppression by disulfiram. J. Pharmacol. exp. Ther. **163**, 84—90 (1968).

SHARE, N.N., MELVILLE, K.I.: Centrally mediated sympathetic cardiovascular responses induced by intraventricular noradrenaline. J. Pharmacol. exp. Ther. **141**, 15—21 (1963).

SHARPE, L.G., MYERS, R.D.: Feeding and drinking following stimulation of the diencephalon of the monkey with amines and other substances. Exp. Brain Res. **8**, 295—310 (1969).

SHARPLESS, S.: The effects of intravenous epinephrine and norepinephrine on a conditioned response in the cat. Psychopharmacologia (Berl.) **1**, 140—149 (1959).

SHERWOOD, S.L.: The response of psychotic patients to intraventricular injections. Proc. roy. Soc. Med. **48**, 855—863 (1955).

SHORE, P.A.: Release of serotonin and catecholamines by drugs. Pharmacol. Rev. **14**, 531—550 (1962).

— BUSFIELD, D., ALPERS, H.S.: Binding and release of metaraminol: mechanism of norepinephrine depletion by α-methyl-*m*-tyrosine and related agents. J. Pharmacol. exp. Ther. **146**, 194—199 (1964).

SIGG, E., OCHS, S., GERARD, R.W.: Effects of the medullary hormones on the somatic nervous system in the cat. Amer. J. Physiol. **183**, 419—426 (1955).

SKOGLUND, C.R.: Influence of noradrenaline on spinal interneuron activity. Acta physiol. scand. **51**, 142—149 (1961).

SKULTETY, F.M.: Changes in caloric intake following brain stem lesions in cats. Arch. Neurol. (Chic.) **14**, 541—552 (1966).

SLANGEN, J.L., MILLER, N.E.: Pharmacological tests for the function of hypothalamic norepinephrine in eating behaviour. Physiol. Behav. **4**, 543—552 (1969).

SMITH, C.B., DEWS, P.B.: Antagonism of locomotor suppressant effects of reserpine in mice. Psychopharmacologia (Berl.) **3**, 55—59 (1962).

SMITH, R.W., MCCANN, S.M.: Aphagia, adipsia and polydipsia following hypothalamic lesions in the rat. Fed. Proc. **20**, 333 (1961).

SMYTHIES, J.R., LEVY, C.K.: The comparative psychopharmacology of some mescaline analogues. J. ment. Sci. **106**, 531—536 (1960).

SNYDER, S.H., GREEN, A.I., HENDLEY, E.D.: Kinetics of H^3-norepinephrine accumulation into slices from different regions of the rat brain. J. Pharmacol. exp. Ther. **164**, 90—102 (1968).

SOMMER, S.R., NOVIN, D., LEVINE, M.: Food and water intake after intrahypothalamic injections of carbachol in the rabbit. Science **156**, 983—984 (1967).

Sourkes, T. L., Murphy, G. F., Chavez, B., Zielinska, M.: The action of some α-methyl and other amino acids on cerebral catecholamines. J. Neurochem. **8**, 109—115 (1961).

Spector, N. H., Brobeck, J. R., Hamilton, C. L.: Feeding and core temperature in albino rats. Changes induced by preoptic heating and cooling. Science **161**, 286—288 (1968).

Spector, S., Mata, R. O., Sjoerdsma, A., Udenfriend, S.: Biochemical and pharmacological effects of iodo-tyrosine, in relation to tyrosine hydroxylase inhibition *in vivo*. Life Sci. **4**, 1307—1311 (1965b).

— Prockop, D., Shore, P. A., Brodie, B. B.: Effect of iproniazid on brain levels of nor-epinephrine and serotonin. Science **127**, 704 (1958).

— Shore, P. A., Brodie, B. B.: Biochemical and pharmacological effect of the monoamine oxidase inhibitor iproniazid, 1-phenyl-2-hydrazinopropane (JB-516), and 1-phenyl-3-hydrazinobutane (JB-835). J. Pharmacol. exp. Ther. **128**, 15—21 (1960).

— Sjoerdsma, A., Udenfriend, S.: Blockade of endogenous norepinephrine synthesis by α-methyl-tyrosine, an inhibitor of tyrosine hydroxylase. J. Pharmacol. exp. Ther. **147**, 86—95 (1965a).

Spooner, C. E., Winters, W. D.: Evidence for a direct action of monoamines on the chick central nervous system. Experientia (Basel) **21**, 256—258 (1965).

— — Mandell, A. J.: DL-norepinephrine-7-H^3 uptake, water content, and thiocyanate space in the brain during maturation. Fed. Proc. **25**, 451 (1966).

Steiner, G., Cahill, G. F.: Brown and white adipose tissue metabolism in cold-exposed rats. Amer. J. Physiol. **207**, 840—844 (1964).

Stjärne, L.: Tyramine effects on catechol amine release from spleen and adrenals in the cat. Acta physiol. scand. **51**, 224—229 (1961).

— Studies of noradrenaline biosynthesis in nerve tissue. Acta physiol. scand. **67**, 441—454 (1966).

— Lishajko, F.: Drug-induced inhibition of noradrenaline synthesis *in vitro* in bovine splenic nerve tissue. Brit. J. Pharmacol. **26**, 398—404 (1966).

— Roth, R. H., Lishajko, F.: Noradrenaline formation from dopamine in isolated subcellular particles from bovine splenic nerve. Biochem. Pharmacol. **16**, 1729—1739 (1967).

Stone, C. A., Ross, C. A., Wenger, H. C., Ludden, C. T., Blessing, J. A., Totaro, J. A., Porter, C. C.: Effect of α-methyl-3,4-dihydroxyphenylalanine (methyldopa), reserpine and related agents on some vascular responses in the dog. J. Pharmacol. exp. Ther. **136**, 80—88 (1962).

Ström, G.: Central nervous regulation of body temperature. In: "Handbook of Physiology, Section I. Neurophysiology, Vol. 2", pp. 1173—1196. Eds. J. Field, H. W. Magoun and V. E. Hall. Washington: Amer. Phys. Soc. (1960).

Stuart, D. G., Kawamura, Y., Hemingway, A.: Activation and suppression of shivering during septal and hypothalamic stimulation. Exp. Neurol. **4**, 485—506 (1961).

Sulser, F., Bickel, M. H., Brodie, B. B.: The action of desmethylimipramine in counter-acting sedation and cholinergic effects of reserpine-like drugs. J. Pharmacol. exp. Ther. **144**, 321—330 (1964).

— Watts, J., Brodie, B. B.: On the mechanism of antidepressant action of imipramine-like drugs. Ann. N. Y. Acad. Sci. **96**, 279—288 (1962).

Svensson, T. H., Waldeck, B.: On the significance of central noradrenaline for motor activity: experiments with a new dopamine β-hydroxylase inhibitor. Europ. J. Pharmacol. **7**, 278 to 282 (1969).

Takagi, H., Satoh, M., Yamatsu, K., Kimura, K., Nakama, M.: Central effects of 3,4-dihydroxyphenylalanine and 5-hydroxytryptophan on tetrabenazine-pretreated rabbits with special reference to the possible role of catecholamine and serotonin in the brain. Int. J. Neuropharmacol. **7**, 265—273 (1968).

Taylor, P. M.: Oxygen consumption in new-born rats. J. Physiol. (Lond.) **154**, 153—168 (1960).

Thoenen, H., Haefely, W., Gey, K. F., Hürlimann, A.: Diminished effects of sympathetic nerve stimulation in cats pretreated with disulfiram; liberation of dopamine as sympathetic transmitter. Life Sci. **4**, 2033—2038 (1965).

— — — — Quantitative aspects of the replacement of norepinephrine by dopamine as a sympathetic transmitter after inhibition of dopamine-β-hydroxylase by disulfiram. J. Pharmacol. exp. Ther. **156**, 246—251 (1967).

Toda, N., Matsuda, Y., Shimamoto, K.: Cardiovascular effects of sympathomimetic amines injected into the cerebral ventricles of rabbits. Int. J. Neuropharmacol. **8**, 451—461 (1969).

Traczyk, W. Z.: Experimental catalepsy produced in dogs by intraventricular administration of adrenaline and noradrenaline. Int. J. Neuropharmacol. **3**, 261—266 (1964).

Trendelenburg, U.: Modification of the effect of tyramine by various agents and procedures. J. Pharmacol. exp. Ther. **134**, 8—17 (1961).

UDENFRIEND, S., CREVELING, C.R.: Localization of dopamine-β-oxidase in brain. J. Neurochem. **4**, 350—352 (1959).
— WYNGAARDEN, J.B.: Precursors of adrenal epinephrine and norepinephrine *in vivo*. Biochim. biophys. Acta (Amst.) **20**, 48—52 (1956).
— ZALTZMAN-NIRENBERG, P.: On the mechanism of norepinephrine release produced by α-methyl-meta-tyrosine. J. Pharmacol. exp. Ther. **138**, 194—199 (1962).
— — Norepinephrine and 3,4-dihydroxyphenethylamine turnover in guinea-pig brain *in vivo*. Science **142**, 394—396 (1963).
— — GORDON, R., SPECTOR, S.: Evaluation of the biochemical effects produced *in vivo* by inhibitors of the three enzymes involved in norepinephrine biosynthesis. Molec. Pharmacol. **2**, 95—105 (1966).
— — NAGATSU, T.: Inhibitors of purified beef adrenal tyrosine hydroxylase. Biochem. Pharmacol. **14**, 837—845 (1965).
UNGERSTEDT, U., BUTCHER, L.L., BUTCHER, S.G., ANDÉN, N.-E., FUXE, K.: Direct chemical stimulation of dopaminergic mechanisms in the neostriatum of the rat. Brain Res. **14**, 461—471 (1969).
VERNADAKIS, A., WOODBURY, D.M.: Cellular and extracellular spaces in developing rat brain. Radioactive uptake studies with chloride and insulin. Arch. Neurol. (Chic.) **12**, 284—293 (1965).
VOGT, M.: Concentration of sympathin in different parts of the central nervous system under normal conditions and after the administration of drugs. J. Physiol. (Lond.) **123**, 451—481 (1954).
— Catecholamines in brain. Pharmacol. Rev. **11**, 483—493 (1959).
VOORHOEVE, P.E.: Autochthonous activity of fusimotor neurones in the cat. Acta physiol. pharmacol, neerl. **9**, 1—43 (1960).
WADA, J.A.: Behavioral and electrographic effects of intraventricular injection of bulbocapnine and other substances in freely moving monkeys. Ann. N.Y. Acad. Sci. **96**, 227—249 (1962).
— WRINCH, J., HILL, D., MCGEER, P.L., MCGEER, E.G.: Central aromatic amine levels and behavior. Arch. Neurol. (Chic.) **9**, 69—80 (1963).
WAELSCH, H.: Blood-brain barrier and gas exchange. In: "Biochemistry of the Developing Nervous System", pp. 187—207. Ed. H. WAELSCH. New York: Academic Press 1955.
WAGNER, J.W., DE GROOT, J.: Changes in feeding behavior after intracerebral injections in the rat. Amer. J. Physiol. **204**, 483—487 (1963).
WEIL-MALHERBE, H.: The passage of catechol amines through the blood-brain barrier. In: "Adrenergic Mechanisms". Ciba Foundation Symposium, pp. 421—423. Eds. J. R. VANE, G.E.W. WOLSTENHOLME and M. O'CONNOR. London: Churchill 1960.
— POSNER, H.S., BOWLES, G.R.: Changes in the concentration and intracellular distribution of brain catecholamines: the effects of reserpine, β-phenylisopropylhydrazine, pyrogallol and 3,4-dihydroxyphenylalanine, alone and in combination. J. Pharmacol. exp. Ther. **132**, 278—286 (1961a).
— WHITBY, L.G., AXELROD, J.: The blood-brain barrier for catecholamines in different regions of the brain. In: "Regional Neurochemistry", pp. 284—292. Eds. S.S. KETY and and J. ELKES. Oxford: Pergamon Press 1961b.
WEISSMAN, A., KOE, B.K.: Behavioural effects of L-α-methyltyrosine, an inhibitor of tyrosine hydroxylase. Life Sci. **4**, 1037—1047 (1965).
— — Contrasting locomotor effects of catecholamine releasers and tyrosine hydroxylase inhibitors in MAO inhibited rats. Psychopharmacologia (Berl.) **11**, 282—286 (1967).
WENTINK, E.: The effects of certain drugs and hormones upon conditioning. J. exp. Psychol. **22**, 150—163 (1938).
WIEGAND, R.E., PERRY, J.E.: Effect of L-DOPA and N-methyl-N-benzyl-2-propynylamine HCl on dopa, dopamine, norepinephrine, epinephrine and serotonin levels in mouse brain. Biochem. Pharmacol. **7**, 181—186 (1961).
WILSON, S.P., TISLOW, R.: Differential antagonism of reserpine eyelid closure by imipramine and amphetamine. Proc. Soc. exp. Biol. (N.Y.) **109**, 847—848 (1962).
WILSON, V.J.: Effect of intra-arterial injections of adrenaline on spinal extensor and flexor reflexes. Amer. J. Physiol. **186**, 491—496 (1956).
WINDLE, F.: Physiology of the fetus. p. 163. Philadelphia: Saunders 1940.
WISE, R.A.: Hypothalamic motivational systems: Fixed or plastic neural circuits? Science **162**, 377—379 (1968).
WURTMAN, R.J., FRANK, M.M., MORSE, W.H., DEWS, P.B.: Studies on behavior. V. Actions of l-epinephrine and related compounds. J. Pharmacol. exp. Ther. **127**, 281—287 (1959).
WYRWICKA, W., DOTY, R.W.: Feeding induced in cats by electrical stimulation of the brain stem. Exp. Brain Res. **1**, 152—160 (1966).
ZHELYASKOV, D.K., LEVITT, M., UDENFRIEND, S.: Tryptophan derivatives as inhibitors of tyrosine hydroxylase *in vivo* and *in vitro*. Molec. Pharmacol. **4**, 445—451 (1968).

Chapter 13

Fundamental Mechanisms in the Release of Catecholamines

A. D. SMITH and H. WINKLER

With 15 Figures

Introduction

In some endocrine tissues, such as the steroid-secreting glands, the release of the hormone is tightly coupled to its rate of biosynthesis because the tissue does not contain a significant store of the hormone (see VOGT, 1943; HOLZBAUER, 1957). The tissues which synthesise and release catecholamines do, however, contain a store of the amines, at least part of which is located in subcellular particles. Although some aspects of the release of catecholamines can be studied without reference to the store, an understanding of the fundamental mechanisms involved requires a detailed study of the nature of the store. Several questions have to be considered, among which are the following:

1. Is the store heterogeneous ? What proportion of the store resides in particles, and are all the particles of the same type ?
2. What proportion of the catecholamines released originates from each of the different storage sites ? Can the entire store be mobilised for release, or only part of it ?
3. What is the relation between the storage and the biosynthesis of the amines ? Can newly synthesised amines be released independently of those in the stores ?
4. Is release brought about by modification of the forces which maintain the high concentration of catecholamines in the store, followed by diffusion of the amines out of the cell, or does the storage particle play a more direct role in the release process ?

Not all of these questions can be answered at present, but in the first part of the chapter we shall describe the evidence provided by biochemical studies on the chromaffin cell and adrenergic neuron which have begun to throw light on some of these problems. Particular attention will be given to recent studies which have established that secretion from the adrenal medulla occurs by exocytosis and which raise the possibility that such a process may also occur in the adrenergic neuron. In the second part of the chapter we shall discuss some of the fundamental mechanisms involved in exocytosis, and the implications this mode of secretion has for the dynamics of the chromaffin cell and the adrenergic neuron.

A. Origin of Catecholamines Released from the Cell

I. Localisation of the Catecholamine Store

1. In the Adrenal Medulla

The discovery in 1953 that a large proportion of the catecholamines in homogenates of adrenal medulla is present in a subcellular particle (BLASCHKO and

WELCH, 1953; HILLARP et al., 1953), was followed by biochemical and morphological studies which have shown that the catecholamine-containing particles (chromaffin granules) can be differentiated from mitochondria, lysosomes and microsomes. These studies have been reviewed in detail recently (SMITH, 1968; SMITH and WINKLER, 1969) and will also be discussed in the chapters by COUPLAND, by VON EULER and by STJÄRNE.

Application of centrifugation methods to homogenates of adrenal medulla has not only led to the conclusion that most of the amines are stored in a specific type of cell particle, it has also enabled the composition of the particle to be determined and has thrown some light on the problem of the heterogeneity of the catecholamine store.

Two approaches can be used to determine the composition of a subcellular particle: first, if the particle in question can be obtained free from significant contamination with other particles, then its chemical composition can be determined directly. Second, the distribution of a substance between different subcellular fractions of the tissue can be compared with that of a known constituent of the particle. Following the original work of HILLARP (1959), the first approach has been most widely applied in studies on the composition of adrenal chromaffin granules. This approach has the advantage that the chemical composition of the particle can be determined by analysis of a single fraction obtained by centrifugation; for example HILLARP (1959) gave the dry weight composition of chromaffin granules as protein (35%), total lipids (22%), catecholamines (20.5%) and ATP (15%). An earlier determination of the composition of a catecholamine-containing fraction (HILLARP and NILSON, 1954a) showed that up to 20% of the dry weight could not be account for as protein, lipid and catecholamine: this led to the search for other components and to the discovery of ATP in the particles (HILLARP et al., 1955; FALCK et al., 1956; BLASCHKO et al., 1956). The major pitfall of this approach is the possibility of contamination of the fraction by particles which do not contain the catecholamines. Contamination of "granule" fractions from bovine adrenal medulla by lysosomes (SMITH and WINKLER, 1966, 1969; LADURON and BELPAIRE, 1968b) is the most likely explanation for the presence of acid phosphatase (HILLARP and FALCK, 1956) and acid nucleases in this fraction (PHILIPPU and SCHÜMANN, 1964; SMITH and WINKLER, 1965). Furthermore, it is likely that most of the RNA present in a "granule" fraction (PHILIPPU and SCHÜMANN, 1963) was due to contamination by lighter particles (PHILIPPU and SCHÜMANN, 1964; KIRSHNER, 1969), which are probably microsomes (SMITH and WINKLER, 1968; WINKLER, 1969).

The isolation of highly purified chromaffin granules depends upon the use of some form of sucrose density gradient centrifugation, which was first applied to chromaffin tissue by BLASCHKO et al. (1957). In a simplified procedure, which avoids making up density gradients (SMITH and WINKLER, 1967a), a chromaffin granule fraction can be obtained in high yield as a pellet. The pellet contains up to 48% of the catecholamines but less than 2% of the mitochondria, 7% of the lysosomes, and 3% of the microsomes (WINKLER, 1969; WINKLER et al., 1970a). Other methods of isolating chromaffin granules have been reported, such as by differential centrifugation (BANKS, 1966b; TAUGNER and HASSELBACH, 1966) and by filtration (OKA et al., 1966; POISNER and TRIFARÓ, 1967) but the purity of the fractions has not always been established by analysis of marker enzymes for all the possible contaminating particles. A recent study has shown that chromaffin granules isolated by a filtration method are heavily contaminated by other particles (TRIFARÓ and DWORKIND, 1970); in the same paper a method for isolating purified chromaffin granules in an iso-osmotic density gradient is described.

The second approach to the identification of constituents of chromaffin granules, in which the distribution of a substance between different fractions is compared with that of the catecholamines, is valuable because it reveals the presence of hitherto unsuspected particles (e.g. the lysosomes) and because it can be used to study the heterogeneity of the catecholamine store. An example of the use of this method to identify a specific component of the chromaffin granules is the analysis of fractions by microcomplement fixation for an acidic protein, now called chromogranin A (BLASCHKO et al., 1967a; SCHNEIDER et al., 1967): the distribution of chromogranin A between fractions obtained by differential centrifugation (KIRSHNER et al., 1967) and sucrose density gradient centrifugation (SAGE et al., 1967) closely paralleled that of the catecholamines. The heterogeneity of the catecholamine store has been revealed by analysis of the different fractions obtained by centrifugation of homogenates. Two types of heterogeneity can be distinguished: in the first, the store may be divided between a particulate and a non-particulate phase; in the second, the particulate store is itself heterogeneous.

a) Is there an Extragranular Store of Catecholamines?

The existence of a particle-free store of amines in the adrenal medulla was discussed by HILLARP (1960a), who reported that, however carefully the adrenals of different animals were homogenised, at least 5—10% of the amines were recovered in the supernatant. He considered that while some of the soluble amines may have been released from chromaffin granules during homogenisation, some may reflect the presence of a small pool of newly synthesised catecholamines in the cytosol. HILLARP's observations showed that the size of the 'free' pool, relative to that of the particulate store, must be very small. If we assume that the presence of macromolecular constituents of the chromaffin granules, such as chromogranin A, in the supernatant is due to release from particles damaged during homogenisation, it should be possible to estimate the size of the 'free' pool. However, this has not so far been achieved. Because of the experimental error involved in the immunochemical assay for chromogranin A, all that can be said is that the ratio of the amount of the protein to that of the catecholamines in the supernatant is not very different from the ratio in chromaffin granules (KIRSHNER et al., 1967). The ratio of dopamine β-hydroxylase activity to catecholamines in a supernatant fraction of bovine adrenal medulla (15.8) was higher than the ratio (8.6) in the large granule fraction (VIVEROS et al., 1968). A similar observation was made on rabbit adrenal medulla (VIVEROS et al., 1969a). Since only half of the total dopamine β-hydroxylase in chromaffin granules is recovered in the soluble lysate after hypo-osmotic shock (DUCH, et al., 1968; BELPAIRE and LADURON, 1968; VIVEROS et al., 1969c; WINKLER et al., 1970a), a ratio of no more than 4.3 would be predicted for the bovine adrenal medulla supernatant if all the dopamine β-hydroxylase and catecholamines in this fraction came from damaged particles. Several possible explanations of the unexpectedly high ratio of dopamine β-hydroxylase to catecholamines in the supernatant have been suggested (VIVEROS et al., 1968; VIVEROS et al., 1969a), two of which are (a) that there is normally a pool of dopamine β-hydroxylase in the cytosol, and (b) that there is a population of chromaffin granules, which is labile to homogenisation, that is rich in dopamine β-hydroxylase but poor in catecholamines.

It has to be concluded that we still have no more information about the size of the particle-free pool of catecholamines in the adrenal medulla than was provided by HILLARP in 1960.

b) Heterogeneity of the Particulate Store of Catecholamines

This has been revealed by analysis of fractions obtained by sucrose density gradient centrifugation. Three types of heterogeneity have so far been identified: 1. particles which contain either adrenaline or noradrenaline, 2. particles containing different proportions of catecholamines and ATP, 3. particles containing different proportions of catecholamines and dopamine β-hydroxylase.

1. The early work of SCHÜMANN (1957) and EADE (1957, 1958) established that the noradrenaline-containing chromaffin granules of chick and ox adrenals, respectively, sedimented to a denser region on a sucrose gradient than did the adrenaline-containing granules. It is not known whether this difference between the granules reflects a fundamental difference in chemical composition, but studies on the noradrenaline-containing granules of pig adrenal medulla have shown that these particles contain the same soluble proteins, and have a similar phospholipid composition to the total chromaffin granule fraction (WINKLER, 1969). Evidence that, in the normal adrenal medulla, noradrenaline and adrenaline are stored in separate cells will be described in the chapter by COUPLAND.

2. HILLARP (1960a) investigated the discrepancy between the molar ratio of catecholamines to adenosine phosphates, which was close to 4 in chromaffin granules obtained from the lower layers of a density gradient, and this ratio in the whole homogenate, which was 6. The apparent deficit of adenine nucleotides (ATP, ADP and AMP) in the homogenate could only partly be accounted for by catabolites, such as hypoxanthine, and when these were allowed for a molar ratio of 4.9

Fig. 1. Sucrose density gradient centrifugation of large granule fraction from ox adrenal medulla (BANKS, 1964)

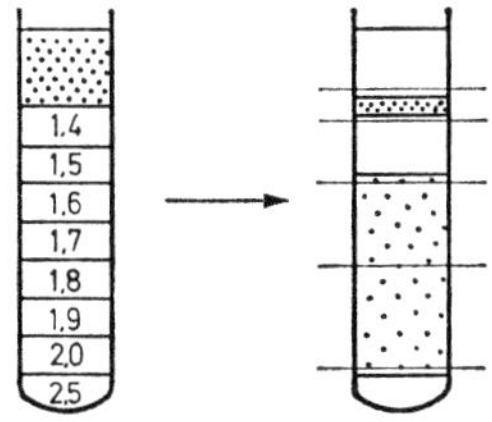

1.4
1.5
1.6
1.7
1.8
1.9
2.0
2.5

Fraction	% Total Catecholamines	% Noradrenaline	% Total ATP	Catecholamines (µmoles): ATP (µmoles)
1	10.1	22	0.2	262
2	5.7	19	1.8	17
3	5.9	20	3.6	9.1
4	41.6	13.5	49.5	4.6
5	34.8	30	42.3	4.5
6	1.8	100	2.4	4.1

was obtained. The deficit of nucleotides was not due to a pool of catecholamines in the cytosol, that was not associated with nucleotides, because the molar ratio of catecholamines to adenine nucleotides in the large granule fraction was also about 5. HILLARP (1960a) proposed, therefore, that there are two pools of granule-bound amines: one in a particle that contains catecholamines and adenine nucleotides in the molar ratio of 4:1, and which is recovered in the lower region of sucrose density gradients; and the other pool in another population of chromaffin granules which contains much less nucleotide, if any, and which must have remained in the upper regions of the density gradient in his previous experiments (HILLARP and THIEME, 1959). Some earlier experiments by SCHÜMANN (1957, 1958a) showed that chromaffin granules from the chicken adrenal contained different amounts of ATP according to their position in a density gradient: in the predominantly adrenaline-containing granules (1.6M — 1.8M — sucrose layer) the molar ratio of amine to ATP was 6.3, whereas in the mixed (adrenaline- and noradrenaline-containing) granules (1.8M — 2.0M — sucrose layer) the ratio was 5.0 (SCHÜMANN, 1958a). Further direct evidence which supports HILLARP's suggestion has been provided by BANKS (1964), who determined the catecholamine and ATP content of six fractions from a sucrose density gradient of the large granules from bovine adrenal medulla: these results are reproduced in Fig. 1. If the value for the particle-free supernatant (fraction 1) is discounted it can be seen that fractions 2 and 3, which contained nearly 12% of the amines, were deficient in ATP and so could well be the second population of particles whose existence was postulated by HILLARP (1960a).

The nature of this type of particle needs to be studied further in order to provide answers to the following questions: a) Is the deficiency of adenine nucleotides in this particle due to their replacement by other nucleotides such as GTP? GTP is present in the large granule fraction (HILLARP, 1960a; HELLE, 1966a). b) Is this particle more labile than the chromaffin granules which are rich in nucleotides, as suggested by some of HILLARP's (1960a) observations? c) Does the particle contain newly synthesised catecholamines, as suggested by HILLARP (1960a), and does it also contain newly synthesised chromogranins? d) Can this particle take up ATP from the cytosol? CARLSSON et al. (1963) found that the large granule fraction took up small amounts of ATP when incubated at 31°.

The ability of a particle to store catecholamines without stoichiometric amounts of ATP is not unique: such particles are present in some phaeochromocytomas (see chapter by WINKLER and SMITH) and in the splenic nerve (see below). However, in these two examples the possibility that other nucleotides were present was not excluded.

3. In the first paper in which dopamine β-hydroxylase activity was measured in density gradients after centrifugation of the large granule fraction, a close correlation was found between the distribution of catecholamines and that of the enzyme (OKA et al., 1967a). However, subsequent studies in which different density gradients were used have shown that in both bovine (LADURON and BELPAIRE, 1968b) and rabbit (VIVEROS et al., 1969a) adrenal medulla the distribution of dopamine β-hydroxylase activity does not exactly parallel that of the catecholamines: the peak of dopamine β-hydroxylase activity is displaced slightly towards a region of lower density. This finding was discussed by VIVEROS et al. (1969a), who made the interesting suggestion that all chromaffin granules contain the same amount of dopamine β-hydroxylase activity but that their catecholamine content varies, and that it is the content of amines which largely determines the density of the particle. Support for this idea came from the finding that rabbit chromaffin granules deficient in adrenaline equilibrated in a region of lower density in a sucrose density gradient (VIVEROS et al., 1969d). It is ,therefore, possible that in the normal adrenal medulla the store of catecholamines is heterogeneous with respect to dopamine β-hydroxylase, but it cannot be excluded that the heterogeneity arose during fractionation, when a proportion of the chromaffin granules may have lost some of their catecholamines but not their dopamine β-hydroxylase.

c) Conclusions

The stores of adrenaline and noradrenaline in the chromaffin cells of the adrenal medulla are mainly located in chromaffin granules which are rich in adenine nucleotides. Perhaps as much as 20% of the store is located in particles which are deficient in adenine nucleotides. The noradrenaline- and adrenaline-containing granules can be distinguished, but both contain the chromogranins. It is possible that the proportion of dopamine β-hydroxylase to catecholamines is not the same in all chromaffin granules. Only a small part, probably less than 5% of the total store, is normally located in the cytosol.

2. In the Sympathetic Nerves

Three years after the discovery that the catecholamines of the adrenal medulla were stored in a cell particle, EULER and HILLARP (1956) reported that some of the noradrenaline in homogenates of bovine splenic nerve, bovine spleen and rat spleen was recovered in a particulate fraction after centrifugation. This finding opened up the possibility of applying biochemical methods to study the nature of the particle(s) which contain the neurotransmitter. Centrifugation experiments have provided information about the following: the proportion of noradrenaline stored in particles; the type of cell particle containing the noradrenaline; the heterogeneity of the particulate store; and the composition of the storage particles. For reviews of this subject the reader is referred to the chapter by EULER and to articles by DE POTTER (1971), GEFFEN and LIVETT (1971) and SMITH (1971b). What may we conclude from these biochemical studies and how far can the conclusions be correlated with the results of morphological studies (see chapter by BLOOM)?

Biochemical evidence concerning the nature of the noradrenaline-containing particles in the central nervous system is meagre. Although it has been shown that noradrenaline is present in synaptosomes and that some of this synaptosomal noradrenaline is in particles within the nerve ending, there is no evidence whether or not the nerve endings contain more than one type of noradrenergic vesicle.

Fig. 2. Distribution of noradrenergic vesicles within the splenic nerve

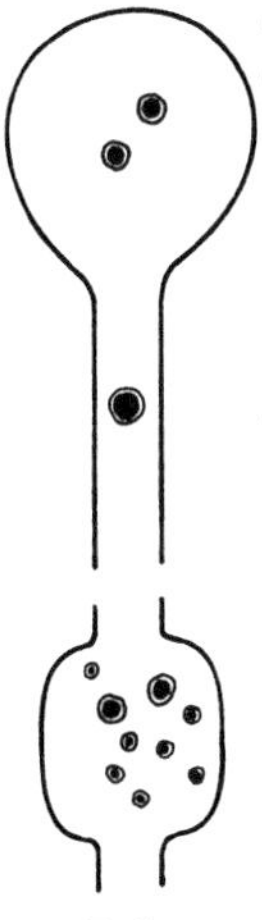

	Type of vesicle			
	Microscopical	Biochemical	Size (1)	Components of vesicle
Cell Body	Large	Heavy	787 Å	Noradrenaline Dopamine β-hydroxylase (2)
Axon	Large	Heavy	700 Å	Noradrenaline Dopamine β-hydroxylase Chromogranin A ATP
Terminal	Large	Heavy	~700 Å	Noradrenaline Dopamine β-hydroxylase
Varicosity	Small	Light	443 Å	Noradrenaline ? Dopamine β-hydroxylase

References: 1. GEFFEN and OSTBERG (1969); 2. W.P. DE POTTER (personal communication).

Much more is known about the noradrenergic vesicles of peripheral sympathetic neurons. Our present knowledge can be summarised as follows:

1. Most of the noradrenaline is stored in particles.
2. The noradrenaline-containing particles of preterminal axons of the splenic nerve can be distinguished from other cell particles, such as mitochondria, lysosomes and membrane fragments.
3. The particulate store is heterogeneous: noradrenaline is found in the 'light' noradrenergic vesicle (possibly identical with the small dense-cored vesicle described by electron microscopists) and in the 'heavy' noradrenergic vesicle (possibly identical with the large dense-cored vesicle).
4. In the cell body and nonterminal axons, the 'heavy' vesicles are the predominant type.

5. In the terminal varicosities both 'heavy' and 'light' noradrenergic vesicles occur, but the latter store most of the noradrenaline.

6. The 'heavy' noradrenergic vesicles of nonterminal axons contain ATP, chromogranin A and dopamine β-hydroxylase. The 'heavy' vesicles in the terminals also contain dopamine β-hydroxylase, but it is not yet certain whether the 'light' vesicles contain this enzyme. There is some evidence that the 'light' vesicles contain ATP.

7. Preliminary observations suggest that the 'heavy' vesicles in the nerve terminals contain a higher concentration of noradrenaline than the 'heavy' vesicles in the nonterminal axons.

A diagram illustrating some of these conclusions in so far as they apply to the splenic nerve is given in Fig. 2.

II. Type of Binding in the Store: Its Relation to the Mechanism of Release

We still do not know how chromaffin granules and noradrenergic vesicles maintain their stores of catecholamines. None of the mechanisms proposed in the literature can account for all the observations, and this led to the suggestion that several factors, not just one, are involved in the binding of catecholamines by these subcellular particles (SMITH, 1968). This subject has been reviewed in detail by STJÄRNE (1964), SMITH (1968) and KIRSHNER (1969) and is also discussed in the chapters by EULER and by STJÄRNE. We shall consider the nature of the binding very briefly in order to formulate in more depth the question raised in the introduction, i. e. is release brought about by modification of the forces which maintain the high concentration of catecholamines in the store?

Two mechanisms have been proposed to account for the ability of catecholamine-containing particles to bind the amines:

1. the participation of the catecholamines in a high molecular weight complex which is unable to diffuse across the vesicle membrane ('storage complex' hypothesis);

2. the uptake of catecholamines from the cytosol, catalysed by an enzyme system located in the periphery of the vesicle ('active uptake' hypothesis).

The important discovery that catecholamines and ATP can form high molecular weight aggregates (micelles) in concentrated aqueous solution containing divalent metal ions (BERNEIS et al., 1969, 1970) has provided the first evidence about the nature of the hypothetical storage complex. However, such micelles are less stable at 37° than at lower temperatures, whereas active uptake is only efficient at body temperature. Accordingly, we suggest that both these mechanisms normally operate in the cell, the one complementing the other.

Possible Modes of Release of Catecholamines from the Store

Most of the catecholamines, in both the adrenal medulla and the sympathetic nerve terminal, are present within membrane-limited vesicles. There are two possible fates for the store in the vesicles:

1. The store may be released from the vesicles into the cytosol, and the amines in the cytosol may then diffuse out of the cell.

2. The store in the vesicles may be the immediate source of the amines released from the cell.

These alternatives are illustrated in Fig. 3. Release of the store into the cytosol could be brought about (a) by destruction of the storage complex, or (b) by inhibition of the active uptake process, or (c) by partial dissolution of the vesicle membrane. Release of the store directly into the extracellular space could be achieved (a) by formation of a 'tight junction' between the membrane of the chromaffin granule and that of the cell, or (b) by expulsion of the intact vesicle from the cell, or (c) by exocytosis.

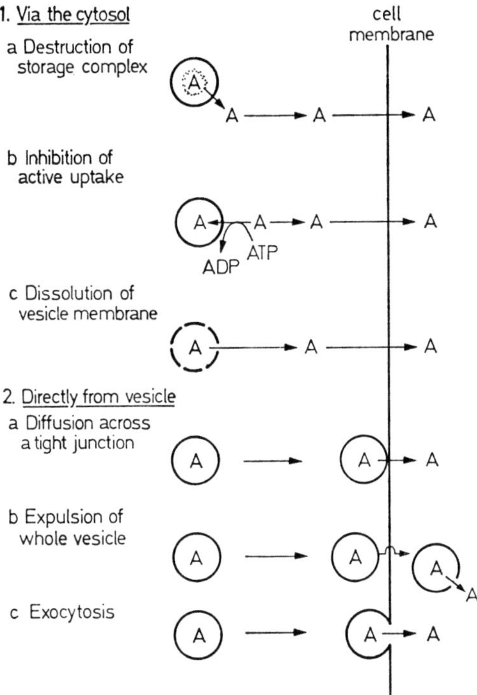

Fig. 3. Possible modes of release of an amine (A) from a vesicle

There are several obvious differences between mechanisms 1 and 2. Firstly, mechanism 2 does not necessarily involve any direct interference with the processes which maintain the high concentration of amines within the vesicle, except that the vesicle membrane must be ruptured in 2b and c. Secondly, mechanism 1 involves diffusion of low molecular weight amines across the cytoplasm, whereas mechanism 2 involves movement of the entire vesicle across the cytoplasm. The other main difference between these mechanisms is that mechanisms 2b and c involve the simultaneous release of other components of the store in addition to the catecholamines, whereas the release of these components is not obligatory in mechanism 1. It has, in fact, proved possible to distinguish the two mechanisms experimentally by virtue of some of these differences. Thus, the liberation of amines into the cytosol exposes them to the monoamine oxidase of mitochondria, with the result that deaminated metabolites of the amines are released (see reviews by Kopin, 1964, 1966). By looking for the release of several components of the vesicle it has been possible to identify release by mechanism 2 and to distinguish 2a from 2b and c. This approach was adopted in early studies on the adrenal medulla by Carlsson and Hillarp (1956); Carlsson et al. (1957) and by Douglas and his colleagues (see review by Douglas, 1966). It has since been applied in many other studies on the adrenal medulla and, more recently, in work on the splenic nerve. By correlating the results obtained using this biochemical approach with features of the ultrastructure of the chromaffin cell revealed by electron microscopy, it has been concluded that most, if not all, of the catecholamines secreted from the adrenal medulla, in response to cholinergic drugs or splanchnic nerve stimulation, are released by exocytosis (see reviews by DOUGLAS, 1968; SMITH, 1968; KIRSHNER, 1969). The evidence upon which this conclusion is based will be considered below, together with recent observations on the splenic nerve which are consistent with the release of some, at least, of the neurotransmitter by a similar mechanism.

III. Fate of Components of the Store Following Stimulation: Biochemical Evidence of Exocytosis in the Adrenal Medulla

Two different experimental approaches have been used in studies on the fate of components of the chromaffin granule, following stimulation of the gland. In the first, the whole gland or a particulate fraction is analysed for catecholamines and for the component being studied; in the second, the perfusate or blood leaving the gland is analysed. The first approach is the easiest to apply for *in vivo* studies, whereas the second approach is well suited to *in vitro* studies. Ideally, the two approaches should be used together, but this has only been done in a few cases. If the first approach is used alone, detailed studies should be made of the time courses of the changes in components of the tissue, since resynthesis of these components may obscure changes initially caused by stimulation of the gland. Exclusive use of the second approach may be satisfactory for short-term experiments, but the tissue will not necessarily have exactly the same properties in a perfused gland as it does *in vivo*. We shall concentrate in this section on the short-term experiments, in which the initial response of the gland to stimulation has been studied. Some of the results of the longer-term experiments will also be mentioned, since these are relevant to the discussion in Section B on the dynamics of the secreting cell.

The fate of three components of the chromaffin granule, in addition to the catecholamines, will be considered: these are, the adenine nucleotides, the proteins (soluble and insoluble), and the lipids.

1. Fate of the Adenine Nucleotides

Studies on adenine nucleotides in the adrenal medulla following stimulation were reported soon after the chromaffin granules and been shown to contain ATP (CARLSSON and HILLARP, 1956; D'IORIO and EADE, 1956); these, and subsequent, studies are summarised in Table 1 (a). STJÄRNE (1964) reported the first experiments in which the composition of perfusates from stimulated adrenal glands was examined; the observations using this approach are summarised in Table 1 (b).

Most of the observations on tissue levels of nucleotides following neurogenic stimulation of the adrenal medulla (e.g. by administration of morphine or insulin) have shown a parallel fall in the concentrations of adenine nucleotides and catecholamines, such that the molar ratio of amines to nucleotides was not markedly changed. However, in rabbits treated with insulin (D'IORIO and EADE, 1956; EADE, 1957) there was a 75% fall in the concentration of adrenaline without a corresponding fall in the ATP content of the adrenal glands. Since BANKS (1964) found that electrical stimulation of the splanchnic nerve of the rabbit led to a parallel decrease in the ATP and adrenaline content of the gland, it is unlikely that the lack of effect of insulin is due to a species difference in the mode of

Table 1. *Fate of adenine nucleotides upon stimulation of the adrenal medulla*

(a) Analysis of the adrenal medulla

Animal	Stimulus	Substance	Control tissue	Stimulated tissue	Percentage decrease	Notes	Ref.
Cat	Morphine HCl (20 mg/kg, s.c.) Time: 20 hr	Catecholamines (mg/g)	8.4	2.41	71		1
		Acid-labile P (mg/g)	3.91	1.23	69		
Rat	Insulin (10 I.U./100 g, s.c.) Time: 2 hr	Catecholamine (mg/g)	10.8	3.12	71	In both control and stimulated glands 76—79 % of the catecholamines were in large granule fraction. Values for acid-labile P refer to large granule fraction	2
		Acid-labile P (mg/g)	0.8	0.23	72		
Rabbit	Insulin (5 I.U./kg) Time: 2.5 hr	Adrenaline (μmoles/mg protein)	31.8	8.0	75	Decrease in ATP was not statistically significant	3
		ATP (μmoles/mg protein)	9.5	6.8	28		
Sheep	Insulin (12 I.U./kg, i.m.) Time: 20 hr	Catecholamines (mg/g)	10.9—12.2	2.55—3.72	66—79	Analysis of large granule fraction showed no increase in ADP, AMP, adenosine or inorganic phosphate. Ultraviolet spectra showed no increase in adenine derivatives in supernatant	4
		Acid-labile P (mg/g)	0.71—0.79		64—68		
Chicken	Insulin (1000 I.U., i.v.) Time: 3 hr	Catecholamines (mg/g)	3.55—4.16	2.19		Figures refer to content of large granule fraction: insulin only decreased catecholamine and ATP content of adrenals in 1 out of 2 birds	5
		ATP (mg/g)	1.69—2.36	1.32			
Chicken	Insulin (2500 I.U./kg, i.v.) Time: 20 hr	Catecholamines (μg/kg body wt.)	327	229	30	Figures are for the total large granule fraction: the same result was obtained on fractions from a sucrose density gradient	6
		ATP (μg/kg body wt.)	156	114	27		
Chicken	Reserpine (1 mg/kg i.v.) Time: 20 hr	Catecholamines (μg/kg body wt.)	327	94	71	Figures refer to large granule fraction	7
		ATP (μkg/kg)	156	53	66		
Rat	Insulin (10 I.U./kg, s.c.) Time: 3—24 hr	Adrenaline (μg/kg body wt.)	220	56—96	56—74	Greatest fall in catecholamines was after 9 hr; levels began to rise after 24 hr. Greatest fall in ATP after 3 hr; levels began to rise after 6 hr	8
		ATP (μg/kg)	160	51—105	35—58		
Rat	Reserpine (1 mg, i.p.) Time: 16 hr	Catecholamines (μmoles/g)	67	14.5	78		9
		ATP + AMP (μmoles/g)	9.7	3.3	66		
Chicken	Insulin (1000 I.U., i.v.) Time: 20 hr	Catecholamines (μmoles/g)	68.5	41.1	40	After 3 days, the catecholamine and adenine nucleoride content had returned to normal	10
		ATP (μmoles/g)	12.7	6.6	48		
		ADP (μmoles/g)	4.3	2.4	44		
		AMP (μmoles/g)	3.1	1.8	42		

Table 1 (continued)

(a) Analysis of the adrenal medulla

Animal	Stimulus	Substance	Control tissue	Stimulated tissue	Percentage decrease	Notes	Ref.
Chicken	Reserpine (30 mg, i.m.) Time: 5 days	Catecholamines (μmoles/g)	68.5	6.5	95	Note that catecholamine content fell disproportionately further than did that of adenine nucleotides; this was also true for the shortest time interval (1 day). Minimum levels of catecholamines and nucleotides were reached after 5—11 days, but levels remained below normal for more than 3 months	11
		ATP (μmoles/g)	11.6	3.5	70		
		ADP (μmoles/g)	4.8	2.4	50		
		AMP (μmoles/g)	3.4	2.2	35		
Chicken	Reserpine (10 mg, i.v.) Time: 1—3 days	Catecholamines			50—65	The same disproportionately greater fall in catecholamine content compared with nucleotides as in experiments of BURACK et al. (1960) was found in a chromaffin granule fraction	12
Rat	Reserpine (10 mg/kg., i.p.) Time: 1 day	Catecholamines (μmoles/g)	46	2.4	95	4 days after reserpine the catecholamine and ATP levels had returned to 50 % of normal. Data given up to 21 days	13
		(ATP (μmoles/g)	1.6	0.075	95		
Sheep	Reserpine (2—4 mg/kg, s.c.) Time: 13—14 hr	Catecholamines (mg/g)	10.25	0.5	95	Figures for adenine nucleotides refer to a large granule fraction. There was no accumulation of nucleotides in the supernatant	14
		ATP (moles/mole of amine)	0.235	0.19	96		
		ADP (moles/mole of amine)	0.032	not detected			
		AMP (moles/mole of amine)	0.012	not detected			
Rabbit	Splanchnic nerve (20 shocks/sec)	Adrenaline (nmoles/left gland)	407	243	40	A similar result was obtained when a chromaffin granule fraction was analysed	15
		ATP (nmoles/left gland)	273	183	33		
Ox	Perfused gland: carbamylcholine	Catecholamines (μmoles/g)	76	28—44	42—64	Molar ratio catecholamines: nucleotides in control glands was 3.1 and 2.8 in stimulated glands	16
		Adenine nucleotides (μmoles/g)	25	10—15	38—58		

References: 1. CARLSSON and HILLARP (1956); 2. CARLSSON and HILLARP (1956); 3. D'IORIO and EADE (1956), EADE (1957); 4. CARLSSON et al. (1957); 5. SCHÜMANN (1957); 6. SCHÜMANN (1958a); 7. SCHÜMANN (1958a); 8. SCHÜMANN (1958a); 9. KIRPEKAR et al. (1958); 10. WEINER et al. (1960); 11. BURACK et al. (1960); 12. BURACK et al. (1961); 13. KIRPEKAR et al. (1963a); 14. HILLARP (1960b); 15. BANKS (1964); 16. BANKS (1965a).

Table 1 (continued)

(b) Analysis of perfusates from the adrenal gland

Animal	Perfusion fluid	Stimulus	Substance	Content in perfusate	Notes	Ref.
Ox	Tyrode's solution (37°) (Retrograde)	Acetylcholine	Catecholamines (μmoles)	22.7	No ATP, ADP or AMP could be detected, but hypoxanthine and an unidentified purine derivative were found	1
Cat	Locke's solution (22°—25°)	(i) Acetylcholine, Carbamylcholine, Nicotine, K^+, Ca^{2+}	Catecholamines (nmoles/min)	101	Efflux of AMP was also obtained when acetylcholine, K^+ or Ca^{2+} were used as stimulants. AMP content of perfusate was significantly correlated with catecholamine content: mean molar ratio of catecholamines to AMP was 6.4, 70% of ATP infused into gland was recovered as AMP	2
			Total P (nmoles/min)	50		
		(ii) Nicotine	Catecholamines (nmoles/min)	98.2		
			ATP (nmoles/min)	0.2		
			ADP (nmoles/min)	0.3		
			AMP (nmoles/min)	14.1		
Cat	Locke's solution (22°—25°)	(i) Splanchnic nerve (30/sec)	Catecholamines (nmoles/min)	56.5	Molar ratio of catecholamines to AMP was 6.1	3
		(ii) Splanchnic nerve (30/sec)	Catecholamines (nmoles/min)	164	Molar ratio of catecholamines to ATP plus catabolites was 4.22 (mean of 2). Time course of AMP release closely paralleled that of amines; measured at 3 sec intervals	
			ATP (nmoles/min)	0.88		
			ADP (nmoles/min)	0.54		
			AMP (nmoles/min)	26.5		
			Adenosine (nmoles/min)	11.1		
		(iii) Acetylcholine	Catecholamines (nmoles/min)	153	Molar ratio of catecholamines to ATP plus catabolites was 4.22 (mean of 4)	
			ATP (nmoles/min)	1.03		
			ADP (nmoles/min)	0.55		
			AMP (nmoles/min)	29.1		
			Adenosine (nmoles/min)	5.18		
Cat	(i) Locke's solution (22°—25°)	Barium chloride	Catecholamines, ATP, AMP		Mean molar ratios: catecholamines/ATP = 1924 catecholamines/AMP = 8.7	4
	(ii) Locke's solution Ca & Mg-free + EDTA (2 mM)	Barium chloride	Catecholamines, ATP, ATP-catabolites		Mean molar ratios: catecholamines/ATP = 11.1 catecholamines/ATP + catabolites = 4.7	
Ox	Tyrode's solution (Retrograde)	Carbamylcholine	(i) Catecholamines (μmoles/min)	13.5	Molar ratio of catecholamines to ATP = catabolites was 5.7 (mean of 3)	5
			AMP (μmoles/min)	1.1		
			Adenosine (μmoles/min)	0.54		
			Inosine (μmoles/min)	0.32		
			Hypoxanthine (μmoles/min)	0.5		
			(ii) Catecholamines, ATP		Molar ratio of catecholamines to ATP ranged from 105—271	
Cat	Locke's solution (22°—25°)	Acetylcholine	Catecholamines, AMP		Molar ratio of catecholamines to AMP = 6.75	6
		Amphetamine	Catecholamines, AMP		Molar ratio of catecholamines to AMP = 6.22	
		Phenylethylamine	Catecholamines, AMP		Molar ratio of catecholamines to AMP = 6.76	

References: 1. Stjärne (1964); 2. Douglas et al. (1965); 3. Douglas and Poisner (1966a); 4. Douglas and Poisner (1966b); 5. Banks (1966a); 6. Rubin and Jaanus (1967).

release. A possible explanation of EADE and D'IORIO's (1956) result, suggested by WEINER et al. (1960), is that in the rabbit the resynthesis of ATP may be very rapid and may precede that of the catecholamines. SCHÜMANN (1958a) found just this in his studies on the rat: the ATP content of the adrenal gland began to rise 6 hr after the administration of insulin, whereas the catecholamine content did not begin to rise until 18 hr later. We can conclude that, in several species, the reflex or direct neural stimulation of the adrenal medulla leads to a parallel decrease in the catecholamine and adenine nucleotide content of the chromaffin granules.

The action of reserpine on the adrenal medulla is complex, since it not only acts directly on the chromaffin cell and indirectly via the central nervous system, but, in addition, the dose required varies according to the species (MUSCHOLL and VOGT, 1958) and according to the strain within a particular species (COUPLAND, 1958). Accordingly, the results of the experiments in which the adenine nucleotide content of the adrenal medulla was analysed, following administration of reserpine, are difficult to interpret. In the chicken, a low dose of reserpine caused a parallel loss of ATP and catecholamines (SCHÜMANN, 1958a) but higher doses caused a greater loss of amines than of nucleotides (BURACK et al., 1960, 1961). Possibly, a low dose of reserpine acts via the nervous system, whereas higher doses act both centrally and directly on the chromaffin cells (see COUPLAND, 1965a). This suggestion is consistent with the action of insulin in the chicken, which causes the reflex stimulation of the adrenal medulla and is associated with a parallel fall in the adrenal catecholamine and ATP content (SCHÜMANN, 1958a; WEINER et al., 1960). In order to distinguish between the direct action of reserpine and that via the nervous system, experiments should be performed in which the animals have been pretreated with potent ganglion-blocking agents. Until such experiments are done, we can only tentatively conclude that when reserpine acts on the adrenal medulla via the central nervous system it causes a parallel fall in adenine nucleotide and catecholamine concentrations, whereas when it acts directly on the gland it tends to release the catecholamines but not the nucleotides from chromaffin granules.

In several of the early studies, it was found that the fall in the concentration of adenine nucleotides after stimulation with insulin was not accompanied by a rise in the ADP, AMP, adenosine, or inorganic phosphate content of the large granule fraction or of any other fraction of the adrenal homogenate. It was suggested, therefore, that "apparently the adenine part of the lost ATP had disappeared from the adrenal medullary cells" (CARLSSON et al., 1957). However, it was not until seven years later that studies on the perfused adrenal gland were described: STJÄRNE (1964) identified hypoxanthine in the perfusates from ox adrenals stimulated with acetylcholine, and also reported the presence of another purine derivative in the perfusate. Quantitative studies by DOUGLAS et al. (1965), DOUGLAS and POISNER (1966a, b) and by BANKS (1966a) established that several catabolites of ATP were present in the perfusates from cat and ox adrenal glands during stimulation. Although the catabolites differed according to the species (probably because the ox gland was perfused at a higher temperature and in a retrograde fashion), it was striking that the molar ratios in the perfusates of catecholamines: ATP + catabolites ranged from 4.22 (cat adrenal) to 5.7 (ox adrenal) which are not far from the ratios of 3.7 (HILLARP and THIEME, 1959) and of 4.0 (HILLARP, 1960a) found in the nucleotide-rich chromaffin granules isolated from the respective glands.

By perfusing the cat adrenal gland with Ca^{2+}- and Mg^{2+}- free Locke's solution containing EDTA, DOUGLAS and POISNER (1966b) showed that, with barium chloride as a stimulant, a considerable amount of unmetabolised ATP was recovered in the perfusate. They suggested that, normally, the ATP released from chromaffin granules is broken down in the blood vessels. This breakdown must be rapid, because the release of AMP upon splanchnic nerve stimulation is simultaneous with the release of catecholamines (DOUGLAS and POISNER, 1966a).

We can conclude that the experiments carried out both *in vivo* and *in vitro* are consistent with the release of most, if not all, of the ATP from the nucleotide-rich chromaffin granules, together with the catecholamines, when the adrenal medulla is stimulated via the splanchnic nerve, by typical cholinergic stimulants (acetylcholine, carbamylcholine, nicotine), by amphetamine or phenylethylamine (which act via cholinoceptors) and by the ions K^+, Ca^{2+} or Ba^{2+}.

2. Fate of the Soluble Proteins (Chromogranins) of Chromaffin Granules

Observations on the proteins (a) of particulate fractions from adrenal medulla and (b) of perfusates from adrenal glands following stimulation are summarised in Table 2. Many of the early studies measured only the total protein content of the large granule fraction, a fraction now known to contain mitochondria and lysosomes in addition to chromaffin granules.

The possibility that changes in the protein composition of these other cell particles may have been caused by stimulation should not, therefore, be forgotten. Indeed, it has been found that small amounts of several lysosomal enzymes are secreted from the ox adrenal gland in response to carbamylcholine (SCHNEIDER, 1968a, b; 1969b, 1970; SMITH, 1969), although the amount of protein represented by these enzymes is likely to be very small. It can be calculated that the amount of a lysosomal enzyme released per minute by carbamylcholine is only about 0.1% of the total amount of the enzyme in the adrenal medulla, whereas about 1% of the total catecholamines are released per minute (SCHNEIDER, 1970).

The chromaffin granules of ox adrenal medulla contain 50% of the protein present in the large granule fraction (calculated from the data of SMITH and WINKLER, 1966) and so any changes in the protein content of the chromaffin granules would be expected to show up in analyses of the large granule fraction. Decreases in the protein contents of the large granule fractions of rat and sheep adrenals following stimulation were reported by CARLSSON and HILLARP (1956) and CARLSSON et al. (1957). The changes observed were not large compared with the decreases in catecholamine content, and were interpreted cautiously: "Although the data so far available argue against a profound damage of the granule membrane, they seem to indicate a certain loss of protein from the granules" (CARLSSON et al., 1957). These authors compared the observed loss of protein with that expected if all the soluble proteins of the chromaffin granules (thought, then, to be 50% of the total) were lost from the granules together with the catecholamines: the figures for three experiments on sheep adrenal medulla, taken from Table 2 of CARLSSON et al. (1957), are given in Table 3. In the right-hand column of the table we have given the calculated loss of protein using more recent data on the protein content of chromaffin granules. A rather striking agreement is revealed between the original observations and the predicted changes calculated from the new data. Such agreement may, of course, be fortuitous but it is entirely consistent with the disappearance from the chromaffin granules of the soluble proteins upon release of the catecholamines. Analyses of fractions from sucrose density gradients which contain the chromaffin granules have shown that both *in vivo* after insulin (SCHÜMANN, 1958a) and *in vitro* after perfusion with acetylcholine (POISNER et al., 1967) the protein content of the fraction falls. These experiments do not tell us anything about the fate of the protein after it leaves the chromaffin granules. Does the protein remain within the cell, free in the cytosol, or is it secreted from the cell? Evidence that the chromogranins are indeed secreted has come from experiments in which more specific methods of assay were used. The amount of dopamine β-hydroxylase in rabbit adrenal glands decreases after stimulation with insulin (see Fig. 4) and the loss was mainly from the soluble moiety of the large granule fraction (VIVEROS et al., 1969b, c). It could always be argued that the decreased activity of dopamine β-hydroxylase in the adrenal gland after stimulation was due

Table 2. *Fate of chromaffin granule proteins upon stimulation of the adrenal medulla*

(a) Analysis of the gland

Animal	Stimulus	Fraction of homogenate	Control tissue	Stimulated tissue	Percentage decrease	Notes	Ref.
Rat	Insulin (10 I.U./100 g, s.c.) 5 hr	6800 g for 60 min sediment	48.7 mg protein/g tissue	42.7	12	71 % depletion of catecholamines	1
Sheep	Insulin (12 I.U./kg, i.m.) 17—20 hr	7000 g for 60 min sediment	22—26 mg protein/g tissue	14.5—19	20—32	66—79 % depletion of catecholamines (see also Table 3)	
Chicken	(i) Insulin (2500 I.U., i.v.) 20 hr	800 g for 10 min supernatant centrifuged at 12000 g for 15 min. sediment on density gradient (1.4 M—2.0 M-sucrose): 142000 g for 30 min:				30 % decrease in catecholamines. Increased amount of protein in less dense layer of gradient compensates for loss in denser layer	3
		2 fractions 1.6—1.8 M layer	29 μg N/kg body wt.	52	(79 % increase)		
		1.8—2.0 M layer	81	58	29		
	(ii) Reserpine (1 mg/kg, i.v.) 20 hr	As above: 2 fractions 1.6—1.8 M	29 μg N/kg	60	(107 % increase)	71 % decrease in catecholamines	
		1.8—2.0 M	81	57	30		
Sheep	Reserpine (2—4 mg/kg, s.c.) 13—14 hr	800 g for 6 min		15.4	43	95 % decrease in catecholamines. Redistribution of protein after reserpine: less recovered in large granule fraction, more in supernatant	4
		supernatant centrifuged at 23000 g for 20 min	27 mg protein/g tissue	15.4			
Chicken	Reserpine (10 mg, i.v.) 1—3 days	800 g for 10 min		35.6	0	No change in proportion of total protein recovered in large granule fraction. Catecholamines depleted by 55—65 %.	5
		supernatant centrifuged at 12000 g for 20 min	34.4 mg protein/g tissue				
Ox	Acetylcholine (perfused gland)	20000 g for 20 min sediment on density gradient (1.4 M—1.8 M-sucrose): 145000 g for 60 min. 1.8 M-sucrose layer analysed	1.2 mg protein/g tissue	0.35	71	Catecholamine content of fraction decreased by about 90 %	6

Table 2 (continued)

(a) Analysis of the gland

Animal	Stimulus	Fraction of homogenate	Control tissue	Stimulated tissue	Percentage decrease	Notes	Ref.
Rabbit	(i) Insulin (40 I.U./kg, i.v.) 3 hr	26000 g for 20 min sediment	Dopamine β-hydroxylase: 61 units/g tissue	38	38	Catecholamine content of fraction was 42 % of normal. 81 % of the decrease in dopamine β-hydroxylase in the gland was accounted for by the loss from the large granule fraction. Data for 3—144 hr given in Fig. 4	7
	(ii) Reserpine (1 mg/kg, i.v.) 24 hr	as above				No change in dopamine β-hydroxylase content of gland or of large granule fraction: catecholamines fell by 70 %	
	(iii) Reserpine (5 mg/kg, i.v.) 24 hr	Whole gland	Dopamine β-hydroxylase: 273 units/g tissue	95	75	Catecholamine content fell by 98 %	
Rabbit	Insulin (40 I.U./kg, i.v.)	26000 g sediment lysed with water to give soluble lysate and insoluble residue	Dopamine β-hydroxylase: 53.5 units/g tissue	32	40	Most of the decrease in dopamine β-hydroxylase occurred from soluble lysate. Similar results after high dose of reserpine could be prevented by administration of ganglion blocker	8
Rabbit	(i) Insulin (40 I.U./kg, i.v.) 4 hr	26000 g sediment on density gradient (1.0 M—2.25 M sucrose). Fraction from 1.6 M—2.5 M sucrose analysed	Dopamine β-hydroxylase: 0.82 units/2 glands	0.1	88	Catecholamine content of the fraction decreased by 84 %, but the ratio of dopamine β-hydroxylase activity to catecholamines in the fraction did not change	
	(ii) Reserpine (1 mg/kg) 24 hr	As above				55 % depletion of catecholamine content of gland, but only 15 % fall in dopamine β-hydroxylase. On the density gradient the peak of amine and enzyme was in a less dense region, and the enzyme to amine ratio was greater than normal	

References: 1. Carlsson and Hillarp (1956); 2. Carlsson et al. (1957); 3. Schümann (1958a); 4. Hillarp (1960b); 5. Burack et al. (1961); 6. Poisner et al. (1967); 7. Viveros et al. (1969b); 8. Viveros et al. (1969c); 9. Viveros et al. (1969d).

Table 2 (continued)

(b) Analysis of perfusate or blood leaving the gland

Animal	Perfusion fluid	Stimulus	Substance	Content in perfusate	Notes	Ref.
Ox	Tyrode's solution (37°) Retrograde perfusion	Carbamylcholine	Catecholamines (μmoles) Protein (mg)	7—15 0.7—2.3	Average of 6.6 μmoles catecholamines secreted per mg protein released. Protein in stimulation period perfusates cross-reacted with antiserum to chromogranin A by immunodiffusion test	1
Ox	Locke's solution (22°—33°) Retrograde (2—4 ml/min)	Acetylcholine and nicotine	Catecholamines (μmoles/min) Chromogranin A (mg/min)	0.12—0.82 0.017—0.084	Mean of ratio catecholamines: protein in stimulation period perfusates was 11.5, and in adrenal glands was 7.1	2
Ox	Locke's solution (30°) Retrograde (2—4 ml/min)	Acetylcholine	Catecholamines (μmoles/min) Chromogranin A (mg/min)	0.3—0.33 0.029—0.032	Chromogranin A in perfusate identified by immunoelectrophoresis and estimated by complement fixation	3
Ox	Locke's solution (30°) Retrograde (2—4 ml/min)	Acetylcholine	Catecholamines (μmoles/min) Chromogranin A (mg/min)	0.012—0.78 0.012—0.094	Slight time lag (c. 1 min) in release of chromogranin A compared with amines. Ca^{2+} was required for acetylcholine and nicotine induced release of amines and chromogranin. Mean of ratio catecholamine: chromogranin A secreted was 9.8, and was 8.75 in large granule fraction of the same glands analysed after perfusion. In control period perfusates the catecholamine: chromogranin A ratio was 17	4
		Nicotine	Catecholamines (μmoles/min) Chromogranin A (mg/min)	0.59—0.72 0.066—0.084		
		$BaCl_2$	Catecholamines (μmoles/min) Chromogranin A (mg/min)	0.84—1.34 0.064—0.142		
Calf	Blood (*in vivo*) (C.10 ml/min)	Splanchnic nerve (30/sec)	Catecholamines (μmoles/ml plasma) Chromogranin A (mg/ml)	0.02—0.07 0.001—0.005	Ratios of catecholamines: chromogranin A ranged from 3.3—11.3. Release of protein continued after that of catecholamines	5
Ox	Tyrode's solution (37°) Retrograde (7—20 ml/min)	Carbamylcholine	Catecholamines (μmoles/min) Total protein (mg/min) Chromogranin A (mg/min)	0.4—3.1 0.02—0.6 0.01—0.3	At a flow rate of 9 ml/min there was a slight time lag in release of protein but not at 13 ml/min. Ca^{2+} was required for release of catecholamines and protein. Mean of ratio catecholamine: total protein secreted was 4.8, compared with 4.8 in soluble lysate of chromaffin granules. Mean of ratio catecholamine: chromogranin A secreted was 11.9, compared with 10.1 in soluble lysate of chromaffin granules. 8 different proteins were identified by starch gel electrophoresis of the perfusate: their mobilities and relative proportions corresponded to those of the chromogranins, Amino acid composition of secreted proteins was similar to that of chromogranins	6

Table 2 (continued)

(b) Analysis of perfusate or blood leaving the gland

Animal	Perfusion fluid	Stimulus	Substance	Content in perfusate	Notes	Ref.
Calf	Locke's solution (25°) 10 ml/min via artery *in situ*	Acetylcholine	Catecholamines (μmoles/min) Protein (mg/min)	0.21—0.72 0.04—0.67	Ratio catecholamine: protein was about 1 (one experiment)	7
Cow	Locke's solution (30°) Retrograde (3.8 ml/min)	Acetylcholine or nicotine	Catecholamines (μmoles/min) Dopamine β-hydroxylase (units/min)	0.53 1032	Control period perfusates contained one third as much catecholamine and dopamine β-hydroxylase. Release of amines and enzyme was inhibited when calcium was left out of perfusion fluid. Mean of ratio dopamine β-hydroxylase: catecholamines in control period perfusate was 1960, in the stimulation period perfusate was 2000, and in large granule fraction from control gland was 1550	8
Ox	Tyrode's solution (37°) Retrograde (10—14 ml/min)	Carbambylcholine β-phenylethylamine	Catecholamines Total protein Chromogranin A		Mean of ratios catecholamines: total proteins in perfusates was 4.81 μmoles/mg (carbamylcholine) and 2.61 (β-phenylethylamine). Mean of ratios catecholamines: chromogranin A was 14.9 μmoles/mg (carbamylcholine) and 13.5 (β-phenylethylamine). Release of amines and proteins by carbachol was abolished in calcium-free media, but the release induced by β-phenylethylamine was only inhibited by 62—71%. Cocaine (30 μg/ml) and hexamethonium (250 μg/ml) prevented release of amines and proteins induced by carbachol	9
Ox	Medulla dissected free of cortex. Tyrode's solution (37°) Retrograde (10—15 ml/min)	Carbamylcholine	Catecholamines Total protein		Confirmed quantitative results of SCHNEIDER et al. (1967) on whole gland. Proteins released has same pattern in polyacrylamide gel electrophoresis as chromogranins.	10
Ox	Tyrode's solution (37°) Retrograde (10—15 ml/min)	$BaCl_2$	Catecholamines (μmoles/min) Total protein (mg/min)	1.3—4.3 0.3—0.85	Mean of ratio catecholamines: protein was 4.73 (cf. 4.8 in soluble lysate of chromaffin granules). Hexamethonium (30 mM) did not prevent release of proteins and amines. Pattern of the released proteins in polyacrylamide gel electrophoresis was identical with that of the chromogranins	11
Ox	Tyrode's solution (37°) Retrograde (5 ml/min)	Carbamylcholine	Catecholamines Proteins		After infusion of radioactive tyrosine or leucine, radioactively labelled proteins were released: these gave the same gel electrophoretic pattern as the chromogranins	12

References: 1. BANKS and HELLE (1965); 2. KIRSHNER et al. (1966); 3. SAGE et al. (1967); 4. KIRSHNER et al. (1967); 5. BLASCHKO et al. (1967a); 6. SCHNEIDER et al. (1967); 7. TRIFARÓ et al. (1967); 8. VIVEROS et al. (1968); 9. SCHNEIDER (1969a); 10. SCHNEIDER (1969b); 11. SMITH and DE POTTER (1969); 12. WINKLER et al. (1970b).

to its inactivation or destruction within the cell, rather than to its secretion from the cell. This can be tested by the direct analysis of perfusates or of the venous blood leaving the adrenal gland.

Table 3. *Loss of protein from large granule fraction of sheep adrenal medullae after stimulation.* In each experiment, the observed difference (CARLSSON et al., 1957) between the control and the insulin-treated animal is given. This value is compared with the calculated loss of protein if the loss of catecholamines is associated with destruction of the chromaffin granule membrane such that the soluble proteins escape. (a) The original calculation of CARLSSON et al. (1957) based on the assumptions that all the protein in the large granule fraction is in chromaffin granules and that 50% of the protein is soluble, (b) A calculation based on the fact that only 50% of the protein in the large granule fraction is in chromaffin granules (SMITH and WINKLER, 1966) and that 77% of the chromaffin granule protein is soluble (HILLARP, 1958)

Experiment No.	Observed Loss	Calculated Loss (a)	Calculated Loss (b)
1	20%	36%	27%
2	23%	34%	26%
3	32%	43%	33%
Mean (± S.D)	25.0±6.2	37.7±4.7	28.7±3.7

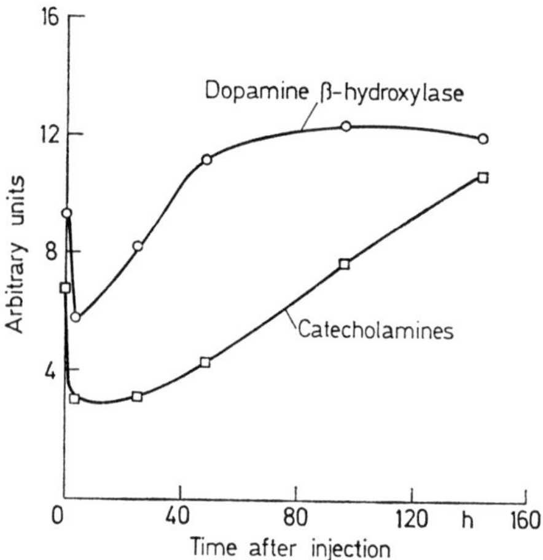

Fig. 4. *Effect of administration of insulin to rabbits on the catecholamine and dopamine β-hydroxylase content of the large granule fraction of adrenal glands.* The graph is plotted from data given by VIVEROS et al. (1969b)

During his studies on the fate of the ATP released upon stimulation of the perfused ox adrenal gland, BANKS noticed that the acidified perfusates collected during stimulation were more turbid then those collected in between periods of stimulation. He showed that this turbidity was due to the presence of increased amounts of protein in the perfusates. The ratio of the amount of catecholamines to that of protein in the perfusates collected during stimulation was quite close to this ratio in the soluble lysate of purified chromaffin granules (BANKS and HELLE, 1965). At the time of these experiments, HELLE (1966b) had just prepared anti-serum to bovine adrenal chromogranin A, and it was found that the protein in the stimulation period perfusates cross-reacted with this antiserum (BANKS and HELLE, 1965). This important discovery opened up the possibility of applying quantitative immunochemical and biochemical methods to compare the protein composition of the perfusate from adrenal glands with that of purified adrenal chromaffin granules.

It was soon shown by KIRSHNER et al. (1966, 1967), who used a complement-fixation method to estimate chromogranin A, that the ratio catecholamines: chromogranin A in perfusates was close to that in whole adrenal glands and in the large granule fraction. After stimulation of the splanchnic nerve in the calf, chromogranin A was found in the adrenal venous blood and the ratio catecholamines: chromogranin A was similar to that in the soluble lysate of chromaffin granules (BLASCHKO et al., 1967a). These studies all show that the release of chromogranin A is not just a result of leakage of small amounts of the protein out of the gland; rather, there is an almost stoichiometric release of this protein from the chromaffin granules. Further work revealed that chromogranin A is not the only protein released: by means of starch gel electrophoresis, eight different proteins (including chromogranin A) were identified in perfusates collected during stimulation of the ox adrenal medulla (SCHNEIDER et al., 1967). These proteins not only had the same mobility as the chromogranins, they were also present in the perfusate in the same relative proportions as they occur in chromaffin granules. We can conclude that the agreement between the ratio catecholamines: total protein in perfusates and this ratio in the soluble lysate of chromaffin granules (BANKS and HELLE, 1965; SCHNEIDER et al., 1967) must be accounted for by the quantitative secretion of the entire soluble protein content of the chromaffin granules.

The enzyme dopamine β-hydroxylase, now known to be present in the soluble lysate as well as in the insoluble residue of chromaffin granules (see Section A. I, 1.), gives rise to the faintly-staining, slowest running band in gel electrophoretograms of the chromogranins (SMITH et al., 1970), and this band was seen (but not then identified) in electrophoretograms of stimulation period perfusates by SCHNEIDER et al. (1967). VIVEROS et al. (1968), using a more sensitive method of assay for dopamine β-hydroxylase activity than in previous work (KIRSHNER et al., 1966, 1967), showed that this enzyme is secreted into the perfusate in response to acetylcholine. The ratio dopamine β-hydroxylase activity: catecholamines in the perfusate was 2000, which is considerably greater than the value of 775 predicted if just the soluble part of the enzymic activity is released from the chromaffin granules. Further studies (N. KIRSHNER, personal communication) showed that this finding was due to the difficulty in measuring the activity of the enzyme in tissues which also contain inhibitors (DUCH et al., 1968; NAGATSU et al., 1967; BELPAIRE and LADURON, 1970): when care was taken to measure the enzyme activity under optimal conditions, the ratios in the perfusates and in the soluble lysate were in good agreement.

The early *in vivo* studies on the protein content of the large granule fraction, and the more recent work on the levels of dopamine β-hydroxylase activity in adrenal glands after stimulation, are clearly consistent with the observations on perfused glands and we can conclude that the chromogranins are secreted, nearly quantitatively, together with the catecholamines when the adrenal medulla is stimulated via the splanchnic nerve, or by cholinergic drugs, or by barium ions.

The action of reserpine on chromaffin granule proteins is more complex and can only be studied *in vivo*. VIVEROS et al. (1969b, c) found that injection of rabbits with low doses of reserpine decreased the catecholamine content of the large granule fraction without changing the amount of dopamine β-hydroxylase; higher doses of reserpine were found to cause a large fall in both the catecholamine and dopamine β-hydroxylase content. The depletion of dopamine β-hydroxylase, but not that of catecholamines, by high doses of reserpine could be prevented by pretreatment of the rabbits with a ganglion blocking agent (chlorisondamine) and so it was suggested (VIVEROS et al., 1969b, c) that low doses of reserpine act directly on the chromaffin cell (by inhibiting the active uptake of catecholamines into the chromaffin granules), and that the higher doses act both directly and via the central nervous system. Although this interpretation seems to be consistent with the observations, it is contrary to much previous work which has led to the conclusion (see COUPLAND, 1965a, pp. 138—140) that low doses of reserpine deplete adrenal catecholamines by a central action, whereas high doses act both centrally and directly. Perhaps the finding (VIVEROS et al., 1969c) that the sensitivity of rabbits to reserpine depends upon their living conditions is related to these contradictory observations.

The fact that, under certain conditions, the action of reserpine on the dopamine β-hydroxylase content of the adrenal gland differed from that of insulin, is consistent with the idea that the direct action of this alkaloid on chromaffin cells is to decrease the ability of the chromaffin granules to store the catecholamines, without at the same time affecting the storage of any macromolecular components of the chromaffin granules. This action of reserpine corresponds to release by mechanism 1 (see Fig. 3). Reserpine may act (a) by decreasing the stability of the 'storage complex' (BERNEIS et al., 1970) and/or (b) by inhibiting the ATP-dependent uptake of catecholamines (KIRSHNER, 1962; CARLSSON et al., 1963; VIVEROS et al., 1969b) and/or (c) by increasing the permeability of the chromaffin granule membrane to catecholamines. Further experimental evidence in favour of this general mechanism, but which does not distinguish between a, b or c, was provided by VIVEROS et al. (1969d) who showed that chromaffin granules from the adrenals of reserpine treated rabbits had lost most of their adrenaline but not their dopamine β-hydroxylase. The decreased content of adrenaline caused the dopamine β-hydroxylase-rich chromaffin granules to equilibrate in a less dense region of the density gradient. It would be of interest to know whether these modified chromaffin granules contained the same amount of ATP as normal granules, since there is some evidence that ATP is not depleted after reserpine treatment (see p. 550).

3. Fate of the Insoluble Proteins and Lipids of Chromaffin Granules

The insoluble residue remaining after lysis of ox chromaffin granules contains 22% of the total protein, all the phospholipids and cholesterol, 50% of the dopamine β-hydroxylase activity, but only traces of chromogranin A (see WINKLER et al., 1970a). The insoluble residue must contain, and may consist entirely of, the chromaffin granule membranes. Knowledge of the composition of the membrane has been used to study the question whether secretion takes place by expulsion of the entire chromaffin granule from the cell (mechanism 2b in Fig. 3) or by a mechanism in which the membrane remains behind in the cell.

Perfusates from the ox adrenal gland contain small amounts of phospholipid and cholesterol but only slight (SCHNEIDER et al., 1967; SCHNEIDER, 1969b) or insignificant (TRIFARÓ et al., 1967) increases in the amounts of these lipids occurred in perfusates collected from glands stimulated with carbamylcholine or acetylcholine. For each μmole of catecholamines in purified ox adrenal chromaffin granules there are 0.18 μmoles of phospholipid and 0.102 μmoles of cholesterol, whereas for each μmole of catecholamines secreted from stimulated glands there were only 0.0012 μmoles of phospholipid and 0.0009 μmoles of cholesterol released into the perfusate (SCHNEIDER et al., 1967). Thus, the increments in the amounts of phospholipid or cholesterol are each less than 1% of what would be expected if the whole chromaffin granule was released into the perfusate.

Analyses of perfused ox adrenal glands stimulated with acetylcholine showed that the cholesterol and phospholipid content of the large granule fraction remained unchanged even when there was a 40% fall in the catecholamine content (POISNER et al., 1967). When this large granule fraction was subjected to density gradient centrifugation, there were decreases of 58% and 46.5%, respectively, in the phospholipid and cholesterol content of the chromaffin granule fraction (1.8 M—2.5 M-sucrose layer); most of the 'lost' lipid was recovered in the upper layers (1.4 M-sucrose) of the gradient (POISNER et al., 1967). The empty membranes of hypo-osmotically shocked chromaffin granules were also recovered in this upper layer after density gradient centrifugation (POISNER et al., 1967). Thus, although the lipids of the chromaffin granule remain in particles which sediment in the large granule fraction, the particles no longer sediment to the dense layers in a sucrose gradient. This may not only be because the particles are less dense than normal chromaffin granules, it could also be because they are smaller and have not reached their equilibrium density.

Annother way of studying the fate of the chromaffin granule membrane is to use the insoluble proteins as markers. These proteins include a cytochrome, a Mg-activated nucleoside triphosphatase and the insoluble dopamine β-hydroxylase (see WINKLER et al., 1970a for further details and references). Dopamine β-hydroxylase is the only protein which has so far been used as a marker. This enzyme is about equally distributed between soluble lysate and insoluble residue of ox adrenal chromaffin granules (DUCH, et al., 1968; BELPAIRE and LADURON, 1968; WINKLER et al., 1970a) and between 22% (VIVEROS et al., 1969a) and 52% (VIVEROS et al., 1969c) is soluble in rabbit chromaffin granules. In their studies on the catecholamine and dopamine β-hydroxylase contents of rabbit adrenal glands, VIVEROS et al., (1969b) found that 3 hr after the injection of insulin the catecholamine content of the large granule fraction had decreased by 58%, whereas the dopamine β-hydroxylase activity had only fallen by 38% (see Fig. 4); the ratio of dopamine β-hydroxylase activity to catecholamines in the large granule fraction was, therefore, greater than in the control animals. This is evidence against the release of intact chromaffin granules. Further studies (VIVEROS et al., 1969c) showed that about 80% of the decrease of dopamine β-hydroxylase in the large granule fraction was caused by loss of the enzyme from the soluble contents of chromaffin granules. Part of the insoluble dopamine β-hydroxylase was recovered in the microsomal fraction, and that which remained in the large granule fraction was recovered in fractions near the top of a sucrose density gradient (1.2 M-sucrose layer), above the layer of residual chromaffin granules (VIVEROS et al., 1969c, d). Since these analyses were done 3—4 hr after insulin administration, it seems unlikely that the changes in distribution of dopamine β-hydroxylase were related to resynthesis of the enzyme (which occurred after 1 day). The most probable interpretation of these results is that the soluble dopamine β-hydroxylase of chromaffin granules is released from the gland, but that all the membrane-bound enzyme remains behind, most being recovered in the upper layers of the density gradient of the large granule fraction, and part in the microsomal fraction.

There has been only one report of electron microscopic studies on fractions isolated from homogenates of stimulated adrenal medulla (MALAMED et al., 1968). These authors used a filtration method (OKA et al., 1966), which supposedly removes particles larger than chromaffin granules, in order to isolate chromaffin granules. Analysis of a fraction from a control perfused gland showed many typical chromaffin granules of diameter up to 450 mμ. Similar fractions obtained from adrenals which had been perfused with acetylcholine, until their catecholamine content was about 20% of normal, contained only a few intact chromaffin granules but many electron-lucent vesicles ranging in diameter from 30—370 mμ. Although no statistical data were reported, it appears from the published micrographs that the fractions from stimulated glands contained a larger proportion of small vesicles than the control. So far, there have been no morphological studies on fractions well characterised by biochemical methods, and so it is only possible to conclude that the fraction which, from normal glands, contained morphologically identifiable chromaffin granules, contained mainly membranous vesicles when isolated from stimulated glands.

4. Correlation of the Biochemical Evidence with Ultrastructural Observations

The ability to separate the chromaffin granule from other cell particles has led to a fairly precise knowledge of its chemical composition. Accordingly, it is possible to make quantitative predictions concerning the fate of the other constituents of the chromaffin granule when the catecholamines are secreted. As a way of summarising this section, we have shown in Fig. 5 what can be predicted about the changes in the composition of stimulated adrenal glands and of the perfusates from stimulated glands on the hypothesis that the entire chromaffin granule passes out of the cell into the perfusate. The predicted changes, which were calculated from changes in the amounts of the catecholamines, are compared with the observations reported in literature which we have described above. The conclusions that can be drawn from Fig. 5 are:

1. The soluble components of the nucleotide-rich chromaffin granules disappear from the gland and are quantitatively recovered in the perfusate.

2. The insoluble (membrane-bound) components of the chromaffin granules are not released into the perfusate, and are quantitatively retained in the gland.

This biochemical evidence shows that the reports by microscopists (CRAMER, 1918; COSTERO et al., 1965; BENEDECZKY, 1966a; see also BACHMANN, 1954) of intact chromaffin granules in the sinusoids of the adrenal gland are unrelated to the *normal* mode of release of the catecholamines. Likewise, the remarkable type of apocrine secretion observed by BENEDECZKY (1966b) in chick embryos which had been refrigerated, does not happen in the gland stimulated by acetylcholine. Although the biochemical evidence excludes the release of intact chromaffin granules into the perfusate, the possibility remains that the chromaffin granules are released into the extracellular space where they might disintegrate, leaving residual membranes which would not penetrate into the blood vessels. With this minor qualification, we can say that the biochemical evidence excludes the release of the intact chromaffin granule (mechanism 2b of Fig. 3).

What morphological evidence can account for the quantitative and nearly simultaneous release of the soluble constituents of the chromaffin granules? The discovery of the release of high molecular weight proteins has narrowed the choice of mechanisms. We can now exclude those in which only low molecular weight substances pass across cell membranes (mechanisms 1a, b of Fig. 3). Three mechanisms remain: dissolution of the chromaffin granule membrane followed by diffusion of the substances across the cytosol (mechanism 1c); diffusion of the substan-

---

Fig. 5. *Fate of components of the chromaffin granule upon stimulation of the adrenal medulla.* The stippled columns give the observed change in the amount of each substance. The open columns indicate the predicted change in the amount of each substance if the intact chromaffin granule is released from the tissue. On the left: changes in the content of stimulated adrenal glands relative to control glands. On the right: composition of perfusates from stimulated adrenal glands relative to the amount of catecholamines. The scale on the right is the amount of each substance relative to 100 μmoles of catecholamines and the units are: ATP (μmoles), protein (mg) dopamine β-hydroxylase (10^{-8} moles of octopamine/15 min), chromogranin A (mg), phospholipid (μmoles), cholesterol (μmoles), lysolecithin (μmoles). With the exeption of the studies on the lipids, all the observations on the composition of the adrenal gland were done following stimulation *in vivo* by administration of insulin. The other experiments were all done on perfused glands which were stimulated by cholinergic drugs (see Table 2 for details). References: (1) CARLSSON and HILLARP (1956), (2) CARLSSON et al. (1957), (3) SCHÜMANN (1958), (4) WEINER et al. (1960), (5) CARLSSON et al. (1957), (6) Viveros et al. (1969c), (7) VIVEROS et al. (1969d), (8) POISNER et al. (1967), (9) DOUGLAS and POISNER (1966a), (10) BANKS (1966a), (11) SCHNEIDER et al. (1967), (12) VIVEROS et al. (1968), (13) KIRSHNER et al. (1967), (14) TRIFARÓ et al. (1967)

ces across a 'tight junction' formed between the chromaffin granule membrane and the cell membrane (mechanism 2a); and exocytosis (mechanism 2c). There is morphological evidence consistent with each of these three mechanisms, and so we shall have to turn again to biochemical studies to see whether a final choice can be made.

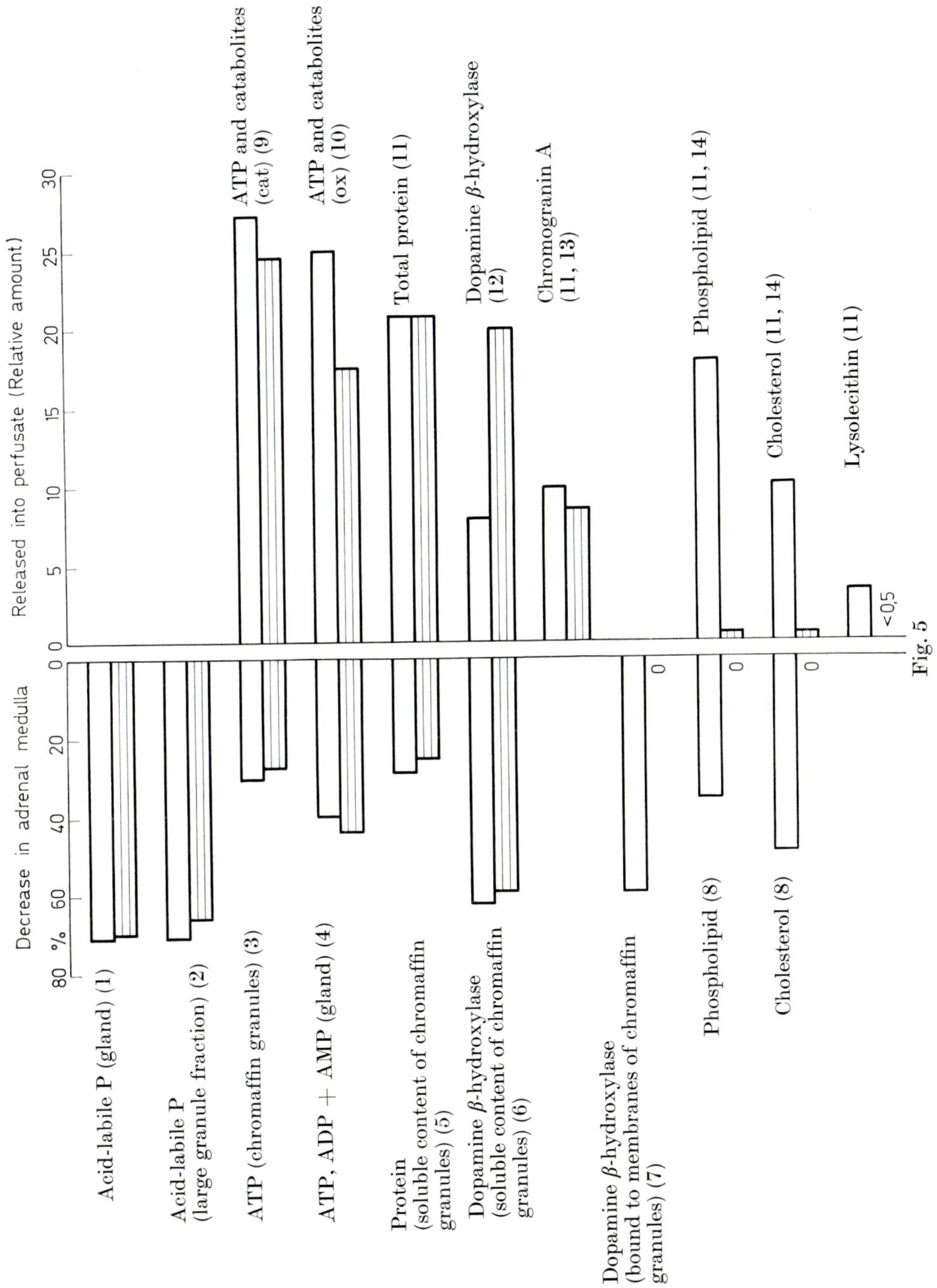

Fig. 5

A mechanism in which discontinuities form in the limiting membrane of the chromaffin granules, as suggested by LEVER and FINDLAY (1966) on the basis of their electron microscopic studies, would allow the chromogranins to enter the cytosol. It is then necessary to postulate either similar discontinuities in the cell membrane, or some specific carriers which might transport the chromogranins across the cell membrane. The discontinuities, or pores, in the cell membrane would have to be large enough to allow the chromogranins to pass through. A molecule of chromogranin A has a large effective hydrodynamic volume which decreases with increasing ionic strength; at an ionic strength of 0.3 the diameter of the molecule is about 120 Å (calculated from the data of SMITH and WINKLER, 1967b). Two lines of evidence argue against a mechanism in which catecholamines and chromogranins free in the cytosol pass through pores in the cell membrane: 1. the lack of release of other proteins normally present in the cytosol, and 2. the nearly simultaneous release of all the soluble components of the chromaffin granule.

1. Upon stimulation of the ox adrenal, there is no detectable release of three enzymes located in the cytosol of the chromaffin cell: tyrosine hydroxylase (VIVEROS et al., 1968), phenylethanolamine-N-methyltransferase (KIRSHNER et al., 1967), and lactate dehydrogenase (SCHNEIDER et al., 1967). Thc significance of these observations depends on the sensitivity of the method of assay, on the size of the protein molecules relative to that of chromogranin A, and on the numbers of molecules of each enzyme in the cytosol relative to that of chromogranin A. The assay method for phenylethanolamine-N-methyltransferase could have detected the enzyme in the perfusate if present in a concentration one tenth of that in the cytosol (KIRSHNER et al., 1967). Knowing the specific activity of lactate dehydrogenase in the cytosol, SCHNEIDER et al. (1967) were able to conclude that if only 1% of the amount of protein secreted upon stimulation had been derived from the cytosol it would have been possible to detect this. The phenylethanolamine-N-methyltransferase purified from ox adrenal medulla has a molecular diameter of 56 Å (CONNETT and KIRSHNER, 1970) and ox lactate dehydrogenase has a molecular diameter of 74 Å; both these protein molecules are, therefore, much smaller than chromogranin A (120 Å). If there is a large excess of molecules of chromogranin A over those of lactate dehydrogenase or phenylethanolamine-N-methyltransferase in the cytosol, then chromogranin A would preferentially pass through pores in cell membrane. However, approximate calculations have shown that there are at least 10^{13} molecules of phenylethanolamine-N-methyltransferase per mg of protein in the cytosol (from the data of CONNETT and KIRSHNER, 1970), but that no more than 10^{12} molecules of chromogranin A (per mg of protein in the cytosol) are released from the gland in one second. It can be concluded that on the basis of the sensitivity of the assay method and from the size and number of the enzyme molecules, it should have been possible to detect increased release of enzymes from the cytosol if chromogranin A was passing through pores in the cell membrane. No such release of enzymes was detected.

2. Quite independent of the above argument is the fact that the release of adenine nucleotides from the cytosol is quantitative and occurs simultaneously with the release of catecholamines (DOUGLAS and POISNER, 1966a), and that the release of chromogranins is almost as rapid, especially when the rate of perfusion is not too low (SCHNEIDER et al., 1967). It is hardly likely that such a simultaneous and quantitative release could occur following diffusion of all these different substances across the cytosol: mechanism 1c can, therefore, be excluded.

Electron microscopists have described the presence of chromaffin granules in the periphery of the cell close to, and sometimes apparently in contact with, the cell membrane (DE ROBERTIS and VAZ FERREIRA, 1957; DE ROBERTIS and SABA-

TINI, 1960; COUPLAND, 1965b; LEVER and FINDLAY, 1966; DINER, 1967; PLATTNER et al., 1969). Although the contact between chromaffin granule and cell membranes may be close, it is not certain whether 'tight junctions' are formed. These regions of close contact could be a site of release (mechanism 2a), or they may simply be a prelude to complete fusion of the two membranes, as occurs in exocytosis (mechanism 2c). Exocytosis (the word comes from DE DUVE, 1963) was proposed as a mechanism for the release of catecholamines by DE ROBERTIS and VAZ FERREIRA (1957) and DE ROBERTIS and SABATINI (1960) on the basis of their electron microscopic studies. The first clear pictures showing continuity of the two interacting membranes were published by COUPLAND (1965b) in his paper on the ultrastructure of the rat adrenal medulla. Unequivocal microscopic evidence of exocytosis in the hamster adrenal medulla was reported by DINER (1967) (see also GRYNSZPAN-WINOGRAD, 1971) who found numerous examples of the dense cores of

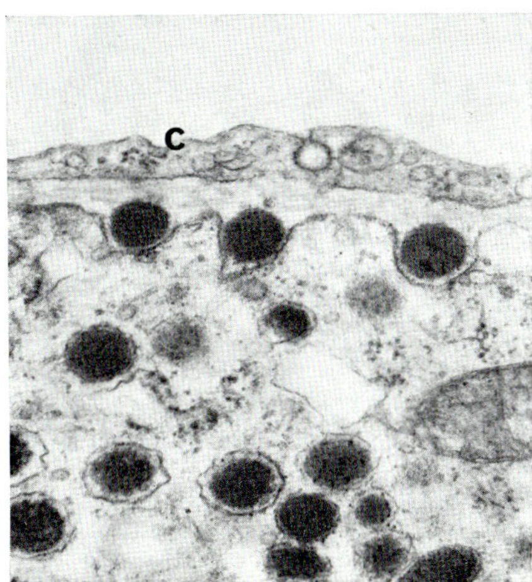

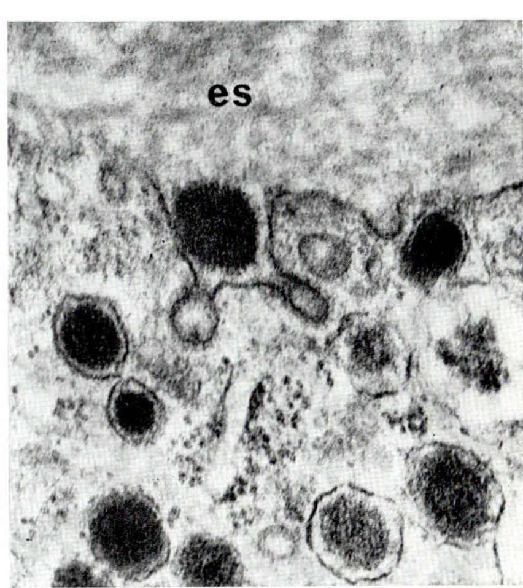

Fig. 6. *Exocytosis in the adrenal medulla of the hamster.* These two electron micrographs show the plasma membrane of adrenaline-containing cells. (fixation: glutaraldehyde; osmium tetroxide). Kindly provided by Dr. O. GRYNSZPAN-WINOGRAD (see DINER, 1967; GRYNSZPAN-WINOGRAD, 1971). Left: The electron-dense contents of three granules are seen outside the cell; each of them is in a pocket resulting from the fusion of the membrane which surrounded it with the plasma membrane. × 28000 (*c*: capillary). Right: Frequently, the pocket which contains the expelled granule possesses "coated pits". Here, two "coated pits" are seen. × 50000 (*es*: extra cellular space occupied by connective fibrils)

chromaffin granules lying outside the cell: one of her pictures is reproduced in Fig. 6. The relation of these observations to the function of the gland is uncertain, since it is not known why the hamster adrenal medulla should be the only one in which, so far, exocytosis can be so readily observed. The hamster adrenal glands studied by DINER (1967) were not deliberately stimulated and there have not yet been any studies like those on the anterior pituitary gland (DE VIRGILIIS et al., 1968; COUCH et al., 1969) and on the corpus cardiacum (NORMANN, 1969), which show an increase in the incidence of exocytotic profiles following stimulation. It may, of course, be because chromaffin granules in the hamster adrenal remain fused with the cell membrane for an unusually long time that exocytosis can be so easily seen in electron micrographs of this tissue.

It is not easy to distinguish experimentally between release across a 'tight junction' and release by exocytosis. Release of a low molecular weight substance across a 'tight junction' seems quite plausible, but release of high molecular weight substances in this way raises certain problems. Using fluorescence histochemical methods, it has been found that molecules no larger than serum albumin (molecular diameter about 72 Å) can cross 'tight junctions' between cells (Kanno and Loewenstein, 1966; Loewenstein, 1966). A molecule of chromogranin A has an effective diameter of 120 Å, and dopamine β-hydroxylase is probably of similar size. How do these large molecules cross the two apposed membranes: by a complex system of carries in each membrane, or through pores in each membrane? If release occurs through pores, then the pores on one membrane must be in line with pores in the second membrane. The resulting situation (see Fig. 7) begins to

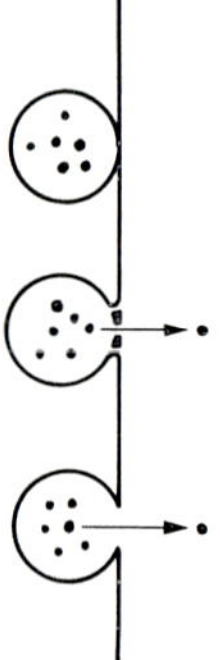

Fig. 7. 'Tight' junction, or exocytosis?

look rather like exocytosis, in which a single large 'pore' is formed following the fusion of the two membranes. We are led to the conclusion that not only is the mechanism of exocytosis supported by much experimental evidence, it also has the advantage that it is the simplest hypothesis consistent with the known facts. Thus, there is no need to postulate specific carriers or pores in membranes for the catecholamines, for ATP, and for each of the chromogranins: in exocytosis the specificity of the release resides in the store, because the store is itself the site from which all these substances are secreted into the extracellular space. There is nothing in the concept of exocytosis to disturb William of Occam (1280—1347): "It is vain to do with more what can be done with fewer".

a) Further Permeability Barriers

Having avoided crossing the cell membrane by passing through a hole in it, how do the contents of the chromaffin granule, in particular the proteins, cross the basement membrane and the capillary endothelium? Coupland (1965b) has reported that the basement membrane opposite a chromaffin granule undergoing exocytosis is less electron dense than usual and may be discontinuous: is one of the components of the chromaffin granule able to dissolve the material of the basement membrane? (This may not, of course, be necessary since the basement membrane of several tissues is freely permeable to ferritin, which has a molecular diameter of 100 Å: for references see Clementi and Palade, 1969). Once across the basement membrane, the proteins presumably cross the endothelium at specialised regions, the capillary fenestrae, which are circular openings in endothelial cells. Elfvin (1965) has described the capillary fenestrae in the rat adrenal medulla: they are about 500 Å in diameter and are bridged by a thin 'membrane' which does not seem to contain lipid. The size and, perhaps, the permeability properties of these fenestrae seem, therefore, to offer no barrier for the passage of protein molecules of the size of chromogranin A into the blood.

b) Resting Secretion

It would be of interest to know whether or not the release of catecholamines from denervated, non-stimulated glands occurs by exocytosis. The presence of chromogranin A and dopamine β-hydroxylase in perfusates from unstimulated glands has been reported: the ratio of catecholamines (μmoles) to chromogranin A (mg) was 17, compared with 8.75 in the large granule fraction of the glands (KIRSHNER et al., 1967). This observation suggests that about half of the resting secretion might occur by exocytosis and half by a mechanism not involving release of the proteins. However, this is not supported by the finding that the ratios of the amounts of catecholamines to dopamine β-hydroxylase activity in control and stimulation period perfusates were almost identical (VIVEROS et al., 1968).

An alternative method of studying 'resting secretion' is to determine the relative proportions of the different catecholamines released during control and stimulation periods. The catecholamines secreted upon stimulation come from the chromaffin granules, whereas those released at rest could come from the cytosol as well. HEMPEL and MÄNNL (1969) found that, one hour after injection of cats with [^{3}H]tyrosine, 14% of the radioactive catecholamine in the adrenal venous blood was dopamine, and 70% was noradrenaline. In rabbits only 3% of the radioactive catecholamine was dopamine. Unfortunately, these authors did not study secretion from the same glands during stimulation. A difficulty in interpreting results with trace amounts of radioactive substances is that some of the radioactive amines released may have come from noradrenergic nerves in the adrenal gland. Further work is clearly required to settle the question of whether all, or only part, of the 'resting secretion' from the adrenal gland occurs by exocytosis. It is possible that the bulk of the catecholamines released from some phaeochromocytomas has diffused across the cytosol (see chapter 18 by WINKLER and SMITH).

IV. The Role of Noradrenergic Vesicles in the Release of Catecholamines from Sympathetic Neurons:

Evidence that Some of the Neurotransmitter Is Released by Exocytosis

In this section we shall not attempt to give a comprehensive review of all the studies on the release of noradrenaline, but will consider the question: is the mechanism of release from neurons the same as that from the adrenal medulla? This possibility has often been discussed (see, for example, POTTER, 1967; DOUGLAS, 1968; KOPIN, 1968) because of similarities between the two tissues. For instance, in both tissues the amines are stored in a membrane-limited particle, and calcium ions are required for the release of the amines from each type of tissue (see Section B, 1).

Is it possible to obtain more direct evidence that the noradrenergic vesicle is the immediate site of origin of the catecholamines released from neurons? Five experimental approaches have been used in an attempt to answer this question: (i) electrophysiological studies on smooth muscle, (ii) estimation of the amount of noradrenaline released per stimulus applied to the nerve, (iii) pharmacological diversion of the noradrenaline store from the vesicle to the cytosol, (iv) pharmacological modification of the type of amines stored in the vesicles, and, (v) biochemical observations on the fate of components of the vesicle.

1. Quantal Release of Noradrenaline

Spontaneous junction potentials have been observed in intracellular recordings from smooth muscle cells of the vas deferens (several species) and of the dog retractor penis (see review by HOLMAN, 1970). These excitatory spontaneous junction potentials are unaffected by concentrations of tetrodotoxin which block nerve impulses and evoked neuromuscular transmission; their frequency in the vas deferens is reduced by reserpine; they are abolished by denervation in the retractor penis; and their frequency in the vas deferens is increased following stimulation of the hypogastric nerve. These observations provide evidence for the release of noradrenaline in discrete multimolecular packets, but it is not yet possible to conclude that such packets are made up from units of constant size. The amplitudes of the spontaneous junction potentials in the vas deferens range from 20 mV to less than 1 mV, most being of low amplitude. Several possible explanations for the variation in amplitude have been discussed by Holman (1970) who concluded with the comment "the possibility that the packets of noradrenaline are not of uniform size must also be considered". Because of the wide variation (from less than 200 Å to more than 1 μ) in the gap between the nerve varicosity and muscle cell membranes in the vas deferens (Burnstock, 1970), it may prove very difficult to correlate the size of the junction potentials with the noradrenaline content of the two types of vesicle in the terminals of the hypogastric nerve. However, these electrophysiological observations are consistent with the release of noradrenaline in quanta rather than molecule by molecule.

2. Amount of Noradrenaline Released per Stimulus

If noradrenaline is released directly from the noradrenergic vesicles, then the amount of noradrenaline released per stimulus from one varicosity should either be equal to that present in one vesicle, or to a multiple of this amount. However, since it is only possible to measure the quantity of noradrenaline released from a piece of tissue containing several hundred varicosities, all that can be calculated is the *average* amount of noradrenaline released from one varicosity. This average amount can then be compared with the amount of noradrenaline present in a vesicle.

The noradrenaline content of a vesicle has been calculated as follows. From biochemical analysis of the amount of noradrenaline per unit of tissue, and histochemical analysis of the number of varicosities per unit of tissue, Dahlström et al. (1966) concluded that the average noradrenaline content of a varicosity in the rat vas deferens is 3.4×10^{-5} pmoles. (This gives a concentration in the varicosity cytoplasm, volume about 2 μ^3, of about 11 mM). The noradrenaline content of a varicosity in the rat iris is 2.4×10^{-5} pmoles and so a mean value of 2.9×10^{-5} pmoles was taken (Dahlström et al., 1966). On the assumptions that all this noradrenaline is stored in vesicles (small dense-cored) and that the concentration in a vesicle is the same as in an adrenal chromaffin granule, Dahlström et al. (1966) calculated that each varicosity contained about 1500 vesicles. Each vesicle would then contain about 10000 molecules of noradrenaline. Folkow et al. (1967) suggested that a varicosity contained about 1000 vesicles, and so each vesicle would then contain about 15000 molecules of transmitter.

These estimates are, of course, only approximate. A possible source of error is in the calculation of the concentration of noradrenaline in a vesicle. The sympathetic nerve terminals are, after all, in a higher state of activity than the adrenal medulla and many vesicles may be present which contain less than the maximum possible content of noradrenaline (see, for example, the electron microscopic studies of Tranzer and Thoenen, 1967). This suggests that the noradrenaline content of a vesicle, may, on average, be less than that calculated by Dahlström et al. (1966) but we cannot yet say how much their value may be in excess. Perhaps a more reliable estimate of the noradrenaline content per vesicle could be obtained by counting the number of vesicles in electron micrographs and comparing this with the noradrenaline content of an average varicosity. However, such tedious experiments have not yet been carried out (see, however, Hökfelt, 1969).

Folkow et al. (1967) argued that it should be possible to calculate the amount of noradrenaline released from each varicosity per stimulus by measuring the overflow of noradrenaline from a tissue while stimulating the nerve in the presence of drugs that inhibit the uptake of noradrenaline into tissues. Observations of this kind, which have been made on four different sympathetically innervated tissues: spleen, calf muscle, pulmonary artery and uterine artery, are summarised in Table 4. The experimental results give the output of noradrenaline as a fraction of the total tissue store, and values for this fraction ranging from 2×10^{-5} to 5×10^{-4} have been reported. If this fraction also applied to release at the level of a varicosity, it would be possible to calculate the amount of noradrenaline released per varicosity. Folkow et al. (1967) assumed that the value of 2.9×10^{-5} pmoles of noradrenaline per varicosity, given by Dahlström et al. (1966) as the mean content of varicosities in rat vas deferens and iris, might apply to varicosities in cat calf-muscle: they then obtained a value of about 400 molecules of noradrenaline released per stimulus from one varicosity. For the sake of comparison, we have calculated the other data in Table 4 making the same assumption as Folkow et al. (1967) and the values are given in parentheses in the last column of the table. Bevan et al. (1969) were able to estimate directly the amount of noradrenaline released per varicosity in the pulmonary artery, without making any assumptions about the noradrenaline content of a varicosity; this was done by counting the number of varicosities per unit of tissue and determining the amount of noradrenaline released per unit. The direct estimate obtained by Bevan et al. (1969) was 2000 molecules released per varicosity per stimulus, compared with the value of 900 molecules calculated on the assumption that a varicosity contains 2.9×10^{-5} pmoles of noradrenaline. A similar direct approach was used by Bell and Vogt (1971) in studies on the uterine artery. The varicosities in this tissue are somewhat richer in noradrenaline than in other smooth muscle tissues; each varicosity was found to contain approximately 20×10^{-5} pmoles of noradrenaline. The average amount of noradrenaline released per varicosity per stimulus was approximately 25000 molecules (Bell and Vogt, 1971).

For three of the four tissues in Table 4, the number of molecules of noradrenaline released per stimulus per varicosity ranged from 400 to 9000. As discussed above, it is believed that the number of molecules of noradrenaline present in one small dense-cored vesicle is no more than 10000—15000. Only in one tissue (uterine artery) did the number of molecules of noradrenaline released per stimulus from each varicosity exceed the content of one vesicle. It could, therefore, be argued, that in the uterine artery the contents of two vesicles are released from some varicosities at each stimulus, and that the content of one vesicle is released from each of the remaining varicosities. Several interpretations of the results in other tissues are possible (assuming for the sake of argument, that each vesicle contains 15000 molecules of noradrenaline), e.g.:

a) Between 2.5% and 60% of the content of one vesicle is released from each varicosity per stimulus.

b) The entire content of one vesicle is released from 2.5% to 60% of the varicosities by each stimulus, or, put in another way, the entire content of one vesicle is released from each varicosity every 2—40 stimuli.

c) Any situation intermediate between (a) and (b).

Folkow et al. (1967), whose data gave the lowest amount (400 molecules) of noradrenaline released, have put forward several arguments against interpretation (b). However, arguments in favour of this interpretation were given by Bevan et al. (1969). These authors made some interesting calculations about the expected concentrations of noradrenaline at distances of 4—8 μ from a varicosity in the

Table 4. *Output of noradrenaline from tissues per nerve impulse*

Tissue	Perfusion fluid	Drugs	Frequency of Stimulation	No. of Stimuli	Output of noradrenaline per stimulus (i) Fraction of total store	(ii) No. of molecules per varicosity	Ref.
Cat spleen	Blood	Phenoxybenzamine	10	200	(10^{-4})[b]	(1750)[a]	1
Cat spleen	Tyrode's solution	Phenoxybenzamine	4	480	$(2.5—5\times10^{-4})$	(4400—9000)[a]	2
Cat spleen	Blood	Phenoxybenzamine	5	240	(4.8×10^{-4})[b]	(8400)[a]	3
Cat spleen	Krebs-bicarbonate	Phenoxybenzamine	5	200	(4.6×10^{-4})[b]	(8000)[a]	4
Cat spleen	Krebs-Henseleit's solution	Phenoxybenzamine or Cocaine + Hydergin	1—10	?	c. 10^{-4}	(1750)[a]	5
Cat spleen	Blood	Phenoxybenzamine Prostaglandin E_1	10	200	(3.6×10^{-4})[b]	(6300)[a]	6
Cat calf muscle	Blood	Desipramine or Lundbeck 3—010	6	2160	2×10^{-5}	400[a]	7
Cat calf muscle	Krebs-Henseleit's solution	Phenoxybenzamine	6	1080	6×10^{-5}	(1050)[a]	8
Rabbit pulmonary artery	Krebs solution	Phenoxybenzamine	10	1200—2400	(5×10^{-5})	2000 (900)[a]	9
Guinea-pig uterine artery	Krebs solution	Phenoxybenzamine	5	3000	2.2×10^{-4}	25000 (3700)[a]	10

References: 1; KIRPEKAR et al. (1963b). 2; HAEFELY et al. (1965). 3; GILLESPIE and KIRPEKAR (1966a). 4; KIRPEKAR and MISU (1967). 5; HEDQVIST and STJÄRNE (1969). 6; BLAKELEY et al. (1969). 7; FOLKOW et al. (1967). 8; STJÄRNE et al. (1969). 9; BEVAN et al. (1969). 10; BELL and VOGT (1971).

The figures in parenthesis were not given in the original papers, but have been calculated either from the original data or as indicated by the superscripts a and b.

[a] calculated from the mean noradrenaline content (2.9×10^{-5} pmoles) of varicosities in rat iris and vas deferens (DAHLSTRÖM et al., 1966).
[b] calculated from the mean noradrenaline content of cat spleen of 50.3 nmoles (DEARNALEY and GEFFEN, 1966).

outermost lamina of the pulmonary artery. (The *minimum* distance between a varicosity and a muscle cell in this tissue is 2 μ). It was tentatively concluded that the concentration of noradrenaline, up to 6 μ from the site of release of the entire contents of one vesicle, would be above the measured threshold of excitation of the muscle, and that "it is more certain that contraction will follow the release of the total contents of a single vesicle than its partial content". BEVAN et al. (1969) found that 2000 molecules of noradrenaline were released per varicosity per stimulus which, by interpretation (b), would be equal to the total contents of one vesicle released from each varicosity every 7—8 pulses. It is, therefore, of interest that a minimum of 6—8 pulses must be applied to the sympathetic innervation of the pulmonary artery before a response is observed (BEVAN and VERITY, 1966; BEVAN and NEDERGAARD, 1968). "This minimum number of pulses is not influenced by pretreatment with sub- or supra-threshold concentrations of noradrenaline. These observations have been interpreted as suggesting that only after the 6th to 8th pulse in a train of pulses after rest is a significant amount of transmitter released. The results presented in this paper [i. e. BEVAN et al. (1969)] suggest that the contents of one vesicle may be released on the average every 7—8 pulses. This is an average figure. A strict release precisely at every 7th to 8th pulse is not envisaged. The number 7 or 8 represents the mode of the hypothetical frequency distribution curve of release and number of preceding pulses not associated with release. Consequently, after a period of rest, although some vesicles may be released prior to the mode, i.e. prior to the 6—8 pulses, only after such a train is a significant number of vesicles released to initiate a detectable effect. This observation supports the hypothesis of periodic release of total vesicle content by any one node." (BEVAN et al., 1969).

One of the assumptions underlying experiments of the kind summarised in Table 4 is that the amount of noradrenaline overflowing from a tissue is the same as that released from the nerve terminals. For tissues with a dense innervation, or in which many varicosities are partly surrounded by Schwann cells (see BURNSTOCK, 1970), the amount of noradrenaline recovered in the perfusate may be considerably less than that released. This is the reason why drugs were used to inhibit the uptake of noradrenaline into nerves. However, it is now recognised that in some organs uptake and metabolism of noradrenaline by extraneuronal tissues is an important phenomenon (see LIGHTMAN and IVERSEN, 1969; LANGER, 1970, and chapter 14 by TRENDELENBURG). Phenoxybenzamine inhibits uptake of noradrenaline into extraneuronal tissues as well as into neurons and so, in most of the experiments in Table 4, the overflow of noradrenaline may be close to the amount which was released from the nerves.

Another possible source of error was pointed out by STJÄRNE et al. (1969) who found that the amount of noradrenaline released per stimulus depended upon the number of stimuli. In the experiments of FOLKOW et al. (1967) the nerve was stimulated for 6 min before the blood was collected for analysis, whereas STJÄRNE et al. (1969) found that the output reached a peak after 3 min and then declined. Fortunately, most of the experiments in Table 4 were done with short periods of stimulation, but the data obtained by FOLKOW et al. may be too low by a factor of 3, as suggested by STJÄRNE et al. (1969).

A third assumption in the calculations, which does not apply to the studies of BEVAN et al. (1969) and of BELL and VOGT (1971), is that the average noradrenaline content of a varicosity in cat calfmuscle and spleen is the same as that in the rat iris and vas deferens. However, a subjective impression obtained by fluorescence histochemistry is that the content of a varicosity in the spleen may be less than that in the vas deferens (WOODS, 1968, quoted by BLAKELEY et al., 1970).

Finally, it should not be forgotten that the comparisons made above, of the number of molecules of noradrenaline released with the amount stored in one vesicle, assumed that the nerve terminals contained predominantly one type of vesicle, the small dense-cored vesicle. However, as discussed in Section A. I 2, up to 20% of the vesicles in varicosities in the spleen may be large dense-cored vesicles, and these vesicles are also common in varicosities in the cat pulmonary artery (VERITY et al., 1966).

It is premature to draw any firm conclusions from the results of this type of experimental approach in view of the uncertainty concerning the average amount of noradrenaline stored in a single vesicle, and all the other assumptions. The results of the more direct method applied by BEVAN et al. (1969), taken together with their physiological studies, are, however, consistent with the hypothesis that the contents of one vesicle are released from each varicosity every few pulses. Further work along these lines in other tissues would be well worthwhile.

The physiological implications of these results cannot be discussed here, but it does appear that release of transmitter from a varicosity of a sympathetic nerve is not so efficient as that from the terminal of a motor neuron, where a single impulse releases several hundred quanta (see ECCLES, 1964).

3. Failure of Nerve Impulses to Release Noradrenaline Stored in the Cytosol

Reserpine depletes tissues of their catecholamines by preventing the uptake and/or binding of the amines by the storage vesicles (see Section A, II and chapter by EULER). In the presence of a monoamine oxidase inhibitor, sympathetically innervated tissues pretreated with reserpine can take up and retain noradrenaline (LINDMAR and MUSCHOLL, 1964). The noradrenaline is taken up into neurons, as shown by fluorescence histochemistry and it has been suggested (MALMFORS, 1965) that most of the noradrenaline taken up under these conditions is not present in vesicles, but is free in the cytosol where it is protected from oxidation by the monoamine oxidase inhibitor. This suggestion has been confirmed by subcellular fractionation studies on the heart (IVERSEN et al., 1965; LUNDBORG, 1968) and vas deferens (POTTER, 1967) which have shown that most of the noradrenaline taken up is not particle-bound. Likewise, electron microscopic observations on nerve terminals in the vas deferens showed no increase in the proportion of vesicles containing dense cores (reduced to 11% of normal by reserpine treatment) even though the noradrenaline content of the tissue and the fluorescence intensity of the nerve fibres had returned to normal levels (VAN ORDEN et al., 1967). Electron microscopic radioautography (TAXI, 1969) has also shown that exogenous noradrenaline can be taken up into neurons in treated animals: the cytoplasm in nerve fibres became labelled but not the vesicles. Thus, nerve terminals from an animal treated with reserpine and a monoamine oxidase inhibitor can take up relatively large amounts of noradrenaline, which is stored in the cytosol. Can this noradrenaline be released by stimulation of the nerve?

VAN ORDEN et al. (1967) found that the response of the vas deferens to stimulation of the hypogastric nerve was almost completely inhibited by this pharmacological diversion of the noradrenaline store from vesicles to cytosol. The surprising observation was also made that this inhibition of the response to nerve stimulation was even greater than that in a vas deferens from an animal treated with reserpine alone. These results can most readily be explained by the work of POTTER (1967), who treated rats with reserpine and then incubated the vasa deferentia with (^{3}H)-noradrenaline in the presence of a monoamine oxidase inhibitor. The amount of (^{3}H-)noradrenaline taken up was almost the same as in the vasa from untreated rats, but only 19% of it was recovered in the microsomal fraction compared with 63% in the controls. The spontaneous rate of release of noradrenaline from the treated vas deferens was three times that from the control vas deferens, but stimulation of the hypogastric nerve only caused a 50% increase in the amount of noradrenaline released from the treated vas deferens compared with a 650% increase in the rate of release from the control tissue. These biochemical experiments, which show an impaired release of noradrenaline by nerve stimulation, account for the inhibition in the response of the treated vas deferens observed by VAN ORDEN et al. (1967). Perhaps the high level of spontaneous release observed by POTTER (1967) might obscure small changes in the response to nerve stimulation, which would provide an explanation of the finding (VAN ORDEN et al., 1967) that the response to nerve stimulation was more severely impaired in animals given reserpine and a monoamine oxidase inhibitor than in animals given reserpine alone.

Experiments described by HÄGGENDAL and MALMFORS (1969) provide further evidence that pharmacological diversion of the noradrenaline store from vesicles to cytosol makes the transmitter unavailable for release upon nerve stimulation. These authors studied the irides and salivary glands of rats which had first been treated with reserpine and a monoamine oxidase inhibitor and had then received an intravenous infusion of noradrenaline. Fluorescence histochemistry showed an accumulation of the exogenous noradrenaline in the nerves of the irides, with the 'smooth' type of fluorescence typical of neurons in animals so treated (MALMFORS, 1965). The intensity of the fluorescence in the irides did not change upon stimulation of the preganglionic nerve trunk; neither was there any physiological response in the diameter of the pupil or degree of protrusion of the eyeball. Biochemical studies showed that the noradrenaline content of the salivary gland had been restored to about 20% of normal, but that there was no change in the amount of noradrenaline in the gland upon stimulation of the nerve.

These studies have shown that exogenous noradrenaline taken up into adrenergic nerve endings, but confined to the cytosol because its uptake into the vesicles is inhibited by reserpine, cannot be released by electrical stimulation of the nerve. It could be argued that the drugs themselves might inhibit release of the transmitter non-specifically (i. e. regardless of whether it is present in the vesicles or in the cytosol). Two recent reports that reserpine *in vitro* inhibits the vasoconstrictor response (DAY and OWEN, 1968) and the muscular response (EULER, 1969) to sympathetic stimulation in the ear artery and vas deferens, respectively, suggest that this drug may under some conditions interfere with the release of transmitter. (The concentrations used in these *in vitro* studies were 0.05—0.5 μg/ml.) However, some experiments described by HÄGGENDAL and MALMFORS (1969) show that, *in vivo*, reserpine and a monoamine oxidase inhibitor do not prevent the release of noradrenaline stored in the vesicles. These authors infused (i.v.) dopamine into rats pretreated with the two drugs and found that the fluorescence was restored in neurons in the iris but that, in contrast to the fluorescence after infusion of noradrenaline, it had the normal varicose appearance. In the animals treated with dopamine, stimulation of the nerve increased the pupil diameter and degree of protrusion of the eyeball and this was accompanied by a decrease in the intensity of fluorescence in the nerves. Likewise, infusion of dopamine partly restored the noradrenaline content of the salivary gland, and this noradrenaline could be released upon stimulation of the gland. HÄGGENDAL and MALMFORS (1969) suggested that dopamine could restore the response to nerve stimulation because it was taken up into the vesicles where it was converted into noradrenaline; the vesicles were assumed to be the "proper site for release". In order to clinch this argument, biochemical studies should be done to show that, in animals treated with reserpine, the noradrenaline formed from dopamine is, indeed, located in noradrenergic vesicles.

The ability of dopamine to restore normal function, where noradrenaline does not, in animals treated with reserpine and a monoamine oxidase inhibitor, may be due to a combination of several factors: the dose of dopamine infused was ten times that of noradrenaline (HÄGGENDAL and MALMFORS, 1969); the uptake mechanism in the vesicles may have a higher affinity for dopamine and occur at a higher rate (compare, adrenal chromaffin granules: LADURON and BELPAIRE, 1968b); and/or the uptake of dopamine into vesicles may occur by a process resistant to reserpine (compare, chromaffin granules: LUNDBORG, 1966).

It can be concluded that noradrenaline diverted from its store in vesicles to the cytosol by the action of reserpine cannot be released by stimulation of the nerve. If this is also true of the noradrenaline present in the cytosol of neurons in untreated animals, then mechanisms of release which involve diffusion of the noradrenaline from the vesicles into the cytosol (type 1 of Fig. 3) can be excluded. The remaining possible mechanisms of release (type 2 of Fig. 3) all involve the vesicle as the immediate source of the transmitter that is secreted.

4. Release of False Adrenergic Transmitters

Enzymes involved in the biosynthesis of noradrenaline, in particular dopadecarboxylase and dopamine β-hydroxylase, do not show a high degree of specificity. Sympathetic nervous tissue can, therefore, convert analogues of dopa into analogues of dopamine and of noradrenaline (see review by KOPIN, 1968). The discovery that α-methylnoradrenaline, formed in the heart following administration of α-methyldopa, is released together with noradrenaline upon stimulation of the nerve (MUSCHOLL and MAÎTRE, 1963) not only opened up a new field of pharmacology, it also led to studies on the subcellular localisation and release of other false transmitter substances. These studies have provided further evidence for the key role of the noradrenergic vesicle in the release of transmitters.

There have been several detailed reviews of this subject (MUSCHOLL, 1966; KOPIN, 1966 and 1968; THOENEN, 1969) and so we shall only summarise the results (see also chapter by MUSCHOLL). The significant findings in relation to mechanisms of release are:

1. Derivatives of phenylethylamine, either formed from amino acids or taken up *in vivo* or *in vitro*, are concentrated by sympathetically innervated tissues. Since these tissues lose most of their ability to retain the amines after denervation, it is likely that the amines are taken up into neurons.

2. Some of these phenylethylamine derivatives are recovered in the microsomal fraction after homogenisation and centrifugation, but others are found in the supernatant.

3. Only those phenylethylamine derivatives which are bound in the microsomal fraction (presumably stored in the noradrenergic vesicles) can be released from the tissue upon stimulation of the nerve. There is a correlation between the amount of the phenylethylamine stored in the microsomal fraction and the amount released upon stimulation (see KOPIN, 1966; POTTER, 1967).

4. The amount of the false transmitter, relative to that of noradrenaline, released upon stimulation is close to the relative proportions of these compounds in the tissue.

5. Compounds, such as tyramine, which are taken up into the nerve but remain in the cytosol are not released.

As has already been pointed out (POTTER, 1967; KOPIN, 1968; THOENEN, 1969), these results provide quantitative evidence that only those amines that can be stored in noradrenergic vesicles are released by nerve stimulation and suggest that the vesicles must release their contents directly into the extracellular space.

More detailed studies on the subcellular localisation of false transmitters would be valuable, especially in a tissue like the spleen which contains a relatively large proportion of 'heavy' noradrenergic vesicles that are rich in dopamine β-hydroxylase. Is it possible that those false transmitters which are formed by the action of dopamine β-hydroxylase might initially be concentrated in the 'heavy' vesicles, and might become redistributed into the 'light' vesicles following release from the nerve and re-uptake? In this connection, it is of interest that the preferential release of newly synthesised noradrenaline, *in vitro*, (KOPIN et al., 1968) and of α-methylnoradrenaline, *in vivo*, (MUSCHOLL, 1968) has been reported. Does release take place preferentially from the 'heavy' noradrenergic vesicles, or are these observations simply a reflection of the different functional states of groups of neurons?

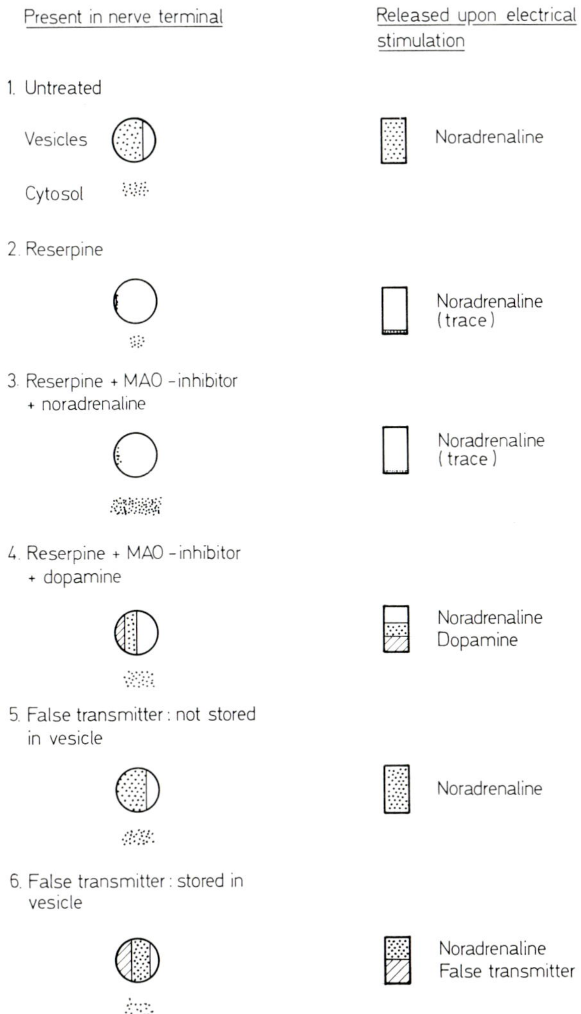

Fig. 8. Drugs which act on stores in Noradrenergic vesicles

It has been shown that studies of adrenergic neurotransmission in animals treated with drugs have provided a lot of valuable information concerning the fundamental mechanisms of release. At the risk of over-simplification, but in order to summarise these studies, we have expressed the results diagrammatically in Fig. 8. The observations all point to the noradrenergic vesicle as the site from which amines are released upon stimulation of the nerve.

5. Release of Proteins from Noradrenergic Vesicles upon Stimulation of the Splenic Nerve

The biochemical studies which established that all the soluble components of the chromaffin granule are released upon stimulation of the adrenal medulla (see Section A, III) opened up the possibility of applying the same approach to the sympathetic neuron. The success of this approach in the work on the adrenal gland depended on the ability to recognise specific components of the chromaffin granule, i.e. ATP and the chromogranins. In the chromaffin cell, the ATP present in the chromaffin granules is greatly in excess of that in the rest of the cell, including the mitochondria (BLASCHKO et al., 1957). However, it is obvious that the ATP present in noradrenergic vesicles of sympathetic nerve terminals in an organ is a mere fraction of the total in the tissue. A search for the release of adenine nucleotides from sympathetically innervated tissues would, therefore, be pointless (see STJÄRNE et al., 1970) unless a purified fraction of noradrenergic vesicles from the tissue was examined. Only one such study has so far been reported: POTTER and AXELROD (1963b) found that the ATP content of a partly purified fraction of 'light' noradrenergic vesicles from rat heart did not decrease 2 hr. after administration of reserpine, although the catecholamine content of the fraction fell by 77%. This interesting observation supports the idea that one of the actions of reserpine is to inhibit uptake of catecholamines into noradrenergic vesicles. No similar studies have yet been reported on the ATP content of a noradrenergic vesicle fraction after sympathetic nerve stimulation.

Whereas ATP is found in all cells, sympathetic neurons must contain some proteins which are specific to the nerve (although these proteins may also be found in chromaffin cells) and we have already described the evidence that the noradrenergic vesicle of splenic nerve contains at least two such proteins: dopamine β-hydroxylase and chromogranin A (see Section A, I, 2). The fate of these two proteins upon stimulation of the splenic nerve has recently been studied. However, before the presence of these proteins in noradrenergic vesicles had been established, LIVETT et al. (1968) found that, following injection of (^{14}C) leucine into the coeliac ganglion, radioactively labelled protein(s) migrated along the splenic nerve (from the ganglion to the spleen) at a rate of about 0.5 cm/hr; this was the same as the rate of migration of radioactive noradrenaline. It was suggested that the rapidly migrating protein(s) might be components of the noradrenergic vesicles (LIVETT et al., 1968), and it was briefly reported (GEFFEN and LIVETT, 1968) that minute amounts of radioactive protein and noradrenaline were released into the venous effluent from the spleen upon stimulation of the nerve. Stimulation of the nerve (at 30 Hz) caused a 300—800% increase in the amounts of (^{14}C) noradrenaline released, and a 20—90% increase in the amounts of (^{14}C) protein released (GEFFEN et al., 1970). Because the radioactive protein may have originated from sites other than the nerve, these workers went on to use immunochemical methods, which enabled them to demonstrate the rapid axonal transport, in sheep splenic nerve, of dopamine β-hydroxylase and chromogranin A (GEFFEN et al., 1969a) and the release of these proteins into the perfusate from sheep spleen, upon stimulation of the splenic nerve (GEFFEN et al., 1969b). The proteins released from the spleen were identified qualitatively by immunodiffusion and by complement fixation (GEFFEN et al., 1970). Independent studies established that dopamine β-hydroxylase activity was released into the splenic perfusate upon stimulation of the splenic nerve (at 30 Hz) of the dog (DE POTTER et al., 1969a) and of the calf (DE POTTER et al., 1969b), and that chromogranin A was released from the spleen of the calf (DE POTTER et al., 1969b). In the latter experiments, the amounts of the proteins in perfusates were estimated by a radiochemical method (dopamine β-hydroxylase) and by complement fixation (chromogranin A): stimulation of the splenic nerve of the calf caused the release of up to 82 nmoles of noradrenaline, 460 units of dopamine-β-hydroxylase activity, and 0.21 μg of chromogranin A. Fig. 9 shows an experiment which illustrates the calcium-dependent release of dopamine β-hydroxylase from the dog spleen. These results have been described in

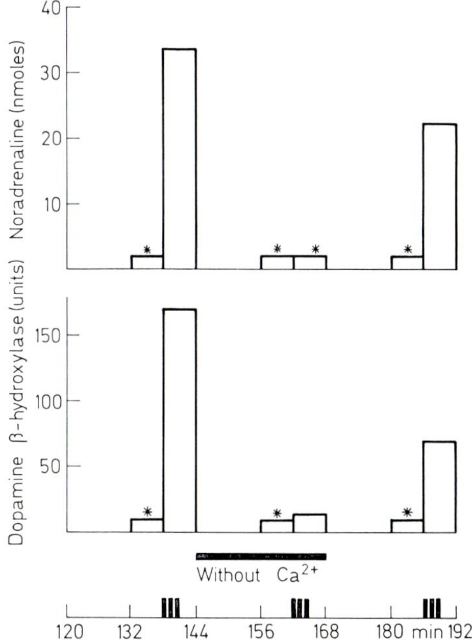

Fig. 9. *Release of dopamine β-hydroxylase from dog spleen: requirement for calcium.* The spleen was perfused with Tyrode's solution, and the splenic nerve was stimulated at the times indicated by thick vertical bars on the abscissa. Frequency of stimulation: 30 Hz. The asterisk above a column indicates that the substance could not be detected, and the height of this column is the smallest amount which could have been measured. The spleen was perfused with Tyrode's solution lacking calcium chloride for the time indicated by the thick horizontal line

detail by SMITH et al. (1970). Dopamine β-hydroxylase activity is also released into the perfusate upon stimulation (30 Hz) of the splenic nerve of the cat (GEWIRTZ and KOPIN, 1970). It has now been shown that the release of the proteins from sheep (GEFFEN et al. 1970) and calf (W. P. DE POTTER, unpublished observations) spleens also occurs at lower (5 Hz—10 Hz), more physiological, frequencies of nerve stimulation.

a) What is the Origin of the Released Proteins?

Before it can be concluded that these proteins are released from the terminal varicosities of the splenic nerve, three other possible sites of origin must be excluded. These are: extra-adrenal chromaffin cells; blood pooled in the sinuses and red pulp; and unidentified sites which might be sensitive to the noradrenaline released from the nerve.

Stimulation of the splenic nerve in the dog causes the release of acetylcholine, as well as of noradrenaline, into the perfusate (LEADERS and DAYRIT, 1965) and so the possibility has to be considered that acetylcholine is causing the release of catecholamines and proteins from chromaffin cells. However, there is no fluorescence histochemical evidence for the presence of chromaffin cells in the spleen of the dog (Dahlström and Zetterström, 1965) or cat (Gillespie and Kirpekar, 1966b; Fillenz, 1970); nor is there any biochemical evidence of chromaffin granules in homogenates of dog spleen (De Potter, 1968; Chubb et al., 1970). The possibility that dopamine β-hydroxylase and chromogranin A came from chromaffin cells in the dog or calf spleen was excluded by adding to the perfusion fluid drugs which block the action of acetylcholine on chromaffin cells (hexamethonium and atropine): the presence of these drugs did not prevent the release by nerve stimulation of the two proteins (De Potter et al., 1969a, b; Smith et al., 1970). (Indeed, in these experiments, hexamethonium (1.4 mM—3.0 mM) actually increased the amounts of noradrenaline and of the two proteins released, suggesting that this drug might have a presynaptic action. Blakeley et al. (1963) have also reported that hexamethonium sometimes increased the overflow of noradrenaline from the spleen.)

In the experiments of De Potter and his colleagues, the spleens were perfused with Tyrode's solution for up to 2 hr. before samples of the perfusate were analysed; nevertheless, some blood was still present in the tissue and some was ejected when the spleen contracted. Since both chromogranin A and dopamine β-hydroxylase are released from the adrenal medulla, it is likely that blood normally contains small amounts of these proteins. It has, in fact, been shown that venous blood from an anaesthetised calf (Blaschko et al., 1967a) and arterial blood from an ox killed in the slaughterhouse (A. D. Smith, unpublished observation) contains material which cross-reacts with antiserum to chromogranin A. Two kinds of experiment have been carried out to exclude the possibility that the chromogranin A and dopamine β-hydroxylase released from the spleen came from blood pooled in the organ. In the first type of experiment, the spleens (dog or calf) were perfused with Tyrode's solution containing phenoxybenzamine; although this drug prevented contraction of the spleen, and the consequent expulsion of blood, it did not affect the release of the two proteins caused by stimulation of the nerve (De Potter et al., 1969b; Smith et al., 1970). The second type of experiment involved causing the calf spleen to contract by the infusion of noradrenaline: some blood was ejected from the spleen but no more than a trace of dopamine β-hydroxylase activity was released (Smith et al., 1970). The last experiment not only shows that the dopamine β-hydroxylase released from the spleen by nerve stimulation does not come from blood, it also excludes its origin from unidentified sites in the organ which are sensitive to the transmitter.

If dopamine β-hydroxylase and chromogranin A are not released from chromaffin cells, from the blood, or from unidentified sites sensitive to noradrenaline, then it is difficult to see where else they could have come from except from the terminals of the splenic nerve. Evidence consistent with this conclusion was the finding that several biochemical properties (pH optimum, mobility in gel electrophoresis, sedimentation rate) of the dopamine β-hydroxylase released from calf spleen were the same as those of the dopamine β-hydroxylase in the soluble lysate of noradrenergic vesicles isolated from ox splenic nerve (Smith et al., 1970). The most direct evidence that the proteins were released from terminals of the splenic nerve was the highly significant correlation between the amounts of each protein and the amounts of noradrenaline in perfusates collected during stimulation of the splenic nerve; this correlation was not only found in spleens perfused with normal Tyrode's solution, but also when release was potentiated by hexamethonium or inhibited by lack of calcium (Smith et al., 1970). As shown by denervation experiments (Euler and Purkhold, 1951; Laduron and Belpaire, 1968c), more than 90%

of the noradrenaline in the spleen is present in the splenic nerve, and so it can be concluded that dopamine β-hydroxylase and chromogranin A are released from the nerve.

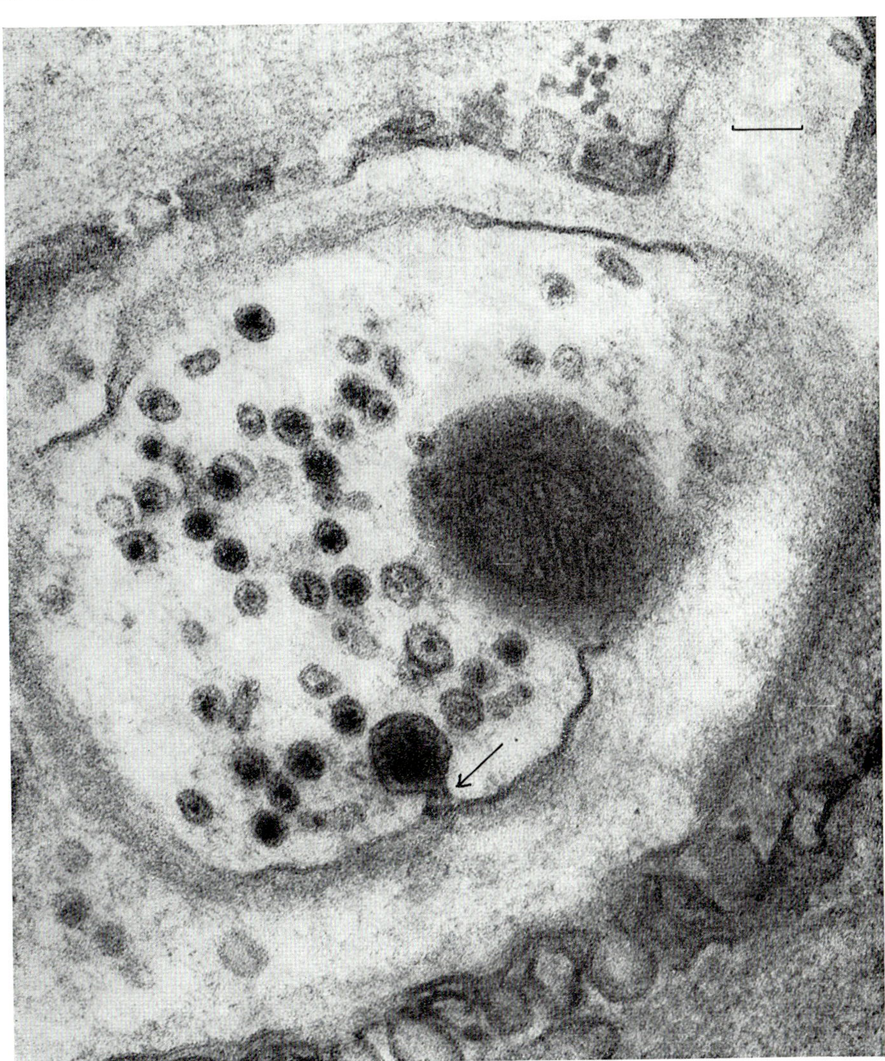

Fig. 10. Axon varicosity in rat vas deferens showing fusion of membrane of large dense-cored vesicle with axon membrane (↑). Acrylic aldehyde in sodium dichromate fixation. Calibration: 0.1 μ. Kindly provided by Dr. M. FILLENZ (see FILLENZ, 1971)

b) How Are the Proteins Released from the Nerve?

It has been shown that all, or nearly all, the chromogranin A and dopamine β-hydroxylase of splenic nerve axons is located in the 'heavy' noradrenergic vesicles (see Section A, I, 2), and so it is likely that the noradrenergic vesicles release their soluble proteins as well as noradrenaline upon nerve stimulation. Evidence that this release is specific, and not due to damage to the axonal membrane caused by perfusion, is that two enzymes present in the cytosol of the splenic nerve, tyrosine hydroxylase and dopa decarboxylase, were not released (De Potter et al., 1969a, b). It was calculated that the method of assay (Laduron and Belpaire, 1968a) was sensitive enough to have detected dopa decarboxylase in the perfusate if as little as 0.5% of the noradrenaline had been released by a process which simultaneously increased the permeability of the nerve cell membrane to a protein the size of dopa decarboxylase (Smith et al., 1970).

As we have already said, in connection with secretion from the adrenal medulla (Section A, II), the release of high molecular weight proteins from a vesicle within a cell may, in theory, occur by one of four mechanisms: transport across the cell membrane by combination with carriers; passage through pores in the cell membrane; release of the intact vesicle; or by exocytosis. The dopa decarboxylase present in the cytosol of the splenic nerve has a lower sedimentation coefficient than the soluble dopamine β-hydroxylase of the noradrenergic vesicles (Smith et al., 1970) and so it is probably a smaller molecule. The fact that dopa decarboxylase is not released, whereas the larger molecules of dopamine β-hydroxylase and chromogranin A are, argues against the release of the two vesicle proteins first into the cytosol, and then through pores in the nerve cell membrane. Evidence against the release of the intact vesicles into the perfusate is that neither of the proteins in the perfusates were present in particles that could have been sedimented at 60000 g for 90 min (Smith et al., 1970); this finding does not, of course, exclude the unlikely possibility of release of intact vesicles followed by their disintegration. Exocytosis is the remaining possible mechanism for the release of the vesicle proteins.

There are only two reports by microscopists of what seems to be exocytosis in sympathetic nerve terminals. One of the micrographs in a paper by Farrell (1968, Fig. 2) shows a nerve terminal from a rat vas deferens in which a large dense-cored vesicle appears to have fused with the cell membrane; the author did not comment on this. The micrograph published by Farrell (1968) was from a rat treated with reserpine, and so may be atypical. However, Fillenz (1971) has seen exocytosis from a large dense-cored vesicle in a nerve terminal of vas deferens from a normal rat, and her micrograph is reproduced in Fig. 10. The continuity between vesicle and cell membrane can be seen, although the dense contents of the vesicle have not yet been released. Thus, it can be said for the first time on the basis of morphological evidence that exocytosis is a mechanism which might be involved in the release of the contents of a large dense-cored vesicle. Dopamine β-hydroxylase and chromogranin A are present in the large dense-cored vesicles of splenic nerve axons, and dopamine β-hydroxylase has also been shown to be present in the 'heavy' noradrenergic vesicles of the nerve terminals in the spleen (see Section A I, 2). The evidence so far discussed is, therefore, consistent with the release of these two proteins by exocytosis from large dense-cored vesicles of the splenic nerve. Can more quantitative evidence of exocytosis from these vesicles be obtained ?

6. Hypothesis: Exocytosis from Large Dense-Cored Vesicles

Exocytosis was established as the mechanism of secretion in the adrenal medulla by the near identity of the proportions of chromaffin granule constituents in the perfusates after stimulation with the proportions in the soluble lysate of isolated chromaffin granules. Smith et al. (1970) used the same approach for the proteins and noradrenaline released from the splenic nerve and compared the relative proportions of these substances in the perfusates with the proportions in soluble lysates of 'heavy' noradrenergic vesicles in splenic nerve axons (De Potter et al., 1970) and terminals (De Potter, 1971). These calculations, together with similar ones made from the data of GEWIRTZ and KOPIN (1970) on the release of dopamine β-hydroxylase from cat spleen, are given in Table 5.

Interpretation of the ratios in perfusates is complicated because the amounts of proteins and of noradrenaline in the perfusates are not necessarily identical with the amounts released from the nerves. This problem was discussed in detail by SMITH et al. (1970) who concluded that the amounts of noradrenaline in the perfusates may have been underestimated by a factor of 2, owing to uptake into neurones and uptake and metabolism by extraneuronal tissues. The amounts of protein were also underestimated by a factor of 2 simply because the release of protein into the perfusate was slower than that of noradrenaline. It was not possible to estimate the loss of proteins, if any, by binding to tissues or by uptake into cells. Accordingly, it was suggested (SMITH et al., 1970) that the actual amounts of noradrenaline and of the proteins released were about twice the amounts measured in the perfusates; the *ratios* of the amount of each protein to that of noradrenaline released are, then, the same as the ratios found in the perfusates.

Table 5. *Relative proportions of chromogranin A, dopamine β-hydroxylase and Noradrenaline (NA) in perfusates from the spleen and in soluble lysates of noradrenergic vesicles from splenic nerve*

Animal	Ratio	Noradrenergic vesicles of preterminal axon[1]	Noradrenergic vesicles (heavy) of terminals[1]	Perfusate[2]
Dog	Dopamine β-hydroxylase: NA	96	9.6	3.2
Calf	Dopamine β-hydroxylase: NA	106	(10.6)	6.8
Cat	Dopamine β-hydroxylase: NA	427	(42.7)	29
Calf	Chromogranin A: NA	0.23	(0.023)	0.002

Units: noradrenaline (nmoles), chromogranin A (μg), dopamine β-hydroxylase activity (pmoles of octopamine formed in 20 min from tyramine).

[1] The figures for the soluble lysate of noradrenergic vesicles of preterminal axons come from DE POTTER et al. (1970) for the ox, SMITH et al. (1970) for the dog and GEWIRTZ and KOPIN (1970) for the cat. The figures for the vesicles in terminals of dog spleen are from DE POTTER (1971) with the assumption that the same proportion of each protein is soluble in the 'heavy' vesicles of the terminals as in the 'heavy' vesicles of preterminal axons. The figures in parenthesis are even more uncertain since they depend upon the latter assumption and also upon the assumption that in the cat and calf, the 'heavy' vesicles in terminals of the splenic nerve contain about ten times as much noradrenaline per unit of dopamine β-hydroxylase activity as the vesicles in preterminal axons: this has, so far, only been demonstrated for the dog splenic nerve (DE POTTER, 1971).

[2] The figures for the ratios in perfusates collected from the spleen during stimulation of the splenic nerve come from SMITH et al. (1970) for dog and calf, and from GEWIRTZ and KOPIN (1970) for cat.

It can be seen from Table 5 that the ratios of dopamine β-hydroxylase activity to noradrenaline in splenic perfusates are 33% (dog), 64% (calf) and 68% (cat) of those calculated for the soluble lysate of 'heavy' noradrenergic vesicles from the respective splenic nerve terminals; the corresponding figure for chromogranin A is 8.5%. (These values depend on the assumption that the proportion of the total dopamine β-hydroxylase, or chromogranin A, which is soluble in the 'heavy' vesicles of the terminals is the same as that found experimentally for the same vesicles in preterminal axons.) However, not all the noradrenaline in terminal varicosities of the splenic nerve is stored in large dense-cored vesicles. Biochemical studies indicate that approximately half the noradrenaline in dog spleen is present in the 'light' noradrenergic vesicles (CHUBB et al., 1970). Thus, if we assume that the noradrenaline released comes equally from both populations of vesicles, we have to multiply the ratios in the perfusates by 2: this gives ratios which are 17% (chromogranin A), 66% (dopamine β-hydroxylase, dog) and 128% (dopamine β-hydroxylase, calf) of the respective ratios in the large dense-cored vesicles of the nerve terminals. We can conclude that, on the assumption that the proteins are released only from the large dense-cored vesicles, the observations show a nearly quantitative secretion of catecholamines and proteins.

The relative deficiency in the amounts of chromogranin A released cannot at present be explained, although Smith et al. (1970) raised the possibility that the amount of this protein reaching the perfusate might be reduced by tissue binding because chromogranin A is highly acidic and has unusual hydrodynamic properties (Smith and Winkler, 1967b; Kirshner and Kirshner, 1969). Experiments should be carried out to see what proportion of chromogranin A and dopamine β-hydroxylase is recovered in the venous effluent after addition of these proteins to the perfusion fluid.

The assumptions made in the argument presented above correspond to a hypothesis which can be experimentally tested. The hypothesis is as follows:

Sympathetic nerves synthesise proteins (including chromogranin A and dopamine β-hydroxylase) which are packaged into large dense-cored vesicles in the perikaryon together with some noradrenaline; these vesicles migrate along the axon towards the terminals where they first become enriched in noradrenaline, and then release their soluble contents by exocytosis. The second population of noradrenergic vesicles (small dense-cored) in the terminals also release noradrenaline, but they do not contain any soluble dopamine β-hydroxylase or chromogranin A.

Some of the evidence which led to this hypothesis will be discussed in Section B II. It has already been pointed out that the noradrenaline content of the large dense-cored vesicles of splenic nerve terminals, relative to the amount of dopamine β-hydroxylase, is higher than that in the vesicles of preterminal axons (De Potter, 1971): it has not, of course, been excluded that this is due to a loss of dopamine β-hydroxylase rather than to a gain in noradrenaline. It has also been mentioned (Section A I, 2) that Chubb et al. (1970) have shown that the 'light' noradrenergic vesicles of the splenic nerve terminals contain little, if any, dopamine β-hydroxylase. The hypothesis predicts, among other things: (i) The dopamine β-hydroxylase and chromogranin A present in the 'heavy' noradrenergic vesicles of the nerve terminals should, in part, be soluble after rupture of the membrane. (ii) If dopamine β-hydroxylase is present in the 'light' noradrenergic vesicles it should be entirely membrane-bound: Potter (1967) has, in fact, reported that the dopamine β-hydroxylase of the 'light' vesicle fraction from rat heart was confined to the membrane. (iii) The amount of dopamine β-hydroxylase released from a nerve will depend upon the relative proportion of large dense-cored to small dense-cored vesicles.

7. Exocytosis from All Vesicles, or only from Some?

Exocytosis is the most likely mode of release for the proteins secreted from the splenic nerve, and we have shown that it can be argued that most of the noradrenaline stored in the large dense-cored vesicles is released in this way. The biochemical observations have not yet provided any information about the mode of release of noradrenaline from the small dense-cored vesicles which do, after all, store the bulk of the transmitter in sympathetic nerve terminals. In order to study this question by biochemical methods, it will first be necessary to see whether the small dense-cored vesicles contain any specific proteins. Fillenz (1971) has, however, reported electron microscopic evidence of exocytosis from small dense-cored vesicles in nerve terminals of the rat vas deferens. The studies we have reviewed on the spontaneous junction potentials in smooth muscle cells, and the estimates of the amount of transmitter released per nerve impulse also do not provide direct evidence of exocytosis: they indicate that release is quantised, but do not show how the quanta are released from the cell. On the other hand, the occurrence of exocytosis predicts that release will occur in multimolecular packets, which may equal in size the entire content of a vesicle. If, however, the vesicle and cell membranes only remain fused for a very short time, it is possible that only part of the contents will be released each time they fuse.

There are, nevertheless, two kinds of observation which make it likely that the mechanism of release from both types of vesicle is fundamentally the same: (i) the requirement for calcium ions in release, and (ii) the inability of nerve impulses to release amines from the cytosol.

Calcium. The release of catecholamines from sympathetic nerves, as well as from the adrenal medulla, requires calcium ions (see Section B, I) and the secretion of dopamine β-hydroxylase (see Fig. 9) and chromogranin A from the splenic nerve was found to be inhibited by lack of calcium (SMITH et al., 1970). It is significant that all the noradrenaline, not just a small part of it, is released by a calcium-dependent process from sympathetic neurons. Calcium must, therefore, be required not just for the release of noradrenaline from large dense-cored vesicles, but also for release from small dense-cored vesicles. A remarkable correlation exists between the occurrence of exocytosis and a requirement for calcium in many different secretory tissues (see reviews by DOUGLAS, 1968; SIMPSON, 1968; STORMORKEN, 1969; SMITH, 1971a). It is, furthermore, likely that release that is not dependent upon calcium, such as the release of noradrenaline from sympathetic nerves which is induced by tyramine, does not occur by exocytosis (see Section B, I). We are prompted to ask the question: if the release of noradrenaline from large dense-cored vesicles normally occurs by exocytosis but the release of noradrenaline from small dense-cored vesicles does not, then can it be shown that calcium plays two entirely different roles in the release of noradrenaline? Is it not more likely that calcium is required because the same fundamental mechanism is involved in release from both types of vesicle? Of course, the requirement for calcium may be in the attachment of the vesicle to the cell membrane, which could be followed either by the formation of a tight junction or by the fusion of membranes leading to exocytosis (see Section B).

Amines in the Cytosol. We have described the evidence (see pages 570—572) which shows that in order for amines to be released from sympathetic nerves they must be stored in the noradrenergic vesicles. These findings are most simply accounted for if the store in the vesicles is released by exocytosis. However, an alternative mode of release, in which the vesicles play a subsidiary role, has been proposed (EULER, 1966; STJÄRNE, 1966; STJÄRNE et al., 1969). The Swedish workers suggested that the noradrenaline released upon stimulation of the nerve comes from a store outside the vesicles (= granules):

"During the normal release process by nerve activation, it appears probable that the depolarization of the axon membrane causes some primary alteration of transmitter binding and/or membrane permeability, allowing the transmitter to become functionally free, leave the axon, and combine with the receptors. This portion may correspond to the loosely bound extra-granular part. Assuming a dynamic equilibrium between the extra-granular and granular stores, a fall in extra-granular transmitter concentration, caused by the release, would induce an increase in the net release rate from the granules." (EULER, 1968, p. 92).

A possible site for the extra-granular store is the nerve cell membrane (EULER, 1966; STJÄRNE, 1966). How is this extra-granular store replenished? STJÄRNE (1966) suggested that it is refilled, in part, by uptake of noradrenaline that had been released but that "the inevitable gradual loss of noradrenaline would have to be compensated for by refilling from nerve granules topographically unrelated to the axonal membrane." However, it is admitted that "if the extra-granular transmitter occurred in a free form it would be highly susceptible to rapid inactivation by the monoamine oxidase present in the axon terminal." (EULER, 1968). Not only will noradrenaline released from vesicles into the cytosol, in order to replenish the extra-granular store, have to run the gamut of mitochondrial monoamines oxidase, it will diffuse in all directions within the cytosol, so that only a fraction (NA/x) of the store in the vesicles will be released (see Fig. 11a). According to the EULER and STJÄRNE hypothesis, noradrenaline in the cytosol can be released following binding to the extra-granular store. However, evidence has been described on p. 570 that noradrenaline and other amines stored in the cytosol cannot be released by nerve impulses.

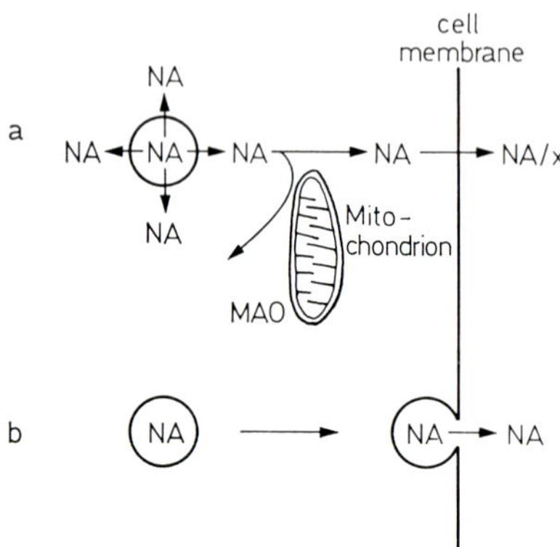

Fig. 11. Release from the cytosol or from the vesicle ?

Release by exocytosis has none of these disadvantages (Fig. 11b): the entire store of transmitter in a vesicle is released without passing *across* any membrane, without passing into the cytosol, and without loss due to diffusion or destruction by monoamine oxidase. Although further experiments are needed before exocytosis is established as the mode of release of noradrenaline from sympathetic nerve terminals, this mechanism has the virtue that it is the simplest explanation of the facts and that it leads to predictions which can be tested experimentally. Most of these arguments also apply to release from vesicles by diffusion of the noradrenaline across a tight junction formed between the vesicle membrane and the nerve cell membrane. If the small noradrenergic vesicles do not contain soluble proteins, whose release could be looked for by biochemical methods, it will be difficult to distinguish secretion by exocytosis from release across a tight junction except by ultrastructural analysis.

B. Subcellular and Molecular Mechanisms of Exocytosis

The recognition that secretion of catecholamines occurs by exocytosis makes it possible to begin an analysis at the subcellular and molecular levels of some of the fundamental mechanisms involved in the response of the secreting cell to a stimulus. In this part of the chapter we shall outline some of the progress that has already been made in this type of analysis, and will raise a few of the many, as yet unanswered, questions posed by the phenomenon of exocytosis. As in part A, we shall concentrate on secretion evoked by nerve stimulation or by cholinergic drugs, and will not discuss in detail the action of other drugs which may cause release of catecholamines by different mechanisms. An exhaustive review has not been attempted.

I. The Cell Membrane as the Site of Stimulus-Secretion Coupling

Douglas and Rubin (1961) coined the phrase 'stimulus-secretion coupling' which "is intended to embrace all the events occurring in the cell exposed to its immediate stimulus that lead, finally, to the appearance of the characteristic secretory product in the extracellular environment" (Douglas, 1968). With emphasis on the word 'immediate' we shall discuss in this section only the final events that are involved in the mobilisation of preformed stores of catecholamines for secretion. Earlier, and subsequent, events involved in secretion will be discussed in section II.

Fig. 12. Stimulus-secretion coupling: the events occurring at the plasma membrane

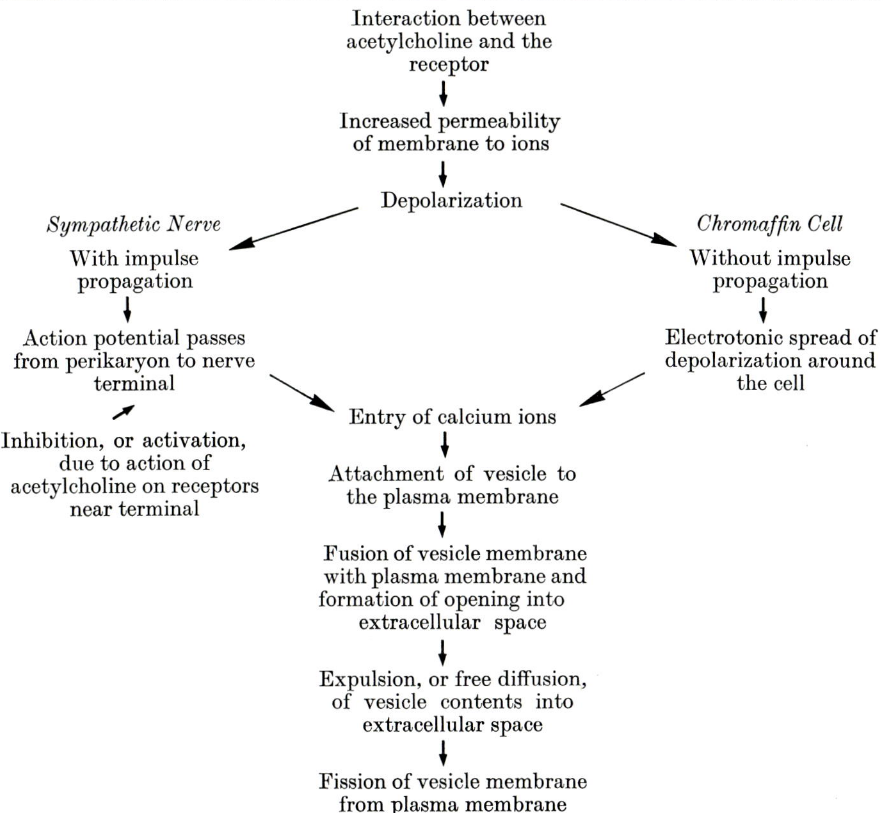

One of the most important consequences of the finding of secretion by exocytosis is that it defines the site, within the cell, of stimulus-secretion coupling. *All the events involved in stimulus-secretion coupling, from the interaction of acetylcholine with receptors to the fusion of vesicle and plasma membranes must occur on, within, or very close to the plasma membrane.* In secretion by exocytosis, there is no need for a signal to pass from the activated receptor on the plasma membrane to storage vesicles deep within the cell, so long as we can assume that there is a high frequency of random collisions between the vesicles and the inner side of the plasma membrane as a result of Brownian motion. A similar assumption has been made in relation to vesicles in motor nerve terminals: "I envisage that the frequency of collisions is very high at all times, but the vast majority of such collisions are unsuccessful and do not lead to transmitter release" (KATZ, 1969). Brownian motion of chromaffin granules has not been observed in living cells, but it has been shown that the neurosecretory granules of neurons in the corpus cardiacum (NORMANN, 1965) and the granules (lysosomes) of polymorphonuclear leucocytes (GLADSTONE and VAN HEYNINGEN, 1967; WOODIN et al., 1963) are in constant motion *in vivo*.

What events take place in the plasma membrane of the cell during stimulus-secretion coupling? It will, eventually, be possible to break down the sequence of events further and further until the molecular and sub-molecular levels are reached but, for the time being, there is still much to discuss, as shown in the 'flow sheet' in Fig. 12.

1. Cholinoceptors

The classical studies of FELDBERG et al. (1934) and FELDBERG and GADDUM (1934) established that acetylcholine is the transmitter released from the splanchnic nerve terminals in the cat adrenal medulla and from the terminals of the cervical sympathetic nerve in the cat superior cervical ganglion.

FELDBERG et al. (1934) found that the action of acetylcholine on the adrenal medulla, although mainly nicotine-like, had a muscarine-like component. This has recently been confirmed for the cat adrenal medulla (DOUGLAS and POISNER, 1965; LEE and TRENDELENBURG, 1967; RUBIN and MIELE, 1968a) and for the dog adrenal medulla (KAYAALP and TÜRKER, 1969; KAYAALP and MCISAAC, 1968, 1969). In the cat adrenal medulla, the distribution of the two types of acetylcholine receptors is not random: the noradrenaline-cells have predominantly nicotinic, and the adrenaline-cells predominantly muscarinic receptors (DOUGLAS and POISNER, 1965; RUBIN and MIELE, 1968a; MIELE, 1969). Such a correlation was not found in studies on the dog (KAYAALP and MCISAAC, 1968). The ox adrenal medulla, perfused with Tyrode's solution *in vitro* (retrogade) did not release catecholamines even when exposed to high concentrations (10^{-4} to 10^{-2} M) of two typical muscarinic stimulants: pilocarpine and methylfurmethide (A.D. SMITH, unpublished observations).

That the perikaryon may not be the only part of an adrenergic neuron which contains cholinoceptors was suggested by the pharmacological studies of COON and ROTHMAN (1940) on the pilomotor response to acetylcholine, and by the discovery of the sympathomimetic response of the spleen to acetylcholine (FARBER, 1936; DALY and SCOTT, 1961; BRANDON and RAND, 1961). FERRY (1963) showed that the sympathomimetic response of the spleen was due to an action of acetylcholine on the post-ganglionic adrenergic C fibres in the splenic nerve, "somewhere near their endings". The presence of cholinergic fibres in post-ganglionic sympathetic nerves led to the suggestion that the cholinoceptors in the terminal region of adrenergic neurons may have a physiological function (BURN and RAND, 1960). Recent electron microscopical studies have shown that acetylcholinesterase-containing (presumably cholinergic) nerve terminals lie very close to noradrenergic nerve terminals in the pancreatic arterioles (GRAHAM et al., 1968). These morphological observations, if confirmed for other tissues, provide support for the idea that locally released acetylcholine may modify the release of noradrenaline by acting on nicotinic receptors (potentiation of release) or on muscarinic receptors (inhibition of release). In the rabbit heart, the latter effect is likely to be of greater physiological significance (LÖFFELHOLZ and MUSCHOLL, 1969). This subject will be considered in more detail in the chapters by KOSTERLITZ and LEES and by HAEFELY.

2. Depolarization

The resting transmembrane potentials of chromaffin cells are of the order of —30 mV (DOUGLAS et al., 1967 a, b; MATTHEWS, 1967) and are lower than the membrane potentials of cells in the adrenal cortex (see Table 6). Acetylcholine, and a number of other chromaffin cell stimulants, depolarize the chromaffin cells of the gerbil in tissue culture, but no action potentials were ever recorded (DOUGLAS et al., 1967 a). Depolarization caused by acetylcholine increases in proportion to the logarithm of the external sodium concentration and, in sodium-free media, is similarly dependent on the external calcium concentration (DOUGLAS et al., 1967 b). These, and other, electrophysiological studies on the chromaffin cell have been reviewed by DOUGLAS (1968). Similar changes in membrane potential presumably occur *in vivo* in response to acetylcholine liberated from the splanchnic nerve. This raises the question whether the depolarization, or ionic movements associated with it, are involved in secretion. For this to be so, the depolarization must occur around the entire cell surface and it should be possible to demonstrate some critical link between depolarization and secretion.

Table 6. *Membrane potentials of adrenal cells*

Animal	Cells	Resting Potential (— mV)	Effect of drugs	Reference
Rabbit	Cortex	66.2	ACTH: no effect except in K^+-free media	MATTHEWS (1967) MATTHEWS and SAFFRAN (1968)
Rat	Cortex	70.5		MATTHEWS (1967)
Kitten	Cortex	71.4		MATTHEWS (1967)
Rabbit	Medulla	24.2	Only slightly affected by changes in $[K]_0$	MATTHEWS (1967)
Rat	Medulla	20.4		MATTHEWS (1967)
Kitten	Medulla	31.7		MATTHEWS (1967)
Gerbil	Medulla	32.8	Depolarized by acetylcholine, nicotine, pilocarpine, histamine, 5-HT, angiotensin, bradykinin	DOUGLAS et al. (1967 a)

There is electron microscopic evidence that, in the hamster adrenal medulla, exocytosis can take place anywhere along the cell surface (DINER, 1967; GRYNSZPAN-WINOGRAD, 1971) and so acetylcholine released from the terminals of the splanchnic nerve must either diffuse around the entire cell, or the local depolarization opposite the nerve terminal must spread to other parts of the cell. Morphological studies (COUPLAND, 1965c; GRYNZSPAN-WINOGRAD, 1969) argue against the first possibility: "Since nerve endings on chromaffin cells often lie in a surface depression and are covered externally by a layer of Schwann cell cytoplasm, it is likely that the acetylcholine released at these endings will exert a largely, if not entirely, local effect on the target cell. This morphological arrangement makes it unlikely that diffusion of the chemical transmitter substance occurs in the adrenal medulla" (COUPLAND, 1965c). The mainly local action of acetylcholine is made even more likely because of the presence of acetylcholinesterase activity on the nerve and chromaffin cell membranes (PALKAMA, 1967; LEWIS and SHUTE, 1969). The lack of any action potentials in chromaffin cells depolarized by acetylcholine (DOUGLAS et al., 1967a) means, therefore, that the local depolarization in the region of the nerve terminals must spread electrotonically. This would readily occur (see HELLERSTEIN, 1968) because chromaffin cells are small (diameter 10 μ—30 μ) and are not markedly elongated (COUPLAND, 1965a, b).

The situation in the adrenergic neuron is, of course, very different because in this cell a propogated impulse results from the action of acetylcholine on the perikaryon. Electrophysiological studies on neurons will be described in the chapter by HAEFELY.

3. Entry of Calcium

Which of the ionic currents associated with depolarization is the vital link in the chain of events leading to secretion? Following the demonstration that calcium is required for the secretion of catecholamines from the adrenal medulla (DOUGLAS and RUBIN, 1961) and the nerve terminals in the heart (HUKOVIC and MUSCHOLL, 1962) a great deal of evidence has been obtained that it is the entry of calcium ions into the cell which provides this link. (For reviews see DOUGLAS, 1968; BANKS, 1970.)

DOUGLAS and RUBIN (1961, 1963) found that omission of either Na^+, K^+, Mg^{2+} or Cl^- from the perfusion fluid did not prevent the release of catecholamines evoked by acetylcholine from the cat adrenal gland; omission of calcium ions, however, completely inhibited the release of catecholamines. The requirement for calcium has since been shown to extend to secretion evoked by such diverse stimuli as potassium ions and angiotensin (see Table 7). Further evidence that sodium ions are not required for secretion is that tetrodotoxin (10^{-7} to 10^{-5} g/ml), which in other tissues blocks the entry of sodium into the cell (KAO, 1966), does not inhibit the release of catecholamines from ox adrenal glands perfused with carbamylcholine (A. D. SMITH, unpublished observation).

The first clue that the action of calcium might depend upon its entry into the cell was the finding of an increased uptake of radioactive calcium into the adrenal gland perfused with acetylcholine (DOUGLAS and POISNER, 1962), although the possibility was not excluded that this might have been due to exchange diffusion (i.e., exchange of radioactive for non-radioactive calcium). What observations of an increased uptake of radioactive calcium (DOUGLAS and POISNER, 1962; RUBIN et al., 1967) do suggest is that acetylcholine increases the permeability of the chromaffin cell membrane to calcium ions. If the concentration of free calcium in chromaffin cells is as low as in other cells (e.g. 10^{-7} M in crab muscle fibres, PORTZEHL et al., 1964; 10^{-5} M in squid nerve, HODGKIN and KEYNES, 1957), then an increase in the permeability of the membrane to calcium will allow extracellular calcium ions (2×10^{-3} M) to run down an electrochemical gradient and enter the cell.

Strong support for this idea has come from electrophysiological studies (DOUGLAS et al., 1967b) which show that although depolarization of the chromaffin cell by acetylcholine is mainly due to an inward sodium current, a small depolarization (about 5 mV) occurs when sodium is absent and this is mainly due to the inward movement of calcium ions. The depolarization due to an inward sodium current was not blocked by tetracaine, whereas that due to the calcium current was prevented by this local anaesthetic (DOUGLAS and KANNO, 1967). That this inward calcium current provides the link with secretion is shown by the fact that the same, or lower, concentrations of tetracaine inhibit the release of catecholamines from the perfused adrenal gland of the gerbil (DOUGLAS and KANNO, 1967) and of the cat (RUBIN et al., 1967). It has been concluded from these, and other, observations that it is the inward movement of calcium ions rather than depolarization *per se*, which is required for secretion (DOUGLAS, 1968). Of course, depolarization will occur in response to acetylcholine *in vivo* because the blood contains sodium ions.

Table 7. *Role of calcium in the release of catecholamines and other vesicle-constituents. Unless stated under 'Notes' the presence of calcium is required for release*

(a) Adrenal medulla (perfused)

Stimulus	Animal	Substances released	Exocytosis (see Tables 1 and 2)	Notes	Reference
Acetylcholine	Cat	Catecholamines	Yes	Release inhibited by Mg^{2+}	DOUGLAS and RUBIN (1961, 1963)
	Ox	Catecholamines	Yes		PHILIPPU and SCHÜMANN (1962, 1966)
	Ox (slices of adrenal)	Catecholamines	(Yes)		OKA et al. (1965a), TRIFARÓ (1969b)
	Rat	Catecholamines	Not known		CESSION-FOSSION (1967)
	Ox	Dopamine β-hydroxylase	Yes		VIVEROS et al. (1968)
	Ox	Chromogranin A	Yes		KIRSHNER et al. (1967)
Carbamylcholine	Ox	Catecholamines	Yes		BANKS (1965b, 1967)
	Ox	Total chromogranins	Yes		SCHNEIDER et al. (1967)
	Ox	Chromogranin A	Yes		SCHNEIDER (1969a)
Methacholine	Cat	Catecholamines	Not known		POISNER and DOUGLAS (1966)
Muscarine	Cat	Catecholamines	Not known		POISNER and DOUGLAS (1966)
Nicotine	Ox	Catecholamines	Yes		KIRSHNER et al. (1967)
		Chromogranin A	Yes		KIRSHNER et al. (1967)
Pilocarpine	Cat	Catecholamines	Not known		POISNER and DOUGLAS (1966)
Histamine	Cat	Catecholamines	Not known		POISNER and DOUGLAS (1966)
5-Hydroxytryptamine	Cat	Catecholamines	Not known		POISNER and DOUGLAS (1966)
Angiotensin	Cat	Catecholamines	Not known		POISNER and DOUGLAS (1966)
Bradykinin	Cat	Catecholamines	Not known		POISNER and DOUGLAS (1966)
Potassium	Cat	Catecholamines	Yes	Release inhibited by Mg^{2+}	DOUGLAS and RUBIN (1961, 1963)
	Ox (slices of adrenal)	Catecholamines	(Yes)		OKA et al. (1965a)
Phenylethylamine	Ox	Catecholamines	Yes, partly	Ca^{2+} not required for release	PHILIPPU and SCHÜMANN (1962)
	Ox	Catecholamines	Yes, partly	Release inhibited 71% without Ca^{2+}	SCHNEIDER (1969a)
	Ox	Chromogranin A	Yes	Release completely dependent on Ca^{2+}	SCHNEIDER (1969a)
	Cat	Catecholamines	Yes	Release inhibited by Mg^{2+} and hexamethonium	RUBIN and JAANUS (1966)
Tyramine	Ox	Catecholamines	Not known	Ca^{2+} not required	PHILIPPU and SCHÜMANN (1966)
	Ox (slices of adrenal)	Catecholamines	Not known	Ca^{2+} not required	OKA et al. (1965a)
	Cat	Catecholamines	Not known	Release inhibited by Mg^{2+}	RUBIN and JAANUS (1966)
	Rat	Catecholamines	Not known		CESSION-FOSSION (1967)
(+) Amphetamine	Cat	Catecholamines	Yes	Release inhibited by Mg^{2+} and hexamethonium	RUBIN and JAANUS (1966)
Metamphetamine	Cat	Catecholamines	Not known		RUBIN and JAANUS (1966)
Phenylpropanolamine	Cat	Catecholamines	Not known	Release inhibited by hexamethonium	RUBIN and JAANUS (1966)
Ephedrine	Cat	Catecholamines	Not known		RUBIN and JAANUS (1966)
	Rat	Catecholamines	Not known		CESSION-FOSSION (1967)
Reserpine	Ox	Catecholamines	Not in rabbit	Ca^{2+} not required	PHILIPPU and SCHÜMANN (1966)
Segontin (Prenylamine)	Ox	Catecholamines	Not known	Ca^{2+} not required Segontin will lyse chromaffin granules *in vitro* (GROBECKER et al., 1968)	PHILIPPU and SCHÜMANN (1966)
Acetaldehyde	Cat	Catecholamines	Not known	Ca^{2+} not required Release not blocked by hexamethonium	AKABANE et al. (1965)

Table 7 (continued)

(b) Sympathetic nerve terminals

Stimulus	Organ perfused	Substance released	Notes	Reference
Nerve at 10 Hz	Rabbit heart	Noradrenaline	Release was inhibited by 68% when Ca^{2+} was 1/8 normal concentration	HUKOVIĆ and MUSCHOLL (1962)
Nerve at 10 Hz	Rabbit ileum	(Not measured)	Low Ca^{2+} inhibited the response to nerve stimulation, but not to added noradrenaline	BURN and GIBBONS (1964)
Nerve at 5—30 Hz	Cat spleen	Noradrenaline	Noradrenaline output/stimulus was linearly related to $\log_{10}(Ca^{2+})$	KIRPEKAR and MISU (1967)
Nerve at 10 Hz	Cat colon	^{3}H Noradrenaline	Lack of Ca^{2+} very slightly increased spontaneous release	BOULLIN (1967)
Nerve at 30 Hz	Dog spleen	Noradrenaline Dopamine β-hydroxylase	See Fig. 9	DE POTTER et al. (1969a); SMITH et al. (1970)
Nerve at 30 Hz	Calf spleen	Noradrenaline Dopamine β-hydroxylase Chromogranin A		DE POTTER et al. (1969b); SMITH et al. (1970)
Excess potassium	Cat heart	Noradrenaline	Lack of Ca^{2+} did not inhibit antidromic discharges in nerves	HAEUSLER et al. (1968)
Excess potassium	Cat spleen	Noradrenaline	Mg^{2+} inhibited the action of potassium	KIRPEKAR and WAKADE (1968)
Excess potassium	Rat vas deferens	Noradrenaline	Mg^{2+} inhibited the action of potassium	BISBY and FILLENZ (1969)
Electrical	Rat heart slices	^{3}H Noradrenaline		BALDESSARINI and KOPIN (1967)
Electrical	Rat brain slices	^{3}H Noradrenaline	Lithium ions inhibited release	BALDESSARINI and KOPIN (1967); KATZ and KOPIN (1969)
Acetylcholine (+ hyoscine)	Rabbit atria	(not measured)	Acetylcholine only accelerated the heart rate in presence of Ca^{2+}.	BURN and GIBBONS (1965)
Acetylcholine (+ atropine)	Rabbit heart	Noradrenaline	Spontaneous release was not affected by changes in Ca^{2+} concentration	LÖFFELHOLZ (1967)
Acetylcholine	Cat hypothalamus	^{14}C Noradrenaline		PHILIPPU et al. (1970)
Acetylcholine	Cat heart	Noradrenaline	Lack of Ca^{2+} did not inhibit antidromic discharges in nerves	HAEUSLER et al. (1968)
Nicotine	Rabbit atria	(Not measured)	Nicotine only accelerated heart rate in presence of Ca^{2+}	BURN and GIBBONS (1965)
DMPP	Rabbit heart	Noradrenaline	Blocked by hexamethonium (LINDMAR and MUSCHOLL, 1961)	LINDMAR et al. (1967)
DMPP	Cat heart	Noradrenaline	Lack of Ca^{2+} did not inhibit antidromic discharges in nerves	HAEUSLER et al. (1968)
Tyramine	Rabbit atria	(Not measured)	Hardly any effect of varying Ca^{2+} concn.	BURN and GIBBONS (1965)
Tyramine	Rabbit heart	Noradrenaline	Ca^{2+} not required Not blocked by hexamethonium (LINDMAR and MUSCHOLL, 1961)	LINDMAR et al. (1967)
Tyramine	Cat irides	^{3}H Noradrenaline	Lack of Ca^{2+} caused small *increase* in spontaneous release and in tyramineinduced release	THOENEN et al. (1969a)
Tyramine	Calf spleen	Noradrenaline	Not known whether Ca^{2+} required No dopamine β-hydroxylase was released	W. P. DE POTTER and I. CHUBB (unpublished observations)

Since the entry of calcium ions is both a necessary and a sufficient stimulus for the release of catecholamines from the adrenal medulla, it is of interest to consider what factors might regulate this process. Four of the possible factors are: the membrane potential; a direct action of acetylcholine or drugs; the presence of ions outside the cell which compete with calcium; the presence of other ions within the cell.

1. Depolarization caused by excess potassium evokes the release of catecholamines (VOGT, 1952) which is calcium dependent (DOUGLAS and RUBIN, 1961). This suggests that depolarization opens a gate to calcium ions, just as electrical depolarization does at the neuromuscular junction (KATZ and MILEDI, 1967). Does a similar event occur in sympathetic nerve terminals? (see chapter by HAEFELY).

2. The action of tetracaine in specifically blocking calcium influx, rather than sodium influx, has already been mentioned. Other local anaesthetics also act in this way (JAANUS et al., 1967) but some act in addition as agonists and antagonists at the cholinoceptors (MIELE and RUBIN, 1968). The ability of local anaesthetics to block calcium-dependent secretion from the adrenal medulla is related to their aromatic character (RUBIN and MIELE, 1968b), rather than to the presence or properties of an alkyl amino group which is involved in their interaction with cholinoceptors (MIELE and RUBIN, 1968). A striking correlation was pointed out (RUBIN and MIELE, 1968b) between the ability of different local anaesthetics to interfere with calcium movement in the adrenal medulla and their ability to block the transport of sodium ions in nerves. It can, then, be predicted that local anaesthetics will have three different actions on sympathetic nerves: they will block impulse propagation in the axon by inhibition of sodium ion movements; they might inhibit release from terminals by blocking calcium ion movements; and they might act as agonists or antagonists at cholinoceptors. There is evidence that tetracaine causes the release of noradrenaline from nerve terminals in the rat vas deferens (VOHRA, 1969) and one possible explanation of this observation is that tetracaine activates nicotinic cholinoceptors in the terminals.

3. Removal of external sodium ions, which causes hyperpolarization of the chromaffin cell (DOUGLAS et al., 1967b), potentiates the release induced by acetylcholine (DOUGLAS and RUBIN, 1963). This raises the possibility that external sodium ions may inhibit the entry of calcium ions. Increasing the concentration of external magnesium ions inhibits the release of catecholamines evoked by acetylcholine and by excess potassium, and this effect of Mg^{2+} can be overcome by increasing the concentration of Ca^{2+} (DOUGLAS and RUBIN, 1963).

4. BANKS (1967) found that ouabain potentiates both the spontaneous release of catecholamines from the perfused adrenal gland, and that induced by carbamylcholine. Further studies on the role of sodium (BANKS et al., 1969b) led to the suggestion that the intracellular concentration of sodium ions may play a part in regulating the influx of Ca^{2+} (see BANKS, 1970).

It should be pointed out that there is at present no evidence to support the idea that, in the adrenal medulla, cyclic AMP is involved in the influx of calcium into the cell, as suggested by RASMUSSEN and TENENHOUSE (1968) for other secreting tissues. Neither cyclic AMP (10^{-2} M) nor its dibutyryl derivative (5×10^{-3} M), nor theophylline (10^{-2} M) evoked the release of catecholamines from the retrogade perfused ox adrenal gland; theophylline (10^{-2} M) inhibited the spontaneous release of catecholamines (A.D. SMITH and W.P. DE POTTER, unpublished observations). KIRSHNER (1969) has reported similar findings and his observation that aminophylline (5×10^{-3} M) evoked a release of amines can be explained by the non-specific action of the ethylenediamine it contains (see SCHNEIDER, 1969a). Experiments should be carried out to see whether derivatives of cyclic AMP, or inhibitors of the phosphodiesterase, modify the action of acetylcholine on the adrenal medulla.

The demonstration that the entry of calcium ions into the cell is required for secretion by exocytosis does not tell us at which stage calcium is involved in stimulus-secretion coupling or, indeed, whether its requirement is specifically related to exocytosis. It could, for example, be argued that calcium is involved in the interaction of acetylcholine with the cell, such as the binding of acetylcholine to the cholinoceptors (see PATON and ROTHSCHILD, 1965). This seems unlikely, however, because calcium is required for secretion evoked by diverse stimuli and, indeed, can itself evoke secretion (DOUGLAS and RUBIN, 1961). Alternatively, calcium may be involved in some change in the property of the cell membrane which occurs in all forms of secretion, not just exocytosis. There is little direct evidence against this possibility, although it has been found that secretion (by ion-pumps?) of water and electrolytes from the salivary gland does not show such a pronounced dependence on calcium as does secretion (by exocytosis: AMSTERDAM et al., 1969) of the proteins from the gland (DOUGLAS and POISNER, 1963).

If calcium is directly involved in exocytosis, then the release of catecholamines by mechanisms other than exocytosis may be (but does not have to be) independent of calcium ions. There are indications (see Table 7) that this is so. The release of catecholamines from the perfused adrenal medulla by reserpine is independent of calcium (PHILIPPU and SCHÜMANN, 1966) and, as described in Section A III, 2, when reserpine acts directly on the adrenal gland it does not cause release by exocytosis. Similarly, the release induced by prenylamine does not require calcium (PHILIPPU and SCHÜMANN, 1966) and this drug has a direct lytic action on the membrane of the chromaffin granule (GROBECKER et al., 1968). Observations on the mode of action of indirectly-acting sympathomimetic amines are particularly interesting. SCHNEIDER (1969a) found that phenylethylamine has two actions on the perfused adrenal gland: the first was dependent upon calcium ions and caused secretion of catecholamines and chromogranin A (i. e. exocytosis); the second was independent of calcium and caused the release of catecholamines but not of chromogranin A. Possibly, the Ca^{2+}-independent release of catecholamines produced by phenylethylamine is a result of the direct action of this amine on chromaffin granules, since SCHÜMANN and PHILIPPU (1962) have shown that phenylethylamine displaces catecholamines from isolated chromaffin granules. The noradrenaline-releasing action of tyramine on sympathetic nerve terminals in the heart (LINDMAR et al., 1967) and irides (THOENEN et al., 1969a) is independent of calcium and so it is noteworthy that this sympathomimetic amine released noradrenaline but not dopamine β-hydroxylase from the terminals of the splenic nerve (W. P. DE POTTER and I. W. CHUBB, unpublished observations). Calcium is, however, required for the release of noradrenaline from sympathetic nerves by electrical stimulation (see Table 7) and for the release of dopamine β-hydroxylase from the splenic nerve stimulated at 30 Hz (see Fig. 9) (DE POTTER et al., 1969a, b).

We can conclude that the evidence for a *specific* role of calcium in exocytosis is mainly indirect. If calcium ions are involved in exocytosis, they might be required just for attachment of the vesicle membrane to the plasma membrane or for the fusion of the two membranes.

4. Attachment of the Vesicle to the Plasma Membrane

The idea that calcium is involved in the attachment of the chromaffin granule to the plasma membrane has often been discussed (see BANKS, 1966b, 1970; DOUGLAS, 1968; SIMPSON, 1968) but there is no direct evidence for this hypothesis. BANKS (1966b) found that calcium ions decreased the net negative charge on chromaffin granules suspended in sucrose solution and suggested that, in the cell, this action of calcium might allow the chromaffin granule to become attached to the cell membrane. A similar observation on the effect of calcium ions on the electrophoretic mobility of 'light' noradrenergic vesicles from rat heart was made by POTTER (1967). Another possibility is that calcium ions, after crossing the membrane, might remain on the inside of the plasma membrane and so form part of a specific attachment site for a negatively charged chromaffin granule. The advantage of the calcium ions remaining on the inner side of the cell membrane, rather than diffusing into the cell, is that fewer ions will be required to enter the cell. Furthermore, if calcium ions do enter the cytosol, they might cause chromaffin granules and other cell particles to agglutinate, as they do *in vitro* (BANKS, 1966b). In their studies on the frog neuromuscular junction, DODGE and RAHAMINOFF (1967) found that the co-operative action of about four calcium ions was necessary for the release of each quantal packet of transmitter, and they suggested that "the probability of release depends on a membrane process in which about four calcium ions must be present simultaneously in a critical position". In view of this suggestion, it is interesting that DOUGLAS and RUBIN (1961) found that the requirement for calcium in the release of catecholamines was not an all-or-none phenomenon: the amount of amine released was greater at higher concentrations of calcium than at lower. Unfortunately, it would be technically very difficult to estimate how many calcium ions are involved in the release of the contents of one chromaffin granule.

Whatever role calcium does play, it seems unlikely that this ion alone is responsible for the specificity of the attachment of the storage vesicle to the cell membrane. Presumably, macromolecules in the plasma membrane and/or in the vesicle membrane are involved in the way the vesicle 'recognises' the attachment site.

Evidence that extracellular calcium can enter the cytosol of chromaffin cells was provided by BOROWITZ (1969) who found that perfusion of the ox adrenal gland with Locke's solution containing ^{45}Ca led to the presence of radioactive calcium in all subcellular fractions. The uptake of ^{45}Ca into each fraction, except the microsomes, occurred about twice as rapidly if the perfusate contained acetylcholine. However, no *net* uptake of calcium could be detected and so it is likely that most of the uptake of radioactive calcium was due to exchange with non-radioactive calcium. The degree of exchange of ^{45}Ca in whole glands, that was caused by acetylcholine, correlated with the amounts of catecholamines released from the glands. BOROWITZ (1969) suggested that this finding supported the hypothesis that calcium acts at an intracellular site to initiate the release process. Another possibility is, however, that acetylcholine was acting on a variable proportion of the cells in different glands. With one exception, the pattern of uptake of ^{45}Ca into the different subcellular fractions was not affected by acetylcholine: in both control and stimulated glands a fraction containing mitochondria and lysosomes had the highest concentration, and the particle-free supernatant had the lowest concentration of ^{45}Ca per weight of protein. The exception was a population of chromaffin granules recovered at the bottom of the sucrose density gradient, which showed a greater increase in ^{45}Ca-content after perfusion of the gland with acetylcholine than did the other cell particles. The population of chromaffin granules in less dense layers of the density gradient did not show this effect. BOROWITZ (1969) argued that the ^{45}Ca taken up into the 'heavy' population of chromaffin granules was not bound superficially but might be bound within the particles. It can be concluded that acetylcholine has two effects, one of which is simply to increase the *rate* of exchange of extracellular calcium with intracellular calcium, an exchange which occurs in the absence of acetylcholine. A second action of acetylcholine is to increase specifically the rate of exchange of extragranular calcium with calcium tightly bound in a certain population, presumably the noradrenaline-containing population (see Fig. 1 and p. 541), of chromaffin granules. A possible explanation of this observation is that the noradrenaline-containing cells are more permeable to Ca^{2+} than the adrenaline-containing cells.

Cogent arguments against the idea (PHILIPPU and SCHÜMANN, 1962, 1966; OKA et al., 1965a) that the role of calcium ions is to release catecholamines directly from chromaffin granules deep in the cell were given by BANKS (1966b, 1970). The chief objections are that such a mechanism does not account for exocytosis, and that the release caused by Ca^{2+} from isolated chromaffin granules (PHILIPPU and SCHÜMANN, 1962; OKA et al., 1965a) is far slower than that from the perfused gland.

What can we Conclude about the Role of Calcium?

The electrophysiological observations show that acetylcholine increases the permeability of the chromaffin cell membrane to calcium, but this effect is transitory and most of the calcium which enters the cell must be pumped out again (see BANKS, 1970) because no net uptake of calcium has been found. The isotopic studies show that acetylcholine promotes an exchange of extracellular with intracellular calcium, and suggest that the calcium which enters the cytoplasm is exchanged with that in all types of cell particle, not just the chromaffin granules. Any action of calcium on chromaffin granules remote from the cell membrane is unlikely to be directly related to secretion of the catecholamines. Some of the calcium which enters the cell may remain at special regions on the inside of the cell membrane, which become the sites of attachment for chromaffin granules. There is no direct evidence from studies on the adrenal medulla for the last suggestion, although a similar hypothesis has been proposed (WOODIN and WIENEKE, 1963, 1964), on the basis of microscopical and biochemical evidence, for the role of calcium in secretion by exocytosis from the granules of polymorphonuclear leucocytes (see WOODIN and WIENEKE, 1970). The chromaffin granule, having become attached to the cell membrane, must, briefly, fuse with the cell membrane in order to secrete its contents. How is this fusion of membranes brought about?

5. Membrane Fusion

In order to understand how two membranes can fuse it is necessary to know what proteins and lipids they contain and how these macromolecules are arranged within the membranes. The arrangement of lipids and proteins in membranes is still only dimly understood (see FINEAN, 1969), and we know only a little about the proteins of the chromaffin granule membrane (HELLE and SERCK-HANSSEN, 1969; WINKLER et al., 1970a; WINKLER, 1971), and even less about the proteins of the plasma membrane of the chromaffin cell. Determination of the lipid composition of the chromaffin granule membrane has, however, provided a clue to one aspect of the fusion process, i.e. how the lipid components of the two interacting membranes might fuse together.

The story begins in 1940 when FELDBERG reported that lysolecithin caused the release of adrenaline from the perfused adrenal gland of the cat. FELDBERG (1940) attributed this to a direct lytic action of the phospholipid on the cells, because he found that lysolecithin released adrenaline from a particulate fraction of the adrenal homogenate. (This was later confirmed by HILLARP and NILSON, 1954b.) FELDBERG did not, of course, have any reason to think that his observations were any more than of pharmacological interest. However, in 1957 HAJDU et al. found that the ox adrenal medulla (but not the cortex) was very rich in a substance which had a digitalis-like action on the heart. This substance was isolated by HAJDU et al. (1957) from ox adrenal medulla and was shown to be lysolecithin (1-palmitoylglycerophosphorylcholine). Perhaps because they were unaware of Feldberg's observations, HAJDU et al. (1957) did not attempt to relate their observation to the physiology of the gland, except to raise the possibility that lysolecithin might be released from the gland in order to act upon the heart.

We now know that insignificant amounts of lysolecithin are released from the adrenal gland (SCHNEIDER et al., 1967) and that the cardiac action of lysolecithin is not due to a direct digitalis-like action, but is the result of the release of noradrenaline from sympathetic nerve terminals (GOVIER and BOADLE, 1967).

Unaware, at the time, of the work of HAJDU et al. (1957) we rediscovered that the adrenal medulla was rich in lysolecithin (BLASCHKO et al., 1966) during studies on the soluble proteins of chromaffin granules (see SMITH and WINKLER, 1967b). DOUGLAS et al. (1966) also reported that lysolecithin was present in the adrenal medulla of cats, dogs and oxen, but the amounts present in the glands were not measured. The striking result of the quantitative studies (BLASCHKO et al., 1966, 1967b; WINKLER et al., 1967) was that although lysolecithin was present in all the subcellular fractions analysed, only small amounts (less than 2% of the total lipid-P) were found in the mitochondrial and microsomal fractions but relatively large amounts (17% of the lipid-P) were found in chromaffin granules. The small amounts present in the other fractions are similar to the amounts found in other tissues, e.g. the phospholipids of rat liver contain 0.9% lysolecithin (SKIPSKI et al., 1964). Almost all the lysolecithin in the adrenal medulla can be quantitatively accounted for by that present in the membranes of chromaffin granules (WINKLER, 1969). Studies on the adrenal medulla of three other species and of chromaffin granules isolated from three different human phaeochromocytomas established that *lysolecithin is a characteristic component of the chromaffin granule membrane* (see Table 8).

A study of the fatty acid composition of lecithin and lysolecithin isolated from chromaffin granules (WINKLER and SMITH, 1968) led to the conclusion that the lysolecithin is entirely in the form of 1-acyl isomer: the main fatty acids present in lysolecithin were stearic acid (43%), palmitic acid (30%) and oleic acid (19%). The problem of the origin and formation of the lysolecithin of chromaffin granules has been discussed previously (WINKLER and SMITH, 1968; SMITH and WINKLER, 1969).

Table 8. *Lysolecithin in chromaffin granules*

Adrenal Gland	Lysolecithin (% of total Lipid-P)	Reference
Ox (English)	16.8	BLASCHKO et al. (1966, 1967b)
Ox (Austrian)	16.8	WINKLER et al. (1967)
Ox (Canadian)	12.9	TRIFARÓ (1969)
Horse	7.1	WINKLER et al. (1967)
Pig	11.3	WINKLER et al. (1967)
Pig (total chr. gran.)	13.5	WINKLER (1969)
Pig (mainly noradrenaline-containing)	19.7	WINKLER (1969)
Human phaeochromocytomas (3)	11.7, 17.8, 23.8	BLASCHKO et al. (1968)
Rat	15.4	WINKLER et al. (1967)

What is the Function of Lysolecithin in Chromaffin Granules?

The rediscovery of lysolecithin in the adrenal medulla came at an opportune moment, for evidence had just been reported indicating that the catecholamines were released by exocytosis. It was natural to think that the lysolecithin in chromaffin granules might be involved in the fusion of the chromaffin granule membrane with the plasma membrane (BLASCHKO et al., 1967b; WINKLER et al., 1967). This suggestion arose out of the well-known membrane-lytic properties of lysolecithin and was no more than an attractive hypothesis until HOWELL and LUCY (1969) were able to demonstrate that lysolecithin can indeed cause biological membranes to fuse. Addition of lysolecithin to suspensions of hen erythrocytes not only caused haemolysis, it caused the formation of multinucleate cells. The syncytia had formed by fusion of the membranes of the individual erythrocyte ghosts (HOWELL and LUCY, 1969). These observations not only demonstrate that lysolecithin can cause the fusion of membranes, they raise the possibility that the presence of lysolecithin in a membrane might be all that is required to bring about fusion. We consider that HOWELL and LUCY's (1969) studies provide strong, though indirect, support for the idea that lysolecithin in chromaffin granule membranes is involved in the process of membrane fusion.

The molecular mechanism of membrane lysis and fusion caused by lysolecithin is probably related to the shape of the molecule. Whereas diacylglycerophosphatides are approximately rectangular in cross-section, their lyso-compounds (monoacylglycerophosphatides) are wedge-shaped because the hydrophilic moiety is broader than the hydrophobic moiety (HAYDON and TAYLOR, 1963). Because of its wedge-shape, a molecule of lysolecithin cannot fit into bimolecular layers of lecithin, and so they break down into globular micelles (HAYDON and TAYLOR, 1963; BANGHAM and HORNE, 1964). A model of how lysolecithin might be involved in membrane fusion was proposed by LUCY (1969). According to this model, only those regions of two interacting membranes which contain a sufficient proportion of lipids in a micellar form will fuse. We are thus left with the question whether the plasma membrane of the chromaffin cell (which is not rich in lysolecithin) contains lysolecithin localised in a few specific sites, or whether it contains a phospholipase A which could form lysolecithin when the cell is stimulated (see WINKLER, 1971, for a more detailed discussion).

There is no evidence, either that the amounts of lysolecithin change, or that it turns over more rapidly than other phospholipids following stimulation *in vitro* (TRIFARÓ, 1969a). In his studies on phospholipid metabolism, TRIFARÓ (1969a) confirmed and extended the original observation of HOKIN et al. (1958) that acetylcholine causes an increased incorporation of radioactivity from ^{32}P-orthophospate into phosphatidic acid, phosphatidylinositol and lecithin. Acetylcholine did not release catecholamines from slices of adrenal medulla incubated in a calcium-free medium, but its action on phospholipid metabolism was unaffected (TRIFARÓ, 1969b). This finding, together with the fact that the metabolic effect of acetylcholine is slower than its action in evoking secretion (TRIFARÓ, 1969a) argue against a direct relation of phospholipid turnover to stimulus-secretion coupling. A similar effect of stimulation on phospholipid metabolism has been found in sympathetic ganglia (HOKIN et al., 1960), where it has been shown to be located postsynaptically (LARRABEE and LEICHT, 1965; LARRABEE, 1968) in the cell bodies of sympathetic neurons (HOKIN, 1965, 1969).

6. Release by Diffusion, or by Active Expulsion, of Vesicle Contents?

Soon after the discovery of chromaffin granules, HILLARP and NILSON (1954b) described detailed studies on the stability of isolated chromaffin granules which established that any procedure that causes damage to the membrane results in the immediate release of catecholamines into solution. The specific disruption of the chromaffin granule membrane that occurs in exocytosis will have the same effect: the micellar storage complex within the granules will be able to diffuse out, and water will be able to diffuse in, through the opening in the membrane. In the extracellular space the micelles will rapidly break down as a result of dilution. It is even possible that their breakdown is favoured by extracellular ions, since BERNEIS et al. (1970) have reported that excess Ca^{2+} caused the micelles to collapse. Proteins present within the chromaffin granule will also be able to diffuse into the extracellular space provided that the opening in the membrane is several times larger than the diameter of the largest protein molecule. In fact, from the micrographs of DINER (1967) and GRYNSZPAN-WINOGRAD (1971) it can be seen that the opening is often large enough to allow the entire contents (the dense-cores) to pass intact into the extracellular space. On the basis of the size of the molecules in chromaffin granules relative to that of the opening formed during exocytosis, we can conclude that there is no reason to postulate active expulsion of the contents since free diffusion will suffice.

Does the chromaffin granule remain fused with the cell membrane for a sufficient length of time to allow its contents to diffuse into the extracellular space? The mean rate of displacement of a molecule of chromogranin A by Brownian motion can be calculated from its diffusion coefficient (SMITH and WINKLER, 1967b) using EINSTEIN's equation: the molecule will diffuse 3000 Å (the diameter of a typical chromaffin granule) in about 10 msec. It is not known how long a chromaffin granule remains fused with the cell membrane, and so we must look at other secreting cells. The fusion and emptying of the granules of polymorphonuclear leucoytes during excoxytosis has been observed by phase contrast microscopy and appears to be complete within about 100—200 msec (HIRSCH, 1962). However, this is two orders of magnitude slower than the synaptic delay found in neuromuscular junctions and in the giant synapse of the squid (KATZ, 1969). The release of transmitter occurs within about 1 msec of the arrival of an action potential in the terminal. If release occurs by exocytosis, this period must be sufficient for the vesicle to fuse with the plasma membrane. This does not, of course, tell us how long the vesicle may remain fused *after* the transmitter has diffused or been expelled, into the synaptic gap.

It could be argued that a chromaffin granule fuses several times with the cell membrane, each time expelling a portion of its contents. If the period of fusion was short (1 msec or less) then the low molecular weight substances would diffuse out of the granule preferentially. The chromaffin granule would then become relatively rich in proteins (including dopamine β-hydroxylase) but would be less dense due to loss of amines and ATP. VIVEROS et al. (1969d) showed that 4 hr after the administration of insulin to rabbits, the adrenaline and dopamine β-hydroxylase which remained in the adrenals were stored in chromaffin granules that had the same density as normal chromaffin granules. Furthermore, the ratio of dopamine β-hydroxylase activity to adrenaline in the chromaffin granules from stimulated adrenals was close to that in normal glands. (In contrast, VIVEROS et al. (1969d) found that the chromaffin granules in the adrenals of rabbits treated with reserpine were less dense than normal and contained much more dopamine β-hydroxylase relative to adrenaline). These experiments show that, in the long term (i.e. hours), following reflex stimulation of the adrenal medulla, the entire content of each chromaffin granule is released. It would, of course, be interesting to know whether the immediate response to a stimulus is the same.

KIRSHNER and VIVEROS (1970) have calculated, from data in the literature, that each stimulus applied to the splanchnic nerve of the cat leads to the release of approximately the same amount of catecholamines, from each chromaffin cell, that is present in one chromaffin granule (2.4×10^6 molecules). This kind of calculation, when applied to a nerve, may give a meaningful result but, even so, many assumptions have to be made (see pp. 566—570). However, a similar approach can hardly be used to provide evidence of quantal release from the adrenal medulla, since the chromaffin cells are stimulated indirectly by acetylcholine released from the splanchnic nerve. There does not yet appear to be any way of calculating whether a chromaffin granule releases its contents all at once, or in series of separate "exocytotic fusions".

An argument against the idea that the contents of a chromaffin granule are released by diffusion alone is that, in the hamster adrenal medulla, the intact dense-core of the chromaffin granule is found in the extracellular space (DINER, 1967; GRYNSZPAN-WINOGRAD, 1971). Such a large particle would take a relatively long time to diffuse out of an opening not much larger than itself. Another argument in favour of the contents of the vesicle being expelled into the extracellular space is that the surface tension in the membrane of a vesicle would tend to make the membrane flatten in line with the cell membrane: this would, presumably, occur almost instantaneously and so might force the contents into the extracellular space (see Fig. 13, below). We can conclude that a combination of free diffusion and surface tension forces should be sufficient to eject the contents of a vesicle that has fused with the cell membrane. The arguments are, however, indirect and the possibility is by no means excluded that there is an active, enzyme catalysed, process which expels the contents.

There are several reports that energy is required for the secretion of adrenal catecholamines evoked by acetylcholine (KIRSHNER and SMITH, 1969; RUBIN, 1969) or by K^+ or Ca^{2+} (RUBIN, 1969). It is likely that ATP, provided either by glycolysis or oxidative phosphorylation, is involved in one or more stages in stimulus-secretion coupling. It is not yet possible to identify which stage(s) require ATP. POISNER and TRIFARÓ (1967) have proposed a model in which ATP present in the cell membrane is involved in the fusion of the chromaffin granule membrane with the cell membrane. In this model, fusion is initiated by the action of the Mg^{2+}- activated ATPase in the chromaffin granule membrane on the ATP bound to the cell membrane. POISNER and TRIFARÓ's hypothesis arose out of their own observations and those of others (OKA et al., 1965b, 1967b, c; LISHAJKO, 1969, 1970; FERRIS et al., 1970) on the effect of ATP on isolated chromaffin granules. Chromaffin granules, when suspended in salt solutions, but not when suspended in sucrose solutions, are slowly lysed when ATP and Mg^{2+} are added. The lysis is accompanied (or preceded ?) by a decrease in the optical density of the suspension (OKA et al., 1967b, c; TRIFARÓ and POISNER, 1967). Some of the drugs which inhibit the Mg^{2+}-dependent ATPase also inhibit lysis of the granules, and inhibit the acetylcholine-evoked release of catecholamines from the perfused gland (FERRIS et al., 1970; KIRSHNER, 1969). The latter effect may be fortuitous, or it might indicate a role for the Mg^{2+}-dependent ATPase in secretion.

It is difficult to correlate observations on the lysis of isolated chromaffin granules with events in stimulus-secretion coupling for three reasons. (i) Secretion by exocytosis involves an interaction between the plasma membrane and the membrane of the chromaffin granule. Is it possible that the chromaffin granule fractions studied are, in fact, contaminated by fragments of plasma membrane ? (ii) The lytic action of ATP and Mg^{2+} seems to occur far too slowly (see OKA et al., 1967b, c; TRIFARÓ and POISNER, 1967; POISNER and TRIFARÓ, 1969; FERRIS et al., 1970) for it to be involved in secretion. (iii) The slowness of the lysis, together with its requirement for chloride ions (LISHAJKO, 1969) suggest that the action of ATP and Mg^{2+} on isolated chromaffin granules is to cause the uptake of an ion (chloride) into the granules, which is followed by the osmotic uptake of water leading to swelling and, eventually, lysis.

7. Membrane Fission

In the early morphological studies on the adrenal medulla which led to the concept of exocytosis (DE ROBERTIS and VAS FEIRRERA, 1957; DE ROBERTIS and SABATINI, 1960) the question of what happens to the chromaffin granule membrane after it has fused with the plasma membrane was left unanswered. It seems, however, to have been assumed by DE ROBERTIS and SABATINI (1960) that the empty membranes of chromaffin granules did not remain permanently incorporated in the cell membrane, but returned to the cytoplasm where they "disappear" (Figs. 6 and 7 of DE ROBERTIS and SABATINI, 1960). Palade pointed out in 1959 (see below), in connection with his demonstration of exocytosis in the exocrine pancreas, that some mechanism must exist to retrieve the membranes of zymogen granules which have fused with the cell membrane. However, there is still very little evidence about how the membrane of any secretion granule is recovered. Two means of retrieval can be distinguished:

1. Non-Specific Membrane Retrieval. The membrane of the secretion granule may remain incorporated in the plasma membrane, but a net increase in the area of the plasma membrane may be avoided by the removal of other parts of the plasma membrane into the cytoplasm. This retrieval might occur by micropinocytosis of plasma membrane giving rise to small vesicles or, alternatively (see HOKIN, 1968) parts of the plasma membrane may return to the cytoplasm following their breakdown into submicroscopic subunits.

2. Specific Retrieval. The membrane of the secretion granule may itself be removed from the plasma membrane by fission at the original site of fusion. Retrieval by this means would avoid "diluting" the plasma membrane with non-specific membrane; it also makes it possible, in theory, for the secretion granule membrane to be refilled with secretory material and used again in a secretion 'cycle', or 'shuttle service' (see Section B II).

It has not yet proved possible to distinguish these mechanisms by electron microscopical methods. Several authors have reported the presence, in stimulated adrenal chromaffin cells, of 'empty membranes' or 'small vesicles' (e.g. DE ROBERTIS and SABATINI, 1960; YATES, 1964; BENEDECZKY et al., 1965; MOPPERT, 1966a; MALAMED et al., 1968; D'ANZI, 1969), but the origin of these vesicles was not established by the use of enzyme markers (e.g. AMPase for plasma membrane: WOOD, 1967). There is no specific marker for the chromaffin granule membrane which could be used in electron microscopy. A similar problem exists in other cells, and was recognised by PALADE (1959) in his studies on the exocrine pancreas:

"It is highly improbable that the membrane [of the zymogen granule] moves only from the centrosphere to the surface. An unidirectional movement would soon result in considerable enlargement of the lumen and exhaustion of the intracellular membranous material. It is reasonable to assume that a concomitant movement, from the surface to the centrosphere region, takes place, and the presence of small 'empty' vesicles below the luminal membrane is compatible with this assumption. We may conclude that we 'see' the centrifugal arc of this circular movement because the membrane is marked for its duration by the characteristically dense content of the zymogen granule. And we may assume that we cannot visualise the centripetal arc because in its case we lack a natural marker".

PALADE's suggestion that small 'empty' vesicles, present below the plasma membrane, might be part of the centripetal flow of membranes has been supported by observations on the parotid gland (AMSTERDAM et al., 1969). It was found that, after the release by exocytosis of the contents of a large proportion of the zymogen granules, the lumen temporarily became enlarged, but that, as the lumen contracted to its original size, a large number of small vesicles appeared in the cytoplasm beneath the luminal membrane (AMSTERDAM et al., 1969). Empty vesicles have, as already pointed out, been observed in stimulated adrenal medullary cells, and an examination of the published micrographs (YATES, 1964; MALAMED et al., 1968) suggests that many of these vesicles are smaller than typical chromaffin granules: D'ANZI (1969) has, in fact, pointed this out from his own studies.

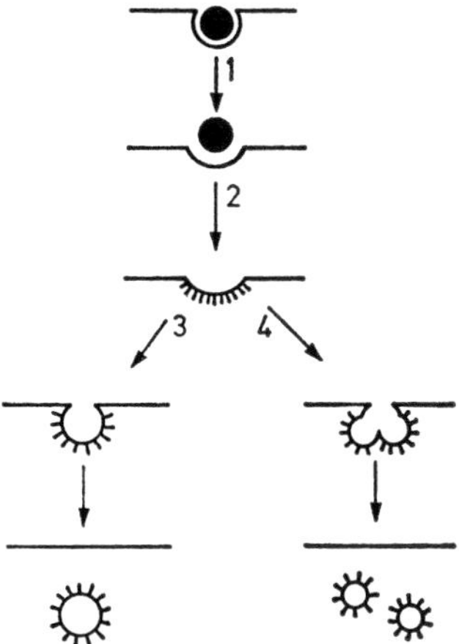

Fig. 13. *Membrane fusion and fission.* 1. Vesicle has just fused with cell membrane and surface tension force tends to flatten vesicle membrane, so expelling the contents into the extracellular space. 2. Bristle coating forms on vesicle membrane. 3. Vesicle membrane is drawn back into sphere, leading to fission of vesicle membrane from cell membrane. A coated vesicle is formed. 4. Vesicle membrane is drawn into two spheres, fission occurs and two small coated vesicles are formed

Is it possible to identify the site of origin of these small vesicles in chromaffin cells? They may be derived from the coated pits observed in the plasma membrane of rat adrenal chromaffin cells by HOLZTMAN and DOMINITZ (1968): this could then, be an example of non-specific retrieval. However, in her studies on the hamster adrenal medulla, DINER (1967) discovered that many of the chromaffin granule membranes which had fused with the cell membrane were no longer smooth in outline, but had one or more coated pits attached to them. This can be seen in one of DINER's micrographs which is reproduced in Figure 6. In further studies, GRYNSZPAN-WINOGRAD (1971), formerly DINER, reported that 30—40% of the chromaffin granule membranes involved in exocytosis had coated pits attached to them. The coated pits formed from chromaffin granule membranes represented about a third of all the coated pits along the plasma membrane,

HOLTZMAN and DOMINITZ (1968) showed that the coated pits along the chromaffin cell membrane gave rise to coated vesicles in the cytoplasm. The presence of a bristle coating on a vesicle attached to a plasma membrane has so often been associated with the fission of the vesicle from the plasma membrane (see FAWCETT, 1965) that we can assume that *the presence of a coating on a membranous pit indicates that it is about to undergo fission and form a vesicle.* DINER's (1967) discovery is, therefore, possibly the clue to how the chromaffin granule membrane is retrieved from the plasma membrane. The presence of the coating may represent a contractile mechanism which is required to overcome the increase in surface tension involved in the fission of a small vesicle from a large surface (see Fig. 13). Could this be one of the functions of the Mg^{2+}-activated ATPase in the chromaffin granule membrane ?. Is this an energy-requiring step ? Perhaps the energy requirement for secretion is, in part, because of the necessity to remove the chromaffin granule membrane after exocytosis so that other chromaffin granules can fuse with the plasma membrane at the (limited number ?) of specific attachment sites. These speculations are offered as hypotheses to be tested by future experimentation.

One of the most promising experimental approaches is to combine ultrastructural and biochemical techniques. If the biochemist can provide the microscopist with a marker for the chromaffin granule membrane, it will be possible to follow the fate of the membrane after secretion. VIVEROS et al. (1969d) have already reported biochemical evidence consistent with the idea that each chromaffin granule membrane disintegrates into several smaller vesicles following secretion: most of the membrane-bound dopamine β-hydroxylase remaining in the rabbit adrenal gland after stimulation was recovered in the microsomal fraction, and so must have been present in lighter (and so, possibly, smaller) particles than intact chromaffin granules. A suggestion has also been made (SMITH, 1970) that the small dense-cored vesicles of sympathetic nerve terminals might originate in a similar way by fission from the membranes of large dense-cored vesicles, following exocytosis (see Section B II).

II. Subcellular Dynamics of Catecholamine-Containing Vesicles

The secretion of proteins, in addition to the catecholamines, from the chromaffin cell and from the sympathetic neuron raises a number of new questions, e.g.: where are the proteins synthesised and where are they packaged into vesicles; what relationship is there between the synthesis of the proteins and that of the catecholamines; how are the vesicles transported to the site of secretion; and, what is the origin and ultimate fate of the membrane of the vesicle ? At present, most of these questions cannot be answered, and all we can do is to make some suggestions on the basis of what is known about other secreting cells.

From the work of Palade and his colleagues a fairly complete picture has been built up of how secretory proteins are synthesised and transported to the extracellular space in the exocrine pancreas cell of the guinea pig (see JAMIESON and PALADE, 1967a, b; 1968a, b and references therein). The proteins are synthesised on ribosomes of the rough endoplasmic reticulum, pass into the cisternae of the endoplasmic reticulum, and are transported to cisternae of the Golgi apparatus by small vesicles which bud off the transitional endoplasmic reticulum. In the Golgi apparatus the proteins are packaged into condensing vacuoles, which mature into zymogen granules. The zymogen granules move to the cell surface where they release their contents by exocytosis. It is likely that the subcellular mechanisms in other protein-secreting cells are similar to those in the exocrine pancreas, but the possibility that other pathways occur should not be excluded (see, for example, RENOLD, 1970).

In this final section we shall outline some of the subcellular pathways of catecholamine-containing vesicles in the chromaffin cell and in the sympathetic neuron. In order to keep the discussion brief we have summarised several possible pathways diagrammatically (Figs. 14 and 15). It should be emphasized that these drawings only represent working hypotheses, and that the arrows indicate directions of movement which have been inferred from biochemical studies or extrapolated from observations on other cells.

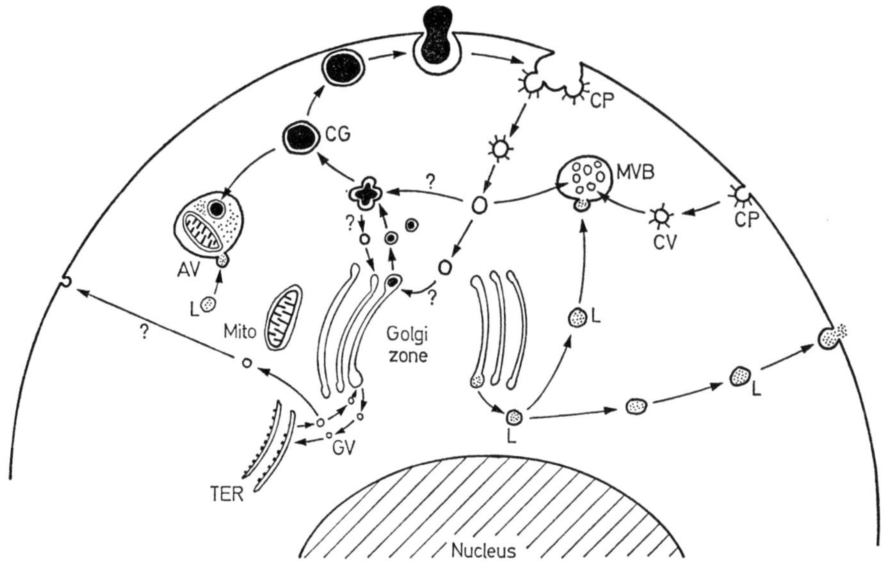

Fig. 14. *Subcellular dynamics of the chromaffin cell.* Key: AV = autophagic vacuole, CG = chromaffin granule, CP = coated membrane pit, CV = coated vesicle, GV = Golgi vesicle, L = Lysosome (primary), MITO = Mitochondrion, MVB = Multivesicular body, TER = Transitional (rough smooth) endoplasmic reticulum

1. Chromaffin Cell (Fig. 14)

a) Origin of the Chromaffin Granules

It is probable that the chromogranins are synthesised in the rough endoplasmic reticulum, which hypertrophies in the chromaffin cells of cold-stressed rats (M. VIOLA-MAGNI, personal communication). Although many electron microscopists have suggested that chromaffin granules originate in the Golgi apparatus (see chapter by COUPLAND), it is not known how the newly synthesised chromogranins are transferred to the cisternae of the Golgi region. One possibility is that small vesicles transfer the proteins from the transitional endoplasmic reticulum to the Golgi cisternae in a 'shuttle service', as occurs in the exocrine pancreas cell. Alternatively, or in addition, chromaffin granules may arise directly from those cisternae of transitional endoplasmic reticulum which lie close to the Golgi apparatus (HOLTZMAN and DOMINITZ, 1968).

It has been pointed out by microscopists that the 'newly formed' chromaffin granules near the Golgi apparatus are smaller than the 'mature' chromaffin granules which lie in the periphery of the cell (DE ROBERTIS and SABATINI, 1960;

COUPLAND, 1965b; RATZENHOFER and MÜLLER, 1967). These small chromaffin granules are particularly prominent in cells that are recovering from a prolonged stimulus (CLEMENTI and ZOCHE, 1963) and in adrenal chromaffin cells after hypophysectomy (POHORECKY and RUST, 1968). (It seems as if hypophysectomy inhibits the formation of mature chromaffin granules in both adrenaline- and noradrenaline-containing cells). How are the small chromaffin granules converted into the more common, larger, chromaffin granules? Perhaps, as indicated in the diagram, several small granules fuse to give a large one. In two electron micrographs published by ALLAMI (1969, Figs. 3 and 4) some chromaffin granules can be seen in the Golgi region whose membranes are not smooth: each chromaffin granule seems to have a smaller vesicle attached to it.

The possibility should be considered that some of the small chromaffin granules which bud off the cisternae of the Golgi apparatus may be able to release their contents by exocytosis. If this is also so for the small chromaffin granules which originate from the transitional endoplasmic reticulum (HOLTZMAN and DOMINITZ, 1968), then a pathway for the release of proteins will be provided that by-passes the Golgi apparatus. Such a pathway has been proposed by RENOLD (1970) in order to account for some aspects of secretion from the β-cells of the pancreas.

Another question which remains to be settled is how the chromaffin granule obtains its membrane. Biochemical analysis has shown that the membrane of the chromaffin granule is chemically distinct from that of other membranes in the cell (see WINKLER et al., 1970a); the only common protein component so far identified is cytochrome b_{559}, which is present both in chromaffin granules and in the microsomal fraction (see BANKS, 1965b). It has not yet proved possible to isolate membranes of the Golgi apparatus in order to see whether they have a similar composition to the membranes of chromaffin granules.

The macromolecular components of the chromaffin granule are synthesised and assembled in the endoplasmic reticulum and/or in the Golgi apparatus. At what stage are the catecholamines and ATP added to the particle? Is the synthesis of catecholamines tightly linked with that of the other components of the chromaffin granule? In animals treated with large doses of insulin the majority of the adrenaline-containing chromaffin cells in the adrenal gland are depleted of their amines: in the adrenals of such animals the resynthesis of ATP (SCHÜMANN, 1958a) and of dopamine β-hydroxylase (see Fig. 4) occurs several hours earlier than resynthesis of the catecholamines. Thus it appears that the catecholamines can be added to the chromaffin granules after the other components. Independent evidence in support of this, is that as early as three minutes after perfusion of the ox adrenal gland with [^{3}H] tyrosine, radioactive catecholamines are found in chromaffin granules isolated by density gradient centrifugation (H. HÖRTNAGL, J. SCHÖPF and H. WINKLER, unpublished observations). Although we can conclude from these results that there is not a *tight* coupling between the synthesis of each of the various components of the chromaffin granule, some signal must tell the cell when to increase the rate of synthesis of catecholamines and other secreted substances following stimulation. Is the signal simply a result of depletion of the store, or does nerve stimulation have an independent action on the chromaffin cell? We have already mentioned an effect of acetylcholine on phospholipid metabolism which is not directly related to secretion (see p. 594); is this a reflection of the turnover of membranes associated with the assembly of chromaffin granules? Particularly interesting is the finding that stimulation increases the amount of tyrosine hydroxylase in adrenal glands (VIVEROS et al., 1969c; THOENEN et al., 1969b), since this enzyme is not present in chromaffin granules (LADURON and BELPAIRE, 1968b).

b) Transport of Chromaffin Granules

The small size of the chromaffin cell makes it likely that diffusion of chromaffin granules as a result of random Brownian motion would be sufficient to carry chromaffin granules from their site of assembly in the Golgi region to the periphery of the cell (for a detailed discussion see MATTHEWS, 1970). This does not exclude the possibility that other mechanisms of migration are also involved. Microtubules are believed to play a role in the active translocation of vesicles, and/or in determining their direction of movement, in several types of cell. Occasional microtubules can be seen in electron micrographs of chromaffin cells (see COUPLAND, 1965b; DINER, 1967), but these tubules are not orientated in any particular direction. Two substances which interact with microtubules, colchicine and vinblastine, reversibly inhibit the secretion of catecholamines evoked by carbamylcholine from the perfused ox adrenal gland (A. D. SMITH, unpublished observations.). However, high concentrations of these drugs (5×10^{-3} M) were required, and their inhibitory action on secretion may have been unrelated to their action on microtubules.

c) Ultimate Fate of Chromaffin Granules

Autophagic vacuoles are found in the chromaffin cells of normal adrenal medulla (HOLTZMAN and DOMINITZ, 1968; AL-LAMI, 1969; YOKOYAMA and TAKAYASU, 1969) and of human phaeochromocytomas (BLASCHKO et al., 1968; YOKOYAMA and TAKAYASU, 1969); these autophagic vacuoles sometimes contain partly digested chromaffin granules. This, then, may be the way in which the cell removes excess chromaffin granules (cf. SMITH and FARQUHAR, 1966). After secretion by exocytosis, the empty membrane of the chromaffin granule remains behind in the cell. Eventually, these membranes will also probably be degraded in autophagic vacuoles. Perhaps multivesicular bodies, which have been seen in chromaffin cells (COUPLAND, 1965b; BENEDECZKY, 1967; HOLTZMAN and DOMINITZ, 1968), represent one of the sites of intracellular digestion of the membranes, since a multivesicular body can become an autophagic vacuole following fusion with a lysosome. Lysosomes of chromaffin cells contain a full complement of hydrolytic enzymes (SMITH and WINKLER, 1966, 1968).

Although the *ultimate* fate of the chromaffin granule membrane is to be destroyed, like other cell components, by autophagy, the possibility should be considered that each membrane can be used more than once. Perhaps, as indicated in Fig. 14, the empty membranes return to the Golgi region where they are used to envelope more secretory products. This would be a kind of 'secretion cycle' or 'shuttle service' similar to that which the small Golgi vesicles operate between the endoplasmic reticulum and the Golgi apparatus in the exocrine pancreas. Studies on the relative rates of turnover of the chromogranins and of the chromomembrins (the specific membrane proteins of chromaffin granules) might throw light on this question (see WINKLER, 1971). Re-use of the chromaffin granule membrane several times, before it is degraded by autophagy, would clearly be very economical for the cell. In secreting cells, such as neurons, which contain much smaller vesicles, an even greater rate of breakdown and synthesis of membrane would be required if the vesicle membrane is not re-used (see discussion by LOCKE and COLLINS, 1968). This is one of the strongest arguments for the re-use of synaptic vesicle membranes in neurons (see below).

2. Sympathetic Neuron (Fig. 15)

One of the main differences between the subcellular dynamics of the neuron and that of the chromaffin cell arises because the nerve terminals are remote from the perikaryon. The perikaryon is the major site of protein synthesis in the neuron (DROZ, 1969). Proteins released from the terminals will, therefore, probably have been synthesised in the perikaryon and transported along the axon to the terminals. However, the terminal does not depend upon the perikaryon for more than a trace (less than 1% per day) of its noradrenaline (GEFFEN and RUSH, 1968). In the nerve terminal the synthesis of noradrenaline is dissociated from that of the secretory proteins: synthesis of the neurotransmitter will continue so long as there are sufficient amounts present of the enzymes required for its biosynthesis (for a review, see GEFFEN and LIVETT, 1971).

a) Origin of Noradrenergic Vesicles

As discussed in Section A I, 2 the distribution of the different types of noradrenergic vesicle in neurons is not uniform. The large dense-cored vesicles are the predominant, or only, type of noradrenergic vesicle in cell bodies and in preterminal axons; but nerve terminals contain mainly the small dense-cored vesicles. It seems reasonable to conclude that the small dense-cored vesicles originate in the terminals, and the possible modes of origin of this type of vesicle will be discussed below in connection with the fate of the large vesicles.

Large dense-cored vesicles probably originate in the Golgi region of the perikaryon (HÖKFELT, 1968, 1969; GEFFEN and OSTBERG, 1969) although the presence of other dense bodies (primary lysosomes) in this region of the cell makes it difficult to be certain.

b) Transport of Noradrenergic Vesicles

The discovery of the rapid proximo-distal flow of noradrenaline in sympathetic nerves (for reviews see DAHLSTRÖM, 1969; GEFFEN and LIVETT, 1971) led to the idea that noradrenergic vesicles were moving along the axon from the cell body to the terminals. This idea was further supported by the demonstration that dopamine β-hydroxylase and chromogranin A, two proteins present in the vesicles (see Section A I, 2), also migrated rapidly along the axon (LADURON and BELPAIRE, 1968c; GEFFEN et al., 1969b). Finally, it has been shown that dense-cored vesicles accumulate on the proximal side of constrictions placed round sympathetic nerves (KAPELLER and MAYOR, 1967, 1969; BANKS et al., 1969c). It was pointed out by GEFFEN and OSTBERG (1969) that the dense-cored vesicles which accumulated were exclusively of the larger type.

The rate of proximo-distal movement of large dense-cored vesicles in nerve axons is high. If we assume that the rate of movement of [^{14}C] noradrenaline in cat splenic nerve (0.5 cm/hr., LIVETT et al., 1968) is the same as that of the vesicles, then a vesicle will be moving at 1.4 μ/sec. Such a rate of movement over a *short* distance is not much greater than that possible by random Brownian motion, although the rate of displacement by Brownian motion depends upon the viscosity of the medium (see SHEA and KARNOVSKY, 1966). If the viscosity of the axoplasm in the splenic nerve is as low as that of the axoplasm in lobster nerve, i.e. about 0.06 poises (HEILBRÜNN, 1956), then a vesicle of radius 500 Å would have a root mean square displacement of 1.2 μ in one second by Brownian motion. What is remarkable about the flow of vesicles in nerves is not so much their *rate* of movement, it is rather the fact that the *movement occurs in one direction, over a large distance.* SHEA and KARNOVSKY (1966) have discussed how Brownian motion could account for the movement of micropinocytotic vesicles from one side of an endothelial cell to another, but here the distance involved is relatively small. It is quite possible that movement in one direction over a large distance can only be achieved by an active process. SCHMITT and SAMSON (1969) suggested that the microtubules orientated longitudinally in nerve axons might be involved in the transport of vesicles, by a mechanism similar to that involved in muscular contraction; and electron microscopic studies have revealed an association between synaptic vesicles and microtubules in axons of the lamprey nerve cord (JÄRLFORS and SMITH, 1969). Colchicine, applied topically to a sympathetic nerve, blocks the transport of noradrenaline (DAHLSTRÖM, 1969).

c) Fate of Large Dense-Cored Vesicles

Terminal varicosities of sympathetic nerves contain predominantly small dense-cored vesicles and look quite unlike the axon above a ligature, which is full of large dense-cored vesicles. It seems, then, that most of the large vesicles which reach the terminal disappear. GEFFEN and OSTBERG (1969) suggested that the large vesicles might be precursors of the small vesicles. This idea would be strongly supported if common structural components (e.g. the membrane proteins) could be demonstrated in both types of vesicle. As we have already discussed (see Section A I, 2) there is still no unequivocal evidence for the presence of dopamine β-hydroxylase in small dense-cored vesicles. POTTER (1967) found this enzyme, bound to membranes, in a highly purified fraction of noradrenergic vesicles (probably of the 'light' type) isolated from rat heart. Subcellular fractionation studies on the vas

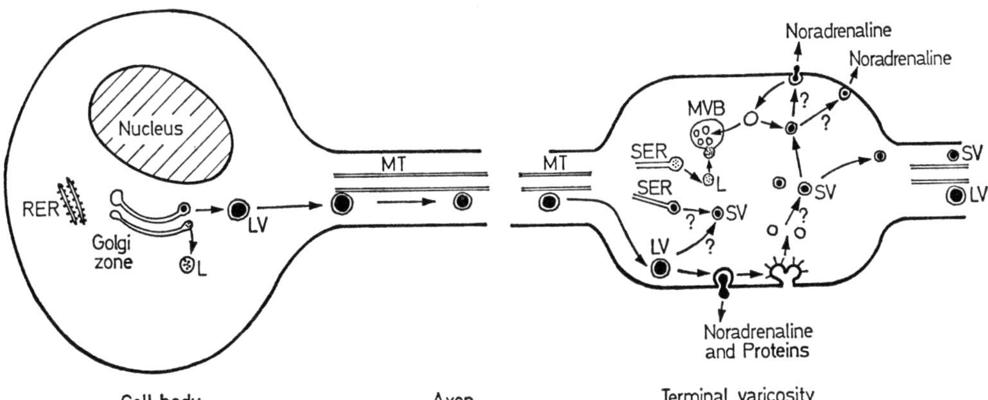

Fig. 15. *Subcellular dynamics of the noradrenergic vesicle in neurons.* Key: L = Lysosome (primary), LV = Large dense-cored vesicle, MT = Microtubule, MVB = Multivesicular body, RER = Rough endoplasmic reticulum (Nissl substance), SER = Smooth endoplasmic reticulum, SV = Small dense-cored vesicle

deferens have also led to the suggestion that the 'light' noradrenergic vesicles contain dopamine β-hydroxylase (M. BISBY, M. FILLENZ and A.D. SMITH, unpublished observations). However, it is less certain that the 'light' vesicles of the terminals of the splenic nerve contain dopamine β-hydroxylase (CHUBB et al., 1970).

We cannot, therefore, at present decide between two possible sites of origin of the small dense-cored vesicles (see Fig. 15): *first*, they may bud off from cisternae of smooth endoplasmic reticulum present in the terminals, in which case they will not necessarily contain dopamine β-hydroxylase; or, *second*, they may come from the large dense-cored vesicles, in which case they will contain dopamine β-hydroxylase.

The formation of the small vesicles from the large dense-cored vesicles would not only account for the origin of the small vesicles, it could explain the relative paucity of large vesicles in the terminal varicosities. What is there, in the terminals, which could cause the large vesicles to be converted into the small vesicles? The terminal is the site of release of the contents of the large vesicles by exocytosis (see p. 574), and it is quite possible that the membrane of the large vesicle is retrieved from the cell membrane by fission into two small vesicles (see SMITH, 1970), just as the chromaffin granule membrane may be (see p. 596). These empty vesicles (see Fig. 15) would contain the membrane-bound dopamine β-hydroxylase of the large dense-cored vesicles (HÖRTNAGL et al., 1969; DE POTTER et al., 1970), and would be able to concentrate and store noradrenaline by virtue of the ATP-dependent uptake process in their membrane (see chapter by EULER). The empty small vesicles formed from large vesicles would, therefore, be able to synthesise noradrenaline from the dopamine; to take up dopamine and noradrenaline from the cytosol; and, because they have the same membrane as the large vesicle, they might be able to release their contents by exocytosis.

This hypothesis, which is an extension of that proposed earlier (see p. 580), is suggested because it can be tested experimentally. Some of the predictions it leads to are given below.

1. In order to distinguish the origin of small vesicles by division of intact large vesicles, from their origin (following exocytosis) by disintegration of the membranes of large vesicles, it will be necessary to see whether the small vesicles contain just the membrane-bound dopamine β-hydroxylase, and not the soluble enzyme.

2. The passage of impulses along the splenic nerve does not seem to affect the rate of transport of noradrenergic vesicles from the perikaryon to the terminals (GEFFEN and RUSH, 1968). Accordingly, the type of vesicles present in the terminals will depend upon the activity of the nerve. In the terminals of a sympathetic nerve whose preganglionic fibre has been cut, there should be an increased number of large dense-cored vesicles; whereas in the terminals of a sympathetic nerve which has been heavily stimulated, there should be a smaller number of large vesicles than normal and an increased number of small vesicles. These predictions could be tested by counting the vesicles in electron micrographs, or by biochemical assays for noradrenaline and dopamine β-hydroxylase.

3. The amount of noradrenaline relative to dopamine β-hydroxylase in small dense-cored vesicles will depend upon their rate of formation (i. e. on the activity of the nerve). Thus, a massive stimulus may give rise to many empty small vesicles (formed from the membranes of large vesicles) which are rich in dopamine β-hydroxylase but which contain little or no noradrenaline. In time, these vesicles will synthesise noradrenaline and will take it up from the cytosol. By analogy with the adrenal chromaffin granule (see VIVEROS et al., 1969d), as the small vesicles become richer in noradrenaline they will sediment to denser regions in a sucrose density gradient. Could this be the explanation of the finding of CHUBB et al. (1970) that the distribution of dopamine β-hydroxylase was not the same as that of the noradrenaline present in 'light' noradrenergic vesicles of the spleen? The laparotomy involved in removing a spleen from an anaesthetized animal is known to produce a massive stimulus to the splenic nerve, leading to a 40% depletion in the noradrenaline content of the spleen (BROWN et al., 1967). This would, on our hypothesis, give rise to a large number of newly formed small vesicles which would have little time to become recharged with noradrenaline.

It is likely that the small dense-cored vesicles are used for many cycles of release, synthesis, and uptake of noradrenaline, otherwise there would be a large turnover of membranes. The microscopic studies of terminal varicosities have not revealed a large number of structures (autophagic vacuoles, multivesicular bodies, myelin figures) which would be involved in membrane turnover. It is not known whether membranes can be synthesised *de novo* in nerve terminals, or assembled from subunits, or whether the terminal depends upon the perikaryon for a supply of preformed membranes. If the vesicles are re-used several times and if, as seems probable (see Section A I, 2), they contain ATP, then an important problem is raised: how do the vesicles obtain their ATP? If the small vesicles release their noradrenaline by exocytosis or across a tight junction, the ATP will also probably be released. It is known that empty small noradrenergic vesicles can take up exogenous catecholamines (see TRANZER and THOENEN, 1967), but can they also take up ATP which has been synthesised in mitochondria? Eventually, after several cycles of re-use, the small noradrenergic vesicles will have to be degraded. Are they degraded in the terminals, in multivesicular bodies (Fig. 15), or do they return to the perikaryon which is rich in lysosomes?

C. Conclusions

Since the discovery of catecholamine-containing particles in 1953, much has been learnt about their chemical composition. The ability to identify components of the chromaffin granule and of the noradrenergic vesicle has led directly to evidence that the release of catecholamines occurs by exocytosis. In the adrenal medulla, exocytosis is the normal mode of release of all the catecholamines. In the sympathetic neuron, it is unlikely that noradrenaline present in the cytosol can be released by nerve impulses; there is, indeed, much evidence that only the noradrenaline present in vesicles can be released. The release of vesicle-proteins from the splenic nerve supports the hypothesis that the release of noradrenaline from large dense-cored vesicles occurs by exocytosis.

The recognition that the chromaffin cell and the sympathetic neuron secrete by exocytosis has solved some problems, but it has also raised many new questions. These questions concern the molecular mechanisms involved in exocytosis, the subcellular events involved in the origin, transport and fate of catecholamine-storing vesicles and, finally, the possible functions of the proteins after their release.

References

Akabane, J., Nakanishi, S., Kohei, H., Asakawa, S., Matsumura, R., Ogata, H., Miyazawa, T.: Studies on sympathomimetic action of acetaldehyde. 2. Secretory response of the adrenal medulla to acetaldehyde: experiment with the perfused cat adrenals. Jap. J. Pharmacol. **15**, 217—222 (1965).

Al-Lami, F.: Light and electron microscopy of the adrenal medulla of Macaca mulata monkey. Anat. Rec. **164**, 317—332 (1969).

Amsterdam, A., Ohad, I., Schramm, M.: Dynamic changes in the ultrastructure of the acinar cell of the rat parotid gland during the secretory cycle. J. Cell Biol. **41**, 753—773 (1969).

Bachmann, R.: Die Nebenniere. In: Handbuch der Mikroskopischen Anatomie des Menschen, **6**, part 5, 1—952 (1954).

Baldessarini, R.J., Kopin, I.J.: The effect of drugs on the release of norepinephrine-^{3}H from central nervous system tissues by electrical stimulation *in vitro*. J. Pharmacol. exp. Ther. **156**, 31—38 (1967).

Bangham, A.D., Horne, R.W.: Negative staining of phospholipids and their structural modification by surface-active agents as observed in the electron microscope. J. molec. Biol. **8**, 660—668 (1964).

Banks, P.: A study of the biochemical pharmacology of the chromaffin cell. D. Phil. Thesis, University of Oxford (1964).

— Effects of stimulation by carbachol on the metabolism of the bovine adrenal medulla. Biochem. J. **97**, 555—560 (1965a).

— The adenosine-triphosphatase activity of adrenal chromaffin granules. Biochem. J. **95**, 490—496 (1965b).

— The release of adenosine triphosphate catabolites during the secretion of catecholamines by bovine adrenal medulla. Biochem. J. **101**, 536—541 (1966a).

— An interaction between chromaffin granules and calcium ions. Biochem. J. **101**, 18C—20C (1966b).

— The effect of ouabain on the secretion of catecholamines and on the intracellular concentration of potassium. J. Physiol. (Lond.) **193**, 631—637 (1967).

— Involvement of calcium in the secretion of catecholamines. In: A Symposium on Calcium and Cellular Function, pp. 148—162. Ed. Cuthbert, A.W. London: MacMillan Ltd. 1970.

— Helle, K.: The release of protein from the stimulated adrenal medulla. Biochem. J. **97**, 40C—41C (1965).

— Helle, K., Mayor, D.: Evidence for the presence of a chromogranin-like protein in bovine splenic nerve granules. Molec. Pharmacol. **5**, 210—212 (1969a).

Banks, P., Biggins, R., Bishop, R., Christian, B., Currie, N.: Sodium ions and the secretion of catecholamines. J. Physiol. (Lond.) **200**, 797—805 (1969b).

— Magnall, D., Mayor, D.: The re-distribution of cytochrome oxidase, noradrenaline and adenosinetriphosphate in adrenergic nerves constricted at two points. J. Physiol. (Lond.) **200**, 745—762 (1969c).

Bell, C., Vogt, M.: Release of endogenous noradrenaline from an isolated muscular artery. J. Physiol. (Lond.) **215**, 509—520 (1971).

Belpaire, F., Laduron, P.: Tissue fractionation and catecholamines. I. Latency and activation properties of dopamine β-hydroxylase in adrenal medulla. Biochem. Pharmacol. **17**, 411—421 (1968).

— — Tissue fractionation and catecholamines. **3**. Intracellular distribution of endogenous inhibitors of dopamine β-hydroxylase in adrenal medulla. Biochem. Pharmacol. **19**, 1323—1331 (1970).

Benedeczky, I.: Electron-microscopic observation of the extracellular catecholamine granules. Acta biol. hung. **17**, 387 (1966a).

— Electron microscopic study on the extracellular catecholamine granules in the adrenal medulla of the chicken. Acta agron. hung. **15**, 107—117 (1966b).

— Ultrastructural analysis of adrenaline resynthesis following insulin treatment. Acta morphol. hung. **15**, 23—37 (1967).

— Puppi, A., Tigyi, A., Lissák, K.: Electron microscopic study of adrenaline and noradrenaline secretion of the adrenal medulla. Acta biol. hung. **15**, 285—298 (1965).

Berneis, K.H., Pletscher, A., Da Prada, M.: Metal-dependent aggregation of biogenic amines: a hypothesis for their storage and release. Nature (Lond.) **224**, 281—283 (1969).

— — — Phase separation in solutions of noradrenaline and adenosine triphosphate: influence of bivalent cations and drugs. Brit. J. Pharmacol. **39**, 382—389 (1970).

Bevan, J.A., Chesher, G.B., Su, C.: Release of adrenergic transmitter from terminal nerve plexus in artery. Agents & Actions (Basel) **1**, 20—26 (1969).

— Nedergaard, O.A.: Abnormal response of the pulmonary artery of the rabbit after high-frequency sympathetic nerve stimulation. Circulat. Res. **22**, 141—147 (1968).

— Verity, M.A.: Postganglionic sympathetic delay in vascular smooth muscle. J. Pharmacol. exp. Ther. **152**, 221—230 (1966).

Bisby, M.A., Fillenz, M.: Effect of perfusion with K-rich solutions on the noradrenaline content of the rat vas deferens. J. Physiol. (Lond.) **204**, 22—23P (1969).

Blakeley, A.G.H., Brown, G.L., Ferry, C.B.: Pharmacological experiments on the release of the sympathetic transmitter. J. Physiol. (Lond.). **167**, 505—514 (1963).

— Dearnaley, D.P., Harrison, V.: The noradrenaline content of the vas deferens of the guinea-pig. Proc. roy. Soc. B. **174**, 491—502 (1970).

Blaschko, H., Born, G.V.R., D'Iorio, A., Eade, N.R.: Observations on the distribution of catecholamines and adenosinetriphosphate in the bovine adrenal medulla. J. Physiol. (Lond.) **133**, 548—557 (1956).

— Comline, R.S., Schneider, F.H., Silver, M., Smith, A.D.: Secretion of a chromaffin granule protein, chromogranin, from the adrenal gland after splanchnic stimulation. Nature (Lond.) **215**, 58—59 (1967a).

— Firemark, H., Smith, A.D., Winkler, H.: Phospholipids and cholesterol in particulate fractions of adrenal medulla. Biochem. J. **98**, 24P (1966).

— — — — Lipids of the adrenal medulla: lysolecithin, a characteristic constituent of chromaffin granules. Biochem. J. **104**, 545—549 (1967b).

— Hagen, J.M., Hagen, P.: Mitochondrial enzymes and chromaffin granules. J. Physiol. (Lond.) **139**, 316—322 (1957).

— Jerrome, D.W., Robb-Smith, A.H.T., Smith, A.D., Winkler, H.: Biochemical and morphological studies on catecholamine storage in human phaeochromocytoma. Clin. Sci. **34**, 453—465 (1968).

— Welch, A.D.: Localization of adrenaline in cytoplasmic particles of the bovine adrenal medulla. Naunyn-Schmiedebergs Arch. exp. Path. Pharmak. **219**, 17—22 (1953).

Borowitz, J.L.: Effect of acetylcholine on the subcellular distribution of ^{45}Ca in bovine adrenal medulla. Biochem. Pharmacol. **18**, 715—723 (1969).

Boullin, D.J.: The action of extracellular cations on the release of the sympathetic transmitter from peripheral nerves. J. Physiol. (Lond.) **189**, 85—99 (1967).

Brandon, K.W., Rand, M.J.: Acetylcholine and the sympathetic innervation of the spleen. J. Physiol. (Lond.) **157**, 18—32 (1961).

Brown, G.L., Dearnaley, D.P., Geffen, L.B.: Noradrenaline storage and release in the decentralised spleen. Proc. roy. Soc. B. **168**, 48—56 (1967).

Burack, W.R., Draskóczy, P.R., Weiner, N.: Adenine nucleotide, catecholamine and protein contents of whole adrenal glands and heavy granules of reserpine-treated fowl. J. Pharmacol. exp. Ther. **133**, 25—33 (1961).

BURACK, W.R., WEINER, N., HAGEN, P.B.: The effect of reserpine on the catecholamine and adenine nucleotide contents of adrenal gland. J. Pharmacol. exp. Ther. **130**, 245—250 (1960).
BURN, J.H., GIBBONS, W.R.: The part played by calcium in determining the response to stimulation of sympathetic postganglionic fibres. Brit. J. Pharmacol. **22**, 540—548 (1964).
— — The release of noradrenaline from sympathetic fibres in relation to calcium concentration. J. Physiol. (Lond.) **181**, 214—223 (1965).
— RAND, M.J.: Sympathetic postganglionic cholinergic fibres. Brit. J. Pharmacol. **15**, 56—66 (1960).
BURNSTOCK, G.: Structure of smooth muscle and its innervation. In: Smooth Muscle, pp. 1—69. Ed. BÜLBRING, E., BRADING, A., JONES, A. and TOMITA, T. London: E. Arnold Ltd. 1970.
CARLSSON, A., HILLARP, N.Å.: Release of adenosine triphosphate along with adrenaline and noradrenaline following stimulation of the adrenal medulla. Acta physiol. scand. **37**, 235—239 (1956).
— — HÖKFELT, B.: The concomitant release of adenosine triphosphate and catechol amines from the adrenal medulla. J. biol. Chem. **227**, 243—252 (1957).
— — WALDECK, B.: Analysis of the Mg^{++}-ATP dependent storage mechanism in the amine granules of the adrenal medulla. Acta physiol. scand. **59**, Suppl. 215, 5—38 (1963).
CESSION-FOSSION, A.: Action des amines sympathicomimétiques a action indirecte sur la médullo-surrénale du rat perfusée "*in vitro*". Arch. int. Physiol. **75**, 303—309 (1967).
CHUBB, I.W., DE POTTER, W.P., DE SCHAEPDRYVER, A.F.: Two populations of noradrenaline-containing particles in the spleen. Nature (Lond.) **228**, 1203—1204 (1970).
CLEMENTI, F., PALADE, G.E.: Intestinal capillaries. 2. Structural effects of EDTA and histamine. J. Cell. Biol. **42**, 706—714 (1969).
— ZOCCHE, G.P.: Morphological and pharmacological effects of reserpine, given alone or after iproniazid, on the catecholamines of the adrenal glands of the rat. J. Cell Biol. **17**, 587—596 (1963).
CONNETT, R.J., KIRSHNER, N.: Purification and properties of bovine phenylethanolamine N-methyltransferase. J. biol. Chem. **245**, 329—334 (1970).
COON, J.M., ROTHMAN, S.: The nature of the pilomotor response to acetylcholine; some observations on the pharmacodynamics of the skin. J. Pharmacol. exp. Ther. **68**, 301—311 (1940).
COSTERO, I., CHÉVEZ, Z.A., PERALTA, L., MONROY, E., RAMÓN, F.: Rhythmic cellular movements in tissue culture of phaeochromocytoma and adrenal medulla. Tex. Rep. Biol. Med. **23**, 213—220 (1965).
COUCH, E.F., ARIMURA, A., SCHALLY, A.V., SOUTO, M., SAVANA, S.: Electron microscopic studies of somatotrophs of rat pituitary after injection of purified growth hormone releasing factor (GRF). Endocrinology **85**, 1084—1091 (1969).
COUPLAND, R. E.: Strain sensitivity of albinorats to reserpine. Nature (Lond.) **181**, 930—931 (1958).
— The Natural History of the Chromaffin Cell, pp. 1—279 London: Longmans 1965a.
— Electron microscopic observations on the structure of the rat adrenal medulla. 1. The ultrastructure and organisation of chromaffin cells in the normal adrenal medulla. J. Anat. (Lond.) **99**, 231—254 (1965b).
— Electron microscopic observations on the structure of the rat adrenal medulla. 2. Normal innervation. J. Anat. (Lond.) **99**, 255—272 (1965c).
CRAMER, W.: Further observations on the thyroid-adrenal apparatus. A histochemical method for the demonstration of the adrenalin granules in the suprarenal gland. J. Physiol. (Lond.) **52**, viii-x (1918).
DAHLSTRÖM, A.: Synthesis, transport and life-span of amine storage granules in sympathetic adrenergic neurons. In: Cellular Dynamics of the Neuron, pp. 153—174. Ed. BARONDES, S. London: Academic Press 1969.
— HÄGGENDAL, J., HÖKFELT, T.: The noradrenaline content of the varicosities of sympathetic adrenergic nerve terminals in the rat. Acta. physiol. scand. **67**, 289—294 (1966).
DAHLSTRÖM, A.B., ZETTERSTRÖM, B.E.M.: Noradrenaline stores in nerve terminals of the spleen: changes during hemorrhagic shock. Science **147**, 1583—1585 (1965).
DALY, M. DE B., SCOTT, M. J.: The effects of acetylcholine on the volume and vascular resistance of the dog's spleen. J. Physiol. (Lond.) **156**, 246—259 (1961).
D'ANZI, F.A.: Morphological and biochemical observations on the catecholamine-storing vesicles of rat adrenomedullary cells during insulin-induced hypoglycemia. Amer. J. Anat. **125**, 381—398 (1969).
DAY, M.D., OWEN, D.A.A.: The interaction between angiotensin and sympathetic vasoconstriction in the isolated artery of the rabbit ear. Brit. J. Pharmacol. **34**, 499—507 (1968).
DEARNALEY, D.P., GEFFEN, L.B.: Effect of nerve stimulation on the noradrenaline content of the spleen. Proc. roy. Soc. B. **166**, 303—315 (1966).

DEDUVE, C.: Endocytosis. In: Lysosomes (Ciba Foundation Symposium). Ed. DE REUCK, A.V.S. and CAMERON, M.P. p. 126. London: Churchill 1963.
DE POTTER, W.P.: Doctoral Thesis, University of Ghent (1968).
— Phil. Trans. roy. Soc. B. **261**, 313—317 (1971). Noradrenaline storage particles in the splenic nerve.
— MOERMAN, E.J., DE SCHAEPDRYVER, A.F., SMITH, A.D.: Release of noradrenaline and dopamine β-hydroxylase upon splenic nerve stimulation. Proc. 4th int. Congr. Pharmac. Abstracts, p. 146. Basel: Schwabe & Co. 1969a.
— DE SCHAEPDRYVER, A.F., MOERMAN, E.J., SMITH, A.D.: Evidence for the release of vesicle-proteins together with noradrenaline upon stimulation of the splenic nerve. J. Physiol. (Lond.) **204**, 102P—104P (1969b).
— SMITH, A.D., DE SCHAEPDRYVER, A.F.: Subcellular fractionation of splenic nerve: ATP, chromogranin A and dopamine β-hydroxylase in noradrenergic vesicles. Tissue & Cell **2**, 529—546 (1970).
DE ROBERTIS, E.D.P.: Adrenergic endings and vesicles isolated from brain. Pharmacol. Rev. **18**, 413—424 (1966).
— SABATINI, D.D.: Submicroscopic analysis of the secretory process in the adrenal medulla. Fedn. Proc. **19**, No. 4, 70—78 (1960).
— VAZ Ferreira: Electron microscope study of the excretion of catechol-containing droplets in the adrenal medulla. Exp. Cell. Res. **12**, 568—574 (1957).
DE VIRGILIIS, G., MELDOLESI, J., CLEMENTI, F.: Ultrastructure of growth-hormone producing cells of rat pituitary after injection of hypothalamic extract. Endocrinology **83**, 1278—1284 (1968).
DINER, O.: L'expulsion des granules de la médullosurrénale chez le hamster. C.R. Acad. Sci. (Paris) **265**, 616—619 (1967).
D'Iorio, A., Eade, N.: Catecholamines and adenosinetriphosphate (ATP) in the suprarenal gland of the rabbit. J. Physiol. (Lond.) **133**, 17P (1956).
DODGE, F.A., RAHAMIMOFF, R.: Co-operative action of calcium ions in transmitter release at the neuromuscular junction. J. Physiol. (Lond.) **193**, 419—432 (1967).
DOUGLAS, W.W.: Calcium dependent links in stimulus-secretion coupling in the adrenal medulla and neuropophysis. In: Mechanisms of Release of Biogenic Amines, pp. 267—289. Ed. EULER, U.S. VON, ROSELL, S. and UVNÄS, B. Oxford: Pergamon Press. 1966.
— Stimulus-Secretion Coupling: the concept and clues from chromaffin and other cells. Brit. J. Pharmacol. **34**, 451—474 (1968).
— KANNO, T.: The effect of amethocaine on acetylcholine-induced depolarization and catecholamine secretion in the adrenal chromaffin cell. Brit. J. Pharmacol. **30**, 612—619 (1967).
— — SAMPSON, S.R.: Effects of acetylcholine and other medullary secretagogues and antagonists on the membrane potential of adrenal chromaffin cells: an analysis employing techniques of tissue culture. J. Physiol. (Lond.) **188**, 107—120 (1967a).
— — — Influence of the ionic environment on the membrane potential of adrenal chromaffin cells and on the depolarizing effect of acetylcholine. J. Physiol. (Lond.) **191**, 107—121 (1967b).
— POISNER, A.M.: On the mode of action of acetylcholine in evoking adrenal medullary secretion: increased uptake of calcium during the secretory reponse. J. Physiol. (Lond.) **162**, 385—392 (1962).
— — Preferential release of adrenaline from the adrenal medulla by muscarine and pilocarpine. Nature (Lond.) **208**, 1102 (1965).
— — Evidence that the secreting adrenal chromaffin cell releases catecholamines directly from ATP-rich granules. J. Physiol. (Lond.) **183**, 236—248 (1966a).
— — On the relation between ATP splitting and secretion in the adrenal chromaffin cell: extrusion of ATP (unhydrolysed) during release of catecholamines. J. Physiol. (Lond.) **183**, 249—256 (1966b).
— — RUBIN, R.P.: Efflux of adenine nucleotides from perfused adrenal glands exposed to nicotine and other chromaffin cell stimulants. J. Physiol. (Lond.) **179**, 130—137 (1965).
— — TRIFARÓ, J.M.: Lysolecithin and other phospholipids in the adrenal medulla of various species. Life. Sci. **5**, 809—815 (1966).
— RUBIN, R.P.: The role of calcium in the secretory response of the adrenal medulla to acetylcholine. J. Physiol. (Lond.) **159**, 40—57 (1961).
— — The mechanism of catecholamine release from the adrenal medulla and the role of calcium in stimulus-secretion coupling. J. Physiol. (Lond.) **167**, 288—310 (1963).
DROZ, B.: Protein metabolism in nerve cells. Int. Rev. Cytol. **25**, 363—390 (1969).
DUCH, D.S., VIVEROS, O.H., KIRSHNER, N.: Endogenous inhibitor(s) in adrenal medulla of dopamine β-hydroxylase. Biochem. Pharmacol. **17**, 255—264 (1968).
EADE, N.: The intracellular localization of the sympathomimetic amines. D. Phil. Thesis, Oxford University (1957).

EADE, N.R.: The distribution of the catechol amines in homogenates of the bovine adrenal medulla. J. Physiol. (Lond.) **141**, 183—192 (1958).
ECCLES, J.C.: The physiology of synapses. Berlin: Springer Verlag 1964.
ELFVIN, L.G.: The ultrastructure of the capillary fenestrae in the adrenal medulla of the rat. J. Ultrastruct. Res. **12**, 687—704 (1965).
EULER, U.S. VON: Twenty years of noradrenaline. Pharmacol. Rev. **18**, 29—38 (1966).
— Some aspects of the mechanisms involved in adrenergic neurotransmission. Perspect. Biol. Med. **12**, 79—94 (1968).
— Acute neuromuscular transmission failure in vas deferens after reserpine. Acta physiol. scand. **76**, 255—256 (1969).
— HILLARP, N.Å.: Evidence for the presence of noradrenaline in submicroscopic structures of adrenergic axons. Nature (Lond.) **177**, 44—45 (1956).
— LISHAJKO, F., STJÄRNE, L.: Catecholamines and ATP in isolated adrenergic nerve granules. Acta physiol. scand. **59**, 495—496 (1963).
— PURKHOLD, A.: Effect of sympathetic denervation on the noradrenaline and adrenaline content of the spleen, kidney, and salivary glands in the sheep. Acta physiol. scand. **24**, 212—217 (1951).
FALCK, B., HILLARP, N.Å., HÖGBERG, B.: Content and intracellular distribution of adenosine-triphosphate in cow adrenal medulla. Acta physiol. scand. **36**, 360—376 (1956).
FARBER, S.: The action of acetylcholine on the volume of the spleen of the dog. Arch. int. Pharmacodyn. **53**, 367—376 (1936).
FARRELL, K.E.: Fine structure of nerve fibres in smooth muscle of the vas deferens in normal and reserpinized rats. Nature (Lond.) **217**, 279—281 (1968).
FAWCETT, D.W.: Surface specialization of absorbing cells. J. Histochem. Cytochem. **13**, 75—91 (1965).
FELDBERG, W.: The action of bee venom, cobra venom and lysolecithin on the adrenal medulla. J. Physiol. (Lond.) **99**, 104—118 (1940).
— GADDUM, J.H.: The chemical transmitter at synapses in a sympathetic ganglion. J. Physiol. (Lond.) **81**, 305—319 (1934).
— MINZ, B., TSUDZIMURA, H.: The mechanism of the nervous discharge of adrenaline. J. Physiol. (Lond.) **81**, 286—304 (1934).
FERRIS, R.M., VIVEROS, O.H., KIRSHNER, N.: Effects of various agents on the Mg^{2+}-ATP stimulated incorporation and release of catecholamines by isolated bovine adrenomedullary storage vesicles and on secretion from the adrenal medulla. Biochem. Pharmacol. **19**, 505—514 (1970).
FERRY, C.B.: The sympathomimetic affect of acetylcholine on the spleen of the cat. J. Physiol. (Lond.) **167**, 487—504 (1963).
FILLENZ, M.: The innervation of the cat spleen. Proc. roy. Soc. Lond. B. **174**, 459—468 (1970).
— Fine structure of noradrenaline storage vesicles in nerve terminals of the rat vas deferens. Phil. Trans. roy. Soc. B. **261**, 319—323 (1971).
FINEAN, J.B.: Biophysical contributions to membrane structure. Quart. Rev. Biophys. **2**, 1—23 (1969).
FOLKOW, B., HÄGGENDAL, J., LISANDER, B.: Extent of release and elimination of noradrenaline at peripheral adrenergic nerve terminals. Acta physiol. scand. Suppl. 307, 1—38 (1967).
GEFFEN, L.B., LIVETT, B.G.: Axoplasmic transport of ^{14}C-noradrenaline and protein and their release by nerve impulses. Proc. int. union physiol. Sci. **7**, 152 (1968).
— — Origin, functions and fate of synaptic vesicles in sympathetic neurones. Physiol. Rev. **51**, 98—157 (1971).
— — RUSH, R.A.: Immunohistochemical localization of protein components of catecholamine storage vesicles. J. Physiol. (Lond.) **204**, 593—605 (1969a).
— — — Immunological localization of chromogranins in sheep sympathetic neurones, and their release by nerve impulses. J. Physiol. (Lond.) **204**, 58—59P (1969b).
— — — Immunohistochemical localization of chromogranins in sheep sympathetic neurones and their release by nerve impulses, pp. 58—72. In: New aspects of storage and release mechanism of catecholamines. (Bayer Symposium II). Eds. H.J. SCHÜMANN and G. KRONEBERG. Berlin: Springer Verlag 1970.
— OSTBERG, A.: Distribution of granular vesicles in normal and constricted sympathetic neurones. J. Physiol. (Lond.) **204**, 583—592 (1969).
— RUSH, R.A.: Transport of noradrenaline in sympathetic nerves and the effect of nerve impulses on its contribution to transmitter stores. J. Neurochem. **15**, 925—930 (1968).
GEWIRTZ, G.P., KOPIN, I.J.: Release of dopamine β-hydroxylase with norepinephrine during cat splenic nerve stimulation. Nature (Lond.) **227**, 406—407 (1970).
GILLESPIE, J.S., KIRPEKAR, S.M.: The uptake and release of radioactive noradrenaline by the splenic nerves of cats. J. Physiol. (Lond.) **187**, 51—68 (1966a).

GILLESPIE, J.S., KIRPEKAR, S.M.: The histological localization of noradrenaline in the cat spleen. J. Physiol. (Lond.) **187**, 69—79 (1966b).
GLADSTONE, G.P., VAN HEYNINGEN, W.E.: Staphylococcal leuocidins. Brit. J. exp. Path. **38**, 123—137 (1957).
GOVIER, W.C., BOADLE, M.C.: The cardiac action of lysolecithin. J. Pharmacol. exp. Ther. **156**, 339—344 (1967).
GRAHAM, J.D.P., LEVER, L.D., SPRIGGS, T.L.B.: An examination of adrenergic axons around pancreatic arteriols of the cat for the presence of acetylcholinesterase by high resolution autoradiographic and histochemical methods. Brit. J. Pharmacol. **33**, 15—20 (1968).
GROBECKER, H., HOLTZ, P., PALM, D., BAK, I.J., HASSLER, R.J.: In vitro lysis of erythrocytes and chromaffine granules by Prenylamine. Experientia (Basel) **24**, 701—703 (1968).
GRYNSZPAN-WINOGRAD, O.: Différences dans l'innervation des "Cellules a adrénaline" et des "Cellules a noradrénaline" de la médullo-surrénale du Hamster. C.R. Acad. Sci. (Paris) **268**, 1420—1422 (1969).
— Morphological aspects of exocytosis in the adrenal medulla. Phil. Trans. roy. Soc. B. **261**, 291—292 (1971).
HAEFELY, W., HURLIMANN, A., THOENEN, H.: Relation between the rate of stimulation and the quantity of noradrenaline liberated from sympathetic nerve endings in the isolated perfused spleen of the cat. J. Physiol. (Lond.) **181**, 48—58 (1965).
HÄGGENDAL, J., MALMFORS, T.: The effect of nerve stimulation on catecholamines taken up in adrenergic nerves after reserpine pretreatment. Acta physiol. scand. **75**, 33—38 (1969).
HAEUSLER, G., THOENEN, H., HAEFELY, W., HURLIMANN, A.: Electrical events in cardiac adrenergic nerves and noradrenaline release from the heart induced by acetylcholine and KCl. Naunyn-Schmiedebergs Arch. Pharmak. exp. Path. **261**, 389—411 (1968).
HAJDU, S., WEISS, H., TITUS, E.: The isolation of a cardiac active principle from mammalian tissue. J. Pharmacol. exp. Ther. **120**, 99—113 (1957).
HAYDON, D.A., TAYLOR, J.: The stability and properties of bimolecular lipid leaflets in aqueous solutions. J. theor. Biol. **4**, 281—296 (1963).
HEDQVIST, P., STJÄRNE, L.: The relative role of recapture and of *de novo* synthesis for maintenance of neurotransmitter homeostasis in noradrenergic nerves. Acta physiol. scand. **76**, 270—283 (1969).
HEILBRÜNN, L.V.: The Dynamics of Living Protoplasm. New York: Academic Press 1956.
HELLE, K.: Some chemical and physical properties of the soluble protein fraction of bovine adrenal chromaffin granules. Molec. Pharmacol. **2**, 298—310 (1966a).
— Antibody formation against soluble protein from bovine adrenal chromaffin granules. Biochim. biophys. Acta (Amst.) **117**, 107—110 (1966b).
— SERCK-HANSSEN, G.: Chromogranin: the soluble and membrane-bound lipoprotein of the chromaffin granule. Pharmacol. Res. Commun. **1**, 25—29 (1969).
HELLERSTEIN, D.: Passive membrane potentials. A generalization of the theory of electrotonus. Biophys. J. **8**, 358—379 (1968).
HEMPEL, K., MÄNNL, H.F.K.: Quantitative Analyse der Catecholamin-Biosynthese des Nebennierenmarks *in vivo* and Ruhesekretion neugebildeter Amine unter besonderer Berücksichtigung des Dopamins. Naunyn-Schmiedebergs Arch. Pharmak. **264**, 363—388 (1969).
HILLARP, N.Å.: Isolation and some biochemical properties of the catecholamine granules in the cow adrenal medulla. Acta physiol. scand. **43**, 82—96 (1958).
— Further observations on the state of the catecholamines stored in the adrenal medullary granules. Acta physiol. scand. **47**, 271—279 (1959).
— Different pools of catecholamines stored in the adrenal medulla. Acta physiol. scand. **50**, 8—22 (1960a).
— Effect of reserpine on the adrenal medulla of sheep. Acta physiol. scand. **49**, 376—382 (1960b).
— FALCK, B.: Localization of acid phosphatase in the adrenal medullary cell. Acta endocr. (Kbh.) **22**, 95—106 (1956).
— LAGERSTEDT, S., NILSON, B.: The isolation of a granular fraction from the suprarenal medulla, containing the sympathomimetic catecholamines. Acta physiol. scand. **29**, 251—263 (1953).
— NILSON, B.: Some quantitative analyses of the sympathomimetic amine containing granules in the adrenal medullary cell. Acta physiol. scand. **32**, 11—18 (1954a).
— — The structure of the adrenaline and noradrenaline containing granules in the adrenal medullary cells with reference to the storage and release of the sympathomimetic amines. Acta physiol. scand. **31**, Suppl. 113, 79—107 (1954b).
— — HÖGBERG, B.: Adenosine triphosphate in the adrenal medulla of the cow. Nature (Lond.) **176**, 1032—1033 (1955).
— THIEME, G.: Nucleotides in the catecholamine granules of the adrenal medulla. Acta physiol. scand. **45**, 328—338 (1959).

HIRSCH, J.G.: Cinemicrophotographic observations on granule lysis in polymorphonuclear leucoytes during phagocytosis. J. exp. Med. **116**, 827—834 (1962).
HODGKIN, A.L., KEYNES, R.D.: Movements of labelled calcium in squid giant axons. J. Physiol. (Lond.) **138**, 399—407 (1957).
HÖKFELT, T.: *In vitro* studies on central and peripheral monoamine neurons at the ultrastructural level. Z. Zellforsch. **91**, 1—74 (1968).
— Distribution of noradrenaline storing particles in peripheral adrenergic neurons as revealed by electron microscopy. Acta physiol. scand. **76**, 427—440 (1969).
HOKIN, L.E.: Autoradiographic localization of the acetylcholine-stimulated synthesis of phosphatidylinositol in the superior cervical ganglion. Proc. nat. Acad. Sci. (Wash.) **53**, 1369—1374 (1965).
— Dynamic aspects of phospholipids during protein secretion. Int. Rev. Cytol. **20**, 187—208 (1968).
— Functional activity in glands and synaptic tissue and the turnover of phosphatidylinositol. Ann. N.Y. Acad. Sci. **165**, 695—709 (1969).
HOKIN, M.R., BENFY, B.G., HOKIN, L.E.: Phospholipids and adrenaline secretion in the guinea pig adrenal medulla. J. biol. Chem. **233**, 814—817 (1958).
— HOKIN, L.E., SHELP, W.D.: The effects of acetylcholine on the turnover of phosphatidic acid and phosphoinositide in sympathetic ganglia, and in various parts of the central nervous system *in vitro*. J. gen. Physiol. **44**, 217—226 (1960).
HOLMAN, M.: Junction potentials in smooth muscle. In: Smooth Muscle, pp. 244—288. Ed. BÜLBRING, E., BRADING, A., JONES, A. and TOMITA, T. London: E. Arnold Ltd. 1970.
HOLTZMAN, E., DOMINITZ, R.: Cytochemical studies of lysosomes, Golgi apparatus and endoplasmic reticulum in secretion and protein uptake by adrenal medulla cells of the rat. J. Histochem. Cytochem. **16**, 320—336 (1968).
HOLZBAUER, M.: The corticosterone content of rat adrenals under different experimental conditions. J. Physiol. (Lond.) **139**, 294—305 (1957).
HOWELL, J.I., LUCY, J.A.: Cell fusion induced by lysolecithin. FEBS Lett. **4**, 147—150 (1969).
HUKOVIĆ, S., MUSCHOLL, E.: Die Noradrenalin-Abgabe aus dem isolierten Kaninchenherzen bei sympatischer Nervenreizung und ihre pharmakologische Beeinflussung. Naunyn-Schmiedeberg's Arch. exp. Path. Pharmak. **244**, 81—96 (1962).
IVERSEN, L.L., GLOWINSKI, J., AXELROD, J.: The uptake and storage of [^{3}H] norepinephrine in the reserpine-pretreated rat heart. J. Pharmacol. exp. Ther. **150**, 173—183 (1965).
JAANUS, S.D., MIELE, E., RUBIN, R.P.: The analysis of the inhibitory effect of local anaesthetics and propranolol on adreno-medullary secretion evoked by calcium or acetylcholine. Brit. J. Pharmacol. **31**, 319—330 (1967).
JAMIESON, J.D., PALADE, G.E.: Intracellular transport of secretory proteins in the pancreatic exocrine cell. 1. Role of the peripheral elements of the Golgi complex. J. Cell. Biol. **34**, 577—596 (1967a).
— — Intracellular transport of secretory proteins in the pancreatic exocrine cell. 2. Transport to condensing vacuoles and zymogen granules. J. Cell. Biol. **34**, 597—615 (1967b).
— — Intracellular transport of secretory proteins in the pancreatic exocrine cell. 3. Dissociation of intracellular transport from protein synthesis. J. Cell. Biol. **39**, 580—588 (1968a).
— — Intracellular transport of secretory proteins in the pancreatic exocrine cell. 4. Metabolic requirements. J. Cell. Biol. **39**, 589—603 (1968b).
JÄRLFORS, U., SMITH, D.S.: Association between synaptic vesicles and neurotubules. Nature (Lond.) **224**, 710—711 (1969).
JONSSON, G., SACHS, C.: Subcellular distribution of ^{3}H-noradrenaline in adrenergic nerves of mouse atrium-effect of reserpine. monoamine oxidase and tyrosine hydroxylase inhibition. Acta physiol. scand. **77**, 344—357 (1969).
KANNO, Y., LOEWENSTEIN, W.R.: Cell-to-cell passage of large molecules. Nature (Lond.) **212**, 629—630 (1966).
KAO, C.Y.: Tetrodotoxin, saxitoxin and their significance in the study of excitation phenomena. Pharmacol. Rev. **18**, 997—1049 (1966).
KATZ, B.: The release of neural transmitter substances, pp. 1—60. Liverpool: Liverpool University Press 1969.
— MILEDI, R.: The timing of calcium action during neuromuscular transmission. J. Physiol. (Lond.) **189**, 535—544 (1967).
KATZ, R.I., KOPIN, I.J.: Release of norepinephrine-^{3}H and serotonin-^{3}H evoked from brain slices by electrical-field stimulation — calcium dependency and the effects of lithium, ouabain and tetrodotoxin. Biochem. Pharmacol. **18**, 1935—1939 (1969).
KAYAALP, S.O., MCISAAC, R.J.: *In vivo* release of catecholamines from the adrenal medulla by selective activation of cholinergic receptors. Arch. int. Pharmacodyn. **176**, 168—175 (1968).

KAYAALP, S. O., MCISAAC, R. J.: Muscarinic component of splanchnic-adrenal transmission in the dog. Brit. J. Pharmacol. **36**, 286—293 (1969).
— TÜRKER, R. K.: Evidence for muscarinic receptors in the adrenal medulla of the dog. Brit. J. Pharmacol. **35**, 265—270 (1969).
KIRPEKAR, S. M., CERVONI, P., COURI, D.: Depletion and recovery of catecholamines and adenosine-triphosphate of rat adrenal medulla after reserpine treatment. J. Pharmacol. exp. Ther. **142**, 71—75 (1963a).
— — Effect of cocaine, phenoxybenzamine and phentolamine on catecholamine output from spleen and adrenal medulla. J. Pharmacol. exp. Ther. **142**, 59—70 (1963b).
— GOODLAND, G. A. J., LEWIS, J. J.: Reserpine depletion of adenosine triphosphate from the rat suprarenal medulla. Biochem. Pharmacol. **1**, 232—233 (1958).
— MISU, Y.: Release of noradrenaline by splenic nerve stimulation and its dependence upon calcium. J. Physiol. (Lond.) **188**, 219—234 (1967).
— WAKADE, A. R.: Release of noradrenaline from the cat spleen by potassium. J. Physiol. (Lond.) **194**, 595—608 (1968).
KIRSHNER, A. G., KIRSHNER, N.: A specific soluble protein from the catecholamine storage vesicles of bovine adrenal medulla. 2. Physical characterization. Biochim. biophys. Acta (Amst.) **181**, 219—225 (1969).
KIRSHNER, N.: Uptake of catecholamines by a particulate fraction of the adrenal medulla. J. biol. Chem. **237**, 2311—2317 (1962).
— Storage and secretion of adrenal catecholamines. Adv. Biochem. Psychopharmacol. **1**, 71—89 (1969).
— SAGE, H. J., SMITH, W. J., KIRSHNER, A. G.: Release of catecholamines and specific protein from adrenal glands. Science **154**, 529—531 (1966).
— — — Mechanism of secretion from the adrenal medulla. 2. Release of catecholamines and storage vesicle protein in response to chemical stimulation. Molec. Pharmacol. **3**, 254—265 (1967).
— SMITH, W. J.: Metabolic requirements for secretion from the adrenal medulla. Life Sci. **8**, (1) 799—803 (1969).
— VIVEROS, O. H.: Quantal aspects of the secretion of catecholamines and dopamine-β-hydroxylase from the adrenal medulla. In: New aspects of storage and release mechanisms of catecholamines (Bayer Symposium II), pp. 78—88. Eds. SCHÜMANN, H. J. and KRONEBERG, H. G. Berlin: Springer 1970.
KOPIN, I. J.: Storage and metabolism of catecholamines: the role of monoamine oxidase. Pharmacol. Rev. **16**, 179—191 (1964).
— Biochemical aspects of release of norepinephrine and other amines from sympathetic nerve endings. Pharmacol. Rev. **18**, 513—523 (1966).
— False adrenergic transmitters. Ann. Rev. Pharmacol. **8**, 377—394 (1968).
— BREESE, G. R., KRAUSS, K. R., WEISE, V. K.: Selective release of newly synthesised norepinephrine from the cat spleen during sympathetic nerve stimulation. J. Pharmacol. exp. Ther. **161**, 271—278 (1968).
LADURON, P., BELPAIRE, F.: A rapid assay and partial purification of dopa decarboxylase. Analyt. Biochem. **26**, 210—218 (1968a).
— — Tissue fractionation and catecholamines — 2. Intracellular distribution patterns of tyrosine hydroxylase, dopa decarboxylase, dopamine β-hydroxylase, phenylethanolamine N-methyltransferase and monoamine oxidase in adrenal medulla. Biochem. Pharmacol. **17**, 1127—1140 (1968b).
— — Transport of noradrenaline and dopamine β-hydroxylase in sympathetic nerves. Life Sci. **7**, 1—7 (1968c).
LANGER, S. Z.: The metabolism of [^{3}H] noradrenaline released by electrical stimulation from the isolated nictitating membrane of the cat and from the vas deferens of the rat. J. Physiol. (Lond.) **208**, 515—546 (1970).
LARRABEE, M. G.: Transynaptic stimulation of phosphatidylinositol metabolism in sympathetic neurons *in situ*. J. Neurochem. **15**, 803—808 (1968).
— LEICHT, W. S.: Metabolism of phosphatidylinositol and other lipids in active neurones of sympathetic ganglia and other peripheral tissues. The site of the inositide effect. J. Neurochem. **12**, 1—13 (1965).
LEADERS, F. E., DAYRIT, C.: The cholinergic component in the sympathetic innervation to the spleen. J. Pharmacol. exp. Ther. **147**, 145—152 (1965).
LEE, F. L., TRENDELENBURG, U.: Muscarinic transmission of preganglionic impulses to the adrenal medulla of the cat. J. Pharmacol. exp. Ther. **158**, 73—79 (1967).
LEVER, J. D., FINDLAY, J. A.: Similar structural basis for the storage and release of secretory material in adrenomedullary and β-pancreatic cells. Z. Zellforsch. **74**, 317—324 (1966).
LEWIS, P. R., SHUTE, C. C. D.: An electron-microscopic study of cholinesterase distribution in the rat adrenal medulla. J. Microscopy **89**, 181—193 (1969).

LIGHTMAN, S.L., IVERSEN, L.L.: The role of uptake in the extraneuronal metabolism of catecholamines in the isolated rat heart. Brit. J. Pharmacol. **37**, 638—649 (1969).

LINDMAR, R. LÖFFELHOLZ, K., MUSCHOLL, E.: Unterschiede zwischen Tyramin and Dimethylphenylpiperazin in der Ca^{2+}-Abhängigkeit und im zeitlichen Verlauf der Noradrenalin-Freisetzung am isolierten Kaninchenherzen. Experientia (Basel) **23**, 933—944 (1967).

— MUSCHOLL, E.: Die Wirkung von Cocain, Guanethidin, Reserpin, Hexamethonium, Tetracain and Psicain auf die Noradrenalin-Freisetzung aus dem Herzen. Naunyn-Schmiedeberg's Arch. exp. Path. Pharmak. **242**, 214—227 (1961).

— — Die Wirkung von Pharmaka auf die Elimination von Noradrenalin aus der Perfusionsflüssigkeit und die Noradrenalinaufnahme in das isolierte Herz. Naunyn-Schmiedeberg's Arch. exp. Path. Pharmak. **247**, 469—492 (1964).

LISHAJKO, F.: Influence of chloride ions and ATP-Mg^{2+} on the release of catecholamines from isolated medullary granules. Acta physiol. scand. **75**, 255—256 (1969).

— Osmotic factors determining the release of catecholamines from isolated chromaffin cell granules. Acta physiol. scand. **79**, 64—75 (1970).

LIVETT, B.G., GEFFEN, L.B., AUSTIN, L.: Proximo distal transport of [^{14}C] noradrenaline and protein in sympathetic nerves. J. Neurochem. **15**, 931—939 (1968).

LOCKE, M., COLLINS, J.V.: Protein uptake into multivesicular bodies and storage granules in the fat body of an insect. J. Cell Biol. **36**, 453—483 (1968).

LÖFFELHOLZ, K.: Untersuchungen über die Noradrenalin-Freisetzung durch Acetylcholin am perfundierten Kaninchenherzen. Naunyn-Schmiedebergs Arch. Pharmak. exp. Path. **258**, 108—122 (1967).

— MUSCHOLL, E.: A muscarinic inhibition of noradrenaline release evoked by postganglionic sympathetic nerve stimulation. Naunyn-Schmiedebergs Arch. Pharmak. **265**, 1—15 (1969).

LOEWENSTEIN, W.R.: Permeability of membrane junctions. Ann. N.Y. Acad. Sci. **137**, 441—472 (1966).

LUCY, J.A.: Lysosomal membrane. In: Lysosomes in Biology and Pathology, pp. 313—341. Ed. DINGLE, J.T. and FELL, H. Amsterdam: North Holland Publishing Company 1969.

LUNDBORG, P.: Uptake of metaraminol by the adrenal medullary granules. Acta physiol. scand. **67**, 423—429 (1966).

— Studies on the uptake and subcellular distribution of catecholamines and their α-methylated analogues. Acta physiol. scand. **72**, Suppl. 302, 1—34 (1968).

MALAMED, S., POISNER, A.M., TRIFARÓ, J.M., DOUGLAS, W.W.: The fate of the chromaffin granule during catecholamine release from the adrenal medulla. III. Recovery of a purified fraction of electron-translucent structures. Biochem. Pharmacol. **17**, 241—246 (1968).

MALMFORS, T.: Studies on adrenergic nerves. The use of rat and mouse iris for direct observations on their physiology and pharmacology at cellular and subcellular levels. Acta physiol. scand. **64**, Suppl. 248, 1—93 (1965).

MATTHEWS, E.K.: Calcium and hormone release. In: A Symposium on Calcium and Cellular Function, pp. 163—182. Ed. CUTHBERT, A.W. London: Macmillan 1970.

— Membrane potential measurement in cells of the adrenal gland .J. Physiol. (Lond.) **189**, 139—148 (1967).

— SAFFRAN, M.: Effect of ACTH on electrical properties of adrenocortical cells. Nature (Lond.) **219**, 1369—1370 (1968).

MIELE, E.: The nicotinic stimulation of the cat adrenal medulla. Arch. int. Pharmacodyn. **179**, 343—351 (1969).

— RUBIN, R.P.: Further evidence for the dual action of local anaesthetics on the adrenal medulla. J. Pharmacol. exp. Ther. **161**, 296—301 (1968).

MOPPERT, J.: Zur Ultrastructur der phaeochromen Zellen im Nebennierenmark der Ratte. Z. Zellforsch. **74**, 32—44 (1966).

MUSCHOLL, E.: Autonomic nervous system: newer mechanisms of adrenergic blockade. Ann. Rev. Pharmacol. **6**, 107—128 (1966).

— Discussion remark. In: *Adrenergic Neurotransmission*, pp. 104—105. Ed. WOLSTENHOLME, G.E.W. and O'CONNOR, M. London: J. & A. Churchill Ltd. 1968.

— MAÎTRE, L.: Release by sympathetic stimulation of α-methylnoradrenaline stored in the heart after administration of α-methyldopa. Experientia (Basel) **19**, 658—659 (1963).

— VOGT, M.: The action of reserpine on the peripheral sympathetic system. J. Physiol. (Lond.) **141**, 132—155 (1958).

NAGATSU, T., KUZUYA, H., HIDAKA, H.: Inhibition of dopamine-β-hydroxylase by sulfhydryl compounds and the nature of the natural inhibitors. Biochim. biophys. Acta (Amst.) **139**, 319—327 (1967).

NORMANN, T.C.: The neurosecretory system of the adult Calliphora erythrocephala. 1. The fine structure of the corpus cardiacum, with some observations on adjacent organs. Z. Zellforsch. **67**, 461—501 (1965).

Normann, T.C.: Experimentally induced exocytosis of neurosecretory granules. Exp. Cell Res. **55**, 285—287 (1969).
Oka, M., Ohuchi, T., Yoshida, H., Imaizumi, R.: The importance of calcium in the release of catecholamine from the adrenal medulla. Jap. J. Pharmacol. **15**, 348—356 (1965a).
— — — — Effect of adenosine triphosphate and magnesium on the release of catecholamines from adrenal medullary granules. Biochim. biophys. Acta (Amst.) **97**, 170—171 (1965b).
— — — — The isolation of catecholamine storage granules from adrenal medulla by the membrane filter technique. Life Sci. **5**, 427—432 (1966).
— Kajikawa, K., Ohuchi, T., Yoshida, H., Imaizumi, R.: Distribution of dopamine β-hydroxylase in subcellular fractions of adrenal medulla. Life Sci. **6**, 461—465 (1967a).
— Ohuchi, T., Yoshida, H., Imaizumi, R.: Structural changes in the catecholamine containing granules of adrenal medulla. Life Sci. **6**, 467—472 (1967b).
— — — — Stimulatory effect of adenosine triphosphate and magnesium on the release of catecholamines from adrenal medullary granules. Jap. J. Pharmacol. **17**, 199—207 (1967c).
Palade, G.E.: Functional changes in the structure of cell components. In: *Subcellular Particles*, pp. 64—83. Ed. Hayashi, T. New York: Ronald Press 1959.
Palkama, A.: Demonstration of adrenomedullary catecholamines and cholinesterases at electron microscopic level in the same tissue section. Ann. Med. exp. Fenn. **45**, 295—301 (1967).
Paton, W.D.M., Rothschild, A.M.: The effect of varying calcium concentration on the kinetic constants of hyoscine and mepyramine antagonism. Brit. J. Pharmacol. **24**, 432—436 (1965).
Philippu, A., Heyd, G., Burger, A.: Release of noradrenaline from the hypothalamus *in vivo*. Europ. J. Pharmacol. **9**, 52—58 (1970).
— Schümann, H.J.: Der Einfluß von Calcium auf die Brenzcatechinaminfreisetzung. Experientia (Basel) **18**, 138—140 (1962).
— — Effect of ribonuclease on the ribonucleic acid, adenosine-triphosphate and catecholamine content of medullary granules. Nature (Lond.) **198**, 795—796 (1963).
— — Ribonucleaseaktivität isolierter Nebennierenmarkgranula. Experientia (Basel) **20**, 547—548 (1964).
— — Über die Bedeutung der Calcium- und Magnesiumionen für die Speicherung der Nebennierenmark-Hormone. Naunyn-Schmiedebergs Arch. exp. Path. Pharmak. **252**, 339—358 (1966).
Plattner, H., Winkler, H., Hörtnagl, H., Pfaller, W.: A study of the adrenal medulla and its subcellular organelles by the freeze-etching method. J. Ultrastruct. Res. **28**, 191—202 (1969).
Pohorecky, L., Rust, J.H.: Studies on the cortical control of the adrenal medulla in the rat. J. Pharmacol. exp. Ther. **162**, 227—238 (1968).
Poisner, A.M., Douglas, W.W.: The need for calcium in adrenomedullary secretion evoked by biogenic amines, polypeptides, and muscarinic agents. Proc. Soc. exp. Biol. (N. Y.) **123**, 62—64 (1966).
— Trifaró, J.M.: The role of ATP and ATPase in the release of catecholamines from the adrenal medulla. 1. ATP-evoked release of catecholamines, ATP, and protein from isolated chromaffin granules. Molec. Pharmacol. **3**, 561—571 (1967).
— — The role of adenosine triphosphate and adenosine triphosphatase in the release of catecholamines from the adrenal medulla. 3. Similarities between the effects of adenosine-triphosphate on chromaffin granules and on mitochondria. Molec. Pharmacol. **5**, 294—299 (1969).
— — Douglas, W.W.: The fate of the chromaffin granule during catecholamine release from the adrenal medulla. II. Loss of protein and retention of lipid in subcellular fractions. Biochem. Pharmacol. **16**, 2101 (1967).
Portzehl, H., Caldwell, P.C., Rüegg, J.C.: The dependence of contraction and relaxation of muscle fibres from the crab *Maia squinidado* on the internal concentration of free calcium ions. Biochim. biophys. Acta (Amst.) **79**, 581—591 (1964).
Potter, L.T.: Storage of norepinephrine in sympathetic nerves. Pharmacol. Rev. **18**, 439—451 (1966).
— Role of intraneuronal vesicles in the synthesis, storage and release of noradrenaline. Circulat. Res. **21**, Suppl. 3, 13—24 (1967).
— Axelrod, J.: Subcellular localization of catecholamines in tissues of the rat. J. Pharmacol. exp. Ther. **142**, 291—298 (1963a).
— — Properties of norepinephrine storage particles of the rat heart. J. Pharmacol. exp. Ther. **142**, 299—305 (1963b).
— Cooper, T., Willman, V.L., Wolfe, D.E.: Synthesis, binding, release and metabolism of norepinephrine in normal and transplated dog hearts. Circulat. Res. **16**, 468—481 (1965).

RASMUSSEN, H., TENENHOUSE, A.: Cyclic AMP, calcium and membranes. Proc. nat. Acad. Sci. (Wash.) **59**, 1364—1369 (1968).

RATZENHOFER, M., MÜLLER, O.: Ultrastructure of adrenal medulla of the prenatal rat. J. Embryol. exp. Morph. **18**, 13—25 (1967).

RENOLD, A.E.: Insulin biosynthesis and secretion — a still unsettled topic. New Engl. J. Med. **282**, 173—182 (1970).

RUBIN, R.P.: The metabolic requirements for catecholamine release from the adrenal medulla. J. Physiol. (Lond.) **202**, 197—209 (1969).

— FEINSTEIN, M.B., JAANUS, S.D., PAIMRE, M.: Inhibition of catecholamine secretion and calcium exchange in perfused cat adrenal glands by tetracaine and magnesium. J. Pharmacol. exp. Ther. **155**, 463—471 (1967).

— JAANUS, S.D.: A study of the release of catecholamines from the adrenal medulla by indirectly acting sympathomimetic amines. Naunyn-Schmiedebergs Arch. Pharmak. exp. Path. **254**, 125—137 (1966).

— — The release of nucleotide from the adrenal medulla by indirectly acting sympathomimetic amines. Biochem. Pharmacol. **16**, 1007—1012 (1967).

— MIELE, E.: A study of the differential secretion of epinephrine and norepinephrine from the perfused cat adrenal gland. J. Pharmacol. exp. Ther. **164**, 115—121 (1968a).

— — The relation between the chemical structure of local anaesthetics and inhibition of calcium-evoked secretion from the adrenal medulla. Naunyn-Schmiedebergs Arch. Pharmak. exp. Path. **260**, 298—308 (1968b).

SAGE, H.J., SMITH, W.J., KIRSHNER, N.: Mechanism of secretion from the adrenal medulla. 1. A microquantitative immunologic assay for bevine adrenal catecholamine storage vesicle protein and its application to studies of the secretory process. Molec. Pharmacol. **3**, 81—89 (1967).

SCHMITT, F.O., SAMSON, F.E.: Neuronal fibrous proteins. In: Neurosciences Research Symposium Summaries, vol. 3, pp. 323—329. Ed. SCHMITT, F.O., MELNECHUK, T., Quarton, G.C. and ADELMAN, G. Cambridge, Mass.: The M.I.T. Press 1969.

SCHNEIDER, F.H.: Observations on the release of lysosomal enzymes from the isolated bovine adrenal gland. Biochem. Pharmacol. **17**, 848—851 (1968a).

— Release of lysosomal enzymes from the isolated bovine adrenal gland. Pharmacologist **10**, 158 (1968b).

— Drug-induced release of catecholamines, soluble protein and chromogranin A from the isolated bovine adrenal gland. Biochem. Pharmacol. **18**, 101—107 (1969a).

— Secretion from the cortex-free bovine adrenal medulla. Brit. J. Pharmacol. **37**, 371—379 (1969b).

— Secretion from the bovine adrenal gland: release of lysosomal enzymes. Biochem. Pharmacol. **19**, 833—847 (1970).

— SMITH, A.D., WINKLER, H.: Secretion from the adrenal medulla: biochemical evidence for exocytosis. Brit. J. Pharmacol. **31**, 94—104 (1967).

SCHÜMANN, H.J.: The distribution of adrenaline and noradrenaline in chromaffin granules of the chicken. J. Physiol. (Lond.) **137**, 318—326 (1957).

— Die Wirkung von Insulin and Reserpin auf den Adrenalin- und ATP-Gehalt der chromaffinen Granula des Nebennierenmarks. Naunyn-Schmiedeberg's Arch. exp. Path. Pharmak. **233**, 237—249 (1958a).

— Über den Noradrenalin- und ATP-Gehalt sympathischer Nerven. Naunyn-Schmiedeberg's Arch. exp. Path. Pharmak. **233**, 296—300 (1958b).

— PHILIPPU, A.: The mechanism of catecholamine release by tyramine. Int. J. Neuropharmacol. **1**, 179—182 (1962).

SHEA, S.M., KARNOVSKY, M.J.: Brownian motion: a theoretical explanation for the movement of vesicles across the endothelium. Nature (Lond.) **212**, 353—355 (1966).

SIMPSON, L.L.: The role of calcium in neurohumoral and neurohormonal extrusion processes. J. Pharm. Pharmacol. **20**, 889—910 (1968).

SKIPSKI, V.P., PETERSON, R.F., BARCLAY, M.: Quantitative analysis of phospholipids by thin-layer chromatography. Biochem. J. **90**, 374—378 (1964).

SMITH, A.D.: Biochemistry of adrenal chromaffin granules. In: *The Interaction of Drugs and Subcellular Components in Animal Cells*, pp. 239—292. Ed. by CAMPBELL, P.N. London: Churchill Ltd. 1968.

— Extracellular release of lysosomal phospholipases from the perfused adrenal gland. Biochem. J. **114**, 72P (1969).

— Proteins of vesicles from sympathetic axons: chemistry, immunoreactivity and release upon stimulation. Neurosci. Res. Prog. Bull. **8**, 377—382 (1970).

— Some implications of the neuron as a secreting cell. Phil. Trans. roy. Soc. B. **261**, 423—437 (1971a).

Smith, A. D.: Subcellular localization of noradrenaline in sympathetic neurons. Pharmacol. Rev. (in press) (1971 b).
— De Potter, W. P.: Unpublished observations (1969).
— — Moerman, E. H., De Schaepdryver, A. F.: Release of dopamine β-hydroxylase and chromogranin A upon stimulation of the splenic nerve. Tissue and Cell **2**, 547—568 (1970).
— Winkler, H.: Acid nucleases of the bovine adrenal medulla. Nature (Lond.) **207**, 634 (1965).
— — The localization of lysosomal enzymes in chromaffin tissue. J. Physiol. (Lond.) **183**, 179—188 (1966).
— — A simple method for the isolation of adrenal chromaffin granules on a large scale. Biochem. J. **103**, 480—482 (1967 a).
— — Purification and properties of an acidic protein from chromaffin granules of bovine adrenal medulla. Biochem. J. **103**, 483—492 (1967 b).
— — Lysosomal phospholipases A_1 and A_2 of bovine adrenal medulla. Biochem. J. **108**, 867—874 (1968).
— — Lysosomes and chromaffin granules in the adrenal medulla. In: Lysosomes in Biology and Pathology, Ed. Fell, H. and Dingle, J. T., **1**, 155—166. Amsterdam: North Holland 1969.
Smith, R. E., Farquhar, M. G.: Lysosome function in the regulation of the secretory processes in cells of the anterior pituitary gland. J. Cell Biol. **31**, 319—347 (1966).
Stjärne, L.: Studies of catecholamine uptake storage and release mechanisms. Acta physiol. scand. **62**, Suppl. 228, 1—60 (1964).
— Storage particles in noradrenergic tissues. Pharmacol. Rev. **18**, 425—432 (1966).
— Hedqvist, P., Bygdeman, S.: Neurotransmitter quantum released from sympathetic nerves in cat's skeletal muscle. Life Sci. **8** (1), 189—196 (1969).
— — Lagercrantz, H.: Catecholamines and adenine nucleotide material in effluent from stimulated adrenal medulla and spleen. Biochem. Pharmacol. **19**, 1147—1158 (1970).
— Lishajko, F.: Comparison of spontaneous loss of catecholamines and ATP *in vitro* from isolated bovine adrenomedullary, vesicular gland, vas deferens and splenic nerve granules J. Neurochem. **13**, 1213—1216 (1966).
— Roth, R. H., Lishajko, F.: Noradrenaline formation from dopamine in isolated subcellular particles from bovine splenic nerve. Biochem. Pharmacol. **16**, 1729—1739 (1967).
Stormorken, H.: The release reaction of secretion. Scand. J. Haemat. Suppl. **9**, 1—24 (1969).
Taugner, G., Hasselbach, W.: Über den Mechanismus der Catecholamin-Speicherung in den "chromaffinen Granula" des Nebennierenmarks. Naunyn-Schmiedebergs Arch. Pharmak. exp. Path. **255**, 266—286 (1966).
Taxi, J.: Morphological and cytochemical studies on the synapses in the autonomic nervous system. Progr. Brain Res. **31**, 5—20 (1969).
Thoenen, H.: Bildung und funktionelle Bedeutung adrenerger Ersatztransmitter. Exp. Med. Path. Klin. **27**, 1—85 (1969).
— Huerlimann, A., Haefely, W.: Cation dependence of the noreadrenaline-releasing action of tyramine. Europ. J. Pharmacol. **6**, 29—37 (1969 a).
— Mueller, R., Axelrod, J.: Trans-synaptic induction of tyrosine hydroxylase. J. Pharmacol. exp. Ther. **169**, 249—254 (1969 b).
Tranzer, J. P., Thoenen, H.: Significance of 'empty vesicles' in postganglionic sympathetic nerve terminals. Experientia (Basel) **23**, 123—124 (1967).
— — Various types of amine-storing vesicles in peripheral adrenergic nerve terminals. Experientia (Basel) **24**, 484—486 (1968).
Trifaró, J.: Phospholipid metabolism and adrenal medullary activity. 1. The effect of acetylcholine on tissue uptake and incorporation of orthophosphate -^{32}P into nucleotides and phospholipids of bovine adrenal medulla. Molec. Pharmacol. **5**, 382—393 (1969 a).
— The effect of Ca^{2+} omission on the secretion of catecholamines and the incorporation of orthophosphate -^{32}P into nucleotides and phospholipids of bovine adrenal medulla during acetylcholine stimulation. Molec. Pharmacol. **5**, 420—431 (1969 b).
— Dworkind, J.: A new and simple method for isolation of adrenal chromaffin granules by means of an isotonic density gradient. Analyt. Biochem. **34**, 403—412 (1970).
— Poisner, A. M.: The role of ATP and ATPase in the release of catecholamines from the adrenal medulla. 2. ATP-evoked fall in optical density of isolated chromaffin granules. Molec. Pharmacol. **3**, 572—580 (1967).
— — Douglas, W. W.: The fate of the chromaffiin granule during catecholamine release from the adrenal medulla. I. Unchanged efflux of phospholipid and cholesterol. Biochem. Pharmacol. **16**, 2095—2100 (1967).
Van Orden, L. S., Bensch, K. G., Giarman, N. J.: Histochemical and functional relationships of catecholamines in adrenergic nerve endings. 2. Extravesicular noradrenaline. J. Pharmacol. exp. Ther. **155**, 428—439 (1967).

VERITY, M.A., BEVAN, J.A., OSTROM, R.J.: Plurivesicular nerve endings in the pulmonary artery. Nature (Lond.) **211**, 537—538 (1966).
VIVEROS, O.H., ARQUEROS, L., CONNETT, R.J., KIRSHNER, N.: Mechanism of secretion from the adrenal medulla. 3. Studies of dopamine β-hydroxylase as a marker for catecholamine storage vesicle membranes in rabbit adrenal glands. Molec. Pharmacol. **5**, 60—68 (1969a).
— — — — Mechanism of secretion from the adrenal medulla. 4. The fate of the storage vesicles following insulin and reserpine administration. Molec. Pharmacol. **5**, 69—82 (1969b).
— — KIRSHNER, N.: Mechanism of secretion from the adrenal medulla. 5. Retention of storage vesicle membranes following release of adrenaline. Molec. Pharmacol. **5**, 342—349 (1969c).
— — — Quantal secretion from adrenal medulla: all-or-none release of storage vesicle content. Science **165**, 911—913 (1969d).
— — — Release of catecholamines and dopamine β-oxidase from the adrenal medulla. Life Sci. **7**, 609—618 (1968).
VOGT, M.: The output of cortical hormone by the mammalian suprarenal. J. Physiol. (Lond.) **102**, 341—356 (1943).
— The secretion of the denervated adrenal medulla of the cat. Brit. J. Pharmacol. **7**, 325—330 (1952).
VOHRA, M.M.: Evidence for the release of endogenous catecholamines by tetracaine. Life Sci. **8** (1), 25—31 (1969).
WEINER, N., BURACK, W.R., HAGEN, P.B.: The effect of insulin on the catecholamines and adenine nucleotides of adrenal glands. J. Pharmacol. exp. Ther. **130**, 251—255 (1960).
WHITTAKER, V.P., MICHAELSON, I.A., KIRKLAND, R.J.: The separation of synaptic vesicles from nerve-ending particles ('Synaptosomes'). Biochem. J. **90**, 293—303 (1964).
WINKLER, H.: Isolierung and Charakterisierung von chromaffinen Noradrenalin-Granula aus Schweine-Nebennierenmark. Naunyn-Schmiedebergs Arch. Pharmak. exp. Path. **263**, 340—357 (1969).
— The membrane of the chromaffin granule. Phil. Trans. roy. Soc. B. **261**, 293—303 (1971).
HÖRTNAGL, H., HÖRTNAGL, H., SMITH, A.D.: Membranes of the adrenal medulla. Behaviour of insoluble proteins of chromaffin granules on gel electrophoresis. Biochem. J. **118**, 303—310 (1970a).
— — — ZUR NEDDEN, G.: Rindernebennierenmark: Synthese und Sekretion von Hormonen und Chromogranin. Naunyn-Schmiedebergs Arch. Pharmak. **266**, 475 (1970b).
— SMITH, A.D.: Lipids of adrenal chromaffin granules: fatty acid composition of phospholipids, in particular lysolecithin. Naunyn-Schmiedebergs Arch. Pharmak. **261**, 379—388 (1968).
— STRIEDER, N., ZIEGLER, E.: Über Lipide, insbesondere Lysolecithin, in den chromaffinen Granula verschiedener Species. Naunyn-Schmiedebergs Arch. Pharmak. exp. Path. **256**, 407—415 (1967).
WOOD, J.G.: The relationship of nucleotidase activity to catecholamine storage sites in adrenomedullary tissue. Amer. J. Anat. **121**, 671—704 (1967).
WOODIN, A.M., FRENCH, J.E., MARCHESI, V.T.: Morphological changes associated with the extrusion of protein induced in the polymorphonuclear leucocyte by staphylococcal leucocidin. Biochem. J. **87**, 567—571 (1963).
— WIENEKE, A.A.: The accumulation of calcium by the polymorphonuclear leucocyte treated with staphylococcal leucocidin and its significance in the extrusion of protein. Biochem. J. **87**, 487—495 (1963).
— — The participation of calcium, adenosine triphosphate and adenosine triphosphatase in the extrusion of the granule proteins from the polymorphonuclear leucocyte. Biochem. J. **90**, 498—509 (1964).
— — Site of protein secretion and calcium accumulation in the polymorphonuclear leucocyte treated with leucocidin. In: A Symposium on Calcium and Cellular Function, pp. 183—197. Ed. CUTHBERT, A.W. London: Macmillan Ltd. 1970.
YATES, R.D.: Fine structural alterations of adreno-medullary cells of the Syrian hamster following intraperitoneal injections of insulin. Tex. Rep. Biol. Med. **22**, 756—763 (1964).
YOKOYAMA, M., TAKAYASU, H.: An electron microscopic study of the human adrenal medulla and phaeochromocytoma. Urol. int. (Basel) **24**, 79—95 (1969).

Chapter 14

Adrenergic False Transmitters

E. Muscholl

I. Introduction

The concept that foreign amines incorporated into the stores which normally hold the physiological transmitter, noradrenaline, may be released as false transmitters was created less than a decade ago. Nevertheless, this idea has aroused great interest and several review articles dealing with various aspects of the subject were previously published (Sourkes, 1965; Muscholl, 1966a; Stone and Porter, 1967; Kopin, 1968a, 1968b; Thoenen, 1969). However, there are recent developments in this field which will be treated below in more detail. These include stereochemical requirements for formation of false transmitters, release of false transmitters by various stimuli, and the quantitative aspects of simultaneous release of a false transmitter and noradrenaline and their actions on adrenoceptors.

The development of the false transmitter concept is intimately connected with the history of the antihypertensive drug, α-methyldopa. In 1954 Sourkes described the amino acid as competitive inhibitor of DOPA decarboxylase. During the following years α-methyldopa was mainly investigated in enzymatic studies, until the discovery of its antihypertensive action by Oates et al. (1960) started a thorough pharmacological research into its mode of action. Carlsson and Lindqvist (1962) then suggested that α-methylated amines, formed in the brain from the amino acid precursor, displaced noradrenaline and dopamine, respectively, and possibly took over their functions. Day and Rand (1963, 1964) modified this idea in two respects. They proposed that α-methylnoradrenaline formed from α-methyldopa was released by the physiological impulse flow from *peripheral* adrenergic fibres and that it behaved as an agonist *weaker* than noradrenaline at the receptors, thus producing incomplete transmission failure.

Kopin (1968a) has defined the criteria which must be met in order to classify a compound as an adrenergic false transmitter. These are analogous to the criteria considered necessary to identify a compound as a neurotransmitter.

1. The false transmitter must be present in adrenergic terminal nerve fibres at the same site as noradrenaline, i.e. in the intraaxonal vesicles.

2. The false transmitter must be released by adrenergic nerve stimulation and depleted by drugs which deplete noradrenaline.

3. In contrast to the requirements for the identification of a physiological neurotransmitter, designation of a false transmitter does not imply that it is as active as noradrenaline. In fact, most false transmitters are less potent at adrenoceptors than noradrenaline.

There are a few compounds which have been shown to be released into perfusates of organs during sympathetic nerve stimulation but yet do not fully meet the criteria for false transmitters outlined above. These include ^{3}H-bretylium (Fischer et al., 1966), ^{3}H-guanethidine (Boullin, 1966) and prostaglandins of the E series (Davies et al., 1967). The following discussion will not be extended to a topic which is closely related to that of false transmitters, namely the subject of "false precursors" giving rise to formation of noradrenaline (cf. Chapter 6, B I 2 by von Euler).

II. Survey of Amines Acting as False Transmitters

1. Structural Requirements for Formation and Metabolism

The four enzymes converting stepwise tyrosine to adrenaline are well known for lack of specificity towards their substrates. This is the reason for the possibility of various amino acids or phenylethylamines to enter the biosynthetic pathway of the natural transmitter, and to give rise to the formation of false transmitters. For instance, tyrosine hydroxylase hydroxylates phenylalanine (Ikeda et al., 1965), α-methyltyrosine (Maître, 1965; Udenfriend et al., 1965, 1966) or metaraminol (Maître and Staehelin, 1965), though at a slower rate than tyrosine.

Furthermore, DOPA decarboxylase (aromatic L-amino acid decarboxylase) forms α-methyldopamine (Weissbach et al., 1960; Carlsson and Lindqvist, 1962; Lovenberg et al., 1962), metatyramine (Blaschko, 1950), α-methyl-metatyramine (Gessa et al., 1962; Lovenberg et al., 1962), α-methyl-5-hydroxy-tryptamine (Weissbach et al., 1960) or noradrenaline (Blaschko et al., 1950; Werle and Sell, 1954) from the corresponding amino acids, α-methyldopa, metatyrosine, α-methyl-metatyrosine, α-methyl-5-hydroxytryptophan, and *threo*-dihydroxyphenylserine. There is an absolute substrate specificity for L-isomers in preference to D-isomers, irrespective of the amino acid concerned. This is true for *in vitro* (Holtz et al., 1938; Lovenberg et al., 1962) as well as for *in vivo* studies (Porter et al., 1961; Sjoerdsma et al., 1963; cf. also the indirect evidence by Kroneberg and Stoepel, 1963; Pettinger et al., 1965).

Several amines other than dopamine are excellent substrates of dopamine-β-hydroxylase *in vitro*, e.g. tyramine, α-methyltyramine, metatyramine, α-methyl-metatyramine and α-methyldopamine (cf. the review by Creveling, 1965). Likewise, *in vivo* formation of β-hydroxylated products of phenylethylamines has been observed by Carlsson and Lindqvist (1962), Maître and Staehelin (1963), Musacchio and Goldstein (1963), Muscholl and Maître (1963), Andén (1964a), Schümann and Grobecker (1964) and Shore et al. (1964). Finally, phenylethanolamine N-methyl transferase purified from adrenal medullary cells has been found to N-methylate not only noradrenaline but, among other amines, also phenylethanolamine, octopamine and *m*-hydroxyphenylethanolamine (Axelrod, 1966). Formation *in vivo* of α-methyladrenaline from α-methylnoradrenaline occurs in the rabbit adrenal medulla (Muscholl, 1965, 1966b) or in frog tissues (Grobecker and Holtz, 1966; Grobecker et al., 1966).

While the enzymes that normally synthesize noradrenaline are equally important for the formation of false transmitters, the enzymes catabolizing the catecholamines may inactivate some of the foreign compounds but may leave others intact. Enzymic destruction by MAO will be discussed first, and its importance is well illustrated in the process of conversion of tyramine to octopamine. Formation of octopamine occurs within the adrenergic neuron (Carlsson and Waldeck, 1963; Kopin et al., 1965) but only 0.3% of the dose of ^{3}H-tyramine administered may be recovered from the rat heart after 4 or 60 min as octopamine (Musacchio et al., 1965a). Since both tyramine and octopamine are good substrates of MAO it is not surprising that inhibition of MAO increased the yield of octopamine from tyramine in the mouse heart about fourfold (Carlsson and Waldeck, 1963) and in the rat salivary gland about tenfold (Kopin et al., 1965). The dependence of ^{14}C-octopamine derived from ^{14}C-tyramine on the activity of intraneuronal MAO has been used as a method to detect possible MAO inhibition by drugs under *in vivo* conditions (WALDECK, 1970). On the other hand, introduction of an α-methyl group into the noradrenaline or dopamine molecule seems to be the simplest means of protecting the resulting compound from MAO (BLASCHKO et al., 1937) without principally changing its similarity to the parent amine as far as vesicular uptake and storage, and affinity to the membrane uptake is concerned (cf. the following section).

Those false transmitters and their precursors which are catechol derivatives are substrates of COMT (see the review by AXELROD, 1966). Accordingly, O-methylated metabolites of the following compounds have been isolated from the urine, from tissues and perfusates of organs: α-methyldopa (BUHS et al., 1964; PORTER and TITUS, 1963; YOUNG and EDWARDS, 1964), α-methyldopamine (GILLESPIE et al., 1962; PORTER and TITUS, 1963; YOUNG and EDWARDS, 1964; PRESCOTT et al., 1966), α-methylnoradrenaline (GJESSING, 1965; STOTT and ROBINSON, 1963, 1967; CARLSSON et al., 1967), 5-hydroxydopamine (THOENEN et al., 1967c) and 3-methoxy-4,5-dihydroxyphenylethylamine (THOENEN et al., 1968).

Since monophenolic compounds are not methylated by COMT (AXELROD, 1966) this route of metabolism does not occur in the case of false transmitter substances such as octopamine, α-methyloctopamine, the meta-hydroxy analogue of octopamine (metaoctopamine) and metaraminol. Among the substances known to be false transmitters metaraminol and α-methyloctopamine are unique in so far as they are resistant to both COMT and MAO.

2. Retention, Storage and Uptake

When the subcellular distribution of amines known to be released as false transmitters was studied it was found that they were retained in the microsomal fraction obtained by high-speed centrifugation of rat heart homogenates (MUSACCHIO et al., 1965b). One hr after injection of labelled tyramine, α-methyltyramine, metatyramine and dopamine only dopamine and the β-hydroxylated derivatives of the injected amines (octopamine, α-methyloctopamine, metaoctopamine, and noradrenaline) were retained in the particulate fraction. Tyramine can enter the microsomal fraction since it was present there 4 min after its injection, provided that β-hydroxylation was inhibited by previous administration of disulfiram. However, after 1 hr the amines lacking both the two phenolic hydroxyl and the β-hydroxyl groups were found almost exclusively in the supernatant fraction, also when β-hydroxylation was blocked. MUSACCHIO et al. (1965a, 1965b) determined the loss of four different amines from the rat heart *in vivo* after a dose of tyramine or guanethidine and observed the following order of decreasing resistance towards depletion: noradrenaline, dopamine, metaoctopamine, octopamine. The same order was obtained when the four amines were ranged according to their ability to be retained in the microsomal fraction. Since the deaminated metabolites are not retained, the amino group is indispensible in this respect.

SMITH and WINKLER (cf. Chapter 13, A IV of this volume) have listed the evidence that incorporation of noradrenaline into the particle-bound store is a prerequisite for the transmitter being released in response to stimulation of the adrenergic nerve. By analogy this should also be true for the release of false transmitters. There is now much evidence supporting this proposal.

Retention of different sympathomimetic amines by the microsomal fraction of tissue homogenates was correlated with the property of these amines to be released during sympathetic nerve stimulation (cf. the review articles by KOPIN, 1966; THOENEN, 1969; THOENEN and TRANZER, 1971). Those non-β-hydroxylated precursors of false transmitters, which are not retained (MUSACCHIO et al., 1965a), are also unable to be released during nerve stimulation (FISCHER et al., 1965). Both dopamine (MUSACCHIO et al., 1965a, 1965b) and α-methyldopamine (MUSACCHIO et al., 1966b) are retained despite lack of a β-hydroxyl group if their β-hydroxylation is blocked by disulfiram; since these catecholamines are released from the cat spleen by nerve stimulation (THOENEN et al., 1965; MUSACCHIO et al., 1966b; THOENEN et al., 1967a, 1967b) the requirement of retention by the microsomal fraction is, likewise, fulfilled. Thus, the presence of a β-hydroxyl group does not seem to be essential for release.

There is no doubt that adrenergic nerves are responsible for the retention of amines that act as false transmitters. Sympathetic postganglionic denervation inhibits the accumulation in rat salivary glands of β-hydroxylated amines derived from labelled precursors such as tyramine (CARLSSON and WALDECK, 1963; ALMGREN et al., 1965; KOPIN et al., 1965), α-methyltyramine (KOPIN et al., 1965) and metatyramine (KOPIN et al., 1965). Uptake and retention of (—)-metaraminol was absent *in vivo* in denervated rat salivary glands (ALMGREN and WALDECK, 1967; ALMGREN et al., 1969) or in hearts of immunosympathectomized rats (SHORE et al., 1964). Likewise, immunosympathectomy greatly inhibited uptake of (—)-metaraminol into rat heart slices (GIACHETTI and SHORE, 1966) or retention by several mouse tissues of ^{3}H-α-methyloctopamine formed from α-methyltyramine (IVERSEN et al., 1966).

Most convincing evidence for uptake and storage of false transmitters in adrenergic nerves comes from histological work. With the fluorescence method of FALCK and HILLARP it was shown that exogenous (—)-α-methylnoradrenaline (MALMFORS, 1965; HAMBERGER, 1967; PATIL and JACOBOWITZ, 1968) is taken up and retained by the terminal and non-terminal parts of the adrenergic neuron in a way similar to noradrenaline. Likewise, α-methylnoradrenaline formed from α-methyldopa *in vivo* is stored in central and peripheral adrenergic neurons (CARLSSON et al., 1965a). Using a microspectrofluorometric method JONSSON and RITZÉN (1966) observed an uptake into adrenergic nerves of metaraminol; this amine cannot be visualized with the conventional fluorescence technique since it causes a fluorescence maximum at a low wave length which is cut off by the secondary filters used by most workers.

With the histofluorescence method PATIL and JACOBOWITZ (1968) studied the uptake and retention, by adrenergic nerves of the rat iris, of a series of corbadrine isomers. In order to abolish the fluorescence of endogenous noradrenaline the rats were pretreated with reserpine. After injection of (—)- and (+)-*erythro*-corbadrine (α-methylnoradrenaline) the fluorescence was essentially similar and more pronounced than after administration of either (+)-α-methyldopamine or ($\pm$)-*erythro*-α-methyladrenaline (dihydroxyephedrine). With high doses of (—)-α-methyldopamine an uptake was demonstrated but ($\pm$)-*threo*-corbadrine and ($\pm$)-*threo*-N-methylcorbadrine (dihydroxypseudoephedrine) were not seen to fluoresce within the terminal nerve fibres. The findings with the latter two amines are difficult to reconcile with the evidence that the *threo*-isomers are taken up, stored and released by sympathetic nerve stimulation (MUSCHOLL and SPRENGER, 1966; LINDMAR et al., 1967; MUSCHOLL and LINDMAR, 1967; WALDECK, 1967; DREWS et al., 1968). Thus, PATIL and JACOBOWITZ (1968) discussed some possible causes for the failure of their method to detect fluorescing *threo*-isomers within the adrenergic nerve fibres of the rat iris. A negative finding of this kind should not distract attention from the impressive evidence which the histofluorescence method has provided for the accumulation within the postganglionic adrenergic nerve fibre of several of the false transmitters.

The localization of false transmitters within the adrenergic terminal axon has been investigated by electron microscopy (cf. the review by THOENEN and TRANZER, 1971). Several amines such as 5-hydroxydopamine, α-methylnoradrenaline, 4-methoxy-3,5-dihydroxyphenylethylamine and 5-hydroxytryptamine have been found to be retained by the storage vesicles. This is in accord with the view that accumulation of false transmitters in the microsomal fraction of tissue homogenates reflects their accumulation by intraaxonal vesicles. It is interesting that exogenous 5-hydroxytryptamine is taken up and retained by the sympathetic nerves of the guinea-pig vas deferens (THOA et al., 1969). Direct evidence for release of 5-hydroxytryptamine by adrenergic nerve stimulation is however lacking.

Studies using α-methylnoradrenaline, metaraminol and related amines, which are resistant to intraaxonal metabolism by MAO, have contributed to the evidence obtained by earlier investigations using noradrenaline (CARLSSON et al., 1963; HAMBERGER et al., 1964; LINDMAR and MUSCHOLL, 1964; IVERSEN et al., 1965; MALMFORS, 1965) that there are two amine concentrating mechanisms: 1. a relatively unspecific mechanism in the neuronal membrane which is blocked by cocaine, tricyclic antidepressants, guanethidine or sympathomimetic amines but not by reserpine and tetrabenazine; and 2. a relatively specific mechanism at the level of the intracellular storage vesicles which is blocked by reserpine and tetrabenazine. Such studies of the two uptake processes were carried out by BERTI and SHORE, 1967a, 1967b; CARLSSON et al., 1965b; CARLSSON and WALDECK, 1965a, 1965b, 1965c, 1966a; GIACHETTI and SHORE, 1966; HAMBERGER, 1967; LINDMAR and MUSCHOLL, 1965; MALMFORS, 1965; MURAD and SHORE, 1966; MUSCHOLL and WEBER, 1965; WEBER and MUSCHOLL, 1965. In the majority of these investigations metaraminol has been used as an experimental tool for the following reasons: There is a sensitive chemical method of its estimation (SHORE and ALPERS, 1964); furthermore, neither MAO, nor amphetamine desaminase (GRAM and WRIGHT, 1965), nor COMT metabolize the amine, and the optical isomers of the compound are available.

It is advantageous to carry out uptake experiments with one isomer rather than with a racemic mixture of two isomers. However, in studies with labelled amines racemates are generally used. Membranal uptake of an amine is measured most precisely by determining its removal from an incubation or perfusion medium; however, much of the work on uptake was done by measuring accumulation by the tissue of an amine, because this procedure is technically easier to carry out (for discussion see LINDMAR and MUSCHOLL, 1964; IVERSEN, 1967). For instance, while (—)- and (+)-metaraminol are transported efficiently by the membrane uptake process (GIACHETTI and SHORE, 1966) only the (—)-isomer is bound to intraaxonal vesicles where it displaces noradrenaline; in contrast, (+)-metaraminol is not bound (as indicated by its low affinity for retention by the particulate fraction, LUNDBORG and STITZEL, 1968a) and rapidly leaves the tissue when the extracellular concentration of the amine levels off (SHORE et al., 1964). Therefore, results of uptake studies obtained with racemic mixtures of amines may be difficult to interpret as long as radiochemical and usually also chemical methods do not differentiate between two optical isomers of an amine.

Uptake (in most cases measured by retention) by adrenergically innervated tissues of α-methylnoradrenaline or metaraminol has been found to be dependent on sodium ions (HAMBERGER, 1967; PATON, 1968, 1971; SUGRUE and SHORE, 1969), potassium ions (HAMBERGER, 1967; PATON, 1968, 1971), on temperature (HAMBERGER, 1967; GIACHETTI and SHORE, 1966) and on metabolic energy sources (HAMBERGER, 1967; PATON, 1968). The inhibition of amine uptake by omission of potassium ions from the incubation medium may be seen only after prolonged time of exposure to a potassium-deficient solution. It is likely that the Na^+ and K^+ activated ATPase may participate in the membrane transport of metaraminol and related amines (BERTI and SHORE, 1967a; PATON, 1971) as has been suggested for the transport of noradrenaline (see Chapter by VON EULER, Section II, B 7).

SUGRUE and SHORE (1969) have recently described a second, sodium-dependent uptake process for metaraminol which operates only at low (20 mM) external concentrations of sodium; in contrast to the membrane uptake mechanism discussed above the second process is optically specific and sensitive to reserpine.

3. Stereochemical Considerations

The structural characteristics facilitating vesicular retention of false transmitters have been discussed in Section II,2. Some of the structural requirements for the formation of false transmitters have also been mentioned in Section II, 1, for instance the substrate specificity of the DOPA decarboxylase for L-isomers.

In many studies α-methylnoradrenaline or metaraminol have been utilized as substitute transmitters. These amines contain two asymmetric carbon atoms (α; β), and therefore four isomeric forms of each compound exist. The absolute configuration of the metabolic products of α-methyldopa and α-MMT has not been determined. Considering the known stereospecificity of the synthetizing enzymes it has been assumed that only one isomer of α-methylnoradrenaline and metaraminol, respectively, is formed biologically from the precursor amino acids, namely that designated as α S : β R (VAN ROSSUM, 1963; VAN ROSSUM and HURKMANS, 1963; LINDMAR and MUSCHOLL, 1965). R (*rectus*) and S (*sinister*) are notations of molecular configuration according to the sequence rule laid down by CAHN et al. (1956). In his review article, VAN ROSSUM (1963) has quoted the evidence derived from rotary dispersion studies which showed that synthetic (—)-corbadrine and (—)-metaraminol both have the configuration α S : β R (also known as the (—)-*erythro* isomer). Further references to chemical work concerning the absolute configuration of α-methylated amines are given by SAARI et al. (1968), TORCHIANA et al. (1968) and PATIL et al. (1970). The (+)-*erythro* isomers of corbadrine and metaraminol have the configuration α R : β S.

The levorotatory corbadrine (SCHAUMANN, 1936; TORCHIANA et al., 1968) or metaraminol (TORCHIANA et al., 1968) is several hundred to several thousand times more active in increasing the arterial blood pressure than the corresponding dextrorotatory isomer. The chemical and biological properties of the α-methylnoradrenaline isolated from organs of animals treated with α-methyldopa were compared with those of the reference compound, (—)-corbadrine. The nearly equivalent replacement of part of the noradrenaline by α-methylnoradrenaline was ascertained by chemical methods (CARLSSON and LINDQVIST, 1962; SCHÜMANN et al., 1965) which do not distinguish between the enantiomorphs, and by biological assays on the pithed rat (MAÎTRE and STAEHELIN, 1963; MUSCHOLL and MAÎTRE, 1963; LINDMAR and MUSCHOLL, 1965; HAEFELY et al., 1967) which do differentiate between the (—)- and (+)-isomers, respectively. If the α-methylnoradrenaline formed in the body after administration of α-methyldopa had been dextrorotatory or racemic rather than levorotatory, the results of the biological estimations would not have precisely agreed with those of the chemical method. Thus, it is safe to assume that the α-methylnoradrenaline formed *in vivo* is levorotatory.

Another line of indirect evidence excluded the possibility that one of the *threo* isomers of α-methylnoradrenaline was formed as a metabolite of α-methyldopa. Rabbits were given a single dose of reserpine in order to deplete the adrenal glands of the adrenaline, and then 2—6 injections of L-α-methyldopa administered in daily intervals (MUSCHOLL, 1966b). The small amounts of α-methyladrenaline which were detected in the adrenals behaved chemically and biologically in a way similar to 3,4-dihydroxyephedrine (*erythro* form), but differed biologically from 3,4-dihydroxypseudoephedrine (*threo* form). Since N-methylation of α-methylnoradrenaline is unlikely to alter the conformation of the parent molecule, this result strongly suggests that α-methylnoradrenaline formed in the body is the (—)-*erythro* isomer, with the absolute configuration α S : β R.

When (±)-*threo*-corbadrine became available as a reference compound it was found that its pressor activity in the pithed rat was only 1/1000 of that of (—)-corbadrine and, conversely, its intensity to fluoresce with the trihydroxyindole procedure was 25 times that of the *erythro* diastereoisomer (MUSCHOLL and RAHN, 1966, 1968). Nuclear magnetic resonance studies have later shown that the *erythro* and *threo* configurations can be assigned to corbadrine and its diastereoisomer (pseudocorbadrine), respectively, (FARRUGIA et al., 1969). The α-methylnoradrenaline excreted in the urine of hypertensive patients continuously treated with L-α-methyldopa was isolated by ion exchange and adsorption chromatography followed by paper chromatography using two different solvent systems. Comparison of the pressor and fluorimetric activities of the isolated α-methylnoradrenaline with the corresponding activities of both the *threo* and *erythro* isomers provided unequivocal evidence that the amine formed was (—)-*erythro*-α-methylnoradrenaline (MUSCHOLL and RAHN, 1968) thus confirming the above considerations.

If biosynthesis leads to α-methylnoradrenaline with the configuration α S : β R, then the intermediate α-methyldopamine has to have the configuration α S (VAN ROSSUM and HURKMANS, 1963). GOLDSTEIN et al. (1964) reported that only the (+)-α-methylated amines (α S) are substrates for the dopamine β-hydroxylase. This was confirmed by TORCHIANA et al. (1968) who incubated both the (+)- and the (—)-isomers of α-methyldopamine and α-methyl-metatyramine, respectively, with purified beef adrenal medullary enzyme and found that only the (+)-isomers were β-hydroxylated. Likewise, in mice formation of α-methylnoradrenaline was observed after injection of (+)-α-methyldopamine but not after injection of (—)-α-methyldopamine (WALDECK, 1968). Similarly, infusion of (+)-α-methyldopamine into rabbits was followed by replacement of 73% of the endogenous noradrenaline by (—)-*erythro*-α-methylnoradrenaline whereas after infusion of (—)-α-methyldopamine no α-methylnoradrenaline could be detected in the hearts, in spite of a large accumulation of the infused amine (KILBINGER et al., 1971).

The substrate stereospecificity of the β-hydroxylase may explain the observations of CARLSSON et al. (1968) who injected tritium-labelled (±)-α-methyldopamine into mice and studied the time course of appearance of α-methylnoradrenaline in the heart. Up to 60 min the concentration of α-methylnoradrenaline steadily increased but 2—4 hr after injection of the precursor it became constant, although there were large amounts of ^{3}H-α-methyldopamine still present in the heart. It was concluded that after 4 hr only the α R isomer of the racemic ^{3}H-α-methyldopamine was left and synthesis of α-methylnoradrenaline necessarily ceased because of lack of precursor.

The stereochemical aspects of the formation of metaraminol *in vivo* have been less thoroughly investigated than those of α-methylnoradrenaline formation. Nevertheless, it is likely that the metaraminol derived from α-MMT is the (—)-

isomer since it remains in the heart for several days (ANDÉN, 1964a; SHORE et al., 1964) as does the reference compound, (—)-metaraminol (SHORE et al., 1964; GRAM and WRIGHT, 1966). In contrast, the (+)-isomer is lost from the heart within a few hours (SHORE et al., 1964; cf. also LUNDBORG and STITZEL, 1968a). The optically active isomers of *threo*-metaraminol have been synthesized and investigated for their sympathomimetic and noradrenaline depleting activities (SAARI et al., 1968). However, metaraminol isolated from tissues after administration of α-MMT does not seem to have been compared with authentic *threo*-metaraminol as a reference compound.

III. Formation of False Transmitters

1. Direct Incorporation of an Amine as False Transmitter

A great number of sympathomimetic amines are concentrated in adrenergic nerve terminals by the membrane uptake mechanism and, in succession, by vesicular retention (cf. Section II, 2). Administration of a false transmitter amine has therefore often been used as a means to incorporate the compound into the amine stores of various tissues. The schedules of pretreatment leading to a given degree of noradrenaline substitution by a false transmitter amine have been tested: (—)-metaraminol (SHORE et al., 1964); (±)-metaraminol (PORTER et al., 1967); dihydroxyephedrine (LINDMAR et al., 1967); dihydroxypseudoephedrine (LINDMAR et al., 1967). Also, changes in the tissue levels of the endogenous noradrenaline and of a false transmitter amine at different times after administration of a single dose of the latter have been studied: (—)-metaraminol (ANDÉN, 1964a; CROUT et al., 1964; SHORE et al., 1964; ANDÉN and MAGNUSSON, 1965; GRAM and WRIGHT, 1966; JOHNSON and MICKLE, 1966); (+)-adrenaline (ANDÉN 1964b); (—)-α-methylnoradrenaline (PHILIPPU and SCHÜMANN, 1965; MUSCHOLL and SPRENGER, 1966); (±)-*threo*-corbadrine (DREWS et al., 1968); (±)-dihydroxyephedrine (MUSCHOLL and SPRENGER, 1966); (±)-dihydroxypseudoephedrine (MUSCHOLL and SPRENGER, 1966). MAÎTRE and STAEHELIN (1967) investigated the time course of noradrenaline depletion in the rat heart during daily administration of (—)-α-methylnoradrenaline for 11 days and determined the myocardial noradrenaline and α-methylnoradrenaline content from 1—11 days after cessation of treatment.

Summing up the results of these different studies it can be stated that repeated administration of a false transmitter amine leads to its progressive accumulation and to increased loss of endogenous noradrenaline. The half-time of loss of (—)-metaraminol or (—)-α-methylnoradrenaline from the heart, when determined 24 hr after their administration, was 2—6 days; the loss of both amines from liver or spleen was more rapid than that from heart.

The *erythro* isomers of both corbadrine (WALDECK, 1967) and dihydroxyephedrine (α-methyladrenaline, MUSCHOLL and SPRENGER, 1966) are retained more efficiently than the corresponding *threo* isomers, *threo*-corbadrine and dihydroxypseudoephedrine, respectively. Since a similar difference in the rate of disappearance of the corbadrine isomers was no longer apparent when the animals had been pretreated with reserpine, WALDECK (1967) concluded that the storage vesicles have a higher affinity for the *erythro* as compared with the *threo* configuration.

Accumulation of dopamine or (+)-α-methyldopamine can be achieved only when intraneuronal β-hydroxylation is blocked, e.g. by disulfiram (MUSACCHIO et al., 1966b; THOENEN et al., 1965, 1967a, 1967b). However, (—)-α-methyldopamine is resistant to β-hydroxylation (see Section II, 3) and was found to persist in the heart for 3 hr after its administration to rabbits. In contrast, after the same time interval only traces of an equivalent dose of (+)-α-methyldopamine were detected (Kilbinger et al., 1971).

Two and even 20 hr after administration of ^{3}H-5-hydroxydopamine to cats some unmetabolized amine was detected in the spleen, in addition to two unidentified β-hydroxylated amines (Thoenen et al., 1967c). Apparently β-hydroxylation of 5-hydroxydopamine proceeds at a much slower rate than that of administered dopamine or (+)-α-methyldopamine.

2. Formation of False Transmitters from Foreign Precursors

a) Formation by a Single Metabolic Step

As pointed out in Section II, 1 various amines are substrates of dopamine β-hydroxylase and thus give rise to formation of false transmitters. Generally speaking, the introduction of a β-hydroxyl group increases retention by vesicular storage sites and facilitates release by adrenergic nerve stimulation (see Section II, 2). Formation of the following false transmitters *in vivo* has been described: Octopamine formed from injected tyramine (Carlsson and Waldeck, 1963; Musacchio and Goldstein, 1963; Chidsey et al., 1964; Masuoka et al., 1964; Almgren et al., 1965; Fischer et al., 1965; Kopin et al., 1965; Musacchio et al., 1965a; Lee et al., 1967). α-Methyloctopamine (*p*-hydroxynorephedrine) formed from α-methyltyramine (*p*-hydroxyamphetamine) (Sjoerdsma and v. Studnitz, 1963; Fischer et al., 1965; Kopin et al., 1965; Musacchio et al., 1965a; Lewander, 1971a). Metaoctopamine formed from metatyramine (Musacchio et al., 1965a, 1965b). α-Methylnoradrenaline formed from (+)-α-methyldopamine (Philippu and Schümann, 1965; Waldeck, 1968; Kilbinger et al., 1971). α-Methylnoradrenaline was formed from (—)-metaraminol by ring-hydroxylation in guinea-pig heart (Maître and Staehelin, 1965; Maier et al., 1967) but not in rat heart (Maier et al., 1967; Porter et al., 1967).

Moreover, formation of false transmitters by a *single* enzymatic step has been observed after administration of a precursor amino acid under conditions which precluded a subsequent β-hydroxylation of the decarboxylation product. For instance, in the presence of disulfiram, which blocks β-hydroxylation, α-methyldopamine is accumulated in heart and spleen of cats treated with α-methyldopa (Thoenen et al., 1967b). Similarly, administration to cats of 4-methoxy-3,5-dihydroxyphenylalanine is followed by accumulation in the spleen of 4-methoxy-3,5-dihydroxyphenylethylamine, an amine that is resistant to β-hydroxylation *in vivo* (Thoenen et al., 1968).

b) Formation of False Transmitters by Several Metabolic Steps

The best known examples of false transmitter amines formed *in vivo* by successive enzymatic steps are those of (—)-metaraminol derived from α-MMT and (—)-α-methylnoradrenaline derived from α-methyldopa, respectively. The first evidence for this route of metabolism of the α-methyl amino acids was provided by the work of Carlsson and Lindqvist (1962). After intraperitoneal injection of 400 mg/kg α-methyldopa into mice the concentrations of 5-hydroxytryptamine and dopamine in the brain decreased by about 50% within 3—6 hr and then rose again to normal values within 24 hr. Noradrenaline was depleted more markedly and for a longer period than dopamine but α-methyldopa could be detected in the brain only for less than 12 hr. Fluorimetric analysis and paper chromatography revealed the presence in the brain of α-methyldopamine; the mean concentration fell from 0.8 μg/g at 3 hr to 0.2 μg/g at 24 hr. In addition, α-methylnoradrenaline was detected by paper chromatography 24 hr after a single dose, or after repeated doses, of α-methyldopa which entirely depleted the mouse brain of its noradrenaline content. Quantitative determinations of the α-methylnoradrenaline formed were not carried out but inspection of the paper chromatograms showed that its amount roughly corresponded to the normal noradrenaline concentration. Furthermore, 24 hr after intraperitoneal injection of 400 mg/kg α-MMT into mice, the brain noradrenaline had disappeared almost completely and there was chromatographic evidence for the storage of metaraminol apparently derived from the precursor amino acid undergoing decarboxylation and β-hydroxylation.

These findings were confirmed and extended by subsequent work in which the α-methylnoradrenaline present in heart, brain, iris and spleen of rats, guinea pigs, rabbits, and cats after administration of α-methyldopa was estimated quantitatively (MAÎTRE and STAEHELIN, 1963; MUSCHOLL and MAÎTRE, 1963; LINDMAR and MUSCHOLL, 1965; SCHÜMANN et al., 1965; HAEFELY et al., 1967; MAÎTRE and STAEHELIN, 1967). In most of these investigations the concentrations in the organs of α-methylnoradrenaline accumulated and noradrenaline lost agreed well; however, after high doses or after repeated administration of α-methyldopa the amount of α-methylnoradrenaline retained often exceeded the loss of noradrenaline (cf. Section V, 1). On the rat and on the guinea-pig heart the time courses of recovery of noradrenaline and disappearance of α-methylnoradrenaline, respectively, after cessation of treatment with α-methyldopa were studied by MAÎTRE and STAEHELIN (1963, 1967). Formation of α-methylnoradrenaline has also been observed on the isolated guinea-pig heart which was perfused with α-methyldopa (PHILIPPU and SCHÜMANN, 1965).

Hospitalized hypertensive patients treated orally with 1—2 g L-α-methyldopa daily were found to excrete amounts of free α-methylnoradrenaline which exceeded the urinary output of free noradrenaline (MUSCHOLL and RAHN, 1966); the same was true in normotensive volunteers who received 1 g of the drug for 2 days (LINDMAR et al., 1968). Formation of α-methylnoradrenaline in man apparently proceeds quite rapidly since the urine of three hypertensive patients receiving a single oral dose of L-α-methyldopa already contained the foreign amine if collected in the 0—2 hr interval after administration of the drug (MUSCHOLL and RAHN, 1968). About 8 hr after administration of α-methyldopa the excretion of α-methylnoradrenaline reached a peak and then declined slowly; urines collected from 56—72 hr after the drug still contained free α-methylnoradrenaline.

Purified beef adrenal tyrosine hydroxylase converts α-methyltyrosine to α-methyldopa (UDENFRIEND et al., 1965). MAÎTRE (1965) found 0.17 μg/g α-methyldopamine and 0.11 μg/g α-methylnoradrenaline in the brain, and 0.32 μg/g α-methylnoradrenaline in the heart, of guinea pigs treated with a single oral dose of 300 mg/kg α-methyl-D,L-tyrosine. As pointed out by the author these concentrations of α-methylated amines are, however, small if compared with those resulting from treatment with an equimolar dose of α-methyldopa. UDENFRIEND et al. (1966) came to the conclusion that the small amount of α-methylnoradrenaline formed in guinea-pig tissues after administration of α-methyltyrosine is not responsible for the noradrenaline depletion observed; rather, the depletion was entirely accounted for by the inhibition of tyrosine hydroxylase exerted by the drug itself. The presence of small amounts of α-methylnoradrenaline in the cat spleen and heart after 3 doses of α-methyltyrosine was revealed by qualitative paper chromatography (THOENEN et al., 1966a). According to AMERY et al. (1969) a dose of α-methyltyrosine (1.5 g daily for 3 weeks) which greatly decreased noradrenaline excretion of a patient with malignant pheochromocytoma also caused a small urinary output of α-methylnoradrenaline (30 μg/24 hr) and a larger one of α-methyldopamine (2.1 mg/24 hr).

In some tissues known to contain a high phenylethanolamine-N-methyl transferase activity α-methyladrenaline (together with its precursor, α-methylnoradrenaline) has been detected after administration of α-methyldopa, e.g. in rabbit adrenal glands (MUSCHOLL, 1965, 1966b) or in frog heart, skin and adrenals (GROBECKER and HOLTZ, 1966; GROBECKER et al., 1966). In view of the possibility that N-methylation of α-methylnoradrenaline also occurred in man, a pooled extract of 20 urine samples of hypertensive patients treated with α-methyldopa was prepared and tested for the presence of α-methyladrenaline (MUSCHOLL and RAHN, 1968). However, no α-methyladrenaline was found although the sensitivity of the method would have permitted the detection of the amine if its urinary concentration exceeded 3% of the concentration of α-methylnoradrenaline.

The time course of alterations of rat brain and heart amine levels after intraperitoneal administration of 400 mg/kg D,L-α-MMT was investigated by ANDÉN (1964a). In both tissues the noradrenaline concentrations decreased by about 80% within 9—12 hr, remained low for another 12 hr and then rose slowly until they reached the control levels on the 5th day. The highest concentrations of α-methyl-metatyramine in brain and heart were observed 6 hr after α-MMT; subsequently, the amine disappeared rapidly from both tissues. In contrast, the metaraminol formed was retained by brain and heart for several days. A similar persistence, after a single injection of α-MMT, of amine, presumably metaraminol, in rat heart and brain or rabbit brain was reported by SHORE et al. (1964). The time course of appearance of both metaraminol and α-methyl-metatyramine in rat brain, heart, spleen and adrenals, and disappearance of noradrenaline (and adrenaline, respectively) from 0—12 hr after administration of 400 mg/kg D,L-α-MMT have been studied by JOHNSON and PUGSLEY (1968, 1970). Metaraminol was also found as a metabolite of α-methylphenylalanine in hearts, brains and adrenal glands of mice, rats and dogs (TORCHIANA et al., 1970).

Another amine that may be released as a false transmitter is *p*-hydroxynorephedrine (THOENEN et al., 1966b). It has been detected in the rat heart after administration of (+)-amphetamine; the intermediary product, *p*-hydroxyamphetamine, seems to be formed mainly in the liver (GOLDSTEIN and ANAGNOSTE, 1965). Two or 12 hr after administration of ^{3}H-amphetamine to cats the injected amine as well as *p*-hydroxynorephedrine and traces of norephedrine and *p*-hydroxyamphetamine were present in spleen and heart (THOENEN et al., 1966b; cf. also LEWANDER, 1971b).

The advantage of using an amino acid precusor as a means of incorporating a false transmitter lies in the fact that usually the amino acid is tolerated much better than the amines derived from it, non-β-hydroxylated or β-hydroxylated. However, formation of the false transmitter via one or two intermediate products necessitates large doses of the precursor to be given. Moreover, the pharmacological analysis of the false transmitter is obscured if performed at a time when precursor amino acid, decarboxylation product and β-hydroxylated amine are simultaneously present in the animal.

3. Formation of False Transmitters by Inhibition of Enzymes Involved in Biosynthesis and Metabolism of Catecholamines

Amines which normally are metabolized at a high rate may accumulate in significant concentrations when their metabolism is effectively inhibited. For example, accumulation of dopamine in heart, spleen, iris and nictitating membrane of cats or heart and spleen of rats was observed after treatment of the animals with large doses of the β-hydroxylase inhibitor, disulfiram (THOENEN et al., 1967a). The decrease of the noradrenaline concentrations was, however, only partially compensated by the accumulation of dopamine.

There are a number of reports showing that administration of a MAO inhibitor causes an accumulation of octopamine in sympathetically innervated organs. In organs of untreated rats (MOLINOFF and AXELROD, 1969) or in rat, rabbit and human urine (KAKIMOTO and ARMSTRONG, 1962) only very small amounts of octopamine were detected. However, treatment of rats with pheniprazine increased the concentration of octopamine 4-fold in salivary glands and 7-fold in the heart, thus producing tissue levels of approximately 0.4 μg/g (MOLINOFF et al., 1969). Administration of iproniazid also caused accumulation of octopamine in brain heart, spleen and kidney of the rabbit (KAKIMOTO and ARMSTRONG, 1962). In cat salivary gland, heart and spleen, endogenous octopamine was not detected but chronic treatment with pheniprazine resulted in octopamine concentrations ranging from 0.2—1.2 μg/g in the various organs (KOPIN et al., 1965). It is therefore not surprising that the tissue levels of octopamine derived from administration of tyramine (see Section III, 2a) can be greatly enhanced by pretreatment of the animals with a MAO inhibitor (CARLSSON and WALDECK, 1963; KOPIN et al., 1965; MOLINOFF et al., 1969).

Only in the paper by KAKIMOTO and ARMSTRONG (1962) has noradrenaline been determined simultaneously with octopamine in rabbit organs; after iproniazid the noradrenaline concentration was increased in brain and heart but decreased in spleen and kidney.

IV. Release of False Transmitters

1. Spontaneous Release (Leakage) of False Transmitters

While the release by nerve stimulation of false transmitters has been comprehensively discussed in the review articles quoted in the Introduction to this chapter, the spontaneous release of false transmitters does not seem to have met with a similar interest. And yet the leakage of false transmitters from the nerve terminals may be a major component of the pharmacological action of this drug category.

There are certain chemical analogies between false transmitters and noradrenaline, and labelled $(\pm)$-noradrenaline may be regarded as one of the closest exogenous congeners of the natural transmitter. It will be shown that much of what was found in the study of false transmitters agrees with previous results which were obtained with labelled noradrenaline. For instance, preferential release from the heart of exogenously administered noradrenaline after its incorporation into the adrenergic neuron has been observed when various kinds of release were studied, namely release occurring spontaneously (CHIDSEY and HARRISON, 1963), after sympathetic nerve stimulation (CHIDSEY and HARRISON, 1963) or after administration of tyramine and other indirectly acting amines (POTTER et al., 1962; CHIDSEY and HARRISON, 1963; POTTER and AXELROD, 1963). However, the preferential release of the labelled noradrenaline was noted only during a limited time interval shortly after its administration. CHIDSEY and HARRISON (1963) compared the specific activity of noradrenaline released into the blood of the dog's coronary sinus with that remaining in the heart. Up to 5 hr after injection of ^{3}H-noradrenaline the specific activity of the amine released by nerve stimulation or tyramine was higher than that of the noradrenaline stores. The highest specific activity was observed in the fraction of amine released spontaneously. At 24 and 48 hr after labelling the amine store, the specific activities of the noradrenaline released spontaneously, by nerve stimulation or by tyramine, did not differ from that of the myocardium. In the rat heart the specific activity of noradrenaline depleted by a dose of tyramine was initially (5—30 min after administration of ^{3}H-noradrenaline) higher and subsequently (1.5—48 hr) lower than that of the noradrenaline remaining in the myocardium (POTTER and AXELROD, 1963).

A preferential spontaneous release of false transmitters such as dihydroxyephedrine and dihydroxypseudoephedrine was observed on isolated perfused hearts taken from rabbits which had received infusions of the above amines for 20 min (LINDMAR et al., 1967). The rabbits were killed 15 min after the end of an infusion and the hearts perfused with Tyrode solution. The proportion of dihydroxyephedrine to noradrenaline (7.7:1) released into the perfusate 40 min after setting up the preparation was much higher than that found in the heart tissue before the perfusion was started (1.4:1) or after its termination (1.7:1). When dihydroxypseudoephedrine was used as a foreign amine the discrepancy of the proportions of amines released spontaneously (2.0:1) and contained in the heart at the end of perfusion (0.5:1) was also noticeable. In addition, there was a preferential release by tyramine of the dihydroxyephedrines which will be discussed in Section IV, 4.

The proportion of a false transmitter released spontaneously depends on the length of time it has been incorporated in the organ. According to CROUT et al. (1964) the spontaneous loss of metaraminol from the perfused cat heart 2 hr after administration of the amine was severalfold higher than that after 17—20 hr. Since the cardiac metaraminol concentration was nearly the same after both time intervals, it was suggested that metaraminol taken up by the heart shifts with time from an "available" to a "less readily available" pool. Similar observations were made when amine release after sympathetic nerve stimulation was studied.

There are only a few studies concerned with the spontaneous release of a false transmitter *in vivo*. Strictly speaking, spontaneous release from an organ can be determined only when the physiological flow of nerve impulses to the organ has been interrupted. Furthermore, when release of the false transmitter is defined as decrease in tissue concentration rather than as quantity of amine carried away with the blood stream, the results are more liable to be influenced by intraneuronal metabolism of the false transmitter.

After administration of ^{3}H-noradrenaline the loss of tritiated amine from the cat superior cervical ganglion was delayed by decentralization and the loss from the rat heart was reduced by long-acting ganglionic blocking agents (HERTTING et al., 1962). ALMGREN and WALDECK (1967) administered ^{3}H-metaraminol to rats and determined its concentration in the salivary glands. Between 10 min and 18 hr the half-time of loss was 12 hr and from 18—144 hr it was 2.5 days. Loss from the decentralized gland occurred only at one exponential rate with a half-time of 4 days. The authors concluded that the early decrease of ^{3}H-metaraminol in the normal glands was due to nervous activity. After 18 hr the amines seemed to be less available for nerve impulses (cf. CROUT et al., 1964, cited above).

The disappearance of a false transmitter from an organ will be delayed by re-uptake. It has been suggested that the long half-life of metaraminol is partly determined by its high affinity to the membrane pump. KRAUSS et al. (1970) made the interesting observation that bretylium is more effective than cocaine and desmethylimipramine (DMI) in depleting metaraminol from the rat heart *in vivo* although it is a less potent inhibitor of ^{3}H-metaraminol uptake. The authors suggested that bretylium enhanced net outward movement of metaraminol by a process not dependent on inhibition of uptake. This phenomenon may be due to a higher cytoplasmic concentration of metaraminol compared with that of noradrenaline or α-methylnoradrenaline since the latter amines were resistant to the depleting effect of bretylium. Nervous activity which may enhance loss of transmitter as discussed above is unlikely to have been greater after bretylium than after cocaine or DMI.

In view of the scanty information available it would be interesting to learn more about the leakage of false transmitters from nerves and about their blood levels in the whole animal. It has been suggested that a constant exposure to foreign amines alters the sensitivity of organs towards various stimuli by postsynaptic mechanisms (see also Section V, 5).

2. Release of False Transmitters by Nerve Stimulation

Of the several criteria an amine must fulfill in order to be classified as a false adrenergic transmitter the property of being released by nerve stimulation is the most obvious one.

As already mentioned in the Introduction the suggestion by CARLSSON and LINDQVIST (1962) that α-methylated amines replacing noradrenaline in the brain may take over the functions of noradrenaline and the hypothesis of DAY and RAND (1963, 1964) that α-methylnoradrenaline acts as a false transmitter with a biological activity inferior to that of endogenous noradrenaline stimulated a great interest in this area.

Indirect evidence in favour of a release by nerve stimulation of α-methylated amines was provided by DAY and RAND (1964). In animals treated with reserpine, responses to sympathetic stimulation were reduced or abolished by reserpine but, depending on the organ investigated, they could be partially restored by an infusion, or by addition to the bath, of solutions of α-methyldopa, α-methyldopamine or α-methylnoradrenaline. Responses to tyramine were similarly restored. In contrast to DAY and RAND (1964), KRONEBERG and STOEPEL (1963) failed to observe restoration of the contraction of the nictitating membrane after nerve stimulation in cats pretreated with reserpine and infused with L-α-methyldopa, although the responses of the blood pressure and the nictitating membrane to tyramine were clearly enhanced. It was realized later that inhibition of vesicular retention (as is caused by reserpine) makes a false transmitter unavailable for release by nerve stimulation (cf. Section II, 2) but does not prevent tyramine from releasing amines, probably from extravesicular cytoplasmic sites (cf. Section IV, 4).

Unequivocal evidence for release of false transmitters by adrenergic nerve stimulation was obtained by using the conventional method of perfusing an isolated organ and estimating the amines appearing in the perfusate. Thus, MUSCHOLL and MAÎTRE (1963) showed that electrical stimulation of the right postganglionic sympathetic nerves to the rabbit heart released a mixture of noradrenaline and α-methylnoradrenaline when the animals had been pretreated with 4 doses of D,L-α-methyldopa. The proportion of both amines in the perfusate (about 1 : 1) equalled the proportion found in the hearts after termination of the experiment. CROUT et al. (1964) injected cats with (—)-metaraminol and isolated the hearts 2 or 17—20 hr later. After both time intervals stimulation of the right sympathetic chain released metaraminol into the perfusate but the amounts were greater at the earlier period (cf. Section IV, 1).

Further examples of false transmitters released by sympathetic nerve stimulation are octopamine or α-methyloctopamine (FISCHER et al., 1965) and α-methyladrenaline (MUSCHOLL, 1965). A survey of the rapidly accumulating list of such false transmitters is given in Table 1.

There are several difficulties in the way of obtaining a true picture of the release patterns of noradrenaline (cf. Chapter 6 by VON EULER, Chapter 16 by TRENDELENBURG) and this will also apply to any false transmitter. The transmitter output from a perfused organ is smaller than the amount released from adrenergic nerves since re-uptake by the nerves, uptake by extraneuronal tissue and enzymic inactivation may occur. Furthermore, output per stimulus is constant only up to a certain frequency of stimulation and then declines. However, low rates of stimulation are insufficient to yield enough amines for the determination. Thus, high rates of stimulation were preferred in the experiments of Table 1. It is not known whether the proportion, noradrenaline to false transmitter, is constant over the whole range of physiological impulse frequencies.

It is, however, well established that the output of false transmitters from organs whose sympathetic supply is stimulated electrically is not caused by the mechanical response to the noradrenaline released concomitantly from the nerve fibres. Stimulation of the sympathetic nerves of the isolated heart of rabbits pretreated with α-methyladrenaline released a mixture of noradrenaline and α-methyladrenaline into the perfusate and increased rate and force of contraction (MUSCHOLL, 1966b). When a similar enhancement of the mechanical performance of the heart was induced by applying electrical shocks (170/min) to the pacemaker region there was no increase in the spontaneous outputs of noradrenaline and α-methyladrenaline, respectively. When CROUT et al. (1964) perfused hearts of cats pretreated with metaraminol a dose of noradrenaline that enhanced myocardial tension to the same level as a series of shocks applied to the sympathetic chain, released much less metaraminol into the perfusate than did nerve stimulation.

On the perfused cat spleen there was no increased output of false transmitters, such as tritiated octopamine or α-methyloctopamine (FISCHER et al., 1965), tritiated α-methyldopamine or α-methylnoradrenaline (after disulfiram, MUSACCHIO et al., 1966b), when a dose of noradrenaline was injected that had a greater vasoconstrictor effect than splenic nerve stimulation; however, stimulation induced release of false transmitter. Levels of tritiated tyramine or α-methyltyramine in the perfusate were also increased by nerve stimulation, but this appeared to be related to splenic contraction which extruded platelets loaded with the amines; after blockade of contraction with phenoxybenzamine the output of amines not hydroxylated in the β-position was not altered by nerve stimulation (FISCHER et al., 1965). Furthermore, intraarterial injection of 1 μg angiotensin into the cat spleen perfused at a constant rate caused an extreme contraction of the organ but did not liberate 5-hydroxydopamine or its β-hydroxylated metabolites which were released by splenic nerve stimulation (THOENEN et al., 1967c).

In support of the findings presented above and in Table 1 the following observations may be taken as indirect evidence for a release of metaraminol by adrenergic nervous impulses. When rats were treated with metaraminol and exposed to cold both the loss of the amine from the heart and its urinary excretion were increased (JOHNSON and MICKLE, 1966). Exposure of rats to cold accelerated the loss of ^{3}H-metaraminol from the heart but not from salivary glands; similarly, cold exposure increased the turnover of ^{3}H-noradrenaline in heart but not that in salivary glands (COSTA et al., 1969). The accelerated loss of metaraminol from the heart may be taken to reflect selective activation of adrenergic nerves that innervate the heart.

Table 1. *Release of false transmitters by adrenergic nerve stimulation*

Species	Organ	False transmitter released[a]	Pretreatment with[a]	[b]	Reference
Cat	spleen	^{3}H-OA	^{3}H-TA	—	Fischer et al. (1965)
Cat	spleen	^{3}H-OA	^{3}H-TA	—	Kopin et al. (1965)
Cat	spleen	^{3}H-α-methyl-OA	^{3}H-α-methyl-TA	—	Fischer et al. (1965)
Cat	spleen	^{3}H-α-methyl-OA	^{3}H-amphetamine	—	Thoenen et al. (1966b)
Cat	heart	metaraminol	metaraminol	—	Crout et al. (1964)
Cat	heart	metaraminol	metaraminol	+	Crout and Shore (1964)
Cat	spleen	DA	dis.	+	Thoenen et al. (1967a)
Cat	spleen	^{14}C-DA	dis. + ^{14}C-DA	—	Musacchio et al. (1966b)
Rabbit	heart	(—)-α-methyl-DA	(—)-α-methyl-DA	+	Kilbinger et al. (1971)
Cat	spleen	^{3}H-α-methyl-DA	dis. + ^{3}H-α-methyl-DA	—	Musacchio et al. (1966b)
Cat	spleen	α-methyl-DA	dis. + α-methyldopa	+	Thoenen et al. (1967b)
Rabbit	heart	α-methyl-NA	α-methyldopa	+	Muscholl and Maître (1963)
Cat	spleen	α-methyl-NA	α-methyldopa	+	Haefely et al. (1967)
Rabbit	heart	(—)-α-methyl-NA	(+)-α-methyl-DA	+	Kilbinger et al. (1971)
Rabbit	heart	*threo*-corbadrine	*threo*-corbadrine	+	Muscholl et al. (1968)
Rabbit	heart	α-methyladrenaline	α-methyladrenaline	+	Lindmar et al. (1967)
Rabbit	heart	DHPE	DHPE	+	Lindmar et al. (1967)
Cat	spleen	^{3}H-5-hydroxy-DA and its 4-methoxy- and 3-methoxy derivatives	^{3}H-5-hydroxy-DA	—	Thoenen et al. (1967c)
Cat	spleen	4-methoxy-3,5-dihydroxy-phenylethylamine	4-methoxy-3,5-dihydroxy-phenylalanine	—	Thoenen et al. (1968)

[a] Abbreviations used: OA, octopamine; TA, tyramine; DA, dopamine; NA, noradrenaline; DHPE, dihydroxypseudoephedrine; dis., disulfiram.

[b] Noradrenaline not determined is indicated by —; +, proportion of endogenous noradrenaline to false transmitter released into the perfusate was determined and found to be the same as proportion of both amines in the organ.

There is also evidence that α-methylnoradrenaline is released from sympathetic nerves in humans treated with 4 oral doses of 250 mg L-α-methyldopa daily for 2 days. Sympathetic reflex responses induced by physical activity caused a parallel increase in the urinary excretions of both noradrenaline and α-methylnoradrenaline (LINDMAR et al., 1968).

In experiments in which both the false transmitter and endogenous noradrenaline were determined in perfusates of heart and spleen it was found that the amines were released in the proportion in which they were stored in the organs (Table 1). As discussed by SMITH and WINKLER in Chapter 13, Section A IV 5, these findings support the hypothesis that nerve stimulation releases adrenergic transmitters by expulsion of the contents of storage vesicles.

3. Release of False Transmitters by Nicotinic Agents

On the perfused rabbit heart infusion of acetylcholine (in the presence of atropine) or of 1,1-dimethyl-4-phenyl piperazine (DMPP) causes a release of noradrenaline which is mediated by stimulation of nicotinic receptors (cf. Chapter 17, Section I C 7, by KOSTERLITZ and LEES). These nicotinic agents have been used to study release of false transmitters, for instance α-methyladrenaline and dihydroxypseudoephedrine (LINDMAR et al., 1967), (—)-α-methyldopamine (KILBINGER et al., 1971), and α-methylnoradrenaline formed from either α-methyldopa (MUSCHOLL and MAÎTRE, 1963) or (+)-α-methyldopamine (KILBINGER et al., 1971). In all these experiments the proportion of false transmitter to endogenous noradrenaline determined in the perfusates after high doses of nicotinic drugs was that in which the amines were found in the hearts. In this respect the simultaneous release of normal and false transmitters by nicotinic agents resembles that after adrenergic nerve stimulation but differs from that caused by indirectly acting amines.

4. Release of False Transmitters by Indirectly Acting Amines

In many studies indirectly acting amines have been used with the intention to mimick the effects of sympathetic nerve stimulation. However, the mode of noradrenaline release produced by these amines differs markedly from that caused by adrenergic nervous impulses.

Indirectly acting amines cause a release of noradrenaline from a store which cannot be acted upon by adrenergic nerve stimulation. This has been demonstrated by showing that exposure to noradrenaline restores the action of tyramine on atria of reserpinized animals but not the effects of adrenergic nerve stimulation (FURCHGOTT et al., 1963; TRENDELENBURG, 1965). In atria from guinea pigs that had been treated with reserpine, inhibition of MAO greatly enhanced the ability of exposures to noradrenaline to restore the response to indirectly acting amines (FURCHGOTT and SANCHEZ GARCIA, 1968). It has been suggested that under these conditions retained noradrenaline can be released from cytoplasmic binding sites of the neuron. In contrast, noradrenaline injected into rats pretreated with reserpine and a MAO inhibitor did not restore the effect of sympathetic nerve stimulation on the iris although it restored the specific fluorescence in the adrenergic fibres of the iris (HÄGGENDAL and MALMFORS, 1969). Similarly, accumulation of exogenous noradrenaline in an extravesicular compartment within the adrenergic nerve terminals of the rat vas deferens treated with reserpine plus iproniazid greatly decreased rather than increased the contractions of the organ on stimulation of the hypogastric nerve (VAN ORDEN et al., 1967). It thus appears that cytoplasmic extravesicular noradrenaline is unavailable for release by adrenergic nerve stimulation (cf. also Chapter 13, Section A 3 b, by SMITH and WINKLER).

The persistence of α-methylated amines due to their resistance towards MAO in the reserpinized animal is illustrated by the following observations. α-Methylnoradrenaline, α-methyldopamine and α-methyldopa were more efficient in restoring the pressor response to tyramine in the rat than their respective natural catechol derivatives. This was true for both duration of the response and dose required to achieve restoration (TORCHIANA et al., 1966). The conclusion was drawn that restoration not only depends on uptake and binding of exogenously administered compounds but also on conversion of precursors to active metabolites. Thus, α-methyldopa was more effective in restoring the response to tyramine in the rat than in the dog; of a given dose 40% was decarboxylated in the rat (PORTER and TITUS, 1963) while only 6% was decarboxylated in the dog (for reference see TORCHIANA et al., 1966).

Similarly, only those phenylethylamines whose chemical structure allows β-hydroxylation have been found to restore the effects of tyramine. Inhibition of this enzymatic step with disulfiram prevents the restoring effect of tyramine on the blood pressure of the rat (WEBER, 1966) or the cat (MUSACCHIO et al., 1966a). Stereospecificity of this effect was demonstrated by TORCHIANA et al. (1968) who found that only the 2 S isomers of α-methyldopamine and α-methyl-metatyramine (both dextrorotatory) and the 1 R : 2 S isomers of α-methylnoradrenaline and metaraminol (both levorotatory) were effective in the rat.

For these reasons there is no clear-cut relationship between inherent sympathomimetic activity of a compound and its activity to restore the response to tyramine. In the rat this was illustrated by the relative efficiency of (+)-α-methyldopamine and (—)-metaraminol to restore the pressor effects of tyramine, in spite of the fact that these amines have little pressor activity themselves (TORCHIANA et al., 1966).

When indirectly acting amines are able to liberate transmitter that is free in the axoplasm, the quantity of a false transmitter released shortly after its uptake into the axon should greatly exceed the quantity of endogenous noradrenaline released simultaneously. The cytoplasmic concentration of noradrenaline is most likely to be lower than that of the agent displacing noradrenaline from vesicular binding sites. The axoplasmic concentration of a false transmitter resistant towards MAO would in any case tend to be higher than that of noradrenaline. In agreement with these predictions, preferential release of α-methyladrenaline compared with that of noradrenaline from the perfused rabbit heart was observed after a dose of tyramine 1.5 hr after the animals had received an infusion of α-methyladrenaline (LINDMAR et al., 1967). Tyramine liberated a mixture of 99% of the foreign amine and 1% noradrenaline into the perfusate whereas sympathetic nerve stimulation released a mixture of 69% α-methyladrenaline and 31% noradrenaline which corresponded to the proportion of exogenous and endogenous amine found in the hearts after the end of perfusion (65% and 35%, respectively). Similar results were obtained 1.5 hr after one or two infusions of dihydroxypseudoephedrine. CROUT and SHORE (1964) injected cats with metaraminol and perfused the hearts which contained approximately equal amounts of noradrenaline and the foreign amine. Sympathetic nerve stimulation caused an output into the perfusate of 43 ng metaraminol and 47 ng noradrenaline. However, injection of 30 μg tyramine released 188 ng metaraminol but only 4 ng noradrenaline, while in hearts of untreated cats this dose of tyramine led to an output of 66 ng noradrenaline.

As an alternative the preferential release of the less firmly bound amine has been suggested (KOPIN, 1968a). This idea is based on experiments with ^{3}H-octopamine which appears to be lost from the rat heart more readily than noradrenaline when one (MUSACCHIO et al., 1965a) or several doses (PÖCH and KOPIN, 1966) of tyramine were administered. CARLSSON and WALDECK (1966b) injected ^{14}C-tyramine into mice and examined 40 derivatives of phenylethylamine for their potency to cause depletion of the ^{14}C-octopamine from the heart. The potency was greatly increased by β-hydroxylation, leading to a levorotatory enantiomer, and by 3-hydroxylation. Yet there were no differences between (—)- or (+)-noradrenaline and (±)-octopamine in the ability to deplete the labelled amine. This seems to contradict the idea of a higher affinity of noradrenaline for the vesicular storage sites. The authors pointed out that factors may operate *in vivo* which neutralize the effects of possible differences in affinities. The amines tested may be metabolized, or taken up by the neuron, at different rates with the result that their affinities for vesicular retention cannot be assessed clearly. It may be added that in the aforementioned studies the disappearance of octopamine from the heart rather than its rate of liberation relative to that of noradrenaline has been examined.

In conclusion, there is direct and indirect evidence for a preferential release of false transmitters by tyramine but the experiments reported are not decisive with regard to the underlying mechanism.

V. Consequences of Incorporation of False Transmitters

1. Depletion of Noradrenaline

A certain degree of noradrenaline depletion from various organs has been observed when sufficiently large doses of sympathomimetic amines or of their precursors giving rise to formation of false transmitters were administered. The depleting action of α-methyldopa or α-MMT was found simultaneously in different laboratories (GOLDBERG et al., 1960; HESS et al., 1961; PORTER et al., 1961; SOURKES et al., 1961). Subsequent papers dealing with incorporation of false transmitters and depletion of noradrenaline have already been discussed (Section III, 1—3).

Several authors have shown that α-methyldopa or α-MMT must be decarboxylated in order to deplete guinea-pig and rat hearts of their noradrenaline since this effect could be antagonized by various decarboxylase inhibitors administered before the amino acid (UDENFRIEND and ZALTZMAN-NIRENBERG, 1962; GESSA et al., 1962; LEVINE and SJOERDSMA, 1964). With respect to noradrenaline depletion from hearts of mice, guinea pigs and rats the two metabolites of α-MMT, α-methylmetatyramine and metaraminol, are more potent than the parent amino acid (PORTER et al., 1961; GESSA et al., 1962; UDENFRIEND and ZALTZMAN-NIRENBERG, 1962). The same holds true for α-methyldopa and α-methyldopamine, respectively (PORTER et al., 1961). These results, and the evidence that the amine metabolites are stored in the tissues for considerable periods of time, favour the view that depletion of noradrenaline is caused by foreign amines displacing the physiological transmitter at its storage sites (CARLSSON and LINDQVIST, 1962; MAÎTRE and STAEHELIN, 1963; MUSCHOLL and MAÎTRE, 1963; ANDÉN, 1964a).

However, it must be kept in mind that a foreign amine may accumulate in a tissue depleted of noradrenaline and that the loss of the transmitter may yet be due to another cause. For instance, α-methyltyrosine decreases the concentration of noradrenaline in guinea-pig heart and brain through inhibition of noradrenaline synthesis at the tyrosine hydroxylase step (SPECTOR et al., 1965). Since α-methylnoradrenaline is formed and stored under these experimental conditions, MAÎTRE (1965) suggested that the depletion of noradrenaline was partly due to its displacement be α-methylnoradrenaline. However, the dissociation in the time course of appearance of α-methylnoradrenaline in the tissues from that of the depletion of noradrenaline observed after α-methyltyrosine (UDENFRIEND et al., 1966) has served as an argument against a role of α-methylnoradrenaline in the effect of the amino acid.

There has been a great deal of discussion on the question of whether false transmitters deplete bound noradrenaline by a mole-for-mole replacement. An earlier proposal that a single equivalent of metaraminol appearing in a tissue depleted more than 30 equivalents of noradrenaline had to be abandoned. ANDÉN (1964a) and CARLSSON (1964) showed that the experiments in favour of this concept were technically inadequate since they utilized a method of metaraminol estimation which failed properly to extract the amine from the tissues. Therefore, the following discussion will be based on those observations only which appear to give technically reliable estimates of the amine concentrations.

A stoichiometric replacement of cardiac noradrenaline by α-methylnoradrenaline was reported by several authors when single or repeated doses of α-methyldopa were injected into rats or guinea pigs (MAÎTRE and STAEHELIN, 1963; SCHÜMANN et al., 1965), rabbits (MUSCHOLL and MAÎTRE, 1963; LINDMAR and MUSCHOLL, 1965) and cats (HAEFELY et al., 1967); the amine concentrations were determined 4—144 hr after the last dose. According to GROBECKER et al. (1966) 62% of the adrenaline of the frog heart was lost 20 hr after the second of two doses of α-methyldopa but was quantitatively replaced by a mixture of α-methyldopamine, α-methylnoradrenaline and, as the main constituent, by α-methyladrenaline. Likewise, treatment of rats with α-MMT may lead after 24—48 hr to almost perfect stoichiometric replacement of the noradrenaline lost from brain stem and heart by metaraminol (ANDÉN, 1964a; ANDÉN and MAGNUSSON, 1965); 7 days after α-MMT the noradrenaline lost from rabbit brain stem was fully replaced by metaraminol (ANDÉN, 1964a; SHORE et al., 1964). Direct incorporation of false transmitter amines also causes mole-for-mole replacement of noradrenaline. This was observed with metaraminol in guinea-pig (ANDÉN, 1964a) and rat heart (SHORE et al., 1964), with α-methyladrenaline and dihydroxypseudoephedrine in rabbit (LINDMAR et al., 1967) and rat heart (MUSCHOLL and SPRENGER, 1966), with *threo*-corbadrine in rat heart and mesentery (DREWS et al., 1968) and with (—)-α-methyldopamine in rabbit heart (KILBINGER et al., 1971).

However, under different experimental conditions either an excess or a deficit of false transmitter, compared with the loss of noradrenaline, may be observed. Especially after repeated administration (11 days) of large doses of D,L-α-methyldopa (300 mg/kg per day orally) the amount of α-methylnoradrenaline retained exceeded the amount of noradrenaline depleted from the rat brain and heart (BRUNNER et al., 1967; MAÎTRE and STAEHELIN, 1967). The same was true for guinea-pig heart, vas deferens and brain after three i.m. injections of 400 mg/kg L-α-methyldopa (PHILIPPU and SCHÜMANN, 1967). JUORIO and VOGT (1967) noticed a slight and apparently insignificant excess of α-methylnoradrenaline over the noradrenaline lost from pigeon hypothalamus 72—168 hr after a single dose of 200 mg/kg L-α-methyldopa, but a large excess 168 hr after 6 doses of 100 mg/kg.

The relationship between the dose of metaraminol administered and the stoichiometric replacement of noradrenaline in the rat heart was studied by PORTER et al. (1967); 18, 44 and 68 hr after 0.24 mg/kg ^{14}C-metaraminol the ventricles contained radioactivity which exactly accounted for the missing noradrenaline, but

42 hr after 3 mg/kg the radioactivity accounted for only 68—83% of the missing noradrenaline. GRAM and WRIGHT (1966) reported that 4—192 hr after an i. v. dose of 1.5 mg/kg metaraminol the noradrenaline deficit in the rabbit heart greatly exceeded the amount of metaraminol retained; the authors discussed the possibility that the difference between this result and those of ANDÉN (1964a) and SHORE et al. (1964) (see above) was related to the lower doses used by these workers (0.05—1.0 mg/kg i.p.). Although this interpretation is plausible (cf. the findings of PORTER et al., 1967), it must be pointed out that GRAM and WRIGHT (1966) used 0.02 N HCl for homogenization, a procedure that does not quantitatively extract metaraminol bound in tissues (CARLSSON, 1964).

Large devations from a mole-for-mole substitution were found when the time course of noradrenaline depletion and appearance of depleting amines were followed at relatively early intervals after administration of the precursor. In the rat heart *in vivo* the concentration of metaraminol 1 hr after 400 mg/kg α-MMT was twice the original noradrenaline concentration; the latter had decreased by 47% (JOHNSON and PUGSLEY, 1968). After 12 hr most of the metaraminol had disappeared and its excess over a stoichiometric replacement of the noradrenaline lost was only 38%. ANDÉN (1964a) observed that 6 hr after α-MMT the sum of metaraminol and α-methyl-metatyramine in the rat heart was 217% of the noradrenaline deficit at this time period. PHILIPPU and SCHÜMANN (1965) perfused guinea-pig hearts with α-methyldopa for 150 min or with α-methyldopamine for 20 min. While the noradrenaline content of the hearts was unaltered after both treatments there was an accumulation of α-methylnoradrenaline comprising about 30% of the endogenous noradrenaline; perfusion with α-methyldopamine additionally caused an accumulation of the latter amine at a concentration exceeding the noradrenaline by 55%.

In a later phase the foreign amine concentration may have decreased as a result of metabolism or leakage from the nerves but the loss of noradrenaline may not have been balanced by re-synthesis (cf. also Section V, 2). Thus, ANDÉN (1964a) noticed that 9—24 hr after α-MMT the loss of dopamine from rat brain was greater than the amount of α-methylated amines accumulated. According to JUORIO and VOGT (1967) the dopamine deficit in the pigeon hypothalamus exceeded the amount of the α-methyldopamine accumulated at 1, 2, 4 and 5 hr after 200—800 mg/kg L-α-methyldopa; only at the 2 hr interval the noradrenaline deficit was not fully balanced.

Another factor which may disturb simple displacement of noradrenaline by the false transmitter formed is environmental temperature. JOHNSON and PUGSLEY (1968) found that there was an approximate mole-for-mole replacement of noradrenaline 4 and 12 hr after a dose of metaraminol administered to rats kept at 27°C, but no correlation between metaraminol storage and noradrenaline loss existed at 4°C. It has been suggested that stoichiometry varies with part of the heart examined (PORTER et al., 1967). These authors found a mole-for-mole replacement of noradrenaline by a small dose of metaraminol in rat ventricle but not in rat atria. However, LINDMAR and MUSCHOLL (1965) observed an equimolar replacement by α-methylnoradrenaline of the noradrenaline lost from rabbit atria as well as from ventricles after 4 doses of 50 mg/kg L-α-methyldopa.

It may be concluded that displacement is the major mechanism leading to noradrenaline depletion and to storage of false transmitters in adrenergically innervated organs. Except for short time intervals and very large cumulative doses of α-methyldopa, α-MMT, α-methylnoradrenaline and metaraminol, the molar ratio, noradrenaline lost: false transmitter stored, does not conspicuously deviate from unity. At short time intervals and high doses possible inhibition of noradrenaline synthesis interferes with assessment of precise stoichiometry. A further complication may arise from administration of racemic rather than isomeric substances since the isomer not entering the biosynthetic or metabolic pathway of the natural precursor or transmitter is likely to behave kinetically quite unlike (—)-noradrenaline.

2. Effects on Noradrenaline Synthesis

The pertinent literature concerning the biosynthesis of the adrenergic transmitter has already been discussed in the chapters by VON EULER and by STJÄRNE; the physiological regulation of noradrenaline synthesis need therefore not be fully discussed. However, the methods used to determine the effect of false transmitters on the rate of noradrenaline synthesis will be mentioned briefly because disagreement as to their validity has been expressed. For example, the method of determination of the rate of synthesis by noradrenaline turnover studies has been criticized by SEDVALL et al. (1968) on the grounds that true synthesis rate exceeds the apparent turnover rate 2—3 fold. On the other hand, the method used by the latter authors (measurement of the accumulation of ^{14}C-noradrenaline after i.v. administration of ^{14}C-tyrosine) has been criticized by NEFF et al. (1969).

Since the work of SOURKES (1954) it is well known that α-methyldopa and α-MMT, which were later shown to be precursors of false transmitters, inhibited DOPA decarboxylase both *in vitro* and *in vivo* (for reviews see SOURKES (1965); HOLTZ and PALM (1966)). However, blockade of noradrenaline formation at the level of DOPA decarboxylase or at the following step, dopamine β-hydroxylase, is unlikely to occur *in vivo* since these enzymes are present in large excess of the requirement of noradrenaline synthesis (CREVELING, 1965; HOLTZ and PALM, 1966; UDENFRIEND et al., 1966). Most authors now believe that displacement of noradrenaline by the amine metabolites of α-methyldopa or α-MMT rather than inhibition of synthesis at the decarboxylase step is the cause of noradrenaline depletion observed after administration of these amino acids (HESS et al., 1961; PORTER et al., 1961; CARLSSON and LINDQVIST, 1962; LEVINE and SJOERDSMA, 1964). This subject has been fully discussed elsewhere (SOURKES, 1965; MUSCHOLL, 1966a; STONE and PORTER, 1967).

False transmitters or their precursors may alter the synthesis of noradrenaline in the adrenergic neuron by exerting end-product inhibition of tyrosine hydroxylase (SPECTOR et al., 1967; UDENFRIEND, 1968) either directly, or indirectly through displacement of noradrenaline from binding sites. Alternatively, or simultaneously, they may compete with dopamine for transport to the site of β-hydroxylation in the storage vesicles (STJÄRNE and LISHAJKO, 1967). After loss of the false transmitter from the axon the ensuing relief from end-product inhibition of tyrosine hydroxylase may increase noradrenaline synthesis until the original level of the transmitter is attained. In the following discussion the evidence for these proposals will be presented.

ANDÉN (1964a) suggested that inhibition of catecholamine synthesis might at least partly account for the depletion of dopamine and noradrenaline from rat brain 9—24 hr after administration of α-MMT; the loss of amines was larger than was expected from simple displacement by the α-methyl-metatyramine plus metaraminol formed.

KOPIN et al. (1969) determined the rate of synthesis of labelled noradrenaline in the rat heart from ^{14}C-tyrosine and ^{3}H-DOPA after metaraminol, α-methyldopa and octopamine. Neither of these compounds significantly inhibited tyrosine hydroxylase or dopamine-β-hydroxylase activities *in vitro*. Thirty min after i.p.

administration of metaraminol (0.5 mg/kg) or α-methyldopa (150 mg/kg) the noradrenaline formation from both tyrosine and DOPA was markedly decreased; 24 hr after either drug the concentration of endogenous noradrenaline was decreased but the formation of noradrenaline from both precursors was only slightly inhibited. Octopamine (10 mg/kg i.m.) caused a decrease of endogenous noradrenaline at 10 min, 2 hr and 5 hr. Formation of noradrenaline from both tyrosine and DOPA was greatly inhibited at 10 min and had nearly returned to normal at 2 hr. After 5 hr the rate of noradrenaline synthesis from tyrosine was increased. Since metaraminol or octopamine, in contrast to (—)-noradrenaline (UDENFRIEND et al., 1965), did not inhibit tyrosine hydroxylase *in vitro*, KOPIN et al. (1969) suggested that the diminished hydroxylation of tyrosine after injection of metaraminol or octopamine was caused by release of noradrenaline from its storage sites into the axoplasm, i.e. by an indirect action. Similarly, the inhibition by tyramine of the noradrenaline formation from tyrosine is thought to be due to intraaxonal release of noradrenaline (WEINER and SELVARATNAM, 1968). The decrease in accumulation of labelled noradrenaline formed from ^{3}H-DOPA found in the experiments of KOPIN et al. (1969) after giving metaraminol, α-methyldopa and octopamine, was attributed to a blockade of the entry of dopamine into the β-hydroxylase-containing vesicles. This represents a mechanism by which a step other than tyrosine hydroxylation becomes rate-limiting in noradrenaline synthesis.

The long-term moderate inhibition of noradrenaline synthesis observed 24 hr after metaraminol seems to be related to its prolonged retention and was explained by decreased β-hydroxylation; this effect persists for a longer time than does inhibition of tyrosine hydroxylase. It has also been noted that chronic treatment with metaraminol did not decrease total catecholamine formation but decreased the conversion of dopamine to noradrenaline (KOPIN and WEISE, 1968). Correspondingly, the rapid removal of octopamine by MAO appears to be the cause for its brief inhibitory effect which is followed (at 5 hr) by an enhancement of noradrenaline synthesis from tyrosine but not from DOPA (KOPIN et al., 1969).

Decreased synthesis of noradrenaline in rats receiving D,L-α-MMT (400 mg/kg i.p.) and exposed to cold is indicated by the finding that the urinary excretion of both noradrenaline and 3-methoxy-4-hydroxyphenylglycol was lower from 0—4 and 4—12 hr after exposure to 4°C if compared with the excretion observed on rats kept at 27°C (JOHNSSON and PUGSLEY, 1968). Conversely, when metaraminol had disappeared from hearts of cold-stressed rats at 12 hr the urinary output of 3-methoxy-4-hydroxyphenylglycol rose markedly between 12 and 24 hr to exceed the quantity excreted by the control animals. The high concentration of α-methyl-metatyramine and metaraminol formed from α-MMT may have elevated the intraaxonal concentration of noradrenaline in analogy to injected metaraminol (KOPIN et al., 1969; see above); this may have led to an inhibition of noradrenaline synthesis. Apart from this mechanism, α-MMT and α-methyl-metatyramine possibly decreased the synthesis of the natural transmitter by entering the biosynthetic pathway of noradrenaline; this should result in less DOPA and dopamine being metabolized to noradrenaline, as suggested by JOHNSSON and PUGSLEY (1970). In the latter paper the authors found that a dose of α-methyltyrosine, which depleted endogenous noradrenaline from rat brain, heart and spleen, increased the formation of metaraminol from α-MMT in these organs at both 27 and 4°C. It was proposed that there is a competition between the synthesis of noradrenaline and that of metaraminol.

However, other authors using experimental conditions with less severe demands for newly synthesized transmitter than exposure to cold failed to note an impairment of noradrenaline synthesis after administration of α-MMT or metaraminol. For example, ANDÉN et al. (1969) obtained evidence that noradrenaline losses from rat spinal cord axons after α-MMT are due to displacement rather than decrease in synthesis. In this study rats with a transection of the spinal cord were used and the body temperature was kept constant. Since all the monoamine neurons to the spinal cord have their cell bodies in the lower brain stem, the nerve impulses reach the terminals which are situated in a position cranial but not caudal to the transection. Drugs causing a depletion of monoamine stores by displacement do so independently of nervous impulses; therefore, noradrenaline is lost from both cranial and caudal sites of the transection. In contrast, inhibitors of noradrenaline synthesis need nerve impulses to lower amine levels; hence, they cause a greater loss of amine at the cranial site of a transection (ANDÉN et al., 1967). Using this technique ANDÉN et al. (1969) found that D,L-α-MMT, contrary to L-α-methyldopa (both 400 mg/kg i.p. 3 hr before sacrifice), did not produce a greater depletion in the cranial part of the spinal cord.

COSTA et al. (1969) determined the turnover rate of cardiac noradrenaline in the rat from the disappearance of ^{3}H-noradrenaline after injection of a tracer dose. The turnover rate, expressed as μg/g per hr, was not significantly changed 20 hr after i.v. injection of 0.1 mg/kg metaraminol which had depleted the endogenous noradrenaline by 62%. A similar depletion was achieved by i.p. injection of 200 mg/kg D,L-α-MMT and again the turnover rate of noradrenaline was unaltered. In view of the proposed feedback control of noradrenaline synthesis the authors expected a low noradrenaline concentration resulting from administration of α-MMT or metaraminol to be associated with an enhanced rate of noradrenaline synthesis. As pointed out by COSTA et al. (1969) the presence of metaraminol in the heart may prevent the usual acceleration of noradrenaline synthesis when the noradrenaline concentrations are low. Since metaraminol does not directly inhibit tyrosine hydroxylase (KOPIN et al., 1969; see above), an alternative explanation may be considered. Shortly after a dose of metaraminol the intraaxonal level of noradrenaline would be greatly increased (because of displacement of noradrenaline from the vesicular uptake sites), but 20 hr after metaraminol most of the free amines may have leaked from the neuron. It is likely that only intraaxonal free amine is able to exert end-product inhibition of noradrenaline synthesis and that the latter is unaltered because at 20 hr the intraaxonal concentration of noradrenaline does not differ from normal (KOPIN et al., 1969).

Thus, a marked decrease in rate of noradrenaline synthesis seems to occur after metaraminol either shortly after its administration when it displaces large amounts of stored noradrenaline or if excessive adrenergic activity leads to a high rate of noradrenaline release and necessitates a rapid synthesis of the transmitter. On the other hand, if metaraminol is still present in the axon 16—24 hr after its injection (though in a tightly bound form, cf. CROUT et al., 1964) the synthesis of noradrenaline is only slightly depressed when compared with that of untreated controls. Removal of a false transmitter from the sympathetic nerves by enzymic destruction (octopamine by MAO) or by enhanced release (metaraminol during cold stress) immediately increases the rate of noradrenaline synthesis.

Though α-methyldopa has also been shown to decrease noradrenaline synthesis (KOPIN et al., 1969; see above), the lack of information as regards the time course of this effect and the individual role played by the amino acid and its metabolites, (+)-α-methyldopamine and (—)-α-methylnoradrenaline, warrants further examination. The following findings provide some indirect evidence for an inhibitory action of α-methyldopa on noradrenaline synthesis. PHILIPPU and SCHÜMANN (1965) suggested that the loss of noradrenaline from guinea-pig hearts *in vivo* after α-methyldopa or α-methyldopamine is caused by inhibition of noradrenaline synthesis rather than by displacement because in their experiments the decline in noradrenaline levels of hearts perfused *in vitro* was not much affected when α-methylnoradrenaline was formed and/or retained during infusions of α-methyldopa, α-methyldopamine, and α-methylnoradrenaline, respectively. Furthermore, isolated heart vesicles incubated with α-methyldopamine or α-methylnoradrenaline accumulated amounts of these amines exceeding several-fold that of endogenous noradrenaline; in spite of this accumulation there was no greater loss of noradrenaline from the vesicles than from vesicles of control preparations (PHILIPPU and SCHÜMANN, 1966). As mentioned above, ANDÉN et al. (1969) observed a greater loss of noradrenaline after α-methyldopa in the spinal cord of the rat cranial than caudal of a transection. The authors suggested that α-methyldopa causes depletion of noradrenaline due to displacement, but inhibition of synthesis is a contributory factor during the early intervals. The diminished urinary excretion of noradrenaline in patients treated with α-methyldopa (MUSCHOLL and RAHN, 1966, 1968) might also be a consequence of decreased noradrenaline synthesis.

3. Diminished Release of Noradrenaline by Sympathetic Nerve Stimulation

It has been stated that substitution of noradrenaline by a foreign amine is followed by a decreased liberation of the natural transmitter in response to nerve stimulation (KOPIN et al., 1965; FISCHER et al., 1965). Although there is direct evidence that noradrenaline and false transmitters are released in the same *proportion* in which they are stored in the organ under study (cf. Section IV, 2), this would lead to a diminished release of noradrenaline only when the *total amount* of amines liberated by nervous impulses after incorporation of the false transmitter did not exceed the original noradrenaline output. From the papers in which this was investigated it appears that incorporation of a false transmitter does not necessarily result in a diminished release of noradrenaline (see Table 2).

Two doses of α-methyladrenaline, infused i.v. at a time interval of 2 hr, decreased the noradrenaline concentration of the rabbit heart to 6% of the normal content while the foreign amine was accumulated at a concentration corresponding to 121% of the original noradrenaline level (LINDMAR et al., 1967). Sympathetic nerve stimulation at a frequency of 10 Hz released a total amount of amines into the perfusate which corresponded to the noradrenaline output of control hearts; consequently, the quantity of noradrenaline released was greatly depressed. After 3 infusions of dihydroxypseudoephedrine the total amine as well as the noradrenaline outputs were depressed. However, after one infusion of α-methyladrenaline or one and two infusions of dihydroxypseudoephedrine the total amount of amines released by nerve stimulation greatly exceeded the quantity of noradrenaline liberated into the perfusate of control hearts; as a result the noradrenaline output did not statistically differ from that of control hearts although 34—65% of the original cardiac noradrenaline had been replaced by the false transmitters. A similar situation exists after incorporation of (—)-α-methyldopamine into the rabbit heart. Sympathetic nerve stimulation released an increased amount of total amines while not altering the output of noradrenaline (KILBINGER et al., 1971). It has been suggested that enhancement of total amine output may be due to inhibition of re-uptake by the nerve terminals when the false transmitter released has a high affinity to the membrane uptake process (cf. Section VI, 2).

There is a surprising lack of information on noradrenaline release by nervous impulses from organs containing metaraminol. Using the observation that treat-

Table 2. *Outputs of noradrenaline and total amines in response to sympathetic nerve stimulation after incorporation of false transmitters*

Pretreatment with [a]	mg/kg[b]	Species	Organ	NA output	Frequency of nerve stimulat. Hz	Total amine output	Response of organ[c]	Determined at Hz[d]	Reference
Pheniprazin + ^{3}H-TA	0.3	cat	spleen	decr.	30	unalt.	decr.	30	Kopin (1968b)
(—)-α-methyl-DA . . .	10	rabbit	heart	unalt.	10	incr.	decr.	0.25—20	Kilbinger et al. (1971)
(+)-α-methyl-DA . . .	30	rabbit	heart	decr.	10	unalt.	unalt.	0.25—20	Kilbinger et al. (1971)
α-methyl-A	1×1.7	rabbit	heart	unalt.	10	incr.	decr.	0.25—1	Lindmar et al. (1967)
							unalt.	5—20	
α-methyl-A	2×1.7	rabbit	heart	decr.	10	unalt.	decr.	0.25—20	Lindmar et al. (1967)
DHPE	1 or 2×1.7	rabbit	heart	unalt.	10	incr.	decr.	0.25—1	Lindmar et al. (1967)
							unalt.	5—20	
DHPE	3×1.7	rabbit	heart	decr.	10	decr.	decr.	0.25—20	Lindmar et al. (1967)
α-methyldopa	3×200	cat	spleen	decr.	6 and 10	unalt.	unalt.	6 and 10	Haefely et al. (1967)
Disulfiram	—	cat	spleen	decr.	6 and 10	—	unalt.	6 and 10	Thoenen et al. (1965)
Disulf. + α-methyldopa	3×200	cat	spleen	decr.	6 and 10	—	decr.	10	Thoenen et al. (1967b)
5-hydroxydopa	3×200	cat	spleen	decr.	6 and 10	—	decr.	6 and 10	Thoenen et al. (1967c)
4-methoxy-3,5-dihydroxyphenylalanine	3×50	cat	spleen	decr.	6 and 10	—	decr.	6 and 10	Thoenen et al. (1968)

[a] Abbreviations used; TA, tyramine; DA, dopamine; A, adrenaline; DHPE, dihydroxypseudoephedrine; NA, noradrenaline; decr., decreased; incr., increased; unalt., unaltered.

[b] Dose of false transmitter or precursor.

[c] On the isolated spleen the parameter tested was the contraction area; on the isolated heart it was rate of beats.

[d] Frequency of nerve stimulation at which response indicated in foregoing column was observed.

ment of animals with α-MMT plus metaraminol causes a 95% replacement of noradrenaline by metaraminol in several tissues, ANDÉN and MAGNUSSON (1965) have questioned the existence of a diminished release of noradrenaline; they reported a single experiment showing unaltered responses of the cat nictitating membrane when the cervical sympathetic trunk was stimulated with pulses of 1—30 Hz. However, HAEFELY et al. (1966) observed a significant inhibition of adrenergic transmission on the nictitating membrane of a group of cats which had received 6 doses of 100 mg/kg α-MMT within 3 days; the transmission failure was obvious from frequency-response curves (0.2—26 Hz) and number of stimuli-response curves (1—27 stimuli).

In Table 2 a few papers are included in which the total amine output after adrenergic nerve stimulation has not been reported but which provide information on noradrenaline output and the responses of the spleen. The functional consequences of a decrease in noradrenaline release will be discussed in Section VI, 3.

4. Differential Depletion of Noradrenaline and False Transmitters by Reserpine and Guanethidine

Work from several laboratories (LINDMAR and MUSCHOLL, 1965; PORTER et al., 1965; SCHÜMANN et al., 1965; MUSCHOLL and SPRENGER, 1966; CARLSSON and WALDECK, 1968) has shown that α-methylnoradrenaline incorporated into the amine stores is less readily depleted by reserpine than is endogenous noradrenaline. When noradrenaline and α-methylnoradrenaline were determined simultaneously in rat heart and spleen (MUSCHOLL and SPRENGER, 1966) or rabbit heart (LINDMAR and MUSCHOLL, 1965) it was found that moderate doses of reserpine (55—75 μg/kg) preferentially depleted noradrenaline but a higher dose (0.3 mg/kg) caused a severe loss of both amines. It was suggested that partial block of the vesicular uptake by the smaller dose of reserpine leads to an increase in the intra-axonal concentrations of both amines and to their exposure to MAO. Since only noradrenaline is metabolized there will be a selective loss of this amine. The higher dose of reserpine, which in control animals depleted 97% of the heart noradrenaline, obviously caused a nearly complete block of vesicular uptake. As a result, retention of both amines is impaired and α-methylnoradrenaline although not deaminated intraaxonally is finally lost by diffusion out of the neuron.

Balance experiments on the isolated heart of rabbits pretreated with reserpine showed that the rates of membranal uptake of noradrenaline and α-methylnoradrenaline were identical but retention of noradrenaline was negligible compared with that of α-methylnoradrenaline. However, inhibition of MAO raised the concentration of noradrenaline retained by the heart to the same level as that of α-methylnoradrenaline when equal doses of either amine were infused (LINDMAR and MUSCHOLL, 1965).

Depletion by reserpine (16 and 64 μg/kg) of α-methylnoradrenaline from hearts of guinea pigs treated with α-methyldopa was much smaller than depletion of noradrenaline from normal guinea-pig hearts by doses of 1—16 μg/kg reserpine (SCHÜMANN et al., 1965). Similarly, incubation with prenylamine more easily depleted noradrenaline from storage vesicles isolated from normal guinea-pig hearts than it depleted α-methylnoradrenaline from heart vesicles of animals pretreated with three doses of α-methyldopa. Since in the latter experiments metabolism of noradrenaline by MAO was excluded, SCHÜMANN et al. (1965) suggested, as an alternative explanation for the differential depletion of the two amines, that α-methylnoradrenaline is more tightly bound than noradrenaline. A similar conclusion was reached by CARLSSON et al. (1965a) who observed a lower tendency of α-methylnoradrenaline, as compared with noradrenaline, to diffuse from adrenergic axons when formaldehyde gas of high humidity was used in their histofluorescence studies. However, a firmer binding of α-methylnoradrenaline than of noradrenaline was apparently ruled out by the following study. LUNDBORG and STITZEL (1967a) injected tritiated noradrenaline (1 μg/kg), α-methylnoradrenaline (100 μg/kg) and metaraminol (40 μg/kg) i.v. into mice and determined the amount of amine retained in the particulate and supernatant fractions of the heart. One hr after injection noradrenaline was found to be present in the particles at a greater percentage (48%) than was either α-methylnoradrenaline (37%) or metaraminol (19%). Inhibition of MAO did not alter the distribution of noradrenaline between the particulate and supernatant fractions. It was concluded that α-methylnoradrenaline was retained less efficiently than noradrenaline. However, the dose of α-methylnoradrenaline administered was 100 times that of noradrenaline and it is possible that the concentration ratio, particles: supernatant, of either amine decreases with increasing cytoplasmic amine levels.

In any case, analysis of differential depletion at the subcellular level is somewhat complicated in view of the observation that metaraminol and, to a lesser degree, α-methylnoradrenaline utilize a *reserpine-resistant* uptake mechanism into adrenergic nerve vesicles, quite in contrast to noradrenaline (CARLSSON et al., 1967; LUNDBORG and STITZEL, 1967a, 1967b, 1968b).

Fractionation of heart homogenates at different time intervals (0.5; 1 and 24 hr) after injection of ^{3}H-metaraminol into mice revealed that the main spontaneous loss of metaraminol was from the supernatant fraction (LUNDBORG and STITZEL, 1967b). Reserpine given 15—45 min before death did not, at any of the times indicated, significantly affect the metaraminol concentration in the supernatant, but depleted metaraminol that was incorporated into the particulate fraction 24 hr before. The authors concluded that metaraminol moves from a site which is resistant towards depletion by reserpine to a site which is sensitive to reserpine. On the other hand, protriptyline caused a preferential loss of metaraminol from the supernatant during the early period after its administration. This agrees with the notion that protriptyline, by blocking the transmembranal uptake of amines (CARLSSON and WALDECK, 1965a; CARLSSON et al., 1967), inhibits the retrieval mechanism and enhances the net loss of metaraminol from the neuron (CARLSSON and WALDECK, 1965b). Comparison of the rate of release of ^{3}H-noradrenaline and ^{3}H-metaraminol from the mouse heart after administration of reserpine showed that metaraminol was depleted almost as readily as noradrenaline (CARLSSON and WALDECK, 1968). In view of the fact that metaraminol is resistant to MAO this was explained with the low affinity of the amine to the vesicular storage mechanism and its ability to escape through the neuronal membrane. Since protriptyline causes a greater potentiation of the rate of release of metaraminol than of noradrenaline, the dependence of metaraminol upon an intact membrane uptake process for its neuronal retention is obvious (CARLSSON and WALDECK, 1965b, 1968).

Differential depletion of noradrenaline and several false transmitters was also observed after guanethidine. Intravenous doses of 1.25—20 mg/kg which depleted 30—70% of the heart noradrenaline of normal or α-methyldopa pretreated rabbits caused significantly smaller losses of the α-methylnoradrenaline which had accumulated in the hearts after four doses of 50 mg/kg L-α-methyldopa (LINDMAR and MUSCHOLL, 1965). Labelled octopamine and its meta-hydroxy analogue retained by the rat heart were depleted more readily than were labelled noradrenaline and dopamine after single doses of reserpine or guanethidine (MUSACCHIO et al., 1965b). Administration of a MAO inhibitor decreased the rate of disappearance of ^{3}H-octopamine by guanethidine but did not affect that of ^{3}H-α-methyloctopamine (KOPIN et al., 1965).

The findings discussed in this section strongly suggest that reserpine or guanethidine more readily deplete a particular amine if the latter is susceptible to metabolism by MAO. Preferential loss occurs also if the amine has a low affinity to vesicular uptake sites and diffuses out of the neuron. The effects of protection of an amine against MAO and facilitation of its diffusion out of the axon may oppose each other in a way that depletion proceeds at a rate similar to the loss of noradrenaline. One example of this is metaraminol (see above) and another one is α-methyladrenaline which is lost from rat heart and spleen after reserpine (13.7—55 μg/kg s.c., 6 hr before death) at approximately the same rate as the endogenous noradrenaline (MUSCHOLL and SPRENGER, 1966).

5. Altered Sensitivity Towards Exogenous Noradrenaline

Depending on species, organ and other factors, chronic treatment with precursors of false transmitters has been shown to produce responses to injected noradrenaline which are either enhanced, unaltered or decreased. After α-methyldopa the pressor response to a single dose of noradrenaline was unaltered in dogs (STONE et al., 1962) and rabbits (SOGANI and SHARMA, 1966). In the cat, different schedules of pretreatment with α-methyldopa did not affect the pressor responses of a large range of noradrenaline doses (HAEFELY et al., 1966, 1967). Similarly, administration of α-MMT did not alter the pressor effect of noradrenaline in the cat (HAEFELY et al., 1966) and dog (STONE et al., 1962). However, treatment of rats for 10 days with α-methyldopa, α-MMT, α-methylnoradrenaline and metaraminol potentiated the pressor effect of noradrenaline (BRUNNER et al., 1967), while treatment with the two amino acids for only two days did not significantly alter the response to noradrenaline (SCHMITT and PÉTILLOT, 1970). Also, 3—6 hr after 400 mg/kg α-methyldopa the pressor effect of noradrenaline in the rat was unaltered (HENNING and SVENSSON, 1968). In normotensive humans a single dose of noradrenaline caused an unaltered pressor effect after 7 days of treatment with α-methyldopa (MCCURDY et al., 1964). However, an increased pressor response to both noradrenaline and α-methylnoradrenaline was found in hypertensive patients when dose-response curves of the amines were obtained before and after administration of α-methyldopa for 3 days (RAHN et al., 1970).

The cat nictitating membrane was sensitized towards injected noradrenaline after administration of α-methyldopa for 3 days, but the sensitivity of the cardiac pacemaker was decreased (HAEFELY et al., 1967). In contrast, in the dog the dose-response curves for the chronotropic actions of both noradrenaline and α-methylnoradrenaline were shifted to the left after 4—5 days of treatment, but they were not affected 3 hr after a single dose of α-methyldopa (SUGARMAN et al., 1968). Pretreatment of guinea pigs with α-methyldopa 24 and 12 hr before isolation of the atria did not alter the effects of noradrenaline or α-methylnoradrenaline on rate and force of contraction (SMITH, 1966). It was suggested that inhibition of amine uptake after incorporation of false transmitters causes the potentiation of injected noradrenaline observed on both the blood pressure (BRUNNER et al., 1967) and on the nictitating membrane (HAEFELY et al., 1967).

On the other hand, the contractions of the nictitating membrane and the pressor effect to noradrenaline were unchanged after pretreatment of cats with 4-methoxy-3,5-dihydroxyphenylalanine (THOENEN et al., 1968) or 5-hydroxydopa (THOENEN et al., 1967c). It has been pointed out by THOENEN et al. (1967b, c; 1968) that only incorporation of false transmitters with α-methyl groups has been found to potentiate the response to injected noradrenaline while those amines lacking an α-methyl group are metabolized by MAO and disappear so quickly from the axoplasm that there is no interference with the inactivation of circulating noradrenaline.

Summarizing these findings it appears that large organ and species differences do exist as far as sensitization to exogenous noradrenaline is concerned. In general, prolonged pretreatment with a precursor of an α-methylated amine or with the amine itself favours development of supersensitivity. Obviously, alteration of sensitivity may occur unnoticed when only the response to a single dose of noradrenaline is tested.

There may be functional consequences of altered sensitivity to *released* noradrenaline. On the cat nictitating membrane the development of *supersensitivity* during prolonged treatment with α-methyldopa interferes with the failure of sympathetic transmission caused by the drug (HAEFELY et al., 1967). However, for reasons at present unknown the supersensitivity seems to be depressed at 4 hr after a dose of α-methyldopa, and this allows the transmission failure to become apparent.

Subsensitivity to the pressor action of noradrenaline has been described as a consequence of infusion of a high dose (1 mg/kg) of metaraminol into reserpine-pretreated spinal cats (BHAGAT and RAGLAND, 1966). Supposedly, metaraminol as a weak agonist occupied most of the adrenoceptors and thus decreased the effect of noradrenaline. This phenomenon requires further examination because in the dog a decreased pressor response to noradrenaline was caused by two injections of 1 mg/kg metaraminol, whereas 2 mg/kg enhanced, and 0.5 mg/kg left unaltered, the response to noradrenaline (STONE et al., 1963). A similar hypothesis (HOLTZ and PALM, 1967), that α-methyldopamine inhibits the action of noradrenaline on adrenoceptors by acting as a competitive partial agonist to the natural transmitter, was tested by FEIN et al. (1967) on the guinea-pig vas deferens. In order to exclude the sensitizing effect that α-methyldopamine exerts by its inhibitory action on amine uptake, the preparations were treated with cocaine. However, α-methyldopamine did not shift the dose-response curve of noradrenaline to the right, and thus did not act as predicted by the above hypothesis.

VI. Consequences of Combined Release of Noradrenaline and False Transmitters

1. Effect of False Transmitters on Adrenoceptors

With the exception of α-methylnoradrenaline and α-methyladrenaline all sympathomimetic amines that are known to be released as false transmitters have much lower potencies than noradrenaline in activating adrenoceptors.

As a vasoconstrictor agent on isolated vessel preparations α-methylnoradrenaline was usually less effective than noradrenaline (rat: MALIK and MUSCHOLL, 1969b; rabbit: PRUSS et al., 1965). This is also true for the pressor effects in conscious rats or in rats anaesthetized with urethane (BRUNNER et al., 1967). According to the majority of investigators the pressor potencies of (—)-α-methylnoradrenaline and (—)-noradrenaline were identical in pithed rats (MAÎTRE and STAEHELIN, 1963; MUSCHOLL and MAÎTRE, 1963; LINDMAR and MUSCHOLL, 1965; TRINKER, 1971), spinal cats (HAEFELY et al., 1966) and anaesthetized dogs (CONRADI et al., 1965; MOHAMMED et al., 1968; TRINKER, 1971). However, a lesser potency of α-methylnoradrenaline in the pithed rat has been reported (DAY and RAND, 1964; SCHMITT and PÉTILLOT, 1970). In cats under urethan-chloralose the diastolic blood pressure was equally enhanced by small doses of noradrenaline and α-methylnoradrenaline (0.4—1×10^{-9}M) but after a larger dose (4×10^{-8}M) the rise in pressure was more pronounced with noradrenaline than with α-methylnoradrenaline (PALM et al., 1967); the different slopes of the dose-response curves of the two amines might have been due to the fact that the vasodilatory, β-receptor stimulating action of α-methylnoradrenaline was ten times that of noradrenaline.

Injected α-methylnoradrenaline may further affect the blood pressure by its strong cardiostimulatory action. The amine did not differ from noradrenaline in causing an increase of heart rate in the dog (CONRADI et al., 1965; SUGARMAN et al., 1968; TRINKER, 1971), spinal cat (HAEFELY et al., 1966) and on isolated atria of guinea pigs (SMITH, 1966; PALM et al., 1967). On the perfused rat heart α-methylnoradrenaline had 1/3 of the positive inotropic action of noradrenaline (BRUNNER et al., 1967). The large contribution of the cardiostimulation by α-methylnoradrenaline to its hemodynamic action is shown by the following study performed on normotensive humans (RAHN et al., 1970). Infusion of 28.8 μg/min α-methylnoradrenaline but only 9.6 μg/min noradrenaline was necessary to increase systolic blood pressure by 30 mm Hg. α-Methylnoradrenaline significantly enhanced cardiac output and decreased total peripheral vascular resistance while noradrenaline mainly acted through an increase of the vascular resistance.

In small doses α-methyladrenaline is a potent vasodilator drug whereas higher doses cause a secondary rise of the blood pressure (SCHAUMANN, 1931; MUSCHOLL and SPRENGER, 1966). Thus, α-methyladrenaline produces effects differing *qualitatively* from those of noradrenaline. The levorotatory isomer has half the inotropic potency of (—)-noradrenaline on guinea-pig auricles (PALM et al., 1967); this agrees with the observation on the perfused rabbit heart that ($\pm$)-α-methyladrenaline has 1/4—1/6 of the potency of (—)-noradrenaline (LINDMAR et al., 1967).

False transmitter amines which on various test organs are approximately one to two orders of magnitude less effective than noradrenaline include octopamine (TRENDELENBURG et al., 1962; KOROL et al., 1968), α-methyloctopamine (TRENDELENBURG et al., 1962), metaraminol (TRENDELENBURG et al., 1962; GRAM and WRIGHT, 1966; HAEFELY et al., 1966; BRUNNER et al., 1967), α-methyldopamine (PALM et al., 1967; KILBINGER et al., 1971), *threo*-corbadrine (MUSCHOLL and LINDMAR, 1967), dihydroxypseudoephedrine (MUSCHOLL and SPRENGER, 1966; LINDMAR et al., 1967) and 4-methoxy-3,5-dihydroxyphenylethylamine (THOENEN et al., 1968). Several of these amines have an indirect action, e.g., (—)-α-methyldopamine on cat blood pressure and guinea-pig heart rate (PALM et al., 1967); octopamine and α-methyloctopamine on cat blood pressure, heart rate and nictitating membrane (TRENDELENBURG et al., 1962); metaraminol on heart rate but not on the nictitating membrane of the cat (TRENDELENBURG et al., 1962) and 4-methoxy-3,5-dihydroxyphenylethylamine on the nictitating membrane and spleen of the cat (THOENEN et al., 1968). Since for the action of false transmitters on adrenoceptors only the direct effects are relevant, the potencies relative to noradrenaline may be as low as 10^{-3} in the case of α-methyloctopamine on the heart rate of the cat (TRENDELENBURG et al., 1962) or 10^{-4} in the case of 4-methoxy-3,4-dihydroxyphenylethylamine on the cat spleen (THOENEN et al., 1968).

2. Effect of False Transmitters on Re-uptake of Amines

There is indirect evidence that the various drugs which are known to inhibit membrane uptake of exogenous noradrenaline also inhibit re-uptake of noradrenaline that is released from nerve fibres (HUKOVIĆ and MUSCHOLL, 1962; THOENEN et al., 1964). A particular amine which is released as a false transmitter may compete with noradrenaline for the uptake process. Accordingly, the potency of an amine to interfere with re-uptake should run parallel to its potency to inhibit the membrane uptake of exogenous noradrenaline that can be determined by conventional methods. The work of BURGEN and IVERSEN (1965) contains such information about nearly all the amines known to be released as false transmitters. From their evidence concerning phenylethylamines the following facts emerge: Introduction of a phenolic hydroxyl group increases, hydroxylation of the β-carbon of the side chain decreases, and methylation of the α-carbon of the side chain increases, the potency of an amine to inhibit noradrenaline uptake. The same relationship between structure and activity was observed when the effects of various sympathomimetic amines on the membrane uptake of α-methylnoradrenaline were determined (MUSCHOLL and WEBER, 1965).

If the affinity of a false transmitter to the membrane uptake process is close to that of noradrenaline one might expect that the proportion of both amines found in the perfusate of an organ after sympathetic stimulation is identical with the proportion of the amines released from the nerve fibres, provided that extraneuronal metabolism does not differentially affect noradrenaline and the false transmitter. The release of α-methylnoradrenaline as a false transmitter may serve as an example for such a situation. On the perfused rabbit heart the cocaine-sensitive neuronal uptake of low concentrations (10 or 20 ng/ml) of exogenous (—)-α-methylnoradrenaline proceeds at the same rate as that of exogenous (—)-noradrenaline (LINDMAR and MUSCHOLL, 1965; WEBER and MUSCHOLL, 1965). When rabbits were pretreated with an infusion of (+)-α-methyldopamine and the hearts isolated after 135 min, sympathetic nerve stimulation caused an output of (—)-α-methylnoradrenaline and noradrenaline into the perfusates; only traces of α-methyldopamine were detected (KILBINGER et al., 1971). The proportion of α-methylnoradrenaline to noradrenaline was identical with the proportion of the amines found in the hearts after termination of the experiment, and the total amounts of both amines in the perfusates were equal to the quantities of noradrenaline determined in the perfusates of normal rabbit hearts after sympathetic nerve stimulation. On the rat heart the affinity to the membrane uptake of (—)-α-methylnoradrenaline was found to be only 1.35 times that of (—)-noradrenaline (BURGEN and IVERSEN, 1965). If in the experiments on the rabbit heart the difference in the relative affinities of both amines was of the same order it may have escaped notice.

However, removal from the α-methylnoradrenaline molecule of the β-hydroxyl group greatly increased the affinity to the uptake sites as shown by a ratio: (±)-α-methyldopamine to (±)-noradrenaline of 3.72 (BURGEN and IVERSEN, 1965). Unfortunately, the inhibition of membrane uptake by (—)-α-methyldopamine has not been investigated so far, but there is indirect evidence that its potency significantly surpasses that of (—)-α-methylnoradrenaline. On rat atria the relative potentiating effect of (—)-α-methyldopamine towards exogenous (—)-noradrenaline was 2.9 times that of (+)-α-methyldopamine and indistinguishable from that of (—)-metaraminol (SWAMY et al., 1969). According to BURGEN and IVERSEN (1965) (—)-metaraminol has an affinity to the membrane uptake 3.5 times that of (—)-noradrenaline, and 2.62 times that of (—)-α-methylnoradrenaline, respectively. In keeping with these observations is the finding that total catecholamine output of the isolated rabbit heart is greatly enhanced when (—)-α-methyldopamine is released by nerve stimulation (KILBINGER et al., 1971). After infusion of the latter amine into rabbits the hearts had lost 66% of the endogenous noradrenaline which was fully replaced by (—)-α-methyldopamine. Nerve stimulation caused an output of noradrenaline plus (—)-α-methyldopamine that was 2.4 times the noradrenaline output of control hearts; however, the proportion of the two amines in the perfusates was identical with that determined in the heart.

Another amine which might enhance total transmitter output if released by nerve stimulation is (—)-metaraminol since it greatly inhibits the membrane uptake process. However, concerning this question no data are available in the literature.

3. Interactions of Noradrenaline and False Transmitters at Adrenoceptors

As to the aim of achieving inhibition of adrenergic transmission it would be advantageous to incorporate an amine that is easily bound by the vesicular storage sites but when released has a much lower potency than noradrenaline. The experiments compiled in Table 2 can be grouped into four categories, and the first one gives several examples for the aim defined above.

1. Sympathetic transmission failure is usually observed when a false transmitter of low potency is released and the noradrenaline output is decreased at the same time (total amine output unaltered or decreased). Release of the following false transmitters was shown to coincide with transmission failure on the organ indicated: Octopamine on spleen (KOPIN, 1968b); α-methyladrenaline and dihydroxypseudoephedrine on heart (LINDMAR et al., 1967); (+)-α-methyldopamine on spleen (THOENEN et al., 1967b); 5-hydroxydopamine on spleen (THOENEN et al., 1967c); 4-methoxy-3,5-dihydroxyphenylethylamine on spleen (THOENEN et al., 1968).

2. Only at low frequencies of stimulation a transmission failure is noticeable when the potency of the false transmitter is lower than that of noradrenaline but release of the latter amine is insufficiently depressed (less than 50%), e.g. after one infusion of α-methyladrenaline or one and two infusions of dihydroxypseudoephedrine (LINDMAR et al., 1967). The unaltered response of the spleen after release of dopamine by stimulation with frequencies as high as 6 and 10 Hz (THOENEN et al., 1965) may be similarly explained.

3. The response to sympathetic nerve stimulation is unaltered in spite of a decrease of noradrenaline release when the total amine output remains constant and the false transmitter has the same potency on the organ as noradrenaline. After administration of (+)-α-methyldopamine to rabbits α-methylnoradrenaline fully compensated for the decrease in noradrenaline output from the heart during nerve stimulation; the frequency-response curves for rate and force of cardiac contraction did not differ from those of the controls (KILBINGER et al., 1971). Release of α-methylnoradrenaline after treatment of cats with α-methyldopa also ensured unimpaired contractile responses of the spleen (HAEFELY et al., 1967).

From these results it can be concluded that transmission failure depends primarily on a large decrease of noradrenaline release; moreover, it is favoured by low rates of nerve stimulation.

4. However, sympathetic transmission may be impaired in spite of an undiminished output of noradrenaline. This was observed on the rabbit heart after release of (—)-α-methyldopamine as a false transmitter (KILBINGER et al., 1971). The cause for the reduced responses is unknown but a postjunctional interference of (—)-α-methyldopamine with the activation of β-receptors by noradrenaline was assumed.

There are several additional observations of the responses to postganglionic stimulation of adrenergic nerves after administration of false transmitters or their precursors which are compatible with the above conclusions. In these experiments the output of amines was not determined. Transmission failure was found after α-MMT on the cat nictitating membrane (HAEFELY et al., 1966), after α-MMT or metaraminol on the dog heart (TORCHIANA et al., 1970), and after α-methyladrenaline or dihydroxypseudoephedrine on the rat mesenteric artery preparation (MALIK and MUSCHOLL, 1969b; MALIK, 1971). Similarly, SCHMITT and PÉTILLOT (1970) observed an inhibition of the effect of vasoconstrictor nerve stimulation in the pithed rat 24 hr after α-MMT and 3 hr after metaraminol, octopamine and α-methyloctopamine; however, 3 hr after α-methylnoradrenaline or 24 hr after α-methyldopa the pressor response was decreased only at low frequencies of stimulation. An unequivocal transmission failure, based on determination of frequency-response curves, after α-methyldopa might be expected only on organs which are less sensitive to α-methylnoradrenaline than to noradrenaline, and this was in fact observed on the cat hindleg resistance and capacitance vessels (KISIN, 1967), on the rat mesenteric arteries (MALIK and MUSCHOLL, 1969a) and on the nictitating membrane of the cat anaesthetized with pentobarbitone and chloralose (DAY and RAND, 1964). However, after repeated doses of α-methyldopa the nictitating membrane of the *spinal* cat developed supersensitivity (HAEFELY et al., 1967); only at a short post-drug interval (4 hr) the supersensitivity disappeared and thus revealed the transmission failure (cf. Section V, 5).

It is questionable whether the transmission failure on the rat eyelid (SALMON and IRESON, 1970) or the dog heart (SUGARMAN et al., 1968) observed 1—2.5 hr after a single i.v. injection of α-methyldopa was due to α-methylnoradrenaline substituting released noradrenaline; alternatively, a neuron-blocking effect of the amino acid has been discussed (SALMON and IRESON, 1970). According to MOHAMMED et al. (1968) treatment of dogs for 3—5 days with α-methyldopa reduced the vascular resistance of the perfused hindleg without impairing the response to nerve stimulation at 50 Hz; on the other hand, the arterial blood pressure was not lowered by the treatment.

Unimpaired transmission after administration of α-methyldopa has been observed on the hearts of dogs (GOLDBERG et al., 1960; frequency not indicated), cats (VARMA and BENFEY, 1963; 10 Hz) and on guinea-pig atria (SMITH, 1966; 0.25—32 Hz). In contrast to the acute effect of α-methyldopa on the dog heart (see above) chronic treatment did not inhibit the chronotropic response to nerve stimulation (0.3—30 Hz) (SUGARMAN et al., 1968). These findings agree with the notion that on the cardiac adrenoceptors α-methylnoradrenaline and noradrenaline are equieffective (cf. Section VI, 1). The significance of the unaltered response of the rat eyelid to preganglionic stimulation of the sympathetic trunk 3—6 hr after α-methyldopa (HENNING and SVENSSON, 1968) cannot be assessed in the context of the present discussion since the relative potencies of noradrenaline and α-methylnoradrenaline on this organ have not been determined.

It appears that there are large differences between test organs as far as their susceptibility to adrenergic blockade by false transmitter mechanisms is concerned. DAY and RAND (1964) have suggested that in man the blood pressure lowering effect of α-methyldopa is caused by a decrease in effectiveness of sympathetic impulses to the blood vessels. This hypothesis has been criticised on the ground that various experiments on well-established sympathetic nerve-muscle preparations have failed to reveal impairment of transmission after α-methyldopa. However, a failure to detect interference with transmission on the nictitating membrane, spleen or eyelid cannot seriously be used to refute a possible impairment at synapses involved in the control of blood pressure. As mentioned above, inhibition of the responses to nerve stimulation was observed on some vascular smooth muscle preparations, although this occurred to a lesser extent than after a high dose of reserpine (Kisin, 1967). Nevertheless, for the hypotensive action of α-methyldopa a peripheral site of attack may be of secondary importance, at least in certain animal species. Henning and associates (reviewed by Henning, 1969) have provided indirect evidence for a centrally mediated hypotensive effect of α-methyldopa which on the rat depends on formation in the CNS of α-methyl-noradrenaline; it was suggested to extend the original false transmitter concept to include central neurones. Since the discussion of the spacious literature on the hypotensive effects of α-methyldopa and related precursors of false transmitters in animals or men is beyond the scope of this chapter the reader is referred to the reviews by Holtz and Palm (1966); Muscholl (1966a); Stone and Porter (1967) and Henning (1969).

References

Almgren, O., Andén, N.-E., Waldeck, B.: Extraneuronal binding as a possible factor of tyramine uptake by sympathetic nerves. Life Sci. **4**, 121—126 (1965).

— Lundborg, P.G., Stitzel, R.E.: Release of ^{3}H-metaraminol from subcellular fractions of rat salivary glands by nerve stimulation. Europ. J. Pharmacol. **6**, 109—114 (1969).

— Waldeck, B.: On the disposition of (^{3}H) metaraminol in the rat salivary gland. J. Pharm. Pharmacol. **19**, 705—708 (1967).

Amery, A., Moerman, E.J., Bossaert, H., de Schaepdryver, A.F.: α-Methyl-p-tyrosine in malignant pheochromocytoma. Pharmacol. Clin. **1**, 174—176 (1969).

Andén, N.-E.: On the mechanism of noradrenaline depletion by α-methyl metatyrosine and metaraminol. Acta physiol. scand. **21**, 260—271 (1964a).

— Uptake and release of dextro- and levo-adrenaline in noradrenergic stores. Acta pharmacol. (Kbh.) **21**, 59—75 (1964b).

— Fuxe, K., Henning, M.: Mechanisms of noradrenaline and 5-hydroxytryptamine disappearance induced by α-methyldopa and α-methyl-metatyrosine. Europ. J. Pharmacol. **8**, 302—309 (1969).

— — Hökfelt, T.: Effect of some drugs on central monoamine nerve terminals lacking nerve impulse flow. Europ. J. Pharmacol. **1**, 226—232 (1967).

— Magnusson, T.: Functional significance of noradrenaline depletion by α-methyl metatyrosine, metaraminol and dextro-adrenaline. In: Pharmacology of Cholinergic and Adrenergic Transmission. Eds. Koelle, G.B., Douglas, W.W., Carlsson, A. 319—328. Oxford: Pergamon Press 1965.

Axelrod, J.: Methylation reactions in the formation and metabolism of catecholamines and other biogenic amines. Pharmacol. Rev. **18**, 95—113 (1966).

Berti, F., Shore, P.A.: A kinetic analysis of drugs that inhibit the adrenergic neuronal membrane amine pump. Biochem. Pharmacol. **16**, 2091—2094 (1967a).

— — Interaction of reserpine and ouabain on amine concentrating mechanisms in the adrenergic neurone. Biochem. Pharmacol. **16**, 2271—2274 (1967b).

Bhagat, B., Ragland, R.: Effect of infusion of metaraminol on the response of reserpine-pretreated spinal cats to tyramine and to noradrenaline. Brit. J. Pharmacol. **27**, 506—513 (1966).

Blaschko, H.: Substrate specificity of amino-acid decarboxylases. Biochim. biophys. Acta (Amst.) **4**, 130—137 (1950).

— Burn, J.H., Langemann, H.: The formation of noradrenaline from dihydroxyphenylserine. Brit. J. Pharmacol. **5**, 431—437 (1950).

— Richter, D., Schlossmann, H.: The oxidation of adrenaline and other amines. Biochem. J. **31**, 2187—2196 (1937).

Boullin, D.J.: A calcium requirement for release of ^{3}H-guanethidine by sympathetic nerve stimulation. J. Pharm. Pharmacol. **18**, 709—712 (1966).

Brunner, H., Hedwall, P.R., Maître, L., Meier, M.: Antihypertensive effects of alpha-methylated catecholamine analogues in the rat. Brit. J. Pharmacol. **30**, 108—122 (1967).

Buhs, R.P., Beck, J.L., Speth, O.C., Smith, J.L., Trenner, N.R., Cannon, P.J., Laragh, J.H.: The metabolism of methyldopa in hypertensive human subjects. J. Pharmacol. exp. Ther. **143**, 205—214 (1964).

Burgen, A.S.V., Iversen, L.L.: The inhibition of noradrenaline uptake by sympathomimetic amines in the rat isolated heart. Brit. J. Pharmacol. **25**, 34—49 (1965).

Cahn, R.S., Ingold, C.K., Prelog, V.: The specification of asymmetric configuration in organic chemistry. Experientia (Basel) **12**, 81—94 (1956).

CARLSSON, A.: Functional significance of drug-induced changes in brain monoamine levels. Progr. Brain Res. **8**, 9—27 (1964).
— DAHLSTRÖM, A., FUXE, K., HILLARP, N.A.: Failure of reserpine to deplete noradrenaline neurons of α-methylnoradrenaline formed from α-methyl DOPA. Acta pharmacol. (Kbh.) **22**, 270—276 (1965a).
— HILLARP, N.A., WALDECK, B.: Analysis of the Mg^{++}-ATP dependent storage mechanism in the amine granules of the adrenal medulla. Acta physiol. scand. **59**, Suppl. 215 (1963).
— LINDQVIST, M.: In-vivo decarboxylation of α-methyl dopa and α-methyl metatyrosine. Acta physiol. scand. **54**, 87—94 (1962).
— — DAHLSTRÖM, A., FUXE, K., MASUOKA, D.: Effects of the amphetamine group on intraneuronal brain amines *in vivo* and *in vitro*. J. Pharm. Pharmacol. **17**, 521—524 (1965b).
— LUNDBORG, P., STITZEL, R., WALDECK, B.: Uptake, storage and release of ^{3}H-α-methylnorepinephrine. J. Pharmacol. exp. Ther. **158**, 175—182 (1967).
— MEISCH, J.-J., WALDECK, B.: On the β-hydroxylation of (±)-α-methyldopamine *in vivo*. Europ. J. Pharmacol. **5**, 85—92 (1968).
— WALDECK, B.: β-Hydroxylation of tyramine *in vivo*. Acta pharmacol. (Kbh.) **20**, 371—374 (1963).
— — Inhibition of ^{3}H-metaraminol uptake by antidepressive and related drugs. J. Pharm. Pharmacol. **17**, 243—244 (1965a).
— — Rapid release of ^{3}H-metaraminol induced by combined treatment with protriptyline and reserpine. J. Pharm. Pharmacol. **17**, 327—328 (1965b).
— — Mechanism of amine transport in the cell membranes of the adrenergic nerves. Acta pharmacol. (Kbh.) **22**, 293—300 (1965c).
— — Release of ^{3}H-metaraminol by different mechanisms. Acta physiol. scand. **67**, 471—480 (1966a).
— — Structure-activity relationships for release of ^{14}C-octopamine from adrenergic nerves by phenethylamines. Acta pharmacol. (Kbh.) **24**, 255—262 (1966b).
— — Different mechanisms of drug-induced release of noradrenaline and its congeners α-methyl-noradrenaline and metaraminol. Europ. J. Pharmacol. **4**, 165—168 (1968).
CHIDSEY, C.A., HARRISON, D.C.: Studies on the distribution of exogenous norepinephrine in the sympathetic transmitter store. J. Pharmacol. exp. Ther. **140**, 217—223 (1963).
— KAISER, G.A., LEHR, B.: The hydroxylation of tyramine in the isolated canine heart. J. Pharmacol. exp. Ther. **144**, 393—398 (1964).
CONRADI, E.C., GAFFNEY, T.E., FINK, D.A., VANGROW, J.S.: Reversal of sympathetic nerve blockade: A comparison of dopa, dopamine, and norepinephrine with their α-methylated analogues. J. Pharmacol. exp. Ther. **150**, 26—33 (1965).
COSTA, E., NEFF, N.H., NGAI, S.H.: Regulation of metaraminol efflux from rat heart and salivary glands. Brit. J. Pharmacol. **36**, 153—160 (1969).
CREVELING, C.R.: Drugs interfering with the formation of adrenergic transmitters. In: Pharmacology of Cholinergic and Adrenergic Transmission. Eds. KOELLE, G.B., DOUGLAS, W.W., CARLSSON, A. 185—204. Oxford: Pergamon Press 1965.
CROUT, J.R., ALPERS, H.S., TATUM, E.L., SHORE, P.A.: Release of metaraminol (aramine) from the heart by sympathetic nerve stimulation. Science **145**, 828—829 (1964).
— SHORE, P.A.: Differential release of metaraminol and norepinephrine from the cat heart. Pharmacologist **6**, 175 (1964).
DAVIES, B.N., HORTON, E.W., WITHRINGTON, P.G.: The occurrence of prostaglandin E_2 in splenic venous blood of the dog following splenic nerve stimulation. J. Physiol. (Lond.) **188**, 38P—39P (1967).
DAY, M.D., RAND, M.J.: A hypothesis for the mode of action of α-methyldopa in relieving hypertension. J. Pharm. Pharmacol. **15**, 221—224 (1963).
— — Some observations on the pharmacology of α-methyldopa. Brit. J. Pharmacol. **22**, 72—86 (1964).
DREWS, E.-F., LINDMAR, R., MUSCHOLL, E.: Noradrenaline depleting and blood pressure lowering activity of threo-corbadrine. Europ. J. Pharmacol. **3**, 167—169 (1968).
FARRUGIA, M.T., HUNTER, W.H., KIRK, G.: The preparation and pharmacological properties of Ψ-corbasil. J. Pharm. Pharmacol. **21**, Suppl. 199S—205S (1969).
FEIN, J., HOLTZ, P., PALM, D.: Beeinflussung des Nervenreizes und der Noradrenalinwirkung am isolierten Hypogastricus-Vas deferens-Präparat des Meerschweinchens durch α-Methyldopamin und andere α-methylierte sympathicomimetische Amine. Naunyn-Schmiedeberg's Arch. Pharmak. exp. Path. **258**, 334—351 (1967).
FISCHER, J.E., HORST, W.D., KOPIN, I.J.: β-Hydroxylated sympathomimetic amines as false neurotransmitters. Brit. J. Pharmacol. **24**, 477—484 (1965).
— WEISE, V.K., KOPIN, I.J.: Release of tritiated bretylium by sympathetic nerve stimulation. Nature (Lond.) **209**, 778—779 (1966).

Furchgott, R.F., Kirpekar, S.M., Rieker, M., Schwab, A.: Actions and interactions of norepinephrine, tyramine and cocaine on aortic strips of rabbit and left atria of guinea pig and cat. J. Pharmacol. exp. Ther. **142**, 39—58 (1963).
— Sanchez Garcia, P.: Effects of inhibition of monoamine oxidase on the actions and interactions of norepinephrine, tyramine and other drugs on guinea-pig left atrium. J. Pharmacol. exp. Ther. **163**, 98—122 (1968).
Gessa, G.L., Costa, E., Kuntzman, R., Brodie, B.B.: On the mechanism of norepinephrine release by a-methyl-metatyrosine. Life Sci. **1**, 353—360 (1962).
Giachetti, A., Shore, P.A.: Studies *in vitro* of amine uptake mechanisms in heart. Biochem. Pharmacol. **15**, 607—614 (1966).
Gillespie, L., Oates, J.A., Crout, J.R., Sjoerdsma, A.: Clinical and chemical studies with a-methyl-dopa in patients with hypertension. Circulation **25**, 281—291 (1962).
Gjessing, L.R.: Studies on urinary phenolic compounds in man. II. Phenolic-acids and -amines during a load of a-methyl-dopa and disulfiram in periodic catatonia. Scand. J. clin. Lab. Invest. **17**, 549—557 (1965).
Goldberg, L.I., Da Costa, F.M., Ozaki, M.: Actions of the decarboxylase inhibitor, a-methyl-3,4-dihydroxyphenylalanine, in the dog. Nature (Lond.) **188**, 502—504 (1960).
Goldstein, M., Anagnoste, B.: The conversion *in vivo* of D-amphetamine to (+)-p-hydroxynorephedrine. Biochim. biophys. Acta (Amst.) **107**, 166—168 (1965).
— McKereghan, M.R., Lauber, E.: The stereospecificity of the enzymatic amphetamine β-hydroxylation. Biochim. biophys. Acta (Amst.) **89**, 191—193 (1964).
Gram, T.E., Wright, H.N.: Lack of metaraminol biotransformation by rabbit tissues *in vitro*. Biochem. Pharmacol. **14**, 1911—1914 (1965).
— — Some factors influencing the action of metaraminol in rabbits. Arch. int. Pharmacodyn. **160**, 294—311 (1966).
Grobecker, H., Holtz, P.: Über die Brenzkatechinamine im Froschherzen und in der Froschhaut vor und nach Verabfolgung von a-Methyldopa. Experientia (Basel) **22**, 42—43 (1966).
— — Müller, H.K.: Die Wirkung von a-Methyldopa und Dopa auf den Brenzcatechinamingehalt des Herzens, der Nebennieren und der Haut des Frosches sowie auf die Melanophoren der Froschhaut. Naunyn-Schmiedeberg's Arch. Pharmak. exp. Path. **255**, 474—490 (1966).
Haefely, W., Hürlimann, A., Thoenen, H.: The effect of stimulation of sympathetic nerves in the cat treated with reserpine, a-methyldopa and a-methylmetatyrosine. Brit. J. Pharmacol. **26**, 172—185 (1966).
— — — Adrenergic transmitter changes and response to sympathetic nerve stimulation after differing pretreatment with a-methyldopa. Brit. J. Pharmacol. **31**, 105—119 (1967).
Häggendal, J., Malmfors, T.: The effect of nerve stimulation on catecholamines taken up in adrenergic nerves after reserpine pretreatment. Acta physiol. scand. **75**, 33—38 (1969).
Hamberger, B.: Reserpine-resistant uptake of catecholamines in isolated tissues of the rat. Acta physiol. scand. **71**, Suppl. 295 (1967).
— Malmfors, T., Norberg, K.-A., Sachs, C.: Uptake and accumulation of catecholamines in peripheral adrenergic neurons of reserpinized animals, studied with a histochemical method. Biochem. Pharmacol. **13**, 841—844 (1964).
Henning, M.: Studies on the mode of action of a-methyldopa. Acta physiol. scand. Suppl. **322** (1969).
— Svensson, L.: Adrenergic nerve function in the anaesthetized rat after treatment with a-methyldopa. Acta pharmacol. (Kbh.) **26**, 425—436 (1968).
Hertting, G., Potter, L.T., Axelrod, J.: Effect of decentralization and ganglionic blocking agents on the spontaneous release of ^{3}H-norepinephrine. J. Pharmacol. exp. Ther. **136**, 289—292 (1962).
Hess, S.M., Connamacher, R.H., Ozaki, M., Udenfriend, S.: The effects of a-methyl-dopa and a-methyl-meta-tyrosine on the metabolism of norepinephrine and serotonin *in vivo*. J. Pharmacol. exp. Ther. **134**, 129—138 (1961).
Holtz, P., Heise, R., Lüdtke, K.: Fermentativer Abbau von l-Dioxyphenylalanin (Dopa) durch Niere. Naunyn-Schmiedeberg's Arch. exp. Path. Pharmak. **191**, 87—118 (1938).
— Palm, D.: Brenzkatechinamine und andere sympathicomimetische Amine. Biosynthese und Inaktivierung, Freisetzung und Wirkung. Ergebn. Physiol. **58**, 1—580. Berlin-Heidelberg-New York: Springer 1966.
— — On the pharmacology of a-methylated catecholamines and the mechanism of the antihypertensive action of a-methyldopa. Life Sci. **6**, 1847—1857 (1967).
Huković, S., Muscholl, E.: Die Noradrenalin-Abgabe aus dem isolierten Kaninchenherzen bei sympathischer Nervenreizung und ihre pharmakologische Beeinflussung. Naunyn-Schmiedeberg's Arch. exp. Path. Pharmak. **244**, 81—96 (1962).

IKEDA, M., LEVITT, M., UDENFRIEND, S.: Hydroxylation of phenylalanine by purified preparations of adrenal and brain tyrosine hydroxylase. Biochem. biophys. Res. Commun. **18**, 482—488 (1965).

IVERSEN, L.L.: The Uptake and Storage of Noradrenaline in Sympathetic Nerves. Cambridge: University Press 1967.

— GLOWINSKI, J., AXELROD, J.: The uptake and storage of ^{3}H-norepinephrine in the reserpine-pretreated rat heart. J. Pharmacol. exp. Ther. **150**, 173—183 (1965).

— — — The physiologic disposition and metabolism of norepinephrine in immunosympathectomized animals. J. Pharmacol. exp. Ther. **151**, 273—284 (1966).

JOHNSON, G.E., MICKLE, D.: The influence of cold exposure on the *in vivo* release of metaraminol. Brit. J. Pharmacol. **28**, 246—254 (1966).

— PUGSLEY, T.A.: The formation and release of metaraminol during exposure to warm or cold environments. Brit. J. Pharmacol. **34**, 267—276 (1968).

— — Studies on the interrelationship between the syntheses of noradrenaline and metaraminol. Brit. J. Pharmacol. **39**, 167—174 (1970).

— RITZÉN, M.: Microspectrofluorometric identification of metaraminol in sympathetic adrenergic neurons. Acta physiol. scand. **67**, 505—513 (1966).

JUORIO, A.V., VOGT, M.: Monoamines and their metabolites in the avian brain. J. Physiol. (Lond.) **189**, 489—518 (1967).

KAKIMOTO, Y., ARMSTRONG, M.D.: On the identification of octopamine in mammals. J. biol. Chem. **237**, 422—427 (1962).

KILBINGER, H., LINDMAR, R., LÖFFELHOLZ, K., MUSCHOLL, E., PATIL, P.N.: Storage and release of false transmitters after infusion of (+)- and (—)-a-methyldopamine. Naunyn-Schmiedeberg's Arch. Pharmak. **271**, 234—248 (1971).

KISIN, I.E.: Der Einfluß von Reserpin, a-Methyldopa und Bretylium auf die Erregungsübertragung von den sympathischen Nerven auf die Gefäße. Verh. dtsch. Ges. exper. Med. **19**, 228—236 (1967).

KOPIN, I.J.: Biochemical aspects of release of norepinephrine and other amines from sympathetic nerve endings. Pharmacol. Rev. **18**, 513—523 (1966).

— False adrenergic transmitters. Ann. Rev. Pharmacol. 8, 377—394 (1968a).

— The influence of false adrenergic transmitters on adrenergic neurotransmission. In: Adrenergic Neurotransmission. Eds. WOLSTENHOLME, G.E.W., O'CONNOR, M. 95—104. London: Churchill 1968b.

— FISCHER, J.E., MUSACCHIO, J.M., HORST, W.D., WEISE, V.K.: "False neurochemical transmitters" and the mechanism of sympathetic blockade by monoamine oxidase inhibitors. J. Pharmacol. exp. Ther. **147**, 186—193 (1965).

— WEISE, V.K.: Effect of reserpine and metaraminol on excretion of homovanillic acid and 3-methoxy-4-hydroxyphenylglycol in the rat. Biochem. Pharmacol. **17**, 1461—1464 (1968).

— — SEDVALL, G.C.: Effect of false transmitters on norepinephrine synthesis. J. Pharmacol. exp. Ther. **170**, 246—252 (1969).

KOROL, B., SOFFER, L., BROWN, M.L.: Some cardiovascular studies on octopamine. Arch. int. Pharmacodyn. **171**, 415—424 (1968).

KRAUSS, K.R., KOPIN, I.J., WEISE, V.K.: The effect of bretylium on amine retention in rat heart. J. Pharmacol. exp. Ther. **172**, 282—288 (1970).

KRONEBERG, G., STOEPEL, K.: Der Einfluß von a-Methyl-Dopa auf die Tyraminwirkung an mit Reserpin vorbehandelten Katzen. Experientia (Basel) **19**, 252—253 (1963).

LEE, F.-L., WEINER, N., TRENDELENBURG, U.: The uptake of tyramine and formation of octopamine in normal and tachyphylactic rat atria. J. Pharmacol. exp. Ther. **155**, 211—222 (1967).

LEVINE, R.J., SJOERDSMA, A.: Dissociation of the decarboxylase-inhibiting and norepinephrine-depleting effects of a-methyl-dopa, a-ethyl-dopa, 4-bromo-3-hydroxy-benzyloxyamine and related substances. J. Pharmacol. exp. Ther. **146**, 42—47 (1964).

LEWANDER, T.: Displacement of brain and heart noradrenaline by p-hydroxynorephedrine after administration of p-hydroxyamphetamine. Acta pharmacol. (Kbh.) **29**, 20—32 (1971a).

— On the presence of p-hydroxynorephedrine in the rat brain and heart in relation to changes in catecholamine levels after administration of amphetamine. Acta pharmacol. (Kbh.) **29**, 33—48 (1971b).

LINDMAR, R., MUSCHOLL, E.: Die Wirkung von Pharmaka auf die Elimination von Noradrenalin aus der Perfusionsflüssigkeit und die Noradrenalinaufnahme in das isolierte Herz. Naunyn-Schmiedeberg's Arch. exp. Path. Pharmak. **247**, 469—492 (1964).

— — Die Aufnahme von a-Methylnoradrenalin in das isolierte Kaninchenherz und seine Freisetzung durch Reserpin und Guanethidin *in vivo*. Naunyn-Schmiedeberg's Arch. exp. Path. Pharmak. **249**, 529—548 (1965).

Lindmar, R., Muscholl, E., Rahn, K.H.: Effects of rest and physical activity on the urinary excretion of noradrenaline and α-methylnoradrenaline in human subjects treated with α-methyldopa. Europ. J. Pharmacol. **2**, 317—319 (1968).
— — Sprenger, E.: Funktionelle Bedeutung der Freisetzung von Dihydroxyephedrin und Dihydroxypseudoephedrin als „falschen" sympathischen Überträgerstoffen am Herzen. Naunyn-Schmiedeberg's Arch. Pharmak. exp. Path. **256**, 1—25 (1967).
Lovenberg, W., Weissbach, H., Udenfriend, S.: Aromatic L-amino-acid decarboxylase. J. biol. Chem. **237**, 89—93 (1962).
Lundborg, P., Stitzel, R.: Uptake of biogenic amines by two different mechanisms present in adrenergic granules. Brit. J. Pharmacol. **29**, 342—349 (1967a).
— — Effect of reserpine and protriptyline on the subcellular distribution of ^{3}H-metaraminol in the mouse heart. Brit. J. Pharmacol. **30**, 379—384 (1967b).
— — Stereospecificity and intracellular binding of metaraminol. Acta physiol. scand. **72**, 392—395 (1968a).
— — Studies on the relationship between adrenergic nerve function and granular uptake mechanisms. Brit. J. Pharmacol. **33**, 98—104 (1968b).
Maier, R., Maître, L., Staehelin, M.: Tyramine induced lipolysis following pretreatment of guinea pigs and rats with metaraminol. Biochem. Pharmacol. **16**, 1509—1515 (1967).
Maître, L.: Presence of α-methyl-Dopa metabolites in heart and brain of guinea pigs treated with α-methyl-tyrosine. Life Sci. **4**, 2249—2256 (1965).
— Staehelin, M.: Effect of α-methyl-DOPA on myocardial catecholamines. Experientia (Basel) **19**, 573—575 (1963).
— — Presence of α-methyl-noradrenaline ('corbasil') in the heart of guinea pigs treated with metaraminol ("Aramine"). Nature (Lond.) **206**, 723—724 (1965).
— — On the norepinephrine replacement by α-methyl-norepinephrine in the rat heart after treatment with α-methyl-DOPA. Experientia (Basel) **23**, 810—811 (1967).
Malik, K.U.: Effect of (±) dihydroxy ephedrine and (±) dihydroxy pseudoephedrine on adrenergic transmission in mesenteric arteries. Brit. J. Pharmacol. **41**, 352—360 (1971).
— Muscholl, E.: The effect of α-methyldopa on the vasoconstrictor responses of the rat mesenteric artery preparation to nerve stimulation. Arzneimittel-Forsch. (Drug Res.) **19**, 1111—1113 (1969a).
— — Effect of sympathomimetic amines on the response of the perfused mesenteric artery preparation to adrenergic nerve stimulation. Arzneimittel-Forsch. (Drug Res.) **19**, 1574 to 1579 (1969b).
Malmfors, T.: Studies on adrenergic nerves. The use of rat and mouse iris for direct observations on their physiology and pharmacology at cellular and subcellular levels. Acta physiol. scand. **64**, Suppl. 248 (1965).
Masuoka, D.T., Alcaraz, A., Hanson, E.: Studies on the formation of octopamine in mice and rats. Biochim. biophys. Acta (Amst.) **86**, 260—263 (1964).
McCurdy, R.L., Prange, Jr., A.L., Lipton, M.A., Cochrane, C.M.: Effects of α-methyldihydroxyphenylalanine, reserpine, and dihydroxyphenylalanine on pressor responses to norepinephrine and tyramine in humans. Proc. Soc. exp. Biol. (N.Y.) **116**, 1159—1163 (1964).
Mohammed, S., Gaffney, T.E., Yard, A.C., Gomez, H.: Effect of methyldopa, reserpine and guanethidine on hindleg vascular resistance. J. Pharmacol. exp. Ther. **160**, 300—307 (1968).
Molinoff, P., Axelrod, J.: Octopamine: normal occurrence in sympathetic nerves of rats. Science **164**, 428—429 (1969).
— Landsberg, L., Axelrod, J.: An enzymatic assay for octopamine and other β-hydroxylated phenethylamines. J. Pharmacol. exp. Ther. **170**, 253—261 (1969).
Murad, J.E., Shore, P.A.: Association between biochemical and behavioral actions of tricyclic antidepressants. Int. J. Neuropharmacol. **5**, 299—304 (1966).
Musacchio, J.M., Bhagat, B., Jackson, C.J., Kopin, I.J.: The effect of disulfiram on the restoration of the response to tyramine by dopamine and α-methyldopa in the reserpine-treated rat. J. Pharmacol. exp. Ther. **152**, 293—297 (1966a).
— Fischer, J.E., Kopin, I.J.: Subcellular distribution and release by sympathetic nerve stimulation of dopamine and α-methyldopamine. J. Pharmacol. exp. Ther. **152**, 51—55 (1966b).
— Goldstein, M.: Biosynthesis of norepinephrine and norsynephrine in the perfused rabbit heart. Biochem. Pharmacol. **12**, 1061—1063 (1963).
— Kopin, I.J., Weise, V.K.: Subcellular distribution of some sympathomimetic amines and their β-hydroxylated derivatives in the rat heart. J. Pharmacol. exp. Ther. **148**, 22—28 (1965a).
— Weise, V.K., Kopin, I.J.: Mechanism of norepinephrine binding. Nature (Lond.) **205**, 606—607 (1965b).

MUSCHOLL, E.: Biosynthese (aus α-Methyldopa), Aufnahme und Freisetzung von α-Methyladrenalin. Naunyn-Schmiedeberg's Arch. exp. Path. Pharmak. **251**, 162—163 (1965).
— Autonomic nervous system: Newer mechanisms of adrenergic blockade. Ann. Rev. Pharmacol. **6**, 107—128 (1966a).
— Release of catecholamines from the heart. In: Mechanisms of Release of Biogenic Amines. Eds. EULER, U.S. VON, ROSELL, S., UVNÄS, B. 247—260. Oxford: Pergamon Press 1966b.
— DREWS, E.-F., LINDMAR, R.: Aufnahme von threo-Corbadrin und seine Freisetzung als falsche sympathische Überträgersubstanz. Naunyn-Schmiedeberg's Arch. Pharmak. exp. Path. **260**, 180—181 (1968).
— LINDMAR, R.: Wirkungen von threo-1-(3,4-Dihydroxyphenyl)-1-hydroxy-2-aminopropan, dem Diastereomeren von Corbadrin. Naunyn-Schmiedeberg's Arch. Pharmak. exp. Path. **257**, 314—315 (1967).
— MAÎTRE, L.: Release by sympathetic stimulation of α-methylnoradrenaline stored in the heart after administration of α-methyldopa. Experientia (Basel) **19**, 658—659 (1963).
— RAHN, K.H.: Nachweis von α-Methylnoradrenalin im Harn von Hypertonikern während einer Behandlung mit α-Methyldopa. Klin. Wschr. **44**, 1412—1413 (1966).
— — Über den Nachweis und die Bedeutung von α-Methylnoradrenalin im Harn von Hypertonikern bei Verabreichung von α-Methyldopa. Pharmacol. Clin. **1**, 19—29 (1968).
— SPRENGER, E.: Vergleichende Untersuchung der Blutdruckwirkung, Aufnahme und Speicherung von Dihydroxyephedrin (α-Methyladrenalin) und Dihydroxypseudoephedrin. Naunyn-Schmiedeberg's Arch. Pharmak. exp. Path. **254**, 109—124 (1966).
— WEBER, E.: Die Hemmung der Aufnahme von α-Methylnoradrenalin in das Herz durch sympathomimetische Amine. Naunyn-Schmiedeberg's Arch. exp. Path. Pharmak. **252**, 134—143 (1965).
NEFF, N.H., NGAI, S.H., WANG, C.T., COSTA, E.: Calculation of the rate of catecholamine synthesis from the rate of conversion of tyramine-^{14}C to catecholamines. Effect of adrenal demedullation on synthesis rate. Molec. Pharmacol. **5**, 90—99 (1969).
OATES, J.A., GILLESPIE, L., UDENFRIEND, S., SJOERDSMA, A.: Decarboxylase inhibition and blood pressure reduction by α-methyl-3,4-dihydroxy-D,L-phenylalanine. Science **131**, 1890—1891 (1960).
PALM, D., LANGENECKERT, W., HOLTZ, P.: Bedeutung der N- und α-Methylierung für die Affinität von Brenzcatechinaminen zu den adrenergischen Receptoren. Naunyn-Schmiedeberg's Arch. Pharmak. exp. Path. **258**, 128—149 (1967).
PATIL, P.N., JACOBOWITZ, D.: Steric aspects of adrenergic drugs. IX. Pharmacologic and histochemical studies on isomers of cobefrin (α-methylnorepinephrine). J. Pharmacol. exp. Ther. **161**, 279—295 (1968).
— LAPIDUS, J.B., TYE, A.: Steric aspects of adrenergic drugs. J. pharm. Sci. **59**, 1205—1234 (1970).
PATON, D.M.: Cation and metabolic requirements for retention of metaraminol by rat uterine horns. Brit. J. Pharmacol. **33**, 277—286 (1968).
— Effects of Na^+ and K^+ on the uptake of metaraminol by rabbit ventricular slices. Brit. J. Pharmacol. **41**, 65—75 (1971).
PETTINGER, W.A., SPECTOR, S., HORWITZ, D., SJOERDSMA, A.: Restoration of tyramine pressor responses in reserpine-treated animals by methyldopa and its amine metabolites. Proc. Soc. exp. Biol. (N.Y.) **118**, 988—993 (1965).
PHILIPPU, A., SCHÜMANN, H.J.: Effect of α-methyldopa, α-methyldopamine, and α-methylnorepinephrine on the norepinephrine content of the isolated heart. Life Sci. **4**, 2039 to 2046 (1965).
— — Aufnahme von α-Methyldopamin und α-Methylnoradrenalin in die Noradrenalin speichernden Herzgranula. Experientia (Basel) **22**, 119—120 (1966).
— — Bildung und Speicherung von α-Methylnoradrenalin. Naunyn-Schmiedeberg's Arch. Pharmak. exp. Path. **256**, 183—195 (1967).
PÖCH, G.R., KOPIN, I.J.: The rôle of octopamine in tachyphylaxis to tyramine. Biochem. Pharmacol. **15**, 210—212 (1966).
PORTER, C.C., TITUS, D.C.: Distribution and metabolism of methyldopa in the rat. J. Pharmacol. exp. Ther. **139**, 77—87 (1963).
— TORCHIANA, M.L., TOTARO, J.A., STONE, C.A.: Displacement of norepinephrine from the rat heart by ^{14}C-metaraminol. Biochem. Pharmacol. **16**, 2117—2124 (1967).
— TOTARO, J.A., BURCIN, A.: The relation between radioactivity and norepinephrine concentrations in the brains and hearts of mice following administration of labelled methyldopa or 6-hydroxydopamine. J. Pharmacol. exp. Ther. **150**, 17—22 (1965).
— — LEIBY, C.M.: Some biochemical effects of α-methyl-3,4-dihydroxyphenylalanine and related compounds in mice. J. Pharmacol. exp. Ther. **134**, 139—145 (1961).
POTTER, L.T., AXELROD, J.: Studies on the storage of norepinephrine and the effect of drugs. J. Pharmacol. exp. Ther. **140**, 199—206 (1963).

POTTER, L.T., AXELROD, J., KOPIN, I.J.: Differential binding and release of norepinephrine and tachyphylaxis. Biochem. Pharmacol. **11**, 254—256 (1962).
PRESCOTT, L.F., BUHS, R.P., BEATTIE, J.O., SPETH, O.C., TRENNER, N.R., LASAGNA, L.: Combined clinical and metabolic study of the effects of α-methyldopa on hypertensive patients. Circulation **34**, 308—321 (1966).
PRUSS, T.P., MAENGWYN-DAVIES, G.D., WURZEL, M.: Comparison of effects of aromatic sympathomimetic amines on rabbit aortic strip and rabbit blood pressure. J. Pharmacol. exp. Ther. **147**, 76—85 (1965).
RAHN, K.H., GILFRICH, H.J., OLBERMANN, M.: Ein Vergleich der Kreislaufwirkungen von Noradrenalin und α-Methylnoradrenalin als Studie über den Wirkungsmechanismus von α-Methyldopa. Verh. dtsch. Ges. inn. Med. **76**, 937—939 (1970).
ROSSUM, J.M., VAN: The relation between chemical structure and biological activity. J. Pharm. Pharmacol. **15**, 285—316 (1963).
— HURKMANS, J.A.T.M.: Reversal of the effect of α-methyldopa by m.a.o. inhibitors. J. Pharm. Pharmacol. **15**, 493—499 (1963).
SAARI, W.S., RAAB, A.W., ENGELHARDT, E.L.: The stereoisomers of α-(1-aminoethyl)-*m*-hydroxybenzyl alcohol. J. Med. Chem. **11**, 1115—1117 (1968).
SALMON, G.K., IRESON, J.D.: A correlation between the hypotensive action of methyldopa and its depression of peripheral sympathetic function. Arch. int. Pharmacodyn. **183**, 60—64 (1970).
SCHAUMANN, O.: Über Oxy-Ephedrine. Naunyn-Schmiedeberg's Arch. exp. Path. Pharmak. **160**, 127—176 (1931).
— Zur Pharmakologie der optischen Isomeren des 3,4-Dioxy-nor-Ephedrins (Corbasil). Medizin und Chemie **3**, 383—392. Leverkusen: Bayer 1936.
SCHMITT, H., PÉTILLOT, N.: Influence du remplacement de la noradrénaline par des faux médiateurs et de l'inhibition de la synthèse sur l'excitabilité sympathique. J. Pharmacol. (Paris) **1**, 183—194 (1970).
SCHÜMANN, H.J., GROBECKER, H.: Nachweis und Lokalisation von α-Methylnoradrenalin in Meerschweinchenorganen nach Vorbehandlung mit α-Methyl-Dopa. Naunyn-Schmiedeberg's Arch. exp. Path. Pharmak. **247**, 297—298 (1964).
— — SCHMIDT, K.: Über die Wirkung von α-Methyl-Dopa auf den Brenzcatechinamingehalt von Meerschweinchenorganen. Naunyn-Schmiedeberg's Arch. exp. Path. Pharmak. **251**, 48—61 (1965).
SEDVALL, G.C., WEISE, V.K., KOPIN, I.J.: The rate of norepinephrine synthesis measured *in vivo* during short intervals; influence of adrenergic nerve impulse activity. J. Pharmacol. exp. Ther. **159**, 274—282 (1968).
SHORE, P.A., ALPERS, H.S.: Fluorometric estimation of metaraminol and related compounds. Life Sci. **3**, 551—554 (1964).
— BUSFIELD, D., ALPERS, H.S.: Binding and release of metaraminol: Mechanism of norepinephrine depletion by α-methyl-*m*-tyrosine and related agents. J. Pharmacol. exp. Ther. **146**, 194—199 (1964).
SJOERDSMA, A., STUDNITZ, W., VON: Dopamine-β-oxidase activity in man, using hydroxyamphetamine as substrate. Brit. J. Pharmacol. **20**, 278—284 (1963).
— VENDSALU, A., ENGELMAN, K.: Studies on the metabolism and mechanism of action of methyldopa. Circulation **28**, 492—502 (1963).
SMITH, C.B.: The role of monoamine oxidase in the intraneuronal metabolism of norepinephrine released by indirectly acting sympathomimetic amines or by adrenergic nerve stimulation. J. Pharmacol. exp. Ther. **151**, 207—220 (1966).
SOGANI, R.K., SHARMA, V.N.: Modification of vascular actions of sympathomimetic drugs by methyldopa. Arch. int. Pharmacodyn. **159**, 135—139 (1966).
SOURKES, T.L.: Inhibition of dihydroxyphenylalanine decarboxylase by derivatives of phenylalanine. Arch. Biochem. Biophys. **51**, 444—456 (1954).
— The action of α-methyldopa in the brain. Brit. med. Bull. **21**, 66—69 (1965).
— MURPHY, G.F., CHAVEZ, B., ZIELINSKA, M.: The action of some α-methyl and other amino acids on cerebral catecholamines. J. Neurochem. **8**, 109—115 (1961).
SPECTOR, S., GORDON, R., SJOERDSMA, A., UDENFRIEND, S.: End-product inhibition of tyrosine hydroxylase as a possible mechanism for regulation of norepinephrine synthesis. Molec. Pharmacol. **3**, 549—555 (1967).
— SJOERDSMA, A., UDENFRIEND, S.: Blockade of endogenous norepinephrine synthesis by α-methyl-tyrosine, an inhibitor of tyrosine hydroxylase. J. Pharmacol. exp. Ther. **147**, 86—95 (1965).
STJÄRNE, L., LISHAJKO, F.: Localization of different steps in noradrenaline synthesis to different fractions of a bovine splenic nerve homogenate. Biochem. Pharmacol. **16**, 1719—1728 (1967).

STONE, C.A., PORTER, C.C.: Biochemistry and pharmacology of methyldopa and some related structures. Advanc. Drug Res. **4**, 71—93 (1967).

— ROSS, C.A., WENGER, H.C., LUDDEN, C.T., BLESSING, J.A., TOTARO, J.A., PORTER, C.C.: Effects of α-methyl-3,4-dihydroxyphenylalanine (Methyldopa), reserpine and related agents on some vascular responses in the dog. J. Pharmacol. exp. Ther. **136**, 80—88 (1962).

— STAVORSKI, J.M., LUDDEN, C.T., WENGER, H.C., ROSS, C.A., TOTARO, J.A., PORTER, C.C.: Comparison of some pharmacological effects of certain 6-substituted dopamine derivatives with reserpine, guanethidine and metaraminol. J. Pharmacol. exp. Ther. **142**, 147—156 (1963).

STOTT, A.W., ROBINSON, R.: Urinary phenols in patients treated with α-methyldopa. J. Pharm. Pharmacol. **15**, 773—774 (1963).

— — The effects of α-methyldopa on excretion of noradrenaline metabolites. J. Pharm. Pharmacol. **19**, 690—693 (1967).

SUGARMAN, S.R., MARGOLIUS, H.S., GAFFNEY, T.E., MOHAMMED, S.: Effect of methyldopa on chronotropic responses to cardioaccelerator nerve stimulation in dogs. J. Pharmacol. exp. Ther. **162**, 115—120 (1968).

SUGRUE, M.F., SHORE, P.A.: The mode of sodium dependency of the adrenergic neuron amine carrier. Evidence for a second, sodium-dependent, optically specific and reserpine-sensitive system. J. Pharmacol. exp. Ther. **170**, 239—245 (1969).

SWAMY, V.C., TYE, A., LA PIDUS, J.B., PATIL, P.N.: Steric aspects of adrenergic drugs. XIII. Norepinephrine potentiating effects of isomers of sympathomimetic amine in rat vas deferens and atria. Arch. int. Pharmacodyn. **182**, 24—31 (1969).

THOA, N.B., ECCLESTON, D., AXELROD, J.: The accumulation of C^{14}-serotonin in the guinea-pig vas deferens. J. Pharmacol. exp. Ther. **169**, 68—73 (1969).

THOENEN, H.: Bildung und funktionelle Bedeutung adrenerger Ersatztransmitter. Berlin-Heidelberg-New York: Springer 1969.

— HAEFELY, W., GEY, K.E., HÜRLIMANN, A.: Diminished effects of sympathetic nerve stimulation in cats pretreated with disulfiram; liberation of dopamine as sympathetic transmitter. Life Sci. **4**, 2033—2038 (1965).

— — — — The effect of α-methyl-tyrosine on peripheral sympathetic transmission. Life Sci. **5**, 723—730 (1966a).

— — — — Quantitative aspects of the replacement of norepinephrine by dopamine as a sympathetic transmitter after inhibition of dopamine-β-hydroxylase by disulfiram. J. Pharmacol. exp. Ther. **156**, 246—251 (1967a).

— — — — Liberation of α-methyldopamine as a "false" sympathetic transmitter after pretreatment of cats with α-methyldopa and disulfiram. Naunyn-Schmiedeberg's Arch. Pharmak. exp. Path. **258**, 181—196 (1967b).

— — — — Diminished effect of sympathetic nerve stimulation in cats pretreated with 5-hydroxydopa; formation and liberation of false adrenergic transmitters. Naunyn-Schmiedeberg's Arch. Pharmak. exp. Path. **259**, 17—33 (1967c).

— — HÄUSLER, G., HÜRLIMANN, A.: Formation of a "false" adrenergic transmitter in cats pretreated with 4-methoxy-3,5-dihydroxyphenylalanine and its effects on postganglionic transmission. J. Pharmacol. exp. Ther. **162**, 70—79 (1968).

— HÜRLIMANN, A., GEY, K.F., HAEFELY, W.: Liberation of p-hydroxynorephedrine from cat spleen by sympathetic nerve stimulation after pretreatment with amphetamine. Life Sci. **5**, 1715—1722 (1966b).

— — HAEFELY, W.: The effect of sympathetic nerve stimulation on volume, vascular resistance, and norepinephrine output in the isolated perfused spleen of the cat, and its modification by cocaine. J. Pharmacol. exp. Ther. **143**, 57—63 (1964).

— TRANZER, J.P.: Functional importance of subcellular distribution of false adrenergic transmitters. Progr. Brain Res. in the press (1971).

TORCHIANA, M.L., PORTER, C.C., STONE, C.A.: Relation between molecular configuration and certain biological actions of α-methyldopamine and α-methyl-meta-tyramine and their β-hydroxylated products α-methylnorepinephrine and metaraminol. Arch. int. Pharmacodyn. **174**, 118—134 (1968).

— — — HANSON, H.M.: Some biochemical and pharmacological actions of α-methylphenylalanine. Biochem. Pharmacol. **19**, 1601—1614 (1970).

— WENGER, H.C., STAVORSKI, J., LUDDEN, C.T., STONE, C.A.: Effect of methyldopa and related agents on pressor responses to tyramine in reserpine-pretreated rats and dogs. J. Pharmacol. exp. Ther. **151**, 242—252 (1966).

TRENDELENBURG, U.: The effect of sympathetic nerve stimulation on isolated atria of guinea pigs and rabbits pretreated with reserpine. J. Pharmacol. exp. Ther. **147**, 313—318 (1965).

— MUSKUS, A., FLEMING, W.W., GOMEZ ALONSO DE LA SIERRA, G.: Modification by reserpine of the action of sympathomimetic amines in spinal cats; a classification of sympathomimetic amines. J. Pharmacol. exp. Ther. **138**, 170—180 (1962).

TRINKER, F.R.: The significance of the relative potencies of noradrenaline and α-methylnoradrenaline for the mode of action of α-methyldopa. J. Pharm. Pharmacol. **23**, 306—308 (1971).

UDENFRIEND, S.: Physiological regulation of noradrenaline biosynthesis. In: Adrenergic Neurotransmission. Eds. WOLSTENHOLME, G.E.W., O'CONNOR, M. 3—11. London: J. & A. Churchill 1968.

— ZALTZMAN-NIRENBERG, P.: On the mechanism of the norepinephrine release produced by α-methyl-meta-tyrosine. J. Pharmacol. exp. Ther. **138**, 194—199 (1962).

— — GORDON, R., SPECTOR, S.: Evaluation of the biochemical effects produced *in vivo* by inhibitors of the three enzymes involved in norepinephrine biosynthesis. Molec. Pharmacol. **2**, 95—105 (1966).

— — NAGATSU, T.: Inhibitors of purified beef adrenal tyrosine hydroxylase. Biochem. Pharmacol. **14**, 837—845 (1965).

VAN ORDEN, L.S., BENSCH, K.G., GIARMAN, N.J.: Histochemical and functional relationships of catecholamines in adrenergic nerve endings. II. Extravesicular norepinephrine. J. Pharmacol. exp. Ther. **155**, 428—439 (1967).

VARMA, D.R., BENFEY, B.G.: Antagonism of reserpine-induced subsensitivity to tyramine by α-methyldopa. J. Pharmacol. exp. Ther. **141**, 310—313 (1963).

WALDECK, B.: On the interaction of threo-^{3}H-α-methylnoradrenaline with the uptake and storage mechanisms of the adrenergic neuron. Europ. J. Pharmacol. **2**, 208—213 (1967).

— On the stereospecificity of the β-hydroxylation of α-methyldopamine. Europ. J. Pharmacol. **5**, 114—116 (1968).

— Failure to demonstrate monoamine oxidase inhibition by glyceryl trinitrate *in vivo*. Acta pharmacol. (Kbh.) **28**, 406—412 (1970).

WEBER, E., MUSCHOLL, E.: Der Einfluß verschiedener Pharmaka auf die Elimination von α-Methylnoradrenalin aus der Perfusionsflüssigkeit des isolierten Kaninchenherzens. Naunyn-Schmiedeberg's Arch. exp. Path. Pharmak. **251**, 161—162 (1965).

WEBER, L.J.: Drug interactions between disulfiram and α-methyldopa and related agents in reserpine-pretreated rats. Proc. Soc. exp. Biol. (N.Y.) **123**, 349—352 (1966).

WEINER, N., SELVARATNAM, I.: The effect of tyramine on the synthesis of norepinephrine. J. Pharmacol. exp. Ther. **161**, 21—33 (1968).

WEISSBACH, H., LOVENBERG, W., UDENFRIEND, S.: Enzymatic decarboxylation of α-methyl amino acids. Biochem. biophys. Res. Commun. **3**, 225—227 (1960).

WERLE, E., SELL, J.: Über die fermentative Decarboxylierung von Mono- und Dioxyphenylserinen. Biochem. Z. **326**, 110—122 (1954).

YOUNG, J.A., EDWARDS, K.D.G.: Studies on the absorption, metabolism and excretion of methyldopa and other catechols and their influence on amino acid transport in rats. J. Pharmacol. exp. Ther. **145**, 102—112 (1964).

Chapter 15

Electrophysiology of the Adrenergic Neuron

W. Haefely

With 14 Figures

Introduction

This chapter deals with two aspects of the adrenergic neuron: a) with its electrical properties in the resting and active state, and b) with electrical events induced in this neuron by chemical agents. This review is restricted to the *(peripheral) sympathetic adrenergic neuron*, since the adrenergic neurons of the central nervous system, whose topography is actually being studied intensively, have, for obvious technical reasons, so far escaped investigations by electrophysiological methods.

The peripheral adrenergic neuron — the last efferent neuron in the sympathetic pathway — usually shares the fate of the motoneuron in being artificially divided into two parts by most biologists. Indeed, an impressive number of physiologists, pharmacologists, biochemists and morphologists is investigating exclusively the most terminal part of the adrenergic neuron and especially its transmitter, noradrenaline. These investigators usually work on tissues and organs rich in adrenergic nerve endings but separated from their proximal axons and cell bodies, the adrenergic ganglion cells. Conversely, many physiologists and pharmacologists interested in the mechanisms of synaptic transmission of nervous impulses are using various preparations of sympathetic ganglia; however, the nerve terminals (and the adrenergic effector organs) serve at best as indicators for the activity of the adrenergic cell bodies. An attempt will be made in this chapter to emphasize the *functional entity of the adrenergic neuron*, although it will be unavoidable to have to treat separately the electrical properties of the soma-dendritic, the axonal and the terminal part of the neuron. It will become clear that electrophysiological studies of the adrenergic nerve terminal are only at their very beginning. The danger had, therefore, to be avoided, to make of the present chapter but another review of the synaptic transmission in autonomic ganglia, a topic on which excellent reviews have appeared in recent years (Gyermek, 1967; Trendelenburg, 1967; Tauc, 1967; Volle, 1966a, b, 1969; Kharkevich, 1967). Hence, in the following pages, fundamental electrophysiological data from autonomic ganglion cells will be treated only as far as they do or may add to our understanding of the actions of chemical agents on this and the other parts of the adrenergic neuron. Whereas the effects of orthodromic stimulation on adrenergic ganglion cells will be treated in some detail, the events taking place in presynaptic structures are not the subject of this review. It will become apparent that there are still enormous gaps in our knowledge of the interaction of chemical agents with the excitable membrane of the adrenergic nerve terminal.

I. The Problem of Identifying Adrenergic Neurons in Electrophysiological Investigations

Electrophysiological investigations are carried out either on a population of neurons (e.g. recordings of potential changes from the surface of sympathetic ganglia, of synchronous compound action potentials form postganglionic sympathetic nerve trunks and of asynchronous orthodromic or antidromic discharges of a varying and mostly unknown number of fibres within such a nerve) or still rather exceptionally on single neurons within a sympathetic ganglion or a postganglionic sympathetic nerve. Electrophysiological studies in mammals have been carried out mostly in the superior cervical, stellate, celiac and hypogastric ganglia and axons arising from these. There is a large body of evidence both from pharmacological studies (e.g. AIKEN and REIT, 1969) and from morphological investigations using chemical (e.g. cholinacetylase determinations: BUCKLEY et al., 1967), histochemical (e.g. cholinesterase staining: MANOCHA and SHANTA, 1969), fluorescence and electron microscopic techniques (HAMBERGER and NORBERG, 1963, 1965; HAMBERGER et al., 1963, 1964, 1965; NORBERG and HAMBERGER, 1964; NORBERG, 1967; JACOBOWITZ and WOODWARD, 1968) that *sympathetic ganglia and so-called postganglionic sympathetic nerves always contain — although to a largely varying degree — also non-adrenergic nerve cell bodies and axons respectively*. Therefore, results obtained with the macroelectrode technique on sympathetic ganglia or nerves are not, in a strict sense, representative of adrenergic neurons. Careful conclusions from such investigations concerning the properties of adrenergic neurons are, however, not invalidated if adrenergic fibres prevail over non-adrenergic ones and if due attention is given to the fact that one is dealing with a mixture of possibly unlike elements. A similar situation is encountered with microtechniques on single cells, which of course can yield more detailed information on bioelectric properties but where the particular cell investigated has never been identified as adrenergic. One possible exception to this may be represented by the sympathetic chain ganglia of frog and toad, where fluorescence microscopy has not revealed the existence of non-adrenergic neurons (NORBERG and MCISAAC, 1967). In this species, however, the adrenergic neurons contain adrenaline instead of noradrenaline (GROBECKER, 1966).

II. Electrophysiological Techniques Used for the Study of Adrenergic Neurons

1. Intraganglionic Part: Soma and Dendrites (SD[1]), Axon Hillock and Initial Segment (IS)

Favoured preparations for studies with the macroelectrode technique are sympathetic ganglia of not too small a size, which are easily accessible and where the pre- and post-ganglionic fibres run in one or several well separated trunks, long enough to be placed on stimulating and recording electrodes. For *in situ* experiments, the existence of ganglia with a separate arterial blood supply are a great advantage, as this permits the addition into the arterial inflow of chemical substances in amounts large enough to reach high concentrations within the ganglion but too small to produce indirect effects on transmission, e.g. by releasing endogenous agents from the rest of the body or producing undesired effects on the whole animal. Separate arterial and venous blood vessels are a prerequisite for setting up a ganglion as an *in situ* perfused preparation. JONES and QUILLIAM (1967) have devised an elegant method for alternate perfusion of the cat's superior cervical ganglion with Locke solution or with the cat's own blood in order to prevent the edema which develops after perfusion with Locke solution for 1 hour. Depending on the special aspect of the problem to be investigated, it is important to work either on ganglia where the afferent nerve contains preganglionic fibres which all end within the ganglion with synaptic contacts or on ganglia transversed by "through fibres" (either preganglionic fibres forming synapses beyond the particular ganglion or postganglionic fibres which have their cell body central to the ganglion). For *in vitro* studies with isolated ganglia maintained in an incubation medium, ganglia of smaller size are preferable where diffusional exchange of solutes between the medium and inner cells enable the latter to survive. Isolated superior cervical ganglia of rats have been successfully used for the simultaneous study of metabolism and electrical activity (LARRABEE, 1958; DOLIVO, 1966; HÄRKÖNEN et al., 1969).

1 Abbreviations see page 715.

a) Extracellular Techniques

A technique used with great success since the pioneering work of J.C. ECCLES (1935 a, b, 1943; see also LLOYD, 1937) for obtaining information on the electrical events taking place in a population of cells within an autonomic ganglion is the recording of potential changes from its surface. With one "non polarizable" electrode on the ganglion surface (either by direct contact or through an electrolyte conductor) and a second similar one on the crushed end of a postganglionic nerve, one obtains a rather selective lead from those cells projecting into the particular postganglionic branch. Direct coupled amplification permits the recording not only of rapid electrical events in the ganglion such as the action potentials, but also of very slow changes of the potential difference between the surface of the ganglion and the inactive end of the postganglionic nerve which are produced by changes in the transmembrane potential of ganglion cells (possibly also of other cells within the ganglion). It is customary to speak of "ganglionic negativity" or "ganglionic depolarization" when the lead from the ganglionic surface becomes negative in respect to the reference electrode on the postganglionic nerve and, conversely, of "ganglionic positivity" or "ganglionic hyperpolarization". The action potential recorded from the surface of the ganglion in response to a synchronous preganglionic or postganglionic volley is virtually identical in its shape and time-course (when allowance is made for the temporal dispersion of individual action potentials due to the different conduction velocities and intraganglionic lengths of fibres) with that recorded from a single ganglion cell with an intracellular microelectrode. With the external recording, the polarity of the electrical signals is the reverse and their amplitude is of course smaller — at best one fifth — of the intracellularly recorded one. The potential changes recorded from the surface of the ganglion can be considered formally as the algebraic sum of the potential changes occurring simultaneously in the large population of individual ganglion cells. Hence, the surface recording technique yields the same qualitative information on bioelectric phenomena in ganglionic cells as does the intracellular technique, as long as the changes occur simultaneously in a large part of the cell population being studied. It remains to be mentioned that surface recordings, similar to those used with autonomic ganglia, are valuable tools for studying potential changes even in much more complex structures, e.g. those occurring in afferent endings and motoneurons of the spinal cord.

A modification of the surface recording technique has been introduced by PASCOE (1956). It consists of using the fluid bathing the isolated ganglion as a *movable fluid surface electrode*. Changing the level of the bathing fluid relative to the ganglion permits the recording of potential changes along the axis of the ganglion.

A further modification of the macroelectrode technique is the adaptation of the *sucrose-gap* arrangement for the isolated sympathetic ganglion (KOSTERLITZ and WALLIS, 1966; KOSTERLITZ et al., 1968; NISHI and KOKETSU, 1968b). Although the amplitudes of the ganglionic action potentials recorded by the sucrose-gap method are not considerably higher than when using conventional surface electrodes, the arrangement has some advantages, e.g. the possibility to study synaptic potentials without the use of ganglionic blocking agents (KOSTERLITZ et al., 1967) and membrane potential changes in the presynaptic arborization (KOKETSU and NISHI, 1968).

Extracellular recording with microelectrodes has been used only exceptionally (THERMAN et al., 1940; SKOK, 1968). This method is unlikely to yield more information on the electrical activity of ganglion cells than the surface macroelectrode but could be helpful in studying presynaptic events within the ganglion.

b) Intracellular Recording

Adrenergic ganglion cells are rather difficult to impale with intracellular microelectrodes because of their small size (see Table 1) and because, in larger ganglia, they are surrounded by a resistant connective tissue. Almost all microelectrode studies have been carried out on isolated ganglia (Table 1). Successful penetrations have been reported in different ganglia of mammals and amphibia.

2. Non-terminal Axon

Conventional macromethods for the recording of monophasic compound action potentials of nerve trunks are useful for measuring conduction velocities in adrenergic nerves. The sucrose-gap method makes it possible to record changes in the resting membrane potential of postganglionic sympathetic nerves (KOSTERLITZ et al., 1968). Extracellular recordings from single fibres in postganglionic sympathetic nerves have been reported (BRONK et al., 1938); they are useful for

Table 1. *Some electrical properties*

Ganglion	Species	Resting pot. (mV)	Time constant (msec)	Cell Resistance (MΩ)	Specific resistance (Ωcm²)	Specific capacitance (μF/cm²)
thoracic chain	frog	48 ± 8.8	12.8 ± 4.7	100 ± 46		4.9
thoracic chain	frog	52		49 ± 19		3.6
thoracic chain	frog	44 (38—55)		47 (30—68)		
lumbar chain	toad	65 (B-cells) 40—50 (C-cells)	8.0 (B-cells) 6.6 (C-cells)	11.5 (B-cells) 16 (C-cells)	414 (B-cells) 151 (C-cells)	21 (B-cells) 47 (C-cells)
lumbar chain	frog	65 (50—80)	10.6	20	456	24
lumbar chain	frog	54 ± 2.8				
superior cervical	rat	45—90	2.7 (1.2—5.7)	39.4 ± 3.2	1800	1.6
superior cervical	guinea-pig	45—90	4.4 (2.5—5.7)	40.6 ± 4.3	2300	2.1
pelvic	guinea-pig	50 (40—70)	8—20	60—160		1—2
pelvic	guinea-pig	40—70	9.6 (6.0—18.0)	124 (50—240)		
thoracic	guinea-pig	50—70	9.11 ± 0.91	55.5 ± 4.8		
superior cervical	rabbit	65—80				
superior cervical	rabbit					
superior cervical*	rabbit	69 (40—110)				
superior cervical	rabbit	40—50				
superior cervical*	rabbit	—68.6 ± 2.2				
stellate	cat	40 50				
ciliary	chick	50—70				
spinal ganglion	frog	72 (57—85)		15.6		
spinal motoneuron	frog	61 (53—77)		2.8		
spinal motoneuron	cat	60—80	2.5	0.8	~ 400	~ 6

* *in situ*

References: 1: HUNT and NELSON (1965), 2: HUNT and RIKER (1966), 3: STONEY and MACHNE (1969), 4: NISHI et al. (1965), 5: NISHI and KOKETSU (1960), 6: BLACKMAN et al. (1963a), 7: PERRI et al. (1970a), 8: PERRI et al. (1970a), 9: BLACKMAN and HOLMAN (1967; HOLMAN et al. (1969), 10: BLACKMAN et al. (1969a), 11: BLACKMAN and PURVES (1969),

the study of the firing rate and pattern of single neurons (GREEN and HEFFRON, 1968), but add little to our knowledge of basic electrical properties of the membrane of adrenergic nerve axons. Intracellular recordings from adrenergic nerve axons have so far not been carried out; accidental impalements of intraganglionic axons have been reported (R.M. ECCLES, 1955).

3. Axon Terminals

The "axon terminal" or "nerve ending" is an ill-defined part of the adrenergic neuron. In the case of the motoneuron, the terminal axon is the morphologically circumscribed short part extending from the point where the axon looses its myelin sheath up to the very thin branchings forming morphologically distinct junctions with the muscle fibre membrane. Microelectrodes can be placed in the region of the end plate under direct vision in the isolated nerve-muscle preparation and can then permit the direct study of electrical events taking place in the motor nerve endings (see KATZ, 1966, 1969). The brilliant studies carried out with this method have provided important information on the electro-secretory coupling mechanism in the motor nerve endings. The possibility to elucidate, by a similar approach, the electrical events responsible for transmitter release at adrenergic nerve "endings" still seems very remote. There are no circumscribed regions in adrenergically innervated end organs where adrenergic neuromuscular junctions are concentrated and toward which microelectrodes could be directed. Morphologically, the junctional sites do not show specialized formations comparable to the motor end-plate complex. It seems that the adrenergic axons form more or less "en passant" contacts, e.g. with smooth muscle fibres. At these sites, the adren-

of sympathetic ganglion cells

Rheobase	Critical threshold depolarization direct	orthodromic	Orthodromic spike amplitude	Spike duration	Maximum cell diameter	Effective membrane area	volume	Ref.
10^{-9} A	(mV)	(mV)	(mV)	(msec)	(μm)	(cm^2)	(cm^3)	
			76 ± 24		largest: 37.5—47.5			1
3.1								2
1.8			66 (45—77)					3
			90 (B-cells)	2.5 (B-cells)	35 (B-cells)			4
			75 (C-cells)	4.5 (C-cells)	18 (C-cells)			4
	25.3 (16—31)	26.1 (18—35)	85			2×10^{-5}		5
		22 ± 3.4	78 ± 1.5					6
1.1		12.2	75.4 ± 1.63 (55—110)	3.6		4.4×10^{-5}		7
1.1		16.9	76.2 ± 1.65	3.0		5.6 ± 10^{-5}		8
2	15—20	15—20						9
	(one cell)							
1.2 (0.5—3)	15.5 (11.5—20)	max. 25	72.25 (67—78)		20—30			10
1—3		10—15	55—90	1.5—2.5			max. 10^{-8}	11
		15—20	70—96	4—7				12
		25—40						13
2.2		20 (5—40)	77 (40—130)	3.1 (0.6—7)				14
								15
								16
			45—78	2—4				17
								18
2.3			100					19
2.4			83					20
	10				~70	5×10^{-4}	2.5×10^{-7}	21

12: ECCLES, R.M. (1955), 13: ECCLES, R.M. (1963), 14: ERULKAR and WOODWARD (1968), 15: LIBET and TOSAKA (1969), 16: WOODWARD et al. (1969), 17: SKOK (1963), 18: STONEY and MACHNE (1969), 19: STONEY and MACHNE (1969), 20: PASCOE (1956), 21: ECCLES (1957).

ergic nerve fibres are enlarged ("varicose") and contain a great number of synaptic vesicles; the Schwann cell processes, which envelop the axon along its whole length, show distinct discontinuities at these varicosities, where transmitter release is therefore reasonably assumed to occur. A single adrenergic nerve axon may possibly form several varicose enlargements along its terminal part and eventually end in a terminal varicosity (BENNETT and MERRILLEES, 1966). *In this chapter, the term "adrenergic nerve ending" will be used to define that terminal part of the axon which forms one or more varicosities and where transmitter release is assumed to occur.*

In view of the difficulties in recording directly from single adrenergic nerve endings, indirect ways have to be sought in order to get at least some insight into the excitable membrane of the endings. Two such approaches are the testing of the electrical and chemical excitability of the endings under physiological conditions and under the influence of drugs. WALL (1958) described a technique which provides information on the electrical excitability of afferent nerve endings within the spinal cord and which allows phases of increased and decreased membrane potentials (hyper- and depolarizations) to be established, generating slow dorsal root potentials and accompanying alterations in synaptic transmission. The method consists of observing the height of antidromic action potentials in dorsal root fibres occurring when short pulses of constant intensity are applied through fine electrodes inserted into the layers of the corresponding afferent terminals. This method has so far not been used for the adrenergic nerve endings; it is questionable whether it would permit the localization of changes in excitability along the adrenergic axon in view of the absence of sufficiently distinct layers of true endings in adrenergically innervated end organs.

The finding that a) chemical agents may excite the terminal part of adrenergic neurons sufficiently to induce the generation of action potentials which propagate centrally and therefore can be recorded in proximal parts of a nerve (FERRY, 1963a), and b) that this antidromic induced activity was absent after treatment with 6-hydroxydopamine (HAEUSLER et al., 1968a) which selectively destroys adrenergic nerve "endings" (TRANZER and THOENEN, 1968), made the determination of chemical excitability of adrenergic nerve endings a useful tool for the study of some of their membrane properties.

III. Electrophysiological Properties of the Adrenergic Nerve Cell Body

1. The Resting Neuron

a) Resting Membrane Potential

Values for resting membrane potential as reported in the literature are summarized in Table 1.

The membrane potential of ganglion cells in different sympathetic ganglia of amphibia and mammals was between 40 and 70 mV, although some cells with higher potentials were occasionally found. Corresponding values in frog and cat spinal motoneurons were usually higher by 10—20 mV; this difference is not necessarily a real one if one considers the greater difficulties encountered with the impalement of the small sympathetic ganglion cells. Small shunts due to incomplete sealing of the penetrated highly resistant membrane around the electrode tip would significantly reduce the measured membrane potential. Therefore, most investigators considered the highest measured values to be closer to the real transmembrane potential of intact cells than the mean of their individual figures.

The dependence of the resting membrane potential on the *external* K^+ concentration was studied in frog sympathetic paravertebral ganglion cells with intracellular electrodes (BLACKMAN et al., 1963b) and in rabbit superior cervical ganglion with the sucrose-gap method (KOSTERLITZ et al., 1968). In both studies, there was a linear and inverse relationship between changes in membrane potential and in the logarithm of the external K^+ concentration above 10 mV. When the external K^+ concentration was reduced below 8 mM or completely omitted, the membrane potential increased only to a small extent. Although it is evident that the membrane potential depends largely on the external K^+ concentration, the experimental observations do not fit satisfactorily to the Nernst equation. The reason why the resting membrane potential is smaller than the K^+ equilibrium potential is not clear. Changes in the leakage resistance around the tip of the microelectrode was considered as a possible explanation in the intracellular study, but the experiments with external electrodes point to another reason.

Sodium and chloride ions do not seem to contribute to the transmembrane potential of frog sympathetic ganglion cells, since replacing Na^+ by a non permeating cation (choline) or by sucrose and substituting Cl^- by another anion had no effect (BLACKMAN et al., 1963b). Ganglion cells maintained in a high Ca^{++} solution, devoid of Na^+, had a considerably higher resting membrane potential and effective membrane resistance (KOKETSU and NISHI, 1969).

WOODWARD et al. (1969) have estimated the *electrolyte distribution in the rabbit superior cervical ganglion*. The calculated concentrations of the main electrolytes in the intracellular and interstitial fluid (µmoles/ml) were:

	Na^+	K^+	Ca^{++}	Mg^{++}	Cl^-
intracellular	37.4	163	—	—	23.5
interstitial	133	4.2	2.8	1.12	111

By substituting E_m by —68.6 mV (the mean resting potential of 50 cells), the relative permeabilities $P_K:P_{Na}:P_{Cl}$ were estimated to be 1.0:0.06:0.02. The calculated Nernst equilibrium potentials were: E_{Na}+33.6 mV; E_K—96.6 mV and E_{Cl} —41.1 mV. It should be borne in mind that it is not possible to distinguish between the electrolyte content of neuronal cell bodies, nerve fibres and satellite cells.

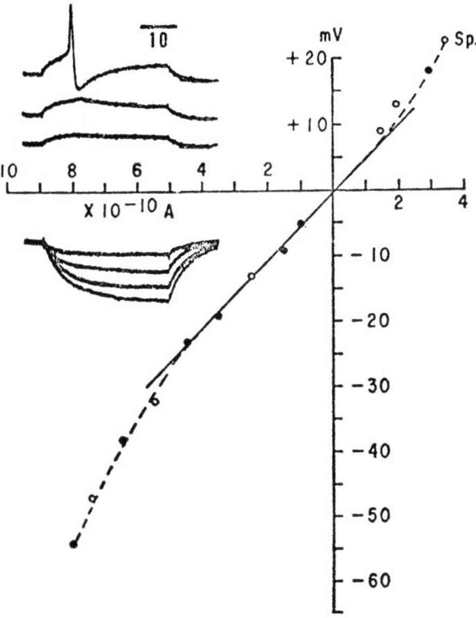

Fig. 1. Plot of the voltage-current relation in a representative frog ganglion cell. The horizontal line corresponds to the resting membrane potential of 50 mV. Decrease (upwards) and increase (downwards) of the membrane potential is indicated on the vertical axis, the strength of the current pulses on the horizontal axis (inward currents on the left, outward currents on the right). Sp indicates the threshold level for initiation of a spike. Examples of electrotonic potentials are also given in the inset (catelectrotonic above, anelectrotonic below horizontal line). The slope resistance in this cell is 52 MΩ (from HUNT and RIKER, 1966)

β) The electric time constant of the membrane (calculated from the time-course of electrotonic potentials produced by rectangular inward and outward current pulses, see Fig. 1) measured by various authors in amphibian and mammalian sympathetic ganglion cells (Table 1) was close to 10 msec, therefore considerably longer than in frog or cat spinal motoneurons.

γ) The cell resistance (calculated from the slope of current-voltage relation obtained with hyperpolarizing currents, a respresentative example of which is given in Fig. 1) varied between 10 and over 100 MΩ (Table 1). Considering the effective membrane area, a *specific membrane resistance* of approximately 400 Ω cm^2 is obtained for amphibian sympathetic B-neurons (cells giving rise to B-fibres) which is identical with that calculated for cat motoneurons; the specific membrane resistance of C-cells (giving rise to postganglionic C-fibres) of toad paravertebral ganglia is less than half this value.

δ) The calculated **specific membrane capacitance** (Table 1) is considerably higher than that of motoneurons. It is especially high in C-cells.

ε) Delayed Rectification. When the strength of short current pulses applied through a microelectrode is plotted against the voltage change across the membrane thus produced (Fig. 1), a fairly linear slope is found in the range of hyperpolarizing currents in frog paravertebral ganglia (NISHI and KOKETSU, 1960; HUNT and NELSON, 1965; HUNT and RIKER, 1966; STONEY and MACHNE, 1969). Similar findings were obtained in thoracic chain ganglia (BLACKMAN and PURVES, 1969a) and in the superior cervical ganglion of the guinea-pig (PERRI et al., 1970a, b), whereas all ganglion cells in the hypogastric nerve (BLACKMAN and PURVES, 1969a) and in the rabbit superior cervical ganglion (CHRIST and NISHI, 1970) showed some degree of anomalous rectification for currents causing hyperpolarization of more than 10 mV (BLACKMAN et al., 1969). With outward (depolarizing) currents, however, the catelectrotonic potential rapidly reached a peak from which it declined after a few msec to a smaller steady value. This delayed rectification was not observed in all cells (NISHI and KOKETSU, 1960) and according to STONEY and MACHNE (1969) usually became pronounced only with currents greater than rheobase, i.e. with current pulses strong enough to initiate an action potential. Frog sympathetic cells differed from frog motoneurons, which showed no evidence of delayed rectification, and from cells of spinal ganglia of the same animal, where delayed rectification was severe before current intensity reached rheobase.

2. Direct Excitation

Subliminal rectangular depolarizing current pulses applied through the intracellular electrode produce local electronic potentials; rising and falling phases have a time constant characteristic for the cell being studied (see III 1b). The threshold for initiation of a propagated impulse by long current pulses *(rheobase)* varies very little in amphibian and mammalian sympathetic ganglion cells (0.5—3.1×10^{-10} A) (Table 1). It corresponds to a critical *threshold depolarization* of 10—20 mV below resting potential.

With long rectangular suprathreshold current pulses, a *repetitive firing* occurs in frog ganglion cells (HUNT and RIKER, 1966; STONEY and MACHNE, 1969; BLACKMAN et al., 1969; BLACKMAN and PURVES, 1969a, b), though it is not maintained for currents exceeding 400 msec in duration. Repetitive firing even to strong and long-lasting current pulses was not observed in rabbit superior cervical ganglion *in situ* (ERULKAR and WOODWARD, 1968). Frog sympathetic ganglion cells behave, in this respect, like motoneurons of the same species but differ from spinal ganglion cells, which are incapable of repetitive firing (STONEY and MACHNE, 1969). The later spikes induced by longer current pulses usually originate from a higher threshold depolarization level than the first one (HUNT and RIKER, 1966; BLACKMAN et al., 1969a; BLACKMAN and PURVES, 1969). The maximum frequency observed was 80/sec in frog paravertebral sympathetic ganglia, 150—170/sec in pelvic ganglia of guinea-pigs, and could be maintained almost indefinitely in most cells (HUNT and RIKER, 1966; BLACKMAN and PURVES, 1969; CROWCROFT et al., 1969). Frog sympathetic ganglion cells were found to be able to fire action potentials at a higher rate than their axons (HUNT and RIKER, 1966). In these ganglia, directly evoked action potentials emerged from a rising electrotonic potential and had *spikes* with overshoot and after-hyperpolarization essentially similar to an antidromic spike; they will, therefore, be discussed in the following paragraph.

Observations made by STONEY and MACHNE (1969) on *accommodation* in frog sympathetic ganglion cells will help to understand some effects of depolarizing agents. These authors studied the response to linearly rising currents. By gradually reducing the rate of current rise, a "minimal current gradient" could be determined below which no excitation occurred, in other words the cells revealed accommodation to slowly rising current flow. The "minimal current gradient" was calculated to be around 5×10^{-9} A/sec or 26 rheobases/sec. Corresponding values were in the same order of magnitude in the rare accommodating motoneurons, distinctly smaller in the non-accommodating motoneurons and considerably higher in spinal ganglion cells which exhibit marked accommodation. STONEY and MACHNE (1969) found that the phenomenon of "minimal current gradient" in frog sympathetic ganglion cells could not be explained solely by delayed rectification but must be due to a marked extent to an increase of the depolarization threshold. The latter could increase to over 200% of its original value. The measurements of changes in threshold current and threshold depolarization were made by applying short (10 msec) depolarizing current pulses superposed at various times on the linearly rising "conditioning" current. The "minimal current gradient" effective for excitation was, therefore, defined as the lowest rate of current rise sufficient to maintain a rate of depolarization exceeding the rate of increasing depolarization threshold. It remains to be shown whether the increase in depolarization threshold is linked to inactivation of the Na^+ carrying system and the delayed rectification to the delayed increase of the K^+ permeability, as found in other nervous tissues.

3. The Invasion of the Adrenergic Nerve Cell Body by Antidromic Impulses

The study of action potentials backfired into the adrenergic cell body is of great importance for several reasons. The antidromic action potential, like that initiated by direct electrical stimulation, is free of the synaptic events which precede and outlast the orthodromic spike. By comparing orthodromic and antidromic potentials, we may, therefore, learn a good deal about the changes induced in the excitable membrane by the synaptic transmitter substance, and it becomes possible to ascribe the slow potential changes which follow the regenerative spike process to either true "afterpotentials" or residues of transmitter action (fast and slow synaptic potentials); it helps to understand the mode and site of action of "ganglionic active" chemical agents and to distinguish between pre- and post-synaptic events underlying the altered synaptic transmission which occurs after several procedures. With the most recent data obtained by the intracellular microelectrode technique in mind, it is surprising to see how many important aspects of our present-day knowledge on fundamental synaptic events were anticipated by ECCLES (1935c, 1937, 1943, 1944) in his early systematic investigations of the interaction of antidromic and orthodromic action potentials in the cat superior cervical ganglion by recording from the ganglionic surface.

In paravertebral ganglia of the frog, the antidromic *spike* amplitude was found to be approximately 90 mV with an overshoot of 25—35 mV (NISHI and KOKETSU, 1960; BLACKMAN et al., 1963a). The time to peak varied between 1.5—3 msec, the duration between 4 and 8 msec (Fig. 2). Shape and time course of antidromic and directly evoked spikes were identical. The rate of rise and the amplitude of the antidromic spike were reduced when Na^+ was partially replaced by choline or sucrose in the absence of changes of the resting membrane potential (BLACKMAN et al., 1963b). The reduction of the amplitude was, however, smaller than could be expected on the basis of the assumption, that at the peak of the overshoot the membrane behaves like a Na^+ electrode. Elevation of K^+ abolished responses to orthodromic stimuli long before antidromic spikes. At K^+ concentrations above 10 mM, the antidromic spike response was attenuated, whereas the orthodromic spike was abolished at K^+ concentrations between 9 and 11 mM. This was ascribed by BLACKMAN et al. (1963b) to the reduced resistance of the cell in high K^+ concentrations and the ensuing short-circuiting of the action potential in the postganglionic axon which is generated across a relatively high resistance.

The same ionic mechanisms underlie the spike potential in ganglion cells and other nervous elements (ECCLES, 1957; HODGKIN, 1964): a) A gradual increase in Na^+ permeability depending on the transmembrane potential (and which, therefore, has a regenerative character) produces the ascending phase; b) Repolarization occurs by the gradual inactivation of the Na^+ carrying mechanism and the delayed transient increase of the K^+ permeability. KOKETSU and NISHI (1968, 1969) provided evidence that Ca^{++} (and Sr^{++}) regulate the activation as well as the inactivation of the spike producing Na^+ mechanism; furthermore, they found

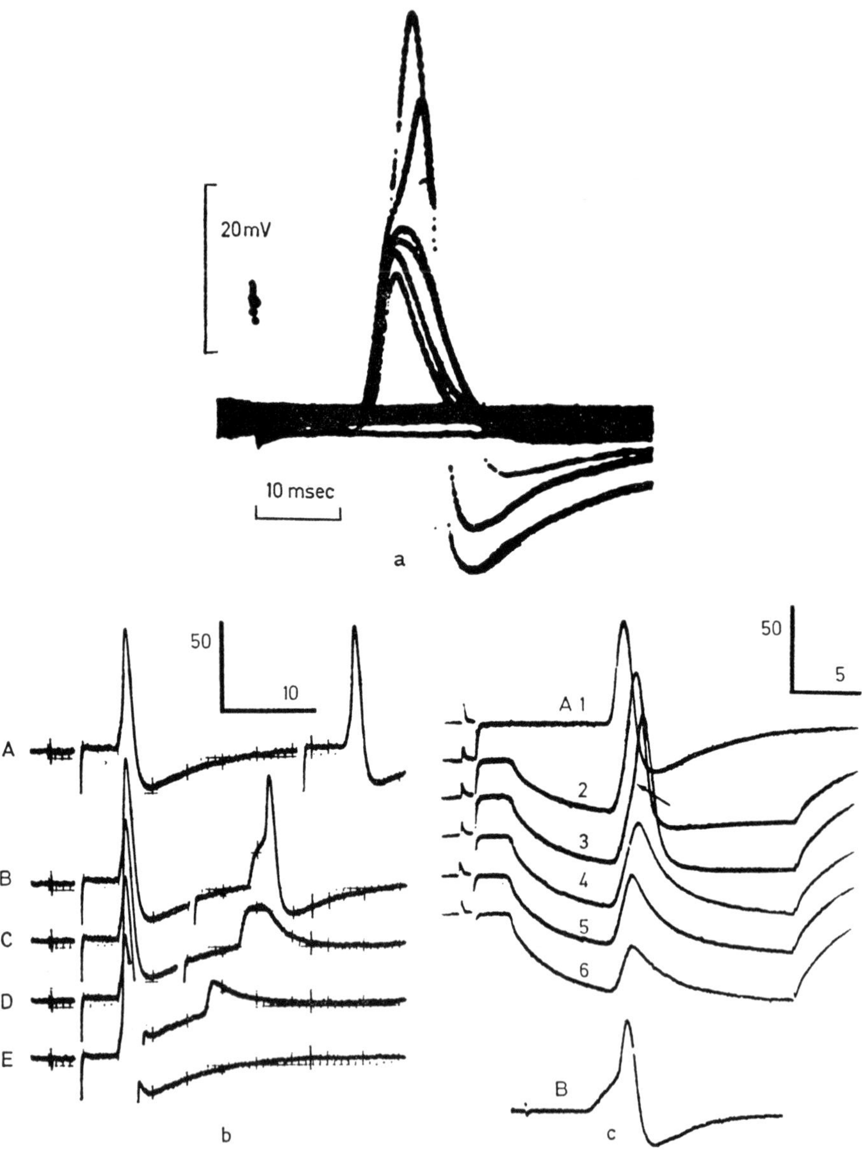

Fig. 2a—c. Intracellularly recorded responses of frog ganglion cells to antidromic stimuli; progressive separation of IS-spike and soma-spike and eventual failure of the latter a) in low external Na^+ concentration (superimposed tracings); b) when diminishing the interval between paired pulses, and c) by hyperpolarizing the cell before antidromic invasion. a) from BLACKMAN et al., 1963; b) and c) from HUNT and RIKER, 1966

that bullfrog sympathetic ganglia are capable of producing spikes in response to direct electrical stimulation in the absence of external Na^+, provided the latter cation is replaced by high concentrations of either Ca^{++}, Sr^{++} or Ba^{++}. "Ca^{++} spikes" had a much higher threshold depolarization than normal "Na^+ spikes" (which explains why Ca^{++}, in spite of being able to act as a current carrier in directly evoked spikes, cannot maintain ganglionic transmission in the absence of Na^+).

It seems evident to pharmacologists that the non-depolarizing ganglion blocking drugs like hexamethonium, mecamylamine and tubocurarine should not affect the antidromic spike at concentrations well above those blocking completely orthodromic transmission; the experimental proof has, however, been provided only recently (BLACKMAN et al., 1963a). On the other hand, tetrodotoxin in small amounts reversibly blocks extracellularly recorded antidromic and orthodromic action potentials without affecting the depolarization induced by K^+ and nicotine-like agents (HAEFELY, 1972b).

Even under apparently normal conditions, an inflexion on the rising phase of the antidromic spike response could sometimes be observed (ECCLES, 1957; NISHI and KOKETSU, 1960; BLACKMAN et al., 1963a; HUNT and RIKER, 1966). This inflexion could be accentuated or unmasked by reducing the Na^+ of the bathing fluid (BLACKMAN et al., 1963b). The same procedure could even lead to a complete separation of two components of the antidromic spike, leaving only a small spike with its peak at the original inflexion point. Similar effects (Fig. 2) could be obtained by gradually decreasing the interval between paired antidromic impulses and by eliciting antidromic spikes during graded hyperpolarization of the cell (NISHI and KOKETSU, 1960; HUNT and RIKER, 1966). It may be assumed, therefore, that the antidromic spike, like that of the motoneuron (ECCLES, 1957), has two components which can be separated under suitable conditions, namely a preceding smaller initial segment *(IS) spike* and a longer soma-dendritic *(SD) spike* (soma spike in amphibian sympathetic ganglion cells, since these have no dendritic processes; PICK, 1963). In some cells it has even been possible to separate a very small depolarization from the IS-spike (NISHI and KOKETSU, 1960), presumably representing the axon spike electrotonically recorded by the intracellular electrode. It seems, therefore, that there are two difficult points for the propagation of the antidromic impulse, the first being the site of sudden enlargement of the axon in the proximity of the cell body or the transition from the myelinated part to the unmyelinated proximal axon in B-cells, the second one being at the axon-soma junction. The safety factor for antidromic invasion of the soma may largely depend on the fine morphology and the relative size of the initial segment (axon hillock, proximal axon) and the proximal axon and hence differ greatly in different species, ganglia and individual cells. The full spike set up by antidromic stimulation is consistently followed by a *hyperpolarizing afterpotential* (after-hyperpolarization, positive afterpotential, postspike positivity). It develops briskly from the descending phase of the spike and reaches its summit very rapidly (Fig. 3). The peak amplitude of this hyperpolarization in frog paravertebral ganglia, measured from the resting base line, is about 25—30% of the spike heigth (NISHI and KOKETSU, 1960; BLACKMAN et al., 1963b). The amplitude of the hyperpolarizing afterpotential is inversely related to the resting membrane potential and reverses its sign at levels of —82 to —97 mV (NISHI and KOKETSU, 1960); by the surface recording method, smaller relative amplitudes of the afterpositivity are usually found (e.g. ECCLES, 1935d). Therefore, it seems likely that intracellular recordings tend to overestimate the size of the hyperpolarizing afterpotential because of the low resting membrane potential of impaled cells. Its duration varied greatly in different cells, total durations between 200 and 400 msec being reported (Blackman et al., 1963a). The hyperpolarizing afterpotential of sympathetic ganglion cells differs from the one which regularly follows the SD spike of mammalian and amphibian motoneurons (Eccles, 1957) by its larger

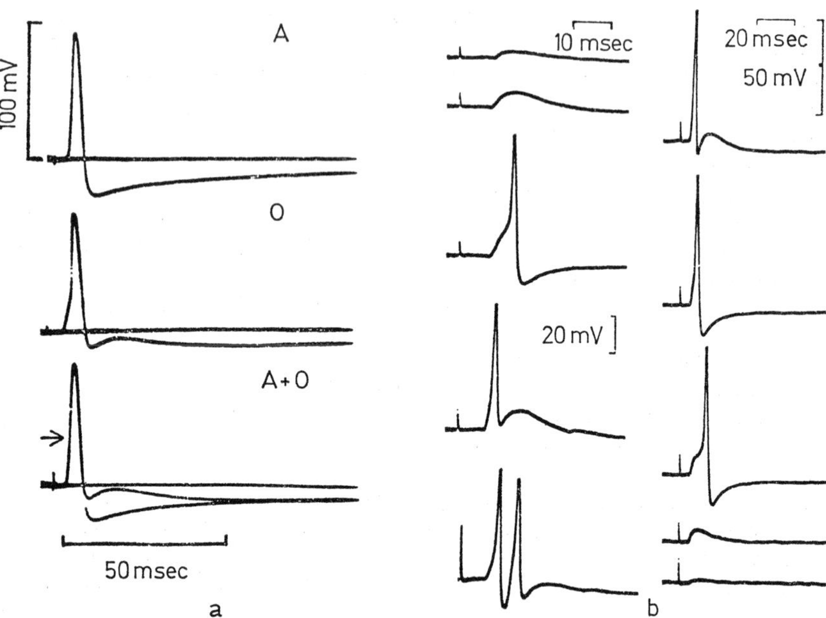

Fig. 3a—b. Intracellular records from cells of frog (a) and guinea-pig (b) paravertebral ganglia. In a) are shown an antidromic (A), and orthodromic (O), and two superimposed antidromic action potentials of which one was timed with an orthodromic stimulus such as synaptic activity started about halfway up the rising phase of the antidromic spike (A+O) (from Blackman et al., 1963a). In b) are shown several orthodromic responses in two different cells. In the cell on the left-hand side, the preganglionic stimulus strength was gradually increased; the first response consisted of a small EPSP, the last one of double spikes. The responses of the other cell (right-hand side) were obtained before and at different intervals after adding hexamethonium to the bath (from Blackman and Purves, 1969a)

amplitude and longer duration and by not being preceded by a depolarizing afterpotential. The hyperpolarizing afterpotential of motoneurons has been ascribed to a net outward diffusion of K^+, due to an increased K^+ conductance of the membrane (Eccles, 1957; Ito and Oshima, 1962). There is much controversy about the *mechanisms responsible for the generation of the hyperpolarizing afterpotential* in adrenergic neurons. It would be of considerable importance if this problem could be solved; the afterpotential is very sensitive to various agents and procedures, and so, alterations in its amplitude and time-course would be helpful in analyzing the mode of action of drugs.

Two essentially different explanations have so far been suggested. According to the first one, the increase in K^+ conductance (P_K) of the membrane would bring the membrane potential closer to the K^+ equilibrium potential. The increase in P_K would set in with a delay after the increase of P_{Na} responsible for the spike and reach its maximum at a time when P_{Na} has already attained the low prespike value ("delayed rectification"). Arguments in favour of this hypothesis are as follows: Reducing K^+ in the bathing fluid to zero did virtually not change the resting membrane potential, but increased the absolute value of the peak of the afterpotential (BLACKMAN et al., 1963b; KOSTERLITZ et al., 1968); increasing external K^+ decreased afterpositivity more than it lowered the membrane potential (KOSTERLITZ et al., 1968); there was a reversal point for the hyperpolarizing afterpotential (NISHI and KOKETSU, 1960). The alternative explanation postulates the involvement of a metabolically supported ion pump which restores the ionic disturbance (gain of intracellular Na^+ and loss of intracellular K^+) induced by the spike. There is no experimental proof for such a mechanism operating after a single spike. However, the marked hyperpolarization which follows a train of repetitive stimuli in unmyelinated nerve fibres has been shown to be due to the activation of an electrogenic Na^+ pump (RANG and RITCHIE, 1968). A similar, very marked posttetanic hyperpolarization (PTH) also occurs in sympathetic ganglion cells. It is tempting to consider this PTH as an exaggerated hyperpolarizing afterpotential. It is furthermore striking that both hyperpolarizing afterpotentials and PTH are the more marked the smaller are the nerve cells or fibres. It seems difficult to understand how the small ganglion cell could get rid of the Na^+ accumulated during the action potential without some increase in the pump activity above the level necessary for maintaining the gradient producing the resting potential in the absence of spike activity. The summation of hyperpolarizing afterpotentials, when paired pulses are fired at short interval, and the gradual increase of PTH, with either increasing train duration or increasing number of impulses within a train, make it difficult to assume that two essentially different mechanisms produce hyperpolarization after a single spike and after a train of pulses. Unfortunately, the suppression of both forms of hyperpolarization by ouabain is of no assistance, since the blockade of the Na^+/Ka^+ activated ATPase results in a loss of intracellular K^+ and increase of Na^+ which would also reduce the hyperpolarizing effect of an increase in P_K. It seems that, as a working hypothesis, the hyperpolarizing afterpotential could be feasibly explained by assuming the involvement of both mechanisms: Increased P_K leading to the rapid and short-lived "undershoot" or "positive phase" of spike and activation of an electrogenic Na^+ pump producing the longer lasting hyperpolarization. Optimal conditions for the activation of a Na^+ pump would be fulfilled at the peak of the "undershoot": Increased intracellular Na^+ and increased K^+ outside the membrane. Up to now, the membrane conductance during the hyperpolarizing afterpotential has not been measured directly in adrenergic ganglion cells, in contrast to the spinal motoneurons (ITO and OSHIMA, 1962), and it remains a matter of speculation whether the same potential change in both types of nerve cells is produced by the same or by different electrogenic mechanisms.

4. Synaptic Excitation

a) The Fast Excitatory Postsynaptic Potential (EPSP)

A single preganglionic volley of insufficient strength for evoking an action potential, or a maximal volley in the presence of a ganglionic blocking agent, induces in ganglion cells a graded, slowly developing, partial depolarization (Fig. 3) which propagates decrementally along the axon, the excitatory postsynaptic potential (EPSP). Several details of this EPSP are known from intracellular studies (Table 2).

The full size of a suprathreshold EPSP induced by a synchronous volley of the total preganglionic input to sympathetic ganglion cells cannot usually be measured, since it is distorted by the initiated spike. Cells belonging to a "subliminal fringe", i.e. cells which cannot be excited to fire an action potential in response to a single volley in their total afferent input

Table 2. *Some characteristics of the EPSP of sympathetic ganglion cells (in vitro)*

Ganglion	Time to peak (msec)	Maximum rate of rise (V/sec)	Time constant of decay (msec)	Total duration (msec)	Equilibrium potential (mV)	References
rabbit sup. cervical	6.4 (4—10)	7.7		29.3 (14—47)		ECCLES, R. M. (1955)
frog paravertebral	2.5—3	30 (25—32)	12 (8—15.5)	40	—14.3 (8—20)	NISHI and KOKETSU (1960)
frog paravertebral					40—55 above resting pot.	BLACKMAN et al. (1963a)
toad paravertebral						
B-cells	1.5—3	40	10.4		—10 (5—15)	NISHI et al. (1965)
C-cells	3 —5	18	13.9		— 7 (3—12)	
frog paravertebral				60—100		TOSAKA et al. (1968)
guinea-pig paravertebral	9.1 (5—15)		11.4 (8.3—15.9)			BLACKMAN and PURVES (1969)
guinea-pig sup. cervical	5.8 ±0.6		8.5 ±0.9			PERRI et al. (1970)
rat sup. cervical	4.7 ±0.6		6.7 ±0.7			PERRI et al. (1970)

without some facilitating procedure, have only exceptionally been encountered in intracellular studies, e.g. in the pelvic plexus of the guinea-pig (BLACKMAN et al., 1969). In these scattered small ganglia, the adrenergic cells seem to be innervated by one single preganglionic fibre, as they respond in an all-or-nothing manner to orthodromic stimuli of varying strength in the form of either an EPSP or a spike. As a rule, however, adrenergic cells in mammalian ganglia are innervated by a varying number of preganglionic fibres, and by increasing the strength of stimulation, the size of the EPSP gradually increases. The various preganglionic fibres differ somewhat in their conduction velocity and/or length of terminal arborization and the EPSP is, therefore, composed of termporarily dispersed "packets"; the EPSP is built up in a series of steps, and discrete potentials may appear in the falling phase (ERULKAR and WOODWARD, 1968; PERRI et al., 1970a).

The size of the EPSP depends on the membrane potential from which it originates; it increases when the cell is hy perpolarized and decreases during depolarizing current pulses (Fig. 9). The relation between the amplitude of the EPSP and the change of the transmembrane potential is almost linear over a wide range (NISHI and KOKETSU, 1960). The *reversal or equilibrium of the EPSP*, i.e. the membrane potential at which the EPSP reverses its polarity, has been found to be —10 to —20 mV in isolated ganglia of the pelvic plexus of the guinea-pig (CROWCRAFT et al., 1969). In amphibia, the equilibrium potential was approximately —10 mV (Table 2) when measured by applying current pulses of different strength or by eliciting an EPSP at the different stages of an antidromic spike. The amplitude of the reversed EPSP at membrane potential values above zero was smaller than that which would have corresponded to the membrane potential and the decay was faster, presumably because of the rectifying property of the membrane.

The *time constant of decay* of the EPSP was consistently found to be higher than the time constant of the cell membrane which is strong evidence that the trans-mitter action outlasts the peak of the EPSP. Synaptic activity is prolonged by cholinesterase inhibitors (BLACKMAN et al., 1963a).

The *electrogenesis of the EPSP* can be explained by assuming that the transmitter, acetylcholine, produces a "shunt" of the resting membrane by increasing non-selectively the permeability of the subsynaptic membrane areas to several cations.

The increase in membrane conductance has been directly demonstrated by the application of constant test current pulses before and during an EPSP (KOBAYASHI and LIBET, 1968). The ions involved in the current flow underlying the EPSP have been studied by KOKETSU (1969). The equilibrium potential of the EPSP of bullfrog sympathetic ganglion cells was not influenced by replacing chloride by glutamate, it was shifted towards the resting membrane potential by a decrease of external Na^+ or K^+ concentration and towards the zero potential by an increase of the external K^+. This indicates that the EPSP — like the end-plate potential (TAKEUCHI and TAKEUCHI, 1960) — is produced mainly by an increased Na^+ conductance of the subsynaptic membrane. Increase and decrease in external Ca^{++} concentrations of the otherwise unchanged Ringer solution shifted the equilibrium potential of the EPSP toward the resting and the zero potential respectively, suggesting that the ratio "Na^+ conductance changes to K^+ conductance changes" during the EPSP were determined by the external Ca^{++} concentration. An equivalent electrical circuit, analogous to that proposed by FATT and KATZ (1951) for other synapses has been presented by BLACKMAN et al. (1963a). The calculations of WOODWARD et al. (1969) indicate that an increase of the Na^+ conductance by a factor of only 4 would already cause a membrane depolarization of 27.3 mV which is the value of an average EPSP.

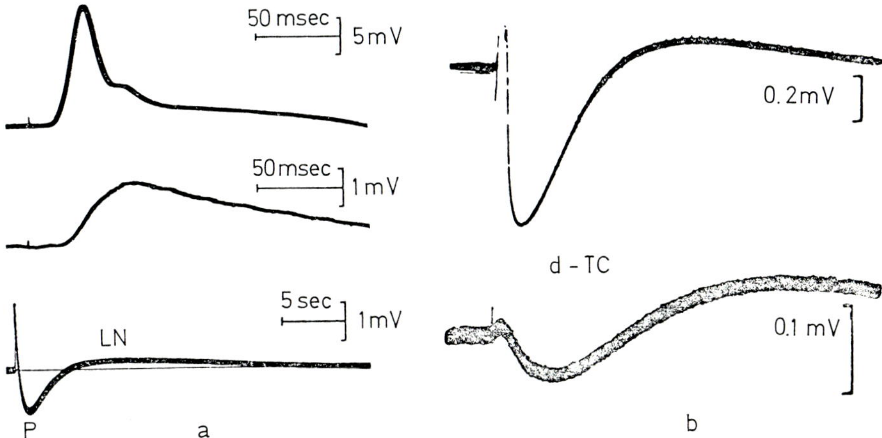

Fig. 4a—b. N-, P- and LN-waves of an isolated rabbit superior cervical ganglion in response to single preganglionic volley. a) Recording with the sucrose-gap method. The upper tracing shows the first part of a compound action potential consisting of a main (S_a cells) and a smaller second spike (S_b cells). In the middle tracing the N-wave and in the lower tracing the N-, P- and LN-waves after exposure to hexamethonium are shown. Note different time and voltage scale (from KOSTERLITZ et al., 1968). b) Recording with conventional external electrodes. Above the compound action potentials (spike off) with a marked post-spike positivity and a faint LN-wave before d-tubocurarine and below N-, P- andLN-waves after addition of d-tubocurarine. Note difference in calibration (from LIBET, 1967)

In the absence of preganglionic stimulation, the occurrence of spontaneous irregular small depolarizations, *spontaneous miniature synaptic potentials* (mEPSP), have been observed in mammalian (BLACKMAN and PURVES, 1969a) and amphibian sympathetic ganglion cells (BLACKMAN et al., 1963c, d; HUNT and NELSON, 1965; NISHI et al., 1967). As at central synapses and neuromuscular junctions, they are thought to be due to the spontaneous liberation of unit packets of the transmitter substance. Calculations of the mean quantum content of synaptic potentials have been reported for sympathetic ganglion cells of the toad (NISHI et al., 1967) and of the guinea-pig (BLACKMAN and PURVES, 1969a).

Non-depolarizing ganglionic blocking agents like tubocurarine, dihydro-β-erythroidine, hexamethonium and mecamylamine, diminish or block the depolarizing action of acetylcholine by competitive interaction at nicotinic receptors. At suitable concentrations, they reduce the amplitude of the EPSP's below the threshold for spike initiation (Figs. 3, 4). This action of ganglionic blocking drugs has been used for recording synaptic potentials from the surface of ganglia (ECCLES, 1943; LAPORTE and LORENTE DE NÓ, 1950b; R.M. ECCLES, 1952b; VOLLE, 1967b; VOLLE and PAPPANO, 1968; DUNANT, 1969). In order to distinguish this "compound" synaptic potential recorded from the whole ganglion from unitary EPSP's, it is usually called the *N-wave*. The amount of ganglionic blocking agents needed to inhibit any spike within a given ganglion reduces, of course, the amplitude of the synaptic potential recorded by external electrodes. This is avoided when spike generation is blocked by placing the distal part of an isolated ganglion in the sucrose chamber of a sucrose gap apparatus (KOSTERLITZ and WALLIS, 1966).

b) The Orthodromic Ganglionic Action Potential

When the EPSP reduces the membrane potential below a critical value, a *spike* is initiated. As can be seen from Table 1, the *critical threshold depolarization*, observed by different authors in cells of various ganglia, is approximately 20 mV below the resting potential (the smaller values seem to be related to lower resting potentials of the respective cells and vice versa). The threshold depolarization for the initiation of an action potential was the same whether depolarization occurred by orthodromic or by direct intracellular stimulation. The critical depolarization level is visible on the rising phase of the spike potential as an inflection, the *synaptic step;* it is especially prominent when the orthodromic impulse is just at threshold strength for the cell (Fig. 3b). The rising phase of the spike is smooth in amphibian ganglion cells, and at a normal membrane potential, a small inflection can only very exceptionally be observed (NISHI and KOKETSU, 1960; NISHI et al., 1965) at a potential level where the soma spike of an antidromic action potential arises from the IS-spike. Some cells of sympathetic ganglia from guinea-pigs, and particularly from rats, revealed a clear separation of IS- and SD-spikes (PERRI et al., 1970a), thus resembling motoneurons where the orthodromic action potential is regularly separated into IS- and SD-spikes (ECCLES, 1957). Presumably, the threshold for spike initiation is not much lower in the IS than in the soma of frog ganglion cells. The maximum slopes in the rising phase were found to be steeper in the rat (mean value 230 V/sec) than in guinea-pig cells (155 V/sec) (PERRI et al., 1970a). Peak amplitudes of orthodromic spikes reported in the literature are given in Table 1. The *overshoot* of the spike is 20—30 mV. The time to peak, measured from the synaptic step, ranges between 1.5 and 3 msec (R.M. ECCLES, 1955), the total duration (time of repolarization to the resting membrane potential) between 1.5 and 7 msec (Table 1); the latter is, therefore, considerably longer than it is in motoneurons (ECCLES, 1957). The decay of the spike was found to be invariably slower than the rise time.

The *slow potential changes following the orthodromic spike* are rather complex and vary not only from cell to cell but even in the same neuron (Fig. 3). Sometimes the orthodromic spike resembles the antidromic one by being followed by a more or less simple hyperpolarizing afterpotential. Usually, however, the orthodromic spike ends with a sudden short-lived *positive phase*, the peak of which may be below or often above the resting membrane potential (and which is called "*undershoot*" by some authors). The positive phase is followed by a slow decrease of the membrane potential for about 50 msec *(after-depolarization);* at its peak, the membrane potential may be below the resting value. Sometimes, however, the afterdepolarization forms only a hump in the *after-hyperpolarization*. The membrane potential returns to the prespike value after 200—500 msec.

The *comparison of orthodromic with antidromic action potentials* and *the study of the influence of synaptic activity on the antidromic response* give much insight into the different phases of the orthodromic action potential (Fig. 3).

The peak of the orthodromic spike usually has a slightly smaller amplitude than that of the antidromic one, and a small hump occurs on the initial falling phase of the orthodromic spike (NISHI and KOKETSU, 1960; BLACKMAN et al., 1963a). BLACKMAN et al. (1963a) could change the shape of an antidromic spike and of its hyperpolarizing afterpotential to become indistinguishable from an orthodromic response by appropriately timing pre- and post-ganglionic volleys, the antidromic action potential invading the cell during the synaptic activity produced by a preganglionic volley. The subsynaptic membrane areas, made less resistant by the transmitter action, shunt the membrane currents underlying spike and afterpotential. It is evident then, that the afternegativity of an orthodromic action potential represents the residual synaptic potential and should not, therefore, be called negative or depolarizing afterpotential. In the late phase — when synaptic activity has subsided — the after-hyperpolarization of the orthodromic action potential becomes identical with the late phase of the hyperpolarizing afterpotential of an antidromic response. The greatly varying shapes and amplitudes of the positive phase, the afterdepolarization and the after-hyperpolarization in different, and even in the same cells, are easily explained by different intensities of synaptic activity. The gradual reduction of the transmitter action, either by decreasing the afferent input to the cell or by adding an antinicotinic agent, produces transition forms of responses from typical orthodromic action potentials with marked afterdepolarization to responses resembling more and more an antidromic action potential (BLACKMAN et al., 1963a; BLACKMAN and PURVES, 1969a; BLACKMAN et al., 1969; SZURSZEWSKI et al., 1969) (Fig. 3b). Conversely, the addition of a cholinesterase inhibitor considerably prolongs the synaptic activity and thereby its influence on the hyperpolarizing afterpotential.

Occasionally two action potentials are fired in response to a single preganglionic volley (ERULKAR and WOODWARD, 1968; LIBET and TOSAKA, 1969; BLACKMAN and PURVES, 1969a; BLACKMAN et al., 1969; PERRI et al., 1970a). The most obvious basis of this phenomenon is the relatively long-lasting synaptic activity which is in part due to a protracted asynchronous transmitter release at the numerous synaptic areas of the soma and of the dendritic arborization of a single ganglion cell. When the synaptic potential is intense enough at the moment the cell recovers from the refractory period (see III 4 e) following the first spike, a second action potential may be initiated. The second spike, initiated by the same synaptic potential (Fig. 3), is usually fired at a higher depolarization level than the first, indicating the occurrence of accommodation as already described for the repetitive firing induced by a constant suprathreshold current pulse. The interval between the two spikes is 10—20 msec. It seems evident that double spikes, in response to a single preganglionic volley, only occur in cells with a very intensive afferent input. It had earlier been observed with surface electrodes that the compound ganglionic spike, induced by an intensive preganglionic volley, is often followed by a small asynchronous discharge (LAPORTE and LORENTE DE NÓ, 1950c; DUNANT, 1967). LAPORTE and LORENTE DE NÓ (1950) c) had postulated two different modes of transmission and synaptic activity to explain the "s" (sudden) and "d" (delayed) discharge. This delayed discharge is observed consistently in the superior cervical ganglion of the cat in response to high-intensity volleys (HAEFELY, unpublished) and is best explained by the firing of a second spike in cells with a rich afferent input.

c) Slow Synaptic Potentials

The slow synaptic potentials to be described open new aspects on the multiple ways in which the excitable membrane of neurons is able to react to chemical agents. Indeed, the response of sympathetic ganglion cells to preganglionic impulses is far more complicated than described in the preceding paragraphs. Thus, besides evoking the EPSP, which triggers an action potential when it reaches a critical amplitude, the transmitter, released from preganglionic nerve endings, induces changes in the postsynaptic membrane after an unusually long delay and which last for a surprisingly long time.

When recording from the surface of the isolated cat stellate ganglion, ECCLES (1943, 1944) had observed that the synaptic potential, which remained after elimination of the action potential by curare, was sometimes followed by a late negativity of the ganglion. LAPORTE and LORENTE DE NÓ (1950b) made an extensive study of a slow positive potential occurring in the isolated turtle superior cervical ganglion, treated with curarine to block the initiation of action potentials. Their early findings have been essentially confirmed and greatly extended by surface recordings from mammalian (R.M. ECCLES, 1952a, b; R.M. ECCLES and LIBET 1961; LIBET, 1964, 1967; DUNANT and DOLIVO, 1967; KOSTERLITZ et al., 1968) and frog sympathetic ganglia (LIBET et al., 1968; KOKETSU and NISHI, 1967; NISHI and KOKETSU, 1967; KOKETSU et al., 1968a; NISHI and KOKETSU, 1968b). Moreover, these slow synaptic potentials could also be recorded with intracellular electrodes in frog (TOSAKA et al., 1968; KOKETSU et al., 1968a) and rabbit isolated sympathetic ganglia (LIBET and TOSAKA, 1969; LIBET and KOBAYASHI, 1969).

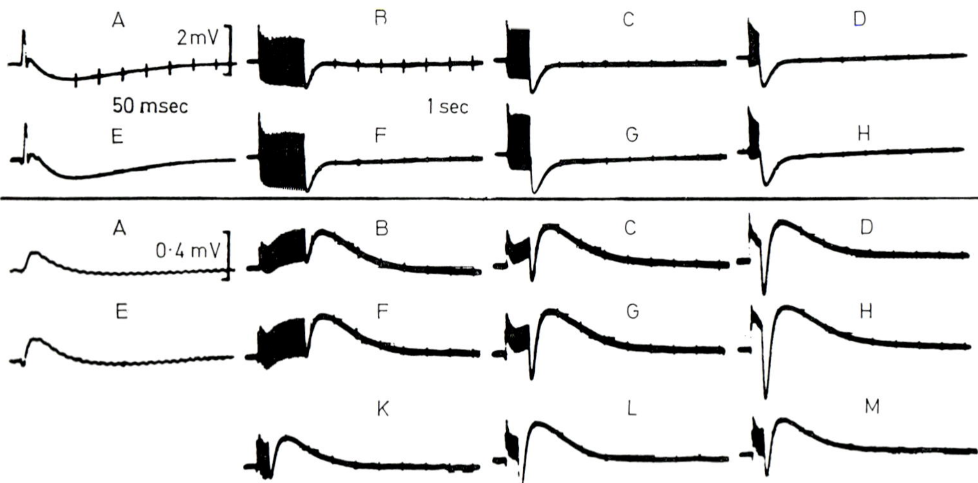

Fig. 5. Isolated rabbit superior cervical ganglion (surface recording). Effect of strength and frequency of stimulation on the size of slow synaptic potentials. The records above the horizontal line were obtained before, those below the line after exposure to dihydro-β-erythroidine. The stimulus strength was submaximal in the uppermost and third row, supramaximal in the second, fourth and fifth row. First column single volley, second column 2 sec trains at 10/sec, third column 1 sec train at 20/sec and fourth column 0.5 sec train at 40/sec (in the bottom row train duration was 0.5 sec throughout). The time scale is 50 msec for the first column and 1 sec for all other columns. Voltage scale: 2 mV before curarization, 0.4 mV after curarization (from R.M. ECCLES and LIBET, 1961)

Briefly, in a slightly curarized preparation (Fig. 4), a single supramaximal preganglionic impulse induces in ganglion cells, after a short synaptic delay (< 1 msec), a depolarization of low amplitude which is decrementally propagated. It is called *EPSP* (or *fast EPSP*) when recorded intracellularly, and synaptic potential or *N-wave* when recorded with external electrodes. In some ganglion cells, this fast excitatory postsynaptic potential may be followed first by a hyperpolarization which, as will be seen later on, has all the characteristics of an inhibitory postsynaptic potential *(IPSP)* and which is called *P-wave* (positive wave) when recorded from the surface. The synaptic delay of the IPSP is approximately

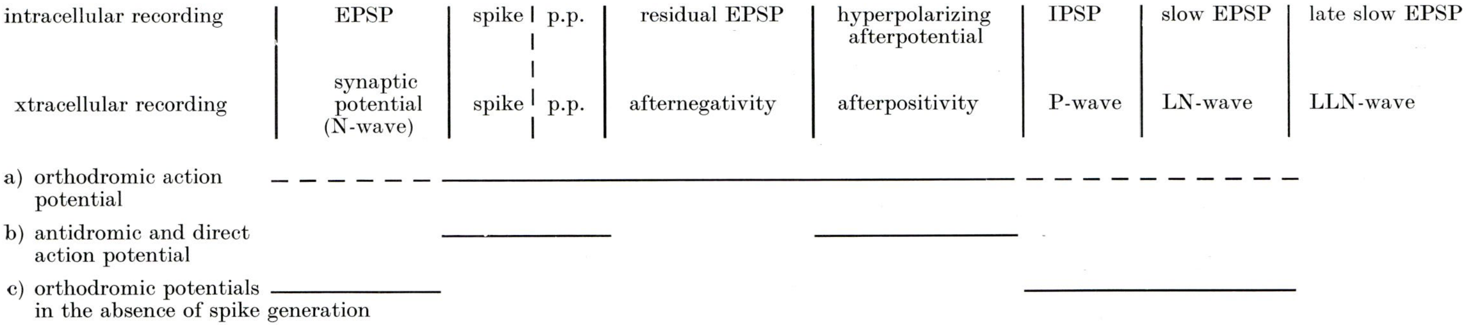

intracellular recording	EPSP	spike	p.p.	residual EPSP	hyperpolarizing afterpotential	IPSP	slow EPSP	late slow EPSP
xtracellular recording	synaptic potential (N-wave)	spike	p.p.	afternegativity	afterpositivity	P-wave	LN-wave	LLN-wave
a) orthodromic action potential	– – –	———	———	———	———	– – –	– – –	
b) antidromic and direct action potential		———	———		———			
c) orthodromic potentials in the absence of spike generation	———					———	———	

Fig. 6. Synopsis of the potential changes in sympathetic ganglia recorded either intracellularly from single cells or extracellularly from the surface of the ganglion. Horizontal line a) indicates the potential changes which can be recorded in response to a supraliminal orthodromic volley (the potential changes above the interrupted line — if present at all — are usually masked by and mixed with the other ones); line b) those recorded in response to direct or antidromic stimulation; line c) those which can be recorded in response to one or several supraliminal orthodromic volleys in the absence of spike generation, e.g. in a slightly curarized ganglion
p. p. signifies positive phase of spike

35 msec, the total duration 200—500 msec (LIBET, 1967). The IPSP or P-wave may be followed by a delayed depolarization, called *slow EPSP* when recorded intracellularly and *LN-wave* (late negative) when recorded extracellularly. The synaptic delay of this slow EPSP is extraordinarily long (200—300 msec), the total duration 2—3 sec. Figure 4 illustrates the synaptic potentials of the isolated rabbit superior cervical ganglion recorded with conventional surface electrodes (LIBET, 1967) and with the sucrose-gap method (KOSTERLITZ et al., 1968).

The intracellularly recorded slow synaptic potentials, in response to a single orthodromic impulse (Fig. 7), are of much lower amplitude than expected from extracellular studies on the whole ganglion (Fig. 4). Obviously, the conditions when using surface electrodes favour the recording of slow potential changes occurring simultaneously in a larger number of cells over very fast potential changes, like the spike. The slow synaptic potentials undergo summation like the fast EPSP and can, therefore, be greatly increased or, if not detectable in response to a single impulse, made visible by using trains of repetitive stimuli (Figs. 5 and 7). Short trains (0.1—1 sec) of stimuli at frequencies between 20 and 100/sec are, therefore, mostly used for the study of slow synaptic potentials. A synopsis of the sometimes confusing terminology of ganglionic potential changes is presented in Fig. 6.

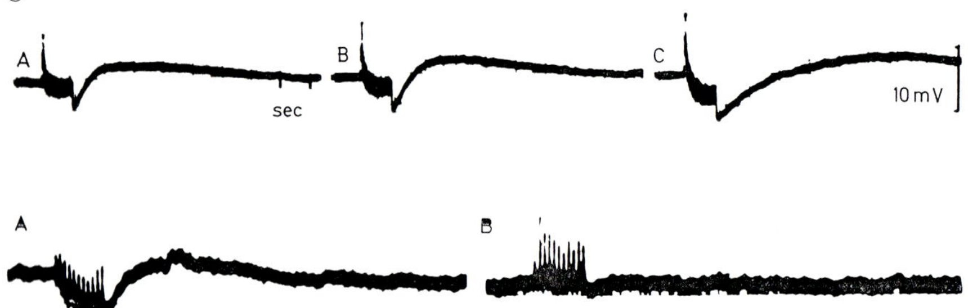

Fig. 7. Intracellular records from two different cells of isolated rabbit superior cervical ganglion. Top row: cell curarized with dihydro-β-erythroidine. Responses to 1 sec trains at 40/sec before (A), 1 min (B) and 2 min (C) after addition of eserine. Bottom row: cell moderately blocked with d-tubocurarine. Responses to 1 sec trains at 40/sec before (left) and after addition of atropine (right) (from LIBET and TOSAKA, 1969)

There is convincing evidence for the true *synaptic nature of the slow synaptic potentials* observed in curarized ganglia:

a) The IPSP and slow EPSP are not afterpotentials, i.e. they are not the consequences of a preceding action potential or of a fast EPSP. Increasing the amount of the curarizing agent decreases or completely abolishes the fast EPSP, but increases, if anything, the amplitude of the slow potentials.

b) They are local potentials of the ganglionic cell body spreading with decrement along the axon (LIBET, 1967) and they are absent in isolated postganglionic axons (LIBET, 1964).

c) They are only observed in response to orthodromic stimuli and do not appear after direct or antidromic stimulation (LIBET, 1964).

d) They are generated by the same transmitter substance which is also responsible for the initial fast EPSP. Inhibition of acetylcholine release from presynaptic endings by a lowered Ca^{++}/Mg^{++} ratio (LIBET, 1964) and botulinum toxin (R.M. ECCLES and LIBET, 1961) reduces both fast and slow synaptic potentials, whereas posttetanic facilitation of transmitter release enhances the amplitude of both.

e) In the ganglion completely blocked by hexamethonium, the P-wave inhibits ganglionic discharges produced e.g. by KCl or pilocarpine; on the other hand the LN-wave generates asynchronous discharges conducted in the postganglionic nerve (Fig. 8) (HAEFELY, 1970, 1972c).

f) The slow synaptic potentials generated in non-curarized ganglia have a modulating influence on the synaptic excitability of ganglion cells (see below).

The special and somewhat complicated conditions under which the slow synaptic potentials were mostly observed (ganglia in *in vitro* conditions, drug-induced blockade of spike generation, usually tetanic stimulation) raise the question of the physiological significance of these unusual postsynaptic changes.

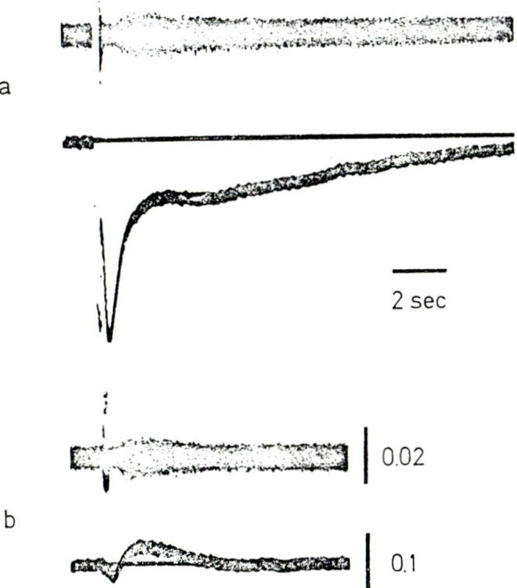

Fig. 8a—b. Cat superior cervical ganglion *in situ*, conditioned by orthodromic tetanic stimulation with 30/sec for 30 sec. Shown are the effect of a 0.25-sec train at 50/sec before (a) and after (b) hexamethonium 10 μmoles. The upper tracing is the recording from the postganglionic external carotid nerve (calibration 20 μV), the lower tracing, the ganglionic surface recording (calibration 100 μV). From HAEFELY (1972c)

Allusion is made in the paper by LIBET (1964) to slow synaptic potentials occurring also in unexcited ganglia; HAEFELY (1970, 1972c) has studied the slow synaptic potentials in the cat superior cervical ganglion *in situ*. He found that short trains of tetanic orthodromic stimuli produced typical P- and LN-waves after complete blockade of nicotinic receptors by either hexamethonium, d-tubocurarine, tetraethylammonium, mecamylamine or chlorisondamine. In contrast to *in vitro* conditions (LIBET, 1964), this particular ganglion *in situ* produced no slow synaptic potentials in response to a single orthodromic volley after blockade by competitive nicotinic antagonists, but did so during the late phase of ganglionic blockade produced by nicotinic agonists (see VI 1 a *a*).

Slow synaptic potentials are generated in ganglia in which nicotinic transmission is intact. This important finding was first made by LIBET (1964). In the isolated rabbit superior cervical ganglion, s small negative wave follows the postspike positivity of a single orthodromic action potential; it disappears after atropine and can be identified as the LN-wave by this fact and by its time-course. A short (0.1—1 sec) train of orthodromic volleys at frequencies between 10 and 100/sec is followed by a posttetanic hyperpolarization. In the decaying phase of this hyperpolarization, a negative hump can usually be seen. Atropine removes this hump, which is clearly a summed LN-wave. When the slow synaptic potentials are blocked by scopolamine, the posttetanic hyperpolarization has a strictly exponential decay (HAEFELY, 1970). The orthodromic tetanus induces asynchronous afterdischarges in the postganglionic axons (Fig. 8). An "early firing" sets in immediately at the end of the tetanus and is followed after a silent period by a late "firing" (HAEFELY, 1972c). The "early firing" coincides with the summed N-wave which outlasts somewhat the tetanus; the silent period is due to the posttetanic hyperpolarization, whereas the "late firing" coincides with the LN-wave which is visible as a negative hump in the decaying hyperpolarization. Scopolamine blocks both the negative hump and the late firing. In the rabbit (LIBET, 1964) and rat (DUNANT and DOLIVO, 1967) superior cervical ganglion *in vitro*, the P-wave seems to intensify the ganglionic postspike positivity.

The occurrence of slow synaptic potentials in an untreated ganglion already suggests that they may be of physiological significance. Although the investigations, designed to prove this, are still scarce, the following observations strongly support the suggestion. Bronk et al. (1938) had described the phenomenon of *recruitment* in sympathetic ganglia, i.e. the progressive increase of the size of postganglionic action potentials during a train of low-frequency orthodromic stimulation. In addition to a presynaptic component (facilitated transmitter release), the LN-wave which builds up during the low-frequency train seems to be causally involved, since atropine, by blocking the LN-wave, greatly reduced or abolished the recruitment in the rabbit superior cervical ganglion *in vitro* (Libet, 1964). Dunant and Dolivo (1967) obtained evidence of a possible physiological inhibitory action of the P-wave in ganglionic excitability. In the rat isolated superior cervical ganglion, a test response to a single supramaximal volley is increased, if it follows by about 50 msec an identical conditioning volley. This *homosynaptic facilitation* must be of presynaptic origin, since it occurs at a time when the postspike positivity of the conditioning action potential should by itself reduce the excitability of the ganglion cells. Removal of the P-wave by atropine, and thereby decreasing the amplitude of the postspike positivity, was found by the authors to increase homosynaptic facilitation. A homosynaptic facilitation is also observed after a conditioning tetanic stimulus train applied to the same preganglionic fibres as the test volley (Larrabee and Bronk, 1947). The conditioning train leads to a posttetanic hyperpolarization which is reduced and shortened by the LN-wave. Suppression of this wave by atropine and the ensuing prolongation and increase of the posttetanic hyperpolarisation reduces posttetanic homosynaptic facilitation in the rabbit (Libet, 1964) and rat (Dunant and Dolivo, 1967) isolated ganglion. *Heterosynaptic facilitation* (conditioning tetanic stimuli and test volleys applied to different afferent inputs of the ganglion) was found by Libet (1964) to be completely blocked by atropine, and he concluded that heterosynaptic facilitation was entirely produced by the LN-wave, whereas homosynaptic facilitation consisted of two components, one being due to the LN-wave and readily blocked by atropine, the other being of presynaptic origin and resistant to atropine. These few examples make it very likely that the level of excitability of ganglion cells, at a given moment, is effectively determined by the amplitude of slow synaptic potentials produced by the preceding preganglionic activity. In fact, considering the usually infrequent activity of autonomic preganglionic fibres, the long-lasting slow synaptic potentials seem better suited than the fast EPSP's for producing the background level of excitability for the integrative action of the ganglion cells.

The *postsynaptic receptors* involved in the generation of the three synaptic potentials are *cholinoceptive*.

There is a striking similarity between the time-course and the sensitivity to drugs of the three synaptic potentials and the triphasic changes of the surface potential induced by exogenous acetylcholine (see VI 1 b, c). Eserine prolongs both P- and LN-waves (Kosterlitz et al., 1968). Curare- and hexamethonium-like agents selectively abolish the fast EPSP, whereas atropine and scopolamine, in doses which have no effect on the latter, abolish both the IPSP and slow EPSP. The receptors mediating these potentials may, therefore, be called "nicotinic" (excitatory), "muscarinic inhibitory" and "muscarinic excitatory" sites. In Volle's terminology (Volle and Pappano, 1968), the receptors are the D-1, the H and the D-2 cholinoceptive sites, D indicating depolarization and H hyperpolarization. Originally, it had been suggested that the generation of the IPSP proceded in two steps, involving a muscarinic excitation of some intraganglionic structure, e.g. of the small chromaffin cells detectable by fluorescence microscopic methods (see e.g. Norberg and Sjöqvist, 1966) which would release catecholamines acting in a second step on adrenergic receptors of ganglion cells. The possible involvement of adrenaline in the generation of the P-wave had already been mentioned by Laporte and Lorente de Nó (1950b) on the basis of a ganglionic inhibitory effect of catecholamines reported by Marrazzi (1939). The arguments for an adrenergic step are almost exclusively based on the action of dibenamine which had been found to reduce the P-wave somewhat more than the N- and LN-wave (R.M. Eccles and Libet, 1961; Libet, 1964; Dunant and Dolivo, 1967). Dibenamine, however, is not a selective adrenolytic agent; it did not antagonize the ganglionic inhibitory action of adrenaline (Matthews, 1956). Moreover, the more selective α-adrenolytic agent, dihydroergotamine, had no effect on the P-wave (R.M. Eccles and Libet, 1961). In the frog paravertebral ganglia, where P-waves and IPSP were observed, histochemical investigations failed to reveal the presence of chromaffin cells (Norberg and McIsaac, 1967). In the superior cervical ganglia of rabbit, rat and cat, the chromaffin cells were found to occur in small scattered clusters; it is difficult to imagine how catecholamines released from there could reach an appreciable number of ganglion cells. On the whole, therefore, the evidence seems to point to a muscarinic receptor mediating the IPSP.

The *electrogenesis of the slow synaptic potentials* is not yet clear.

Neither the IPSP nor the slow EPSP of rabbit and frog sympathetic ganglion cells were found to be accompanied by an increment of the membrane conductance which is typical of the fast EPSP (KOBAYASHI and LIBET, 1968; NISHI et al., 1969). In fact, WEIGHT and VOTAVA (1970) observed a significant increase of the membrane resistance during the slow EPSP of frog sympathetic ganglion cells. Furthermore, changing the membrane potential by the application of steady depolarizing or hyperpolarizing currents across the membrane (Fig. 9) had not the effect on the amplitude of the slow synaptic potentials which one would expect if these were generated by changes in the ionic conductance of the membrane and the resulting ion flow tending to shift the membrane potential in the direction of the equilibrium potential for the respective ion. Thus, moderate depolarization increased and strong depolarization reduced the amplitude of the slow EPSP, whereas hyperpolarization depressed it (KOBAYASHI and LIBET, 1968; KOKETSU, 1969). WEIGHT and VOTAVA (1970) found an identical reversal potential for the slow EPSP and the after-hyperpolarization of the antidromic action potential (index of the K^+ equilibrium potential). They concluded that the slow EPSP in frog sympathetic ganglion cells was generated by a decrease or inactivation of the resting K^+ conductance. Accordingly, this slow EPSP would be the first example of a postsynaptic potential generated by an inactivation of the membrane conductance. The IPSP of cells in the superior cervical ganglion of the rabbit was depressed and eventually abolished by progressive depolarization, but was increased by moderate and depressed by strong hyperpolarization (KOBAYASHI and LIBET, 1968). Essentially identical results were obtained for the P-wave of frog paravertebral

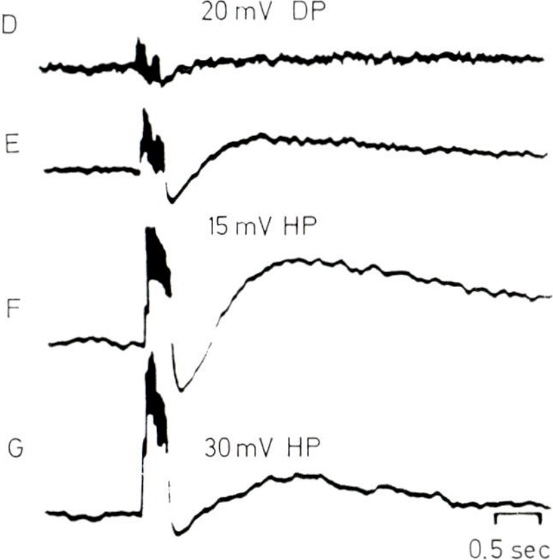

Fig. 9. Intracellular records from an isolated curarized rabbit superior cervical ganglion. Responses to 0.25-sec trains of preganglionic stimuli at 40/sec at the resting potential of 45 mV (2nd tracing) and during depolarization (DP) by 20 mV and hyperpolarization (HP) by 15 and 30 mV respectively. Note the decrease of the summed fast EPSP's with decreasing membran potential and the reduction of IPSP's and slow EPSP's with both strong reduction (20 mV DP) and increase (30 m HP) of the membrane potential (from KOBAYASHI and LIBET, 1968)

ganglia (NISHI and KOKETSU, 1968b; KOKETSU, 1969). The IPSP or P-wave thus behaves quite differently from the postspike positivity. The P-wave of bullfrog ganglia was not affected by changes in external K^+, Cl^- and Ca^{++}, in a way compatible with a role of conductance changes for these ions (KOKETSU and NISHI, 1967). NISHI and KOKETSU (1967) found the P-wave very sensitive to the metabolic inhibitors, dinitrophenol and sodium cyanide, to ouabain and to a lowering of the temperature; increasing the intracellular Na^+ enhanced the P-wave (KOKETSU, 1969). Intracellular studies of KOBAYASHI and LIBET (1968), however, seem to rule out a selective depressant action of ouabain or metabolic inhibitors on the IPSP; moreover, these authors did not find a selective depressant effect of reduced external K^+ on the P-wave, and metabolic inhibitors seemed to depress the slow EPSP long before the IPSP and the fast EPSP. Thus, the information available at present clearly indicates that the slow synaptic potentials differ from both the EPSP of ganglion cells and of the motor end plate as well as from the IPSP studied in central neurons (ECCLES, 1957) and in crustacean skeletal muscles (FATT and KATZ, 1953) in not being generated by increments of the ionic conductance of the membrane. Arguments for (KOKETSU, 1969) and against (KOBAYASHI and LIBET, 1968) the involvement of an electrogenic Na^+/K^+ pump in the production of the P-wave have been reported. Some kind of metabolic process does not seem to be an unlikely cause (KOBAYASHI and LIBET, 1968) and could explain the unusually long synaptic delay.

It should be noted that in the isolated bullfrog lumbar sympathetic ganglia, a third slow synaptic potential has been described (Nishi and Koketsu, 1966, 1968a), the *late slow EPSP* or *LLN* (late late slow wave). When stimulating both preganglionic B- and C-fibres with long trains of tetanic stimuli, afterdischarges were observed in the postganglionic nerves, beginning during the train of stimuli and outlasting it by up to 2 min. These discharges were found to be accompanied by a slow depolarization, detectable by surface recording with the sucrose-gap method and by intracellular electrodes. The so-called early afterdischarge (EAD), obviously produced by the slow EPSP (LN-wave), could be separated from the longer lasting "late afterdischarge" (LAD) ascribed to a late slow EPSP (LLN), by the use of atropine, since this agent abolished the former but did not influence the latter. It was suggested that the LLN-wave was of non-cholinergic nature and that the transmitter generating the LLN-wave and the LAD was released only from preganglionic C-fibres. LLN-waves and LAD have not yet been described in mammalian ganglia. The ionic mechanism underlying the late slow EPSP was found to be similar to those producing the fast EPSP (increment in ionic conductance).

d) Ganglionic Transmission through Muscarinic Receptors and Slow Synaptic Potentials

Hilton and Steinberg (1966) found that the neurogenic vasoconstriction occurring in the dog in response to elevation of the intracranial fluid pressure could not be fully suppressed by the nicotinic receptor blocking agent, chlorisondamine, but that the remaining vasoconstriction was abolished by a small dose of atropine which, in the absence of chlorisondamine, had no effect. It was concluded that transmission through sympathetic ganglia could, in part, be supported by muscarinic receptors during blockade of the classical nicotinic pathway. This investigation is especially interesting as it used natural stimulation of the ganglia. Further evidence for ganglionic transmission of preganglionic impulses through muscarinic receptors was provided by Trendelenburg (1966b); after nicotinic transmission in the superior cervical ganglion of the spinal cat had been completely blocked by repeated high doses of nicotine, a train of repetitive preganglionic volleys produced a moderate, greatly delayed and long-lasting contraction of the nictitating membrane which had all the characteristics of the response to muscarinic ganglionic stimulants.

The only available electrophysiological data on the orthodromic adrenergic neuron activation through muscarinic receptors are supplied by A.M. Brown (1967), Nishi and Koketsu (1968a) and Haefely (1970, 1972c). The first mentioned author found that even high doses of hexamethonium did not completely abolish the rise in blood pressure produced by stimulation of the thoracic sympathetic trunk. Recordings from the inferior cardiac nerve revealed that although hexamethonium completely abolished the compound action potential of C-fibres to single stimuli, a 10-sec train of preganglionic impulses at 20/sec produced an asynchronous discharge in adrenergic nerves, originating in the stellate ganglion. The discharge set in with a delay of about 1 sec and did not reach its peak until 5 sec after the start of the train; it persisted at a slowly decreasing amplitude for up to 4 min after the end of the tetanus. Small doses of atropine abolished postganglionic firing as well as the rise in blood pressure and the tachycardia. In the cat superior cervical ganglion *in situ* blocked by hexamethonium-like agents, only a very small discharge is conducted along postganglionic nerves during the LN-wave induced by a short train of repetitive preganglionic volleys (Haefely, 1970, 1972c). The "muscarinic" pathway is relatively unimportant in this ganglion, but the postganglionic discharge accompanying the LN-wave can be enhanced by drugs and procedures known to increase the ganglionic stimulant action of muscarinic agents such as by isoproterenol, KCl, nicotinic stimulants and orthodromic tetanization (Haefely, 1970, 1972c). It should be noted that

BRONK and PUMPHREY (1935) had already observed, in the cat stellate ganglion, that synchronous postganglionic action potentials progressively decreased during preganglionic stimulation at high frequency (60/sec) whereas asynchronous discharges appeared. They already suggested two types of synaptic transmission.

The findings of A.M. BROWN were confirmed and greatly extended by careful quantitative studies of the transmission through the stellate ganglion of the pithed dog by FLACKE and GILLIS (1968), GILLIS et al. (1968), FLEISCH et al. (1969). They found that the curve relating the frequency of preganglionic sympathetic stimulation to the increase in heart rate was shifted in a parallel manner toward higher stimulation frequencies by hexamethonium. The maximum obtainable chronotropic effect was not depressed. Very small doses of atropine or scopolamine, which had no effect whatsoever in the absence of hexamethonium, virtually abolished the hexamethonium-resistant ganglionic transmission. On the other hand, hexamethonium abolished the effect of stimulation following small doses of atropine. Cholinesterase inhibitors markedly enhanced transmission through muscarinic receptors but had no effect on nicotinic transmission in the dog stellate ganglion. The existence of two cholinoceptive sites for excitation and their different sensitivity to drugs could also be demonstrated in the same ganglion using intraarterial injections of acetylcholine. There were small differences between the blockade of chronotropic effects produced by orthodromic stimuli and that of the responses to exogenous acetylcholine (FLEISCH et al., 1969) which points to the important role of the way by which acetylcholine reaches the ganglion cell in determining its interaction with either nicotinic or muscarinic receptors. There seems to be little doubt that the hexamethonium-resistant synaptic excitation of adrenergic ganglion cells operates through the slow EPSP and perhaps also the late slow EPSP (sometimes atropine did not abolish completely transmission). Recent results of CHEN (1969) with the late contractions of dog and cat nictitating membrane in response to high frequency trains of orthodromic stimulation point in the same direction.

e) Post-activation Phenomena

Grouped under this heading are several changes of the electrical and chemical excitability of the ganglion cell which result from the firing of a single or of a train of action potentials (direct, antidromic or orthodromic). These phenomena include changes of the membrane potential and especially of responses to a test volley (direct, antidromic or orthodromic) and to chemical agents following "conditioning" with single or repetitive volleys. Most of the postactivation phenomena have been studied with external macroelectrodes.

The most marked effect is the absolute and relative *refractory period* due to the inactivation and gradual recovery of the Na^+ carrying mechanism. In toad sympathetic B-ganglion cells the absolute refractory period is less than 10 msec (NISHI, et al. 1965), as measured by direct intracellular test volleys. Recovery then sets in very rapidly (leading to "subnormality"), almost complete excitability being attained after 40 msec. Thereafter, recovery becomes slow and full excitability is not observed until 150—250 msec in B-cells or 500—600 msec in C-cells. Obviously, this late phase is linked to the hyperpolarizing afterpotential (SKOK, 1968). In C-cells, the residual synaptic potential leads to a short "*supernormality*" of the cell body. The amplitude of the compound postganglionic action potential in response to a maximal orthodromic test volley is depressed after a *supramaximal antidromic conditioning action potential* (LORENTE DE NÓ and LAPORTE, 1950b). The recovery curve clearly follows the time curve of the hyperpolarizing afterpotential (ECCLES, 1937; JOB and LUNDBERG, 1953). At the peak of the latter, the postganglionic action potential may be depressed by as much as 50%, indicating that half of the stimulated ganglion cells fail to initiate a propagated spike (cat stellate ganglion, JOB and LUNDBERG, 1953).

Orthodromic transmission following an orthodromic *homosynaptic or heterosynaptic conditioning* volley is altered in a rather complex way and differently in the various ganglia. As a rule, the postspike depression is less marked after orthodromic than after antidromic conditioning (JOB and LUNDBERG, 1953). In the cat superior cervical ganglion *in situ*, the homosynaptic depression is quite considerable (ECCLES, 1937; LLOYD, 1939; GEBBER and VOLLE, 1966). However, a normal or even facilitated response may occur, since the direction and extent of the changes depend on the extent of presynaptic facilitation, the degree of occlusion present in the given ganglion and the postspike negativity and positivity produced by the conditioning volley. The degree of presynaptic facilitation and the size and time-course of postspike potentials and, therefore, the intensity of orthodromic facilitation and/or depression can be substantially affected by drugs. Thus, e.g. the removal of the postspike positivity of the conditioning action potential in the cat superior cervical ganglion by nicotine (ECCLES, 1935c) and by ouabain (GEBBER and VOLLE, 1966), abolishes the depression of the amplitude of a homosynaptic test response elicited some 150 msec after the conditioning one. The same homosynaptic interaction experiment in the isolated rat superior cervical ganglion reveals no overall depression of transmission by the afterpositivity, obviously because this particular ganglion contains a large subliminal fringe, and occlusion is less marked (DUNANT, 1967). Therefore, many cells are only subliminally excited by the conditioning volley (and do not produce hyperpolarizing afterpotentials), but they respond to the test volley because of presynaptic facilitation. That heterosynaptic facilitation (III 4 c) can be explained by the production of the LN-wave (LIBET, 1964) has already been mentioned.

Posttetanic hyperpolarization and depression. Following a train of repetitive action potentials, a very marked hyperpolarization sets in (ECCLES, 1944). It may last up to several minutes after a high frequency burst of activity. During the posttetanic hyperpolarization produced by antidromic stimulation, orthodromic transmission is depressed parallel to the increased membrane potential (LARRABEE and BRONK, 1938a, b; BRONK, 1939). The posttetanic hyperpolarization following a train of orthodromic stimuli may contain the slow synaptic potentials as already discussed. Due to the concomitant slow EPSP and to posttetanically facilitated transmitter release from presynaptic nerve endings, the depression of orthodromic transmission is less marked after an orthodromic than after an antidromic tetanus or may even be replaced by a facilitation (LARRABEE and BRONK, 1947; PAŠIĆ and SAVIĆ 1969). The latter is the rule in the cat superior cervical ganglion. Irrespective of facilitation or depression, the orthodromic ganglionic action potentials elicited during posttetanic hyperpolarization show all the changes which are characteristic for action potentials arising from an elevated membrane potential, namely increased amplitude of postspike negativity and reduced amplitude of postspike positivity. The posttetanic hyperpolarization is reduced by small amounts of ouabain (GEBBER and VOLLE, 1966; HAEFELY et al., 1967) which have no depressant effect on the transmission of single orthodromic stimuli. Doses of ouabain which completely block posttetanic hyperpolarization, also reduce the postspike positivity of single orthodromic action potentials and produce some depolarization of the ganglion. The posttetanic hyperpolarization in adrenergic ganglion cells greatly resembles the hyperpolarization occurring after frequent firing in other nerve cells, e.g. in snail nerve cells (KERKUT and THOMAS, 1965), crayfish stretch receptors (NAKAJIMA and TAKAHASHI, 1966), sensory neurons of leech ganglia (NICHOLLS and BAYLOR, 1968) and especially the hyperpolarization occurring in adrenergic (BROWN and HOLMES, 1956) and vagal C-fibres (RITCHIE and STRAUB, 1957; STRAUB, 1961; CONELLY, 1962; HOLMES, 1962). The posttetanic hyperpolarization of mammalian C-fibres has been shown by RANG and RITCHIE (1968), to be due to the activation of an electrogenic Na^+ pump by the accumulation of intracellular Na^+ during the tetanus, and evidence for such an underlying mechanism has also been obtained for the above-mentioned neurons in lower animals. The arguments for the involvement of an active Na^+ extrusion in posttetanic hyperpolarization in sympathetic ganglia are its abolition by ouabain (GEBBER and VOLLE, 1966) and by replacement of external sodium by lithium (JARAMILLO and VOLLE, 1968b) as well as its enhancement by caesium ions (HANCOCK and VOLLE, 1969b).

Evidence for inconstant small *posttetanic afterdischarges* after orthodromic stimulation in eserine-treated cats had been derived by ECCLES (1935a) when comparing contractions of the nictitating membrane produced by identical trains of tetanic stimuli at 40/sec applied either to the preganglionic or the postganglionic cervical sympathetic (see also CHEN, 1969). By recording from postganglionic nerve, it became possible to study directly the asynchronous postganglionic firing invariably set up immediately after short bursts of orthodromic volleys of high frequency (LARRABEE and BRONK, 1938a, b, 1946, 1947; BRONK, 1939; ECCLES, 1944; HAEFELY, 1972c). The afterdischarge is short-lived and ceases with the initiation of the posttetanic hyperpolarization (BRONK, 1939) (see Fig. 8). The afterdischarge is presumably initiated by the residual synaptic potentials built up during the tetanic burst, since it is blocked by curare (ECCLES, 1944); it differs in its time-course and its sensitivity to drugs from the discharge accompanying the slow EPSP and the late slow EPSP in curarized ganglia.

Long-lasting Changes Following Repetitive Activity. Trains of repetitive orthodromic impulses not only induce in the adrenergic nerve cell the changes, lasting less than 1 min just described, but they may also alter the reactivity to chemical agents for many hours (VOLLE, 1962a, b; TRENDELENBURG and JONES, 1965; TRENDELENBURG, 1966a). The ganglionic responses to acetylcholine, tetramethylammonium, carbachol, to the muscarinic drugs methacholine and McN-A-343, to histamine and to angiotensin and bradykinin are enhanced, those to nicotine little affected and those to KCl unaltered by orthodromic repetitive stimulation. Surprisingly, hexamethonium given after the orthodromic tetanus does not prevent the enhanced responses. The mechanism underlying the prolonged enhanced responsiveness induced by repetitive stimulation is completely unknown. Antidromic tetanic stimulation was found to be ineffective. Hexamethonium given before the orthodromic tetanus in doses producing complete blockade of orthodromic transmission is unable to prevent the posttetanic long-lasting enhancement of drug-responsiveness (TRENDELENBURG and JONES, 1965). The latter cannot, therefore, be due to the repetitive firing of spikes; a synaptic event must clearly be involved. GEBBER (1968a) observed that repetitive orthodromic stimulation at frequencies below 4/sec produced a long-lasting enhancement of the atropine-sensitive firing induced by methacholine and tetramethylammonium and unmasked an atropine-sensitive "late" component of the acetylcholine firing. The hexamethonium-sensitive "early" firing of acetylcholine was not increased. When frequencies above 4/sec were used as conditioning tetani, the postspike positivity of single orthodromic action potentials was markedly reduced for many hours. The reduction of the postspike positivity coincided with an enhancement of the hexamethonium-sensitive firing produced by acetylcholine. Changes of the contour of the action potential and of the drug sensitivity occurred even when the conditioning tetanus was applied during complete transmission block by hexamethonium. The importance of elucidating the nature of these two types of long-lasting posttetanic alterations of the adrenergic neuron can hardly be overestimated in view of the current interest in the neuronal mechanisms underlying learning and "memory".

Electrical impedance changes of ganglionic tissue were studied by BIRZIS and CARREGAL (1966) by means of two fine nichrome or platinum electrodes inserted into the cat superior cervical ganglion through which a low excitation current with a frequency of 17.5 kc was passed. An initial drop of the impedance baseline occurred with trains of orthodromic stimuli, tentatively related to presynaptic events, followed by a long-lasting increase. The impedance changes were interpreted in terms of changes in the relative size of the extracellular fluid compartment, the phase of rising impedance presumably signalling the passage of fluid back into the cells, e.g. cellular hydration. It would be interesting to correlate these impedance changes with other electrical phenomena which follow a train of impulses.

f) Patterns of Innervation and Integrative Activity of Adrenergic Neurons

The way by which adrenergic neurons are connected to the central nervous system and the changes which the signals, arriving over the preganglionic fibres, undergo at the ganglionic synapse should be briefly mentioned.

In the larger sympathetic ganglia of mammals, e.g. in the superior cervical ganglia of cats, rats and rabbits, the adrenergic neurons obtain a *multiple innervation;* there is *convergence* of the input from many preganglionic fibres onto one ganglion cell. On the other hand, the number of postganglionic fibres leaving a ganglion is considerably higher than that of the preganglionic fibres ending in the ganglion (BILLINGSLEY and RANSON, 1918a, b; SANBE, 1961); there is *divergence* of impulses from one preganglionic fibre to a number of ganglionic cells. In most adrenergic ganglion cells, a volley in a single preganglionic fibre does not induce sufficient synaptic activity to initiate an action potential. In order to reach the critical depolarization level, the EPSP has to be built up by the simultaneous activity of a number of afferent fibres (*spatial summation*) or by the repetition at suitable intervals of the submaximal input (*temporal summation*); facilitated transmitter release from presynaptic endings may even be necessary. A single synchronous volley in the total afferent input of an adrenergic ganglion cell is very unlikely to occur under physiological conditions. The asynchronous action potentials running down the preganglionic nerve to a ganglion under physiological conditions will not evoke (after a latency due to pre- and post-ganglionic conduction and synaptic delay) an identical firing pattern in the postganglionic nerve. Most ganglia are not simply relay stations where one preganglionic impulse is transmitted to one or more sympathetic ganglion cells. The adrenergic ganglion cells act rather as small *integrative centres*, and the initiation or absence of a propagated spike in response to an impulse in one afferent fibre depends on the previous activity of the same fibre and on the preceding or simultaneous activity in other preganglionic fibres. Some mammalian ganglion cells behave differently, e.g. in the small scattered ganglia in the hypogastric plexus of the guinea-pig, where adrenergic neurons seem to receive inputs from only one preganglionic fibre (BLACKMAN et al., 1969). These neurons, however, differ in many respects from the usual type of adrenergic neuron: they have poorly developed dendrites and relatively short axons, they are more resistant to immunological and chemical denervation and to reserpine and their activation is not more or less continuous, but occurs in relatively rare bursts (vas deferens).

In the larger sympathetic ganglia, the adrenergic nerve cells have been found to give rise to either small myelinated or unmyelinated axons and are, therefore, designated as B- or C-cells respectively. The afferents of adrenergic neurons in the cat superior cervical ganglion are almost exclusively small myelinated B-fibres (FOLEY, 1943; JÄNIG and SCHMIDT, 1970). In the cervical sympathetic trunk of the rat, unmyelinated C-fibres are present (FOLEY and DUBOIS, 1940), but have no excitatory action on ganglion cells (DUNANT, 1967). Cells in the rabbit superior cervical ganglion receive inputs from both preganglionic B- and C-fibres (BISHOP and HEINBECKER, 1932; R.M. ECCLES, 1952a; R.M. ECCLES and LIBET, 1961; LIBET and TOSAKA, 1969). The same has been found in the superior cervical ganglion of turtles (LAPORTE and LORENTE DE NÓ, 1950a). In amphibian paravertebral ganglia, adrenergic B- and C-fibres are present, the former innervated by preganglionic B-fibres, the latter by preganglionic C-fibres (NISHI et al., 1965). It should be noted that adrenergic neurons seem to receive afferent inputs not only from the central nervous system through the classical preganglionic fibres originating in the spinal cord but also from sensory neurons located more peripherally than the ganglia or possibly also within them. Histological and electrophysiological evidence for such pathways have been obtained in prevertebral ganglia (KUNZ and SACCOMONO, 1944; BROWN, G.L. and PASCOE, 1952; BROWN, G.L. and PASCOE, 1954; JOB and LUNDBERG, 1952; MCLENNAN and PASCOE, 1954; CROWCRAFT et al., 1970; UNGVÁRI and LÉRÁNTH, 1970); they could explain the occurrence of viscero-visceral reflexes after such ganglia have been surgically separated from the central nervous system.

5. Changes of Electrical Properties of Adrenergic Ganglion Cells Following Denervation and Axotomy

a) Chronic denervation of adrenergic ganglion cells is widely used in experiments designed to differentiate between pre- and post-synaptic sites of action of ganglionic active drugs and to answer the question whether the elimination of the presynaptic input (in this type of experiment always combined with degeneration of presynaptic elements) induces changes of the true sensitivity to chemical agents of the excitable membrane of ganglion cells. The literature on the latter problem is rather confusing with regard to both the methods used and the results obtained (see e.g. VOLLE, 1966b, and TRENDELENBURG, 1967). The alteration of ganglionic response to drugs induced by chronic denervation will not be dealt with here in detail. Some elementary facts (in addition to those found in the reviews of VOLLE, 1966b, and TRENDELENBURG, 1967) will be mentioned, however, which should be considered when studying the sensitivity of denervated ganglia and which arise from the preceding electrophysiological discussions. It is obvious that full dose-response curves (providing also the maximum obtainable effect) of chemical agents will provide more information than the determination of threshold doses or responses to a fixed dose. The "effect" of a stimulant agent may be measured as ganglionic depolarization, postganglionic firing or the response of an effector organ, e.g. the contraction of the nictitating membrane. The ideal means of quantifying the effect of a given dose of a stimulant agent would be the measurement of the total number of action potentials elicited in the ganglion and conducted along the postganglionic nerve(s). The total electrical activity in a thin postganglionic nerve can be estimated in a given preparation, but it is impossible to compare it with that occurring in another preparation, because the number of fibres in a postganglionic nerve varies greatly in different animals and the recording conditions cannot be standardized sufficiently. It is, therefore, maintained by many authors, that the easily quantifiable response of an adrenergic effector organ will give more reliable information than electrophysiological techniques. It should be kept in mind, however, that the simplicity of the experimental set-up (e.g. recording of the amplitude of nictitating membrane contractions) is inadequate in comparison with the complexity of the problem. The same amplitude of contraction of the nictitating membrane can be obtained by either a short train (small number of impulses) of postganglionic volleys at a high frequency or a longer train at a much lower frequency. The contractile response of a smooth muscle to impulses in its adrenergic nerve supply (especially to asynchronous ones) obeys very complex laws of spatial and temporal summation and cannot, therefore, provide information about the number of nerve fibres firing, the total number of action potentials or their temporal distribution within an adrenergic nerve. A further point worthy of consideration is the fact that chronically denervated ganglia differ from innervated or acutely denervated ones, not only by a substantial loss of presynaptic cholinesterase, and the individual cells not only by the absence of continuously impinging presynaptic impulses, but also by marked structural alterations; a considerable part of the surface in normal ganglion cells is covered by presynaptic knobs forming intimate connections with the subsynaptic area. In denervated ganglia, the presynaptic terminal knobs are replaced by proliferating Schwann cells (TAXI, 1961; HUNT and NELSON, 1965). The access of exogenous chemical agents to these formerly subsynaptic areas may consequently be substantially altered and, therefore, invalidate conclusions concerning the "sensitivity" of the postsynaptic membrane. It seems that we are far from a definite acceptance or rejection of Cannon's law of denervation in the case of adrenergic nerve cells.

Elementary electrical properties of ganglion cells following chronic denervation have only been studied in frog paravertebral ganglia (HUNT and NELSON, 1965). These ganglion cells were found to have an increased membrane resistance, a finding which, in the absence of changes in the membrane capacitance and cell diameter, has to be ascribed to an *increase of the specific membrane resistance*. It is interesting that an increased membrane resistance was also found in denervated skeletal muscles (NICHOLLS, 1956; MILEDI, 1960), where it could be correlated with a fall of the K^+ conductance of the membrane (HUBBARD, 1963). The resting membrane potential of denervated ganglion cells was not significantly altered and antidromic action potentials appeared normal. It may be mentioned that earlier investigators had already postulated an involvement of K^+ in some denervation characteristics (PERRY and REINERT, 1954; GERTNER and REINERT, 1957).

β) Axotomy of adrenergic neurons induces marked but usually reversible retrograde degenerative alterations in the cell body ("axonal response") (BARTON and CAUSEY, 1958). Orthodromic transmission is depressed or fails some days after axotomy (BROWN and PASCOE, 1954; McLENNAN, 1954), recovery sets in after 3 weeks and is complete between 72 and 100 days following axotomy (ACHESON and REMOLINA, 1955). An intracellular study of axotomised cells in the frog paravertebral ganglia has been carried out by HUNT and RIKER (1966). Beginning on the third day after axotomy, the cells showed a progressive fall in the resting membrane potential associated with a reduction in the cell resistance. The amplitude of orthodromic action potentials was reduced and its time-course increased. The threshold for initiation of impulses by direct stimulation was not significantly increased; axotomized cells, however, failed to respond with repetitive spikes to a strong depolarizing current. The number of cells which were invaded by an antidromic impulse was much reduced. The spike responses to antidromic impulses often had no overshoot, the rate of rise was reduced and the time-course prolonged and they thus resembled antidromic action potentials recorded during hyperpolarization in normal cells. Synaptic potentials — usually suprathreshold in normal cells — were reduced in amplitude and many cells failed to respond with a spike to supramaximal preganglionic volleys. The reduced amplitude of EPSP's may explain the marked posttetanic potentiation of transmission occurring in axotomized cells, which is normally small or absent in normal cells.

Investigations with extracellular electrodes in mammalian ganglia (BROWN and PASCOE, 1954; ACHESON and REMOLINA, 1955) have provided additional information. Thus, the axons between the site of section and the ganglion cell body conducted normally during the degenerative changes observed in the cells. Moreover, a marked subsensitivity to acetylcholine accompanied the "axonal response", of ganglion cells. The first sign of axotomy was a prolongation of the relative refractory period and, therefore, the failure of the ganglion to transmit trains of impulses. Recordings from the ganglionic surface revealed a depression or even absence of slow potentials; posttetanic hyperpolarization was reduced (BROWN and PASCOE, 1954).

On the whole, the retrograde degenerative changes in ganglion cells after axotomy seem to be similar to changes observed in other neurons following section of their axons. There is, unfortunately, no information from the available literature, whether retrograde degeneration differs in adrenergic B- and C-cells. It is, furthermore, not known, how far away from the ganglion cell axotomy can be performed without leading to detectable alterations in the cell body.

IV. Electrical Properties of the Adrenergic Cell Axon

1. Conduction Velocity

Electrophysiological investigations have confirmed earlier morphological studies (HUBER, 1900; RANSON and BILLINGSLEY, 1918) indicating that adrenergic nerve axons are of two types, namely small *myelinated B-fibres* and *unmyelinated C-fibres*. The composition of postganglionic sympathetic nerves varies greatly. In the main efferent nerve of the cat superior cervical ganglion, the internal carotid nerve, ECCLES (1935b) distinguished four groups of fibres with average conduction velocities of 6, 3.4, 2 and 1 m/sec. KOSTERLITZ et al. (1964) studied the fibre composition of the small branch arising from the infratrochlear nerve and innervating the medial smooth muscle of the cat nictitating membrane. This nerve branch usually contained four groups of fibres with conduction velocities between slightly less than 1 m/sec and 13 m/sec. After removal of the superior cervical ganglion some 14 days previously, a large group of fibres conducting at 1.7—3.8m/sec disappeared and, therefore, represent the adrenergic B-fibres innervating the nictitating membrane. A histological control revealed that these axons were very fine medullated fibres. HEINBECKER (1930), HEINBECKER and BISHOP (1929), BISHOP and HEINBECKER (1930, 1932) had already concluded from measurements of conduction velocities and thresholds of excitation that postganglionic sympathetic nerves were composed of B- and C-fibres and that the fibres innervating the orbital region were myelinated; adrenergic vasomotor fibres, however, were assumed to be mainly slowly conducting unmedullated axons. In the inferior cardiac nerve of the cat, arising from the stellate ganglion, the fibres were found to conduct at 0.6—1.4 m/sec (BRONK et al., 1938) and 0.8 m/sec (BRONK, 1939). The splenic nerves of the cat contain a large number of unmyelinated C-fibres conducting at approximately 1 m/sec which are, for the most part, adrenergic (FERRY, 1963a; HAEUSLER et al., 1969). DOUGLAS and RITCHIE (1956) found postganglionic fibres in the rabbit cervical sympathetic trunk which conducted at 0.6 m/sec. Postganglionic fibres of the rabbit inferior mesenteric ganglion conduct at about 0.45 m/sec (G.L. BROWN and PASCOE, 1952). Nerve fibres in the vas deferens nerve of the guinea-pig are slowly conducting unmyelinated fibres (FERRY, 1963b, 1967). Adrenergic B- and C-fibres were also found in rats (DUNANT, 1967), in turtles (LAPORTE and LORENTE DE NÓ, 1950a; LORENTE DE NÓ and LAPORTE, 1950a) and in the toad (NISHI et al., 1965). The distance from the effector cells, at which the adrenergic B-fibres lose their myelin sheath, is unknown.

2. Action Potential

Postganglionic axons have not been studied systematically with intracellular electrodes. Accidental impalements of such axons have been reported by R.M. ECCLES (1955); the action potentials differed from those of ganglion cell bodies by the absence of a synaptic step (III 4 b) and the shorter total duration. Values for the resting potential are not available, but they may be reasonably assumed not to be significantly different from that of the cell bodies. This is supported by the experiments of KOSTERLITZ et al. (1968) who found, with the sucrose-gap method, that K^+ depolarized the proximal axons of the rabbit superior cervical ganglion to the same degree as the ganglion itself.

3. Posttetanic Hyperpolarization

BROWN and HOLMES (1956) studied the monophasic action potentials of various mammalian sympathetic postganglionic nerves after dc amplification. The mass action potential of adrenergic C-fibres resembled the antidromic ganglionic action potential, both being composed of a distinct hyperpolarizing afterpotential of 100—200 msec duration. In the axons, however, the repolarization was less steep and contained a small depolarizing afterpotential. BROWN and HOLMES (1956) confirmed the findings of GRUNDFEST and GASSER (1938) showing that repetitive activity increased the amplitude of action potentials through hyperpolarization. The marked posttetanic hyperpolarization occurred only in fibres conducting at less than 1.1 m/sec and increased the spike height by up to three times. The augmenting effect of a tetanic train on the size of action potentials could be simulated by artificial hyperpolarization of the nerves under the recording electrode. The posttetanic changes were dependent upon the temperature and occurred in all C-fibres studied, whether adrenergic or non-adrenergic; they seem, therefore, to be a general property of unmedullated fibres. It may, consequently, be assumed that the mechanisms underlying this important phenomenon are the same in the different axons and nerve cell bodies, where it has so far been observed and especially in vagal C-fibres, where it has recently been studied most intensively. The fact is generally agreed upon that the posttetanic hyperpolarization must be related to metabolic processes during the recovery after repetitive activity (GREENGARD and STRAUB, 1962; DEN HERTOG et al., 1969; DEN HERTOG and RITCHIE, 1969) and more specifically to the activity of the Na^+ pump which is increased by the Na^+ accumulated intracellularly during repetitive activity. Two ways were proposed by which increased activity of the Na^+ pump could produce hyperpolarization, namely by depletion of K^+ in the periaxonal space as the result of its accelerated uptake, the pump being electroneutral (RITCHIE and STRAUB, 1957), and on the other hand by a direct electrogenic effect of an uncoupled Na^+/K^+ pump (STRAUB, 1961). RANG and RITCHIE (1968) have recently provided conclusive evidence for the latter explanation. They have also worked out a mathematical model of this electrogenic pump in which: a) the "rate of extrusion of Na^+ depends on the degree to which a pool of carrier molecules on the inside surface of the membrane is combined with Na^+"; b) "each carrier molecule transfers three Na^+ at a time" and c) "the rate constant for extrusion of Na^+ also depends on the presence externally of K^+ which combine with some sites of the external surface of the membrane". Posttetanic hyperpolarization was greatly enhanced by replacing external Cl^- by sulphate or by isethionate which removed the short-circuiting effect of internal Cl^-. Small anions such as chloride, nitrate, ioide, bromide and thiocyanate were able to short-circuit the electrogenic pump, while larger anions like sulphate and isothianate could not. Hyperpolarization declined rapidly to a small value when the external K^+ concentration was reduced to zero. Subsequent addition of K^+ caused a marked redevelopment of posttetanic hyperpolarization. This activating response was also obtained with other cations, thallium being even more effective than, and rubium as effective as K^+, whereas caesium and ammonium were 1/10 and lithium 1/30 as effective as K^+. Reduction of external Na^+ increased the size of hyperpolarization, whereas this was little affected by changes of the membrane potential. On the basis of the information available at present, it is not yet possible to decide whether the posttetanic hyperpolarization is due to an electrogenic Na^+ pump distinct from the neutral Na^+/K^+ pump operating at rest, or whether the same pump can operate both in a neutral and electrogenic manner and which are the factors determining the coupling ratio between the two modes of Na^+ extrusion. The experiments of RANG and RITCHIE (1968) suggest that the coupling ratio may not be fixed.

The posttetanic hyperpolarization of the isolated cardiac sympathetic nerve differs from that of the stellate ganglion by the absence of the negative hump produced by the LN-wave and, therefore, by being unaffected by atropine (LIBET, 1964).

4. Possible Interaction of Neighbouring Fibres During Activity

MARRAZZI and LORENTE DE NÓ (1944) have reinvestigated the changes in the excitability of resting myelinated nerve fibres induced by impulses travelling in neighbouring axons in the frog sciatic nerve. They found that the active fibres produced changes in excitability and conduction velocity in neighbouring inactive fibres by the flow of current during the action potential and the recovery phase.

No such investigations have been carried out in adrenergic fibres. In view of the well known fact that the unmedullated adrenergic fibres are often found to be enveloped in groups by a Schwann sheath, electrotonic interaction between these small fibres is very likely to play a more important role than in myelinated fibres. Consideration should be given to this possible interaction in future experiments.

V. Electrical Properties of the Adrenergic Nerve Terminals; Electrical Events Involved in Transmitter Release

The electrical properties of adrenergic nerve endings are virtually unknown, because it is so difficult to study these small terminals by direct electrophysiological methods (see II 3). Nevertheless it would appear worthwile to consider some problems of primary importance.

1. Invasion of Terminal Varicosities by the Action Potential

The question whether or not the action potential invades the terminal varicosities cannot be answered at present. The situation may be similar either to the mammalian and frog motor nerve terminals, where there is good reason to believe that the action potential is propagated actively into the smallest endings (HUBBARD and SCHMIDT, 1963; KATZ and MILEDI, 1964, 1968), or to the crustacean motor nerve, where the very endings seem to be depolarized only electrotonically by the action potential, propagation being blocked at some distance from the ending (DUDEL, 1965). The fine morphology of the adrenergic nerve terminals differs noticeably from that of motor nerve endings; the sudden enlargement of the otherwise very fine fibres at the "varicosities" may create a situation like that encountered by the antidromic action potential when it invades the large cell body and which has been shown above (III 3) to present a critical site for the propagation of the impulse especially under certain conditions, e.g. during hyperpolarization. One can imagine that during repetitive activity, an orthodromic impulse could be blocked at the most proximal "varicosity" which would be electrotonically depolarized, whereas not even passive depolarization would reach the more peripheral "varicosities". One would then expect that successive orthodromic impulses would not necessarily "excite" all the varicosities of a given adrenergic fibre.

2. Electrosecretory Coupling at Adrenergic Nerve Endings

The mechanisms leading to the release of noradrenaline from the adrenergic nerve ending in response to an orthodromic impulse are without doubt initiated by the depolarization of the membrane at the sites, where the transmitter is stored, presumably the "varicosities". That this depolarization must not necessarily be brought about by an action potential has been shown by HAEUSLER et al. (1968a, b, 1969). In the isolated perfused cat heart, acetylcholine and KCl depolarize the adrenergic nerve endings and thereby initiate action potentials which are conducted antidromically along the inferior cardiac nerve; noradrenaline is liberated by both agents into the perfusate. Tetrodotoxin which blocks the generation of action potentials by inhibiting the Na^+ carrying mechanism, abolishes the antidromic firing induced by acetylcholine and KCl but does not prevent the release of noradrenaline by these agents. Since tetrodotoxin blocks the initiation of action potentials in adrenergic ganglion cells but not the depolarization by injected acetylcholine or KCl (HAEFELY, 1972c), it may be assumed that, at the terminals, noradrenaline release was initiated by depolarization even in the absence of action potentials. Evidence was further obtained that depolarization — either by action potentials or electrotonically — was important for the initiation of transmitter release only in so far as it led to an influx of Ca^{++} into the nerve ending. Tetracaine, which at a critical concentration blocks influx of Ca^{++} but not of Na^+ (DOUGLAS and KANNO, 1967), abolished the release of noradrenaline but not the antidromic firing in response to acetylcholine and KCl (HAEUSLER et al., 1969). Omission of Ca^{++} from the perfusion fluid enhanced the antidromic firing induced by the two agents but blocked the release of noradrenaline produced by them and by orthodromic stimuli (see also KIRPEKAR and MISU, 1967). The electrosecretory coupling at adrenergic nerve endings seems, therefore, to be essentially similar to that previously found at motor nerve endings (see KATZ, 1969), and in the adrenal medulla (DOUGLAS and RUBIN, 1963).

3. Facilitated Transmitter Release and Hyperpolarizing Afterpotential

The amount of noradrenaline liberated from the adrenergic nerve endings in the cat isolated perfused spleen was estimated by HAEFELY et al. (1965) during blockade of neuronal and extraneuronal uptake. It was found that the calculated transmitter release per impulse was not constant but increased in the range of frequencies between 0.5/sec and 2/sec. A rate-dependent mechanism facilitating the release of noradrenaline was postulated by these authors as well as by BURNSTOCK et al. (1964) who observed a progressive increase of the junction potential size in guinea-pig vas deferens smooth muscle cells when the sympathetic nerve was stimulated repetitively at frequencies between 0.1/sec and 2/sec. This facilitation of transmitter release appears less obscure in the light of recent investigations carried out at other neuromuscular junctions and at various synapses. The only synapse where it has been possible to record simultaneously by intracellular electrodes the amplitude of the presynaptic depolarization in nerve endings and the amount of transmitter released by it (by measuring the amplitude of the EPSP initiated in the postsynaptic cell) is the giant synapse of the squid. KATZ and MILEDI (1966) produced graded local depolarizations (recorded by a first intracellular electrode) of the presynaptic axons by intracellular injection of current (through a second microelectrode) and recorded the height of the EPSP in the postsynaptic cell in the presence of tetrodotoxin preventing the initiation of action potentials both pre- and post-synaptically. The postsynaptic response was clearly related to the level of presynaptic depolarization. At the squid giant synapse, too, TAKEUCHI and TAKEUCHI (1962) had found that the facilitation of the second of twin pulses was accompanied by an increased amplitude of the presynaptic action potential. These results corroborate findings obtained by less direct methods at the neuromuscular junction and in spinal cord synapses (ECCLES and KRNJEVIĆ, 1959) which indicate clearly that the amount of transmitter released from a nerve ending depends on the amplitude (and duration) of the action potential. Now, BROWN and HOLMES (1956) observed (III 3) that the amplitude of the individual action potentials in adrenergic C-fibres increases during trains of repetitive stimulation. There is no reason to doubt the occurrence of such a phenomenon in the adrenergic nerve terminals as well; it would easily explain, at least in part, the facilitated transmitter release occurring at certain frequencies of stimulation.

4. Posttetanic Changes in Adrenergic Nerve Endings

Following a train of repetitive activity, a marked hyperpolarization occurs in adrenergic ganglion cells and adrenergic nerve axons. It is not known whether adrenergic nerve endings respond in the same way to a burst of activity. Motor nerve terminals in the rat isolated phrenic nerve-diaphragm preparation have been shown to develop posttetanic hyperpolarization by GAGE and HUBBARD (1964) using WALL's (1958) technique (II 3) to measure the excitability of the endings.

VI. Electrical Changes Induced in the Adrenergic Neuron by Various Chemical Agents

It is beyond the scope of this review to describe all the actions on the adrenergic neuron of an immense number of chemical agents, either on its soma-dendritic, axonal or terminal part, even when restricted to investigations carried out with electrophysiological methods. A comprehensive treatment of ganglionic active agents, covering also the older literature, can be found in the reviews by TRENDELENBURG (1967), GYERMEK (1967) and KHARKEWICH (1967). Here, the main effects of some representative agents will be described and an attempt will be made to explain their mode of action on the excitable membrane of the adrenergic neuron. As far as distinct receptive sites are involved in their action, a topography of pharmacological receptors on the neuronal membrane will be attempted. The discussion of the effects of the different classes of substances will be in the order of soma-dendritic, axonal and terminal site of action.

1. Cholinoceptors

From a foregoing paragraph (III 4) dealing with the postsynaptic processes occurring at the soma-dendritic membrane of the adrenergic neuron, the existence of three distinct cholinoceptors has already emerged: the "nicotinic" (excitatory, depolarizing), the "muscarinic inhibitory" (hyperpolarizing) and "muscarinic excitatory" (depolarizing) receptors. This terminology is preferred to the use of abbreviations which are quite convenient for the workers highly familiar with this, altogether restricted, area of pharmacology, but which on the whole tend to create confusion.

a) Nicotinic Receptors

α) Soma-dendritic Part

Depolarization. The direct experimental proof for the depolarizing action on sympathetic ganglion cells of exogenous acetylcholine as well as of nicotine and tetramethylammonium has been provided by PATON and PERRY (1953) who recorded the surface potential of the cat superior cervical ganglion *in situ*. Injections of these drugs into the carotid artery produced depolarization after a very short delay, demonstrating the easy access of these drugs to their receptors. The depolarization is a local response of the ganglion cells and spreads decrementally along the postganglionic trunk, as confirmed by PASCOE (1956). In isolated ganglia, very high concentrations of acetylcholine are necessary for the induction of depolarization in the absence of a cholinesterase inhibitor (PASCOE, 1956; MASON, 1962; D.A. BROWN, 1966a, b, 1969; WATSON, 1970). The depolarization in the absence of anticholinesterases is mainly due to choline (KOSTERLITZ et al., 1968). The depolarizing action of acetylcholine, carbachol, nicotine and tetramethylammonium has also been demonstrated by intracellular recording in frog paravertebral sympathetic ganglia by BLACKMAN et al. (1963a), GINSBORG and GUERRERO (1964), RIKER (1967, 1968), KOKETSU et al. (1968b) and in pelvic sympathetic ganglion cells by MUIR and YONEMURA (1969). The depolarizing action of the nicotinic stimulants is specifically prevented by tubocurarine and hexamethonium, to mention only two antagonists. Hexamethonium (but not tubocurarine), although usually classified as "non-depolarizing" ganglionic blocker, produces a faint, transient depolarization in the isolated rat (SHAND, 1965) and in the cat superior cervical ganglion *in situ* (HAEFELY, unpublished); it is, therefore, a competitive antagonist with a very weak agonistic component. "Nicotinic" depolarizing activity is found in a large number of compounds, as e.g. choline (KOSTERLITZ et al., 1968), carbachol (D.A. BROWN, 1966a, b); WATSON, 1970), DMPP (HAEFELY et al., 1967; JARAMILLO and VOLLE, 1968a; MACHOVÁ and BOŠKA, 1969; WATSON, 1970), lobeline (JARAMILLO and VOLLE, 1968a; HAEFELY, 1972b), neostigmine (MASON, 1962; see however TAKESHIGE and VOLLE, 1963b; WATSON, 1970), piperidine, cytisine, anabasine, coniine (HAEFELY, 1972b), amphetamine (REINERT, 1960; HAEFELY, 1972b) and a series of other primary, secondary, tertiary and quaternary phenethylamines (HAEFELY, unpublished).

The depolarization initiated by "nicotinic" agents is the consequence of an unselective increase of the permeability of the membrane areas fitted with nicotinic receptors. This conclusion is based on studies of the synaptic potential and is corroborated by investigations with exogenous acetylcholine and carbachol. During depolarization with the latter agent, the membrane conductance of frog ganglion cells was found to be greatly increased (GINSBORG and GUERRERO, 1964). The peak amplitude of depolarization by acetylcholine, iontophoretically applied to bullfrog ganglion cells, increased when the cell membrane was hyperpolarized and decreased when the membrane potential was reduced by outward current pulses (KOKETSU, 1969). A discrepancy was found between the equilibrium potential of the EPSP and of the "fast (nicotinic)" acetylcholine depolarization by NISHI et al. (quoted in KOKETSU, 1969) which could be due to interactions of changes induced through "muscarinic" receptors, since GINSBORG and GUERRERO (1964) obtained with high concentrations of acetylcholine, carbachol and tetramethylammonium a maximum reduction of the frog ganglion cell membrane potential to —10 mV, the value of the equilibrium potential for the EPSP (NISHI and KOKETSU, 1960; BLACKMAN et al., 1963a). Although Na^{+} flow is the main event during nicotinic depolarization, Ca^{++} participates at least partially under normal conditions and may support the depolarization in the absence of external Na^+ (Pappano and Volle, 1966a; Koketsu et al., 1968b; Koketsu and Nishi, 1969). Li^+ can replace Na^+, though only for short times; because of the intracellular accumulation of Li^+ (which is extruded more slowly than Na^+), nicotinic depolarization fails after longer periods of perfusion of ganglia with Li^+ (Pappano and Volle, 1966b, 1967). Tetrodotoxin, in doses which completely block the generation of action potentials in a ganglion, does not reduce the depolarization by nicotinic drugs in the cat superior cervical ganglion (Haefely, 1972a); this finding is of interest, as it demonstrates that the ganglionic negativity, recorded with surface electrodes, reveals the true polarization of the ganglion cell population unaffected by the simultaneously fired action potentials. When ganglionic depolarization produced by nicotinic agents injected into the cat superior cervical ganglion was plotted against the dose, typical S-shaped dose-effect curves were obtained (Haefely, 1972b). In view of the impossibility of identical recording conditions in different *in vivo* preparations, the depolarization was expressed in this study as percentage of the complete depolarization, obtained by perfusing the individual ganglia for 2—3 min with isotonic KCl-solution. Apparent "affinities" and "intrinsic activities" of different agents could thereby be calculated. Nicotine, DMPP and acetylcholine (in the presence of scopolamine) had identical "intrinsic activities", while the apparent "intrinsic activity" for other nicotinic agents (e.g. lobeline, amphetamine) was appreciably smaller, most probably because of an unspecific local anaesthetic (membrane stabilizing) action with the higher doses (Haefely, 1972b).

The distribution of nicotinic receptors on the soma-dendritic membrane is unknown. It seems logical to assume an especially dense accumulation of receptors at the subsynaptic membrane areas, but there is no experimental support for or against the occurrence of circumscribed receptor areas separating the cell surface distinctly into chemically excitable and non-excitable membrane areas as in the innervated skeletal muscle; nor has an attempt been made to estimate the number of nicotinic receptors on the ganglion cell, e.g. with a technique used for the motor end plate (Waser, 1962, 1963).

Late Hyperpolarization. While the essential ionic mechanisms leading to depolarization of the ganglion cell when nicotinic agonists combine with nicotinic receptors have been fairly well studied, the processes initiated by this depolarization in the ganglion cell are less well known. The short-circuiting effect of nicotinic receptor activation leads to an accumulation of Na^+ intracellularly and a loss of intracellular K^+. It is very likely that the cells already attempt to restore this altered ionic distribution during the action of the nicotinic agents; such restorative mechanisms should manifest themselves by electrical phenomena and they can, indeed, be observed. Although the authors made no allusion to it, a ganglionic hyperpolarization can be seen in the paper by Paton and Perry (1953) to follow the depolarization produced by an intraarterial injection of tetramethylammonium to the cat superior cervical ganglion. In the isolated superior cervical ganglion, Pascoe (1956) observed a "positive overswing" of the ganglionic surface potential when depolarizing drugs like acetylcholine, tetramethylammonium and nicotine were washed out. Similar observations were made by Mason (1962), D.A. Brown (1966a, b) and Watson (1970). D.A. Brown (1966a) observed that the ganglionic hyperpolarization was clearly related to the degree of initial depolarization; the height of the secondary hyperpolarization could attain that of the initial depolarization. Similar findings were recently reported by Kosterlitz et al. (1968). The late hyperpolarization following depolarization by nicotinic drugs can easily be studied in the most "physiological" preparation, namely the blood-perfused superior cervical ganglion *in situ* by rapidly injecting the agents into its blood supply. Using this technique, tetramethylammonium depolarization, when strong enough, was found to be followed by hyperpolarization (GEBBER and VOLLE, 1966, VOLLE, 1967a). The two phases of polarization are, however, most regular and pronounced with DMPP (HAEFELY et al., 1967; JARAMILLO and VOLLE, 1968a; MACHOVÁ and BOŠKA, 1969; HAEFELY, 1972a), whereas a late hyperpolarization is not always observed with the longer acting nicotine (HAEFELY, 1972b) and is regularly absent with lobeline (JARAMILLO and VOLLE, 1968a; HAEFELY, 1972b). There is now ample evidence that the late hyperpolarization is due to the activity of a Na^+ pump: It is diminished or blocked by ouabain (GEBBER and VOLLE, 1966; HAEFELY et al., 1967; HAEFELY, 1972a), by dinitrophenol (D.A. BROWN et al., 1969), by perfusion with lithium (JARAMILLO and VOLLE, 1968b) and by low temperature (PASCOE, 1956). It is enhanced when chloride is replaced by the non-permeant isethionate (D.A. BROWN et al., 1969) and it is still present when the membrane potential approaches the equilibrium potential for K^+ (KOSTERLITZ et al., 1968). The electrogenic extrusion of Na^+ is evidently dependent on extracellular K^+, since the late hyperpolarization is reduced by lowered external K^+, while addition of K^+ in this situation greatly enhances the hyperpolarization (KOSTERLITZ et al., 1970). A similar activation of the Na^+ pump is also obtained with caesium ions given during the hyperpolarization (HANCOCK and VOLLE, 1969b). All the arguments mentioned for the electrogenesis of the late hyperpolarization by nicotinic drugs apply also to the posttetanic hyperpolarization in ganglion cells or C-fibres (see IV 3). The late hyperpolarization can, therefore, be reasonably explained by the activity of an electrogenic Na^+ pump which is triggered by the simultaneous accumulation of Na^+ intracellularly and of K^+ extracellularly during nicotinic depolarization. The question remains, why the amplitude and time-course of the late hyperpolarization differs with the various "nicotinic" stimulants and is even absent with some of these agents (e.g. lobeline, amphetamine). Based on a comparative study in the cat superior cervical ganglion, HAEFELY (1971b) suggested the following explanation: The activation of the Na^+ pump sets in very early during the initial depolarization; the arguments for this are the occurrence of changes in the contour of ganglionic action potentials characteristic for hyperpolarization at a time when depolarization was not completely worn off, and the finding that the blockade of nicotinic receptors in an early phase of depolarization by a sufficiently high dose of hexamethonium or a similar agent immediately reverses depolarization, produced by any "nicotinic stimulant", into hyperpolarization (Fig. 13). As reported very recently, hexamethonium has the same effect in the isolated rat superior cervical ganglion (D.A. BROWN and SCHOLFIELD, 1970). On the one hand, the early activation of the Na^+ pump may be partly responsible for the waning of depolarization, on the other hand, the tendency of the pump to increase the membrane potential is partially masked by the increase of the membrane conductance which is maintained by the presence of the stimulant drug at the nicotinic receptors. This view is fully supported by the finding that as late as 10 min after the injection of a dose of nicotine — when the ganglionic surface potential has reached the preinjection level and ganglionic transmission block is still very marked — the injection of hexamethonium promptly induces hyperpolarization. The late hyperpolarization is observed regularly and its amplitude is marked with drugs like acetylcholine and DMPP which produce a strong depolarization and disappear rapidly from the ganglionic receptors. It is less pronounced with tetramethylammonium which causes a longer lasting depolarization and may sometimes be absent with nicotine which remains for a much longer time in the ganglion (perhaps because of its higher lipophilic property and hence intracellular accumulation). With nicotine, depolarization decays very slowly (in other words, the membrane conductance slowly returns to its normal value) and thereby the disturbed ionic distribution triggering the pump activity is also gradually restored; there is, therefore, no reason for the increased pump activity to outlast the normalization of the membrane conductance. For some long-lasting nicotinic stimulants which produced no late hyperpolarization (e.g. lobeline, amphetamine), an additional action was shown. These drugs have a weak apparent "intrinsic activity" for depolarization and the curve relating peak amplitudes of depolarization with the doses is bell-shaped. The agents are more potent blockers of impulse conduction in isolated nerves than is nicotine (HAEFELY, unpublished) and their depolarizing action of higher doses is depressed by their membrane stabilizing action. With injections of appropriate mixtures of DMPP or nicotine with procaine, similar dose-depolarization curves were obtained and late hyperpolarization was prevented. With K^+, depolarization is never followed by a late hyperpolarization, and the contours of the action potentials reappearing at the end of the falling phase of depolarization give no indication of an increased activity of the Na^+ pump; a K^+ depolarized cell and one depolarized by a nicotinic stimulant agent seem to differ appreciably in their ionic gradients.

Depolarization and Initiation of Action Potentials. The injection of a nicotinic stimulant into the blood supply of a ganglion initiates a number of action potentials which can be recorded from a postganglionic nerve as a burst of more or less asynchronous firing which is of very low amplitude when compared with the height of a synchronous mass action potential. The simultaneous recording of the ganglionic surface potential with the postganglionic discharge shows that, with low doses, the firing occurs throughout the whole duration of depolarization, the amplitude of both being correlated. With increasing doses, the discharge reaches a higher peak amplitude but the discharge is shorter, and with the highest doses, it may be visible only during a very short time of the ascending phase of depolarization. This indicates that more cells are firing simultaneously shortly after the injection but that discharges cease even before the peak depolarization is attained. The dose-dependent discharge pattern provides a good explanation for the bell-shaped dose-response curves obtained when plotting the doses of stimulant drugs against the intensity of responses of a neuro-effector organ (TRENDELENBURG, 1967). The shortening of discharge will be explained below. It is not difficult to understand the initiation of action potentials by the depolarizing nicotinic agents when remembering how spikes are triggered by orthodromic stimuli. Figure 10 shows intracellular records from 3 different cells in a frog paravertebral ganglion (GINSBORG and GUERRERO, 1964). The two lower concentrations of carbachol produced a small and slowly developing depolarization and failed to initiate spikes. Although the critical depolarization level was obviously reached after several seconds with both 0.1 and 1 mM, spikes were not initiated, most probably because the slowly rising depolarization, like the linearly rising outward current (see III 2), produced accommodation. The depolarization in response to 5 mM carbachol rose much more rapidly and initiated 15 spikes at a frequency of approximately 20/sec. The pattern of firing observed in a postganglionic nerve finds an adequate explanation in the variable number of cells initiating a variable number of spikes at different frequencies at varying times after drug administration. An intracellular study by RIKER (1967, 1968) of acetylcholine depolarization and spike initiation in an isolated paravertebral frog ganglion confirmed that a relatively small percentage of cells produced spikes in response to a constant concentration of acetylcholine. Furthermore, he found that action potentials initiated by acetylcholine resembled antidromic potentials rather than orthodromic ones in their form. RIKER's conclusions may create some confusion with regard to the identity of the action of endogenous presynaptically released and exogenously applied acetylcholine. Those interested in this problem and that of the possible additional presynaptic site of action of nicotinic stimulants are referred to the critical discussion given in the review by VOLLE (1969). Suffice it to say here that it cannot seriously be expected that bathing a ganglion in acetylcholine or injection of it into the blood supply of a ganglion should simulate orthodromic stimulation in every respect. There are too marked differences in the time-course of accumulation of acetylcholine at the sites of the ganglion cell membrane acted upon. It seems logical that the action of exogenous acetylcholine should be rather similar to a steady depolarization by intracellularly injected currents.

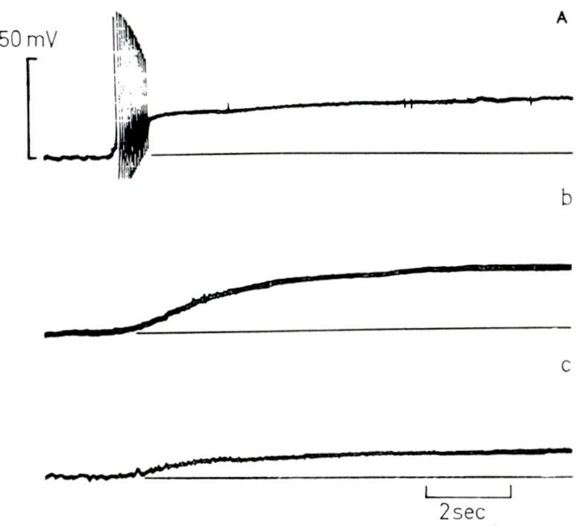

Fig. 10a—c. Intracellular records from 3 cells of a frog paravertebral ganglion *in vitro*. Effects of carbachol added to the bathing fluid in a final concentration of 5 mM (a), 1 mM (b) and 0.1 mM (c). For explanation see text (from GINSBORG and GUERRERO, 1964)

Polarization Changes and Orthodromic Transmission. The first visible effect of low doses of nicotinic stimulant is facilitation of synaptic transmission. The mechanism of facilitation clearly seems to be a slight decrease of the membrane potential which enables those cells with subliminal synaptic activity to reach the critical firing level. Small amounts of nicotine, which do not depress ganglionic transmission, have marked effects on the slow components of orthodromic and antidromic action potentials (ECCLES, 1935b, d; OBRADOR and ODORIZ, 1936; LLOYD, 1939; PATON and PERRY, 1953; R.M. ECCLES, 1956); the postspike negativity is reduced, the postspike positivity becomes more pronounced but shortened. These effects can be ascribed to depolarization, since cathodal current pulses produce similar changes. In the isolated curarized rabbit superior cervical ganglion, nicotine in low concentrations reduced the time of decay of the N-wave (synaptic potential) and in higher concentrations also decreased its amplitude (R.M. ECCLES, 1956); an explanation of this is presumably provided by the increase in the membrane conductance (decrease in the time constant of the membrane).

The complex sequence of events following the administration of higher doses of nicotinic stimulants is best investigated in an *in situ* ganglion preparation in which single doses are injected into the ganglionic blood supply during the continuous recording of ganglionic and postganglionic potentials and during preganglionic stimulation at a low rate (Figs. 10, 11, 12). By this method, PATON and PERRY (1953) and LUNDBERG and THESLEFF (1953) observed that the block of transmission produced by nicotinic stimulants outlasted the period of depolarization. The authors suggested that transmission block by nicotine proceeded in two phases, initially by depolarization and later on by a competitive block of nicotinic receptors. Surprisingly, a causal relationship between depolarization and transmission block has been accepted by pharmacologists without attempts to explain it by electrophysiological considerations; the relationship has recently been challenged (RIKER, 1967, 1968; GEBBER, 1968b). How does depolarization block the initiation of action potentials? Intracellular studies have shown that spike generation is blocked by cathodal current pulses of sufficient strength,

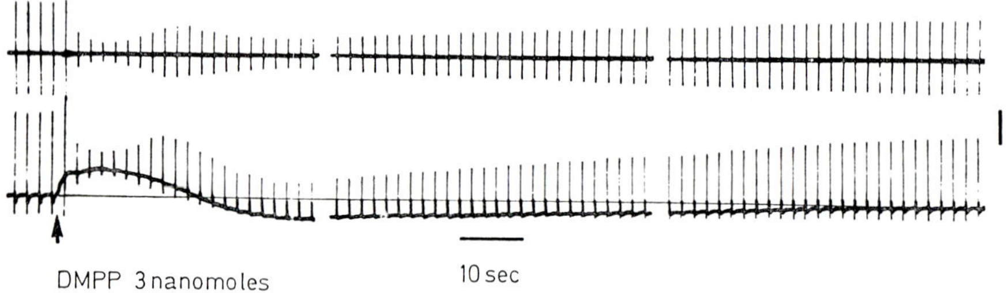

Fig. 11. Postganglionic action potentials of the external carotid nerve (upper beam) and ganglionic potentials (lower beam) of the cat superior cervical ganglion *in vivo* in response to preganglionic volleys of half-maximum strength applied every 2 sec. Biphasic depression of ganglionic transmission separated by a transitory recovery phase in response to the intra-arterial injection of DMPP (3 nanomoles). Calibration: 0.2 mV for postganglionic, 0.5 mV for ganglionic record (HAEFELY, 1972a)

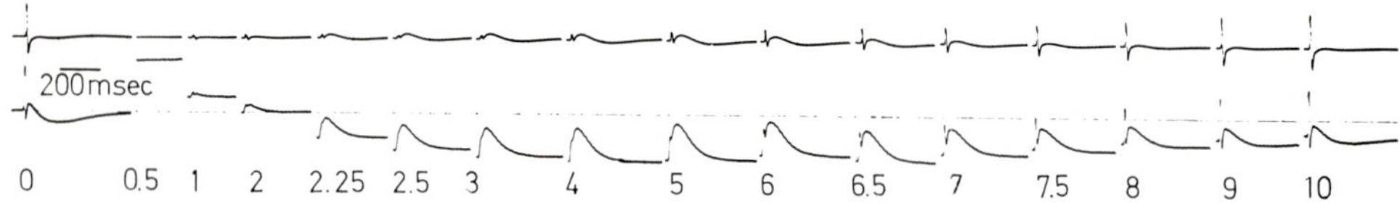

Fig. 12. Biphasic block of ganglionic transmission by DMPP (30 nmoles) injected into the carotid artery of the cat. Shown are postganglionic (upper beam) and ganglionic (lower beam) action potentials in response to supramaximal preganglionic volleys. The first record on the left is the control response immediately before injection of DMPP. The other records were taken at the indicated time (in minutes) after the injection. Note the appearance of almost pure synaptic potentials at the peak of the hyperpolarizing phase and the gradual recovery of the postganglionic spike height with decaying hyperpolarization and normalization of the contour of ganglionic action potentials. The horizontal line indicates reference level of ganglionic polarization. The control ganglionic spike height is 2 mV (from HAEFELY, 1972a)

simulating nicotinic depolarization. From the fundamental studies on the giant axon, this can reasonably be ascribed to the inactivation of the Na^+ carrying mechanism; moreover, delayed rectification and increase of the threshold firing level, described under accommodation (see III 2), may play a role. The explanation of the late phase of transmission block by competitive antagonism at the nicotinic receptors is no longer tenable. Theoretically, a competitive block by the highly potent agonist nicotine could satisfy neither the "occupation" nor the "rate" theory of drug-receptor interaction. In practice, TRENDELENBURG (1957, 1966b) found that the stimulant action of nicotinic drugs was inhibited non-competitively during the late phase of block and proposed the term "non-depolarizing phase" of block.

Ganglionic transmission is also depressed or blocked during both a depolarizing and a non-depolarizing phase with tetramethylammonium (GEBBER and VOLLE, 1966; JARAMILLO and VOLLE, 1968a), DMPP (HAEFELY et al., 1967; JARAMILLO and VOLLE, 1968b; GUMULKA and SZRENIAWSKI, 1968; MACHOVÁ and BOŠKA, 1969; HAEFELY, 1972a), lobeline (JARAMILLO and VOLLE, 1968a) and amphetamine (HAEFELY et al., 1967). From these studies and a systematic investigation of several nicotinic stimulants (HAEFELY, 1972a, b), the following conclusions can be drawn (whereby the two phases of ganglionic depression are best illustrated by the short acting DMPP, Figs. 11, 12): With threshold doses (1 nmole or less into the carotid artery), the initial effect is a facilitation of transmission coinciding with a low-amplitude depolarization. This phase lasts several seconds, depending mainly on the circulatory conditions of the ganglion, and is often followed by a depression of the postganglionic spike amplitude; this second phase is accompanied by a ganglionic hyperpolarization. The contour of ganglionic action potentials is characteristically altered, postspike negativity being enhanced and postspike positivity decreased. This second phase is at least twice as long as the primary, depolarizing phase. Gradual restoration of the contour of the ganglionic action potentials and of the ganglionic surface potential are strongly correlated. With increasing doses, the initial depolarization increases in amplitude and duration, and transmission is completely blocked. Action potentials reappear when depolarization decays and, in exceptional instances, transmission may be completely restored when the ganglionic steady potential reaches the pre-injection level. The ganglionic surface potential then swings in the positive direction to reach a peak of hyperpolarization 10—20 sec later. When the ganglionic surface potential crosses the pre-injection level or even slightly before this, the amplitude of the postganglionic action potentials decreases again and ganglionic transmission may again be completely blocked at the peak of hyperpolarization. At this moment, only a synaptic potential (N-wave) can often be recorded from the ganglionic surface (Fig. 12); this synaptic potential has a greater amplitude than one obtained after blockade of spike generation by hexamethonium but it does not, of course, reach the absolute level of the peak postspike negativity in the absence of the drug. With gradually decreasing hyperpolarization, spikes reappear in ganglionic and postganglionic records, but the ganglionic postspike waves show the characteristic changes until the pre-injection level of the ganglionic steady potential is attained. With medium doses of DMPP, tetramethylammonium and nicotine, the two phases of ganglionic block are clearly separated by the transient partial restoration of ganglionic transmission. This intermediate phase is usually absent with high doses of DMPP and tetramethylammonium and is never very marked with nicotine. The late hyperpolarization is often absent with nicotine (Fig. 13), especially in ganglia in which the initial depolarization has an extremely long duration. The separation of the two phases is at that time not very sharp; nevertheless, at the time when there is only a small residual depolarization or when the pre-injection level of the ganglionic steady potential has been reached, the ganglionic action potentials reveal the changes of postspike waves characteristic of hyperpolarization. Whether the second non-depolarizing phase of depression by nicotinic agents is causally related to the hyperpolarization is still a matter of controversy. HAEFELY (1972a, b) proposed that it was not the hyperpolarization *per se* which caused the late phase but rather the recovery processes triggered by the depolarization. As already explained, the activity of the electrogenic Na^+ pump can only lead to hyperpolarization if the ionic conductance changes induced by nicotinic stimulants wear off rather suddenly. It seems plausible, however, that the electromotive force of the electrogenic Na^+ pump may reduce the transmitter action even in the absence of an increased membrane potential by counteracting the net Na^+ influx. The inhibitory effect of the electrogenic pump may be similar to that of the IPSP in cells where the resting membrane potential is close to or at the equilibrium potential for the IPSP, e.g. in the crustacean skeletal muscle; the IPSP produces no hyperpolarization in this situation, and its presence

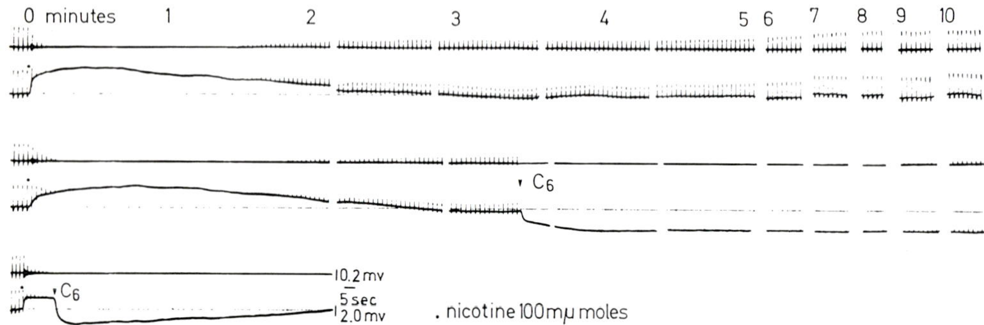

Fig. 13. Cat superior cervical ganglion *in situ*. Recording from the postganglionic external carotid nerve (upper beam) and from the surface of the ganglion (lower beam). Continuous stimulation of the preganglionic cervical sympathetic trunk with supramaximal shocks at a rate of 0.5/sec. The upper pair of tracings shows the effect of nicotine (100 nmoles) injected into the carotid artery. The figures above the top tracings indicate time in minutes after the injection. Note that the late block produced by nicotine was accompanied only by questionable hyperpolarization between 3 and 4 min after injection. The middle pair of tracings illustrates the effect of the same dose of nicotine injected after recovery of transmission from the depression induced by the first dose; hexamethonium injected at the peak of the late phase of transmission block produced an immediate marked hyperpolarization lasting over 10 min. In the bottom pair of tracings, the nicotine injection was repeated and hexamethonium given at the peak of depolarization. The abrupt marked hyperpolarization lasted for 2 min (from HAEFELY, 1972b)

can only be established by its inhibitory effect on excitatory events or by the unmasking of its hyperpolarizing effect during artificial depolarization (FATT and KATZ, 1953; DUDEL and KUFFLER, 1961). Until the proposed mechanism leading to the late phase of block has been properly identified, it seems preferable to call this phase the late non-depolarizable phase, as suggested by TRENDELENBURG (1967). In the late phase of ganglionic block observed with some nicotinic stimulants, there are certainly additional processes involved. Thus it has been shown (HAEFELY, 1972b) that e.g. lobeline and amphetamine have a pronounced local anesthetic component and the late block by these agents closely resembles that produced by procaine. The comparative study by HAEFELY (1972b) has demonstrated the inaccuracy of the statement, often encountered, that DMPP is a stronger ganglionic stimulant but a weaker ganglionic blocking agent than nicotine. In fact, both agents are equipotent in their depolarizing, stimulant and blocking effect, but the duration of the three effects is considerably shorter with DMPP. The interesting aspect of the late phase of block by nicotinic agents is the fact that this pronounced alteration of ganglionic transmission is not due to the presence of the drug but to its previous interaction with the excitable membrane. It must be mentioned that the involvement of some presynaptic events, in addition to the postsynaptic ones, cannot definitely be ruled out. It remains, for example, difficult to explain the transitory remission of transmission between the two phases of synaptic depression. By injecting acetylcholine, DMPP or KCl at different times after a dose of DMPP producing the typical biphasic changes of the ganglionic surface potential, it was found that the test doses were without effect during the peak of depolarization, as was expected, but unexpectedly during the transitory remission phase as well. During the late hyperpolarizing phase, test doses of acetylcholine and even more clearly of KCl produced depolarization of greater amplitude than normally but discharges were greatly depressed. The same was found in the case of 5-hydroxytryptamine by JARAMILLO and VOLLE (1968a) and of angiotensin and bradykinin by HAEFELY (1970a). Differentiation of the depolarizing and non-depolarizing phases of nicotinic block by recording effector responses to injected K^+, as proposed by TRENDELENBURG (1967), is of questionable value on the basis of the electrophysiological investigations just mentioned. Moreover, the estimation of the degree of depolarization produced by repeated injections or by prolonged infusion of nicotine, by measuring the relief from depolarization ("repolarization") by the injection of tubocurarine, as proposed by GEBBER (1968b), is untenable, since hexamethonium and tubocurarine in addition to remove the depolarization also unmask the hyperpolarizing action of the electrogenic Na^+ pump (HAEFELY, 1972b). This inappropriate means to estimate the degree of ganglionic polarization led GEBBER (1968b) to deny a causal relationship between blockade of transmission and depolarization when nicotine is infused in low concentrations over 1 hour into the arterial supply of the cat superior cervical ganglion. Admittedly the relationship between both phenomena is not as clear when the ganglion is exposed over a long period to a constant concentration of a drug, as when single injections of nicotinic stimulants are used. The proper effect of the drug on membrane conductance and the compensatory mechanisms, initiated by the ensuing ionic changes, may be mixed together in a hardly discernible manner. Phenomena observed in such experimental situations, e.g. the waning of depolarization in spite of the presence of constant drug concentrations (PASCOE, 1956) or the restoration of transmission in spite of maintained depolarization (KRIVOY and WILLS, 1956) in a ganglion bathed in a constant acetylcholine concentration await an explanation.

β) Axonal Part. As shown by KOSTERLITZ et al. (1968), the axonal part of adrenergic neurons contains nicotinic receptors mediating depolarization. The internal carotid nerve of the rabbit superior cervical ganglion, exposed in the sucrose-gap apparatus to choline or acetylcholine, is depolarized. The peak depolarization with these two agents is less than with K^+ and less than that obtained in the ganglion with both acetylcholine and choline. Thus, nicotinic receptors are either less concentrated on the axonal surface than on the soma-dendritic surface or less accessible to the agonists. In contrast to the ganglion, washing out the depolarizing agent was not followed by hyperpolarization in the adrenergic nerve. This may be due to the fact that the peak depolarization was less than half that observed in the ganglion. The effect of axonal depolarization on the conduction of action potentials has not been studied in adrenergic nerves. However, in mammalian non-medullated fibres of the vagus, ARMETT and RITCHIE (1961) found that blockade of conduction occurred with depolarization by acetylcholine, nicotine, tetramethylammonium and lobeline. Similar results were obtained by HANCOCK and VOLLE (1969a) in the cat vagus *in situ* when the agents just mentioned and DMPP were injected into the blood supply of the nodose ganglion; a drug-induced firing was not observed. A late phase of auto-inhibition by nicotinic drugs of a still unknown nature was described. The ionic mechanisms underlying acetylcholine-depolarization have been studied by ARMETT and RITCHIE (1963) in non-medullated fibres of the rabbit vagus and the cat hypogastric nerve. They found that acetylcholine increases the permeability of the membrane to Na^+ and Ca^{++}.

γ) Terminal Part. Acetylcholine (FERRY, 1963a, 1967; CABRERA et al., 1966; HAEUSLER et al., 1968a), DMPP (HAEUSLER et al., 1968a), nicotine (HAEUSLER, personal communication), amphetamine and some other phenethylalkylamines (HAEFELY et al., 1966b) depolarize adrenergic nerve terminals by excitation of nicotinic receptors and thereby induce the firing of action potentials which are conducted antidromically along the adrenergic nerve axon. These nicotinic agents seem to act similarly on the terminal and soma-dendritic part: Injection or infusion of low doses into the blood supply of an adrenergic effector organ induces a prolonged discharge. With increasing doses, the amplitude of the discharge is increased immediately after the arrival of the agents at the terminals, but it then decreases, or firing ceases completely in spite of further infusion. Blockade of KCl-induced firing during this phase of electrical silence leaves no doubt that the terminals are depolarized. Whether at the end of infusion, the depolarization turns into hyperpolarization, as it does at the soma-dendritic part, cannot be decided, since KCl-induced firing in the ganglion is also depressed during hyperpolarization. The nicotinic excitation is greatly increased by reduced Ca^{++}-concentrations and blocked by high concentrations of Ca^{++}; it has already been shown that the noradrenaline release is inversely correlated with the amplitude of discharges in low and high Ca^{++}-concentrations. Nicotinic excitation of adrenergic nerve endings is specifically inhibited by hexamethonium (HAEUSLER et al., 1968a; DAVEY et al., 1968) and d-tubocurarine (CABRERA et al., 1966), and unspecifically by general anaesthetics, like ether, pentobarbitone and chloralose (CABRERA et al., 1966).

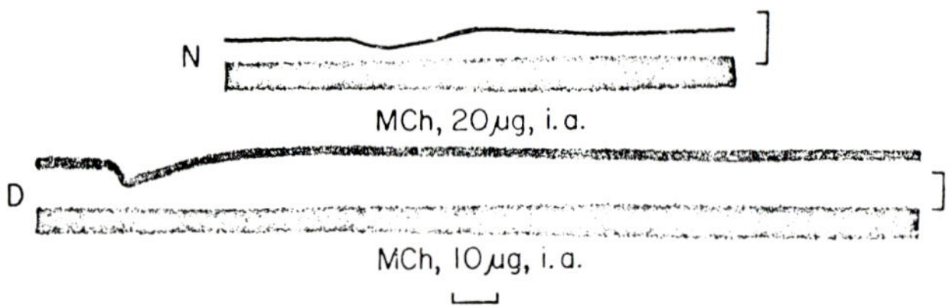

Fig. 14. Changes of the ganglionic surface potential (upper beam) and indication of postganglionic firing (lower beam) in the cat superior cervical ganglion in response to methacholine (MCh). Above (N), response of a normall innervated ganglion to 20 μg, below (D), response of a chronically denervated ganglion to 10 μg methacholine. The horizontal calibration is 2 sec; the vertical calibration refers to the top record of each pair and is 0.5 mV (from TAKESHIGE et al., 1963)

b) Muscarinic Inhibitory Receptors

α) Soma-dendritic Part. Muscarine (D.A. BROWN, 1966c; JARAMILLO and VOLLE, 1967a), methacholine (acetyl-β-methylcholine, TAKESHIGE et al., 1963), oxotremorine (JARAMILLO and VOLLE, 1967a), as well as acetylcholine and carbachol in the presence of hexamethonium (D.A. BROWN, 1966c) injected into the blood supply of the cat superior cervical ganglion produce a biphasic change of the ganglionic surface potential, characterized by an initial hyperpolarization of 2—4 sec followed by a longer lasting low-amplitude depolarization (Fig. 14). The initial hyperpolarization is accompanied by depression of ganglionic transmission (PAPPANO and VOLLE, 1962), whereas during the late depolarization, a low-amplitude asynchronous discharge occurs in the postganglionic nerve. Both effects are best obtained after a conditioning preganglionic tetanus, the injection of a cholinesterase-inhibitor, conditioning with repeated injections of KCl or isoproterenol in innervated ganglia or by chronic denervation. They are blocked by small doses of atropine or scopolamine but resistant to hexamethonium. The similarity of these "muscarinic potentials" to the P- and LN-wave has already been mentioned. The presence of "muscarinic inhibitory" and "muscarinic excitatory" receptors is thus well established.

No selective antagonist at either the inhibitory or excitatory receptors is known at present, whereas pilocarpine seems to be a selective agonist for "muscarinic excitatory" receptors (TAKESHIGE and VOLLE, 1964). The hyperpolarization mediated through muscarinic receptors has probably sometimes been confused with the hyperpolarization following nicotinic depolarization (D.A. BROWN, 1966c) which is blocked by hexamethonium but resistant to atropine. Intracellular studies in frog paravertebral ganglia (GINSBORG, 1965) did not reveal a muscarinic hyperpolarization by methacholine; furthermore, in this species, depolarization by methacholine was blocked by both hexamethonium and atropine (used in very high concentrations, as it blocked synaptic transmission). It is questionable whether an action on muscarinic inhibitory receptors — even if these were present in the frog — could be observed in isolated ganglia. The data available on the electrogenesis of muscarinic hyperpolarization were discussed in the paragraph on slow synaptic potentials (see III 4 c).

β) Axonal Part. It is not known whether muscarinic inhibitory receptors are present on the axonal membrane.

γ) Terminal Part. The muscarinic receptor(s) of the adrenergic nerve terminals will be discussed in the next paragraph.

c) Muscarinic Excitatory Receptors

α) Soma-dendritic Part. A characteristic feature of the depolarization induced through activation of muscarinic receptors is its weak amplitude (WATSON, 1970) which is not greater than about 10% of a maximal nicotinic depolarization (HAEFELY, unpublished) and its peculiar electrogenesis which has already been shown (see III 4 c) to be essentially different from that of the nicotinic depolarization. It cannot be decided yet whether the number of muscarinic excitatory receptors is too low to induce a more marked depolarization or whether the ionic mechanisms producing this allow only a small reduction of the membrane potential. It has been speculated that muscarinic receptors may be located outside the subsynaptic areas, but conclusive evidence is not yet available. An intriguing property of muscarinic depolarization and firing is their small size in a normal ganglion and the need of some facilitatory mechanism, which has already been alluded to (VOLLE, 1962a, b, c; TRENDELENBURG and JONES, 1965), in order to make it manifest. Consistent with the "sensitizing" effect of "membrane labilizing" processes on muscarinic phenomena in ganglion cells, is the ease with which these can be blocked by "membrane stabilizers" such as Ca^{++}, atropine and cocaine (TAKESHIGE and VOLLE, 1964; VOLLE and PAPPANO, 1968) and by unspecific agents such as morphine and methadone (TRENDELENBURG, 1957; JONES, 1963). It is also interesting that muscarinic phenomena are not observed in the cat superior cervical ganglion perfused with Locke solution (VOLLE and PAPPANO, 1968; see, however, FEHÉR and BOKRI, 1959, 1961) and that in the rat superior cervical ganglion, the specificity of muscarinic receptors is altered by perfusion (HANCOCK et al., 1969). Asynchronous discharges, induced by activation of excitatory muscarinic receptors, are found with acetylcholine (TAKESHIGE and VOLLE, 1962, 1963a; DOLIVO and KOELLE, 1970), acetyl-β-methacholine (TAKESHIGE et al., 1963), muscarine (SANGHVI et al., 1963; GYERMEK, et al., 1963; JARAMILLO and VOLLE, 1967a), cholinesterase inhibitors (VOLLE, 1962b;

TAKESHIGE and VOLLE, 1963b), pilocarpine (TAKESHIGE and VOLLE, 1964; MURAYAMA and UNNA, 1963; HAEFELY, 1971c), the synthetic compound McN-A-343* (MYRAYAMA and UNNA, 1963; JARAMILLO and VOLLE, 1967b), choline, propinylcholine, butyrylcholine (GEBBER and VOLLE, 1965) and oxotremorine (DE GROAT and VOLLE, 1963; JARAMILLO and VOLLE, 1967a). It is most interesting that, whereas discharges induced by single injections of tetramethylammonium and acetylcholine in unconditioned ganglia were completely blocked by hexamethonium and unaltered by atropine, the infusion of constant small amounts of both agents induced discharges more resistant to hexamethonium than to atropine (GEBBER and SNYDER, 1968). The interaction between nicotinic and muscarinic excitatory mechanisms will be dealt with below. From an intracellular study on isolated frog sympathetic ganglia, GINSBORG (1965) concluded that the muscarinic agents pilocarpine, acetyl-β-methylcholine and McN-A-343 had actions quite different from those in mammalian ganglia. However, the drug concentrations used by the author were extremely high and his experiments should be repeated in mammalian ganglia *in vitro* before a species difference can be accepted.

Not all investigators using atropine in studies of nicotine and muscarinic stimulation of ganglion cells took into consideration that this alkaloid unspecifically blocks all ganglionic activity in higher concentrations. Thus, the finding that atropine, applied iontophoretically to cells of pelvic ganglia of the guinea-pig, blocked orthodromic transmission as well as the effects of acetylcholine and nicotine (MUIR and YONEMURA, 1969), has to be interpreted with caution.

β) Axonal Part. Muscarinic agents have not so far been studied in the adrenergic axon, but vagal C-fibres were not depolarized by methacholine, bethanechol, arecoline and pilocarpine, as opposed to acetylcholine (ARMETT and RITCHIE, 1961).

γ) Terminal Part. LÖFFELHOLZ et al. (1967) and LINDMAR et al. (1968) discovered the presence of muscarinic receptors at adrenergic nerve endings which inhibited the noradrenaline-release through activation of nicotinic receptors by acetylcholine and DMPP. This interaction between muscarinic and nicotinic receptors was investigated with electrophysiological methods by HAEUSLER et al. (1968a). They confirmed the findings of the previously mentioned authors and observed that atropine reduced the antidromic discharges in the inferior cardiac nerve induced by the infusion of acetylcholine through the isolated cat heart and they obtained indirect evidence that this effect of atropine was due to a more marked depolarization of adrenergic terminals caused by acetylcholine. Conversely, muscarinic agents, like methacholine and pilocarpine, allowed the maintenance of a more continuous discharge during the simultaneous infusion of acetylcholine and at the same time reduced the amount of noradrenaline released. The authors concluded that activation of muscarinic receptors at the terminals depressed the depolarizing potency of nicotinic agents. These muscarinic receptors may be called "inhibitory" with regard to their effect on noradrenaline release and nicotinic depolarization; whether they correspond to the muscarinic hyperpolarizing receptors or to the muscarinic depolarizing receptors of the soma-dendritic membrane remains open. The effect of muscarinic agents on nicotinic discharge and depolarization could have a reasonable explanation if these mediated a membrane hyperpolarization. This hypothetical hyperpolarizing action is, however, difficult to reconcile with the recent finding by LÖFFELHOLZ and MUSCHOLL (1969) that muscarinic agents also reduce the amount of noradrenaline

* 4-(m-chlorophenylcarbamoyloxy)-2-butynyltrimethyl-ammonium chloride.

liberated by orthodromic action potentials if we assume that hyperpolarization increases the amplitude of the action potential (provided it is conducted in the varicosities) and thereby the amount of transmitter released. Of course, the hyperpolarization induced in the terminals through muscarinic receptors could differ in its effect on the spike amplitude from that of a hyperpolarizing current pulse. Moreover, hyperpolarization of the membrane of adrenergic varicosities could impede the invasion of the varicosities by the incoming action potential in a manner similar to the block of invasion of the soma by an antidromic spike. In conclusion, the electrogenesis of the muscarinic induced inhibition in the adrenergic nerve terminals remains obscure.

d) Interaction Between Nicotinic and Muscarinic Receptors

There is an easily understandable interaction between two receptor-mediated processes when these are of opposite electrical sign; thus, nicotinic and muscarinic induced depolarizations and hyperpolarizations may appear in a purer form after either hexamethonium or atropine. A more interesting topic is, however, the unmasking or "sensitization" of muscarinic manifestations by nicotinic receptor activation. Evidence for such an interaction was provided by the finding of TRENDELENBURG (1966a) that repeated administration of nicotine augments the ganglionic effects of muscarinic stimulants. This "potentiation" is not very specific, since it also affects the actions of the non-nicotinic stimulants histamine, 5-hydroxytryptamine and angiotensin. It is possible that the usually small significance of non-nicotinic stimulation is increased simply by depolarization. Similar effects of repeated KCl-injections and of the depolarizing isoprenaline and the prompt disappearance of nicotine-induced sensitization after hexamethonium are in favour of this hypothesis. The findings of GEBBER and SNYDER (1968) with infusions of acetylcholine and tetramethylammonium may have a similar basis. One is reminded of the finding made by KOBAYASHI and LIBET (1968) and KOKETSU (1969) that the slow EPSP is increased by weak depolarizations.

2. Adrenoceptors of the Adrenergic Neuron

The adrenergic neuron is not unique in being sensitive to the substance which it synthetizes itself and which it releases as a transmitter during activity. The investigations of DE GROAT and VOLLE (1966a, b) established the existence of adrenergic α- and β-receptors in sympathetic ganglia (for the earlier literature on ganglionic effects of sympathomimetic agents, see also TRENDELENBURG, 1967, and HAEFELY, 1969a).

The soma-dendritic membrane of at least part of the adrenergic neurons contains *α-adrenergic receptors* which lead to an increase in the resting membrane potential when activated. Intracellular studies have revealed a low-amplitude hyperpolarization of rabbit superior cervical ganglion cells *in vitro* under the influence of noradrenaline (LIBET and KOBAYASHI, 1969); this increase in the transmembrane potential was not accompanied by changes in the membrane resistance and was depressed by steady depolarizing currents. In cells of frog paravertebral ganglion cells, adrenaline produced no hyperpolarization in spite of depressed transmission in the experiments of CHRIST and NISHI (1969), but did do so according to TOSAKA et al. (1968). In the cat superior cervical ganglion *in situ*, HAEFELY (1969a) observed that α-adrenergic agents produced an inconsistent ganglionic hyperpolarization, the amplitude of which was not correlated with the degree of depression of orthodromic transmission; he concluded that depression of ganglionic transmission mediated through α-adrenergic receptors was mainly presynaptic by reduction of the acetylcholine release. This view is supported by the fact that α-adrenergic stimulants did not inhibit discharges induced by nicotinic stimulants; firing induced through muscarinic stimulation is, however, depressed (DE GROAT and VOLLE, 1966b).

Stimulation of *β-adrenergic receptors* of the soma-dendritic membrane induces a low-amplitude depolarization (DE GROAT and VOLLE, 1966a, b; HAEFELY, 1969a). The electrogenesis of this depolarization is not established. However, some findings, e.g. the depression of K^+-induced depolarization and firing may be explained by a reduction in the K^+ permeability as postulated by DE GROAT and VOLLE (1966b). It should be noted that isoprenaline does not induce discharges of ganglion cells, although it produces a more marked depolarization than some ganglionic stimulant agents, e.g. the polypeptides angiotensin and bradykinin (HAEFELY, 1970). Isoprenaline and adrenaline (in the presence of α-adrenolytic agents) facilitate transmission, have no effect on nicotine-induced discharges and diminish K^+ depolarization and firing. However, they enhance or unmask discharges induced by muscarinic stimulants (DE GROAT and VOLLE, 1966b) and by the peptides, angiotensin and bradykinin (HAEFELY, 1970a). The possibility that catecholamines, released within the ganglion from either adrenergic nerve endings, chromaffin cells, recurrent collaterals from adrenergic axons or from the adrenergic cell body itself, may have a physiological role in modulating ganglionic transmission has been disproved by HAEFELY (1969a) for the cat superior cervical ganglion; a possible physiological role of catecholamines in other sympathetic and mainly in parasympathetic ganglia is thereby not excluded.

There is no evidence for the existence of adrenergic receptors in the axonal part of the adrenergic nerve axon. GOFFART and HOLMES (1962) described a hyperpolarizing effect of adrenaline in isolated mammalian A- and C-fibres.

The existence of adrenergic receptors at the adrenergic nerve terminals was investigated by HAEFELY et al. (1966b) by studying possible changes in the antidromic firing pattern in splenic adrenergic nerves induced by intraarterial injections of acetylcholine and KCl into the isolated cat spleen. A depression of this firing occurred with high doses of catecholamines which was, however, considered inconclusive because of concomitant alterations in the circulation.

3. 5-Hydroxytryptamine (5-HT)-Receptors

The first report on ganglionic stimulant actions of 5-hydroxytryptamine (5-HT) was made by ROBERTSON (1953); PAGE and MCCUBBIN (1953) had only observed depression with high doses of 5-HT in the ciliary ganglion of the dog. The pharmacological evidence suggests (TRENDELENBURG, 1967) that the 5-HT-receptors of adrenergic ganglion cells belong to the "M"-type according to GADDUM's (1953) terminology and are blocked by atropine, morphine, methadone and cocaine. In the cat superior cervical ganglion and other ganglia, 5-HT induces a depolarization with rapid onset lasting only a few seconds which is accompanied by asynchronous discharges in postganglionic nerves (REINERT, 1960; R. M. ECCLES and LIBET, 1961; HERTZLER, 1961; GYERMEK and BINDLER, 1961; JARAMILLO and VOLLE, 1968a; WATSON, 1970). The 5-HT-induced depolarization is not prevented by methysergide (WATSON, 1970). According to MACHOVÁ and BOŠKA (1969), higher doses of 5-HT produce a triphasic wave of ganglionic potentials, the primary depolarization being followed by a short hyperpolarization and a longer lasting low-amplitude depolarization. Similar changes were observed by HAEFELY (unpublished), but it remains to be shown how far circulatory effects of 5-HT may be involved. A series of other indole alkylamines have ganglionic stimulant actions (Gyermek and Bindler, 1962). The ionic mechanisms underlying 5-HT depolarization are unknown. During the depolarization produced by small and medium doses, transmission is facilitated; at the end of depolarization, a moderate depression is usually observed and may last for several minutes (Haefely, unpublished). Depression of ganglionic transmission occurs regularly with higher doses fo 5-HT (Reinert, 1960; Machová and Boška, 1969). In an experimental situation differing from the previously mentioned ones, namely when incubating the isolated rat superior cervical ganglion for hours in high concentrations of 5-HT or 5-hydroxytryptophan, de Kalbermatten (1962) and Jéquier (1965) observed a weak depressant effect on orthodromic transmission and an antagonism of the facilitation induced by acetylcholine, choline and carbachol. The authors concluded that, in this situation, 5-HT presumably acted intracellularly and decreased the membrane permeability for K^+.

There is no information on the presence or absence of 5-HT-receptors in the axonal membrane of the adrenergic neuron.

Literature seems to provide no indication of an effect of 5-HT on adrenergic nerve terminals. Haeusler (personal communication) did not observe antidromic discharges in the inferior cardiac nerve when injecting 5-HT into the perfusion fluid of the isolated cat heart. This is surprising in view of the finding that afferent C-fibres in the rabbit vagus and aortic nerve (Douglas and Ritchie, 1957) and in hepatic nerves (Andrews, 1968) were excited by 5-HT. McCubbin et al. (1956) found 5-HT to be a stimulant more potent than lobeline on chemoreceptors of the dog's carotid sinus.

4. Histamine Receptors

Histamine was found to have a very weak and inconsistent stimulant effect in the perfused cat superior cervical ganglion, but to potentiate regularly responses to acetylcholine, choline, nicotine and K^+ (Konzett, 1952). A historical review of the investigations concerned with the ganglionic effects of histamine is given by Trendelenburg (1957). Electrophysiological data are very scarce. Histamine resembles the polypeptides angiotensin and bradykinin in the superior cervical ganglion in that it elicits a delayed depolarization of very low amplitude accompanied by a low-amplitude discharge (Haefely, 1966, unpublished results). In the isolated rat superior cervical ganglion the histamine-induced depolarization was inconsistent (Watson, 1970). The stimulant action of histamine is enhanced by conditioning preganglionic tetanic stimulation (Trendelenburg and Jones, 1965; Iorio and McIsaac, 1966) and by chronic denervation. Antihistaminic drugs inhibit the ganglionic histamine action (Trendelenburg, 1954, 1955). The ionic basis underlying the histamine effect is unknown.

Neither on the axonal nor on the terminal part of the adrenergic neuron has the existence of histamine-receptors been reported.

5. Polypeptides

Angiotensin and bradykinin were shown by Lewis and Reit (1965) to stimulate the cat superior cervical ganglion and thereby to contract the nictitating membrane. In the unconditioned ganglion, the stimulant effect was very inconsistent and small, whereas facilitation of ganglionic transmission and enhancement of acetylcholine-induced stimulation was a regular finding (Haefely et al., 1966a; Trendelenburg, 1966a). After repeated injections of nicotine, the stimulant effect of angiotensin was enhanced and that of bradykinin depressed. These changes disappeared after hexamethonium (Trendelenburg, 1966a). These observations and those of LEWIS and REIT (1965) on the absence of crossed tachyphylaxis between the actions of the two peptides point to a difference in the receptors involved. Electrophysiological investigations with peptides were reported by HAEFELY et al. (1966a), MACHOVÁ and BOŠKA (1967), WATSON (1970) and HAEFELY (1970a). The latter described the effect of angiotensin and bradykinin as consisting in a delayed low-amplitude discharge accompanied inconsistently by a very lowamplitude ganglionic depolarization. Physalaemin and eledoisin — polypeptides with circulatory actions very similar to those of bradykinin — had virtually no effect. The stimulant effect of angiotensin and bradykinin is enhanced by preganglionic stimulation, by injections of isoprenaline and, less consistently, by chronic denervation. During the late hyperpolarizing phase following the injection of DMPP, both polypeptides produced a clear-cut depolarization; postganglionic discharges were, however, depressed or abolished. It was postulated that the ionic mechanisms underlying the ganglionic actions of the polypeptides were different from those involved in nicotinic stimulation. It is not known whether all adrenergic ganglion cells have receptors for polypeptides.

Effects of polypeptides on the axonal membrane have not been reported.

There is no electrophysiological evidence of polypeptide receptors in adrenergic terminals, although an interaction of these agents with noradrenaline release has repeatedly been reported.

6. Amino Acids

It has been suggested or shown that several naturally occurring amino acids act as neuro-chemical transmitters in peripheral (crustacean) neuro-effector junctions and central synapses.

Gamma-amino-butyric acid (GABA), an inhibitory substance at many sites, was reported by MATTHEWS and ROBERTS (1961) as slightly depressing transmission in the cat inferior mesenteric ganglion in high doses but as being ineffective in the superior cervical ganglion. However, DE GROAT (1970) observed a dose-dependent depolarization of the cat superior cervical ganglion with doses of GABA between 0.02 and 500 μg injected intraarterially. The depolarization lasted 20—90 sec. It was never accompanied by discharges of ganglion cells. GABA, in depolarizing doses, inhibited, but never completely blocked, ganglionic transmission. Moreover, it reduced the ganglionic stimulant effect of muscarinic agents as well as that of 5-HT and KCl. The ionic mechanism underlying GABA-induced ganglionic depolarization is unknown. The receptor sites involved in its effect differ from those on which other depolarizing agents are acting. Picrotoxin, but not strychnine, could partially antagonize all the actions of GABA on the superior cervical ganglion. Of the other amino acids studied by DE GROAT (1970), γ-amino-β-hydroxybutyric acid, 3-amino-1-propansulfonic acid, δ-amino-n-valeric acid, guanido-acetic acid, and β-alanine were less potent than GABA, whereas cysteine and glycine, potent inhibitory amino acids in the spinal cord, were completely inactive.

A series of amino acids with a depolarizing action at various postsynaptic sites were studied by SZRENIAWSKI and GUMULKA (1967) in the cat superior cervical ganglion. Ganglionic depolarization was observed with DL-homocysteate. A facilitation of ganglionic transmission, which appeared to be unrelated to changes in membrane potential, occurred for up to 20 min following the intra-arterial injection. Similar effects were obtained with DL-aspartate and DL-cysteate, whereas L-glutamate depressed transmission. DL-homocysteate was found to be devoid of action in the cat superior cervical ganglion by HAEFELY (unpublished); the ganglionic actions of amino acids clearly need to be further investigated.

There seem to be no reports on actions of amino acids on the axonal and terminal part of the adrenergic neuron.

7. Prostaglandins

No effects of prostaglandin E_1 and E_2 on the cat superior cervical ganglion have been observed by KAYAALP and McISAAC (1968). Electrophysiological studies, designed to explain the interaction of prostaglandins and noradrenaline release from adrenergic terminals (VON EULER and HEDQVIST, 1969), appear not to have been carried out. Information on this point would be of special interest, as prostaglandins are released together with noradrenaline when splenic nerves are stimulated (DAVIES et al., 1967).

8. Tetraethylammonium (TEA)

TEA has a large spectrum of actions on excitable membranes. The best known is its hexamethonium-like blocking effect on ganglionic transmission which occurs in the absence of changes in the resting membrane potential of ganglion cells (PATON and PERRY, 1953; RIKER, 1965). Actions of TEA on presynaptic structures will not be dealt with here.

Besides blocking nicotinic receptors of the ganglion cell, TEA decreases the threshold for direct stimulation and prolongs the duration of the action potential of the ganglion cell elicited by direct antidromic stimulation (RIKER, 1964). The latter effect is strictly dose-dependent and affects only the decaying phase of the spike. In small concentrations, TEA progressively prolongs the falling phase and in increasing doses, a hump appears and the full effect is characterized by a marked plateau, the ganglionic action potential then closely resembling the action potential of cardiac muscle fibres. The plateau duration may become more than 10 times longer than the normal action potential. The overshoot was often enhanced, the amplitude of the postspike-positivity (undershoot) reduced. Membrane potential, resting membrane resistance and time constant and rate of rise of the action potential were unaltered. The absolute refractory period was greatly prolonged parallel to the increased duration of the action potential. The duration of the plateau was gradually reduced by inward (hyperpolarizing) current pulses delivered during various stages of the plateau, whereas outward (depolarizing) currents had the opposite effect. The action potentials prolonged by TEA were correspondingly shortened or prolonged when they were elicited during steady hyperpolarization or depolarization of the cell respectively. Hyperpolarizing and depolarizing current pulses retained their effect on the action potentials prolonged by TEA, when delivered less than 100 msec before initiation of the spike, even when the resting membrane potential had reached its normal value. A preceding antidromic tetanus reduced the duration of TEA-prolonged action potentials. TEA lowered the current strength required to depolarize the membrane to the critical threshold depolarization level for initiation of a spike and this threshold depolarization level was simultaneously decreased. In high TEA concentrations, the cells fired spontaneous action potentials rhythmically, singly or in bursts. These spontaneous action potentials appeared identical with antidromically evoked ones, most conspicuously, they arose from the resting potential without preceding slow depolarization. RIKER (1964) explained his results on the frog paravertebral ganglion by the presumed mode of action of TEA on other excitable structures, namely by a delaying effect on the inactivation of the increased

Na^+-permeability occurring normally at the peak of the spike and by its interference with the increased K^+-permeability, normally following the increase of the Na^+-permeability. RIKER also discussed the possibility that TEA may produce the effects mentioned by displacing Ca^{++} from its membrane sites.

THOENEN et al. (1967) observed that TEA increased the amount of noradrenaline released into the perfusate of the isolated cat spleen during and following stimulation of sympathetic splenic nerves. This was the first demonstration of an increased adrenergic transmitter overflow not related to diminished inactivation of neurally released noradrenaline. The authors provided evidence that the increased transmitter release was caused by prolongation of action potentials in splenic adrenergic nerves: TEA increased the duration of the compound action potential of isolated splenic nerves and the increased transmitter overflow was more marked with low than with high frequency trains of stimulation. Evidence was also obtained that prolongation of action potentials occurred mainly in the terminal part of the adrenergic neurons.

9. Local Anaesthetics and Tetrodotoxin

Local anaesthetics (procaine, tetracaine) block ganglionic transmission and the induction of discharges by ganglionic stimulants without affecting the resting membrane potential; they have no selective action on the synapse but block pre- and post-synaptic structures in parallel (QUILLIAM and SHAND, 1964). These agents also reduce and finally abolish, in a dose-dependent manner, ganglionic depolarization caused by nicotinic stimulants and K^+. Evidence has been obtained that some nicotinic stimulants (e.g. lobeline, amphetamine) have a local anaesthetic component which is responsible for the reduction in the peak amplitude of depolarization obtainable with higher doses (HAEFELY, 1971b). Presumably, local anaesthetics act through the same mechanisms in the soma-dendritic membrane of the adrenergic neuron as they do at other excitable membranes (SHANES, 1958), namely by preventing permeability changes of the membrane normally induced by current pulses or chemical agents. Tetrodotoxin in low concentrations differs from the usual local anaesthetics by selectively blocking the increase in the Na^+ conductance (Na^+ carrying mechanism) underlying the spike generation. Consistent with this view is the finding that tetrodotoxin does not inhibit the ganglionic depolarization induced by nicotinic stimulants and K^+ but prevents the initiation of discharges by these substances (HAEFELY, 1971b).

The effects of local anaesthetics and of tetrodotoxin were found to be identical at the ganglion cells and at the adrenergic nerve terminals. The results obtained by HAEUSLER et al. (1968b, 1969) with tetracaine and tetrodotoxin have already been discussed in the paragraph on electrosecretory coupling at adrenergic nerve endings (see V 2).

10. Adrenergic Neuron Blocking Agents

Bretylium and guanethidine depress ganglionic transmission and inhibit the effect of ganglionic stimulants in a manner similar to local anaesthetics. Relatively high doses are necessary; QUILLIAM and SHAND (1964) found bretylium to be one third as potent as procaine. The same authors observed a certain selectivity of bretylium for postganglionic axons as compared with preganglionic ones.

The mode of action of bretylium, guanethidine and debrisoquin at adrenergic nerve endings has been the object of recent investigations by HAEUSLER et al. (1968c, 1969) and HAEUSLER (personal communication). The effects of these adrenergic neuron blocking agents and of tetracaine at the endings of sensory and adrenergic nerves were compared, using as parameters, in the former, the firing in the afferents from carotid baroreceptors induced by carotid pressure changes and injected acetylcholine and, in the latter, the antidromic firing in the inferior cardiac nerve of the cat induced by intracardial injections of acetylcholine and KCl as well as the noradrenaline released by acetylcholine and sympathetic nerve stimulation. At the sinus nerve afferents, both groups of agents had a qualitatively identical stabilizing effect which set in relatively rapidly during constant infusion and which was readily washed out; bretylium had only 1/1000 the potency of tetracaine. At the cardiac adrenergic nerve terminals, the end effect of both groups of agents was a parallel depression of acetylcholine- and KCl-induced antidromic firing and of the noradrenaline released by acetylcholine and cardiac sympathetic nerve stimulation. There were, however, important differences between tetracaine and the adrenergic neuron blocking agents. With tetracaine, infusions of different concentrations rapidly led to a steady stabilizing effect, the effective concentrations being similar at sensory and adrenergic nerve terminals; moreover, the effect of tetracaine was rapidly reversed by drug-free perfusion. With the adrenergic neuron blocking agents, the stabilizing effect increased with the time of infusion (in sharp contrast to its development at sensory nerve endings) and could only partially be reversed by long-lasting drug-free perfusion. Blockade of all parameters was obtained with smaller concentrations of bretylium than were necessary with tetracaine. The conclusions were that the adrenergic neuron blocking agents can be considered as very weak local anaesthetics at sensory nerves and that their rather selective blockade of adrenergic nerve terminals was due to their intraneuronal accumulation in these endings leading to membrane stabilization by the build-up of the necessary concentration in the terminal membrane. Results obtained with bretylium by DAVEY et al. (1968) in the cat spleen were interpreted by the authors in a different way, but according to HAEUSLER et al. (1969) do not contradict the above-mentioned conclusion.

11. Veratrum Alkaloids

Several veratrum alkaloids have two main effects on various excitable membranes: They retard the inactivation of the Na^+ carrying system responsible for the ascending phase of the spike and thereby produce large increases of the negative afterpotentials and (at higher concentrations) they reduce the resting membrane potential by increasing the Na^+-(and K^+-) permeability (see ULBRICHT, 1969).

The characteristic effect of veratrine injected into the blood supply of the cat superior cervical ganglion was an increase in amplitude and duration of the post-spike negativity of orthodromic ganglionic action potentials (LLOYD, 1939). Higher doses of veratrine produced a complete but transient blockade of ganglionic transmission (KOMALAHIRANYA and VOLLE, 1962). Postganglionic firing induced by acetylcholine was enhanced by veratrine which, by itself, did not provoke discharges. The alkaloid furthermore enhanced the persistent postganglionic firing induced by diisopropylphosphorofluoridate in acutely denervated ganglia. The effects of veratrine were blocked by atropine in very low doses.

α-Veratrine and veratrine infused through the isolated cat heart induced repetitive antidromic firing in the inferior cardiac nerve and released noradrenaline into the perfusate (HAEUSLER, personal communication).

Concluding Remarks

The large number of data accumulated mainly during the last 15 years and especially the information provided by the intracellular recording technique made it desirable to devote a review to the electrical properties of the adrenergic neuron and to attempt to explain the action of a series of chemical agents and procedures on the basis of electrical changes of the excitable membrane at the soma-dendritic, axonal and terminal part. With the adrenergic nerve cell, nature provides us with a neuron which is the most accessible to many kinds of studies. The peripheral adrenergic neuron is unique in the vertebral nervous system in respect to the following main points: Relatively simply organized and easily accessible afferent input; established nature of the chemical transmitter substance acting upon the adrenergic nerve cell; anatomical organization permitting the application of drugs selectively either to the soma-dendritic, axonal or terminal part; highly advanced state of knowledge on synthesis, uptake, storage, release, inactivation and action of the adrenergic transmitter substance together with the availability of a large arsenal of chemical agents interfering with any one of these steps; possibility to identify in the light and even in the electron microscope, the adrenergic axons and terminals by the characteristic reactivity of the transmitter substance. It is no exaggeration to say that the peripheral adrenergic neuron is the best known type of neuron in vertebrates.

The essential mechanism of synaptic excitation of the adrenergic neuron by presynaptically released acetylcholine is very similar to that underlying neuromuscular transmission of the motor end plate (DEL CASTILLO and KATZ, 1954). Similarities also exist between the electrical events occurring at the adrenergic nerve cell and at the motoneuron (where the excitatory transmitter is unknown and different from acetylcholine). Some peculiarities of the postsynaptic events at the adrenergic nerve cells may be explained by the relatively small size (large surface to volume ratio), e.g. the marked postspike positivity. A striking peculiarity of postsynaptic events is due to the presence in the adrenergic cell of three types of receptor sites for acetylcholine, mediating three different kinds of changes of the membrane properties. Muscarinic receptors have also been demonstrated by the microelectrophoretic technique and extracellular recording at single neurons of most parts of the mammalian central nervous system (see CURTIS and CRAWFORD, 1969). The slow synaptic potentials and their modulating influence on synaptic events demonstrate the vast possibilities of responses to a single substance provided by the differentiation of the cell membrane sites. The presence of specific inhibitory connections between the adrenergic ganglion cell and the CNS or the periphery has not been demonstrated and seems highly unlikely. In spite of this, the adrenergic neuron displays a high degree of integrative capacity and may, therefore, serve as a valuable model for central neurons, especially since adrenergic neurons are also present in the central nervous system.

The responsiveness of the adrenergic neuron to a series of endogenous substances such as 5-hydroxytryptamine, catecholamines, histamine and polypeptides is interesting. Surprisingly, the adrenergic neuron is rather insensitive to amino acids with potent excitatory actions in the central nervous system.

The easy access of chemical agents to all parts of the adrenergic neuron made it possible to attempt a topography of receptive sites on the soma-dendritic, axonal and terminal part of the neuron. Some drug effects on the terminal part of the adrenergic neuron have been elucidated by electrophysiological investigations. The easily performed exposure of the adrenergic neuron to transient or constant concentrations of chemical agents provided interesting insights into electrical manifestations which are in part the consequence of secondary compensatory mechanisms of the cell rather than of the primary changes of membrane properties following the drug-receptor interaction.

Abbreviations used in this chapter:

DMPP = 1,1-dimethyl-4-phenyl-piperazinium
5-HT = 5-hydroxytryptamine (serotonin)
TEA = tetraethylammonium
EPSP = excitatory postsynaptic potential
IPSP = inhibitory postsynaptic potential
N-wave = negative wave
P-wave = positive wave
LN-wave = late negative wave
LLN-wave = late late negative wave
IS-spike = initial segment spike
SD-spike = soma-dendritic spike
PTH = post-tetanic hyperpolarization
EAD = early afterdischarge
LAD = late afterdischarge

Only publications available by the end of December, 1970, have been included.

References

Acheson, G.H., Remolina, J.: The temporal course of the effects of postganglionic axotomy on the inferior mesenteric ganglion of the cat. J. Physiol. (Lond.) **127**, 603—616 (1955).

Aiken, J.W., Reit, E.: A comparison of the sensitivity to chemical stimuli of adrenergic and cholinergic neurons in the cat stellate ganglion. J. Pharmacol. exp. Ther. **169**, 211—223 (1969).

Andrews, W.H.H.: Afferent impulses in the hepatic nerve of perfused livers elicited by 5-hydroxytryptamine and other substances. Brit. J. Pharmacol. **32**, 421P—422P (1968).

Armett, C.J., Ritchie, J.M.: The action of acetylcholine and some related substances on conduction in mammalian non-myelinated nerve fibres. J. Physiol. (Lond.) **155**, 372—384 (1961).

— — The ionic requirements for the action of acetylcholine on mammalian non-myelinated fibres. J. Physiol. (Lond.) **165**, 141—159 (1963).

Barton, A.A., Causey, G.: Electron microscopic study of the superior cervical ganglion. J. Anat. (Lond.) **92**, 399—407 (1958).

Bennett, M.R., Merrillees, N.C.R.: An analysis of the transmission of excitation from autonomic nerves to smooth muscle. J. Physiol. (Lond.) **185**, 520—535 (1966).

Billingsley, P.R., Ranson, S.W.: On the number of nerve cells in the ganglion cervicale superius and of nerve fibers in the cephalic end of the truncus sympathicus in the cat and on the numerical relations of preganglionic and postganglionic neurones. J. comp. Neurol. **29**, 359—366 (1918a).

— — Branches of the ganglion cervicale superius. J. comp. Neurol. **29**, 367—384 (1918b).

Birzis, L., Carregal, E.J.A.: Electrical impedance and vasomotor changes accompanying synaptic transmission in sympathetic ganglia. Exp. Neurol. **15**, 1—17 (1966).

Bishop, G.H., Heinbecker, P.: Differentiation of axon types in visceral nerves by means of the potential records. Amer. J. Physiol. **94**, 170—200 (1930).

— — A functional analysis of the cervical sympathetic nerve supply to the eye. Amer. J. Physiol. **100**, 519—532 (1932).

Blackman, J.G., Crowcroft, P.J., Devine, C.E., Holman, M.E., Yonemura, K.: Transmission from preganglionic fibres in the hypogastric nerve to peripheral ganglia of male guinea-pigs. J. Physiol. (Lond.) **201**, 723—743 (1969).

— Ginsborg, B.L., Ray, C.: Synaptic transmission in the sympathetic ganglion of the frog. J. Physiol. (Lond.) **167**, 355—373 (1963a).

— — — Some effects of changes in ionic concentration on the action potential of sympathetic ganglion cells in the frog. J. Physiol. (Lond.) **167**, 374—388 (1963b).

— — — Spontaneous synaptic activity in sympathetic ganglion cells of the frog. J. Physiol. (Lond.) **167**, 389—401 (1963c).

— — — On the quantal release of the transmitter at a sympathetic synapse. J. Physiol. (Lond.) **167**, 402—415 (1963d).

— Holman, M.E.: Intracellular recordings from mammalian sympathetic ganglion cells. Proc. Univ. Otago med. Sch. **45**, 52—53 (1967).

— Purves, R.D.: Intracellular recordings from ganglia of the thoracic sympathetic chain of the guinea-pig. J. Physiol. (Lond.) **203**, 173—198 (1969a).

— — Recordings from single cells of mammalian autonomic ganglia. Aust. J. exp. Biol. med. Sci. **47**, 3 (1969b).

Bronk, D.W.: Synaptic mechanisms in sympathetic ganglia. J. Neurophysiol. **2**, 380 (1939).
— Pumphrey, R.J.: Response of a sympathetic ganglion to high frequency stimulation. Proc. Soc. exp. Biol. (N.Y.) **32**, 1661—1663 (1935).
— Tower, S.S., Solandt, D.Y., Larrabee, M.G.: The transmission of trains of impulses through a sympathetic ganglion and in its postganglionic nerves. Amer. J. Physiol. **122**, 1—15 (1938).
Brown, A.M.: Cardiac sympathetic adrenergic pathways in which synaptic transmission is blocked by atropine sulphate. J. Physiol. (Lond.) **191**, 271—288 (1967).
Brown, D.A.: Depolarization of normal and preganglionically denervated superior cervical ganglia by stimulant drugs. Brit. J. Pharmacol. **26**, 511—520 (1966a).
— Effects of hexamethonium and hyoscine on the drug-induced depolarization of isolated superior cervical ganglia. Brit. J. Pharmacol. **26**, 521—537 (1966b).
— Electrical responses of cat superior cervical ganglia in vivo to some stimulant drugs and their modification by hexamethonium and hyoscine. Brit. J. Pharmacol. **26**, 538—551 (1966c).
— Responses of normal and denervated cat superior cervical ganglia to some stimulant compounds. J. Physiol. (Lond.) **201**, 225—236 (1969).
— Brownstein, M.J., Scholfield, C.N.: On the nature of the drug-induced after-hyperpolarization in isolated rat ganglia. Brit. J. Pharmacol. **37**, 511P—513P (1969).
— Scholfield, C.N.: Potentials in isolated rat superior cervical ganglia produced by nicotine. Brit. J. Pharmacol. **40**, 559P—561P (1970).
Brown, G.L., Holmes, O.: The effects of activity on mammalian nerve fibers of low conduction velocity. Proc. roy. Soc. B. **145**, 1—14 (1956).
— Pascoe, J.E.: Conduction through the inferior mesenteric ganglion of the rabbit. J. Physiol. (Lond.) **118**, 113—123 (1952).
— — The effect of degenerative section of ganglionic axons on transmission through the ganglion. J. Physiol. (Lond.) **123**, 565—573 (1954).
Buckley, G., Consolo, S., Giacobini, E., Sjöqvist, F.: Cholinacetylase in innervated and denervated sympathetic ganglia and ganglion cells of the cat. Acta physiol. scand. **71**, 348—356 (1967).
Burnstock, G., Holman, M.E., Kuriyama, H.: Facilitation of transmission from autonomic nerve to smooth muscle of guinea-pig vas deferens. J. Physiol. (Lond.) **172**, 31—49 (1964).
Cabrera, R., Torrance, R.W., Viveros, H.: The action of acetylcholine and other drugs upon the terminal parts of the postganglionic sympathetic fibre. Brit. J. Pharmacol. **27**, 51—63 (1966).
Chen, S.S.: Late contraction of nictitating membrane of the dog. Amer. J. Physiol. **217**, 1205—1210 (1969).
Christ, D.D., Nishi, S.: Presynaptic action of epinephrine on sympathetic ganglia. Life Sci. **8**, 1235—1238 (1969).
— — Anomalous rectification of the sympathetic ganglion cell membrane. Fed. Proc. **29**, 796 (1970).
Conelly, C.M.: Metabolic and electrochemical events associated with recovery from activity. Proc. XXII Int. Congr. Physiol. Lectures and Symposia, **1**, 600—602 (1962).
Crowcroft, P.J., Holman, M.E., Szurszewski, J.H.: Excitatory input from the colon to the inferior mesenteric ganglion. J. Physiol. (Lond.) **208**, 19P—20P (1970).
— Muir, T.C., Szurszewski, J.H.: Response of pelvic ganglion cells of male guinea-pigs to large currents. Aust. J. exp. Biol. med. Sci. **47**, 6P (1969).
Curtis, D.R., Crawford, J.M.: Central synaptic transmission — microelectrophoretic studies. Ann. Rev. Pharmacol. **9**, 209—240 (1969).
Davey, M.J., Hayden, M.L., Scholfield, P.C.: The effects of bretylium on C fibre excitation and noradrenaline release by acetylcholine and electrical stimulation. Brit. J. Pharmacol. **34**, 377—387 (1968).
Davies, B.N., Horton, E.W., Withrington, P.G.: The occurrence of prostaglandin E_2 in splenic venous blood of the dog following splenic nerve stimulation. J. Physiol. (Lond.) **188**, 38P—39P (1967).
De Groat, W.C.: The actions of γ-aminobutyric acid and related amino acids on mammalian autonomic ganglia. J. Pharmacol. exp. Ther. **172**, 384—396 (1970).
— Volle, R.L.: Ganglionic actions of oxotremorine. Life Sci. **8**, 618—623 (1963).
— — The actions of the catecholamines on transmission in the superior cervical ganglion of the cat. J. Pharmacol. exp. Ther. **154**, 1—13 (1966a).
— — Interactions between the catecholamines and ganglionic stimulating agents in sympathetic ganglia. J. Pharmacol. exp. Ther. **154**, 200—215 (1966b).
De Kalbermatten, J.P.: Effet de la sérotonine sur l'hypersensibilité de dénervation du ganglion sympathique cervical isolé du rat. Helv. physiol. pharmacol. Acta. **20**, 293—315 (1962).

Del Castillo, J., Katz, B.: The membrane change produced by the neuromuscular transmitter. J. Physiol. (Lond.) **125**, 546—565 (1954).
Den Hertog, A., Greengard, P., Ritchie, J.M.: On the metabolic basis of nervous activity. J. Physiol. (Lond.) **204**, 511—521 (1969).
— Ritchie, J.M.: A comparison of the effect of temperature, metabolic inhibitors and of ouabain on the electrogenic component of the sodium pump in mammalian non-myelinated nerve fibres. J. Physiol. (Lond.) **204**, 523—538 (1969).
Dolivo, M.: Esquisse des relations entre le métabolisme et le fonctionnement du tissu nerveux isolé des vertébrés. J. Physiol. (Paris) **58**, 127—194 (1966).
— Koelle, G.B.: Properties of nicotinic and muscarinic receptors of isolated rat ganglion. Experientia (Basel) **26**, 679 (1970).
Douglas, W.W., Kanno, T.: The effect of amethocaine on acetylcholine induced depolarization and catecholamine secretion in the adrenal chromaffin cell. Brit. J. Pharmacol. **30**, 612—619 (1967).
— Ritchie, J.M.: The conduction of impulses through the superior cervical and accessory cervical ganglia of the rabbit. J. Physiol. (Lond.) **133**, 220—231 (1956).
— — On excitation of non-medullated afferent fibres in the vagus and aortic nerves by pharmacological agents. J. Physiol. (Lond.) **138**, 31—43 (1957).
— Rubin, R.P.: The mechanism of catecholamine release from the adrenal medulla and the role of calcium in stimulus-secretion coupling. J. Physiol. (Lond.) **167**, 288—310 (1963).
Dudel, J.: Potential changes in the crayfish motor nerve terminal during repetitive stimulation. Pflügers Arch. ges. Physiol. **282**, 323—337 (1965).
— Kuffler, S.W.: Presynaptic inhibition at the crayfish neuromuscular junction. J. Physiol. (Lond.) **155**, 543—562 (1961).
Dunant, Y.: Organisation topographique et fonctionnelle du ganglion cervical supérieur chez le rat. J. Physiol. (Paris) **59**, 17—38 (1967).
— Presynaptic spike and excitatory postsynaptic potential in sympathetic ganglion. Their modifications by pharmacological agents. Progr. in Brain Res. **31**, 131—139 (1969).
— Dolivo, M.: Relations entre les potentiels synaptiques lents et l'excitabilité du ganglion sympathique chez le rat. J. Physiol. (Paris) **59**, 281—294 (1967).
Eccles, J.C.: After-discharge from the superior ganglion. J. Physiol. (Lond.) **84**, 50P—52P (1935a).
— The action potential of the superior cervical ganglion. J. Physiol. (Lond.) **85**, 179—206 (1935b).
— Facilitation and inhibition in the superior cervical ganglion. J. Physiol. (Lond.) **85**, 207—238 (1935c).
— Slow potential waves in the superior cervical ganglion. J. Physiol. (Lond.) **85**, 464—501 (1935d).
— The actions of antidromic impulses on ganglion cells. J. Physiol. (Lond.) **88**, 1—39 (1937).
— Synaptic potentials and transmission in sympathetic ganglion. J. Physiol. (Lond.) **101**, 465—483 (1943).
— The nature of synaptic transmission in a sympathetic ganglion. J. Physiol. (Lond.) **103**, 27—54 (1944).
— The physiology of nerve cells. Baltimore: J. Hopkins Press 1957.
— Krnjević, K.: Presynaptic changes associated with posttetanic potentiation in the spinal cord. J. Physiol. (Lond.) **149**, 274—287 (1959).
Eccles, R.M.: Action potentials of isolated mammalian sympathetic ganglia. J. Physiol. (Lond.) **117**, 181—195 (1952a).
— Responses of isolated curarized sympathetic ganglia. J. Physiol. (Lond.) **117**, 196—217 (1952b).
— Intracellular potentials recorded from a mammalian sympathetic ganglion. J. Physiol. (Lond.) **130**, 572—584 (1955).
— The effect of nicotine on synaptic transmission in the sympathetic ganglion. J. Pharmacol. exp. Ther. **118**, 26—38 (1956).
— Orthodromic activation of single ganglion cells. J. Physiol. (Lond.) **165**, 387—391 (1963).
— Libet, B.: Origin and blockade of the synaptic responses of curarized sympathetic ganglia. J. Physiol. (Lond.) **157**, 484—503 (1961).
Erulkar, S.D., Woodward, J.K.: Intracellular recording from mammalian superior cervical ganglion in situ. J. Physiol. (Lond.) **199**, 189—203 (1968).
Euler, U.S. von, Hedqvist, P.: Inhibitory action of prostaglandins E_1 and E_2 on the neuromuscular transmission in the guinea-pig vas deferens. Acta physiol. scand. **77**, 510—512 (1969).
Fatt, P., Katz, B.: An analysis of the end-plate potential recorded with an intracellular electrode. J. Physiol. (Lond.) **115**, 320—370 (1951).
— — The effect of inhibitory nerve impulses on a crustacean muscle fibre. J. Physiol. (Lond.) **121**, 374—389 (1953).

FEHÉR, O., BOKRI, E.: Über die Acetylcholinreceptoren der sympathischen Ganglien. Pflügers Arch. ges. Physiol. **269**, 68—76 (1959).
— — Contributions to the kinetics of the acetylcholine-receptor function. Pflügers Arch. ges. Physiol. **272**, 553—561 (1961).
FERRY, C.B.: The sympathomimetic effect of acetylcholine on the spleen of the cat. J. Physiol. (Lond.) **167**, 487—504 (1963a).
— The post-ganglionic fibres of the vas deferens in the guinea-pig. J. Physiol. (Lond.) **169**, 72P (1963b).
— The innervation of the vas deferens of the guinea-pig. J. Physiol. (Lond.) **192**, 463—478 (1967).
FLACKE, W., GILLIS, R.A.: Impulse transmission via nicotinic and muscarinic pathways in the stellate ganglion of the dog. J. Pharmacol. exp. Ther. **163**, 266—276 (1968).
FLEISCH, J.H., FLACKE, W., GILLIS, R.A.: Nicotinic and muscarinic receptors in the cardiac sympathetic ganglia of the dog. J. Pharmacol. exp. Ther. **168**, 106—115 (1969).
FOLEY, J.O., DU BOIS, F.S.: A quantitative and experimental study of the cervical sympathetic trunk. J. comp. Neurol. **72**, 587—603 (1940).
— Composition of the cervical sympathetic trunk. Proc. Soc. exp. Biol. (N.Y.) **52**, 212—214 (1943).
GADDUM, J.H.: Tryptamine receptors. J. Physiol. (Lond.) **119**, 363—368 (1953).
GAGE, P.W., HUBBARD, J.I.: Ion changes responsible for post-tetanic hyperpolarization. Nature (Lond.) **203**, 653—654 (1964).
GEBBER, G.L.: Prolonged ganglionic facilitation and the positive afterpotential. Int. J. Neuropharmacol. **7**, 195—205 (1968a).
— Dissociation of depolarization and ganglionic blockade induced by nicotine. J. Pharmacol. exp. Ther. **160**, 124—134 (1968b).
— SNYDER, D.W.: Observations on drug-induced activation of cholinoceptive sites in a sympathetic ganglion. J. Pharmacol. exp. Ther. **163**, 64—74 (1968).
— VOLLE, R.L.: Ganglionic stimulating properties of aliphatic esters of choline and thiocholine. J. Pharmacol. exp. Ther. **150**, 67—74 (1965).
— — Mechanisms involved in ganglionic blockade induced by tetramethylammonium. J. Pharmacol. exp. Ther. **152**, 18—28 (1966).
GERTNER, S.B., REINERT, H.: The role of potassium ions and amino acid anions in the reaction of denervated ganglion cells. Naunyn-Schmiedeberg's Arch. exp. Pathol. Pharmak. **230**, 347—357 (1957).
GILLIS, R.A., FLACKE, W., GARFIELD, J.M., ALPER, M.H.: Actions of anticholinesterase agents upon ganglionic transmission in the dog. J. Pharmacol. exp. Ther. **163**, 277—286 (1968).
GINSBORG, B.L.: The actions of McN-A-343, pilocarpine and acetyl-β-methylcholine on sympathetic ganglion cells of the frog. J. Pharmacol. exp. Ther. **150**, 216—219 (1965).
— GUERRERO, S.: On the action of depolarizing drugs on sympathetic ganglion cells of the frog. J. Physiol. (Lond.) **172**, 189—206 (1964).
GOFFART, M., HOLMES, D.: The effect of adrenaline on mammalian C and A nerve fibres. J. Physiol. (Lond.) **162**, 18P—19P (1962).
GREEN, J.H., HEFFRON, P.F.: Studies upon patterns of activity in single post-ganglionic sympathetic fibres. Arch. int. Pharmacodyn. **173**, 232—243 (1968).
GREENGARD, P., STRAUB, R.W.: Metabolic studies on the hyperpolarization following activity in mammalian non-myelinated nerve fibres. J. Physiol. (Lond.) **161**, 414—423 (1962).
GROBECKER, H.: Brenzcatechinamingehalt des Froschherzens und seine Beeinflussung durch α-Methyldopa. Naunyn-Schmiedeberg's Arch. exp. Path. Pharmak. **253**, 38 (1966).
GRUNDFEST, H., GASSER, H.S.: Properties of mammalian nerve fibers of slowest conduction. Amer. J. Physiol. **123**, 307—318 (1938).
GUMULKA, W., SZRENIAWSKI, Z.: The effect of 1,1-dimethyl-4-phenylpiperazinium iodide on transmission in the superior cervical ganglion of the cat. Int. J. Neuropharmacol. **7**, 511—515 (1968).
GYERMEK, L.: Ganglionic stimulant and depressant agents. In: BURGER, A. (ed.): Drugs affecting the peripheral nervous system. **1**, 149—326. New York: Marcel Dekker Inc. 1967.
— BINDLER, E.: Blockade of the ganglionic stimulant action of 5-hydroxytryptamine. J. Pharmacol. exp. Ther. **135**, 344—348 (1961).
— — Action of indole alkylamines and amidines on the inferior, mesenteric ganglion of the cat. J. Pharmacol. exp. Ther. **138**, 159—164 (1962).
— SIGG, E.B., BINDLER, E.: Ganglionic stimulant action of muscarine. Amer. J. Physiol. **204**, 68—70 (1963).
HAEFELY, W.: Effects of catecholamines in the cat superior cervical ganglion and their postulated rôle as physiological modulators of ganglionic transmission. Progr. in Brain Res. **31**, 61—72 (1969).
— Some actions of bradykinin and related peptides on autonomic ganglion cells. In: Bradykinin and related kinins, pp. 591—599. Plenum Press 1970a.

HAEFELY, W.: Slow synaptic potentials in the cat superior cervical ganglion (SCG) in situ. Experientia (Basel) **26**, 690 (1970b).

— The effects of DMPP in the cat superior cervical ganglion. 1972a (to be published).

— The effects of various nicotine-like agents in the cat superior cervical ganglion. 1972b (to be published).

— Muscarinic postsynaptic events in the cat superior cervical ganglion in situ. 1972c (to be published).

— HUERLIMANN, A., THOENEN, H.: Relation between the rate of stimulation and the quantity of noradrenaline liberated from sympathetic nerve endings in the isolated perfused spleen of the cat. J. Physiol. (Lond.) **181**, 48—58 (1965).

— — — The effect of bradykinin and angiotensin on ganglionic transmission. In: ERDÖS, E.G., N. BACK, F. SICUTERI, and A.F. WILDE (eds.): Hypotensive polypeptides, pp. 314—327. Berlin-Heidelberg-New York: Springer 1966a.

— — — Wirkungen von Nikotin, DMPP, TMA, Amphetamin und KCl auf das Demarkationspotential des Ganglion cervicale superius und die ganglionäre Transmission. Helv. Physiol. Acta **25**, CR418—CR419 (1967).

— STAEHELIN, H., THOENEN, H.: Pharmakologische Rezeptoren für sympathomimetische Amine an der sympathischen Ganglienzelle und deren peripheren Nervenendigungen. Helv. Physiol. Acta **24**, C90—C92 (1966b).

HAEUSLER, G., HAEFELY, W., HUERLIMANN, A.: On the mechanism of the adrenergic nerve blocking action of bretylium. Naunyn-Schmiedeberg's Arch. Pharmak. **265**, 260—277 (1969).

— THOENEN, H., HAEFELY, W., HUERLIMANN, A.: Electrical events in cardiac adrenergic nerves and noradrenaline release from the heart induced by acetylcholine and KCl. Naunyn-Schmiedeberg's Arch. Pharmak. exp. Path. **261**, 389—411 (1968a).

— — — — Elektrosekretorische Koppelung bei der Noradrenalinfreisetzung aus adrenergen Nervenfasern durch nikotinartig wirkende Substanzen. Naunyn-Schmiedeberg's Arch. Pharmak. exp. Path. **263**, 217—218 (1968b).

— — — — Durch Acetylcholin hervorgerufene antidrome Aktivität im kardialen Sympathicus und Noradrenalinfreisetzung unter Guanethidin. Helv. Physiol. Acta **26**, CR352—CR354 (1968c).

HAMBERGER, B., NORBERG, K.-A.: Monoamines in sympathetic ganglia, studied with fluorescence microscopy. Experientia (Basel) **19**, 580 (1963).

— — Studies on some systems of adrenergic synaptic terminals in the abdominal ganglia of the cat. Acta physiol. scand. **65**, 235—242 (1965).

— — SJÖQVIST, F.: Cellular localization of monoamines in sympathetic ganglia of the cat. Life Sci. **9**, 659—661 (1963).

— — — Evidence for adrenergic nerve terminals and synapses in sympathetic ganglia. Int. J. Neuropharmacol. **2**, 279—282 (1964).

— — UNGERSTEDT, U.: Adrenergic synaptic terminals in autonomic ganglia. Acta physiol. scand. **64**, 285 (1965).

HANCOCK, C., KOSERSKY, D.S., VOLLE, R.L.: Cholinoceptive sites in the rat superior cervical ganglion. Pharmacologist **11**, 286 (1969).

— VOLLE, R.L.: Blockade of conduction in vagal fibers by nicotinic drugs. Arch. int. Pharmacodyn. **178**, 85—98 (1969a).

— — Enhancement by cesium ions of ganglionic hyperpolarization induced by dimethylphenylpiperazinium (DMPP) and repetitive preganglionic stimulation. J. Pharmacol. exp. Ther. **169**, 201—210 (1969b).

HÄRKÖNEN, M.H., PASSONNEAU, J.V., LOWRY, O.H.: Relationships between energy reserves and function in rat superior cervical ganglion. J. Neurochem. **16**, 1439—1450 (1969).

HEINBECKER, P.: The functional analysis of a sympathetic ganglion of the turtle by the cathode ray oscillograph. Amer. J. Physiol. **93**, 384—397 (1930).

— BISHOP, G.H.: Differentiation between types of fibers in certain components of involuntary nervous system. Proc. Soc. exp. Biol. (N.Y.) **26**, 645—647 (1929).

HERTZLER, E.C.: 5-hydroxytryptamine and transmission in sympathetic ganglia. Brit. J. Pharmacol. **17**, 406—413 (1961).

HILTON, J.G., STEINBERG, M.: Effects of ganglion- and parasympathetic-blocking drugs upon the pressor response elicited by elevation of the intracranial fluid pressure. J. Pharmacol. exp. Ther. **153**, 285—291 (1966).

HODGKIN, A.L.: The conduction of the nervous impulse. Liverpool: University Press 1964.

HOLMAN, M.E., CROWCROFT, P.J., OSTBERG, A., SZURSZEWSKI, J.H.: Electric properties of pelvic ganglion cells of male guinea-pigs. Aust. J. exp. Biol. med. Sci. **47**, P 14—P 15 (1969).

HOLMES, O.: Effects of pH, changes in potassium concentration and metabolic inhibitors on the after-potentials of mammalian non-medullated nerve fibres. Arch. int. Physiol. **70**, 211—245 (1962).

HUBBARD, J.I., SCHMIDT, R.F.: An electrophysiological investigation of mammalian motor nerve terminals. J. Physiol. (Lond.) **166**, 145—167 (1963).
HUBBARD, S.J.: The electrical constants and the component conductances of frog skeletal muscle after denervation. J. Physiol. (Lond.) **165**, 443—456 (1963).
HUBER, G.C.: A contribution on the minute anatomy of the sympathetic ganglia of the different classes of vertebrates. J. Morph. **16**, 27—90 (1900).
HUNT, C.C., NELSON, P.G.: Structural and functional changes in the frog sympathetic ganglion following cutting of the presynaptic nerve fibres. J., Physiol. (Lond.) **177**, 1—20 (1965).
— RIKER, W.K.: Properties of frog sympathetic neurons in normal ganglia and after axon section. J. Neurophysiol. **29**, 1096—1114 (1966).
IORIO, L.C., MCISAAC, R.J.: Comparison of the stimulating effects of nicotine, pilocarpine and histamines on the superior cervical ganglion of the cat. J. Pharmacol. exp. Ther. **151**, 430—437 (1966).
ITO, M., OSHIMA, T.: Temporal summation of after-hyperpolarization following a motoneuron spike. Nature (Lond.) **195**, 910—911 (1962).
JACOBOWITZ, D., WOODWARD, J.K.: Adrenergic neurons in the cat superior cervical ganglion and cervical sympathetic nerve trunk. A histochemical study. J. Pharmacol. exp. Ther. **162**, 213—226 (1968).
JAENIG, W., SCHMIDT, R.F.: Single unit responses in the cervical sympathetic trunk upon somatic nerve stimulation. Pflügers Arch. **314**, 199—216 (1970).
JARAMILLO, J., VOLLE, R.L.: Ganglion blockade by muscarine, oxotremorin and AHR-602. J. Pharmacol. exp. Ther. **158**, 80—88 (1967a).
— — Nonmuscarinic stimulation and block of a sympathetic ganglion by 4-(m-chlorophenylcarbamoyloxy)-2-butynyltrimethylammonium chloride (McN-A-343). J. Pharmacol. exp. Ther. **157**, 337—345 (1967b).
— — A comparison of the ganglionic stimulating and blocking properties of some nicotinic drugs. Arch. int. Pharmacodyn. **174**, 88—97 (1968a).
— — Effects of lithium on ganglionic hyperpolarization and blockade by dimethylphenylpiperazinium. J. Pharmacol. exp. Ther. **164**, 166—175 (1968b).
JÉQUIER, E.: Effet de la sérotonine sur la transmission synaptique dans le ganglion sympathique cervical isolé du rat. Helv. Physiol. Acta **23**, 163—179 (1965).
JOB, C., LUNDBERG, A.: Reflex excitation of cells in the inferior mesenteric ganglion on stimulation of the hypogastric nerve. Acta physiol. scand. **26**, 366—382 (1952).
— — On the significance of post- and pre-synaptic events for facilitation and inhibition in the sympathetic ganglion of the cat. Acta physiol. scand. **28**, 14—28 (1953).
JONES, A.: Ganglionic actions of muscarinic substances. J. Pharmacol. exp. Ther. **141**, 195—205 (1963).
JONES, K.B., QUILLIAM, J.P.: Perfusion of the superior cervical ganglion of the cat alternately with Locke solution and with the cat's own blood. J. Physiol. (Lond.) **189**, 11P—13P (1967).
KATZ, B.: Nerve, muscle and synapse. New York: McGraw-Hill 1966.
— The release of neural transmitter substances. Liverpool: University Press 1969.
— MILEDI, R.: Propagation of electric activity in motor nerve terminals. Proc. roy. Soc. B **161**, 453—482 (1964).
— — Input-output relation of a single synapse. Nature (Lond.) **212**, 1242—1245 (1966).
— — The effect of local blockade of motor nerve terminals. J. Physiol. (Lond.) **199**, 729—741 (1968).
KAYAALP, S.O., MCISAAC, R.J.: Absence of effects of prostaglandins E_1 and E_2 on ganglionic transmission. Europ. J. Pharmacol. **4**, 283—288 (1968).
KERKUT, G.A., THOMAS, R.C.: An electrogenic sodium pump in snail nerve cells. Comp. Biochem. Physiol. **14**, 167—183 (1965).
KHARKEVICH, D.A.: Ganglion-blocking and ganglion-stimulating agents. Oxford: Pergamon Press 1967.
KIRPEKAR, S.M., MISU, Y.: Release of noradrenaline by splenic nerve stimulation and its dependence on calcium. J. Physiol. (Lond.) **188**, 219—234 (1967).
KOBAYASHI, H., LIBET, B.: Generation of slow postsynaptic potentials without increases in ionic conductance. Proc. nat. Acad. Sci. (Wash.) **60**, 1304—1311 (1968).
KOKETSU, K.: Cholinergic synaptic potentials and the underlying ionic mechanisms. Fed. Proc. **28**, 101—112 (1969).
— NISHI, S.: Characteristics of the slow inhibitory postsynaptic potential of bullfrog sympathetic ganglion cells. Life Sci. **6**, 1827—1836 (1967).
— — Calcium spikes of nerve cell membrane: role of calcium in the production of action potentials. Nature (Lond.) **217**, 468—469 (1968a).
— — Cholinergic receptors at sympathetic preganglionic nerve terminals. J. Physiol. (Lond.) **196**, 293—310 (1968b).

KOKETSU, K., NISHI, S.: Calcium and action potentials of bullfrog sympathetic ganglion cells. J. gen. Physiol. **53**, 608—623 (1969).
— — NODA, Y.: Effects of physostigmine on the afterdischarge and slow postsynaptic potentials of bullfrog sympathetic ganglia. Brit. J. Pharmacol. **34**, 177—188 (1968a).
— — SOEDA, H.: Calcium and acetylcholine-potential of bullfrog sympathetic ganglion cell membrane. Life Sci. **7**, 955—963 (1968b).
KOMALAHIRANYA, A., VOLLE, R.L.: Actions of inorganic ions and veratrine on asynchronous postganglionic discharge in sympathetic ganglia treated with disopropyl-phosphorofluoridate (DFP). J. Pharmacol. exp. Ther. **138**, 57—65 (1962).
KONZETT, H.: The effect of histamine on an isolated sympathetic ganglion. J. Mt. Sinai Hosp. **19**, 149—153 (1952).
KOSTERLITZ, H.W., LEES, G.M., WALLIS, D.I.: Potentials recorded from the isolated superior cervical ganglion of the rabbit. J. Physiol. (Lond.) **188**, 11 P (1967).
— — — Resting and active potentials recorded by the sucrose-gap method in the superior cervical ganglion of the rabbit. J. Physiol. (Lond.) **195**, 39—53 (1968).
— — — Further evidence for an electrogenic sodium pump in a mammalian sympathetic ganglion. Proc. Brit. Pharmacol. Soc., January 1970.
— THOMPSON, J.W., WALLIS, D.I.: The compound action potential in the nerve supplying the medial smooth muscle of the nictitating membrane of the cat. J. Physiol. (Lond.) **171**, 426—433 (1964).
— WALLIS, D.I.: The use of the sucrose-gap method for recording ganglionic potentials. J. Physiol. (Lond.) **183**, 1 P—3 P (1966).
KRIVOY, W.A., WILLS, J.H.: Adaptation to constant concentrations of acetylcholine. J. Pharmacol. exp. Ther. **116**, 220—226 (1956).
KUNTZ, A., SACCOMANNO, G.: Reflex inhibition of intestinal motility mediated through decentralized prevertebral ganglia. J. Neurophysiol. **7**, 163—170 (1944).
LAPORTE, Y., LORENTE DE NÓ, R.: Properties of sympathetic B ganglion cells. J. cell. comp. Physiol. **35**, Suppl. 41—60 (1950a).
— — Potential changes evoked in a curarized sympathetic ganglion by presynaptic volleys of impulses. J. cell. comp. Physiol. **35**, Suppl. 61—107 (1950b).
— — Dual mechanism of synaptic transmission through a sympathetic ganglion. J. cell. comp. Physiol. **35**, Suppl. 107—153 (1950c).
LARRABEE, M.G.: Oxygen consumption of excised sympathetic ganglia at rest and in activity. J. Neurochem. **2**, 81—101 (1958).
— BRONK, D.W.: Long-lasting effects of activity on ganglionic transmission. Amer. J. Physiol. **123**, 126 (1938a).
— — Persistent discharge from sympathetic ganglion cells following preganglionic stimulation. Proc. Soc. exp. Biol. (N.Y.) **38**, 921—922 (1938b).
— — After discharge from sympathetic ganglion cells following preganglionic nerve stimulation. Fed. Proc. **5**, 60—61 (1946).
— — Prolonged facilitation of synaptic excitation in sympathetic ganglia. J. Neurophysiol. **10**, 137—154 (1947).
LEWIS, G.P., REIT, E.: The action of angiotensin and bradykinin on the superior cervical ganglion of the cat. J. Physiol. (Lond.) **179**, 538—553 (1965).
LIBET, B.: Slow synaptic responses and excitatory changes in sympathetic ganglia. J. Physiol. (Lond.) **174**, 1—25 (1964).
— Long latent periods and further analysis of slow synaptic responses in sympathetic ganglia. J. Neurophysiol. **30**, 494—514 (1967).
— CHICHIBU, S., TOSAKA, T.: Slow synaptic responses and excitability in sympathetic ganglia of the bullfrog. J. Neurophysiol. **31**, 383—395 (1968).
— KOBAYASHI, H.: Generation of adrenergic and cholinergic potentials in sympathetic ganglion cells. Science **169**, 1530—1532 (1969).
— TOSAKA, T.: Slow inhibitory and excitatory postsynaptic responses in single cells of mammalian sympathetic ganglia. J. Neurophysiol. **32**, 43—50 (1969).
LINDMAR, R., LÖFFELHOLZ, K., MUSCHOLL, E.: A muscarinic mechanism inhibiting the release of noradrenaline from peripheral adrenergic nerve fibres by nicotinic agents. Brit. J. Pharmacol. **32**, 280—294 (1968).
LLOYD, D.P.C.: The transmission of impulses through the inferior mesenteric ganglia. J. Physiol. (Lond.) **91**, 296—313 (1937).
— The excitability states of inferior mesenteric ganglion cells following preganglionic activation. J. Physiol. (Lond.) **95**, 464—475 (1939a).
— The origin and nature of ganglion after-potentials. J. Physiol. (Lond.) **96**, 118—129 (1939b).
LÖFFELHOLZ, K., LINDMAR, R., MUSCHOLL, E.: Der Einfluß von Atropin auf die Noradrenalin-Freisetzung durch Acetylcholin. Naunyn-Schmiedeberg's Arch. Pharmak. exp. Path. **257**, 308 (1967).

Löffelholz, K., Muscholl, E.: A muscarinic inhibition of the noradrenaline release evoked by postganglionic sympathetic nerve stimulation. Naunyn-Schmiedeberg's Arch. Pharmak. **265**, 1—15 (1969).
Lorente de Nó, R., Laporte, Y.: Properties of postganglionic B fibers. J. cell. comp. Physiol. **35**, Suppl. 9—40 (1950a).
— — Refractoriness, facilitation and inhibition in a sympathetic ganglion. J. cell. comp. Physiol. **35**, Suppl. 155—192 (1950b).
Lundberg, A., Thesleff, S.: Dual action of nicotine on the sympathetic ganglion of the cat. Acta physiol. scand. **28**, 218—223 (1953).
Machová, J., Boška, D.: A study of the action of angiotensin on the superior cervical ganglion in comparison with other ganglion stimulating agents. Europ. J. Pharmacol. **1**, 233—239 (1967).
— — The effect of 5-hydroxytryptamine, dimethylphenylpiperazinium and acetylcholine on transmission and surface potential in the cat sympathetic ganglion. Europ. J. Pharmacol. **7**, 152—158 (1969).
Manocha, S.L., Shanta, T.R.: Enzyme histochemistry of the nervous system. In: Bourne, G.H. (ed.): The structure and function of the nervous tissue. **2**, 184—187. New York: Academic Press 1969.
Marrazzi, A.S.: Electrical studies on the pharmacology of autonomic synapses. II. The action of a sympathomimetic drug (epinephrine) on sympathetic ganglia. J. Pharmacol. exp. Ther. **65**, 395—404 (1939).
— Lorente de Nó, R.: Interaction of neighboring fibers in myelinated nerve. J. Neurophysiol. **7**, 83—102 (1944).
Mason, D.F.J.: Depolarizing action of neostigmine at an autonomic ganglion. Brit. J. Pharmacol. **18**, 572—587 (1962).
Matthews, R.J.: The effect of epinephrine, levarterenol, and dl-isoproterenol in transmission in the superior cervical ganglion of the cat. J. Pharmacol. exp. Ther. **116**, 437—443 (1956).
— Roberts, B.J.: The effect of gamma-aminobutyric acid on synaptic transmission in autonomic ganglia. J. Pharmacol. exp. Ther. **132**, 19—22 (1961).
McCubbin, J.W., Green, J.H., Salmoiraghi, G.C., Page, I.H.: The chemoreceptor stimulant action of serotonin in dogs. J. Pharmacol. exp. Ther. **116**, 191—197 (1956).
McLennan, H.: Acetylcholine metabolism of normal and axotomized ganglia. J. Physiol. (Lond.) **124**, 113—116 (1954).
— Pascoe, J.E.: The origin of certain non-medullated nerve fibres which form synapses in the inferior mesenteric ganglion of the rabbit. J. Physiol. (Lond.) **124**, 145—156 (1954).
Miledi, R.: The acetylcholine sensitivity of frog muscle fibres after complete or partial denervation. J. Physiol. (Lond.) **151**, 1—23 (1960).
Muir, T.C., Yonemura, K.: Iontophoretic application of cholinergic drugs and their antagonists to guinea-pig sympathetic ganglia. Aust. J. exp. Biol. med. Sci. **47**, P 24 (1969).
Murayama, S., Unna, K.R.: Stimulant action of 4-(m-chlorophenylcarbamoyloxy)-2-butynyltrimethylammonium chloride (McN-A-343) on sympathetic ganglia. J. Pharmacol. exp. Ther. **140**, 183—192 (1963).
Nakajima, S., Takahashi, K.: Post-tetanic hyperpolarization and electrogenic Na^+-pump in stretch receptor neurone of crayfish. J. Physiol. (Lond.) **187**, 105—127 (1966).
Nicholls, J.G.: The electrical properties of denervated skeletal muscle. J. Physiol. (Lond.) **131**, 1—12 (1956).
— Baylor, D.A.: Long-lasting hyperpolarization after activity of neurons in leech central nervous system. Science **162**, 279—281 (1968).
Nishi, S., Koketsu, K.: Electrical properties and activities of single sympathetic neurons in frogs. J. cell. comp. Physiol. **55**, 15—30 (1960).
— — Late after-discharge of sympathetic postganglionic fibers. Life Sci. **5**, 1991—1997 (1966).
— — Origin of ganglionic inhibitory postsynaptic potential. Life Sci. **6**, 2049—2055 (1967).
— — The early and late afterdischarges of amphibian sympathetic postganglionic fibers. J. Neurophysiol. **31**, 109—121 (1968a).
— — Analysis of slow inhibitory postsynaptic potential of bullfrog sympathetic ganglion. J. Neurophysiol. **31**, 717—728 (1968b).
— Soeda, H., Koketsu, K.: Studies on sympathetic B and C neurons and patterns of preganglionic innervation. J. cell. comp. Physiol. **66**, 19—32 (1965).
— — — Release of acetylcholine from sympathetic preganglionic nerve terminals. J. Neurophysiol. **30**, 114—134 (1967).
— — — Unusual nature of ganglionic slow EPSP studied by a voltage-clamp method. Life Sci. **8**, 33—42 (1969).

NORBERG, K.-A.: Transmitter histochemistry of the sympathetic adrenergic nervous system. Brain Res. **5**, 125—170 (1967).

— HAMBERGER, B.: The sympathetic adrenergic neuron. Acta physiol. scand. **63**, Suppl. 238 (1964).

— McISAAC, R.J.: Cellular localization of adrenergic amines in frog sympathetic ganglia. Experientia (Basel) **23**, 1052 (1967).

— SJÖQVIST, F.: New possibilities for adrenergic modulation of ganglionic transmission. Pharmacol. Res. **18**, 743—751 (1966).

OBRADOR, S., ODORIZ, J.B.: Transmission through a lumbar sympathetic ganglion. J. Physiol. (Lond.) **86**, 269—276 (1936).

PAGE, I.H., McCUBBIN, J.W.: The variable arterial pressure response to serotonin in laboratory animals and man. Circulat. Res. **1**, 354—362 (1953).

PAPPANO, A.J., VOLLE, R.L.: The reversal by atropine of ganglionic blockade produced by acetylcholine. Life Sci. **12**, 677—682 (1962).

— — Observations on the role of calcium ions in ganglionic responses to acetylcholine. J. Pharmacol. exp. Ther. **152**, 171—180 (1966a).

— — Lithium's failure to replace sodium in mammalian sympathetic ganglia. Science **152**, 85—87 (1966b).

— — Actions of lithium ions in mammalian sympathetic ganglia. J. Pharmacol. exp. Ther. **157**, 346—355 (1967).

PASCOE, J.E.: The effects of acetylcholine and other drugs on the isolated superior cervical ganglion. J. Physiol. (Lond.) **132**, 242—255 (1956).

PAŠIĆ, M., LJ. SAVIĆ, V.: Facilitation and post-tetanic potentiation in autonomic ganglia of the rat. Jug. Physiol. Pharmacol. Acta **5**, 249—255 (1969).

PATON, W.D.M., PERRY, W.L.M.: The relationship between depolarization and block in the cat's superior cervical ganglion. J. Physiol. (Lond.) **119**, 43—57 (1953).

PERRI, V., SACCHI, O., CASELLA, C.: Electrical properties and synaptic connections of the sympathetic neurons in the rat and guinea-pig superior cervical ganglion. Pflügers Arch. **314**, 40—54 (1970a).

— — — Synaptically mediated potentials elicited by the stimulation of post-ganglionic trunks in the guinea-pig superior cervical ganglion. Pflügers Arch. **314**, 55—67 (1970b).

PERRY, W.L.M., REINERT, H.: The effects of preganglionic denervation on the reactions of ganglion cells. J. Physiol. (Lond.) **126**, 101—115 (1954).

PICK, J.: The submicroscopic organization of the sympathetic ganglion in the frog (rana pipiens). J. comp. Neurol. **120**, 409—419 (1963).

QUILLIAM, J.P., SHAND, D.G.: The selectivity of drugs blocking ganglionic transmission in the rat. Brit. J. Pharmacol. **23**, 273—284 (1964).

RANG, H.P., RITCHIE, J.M.: On the electrogenic sodium pump in mammalian non-myelinated nerve fibres and its activation by various external cations. J. Physiol. (Lond.) **196**, 183—221 (1968).

RANSON, S.W., BILLINGSLEY, P.R.: The superior cervical ganglion and the cervical portion of the sympathetic trunk. J. comp. Neurol. **29**, 313—358 (1918).

REINERT, H.: The depolarizing and blocking action of amphetamine in the cat's superior cervical ganglion. In: VANE, WOLSTENHOLME and O'CONNOR (eds.): Adrenergic mechanisms. CIBA Foundation Symposium, pp. 373—379. London: Churchill Ltd. 1960.

RIKER, W.K.: Effects of Tetraethylammonium chloride on electrical activities of frog sympathetic ganglion cells. J. Pharmacol. exp. Ther. **145**, 317—325 (1964).

— Effects of tetraethylammonium on synaptic transmission in the frog sympathetic ganglion. J. Pharmacol. exp. Ther. **147**, 161—171 (1965).

— The basis of the low-amplitude discharge produced by acetylcholine injections in sympathetic ganglia. J. Pharmacol. exp. Ther. **155**, 203—210 (1967).

— Ganglion cell depolarization and transmission block by ACh: independent events. J. Pharmacol. exp. Ther. **159**, 345—352 (1968).

RITCHIE, J.M., STRAUB, R.W.: The hyperpolarization which follows activity in mammalian non-medullated fibres. J. Physiol. (Lond.) **136**, 80—97 (1957).

ROBERTSON, P.A.: An antagonism of 5-hydroxytryptamine by atropine. J. Physiol. (Lond.) **121**, 54 P—55 P (1953).

SANBE, S.: Studies on the incoming and outgoing myelinated nerve fibers of the sympathetic superior cervical ganglion. Fukushima J. med. Sci. **8**, 109—129 (1961).

SANGHVI, I., MURAYAMA, S., SMITH, C.M., UNNA, K.R.: Action of muscarine on the superior cervical ganglion of the cat. J. Pharmacol. exp. Ther. **142**, 192—199 (1963).

SHAND, D.G.: The mode of action of drugs blocking ganglionic transmission in the rat. Brit. J. Pharmacol. **24**, 89—97 (1965).

SHANES, A.M.: Electrochemical aspects of physiological and pharmacological action in excitable cells. Pharmacol. Rev. **10**, 59—273 (1958).

SKOK, V.I.: Intracellular electric potentials of sympathetic ganglion neurons. Fed. Proc. **22**, T 990—T 993 (1963).
— Origin of the after-depression of the sympathetic ganglion. Neurosci. Transl. **1**, 40—46 (1967/1968).
STONEY, S.D., MACHNE, X.: Mechanisms of accommodation in different types of frog neurons. J. gen. Physiol. **53**, 248—262 (1969).
STRAUB, R.W.: On the mechanism of post-tetanic hyperpolarization in myelinated nerve fibres from the frog. J. Physiol. (Lond.) **159**, 19P—20P (1961).
SZRENIAWSKI, Z., GUMULKA, W.: Influence of depolarizing amino acids on ganglionic conduction in cats. Diss. Pharmaceut. et Neurol. **19**, 613—618 (1967).
SZURSZEWSKI, J.H., CROWCROFT, P.J., HOLMAN, M.E.: Intracellular studies on ganglia of the pelvic plexus of male guinea-pigs. Aust. J. exp. Biol. med. Sci. **47**, P 26 (1969).
TAKESHIGE, C., PAPPANO, A.J., DE GROAT, W.C., VOLLE, R.L.: Ganglionic Blockade produced in sympathetic ganglia by cholinomimetic drugs. J. Pharmacol. exp. Ther. **141**, 333—342 (1963).
— VOLLE, R.L.: Bimodal response of sympathetic ganglia to acetylcholine following eserine or repetitive preganglionic stimulation. J. Pharmacol. exp. Ther. **138**, 66—73 (1962).
— — Cholinoceptive sites in denervated sympathetic ganglia. J. Pharmacol. exp. Ther. **141**, 206—213 (1963a).
— — Asynchronous postganglionic firing from the cat superior cervical sympathetic ganglion treated with neostigmine. Brit. J. Pharmacol. **20**, 214—220 (1963b).
— — Modification of ganglionic responses to cholinomimetic drugs following preganglionic stimulation, anticholinesterase agents and pilocarpine. J. Pharmacol. exp. Ther. **146**, 335—343 (1964).
TAKEUCHI, A., TAKEUCHI, N.: On the permeability of end-plate membrane during the action of transmitter. J. Physiol. (Lond.) **154**, 56—67 (1960).
— — Electrical changes in pre- and postsynaptic axons of giant synapse of Loligo. J. gen. Physiol. **45**, 1181—1193 (1962).
TAUC, L.: Transmission in invertebrate and vertebrate ganglia. Physiol. Rev. **47**, 521—593 (1967).
TAXI, J.: Etude de l'ultrastructure des zones synaptiques dans les ganglions sympathiques de grenouille. C. R. Acad. Sci. (Paris) **252**, 174—176 (1961).
THERMAN, P.O., FORBES, A., GALAMBOS, R.: Electric responses derived from the superior cervical ganglion with micro-electrodes. J. Neurophysiol. **3**, 191—200 (1940).
THOENEN, H., HAEFELY, W., STAEHELIN, H.: Potentiation by tetraethylammonium of the response of the cat spleen to postganglionic sympathetic nerve stimulation. J. Pharmacol. exp. Ther. **157**, 532—540 (1967).
TOSAKA, T., CHICHIBU, S., LIBET, B.: Intracellular analysis of slow inhibitory and excitatory postsynaptic potentials in sympathetic ganglia of the frog. J. Neurophysiol. **31**, 396—409 (1968).
TRANZER, J.P., THOENEN, H.: An electron-microscopic study of selective, acute degeneration of sympathetic nerve terminals after administration of 6-hydroxydopamine. Experientia (Basel) **24**, 155—156 (1968).
TRENDELENBURG, U.: The action of histamine and pilocarpine on the superior cervical ganglia and the adrenal glands of the cat. Brit. J. Pharmacol. **9**, 481—487 (1954).
— The potentiation of ganglionic transmission by histamine and pilocarpine. J. Physiol. (Lond.) **129**, 337—351 (1955).
— Reaktion sympathischer Ganglien während der Ganglienblockade durch Nicotin. Naunyn-Schmiedeberg's Arch. exp. Pathol. Pharmak. **230**, 448—456 (1957).
— Observations on the ganglion-stimulating action of angiotensin and bradykinin. J. Pharmacol. exp. Ther. **154**, 418—425 (1966a).
— Transmission of preganglionic impulses through the muscarinic receptors of the superior cervical ganglion of the cat. J. Pharmacol. exp. Ther. **154**, 426—440 (1966b).
— Some aspects of the pharmacology of autonomic ganglion cells. Ergebn. Physiol. **59**, 1—85 (1967).
— JONES, A.: Facilitation of ganglionic responses after a period of preganglionic stimulation. J. Pharmacol. exp. Ther. **147**, 330—335 (1965).
ULBRICHT, W.: The effect of veratridine on excitable membranes of nerve and muscle. Ergebn. Physiol. **61**, 18—71 (1969).
UNGVÁRY, G., LÉRÁNTH, C.: Termination in the prevertebral abdominal sympathetic ganglia of axons arising from the local (terminal) vegetative plexus of visceral organs. Z. Zellforsch. **110**, 185—191 (1970).
VOLLE, R.L.: Potentiation of postganglionic responses to stimulating agents following repetitive preganglionic stimulation. Int. J. Neuropharmacol. **1**, 209—211 (1962a).

VOLLE, R. L.: The actions of several ganglion blocking agents on the postganglionic discharge induced by diisopropyl phosphorofluoridate (DFP) in sympathetic ganglia. J. Pharmacol. exp. Ther. **135**, 45—53 (1962b).
— Enhancement of postganglionic responses to stimulating agents following repetitive preganglionic stimulation. J. Pharmacol. exp. Ther. **136**, 68—74 (1962c).
— Muscarinic and nicotinic stimulant actions at autonomic ganglia. International Encyclopedia of Pharmacology and Therapeutics, Section 12, Vol. 1, Pergamon Press 1966a.
— Modification by drugs of synaptic mechanisms in autonomic ganglia. Pharmacol. Rev. **18**, 839—869 (1966b).
— Hyperpolarization and blockade of ganglionic transmission. Arch. int. Pharmacodyn. **169**, 35—43 (1967a).
— On the mechanism of ganglionic blockade by methacholine. J. Pharmacol. exp. Ther. **158**, 66—72 (1967b).
— Ganglionic transmission. Ann. Rev. Pharmacol. **9**, 135—146 (1969).
— PAPPANO, A. J.: Some relationships between drugs and ions at a ganglionic synapse. Fed. Proc. **27**, 110—114 (1968).
WALL, P. D.: Excitability changes in afferent fibre terminations and their relation to slow potentials. J. Physiol. (Lond.) **142**, 1—21 (1958).
WASER, P. G.: Die cholinergischen Receptoren der Muskelendplatten. Pflügers Arch. ges. Physiol. **274**, 431—446 (1962).
— Nature of the cholinergic receptor. Proc. first internat. pharmacol. meeting, **7**, 101—115, Pergamon Press 1963.
WATSON, P. J.: Drug receptor sites in the isolated superior cervical ganglion or the rat. Europ. J. Pharmacol. **12**, 183—193 (1970).
WEIGHT, F. F., VOTAVA, J.: Slow synaptic excitation in sympathetic ganglion cells: Evidence for synaptic inactivation of potassium conductance. Science **170**, 755—758 (1970).
WOODWARD, J. K., BIANCHI, C. P., ERULKAR, S. D.: Electrolyte distribution in rabbit superior cervical ganglion. J. Neurochem. **16**, 289—299 (1969).

Chapter 16

Factors Influencing the Concentration of Catecholamines at the Receptors

U. TRENDELENBURG

With 6 Figures

I. Introduction

There are no methods available for the direct determination of the concentration of noradrenaline in the "biophase", i.e., in the very small part of the extracellular space in the immediate neighbourhood of the receptors of adrenergically innervated organs. Hence, any discussion of the factors influencing the concentration of the amine at the receptors has to be based on indirect evidence. If the direct approach is impossible, one can gain some insight from recording responses (or changes in responses) of the effector organ to known concentrations of noradrenaline. However, any interpretation involves two crucial assumptions, namely that, in the absence of conclusive evidence to the contrary, the interaction between drug and receptor as well as the function of the link between receptor activation and eventual response remains unaffected by the change in experimental conditions which is being studied. In many experimental situations the validity of these assumptions remains questionable, since it has not been possible to obtain positive evidence.

In one case, namely in decentralization supersensitivity, a considerable body of evidence indicates that a change in response is indeed due to a postjunctional event. After chronic parasympathetic or sympathetic decentralization, smooth muscles or glands respond more strongly to a given dose or concentration of agonists because the responsiveness of the effector cells is increased, not the concentration of the agonists at the receptors. This postjunctional type of supersensitivity is believed to be due to an increase in the population of the receptors or to an improvement in the function of the link between receptor activation and final response (TRENDELENBURG, 1963; GREEN and FLEMING, 1967; LANGER and TRENDELENBURG, 1968; PLUCHINO and TRENDELENBURG, 1968). Thus, decentralization supersensitivity has to be excluded from the present discussion, since there is good evidence that the assumptions stated above are not fulfilled. In other words, although decentralization leads to supersensitivity to various agents, it does not seem to influence the concentration of these agents at the receptors.

Since vasodilator drugs potentiate the effect of intra-arterial injections of noradrenaline on the cat's nictitating membrane, and since this effect is less pronounced after decentralization, CERVONI et al. (1970) suggested that decentralization supersensitivity is due to the vasodilatation that must occur in the nictitating membrane after section of the preganglionic nerves. However, it is unlikely that this suggestion provides a full explanation. The vasodilatation should be most pronounced soon after section of the preganglionic nerves, and decentralization supersensitivity should be maximally developed at that time.

However, it is well documented that decentralization supersensitivity requires more than 48 hours in order to become measurable and that it continues to increase for at least 4 weeks after the operation (LANGER et al., 1967b). This time course of the development of decentralization supersensitivity is not consistent with its being due to vasodilatation; the vascular theory of decentralization supersensitivity remains doubtful.

Other types of supersensitivity have to be considered here, since there is either no evidence for any postjunctional effects or the evidence is conflicting. For instance, on the nictitating membrane of the cat, cocaine seems to cause supersensitivity to noradrenaline entirely through a prejunctional effect (i.e., through an impairment of the neuronal amine uptake; TRENDELENBURG, 1963, 1966a).On other organs cocaine seems to be able to exert, in addition, postjunctional effects (vas deferens of the rat: KASUYA and GOTO, 1968; rabbit aortic strips: KALSNER and NICKERSON, 1969b). This contradictory evidence (which will be discussed below in more detail) serves to illustrate the difficulties encountered in the analysis of the factors influencing the concentration of noradrenaline at the receptors.

In order to discuss the topic in a meaningful way, it will be assumed that agents and procedures used have no postjunctional effects unless there is conclusive evidence to the contrary. Moreover, the discussion will be based on the uptake theory of denervation and cocaine supersensitivity. This hypothesis postulates that, on exposure of the tissue to noradrenaline, there exists a concentration gradient from the circulating plasma (*in vivo*) or the medium (*in vitro*) to the vicinity of the receptors and that the main factor responsible for this concentration gradient is neuronal uptake of noradrenaline. Any impairment of the neuronal uptake (*e.g.*, after denervation or cocaine) decreases the concentration gradient. Thus, for a given amine concentration in the plasma or in the medium, an increased concentration is achieved at the receptors, and supersensitivity ensues.

The uptake theory of denervation and cocaine supersensitivity is preferred to other hypotheses because of its predictive value. There is a nearly unlimited number of drugs or procedures which can interfere with uptake; hence, it is possible to test this hypothesis in a multitude of ways. This does not apply to other hypotheses that have been proposed to account for the effects of either denervation or cocaine. For instance, cocaine has been proposed to cause supersensitivity by deforming receptors (i.e., by changing the interaction between drug and receptor) (MAXWELL et al., 1959; VARMA, 1966; REIFFENSTEIN, 1968). Since the properties of a deformed receptor are unpredictable, the concept does not lead to experiments with which to test the hypothesis. Basically, the hypothesis simply states that certain observations do not seem to agree with the uptake theory of cocaine supersensitivity; hence, a postjunctional site of action of cocaine is postulated. Negatively oriented postulates then have to be countered by reinvestigations with the aim to show that the observations do not disagree with the uptake theory. Such doubly negative studies cannot prove the uptake theory right; they simply serve to show that the objections to the uptake theory were not correct. For an example the reader is referred to the study of VARMA (1966) and subsequent work of others (GREEN and FLEMING, 1967; LANGER and TRENDELENBURG, 1968).

There is a second reason for basing this discussion on the concept that neuronal uptake is the most important mechanism influencing the concentration of noradrenaline at the receptors: it is the most comprehensive hypothesis, since the large majority of observations relevant to our topic is in agreement with this hypothesis. Moreover, as contributory factors are recognized, apparent disagreements with the hypothesis are being resolved. For instance, it has been puzzling for very long why the sensitizing effect of cocaine differs quantitatively from organ to organ. Recent morphological studies have resolved this problem very satisfactorily by demonstrating important differences in the distance between nerve endings and effector cells. These studies have not only removed doubts about the validity of the uptake theory, they actually provided additional circumstantial evidence in favor of it.

II. Methods

The evidence discussed below is based on various types of experiments, the most important of which might be briefly characterized.

1. Sensitivity Studies. Studies of the effect of various agents or procedures on the sensitivity of organs to noradrenaline (or related amines) can yield information on possible changes in the concentration of the amine at the receptors. Optimally, such studies should be done under steady-state conditions, they should consist of determinations of full dose-response curves (to define the ED50 as well as the maximum response and the slope of the dose-response curve), and changes in sensitivity should be expressed as ratios of equieffective doses (TRENDELENBURG, 1963). Care must be taken not to confuse supersensitivity with additive effects (see section XI).

2. Accumulation Studies. Because of neuronal (and possibly of extraneuronal) uptake, adrenergically innervated organs accumulate exogenous noradrenaline.In the interpretation of experiments of this kind, it has to be remembered that accumulation is the consequence not only of uptake through the neuronal membrane but also of neuronal (usually vesicular) retention. Hence, a decrease in accumulation of exogenous amine may be due either to a decrease in membranal uptake or in intraneuronal retention. For the concentration of noradrenaline at the receptors, uptake through the nerve membrane is of decisive importance.

3. Elimination Studies. Organs perfused with noradrenaline are well known to remove a considerable percentage of the amine from the perfusion fluid. This removal seems to be mainly due to the net uptake across the axonal membrane (LINDMAR and MUSCHOLL, 1964). This method for determinations of net uptake through the nerve membrane has the great advantage of being largely independent of the eventual intraneuronal fate of the amine after its uptake.

The removal of noradrenaline can also be measured for organs which cannot be perfused. When incubated with a small volume of medium containing a low concentration of noradrenaline, the isolated nictitating membrane of the cat removes the amine from the medium. Removal seems to be mainly a neuronal event, since it is sensitive to cocaine (GRAEFE and TRENDELENBURG, 1970). The inevitable disadvantage of this method lies in the fact that the concentration of the amine in the medium falls with time.

4. Inactivation Studies. Determinations of the metabolism of exogenous or endogenous noradrenaline have greatly contributed to our knowledge of possible mechanisms of inactivation (and hence, possible factors influencing the concentration of the amine at the receptors). An elegant new method has been introduced by KALSNER and NICKERSON (1968) who incubated tissue with noradrenaline (or related amines) and then immersed it in mineral oil to prevent diffusion out of the tissue. The ensuing slow relaxation is taken as a measure of the rate of inactivation of the amine.

III. Morphological Relation between Adrenergic Nerve Endings and Effector Cells

Both histochemical and electron microscopic studies of recent years have shown that the morphology of the adrenergic innervation differs very much from organ to organ. There are at least three important differences: in density of innervation, in symmetry of innervation and in the distance from nerve endings to effector cells (i.e., in neuro-muscular distance). Although there cannot be any doubt as to the existence of these differences, it is not yet possible to state with certainty which are most important. For the present discussion, organs may be subdivided into two groups; while many organs have a more or less homogeneous adrenergic innervation, others have an asymmetrical one.

a) The Neuro-muscular Interval

Fluorescence microscopy shows that in organs like the nictitating membrane, the heart, the spleen capsule and the vas deferens, adrenergic fibers and their varicosities spread throughout the muscle. This does not necessarily mean that adrenergic nerve endings penetrate each bundle of muscle fibers, but the network of nerve terminals is rather evenly distributed. Moreover, in most cases there seems to be a rather close contact between nerve terminals and effector cells; the minimal neuro-muscular distance is about 200—300 Å in the nictitating membrane (Van Orden et al., 1967; Esterhuizen et al., 1968) and the vas deferens (Merrilees et al., 1963). Because of the short neuro-muscular distance, the exogenous noradrenaline which diffuses into the tissue comes into the vicinity of both effector cells and adrenergic nerve endings. Hence, a considerable concentration gradient results from the removal of the amine by the nerve endings. The magnitude of the difference between the concentration in the medium and that at the receptors of effector cells in the center of the tissue should depend on the density of the innervation as well as on the thickness of the tissue.

One example for the importance of the density of innervation is provided by the nictitating membrane of the cat which has two adrenergically innervated smooth muscles, the medial and the inferior (Acheson, 1938). *In vitro* the two muscles do not differ in maximum tension development or in the proportion of muscle protein/non-muscle protein. Although they seem to represent about equal mixtures of muscular and connective tissue, the noradrenaline content of the medial muscle is nearly twice that of the inferior (Trendelenburg et al., 1969). The two muscles differ in two other respects:

1. On incubation of the isolated muscles with noradrenaline-H^3 the accumulation of the amine by the more densely innervated medial muscle is about twice that of the less densely innervated inferior muscle. The difference is seen only when accumulation is related to the weight of the tissue; it disappears when accumulation is related to the content of endogenous noradrenaline. Apparently, accumulation per nerve ending is identical in both muscles; the muscles differ in density of innervation only.

2. The sensitivity of the more densely innervated medial muscle to noradrenaline or adrenaline is lower than that of the inferior muscle. The difference in sensitivity disappears after denervation, and no difference in sensitivity is observed to amines which are not taken up by adrenergic nerve endings. Hence, sensitivity to amines which are taken up by adrenergic nerve endings is inversely related to the density of the innervation (Trendelenburg et al., 1969).

Differences in density of adrenergic innervation cannot be entirely separated from differences in neuro-muscular distances. If the smooth muscle cells of the two muscles have similarly distributed adrenoceptors, a decrease in the density of adrenergic innervation should be equivalent to an increase in the average neuro-muscular distance. Since the influence of the neuronal uptake on the concentration of noradrenaline at the receptors is inversely related to the neuro-muscular distance, part of the difference in sensitivity to noradrenaline (between the medial and the inferior muscle, see above) may have to be attributed to differences in neuro-muscular distance rather than exclusively to differences in the density of innervation.

Moreover, if density of innervation were the only determinant of the postulated concentration gradient, one would have to expect that the degree of supersensitivity after denervation or cocaine were directly related to the noradrenaline content of various organs. However, this postulate is not in agreement with experimental observations (Table 1). Thus, although there is good evidence to support the view that the density of adrenergic innervation is an important determinant of the postulated concentration gradient, there must be other determinants as well.

Table 1. *Sensitizing effect of cocaine (or denervation) in various tissues*

Tissue	noradrenaline content (μg/g)	sensitization to (—)-noradrenaline	by[12]
guinea-pig vas deferens	11.1[1]	10-fold[1]	denervation
rat vas deferens	8.6[1]	16-fold[1]	denervation
cat nictitating membrane	8.6[2]	20-fold[3]	cocaine
guinea-pig atria	2.7[4]	rate: 14-fold[5]	cocaine
		force: 27-fold[6]	cocaine
guinea-pig aorta	2.4[7]	2.5-fold[7]	cocaine
cat spleen capsule	2.0[8]	20-fold[9]	cocaine
guinea-pig trachea	very low[10]	47-fold[11]	cocaine

1. taken from BIRMINGHAM (1970); 2. taken from TRENDELENBURG et al. (1969); 3. taken from LANGER and TRENDELENBURG (1969); 4. taken from SMITH (1966); 5. taken from TRENDELENBURG (1968); 6. taken from FURCHGOTT et al. (1963); 7. taken from SCHÜMANN and GÜTHER (1967); 8. taken from GREEN and FLEMING (1968); 9. taken from BRIMIJOIN et al. (1970); 10. According to HOLLANDS and VANOV (1965) the density of adrenergic innervation of the guinea-pig trachea is very low indeed, since "the trachea showed less specific fluorescence than all other tissues examined" (such as, for instance, guinea-pig atria); 11. taken from FOSTER (1967); 12. The concentration of cocaine was about 10 μg/ml except in experiments with guinea-pig aorta (2 mg/ml).

b) The Density of Adrenergic Innervation

Arterial smooth muscle does not receive a homogeneous adrenergic innervation; the nerve endings are arranged asymmetrically, since they are located almost exclusively along the adventitio-medial border (EHINGER et al., 1967; VERITY and BEVAN, 1968). As a consequence of this morphological arrangement, the neuro-muscular distance is great. For instance, for the pulmonary artery the average neuro-muscular distance (19000 Å) is very much greater than that for nictitating membrane or vas deferens (VERITY and BEVAN, 1968).

Exact determinations of average neuro-muscular distances must be based on a three-dimensional approach which would involve an inordinate amount of work. Hence, reliable values are obtained only for *minimal* neuro-muscular distances. Moreover, there is an additional reason why the most painstaking morphological study cannot resolve the problem. For a variety of smooth muscles it has been shown that neighbouring cells are electrically coupled (HOLMAN, 1969; FURNESS, 1970). If electric coupling via low resistance connections provides a means of spreading excitation, the average neuro-muscular distance is not a biologically meaningful parameter. However, even if only minimal neuro-muscular distances are considered, they are much greater for arterial smooth muscle than for muscles like the nictitating membrane or the vas deferens (4000 Å for pulmonary artery; VERITY and BEVAN, 1968).

Since the importance of neuronal uptake for the concentration of noradrenaline at the receptors is inversely related to the neuro-muscular distance, the magnitude of the sensitizing effect of cocaine should be inversely related to the neuro-muscular distance. VERITY (1971) prepared a summary of those studies in which cocaine-induced supersensitivity to noradrenaline was determined in organs with known neuro-muscular distances (Fig. 1). The agreement between observations and expectations is good, and neuronal uptake seems drastically to lose its

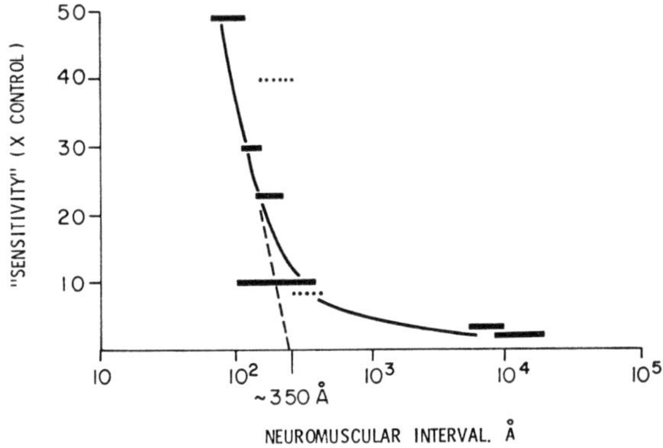

Fig. 1. Relation between the magnitude of the neuromuscular interval and the degree of cocaine-induced supersensitivity to (—)-noradrenaline. Ordinates: increase in sensitivity to (—)-noradrenaline induced by cocaine (linear scale). Abscissae: magnitude of neuromuscular interval (in Å). The broken line gives a rough estimate of maximal neuromuscular interval which permits an influence of the nerve endings on the concentration of (—)-noradrenaline at the receptors. Results were taken from studies of FURCHGOTT et al. (1963), MERRILLEES et al. (1963), TRENDELENBURG (1965), URSILLO and JACOBSON (1965), PICK (1967), BENNET and ROGERS (1967), BEVAN and VERITY (1967), VERITY and BEVAN (1968) and GOVIER et al., (1969). Taken from VERITY (1971) with the kind permission of the author and the publishers

importance (for the concentration of noradrenaline at the receptors) when the neuro-muscular distance approaches 1000 Å. In fact, it is possible that at least some of the very weak sensitizing effects of cocaine observed in organs with very large neuro-muscular distances (right half of Fig. 1) are unrelated to the ability of cocaine to block neuronal uptake. These possibly postjunctional effects of cocaine will be discussed below (section IVd). Cocaine fails to cause supersensitivity to noradrenaline in tissues which are devoid of any adrenergic innervation (human umbilical cord artery and vein; SOMLYO et al., 1965).

It was mentioned above that density of innervation is interrelated with the neuro-muscular distance. This applies also to the results of Fig. 1. On the one hand, one may regard the media of an asymmetrically innervated vessel as a smooth muscle with an innervation of very low density. On the other hand, it so happens that the more densely innervated organs appear in the left half of Fig. 1, the less densely innervated ones in the right half, Thus. part of the correlation between degree of cocaine-induced supersensitivity and neuro-muscular distance may in fact be due to differences in density of innervation.

In an asymmetrically innervated blood vessel, the experimental conditions determine whether or not the neuro-muscular distance is of importance. This was elegantly demonstrated by DE LA LANDE and WATERSON (1967) and DE LA LANDE et al. (1967) from whose results a schematic representation was made (Fig. 2). When noradrenaline is administered into the lumen of the perfused ear artery of the rabbit, it reaches the sites of uptake only after having passed the site of action. Because of the considerable neuro-muscular distance, the concentration gradient is not steep, and cocaine or denervation cause only a two-fold increase in sensitivity (Fig. 2A). However, when administered extraluminally, noradrenaline has to

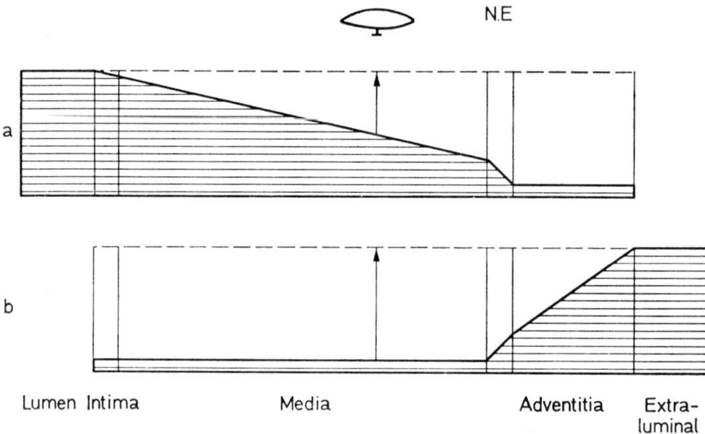

Fig. 2a and b. Schematic representation of the concentration gradient of noradrenaline administered intraluminally (a) or extraluminally (b) to the rabbit ear artery (drawn from the results of DE LA LANDE et al., 1967). The vessel is asymmetrically innervated, the nerve endings (N.E.) being restricted to the adventitio-medial border. If it is assumed that adrenergic nerve endings are the only site of inactivation (through uptake) of noradrenaline, and that neuronal uptake removes 90% of the amine, the smooth muscle of the media is exposed to about half the intraluminal concentration (in a) and to only 1/10 the extraluminal concentration (in b). Since cocaine or denervation prevent neuronal uptake, they abolish the concentration gradient. The consequent increase in concentration of noradrenaline at the receptors is indicated by vertical arrows. Cocaine or denervation cause a two-fold increase in sensitivity in a, a ten-fold increase in b. Note that the slope of the concentration gradient in the adventitio-medial region was set arbitrarily and that the effect of radial diffusion was disregarded

pass the sites of uptake before reaching the site of action; in this case the neuro-muscular distance is of no importance, since the asymmetry of innervation is the decisive factor. Supersensitivity after cocaine or denervation is then very pronounced (about 10-fold) (Fig. 2B). In the absence of cocaine, the sensitivity of the artery to intraluminal noradrenaline is higher than to extraluminal; however, after cocaine or denervation the sensitivity to noradrenaline is uniformely high and independent of the mode of administration.

Similar results were obtained with the tail artery of the rat: desipramine increased the sensitivity to noradrenaline after extraluminal but not after intraluminal administration of the amine; moreover, a decrease of the accumulation of noradrenaline-H^3 was caused by desipramine only when the amine was administered extraluminally (BONACCORSI et al., 1970).

The results are in good agreement with the postulated role of the uptake mechanism. Moreover, they illustrate that the complexity of the morphology of the innervation has to be taken into account. While there is good evidence to show that each of the factors mentioned here (i.e., density of innervation, neuromuscular distance, and symmetry or asymmetry of innervation) is important, it is not yet possible to rank them in order of importance.

IV. The Role of Neuronal Uptake

a) Surgical Denervation

Chronic denervation of adrenergically innervated organs leads to a degree of supersensitivity to various amines which differs markedly from amine to amine. A comparison of the effect of denervation of the cat's nictitating membrane with that of either cocaine or decentralization, shows that denervation supersensitivity consists of two components (Fig. 3): a cocaine-like component develops as rapidly

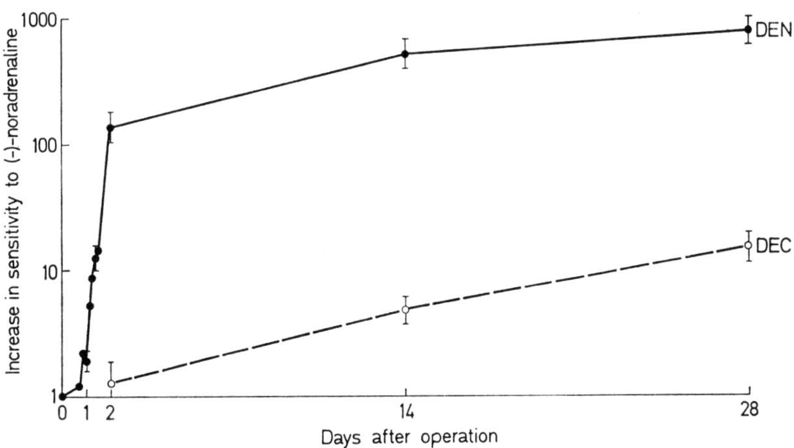

Fig. 3. Development of supersensitivity to noradrenaline in the nictitating membrane of the pithed cat after denervation (solid line) or decentralization (broken line). Note very rapid development of denervation supersensitivity during second postoperative day (prejunctional type of supersensitivity) and the slow subsequent increase in sensitivity to the 28th postoperative day (postjunctional type of supersensitivity which is very similar for both denervation and decentralization). Shown are means of groups of about 5 cats each (with S.E. as vertical bars). Taken from the results of LANGER et al. (1967b)

as the adrenergic fibers degenerate, while a second component, akin to decentralization, develops much more slowly (TRENDELENBURG, 1963, 1966a; LANGER et al., 1967b). The cocaine-like component of supersensitivity is characterized not only by this difference in time course but also by being restricted to amines which are taken up by adrenergic nerve endings. The decentralization type of supersensitivity extends not only to all sympathomimetic amines (irrespective of rate of uptake and of direct or indirect action) but also to other agents which elicit contractions of the nictitating membrane (acetylcholine: TRENDELENBURG and WEINER, 1962; 5-hydroxytryptamine: PLUCHINO, 1972). Since decentralization supersensitivity seems to be due to postjunctional changes in the effector organ which are the consequence of prolonged inactivity of the decentralized effector organ (EMMELIN, 1961; TRENDELENBURG, 1963), it is not surprising that a similar inactivity after denervation should lead to similar changes. The two components of denervation supersensitivity can be separated, since the cocaine-like component is fully developed before the slowly developing decentralization-like component is detectable; in the nictitating membrane of the cat the optimal time for this type of experiment is 2—3 days after denervation (Fig. 3). In the following, the term denervation supersensitivity will be used to denote exclusively the cocaine-like (or prejunctional) component of supersensitivity. The importance of the correct choice of the time interval between operation and experiment is illustrated by the finding that chronic denervation (of 4 weeks) leads to supersensitivity to agents to which there is no denervation supersensitivity (as defined above, i.e., after 2 or 3 days) (PLUCHINO and TRENDELENBURG, 1968; TRENDELENBURG et al., 1970).

The essential feature of denervation supersensitivity is the absence of uptake into neurones. As a consequence, the postulated concentration gradient is reduced and the concentration at the receptors (for any given concentration in the medium) is increased. This view is supported by the observation that the degree of denervation supersensitivity is directly proportional to the rate of uptake of those amines for which information on rates of uptake is available. For the isolated nictitating membrane, degrees of denervation supersensitivity are: (—)-noradrenaline > (—)-adrenaline > (±)-isoprenaline = (±)-methoxamine = zero; rates of uptake by innervated muscles are: (±)-noradrenaline > (±)-adrenaline > (±)-isoproterenol (DRASKÓCZY and TRENDELENBURG, 1970). For rabbit aortic strips the following rates were determined: (±)-noradrenaline > (±)-isoprenaline = (±)-methoxamine (TRENDELENBURG et al., 1970).

When results from spinal cats are used for such comparisons, it should be realized that, because of the neuronal activity dependent on the functioning of the remaining spinal cord, they have high catecholamine plasma levels. After pithing (i.e., destruction of the entire spinal cord) catecholamine levels are low (LANGER et al., 1967b). As a consequence, the highly supersensitive denervated nictitating membrane of the spinal cat is in a state of partial contraction (LANGER, 1966b) which distorts dose-response curves and results in underestimates of the degree of denervation supersensitivity. Thus, quantitative values for degrees of supersensitivity observed in spinal cats should be accepted with caution, while determinations in pithed cats are reliable.

If denervation supersensitivity to noradrenaline is causally related to the loss of the neuronal uptake mechanism, a strict temporal relationship should exist between the loss of the uptake capability and the development of denervation supersensitivity. Observations with nictitating membranes of spinal cats are in agreement with this postulate. During the first 24 postoperative hours, both the ability to retain intravenously administered noradrenaline-H^3 and the sensitivity remain unchanged; during the subsequent 24 hours the ability to retain exogenous noradrenaline declines and supersensitivity develops (LANGER and TRENDELENBURG, 1966; SMITH et al., 1966). Parallel morphological studies showed that degeneration of the adrenergic nerve endings also has a lag period of about 24 hours and is very pronounced 48 hours after the operation (VAN ORDEN et al., 1967).

Since the presence of a sustained contraction of the denervated nictitating membrane of spinal cats (LANGER, 1966b) was discovered after completion of the work discussed in the preceding paragraph, experiments were repeated in pithed cats (LANGER et al., 1967b). Reliable determinations of denervation supersensitivity were obtained; they represent a very good agreement between changes in sensitivity, changes in the retention of noradrenaline-H^3 and degenerative changes in the adrenergic nerves.

The main difficulty in the interpretation of our experiments with nictitating membranes lies in the fact that retention of noradrenaline-H^3 cannot be equated with its uptake into the neurones. The results do not exclude the possibility that retention of the amine declined because of a loss of the mechanism responsible for vesicular storage rather than that responsible for membranal uptake. This uncertainty can be resolved by experiments with organs perfused with low concentrations of noradrenaline. According to LINDMAR and MUSCHOLL (1964) the removal of noradrenaline from the perfusion fluid is a measure of net neuronal uptake; it is independent of intraneuronal events (vesicular storage as well as intracellular deamination). When cat spleens were perfused with 25 ng/ml of (—)-noradrenaline at various time intervals after denervation, uptake remained essentially unchanged in experiments begun not later than 48 hours after the operation; uptake fell during the 3rd and 4th postoperative day and reached very low levels thereafter. Parallel determinations of the sensitivity of isolated splenic strips to (—)-noradrenaline revealed no change in sensitivity during the first two postoperative days, a gradual development of supersensitivity during the 3rd and 4th day, and maximum supersensitivity (which was no further increased by the addition of cocaine) at the end of the 4th day (BRIMIJOIN et al., 1970). Thus, changes in sensitivity correlate well with changes in the net movement of noradrenaline across the neuronal membrane, in full agreement with the uptake theory of denervation supersensitivity.

While the degenerating nerve endings of the nictitating membrane lose their transmitter, a "degeneration contraction" of the denervated membrane is observed in conscious cats (LANGER, 1966a). If an adrenergic neurone-blocker (β-TM10, 10 mg/kg) is injected at the beginning of this contraction, the contraction is shortened and, after 6—8 hours, it is followed by a second one. During the interval of quiescence between the two degeneration contractions, the loss of endogenous noradrenaline is interrupted. However, there is no interruption by β-TM10 of the progression of morphological degeneration of the nerve endings as well as of the development of supersensitivity to noradrenaline (PLUCHINO et al., 1970). Thus, although β-TM10 delays some of the phenomena which occur after denervation (i.e., the end of the degeneration contraction and the loss of transmitter), the strict parallelism between degeneration of nerve endings and development of supersensitivity is preserved. This is further circumstantial evidence in favor of a causal relationship between the latter phenomena.

A few quantitative considerations may be useful. If denervation results in a 20-fold increase in sensitivity to noradrenaline (isolated nictitating membrane: TRENDELENBURG et al., 1969; isolated cat's spleen: BRIMIJOIN et al., 1970), the receptors of innervated muscles should be exposed to only 1/20 of the concentration of noradrenaline achieved at the receptors of denervated muscles (for equal bath concentrations). Thus, when the uptake mechanism is unimpaired, 95% of the noradrenaline molecules diffusing to the region of the receptors must be assumed to be taken up, while only 5% contribute to the effective concentration at the receptors. Such considerations indicate that neuronal uptake must be very effective. Indeed, the question arises whether the maintenance of such a steep gradient is feasible.

HERTTING et al. (1967) perfused normal and denervated spleens with various concentrations of noradrenaline and determined both the response of the spleen and the concentration of noradrenaline in the venous effluent. The increase in sensitivity after denervation equalled the increase in venous concentration of the amine. Therefore, they concluded that the concentration in the venous effluent equals the concentration at the receptors. Although the experimental results agree with the postulate, it is questionable whether generalizations of this kind are permissible. For instance, the isolated rabbit heart removes only 40% of the perfused noradrenaline (LINDMAR and MUSCHOLL, 1964). If it is correct that the concentration of noradrenaline in the venous effluent is equal to that at the receptors, complete block of uptake should cause a maximum increase in sensitivity by a factor of 2.5. Or to reverse the argument: since denervation increases the sensitivity of the isolated nictitating membrane to noradrenaline 20-fold, the organ should be able to remove 95% of the perfused amine (if perfusion were possible). As will be discussed below (section VIII), block of COMT causes a further 5-fold increase in the sensitivity of the denervated membrane. To account for this 100-fold increase in sensitivity (denervated muscle after block of COMT *versus* normal muscle), the perfused organ would have to remove 99% of the perfused noradrenaline before, and none after the combination of denervation and block of COMT. Although such figures are of purely speculative value, they serve to emphasize that it is rather unlikely that the concentration of noradrenaline in the venous effluent always equals that at the receptors. Two possibilities have to be considered. First, because of arterio-venous shunts the concentration of noradrenaline in the venous effluent may be considerably higher than that in the venules close to the receptors; the latter may well be equal to the concentration at the receptors. Second, a considerable portion of the concentration gradient is established between the blood vessels and the effector cells rather than between arteriole and venule. The postulate of HERTTING et al. (1967) may well apply to organs in which denervation supersensitivity does not exceed the factor of 2 or 3.

The relation between uptake and sensitivity can be calculated from a very simple biophase model (BRIMIJOIN et al., 1970). For the model, the following assumptions are made: 1. uptake and sensitivity are measured under steady-state conditions; 2. the distribution of noradrenaline between bath and biophase is determined by passive diffusion and active neuronal uptake; 3. uptake in the spleen is a saturable process with a kinetic constant similar to that determined for the perfused heart (IVERSEN, 1963); 4. the kinetics of uptake by degenerating nerves change mainly by a reduction of the maximal rate of uptake; 5. equal responses of the organ correspond to equal drug concentrations in the biophase. From the observed rates of uptake (determined in normal spleens and at various times after denervation) and the maximum degree of supersensitivity (BRIMIJOIN et al., 1970), and on the basis of the assumptions listed above, an equation was derived which predicts the degree of supersensitivity for any given degree of impairment of uptake. The agreement between theoretical and observed values is very good. The reader is referred to the original paper for details. It is worth emphasizing that the close agreement between experimental observations and predictions derived from a simple model, represents strong evidence in favor of the uptake theory of denervation supersensitivity.

Starting from a slightly different model of the biophase, MAXWELL et al. (1966) compared the theoretical and the observed relationship between decrease in uptake of (±)-noradrenaline-H^3 and increase in sensitivity to the amine as determined in isolated aortic strips of rabbits. The agreement between theoretical and observed values was poor. The most likely explanation for this disagreement is found in the ability of cocaine to produce, in rabbit aortic strips, a postjunctional type of supersensitivity which is not related to block of uptake (see section IV d).

b) Chemical Denervation

Electron microscopy shows that high doses of 6-hydroxydopamine cause a selective destruction of adrenergic nerve endings. This change is accompanied by a loss of the transmitter and of the ability of the tissue to take up and retain (±)-noradrenaline-H^3 (THOENEN and TRANZER, 1968). Parallel sensitivity studies indicate that the ensuing supersensitivity of the nictitating membrane to noradrenaline is of a magnitude similar to that observed after surgical denervation (HAEUSLER et al., 1969).

A detailed study of the events following surgical and chemical denervation revealed striking similarities. 6-Hydroxydopamine elicits a contraction of the nictitating membrane of the conscious cat which is equivalent to the "degeneration contraction" observed in the conscious cat some 24 hours after surgical denervation. Just as supersensitivity to (—)-noradrenaline develops during the degeneration contraction seen after surgical denervation, it also develops in a quantitatively similar way during that seen after 6-hydroxydopamine. For instance, in both cases supersensitivity to (—)-noradrenaline is half maximal when the degeneration contractions have reached the stage of half relaxation (WAGNER and TRENDELENBURG, 1971). These observations are consistent with the view that there is a causal relationship between the degeneration of the nerve endings (after either surgical or chemical denervation) and the development of supersensitivity to (—)-noradrenaline.

c) Immunosympathectomy

Immunosympathectomy provides another experimental approach which allows one to assess the importance of the uptake mechanism for the concentration of noradrenaline at the receptors. Neuronal uptake in the rat heart is greatly impaired, and supersensitivity of this organ to noradrenaline is present in immunosympathectomized rats (BRODY, 1964; ZAIMIS, 1965). However, no attempt has been made quantitatively to compare the supersensitivity induced by immunosympathectomy with that produced by surgical denervation.

d) Cocaine

As noted by various workers (FLECKENSTEIN and BURN, 1953; FLECKENSTEIN and BASS, 1953; INNES and KOSTERLITZ, 1954; FLECKENSTEIN and STÖCKLE, 1955; TRENDELENBURG et al., 1962), cocaine-induced supersensitivity of the nictitating membrane to various amines is very similar to that produced by 2—3 days of denervation. Cocaine does not produce supersensitivity to agents to which decentralization supersensitivity develops but which are not sympathomimetic amines (acetylcholine: TRENDELENBURG, 1962; 5-hydroxytryptamine: PLUCHINO, 1972). Cocaine also fails to cause supersensitivity of the nictitating membrane to a sympathomimetic amine which is not taken up by adrenergic nerves (methoxamine: TRENDELENBURG et al., 1970). Likewise, isoprenaline is not taken up by adrenergic nerves (HERTTING, 1964; ANDÉN et al., 1964; HARDMAN et al., 1965; ROSS and RENYI, 1966; DRASKÓCZY and TRENDELENBURG, 1970) and cocaine does not potentiate its effects on a variety of organs (HEBB and KONZETT, 1949; HARDMAN et al., 1965; BHAGAT et al., 1967; MCNEILL and BRODY, 1968).

Further support for a causal relationship between impairment of neuronal uptake and cocaine-induced supersensitivity is provided by the following observations: *First*, a quantitative correlation between these two events was obtained by MUSCHOLL (1961) who determined, in the same preparation, the uptake of noradrenaline in the rat heart and the change in the pressor response to this amine.

Second, cocaine fails to affect the sensitivity of the denervated nictitating membrane if it is administered after complete degeneration of the adrenergic nerves (KUKOVETZ and LEMBECK, 1962; LANGER et al., 1967b); however, some sensitizing effect is retained when cocaine is administered before degeneration is complete (LANGER et al., 1967b). *Third*, a large variety of agents has been found to impair the neuronal uptake of noradrenaline; provided these agents do not block α-receptors, they all cause supersensitivity to noradrenaline (for review, see TRENDELENBURG, 1966a). Equally important, α-cocaine neither blocks neuronal uptake nor causes supersensitivity to noradrenaline (MUSCHOLL, 1961).

The evidence in support of the uptake theory of cocaine supersensitivity does not necessarily rule out the possibility that cocaine exerts additional, postjunctional effects. For instance, on the isolated rat vas deferens, cocaine has not only the expected prejunctional effect (which results in a shift of the dose-response curve for noradrenaline to the left) but also causes an increase in submaximal or maximal responses to a variety of agents; this effect is dependent on the calcium concentration of the medium (KASUYA and GOTO, 1968). The authors suggest that cocaine has a calcium-mobilizing effect in addition to impairing neuronal amine uptake. Responses of isolated rabbit aortic strips to methoxamine are increased by cocaine (KALSNER and NICKERSON, 1969b). Since the neuronal uptake of methoxamine is negligible (TRENDELENBURG et al., 1970), cocaine must have a postjunctional site of action. It is of interest that experiments with isolated nictitating membranes failed to reveal a potentiation of methoxamine by cocaine (TRENDELENBURG et al., 1970). Thus, the small postjunctional effects of cocaine appear to be organ and/or species dependent. The clearly negative evidence for the nictitating membrane indicates that the generalization, that postjunctional effects by cocaine are exerted on *all* organs, is unwarranted. Moreover, the relative magnitude of the pre- and postjunctional effects of cocaine should be borne in mind. While cocaine shifts the noradrenaline dose-response curve for the isolated nictitating membrane by 1.3 log units to the left (prejunctional effect; LANGER and TRENDELENBURG, 1969), the corresponding shift for rabbit aortic strips (at least partly a postjunctional effect) amounts to 0.3 units (KALSNER and NICKERSON, 1969b).

The concept of a predominantly prejunctional action of cocaine has been challenged by VARMA and MCCULLOUGH (1969) who measured cocaine-induced supersensitivity to noradrenaline in various organs before and after storage in the cold for 7 days. Depending on the organ, cold storage either did not affect or slightly reduced the sensitizing effect of cocaine. Since cold-stored organs have lost most of their endogenous noradrenaline and since their ability to retain exogenous noradrenaline is markedly reduced, cocaine-induced supersensitivity after cold storage was concluded to be due to a postjunctional effect. However, some quantitative aspects of this study are questionable. Since cocaine causes a contraction of the normal nictitating membrane before but not after cold storage, the sensitizing effect of cocaine must have been underestimated for fresh (but not for cold-stored) muscles. This has been verified in our own experiments which show that cold storage decreases the sensitizing effect of cocaine by about 50% (GRAEFE and TRENDELENBURG, 1970). VARMA and MCCULLOUGH (1969) found cocaine unable to reduce the accumulation of noradrenaline-H^3 in cold-stored aorta, spleen and vas deferens. However, since retention of the amine was measured rather than its uptake across the neuronal membrane, it is possible that an impairment of the retention of the amine in cold-stored tissues masks the inhibitory effect of cocaine on neuronal uptake. When the ability of the isolated nictitating membrane to remove noradrenaline from a small incubation medium was determined, cocaine was found to reduce removal in fresh as well as in cold-stored preparations (GRAEFE and TRENDELENBURG, 1970). The results were consistent with the view that storage of the nictitating membrane in the cold destroyed about 50% of the adrenergic neurons (as evidenced by a 50% decrease in endogenous noradrenaline and in response to tyramine) without impairing the ability of cocaine to block neuronal uptake. Since storage in the cold failed to alter the relation between cocaine-induced supersensitivity and cocaine-induced reduction in neuronal uptake, the conclusions of VARMA and MCCULLOUGH (1969) cannot be accepted as a valid argument against the uptake theory of cocaine supersensitivity.

e) Sympathomimetic Amines

The available evidence indicates that all those amines which are taken up by adrenergic nerve endings are able to reduce the uptake of noradrenaline by competition for the uptake mechanism (for review, see IVERSEN, 1967). This also applies to (+)-noradrenaline. In the isolated rabbit heart the uptake mechanism is not stereospecific. Supersensitivity to (—)-noradrenaline (i.e., a shift of the dose-response curve to the left) is obtained in the presence of 0.3—1 μg/ml of the less potent (+)-isomer. However, this effect is not seen in the presence of cocaine (DRASKÓCZY and TRENDELENBURG, 1968). A potentiation of the effects of (—)-noradrenaline by higher concentrations of the (+)-isomer has also been seen when the phosphorylase activity of the rat heart was determined (MCNEILL and BRODY, 1969). Apparently, (+)-noradrenaline can potentiate the affects of the (—)-isomer by impairing its neuronal uptake.

f) Supersensitivity Induced by Nerve Stimulation

When adrenergic neurones are stimulated electrically at a high rate, net neuronal uptake should be reduced either because depolarization of the nerve endings might prevent uptake or because re-uptake of the released transmitter is followed immediately by renewed release. This experimental model can be tested on the nictitating membrane of reserpine-pretreated cats, since depletion of the transmitter stores prevents any marked responses to the nerve stimulation. A pronounced shift of the dose-response curve for noradrenaline to the left was observed, while responses to acetylcholine remained unchanged (TRENDELENBURG, 1966b). Again, the evidence is in favor of a causal relation between decrease in net uptake and increase in the concentration of noradrenaline at the receptors.

g) Reserpine

Although pretreatment with reserpine impairs the uptake and storage of noradrenaline by the storage vesicles of adrenergic nerves, it does not impair the movement of noradrenaline across the neuronal membrane (LINDMAR and MUSCHOLL, 1964). It is entirely consistent with this observation that pretreatment with reserpine fails to cause a cocaine-like supersensitivity of the nictitating membrane to noradrenaline (FLEMING and TRENDELENBURG, 1961). This statement should not be interpreted as meaning that pretreatment with reserpine is unable to change the sensitivity of various organs to noradrenaline. Postjunctional subsensitivity can be observed after very large doses of resperine (FLEMING and TRENDELENBURG, 1961; WESTFALL and FLEMING, 1968), while the prolonged treatment of animals with reserpine can lead to the decentralization type of (postjunctional) supersensitivity (FLEMING and TRENDELENBURG, 1961; TRENDELENBURG and WEINER, 1962). However, a cocaine-like (prejunctional) supersensitivity has not been observed after treatment with reserpine. More subtle effects of pretreatment with reserpine on the neuronal uptake mechanism will be discussed below (section V).

h) Conclusions

Most of the evidence discussed in this section is compatible with the view that neuronal uptake exerts a very strong influence on the concentration of exogenous sympathomimetic amines at the receptors provided that 1. the rate of neuronal uptake of the amine is high, and 2. the morphology of the adrenergic innervation favours uptake (i.e., that there is a dense innervation with short neuro-muscular distances). The agreement between postulates derived from the uptake theory of supersensitivity is good as long as the importance of the morphology of this system as well as that of the weak postjunctional effects of cocaine is realized.

V. The Importance of Vesicular Uptake and of Monoamine Oxidase for the Net Uptake across the Neuronal Membrane

While there is agreement that the rate of neuronal uptake depends on the K_m and the concentration of the amine outside the nerve endings, a third factor must be considered: the concentration of free amine in the cytoplasm of the nerve endings. TRENDELENBURG and DRASKÓCZY (1970) proposed that the rate of neuronal net uptake is reduced by an increase in the cytoplasmic noradrenaline concentration; the latter should increase whenever the intraneuronal mechanisms of inactivation (vesicular storage and monoamine oxidase, MAO) are impaired or exhausted.

The results presented in Table 2 support the hypothesis. Isolated rabbit hearts were perfused with 200 ng/ml of (—)- or (+)-noradrenaline, and arterio-venous differences were measured after perfusions with noradrenaline for 10 and 15 min. The net removal of (—)-noradrenaline declined after pretreatment with reserpine, but that of the (+)-isomer did not. Since vesicular retention is stereospecific (STJÄRNE and EULER, 1965), the differential effect of the pretreatment is consistent with the view that (in the absence of reserpine) the cytoplasmic concentration of (—)-noradrenaline is kept low by vesicular uptake and retention, while that of the (+)-isomer is less effectively lowered. The inhibitory effect of pretreatment with reserpine is observed only when the concentration of (—)-noradrenaline is not below 200 ng/ml; the net removal of the amine from the perfusion fluid is *not* reduced by pretreatment, if the amine concentration is 40 or 60 ng/ml (LINDMAR and MUSCHOLL, 1964; GRAEFE et al., 1971).

Table 2. *Removal of the isomers of noradrenaline from a perfusion (200 ng/ml) through isolated rabbit hearts*

	(—)-noradrenaline	(+)-noradrenaline	P
controls	14.3 ± 1.54	7.9 ± 1.42	<0.01
after pretreatment with reserpine (1 mg/kg, 24 hr)	8.4 ± 1.45	9.2 ± 2.88	N.S.
after pretreatment with pargyline (100 mg/kg, 16 hr)	6.6 ± 2.50	2.6 ± 1.24	N.S.
after pretreatment with reserpine and pargyline	2.0 ± 0.78	3.1 ± 1.45	N.S.

Shown are means (± S.E.) of 100 (A—V)/A, where A = inflow concentration and V = outflow concentration. Measurements were made 10—15 min after beginning of perfusion. Each group consisted of 6—14 hearts. P refers to significance of difference between the isomers. N.S. = not significant. Taken from TRENDELENBURG and DRASKÓCZY (1970).

Pretreatment with pargyline (to block MAO) decreased the net removal of both isomers (Table 2). Apparently, deamination by MAO influences the cytoplasmic concentration of both isomers. The combined pretreatment reduced the net removal of the (—)-isomer to the very low rates observed for the (+)-isomer after pretreatment with pargyline only (Table 2). Evidently, inhibition of one or both of the intraneuronal mechanisms of inactivation decreases net uptake across the neuronal membrane, probably because of an accumulation of the free amine in the neuronal cytoplasm.

Further support for this view comes from a study of the time course of the net removal of the amine during prolonged perfusions with 60 ng/ml of (—)-noradrenaline (GRAEFE et al., 1971). In normal and in reserpine-pretreated hearts a steady-state of net removal was obtained within less than 10 min, and net removal thereafter remained constant for up to 90 min. However, inhibition of MAO by pargyline caused a progressive decline of the net removal of the amine throughout the perfusion; removal reached values close to zero after 90 min (Fig. 4). Experiments

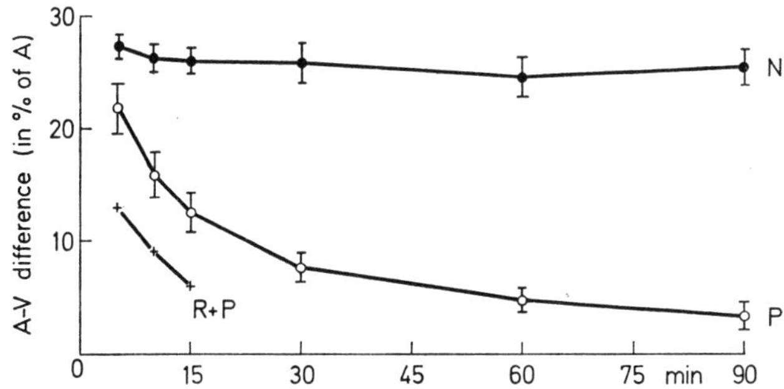

Fig. 4. Removal of noradrenaline from the fluid perfused through isolated rabbit hearts for up to 90 min. Ordinates: arterio-venous difference in per cent of the arterial concentration (60 ng/ml (—)-noradrenaline). Abscissae: time after beginning of perfusion with (—)-noradrenaline. Shown are means (± S.E. as vertical bars) of 5 experiments for N and P, and of 2 experiments for R+P. N = untreated hearts; P = 16 hr after pretreatment with 100 mg/kg pargyline s.c.; R+P = 24 hr after pretreatment with 1 mg/kg reserpine s.c. plus pretreatment with pargyline. Note steady-state conditions for normal hearts and the time-dependent decline in net removal of noradrenaline after pretreatment with pargyline or reserpine plus pargyline (GRAEFE et al., 1971)

with 20 ng/ml of l-noradrenaline showed that the rate of decline of net removal (after pretreatment with pargyline) was directly related to the concentration of the amine in the perfusion fluid; moreover, it was increased by the additional pretreatment with reserpine. Apparently, the vesicular storage capacity is exhausted with time if MAO is blocked; consequently, the cytoplasmic concentration of free noradrenaline rises with time, and net uptake decreases. Experiments with labelled noradrenaline showed that this gradual decline in removal (after pretreatment with pargyline) is due to a gradual increase in efflux of the amine rather than to a decrease in gross influx. It is justified to regard the adrenergic neuron as the site responsible for the changes in net removal discussed here, since cocaine virtually abolished the net removal of noradrenaline by pargyline-pretreated hearts (GRAEFE et al., 1971).

LÖFFELHOLZ et al. (1971 and personal communication) determined the washout of noradrenaline from isolated rabbit hearts after termination of a perfusion with 200 ng/ml of (—)-noradrenaline. With or without pretreatment with reserpine noradrenaline leaves the heart with a short half time. However, after block of

MAO, some of the noradrenaline leaves the heart very slowly (half time about 40 min). It is very likely that the neuronal cytoplasm represents the compartment responsible for this slow washout.

If these findings are applicable to other adrenergically innervated organs, supersensitivity to noradrenaline should be observed after block of MAO (and especially after additional pretreatment with reserpine). Organs with large neuromuscular distances (FURCHGOTT et al., 1955) may show this effect poorly, since neuronal uptake is of little importance for the concentration of the amine at the receptors (see above). For other organs (e.g. nictitating membrane) some authors reported potentiation of the effects of noradrenaline (VARAGIĆ, 1958; FREY, 1963), while others obtained negative results (BALZER and HOLTZ, 1956; SCHMITT and GONNARD, 1956). However, all these studies were carried out *in vivo*, while the results mentioned above were obtained with prolonged exposures of the tissue to a constant concentration of noradrenaline. Thus, more relevant are the observations of TSAI (1968) who found that the isolated nictitating membrane takes much longer to reach the maximum of a response after block of MAO than without this intervention; furthermore, after pretreatment with pargyline the sensitivity of the isolated muscle to noradrenaline increased, while that to α-methyl-noradrenaline (which is not a substrate of MAO) did not. The same phenomenon was observed by FURCHGOTT and SANCHEZ-GARCIA (1968) in experiments with isolated guinea-pig atria: normal and MAO-inhibited atria responded to noradrenaline with a quickly developing increase in force of contraction which was of the same magnitude for both types of preparations; while a steady response was observed thereafter for normal atria, the response of MAO-inhibited atria continued to increase slowly for a considerable period. The authors coined the term "secondary sensitization". Similar observations were made by GRAEFE et al. (1971) on isolated rabbit atria exposed to concentrations of noradrenaline similar to those used for the perfusion experiments discussed above, and by DE LA LANDE and JELLETT (1971) on the isolated ear artery of the rabbit. It is of interest that a slowly increasing response to noradrenaline (after block of MAO) was observed only for the extraluminal administration of the amine (i.e., when the amine was applied close to the nerve endings which are located at the medio-adventitial border) and not on intraluminal administration.

The phenomenon of a slowly increasing response has been demonstrated for the isolated nictitating membrane for noradrenaline, adrenaline and phenylephrine (which are substrates of MAO) but not for ($\pm$)-methoxamine (which is not a substrate) (TRENDELENBURG, 1971). Responses to noradrenaline were found to require more than 70 min to reach a steady state after treatment with pargyline. The degrees of supersensitivity induced by the various pretreatments had the same ranking order as that of the results presented in Table 2: normal $<$ reserpine $<$ pargyline $<$ reserpine+pargyline $=$ denervation. It is of interest that the combined pretreatment with reserpine and pargyline produced a degree of supersensitivity which was comparable with that seen after denervation. However, denervated muscles and those pretreated with both reserpine and pargyline differed in one important aspect: while the full response of the denervated muscle is quick, that of the pretreated innervated muscle is very slow (Fig. 5). Extraneuronal MAO does not seem to be involved in the phenomena discussed here, since pretreatment with pargyline failed to affect the sensitivity of denervated muscles (TRENDELENBURG, 1971).

These observations demonstrate that the effect of block of MAO on the sensitivity to noradrenaline can be observed only when responses are recorded for long periods. It is very likely that earlier reports of a failure of block of MAO to affect the sensitivity of isolated atria to noradrenaline (BURFORD et al., 1960) are due to an insufficient length of period for which responses were recorded.

There is an interesting counterpart to the phenomenon discussed here: while normal or reserpine-pretreated muscles relax quickly and completely soon after the removal of noradrenaline from the bath, pargyline-pretreated muscles show two phases of relaxation: after the initial quick relaxation there is a very slow rate of

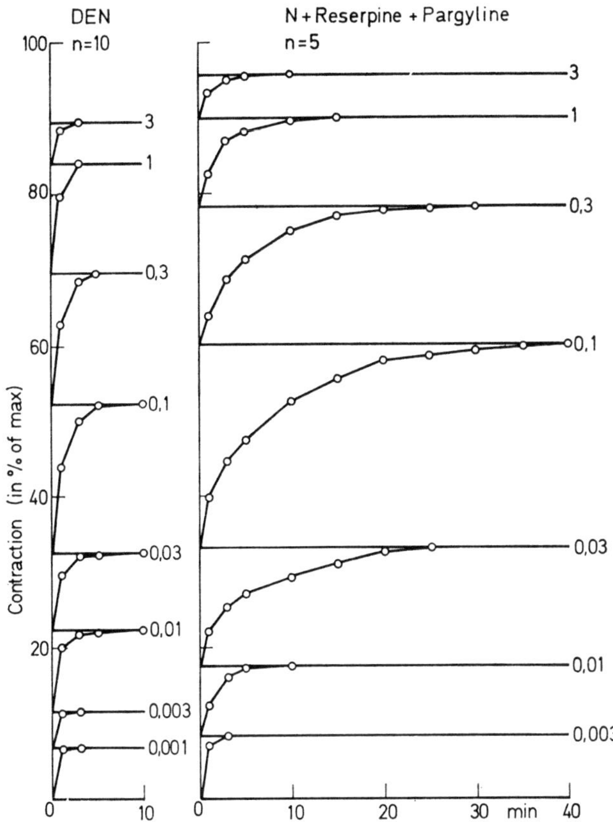

Fig. 5. Time course of contraction of isolated nictitating membrane in response to (—)-phenylephrine. Ordinates: contraction in percent of maximal response. Abscissae: minutes after administration of (—)-phenylephrine. Shown are mean responses determined 1, 3, 5, 10, 15, 20, 25, 30, 35 and 40 min after the administration of the drug. Results are taken from cumulative dose-response curves; the final concentration in the bath was increased as soon as a steady response was observed. Horizontal lines indicate level of steady-state response to the indicated concentrations (in μg/ml). Left: responses of 10 denervated muscles (no pretreatment); right: responses of 5 innervated muscles obtained from reserpine-pretreated cats and incubated with 100 μg/ml of pargyline for 30 min (followed by wash out). Note difference in time required to reach steady state responses

relaxation (isolated nictitating membrane: TRENDELENBURG, 1971; isolated ear artery after extraluminal administration of noradrenaline: DE LA LANDE and JELLETT, 1971). Obviously, this phenomenon is the consequence of the slow washout of noradrenaline mentioned above.

If cytoplasmic noradrenaline leaves the neuron in order to reach the receptors (when MAO is blocked), the very slow relaxation observed after block of MAO (e.g., KALSNER and NICKERSON, 1969a, after immersion in oil) may well be partly due to this redistribution of the amine within the compartments of the tissue rather than solely to the slowing of the inactivation of the amine (as postulated by KALSNER and NICKERSON, 1969a). Experiments with measurements of the rate of relaxation may well have to be re-interpreted.

Conclusions

The evidence is compatible with the hypothesis formulated at the beginning of this section. It is very likely that any impairment or exhaustion of the intraneuronal mechanisms of inactivation leads to an increase in the cytoplasmic concentration of free noradrenaline which, in turn, reduces the net uptake across the neuronal membrane. As a consequence, block of MAO leads to slowly developing changes in sensitivity. Moreover, when MAO is inhibited, cytoplasmic noradrenaline can leave the neuron and interact with the receptors. If this occurs, the nerve endings cease to be a permanent site of loss.

VI. Saturation of Neuronal Uptake

The neuronal uptake mechanism for (—)-noradrenaline is known to obey Michaelis-Menten kinetics; it is saturable and, in the rat heart, has a K_m of about 2×10^{-7}M (IVERSEN, 1963). In the absence of saturation, the rate of neuronal uptake is linearly related to the concentration of the amine in the medium; hence, the magnitude of the postulated concentration gradient (from the medium to the receptors) should be independent of the bath concentration. However, saturation should decrease the concentration gradient, since it is equivalent to a decline in the ability of the nerve endings to remove noradrenaline from the region of the receptors.

a) Slopes of Dose-Response Curves

When (with low concentrations of noradrenaline) there is a linear relation between the bath concentration and the rate of neuronal uptake, a given increase in the bath concentration should cause an identical increase in the concentration at the receptors. However, when the concentration of noradrenaline is increased so much that partial saturation of the uptake mechanism ensues, the increase in the concentration at the receptors should be disproportionately greater than the increase in the bath concentration. Once the uptake mechanism is fully saturated, there should again be a strict proportionality between bath concentration and that at the receptors. A more detailed description of the model is given by LANGER and TRENDELENBURG (1969) and a mathematical analysis by WAUD (1969).

In agreement with these considerations, dose-response curves for (—)-noradrenaline (determined on isolated normal nictitating membranes) were found to have increased slopes when determined in the presence of low concentrations of phentolamine (which shift the dose-response curves into the region of partial saturation of uptake) and to revert to the original slope in the presence of high concentrations of this competitive blocker of α-receptors. Presumably, pharmacologically effective concentrations of noradrenaline then cause nearly complete saturation of uptake. These changes in slopes of dose-response curves are observed only when the neuronal uptake mechanism is intact; they are not observed after cocaine or after denervation (Fig. 6) (LANGER and TRENDELENBURG, 1969). Moreover, the phenomenon is not observed with agents which are not taken up into adrenergic nerve endings: increasing concentrations of phentolamine cause parallel shifts of dose-response curves for methoxamine (with no changes in slopes) (TRENDELENBURG et al., 1970), and the same was observed with acetylcholine in the presence of increasing concentrations of atropine (LANGER and TRENDELENBURG, 1969). Apparently, the changes in slopes of dose-response curves are observed only when 1. the agonist can be taken up by nerve endings, and 2. the uptake mechanism is intact.

Supporting evidence indicates that this phenomenon can be observed under a variety of conditions and in various (but not all)tissues. LANGER and TRENDELENBURG (1969) observed changes in slopes of dose-response curves under the influence of phentolamine on innervated nictitating membranes of spinal or pithed cats (i.e., *in vivo*) for a large number of sympathomimetic amines. HAEUSLER et al. (1969) found chemical denervation (after 6-hydroxydopamine) to be as effective as surgical denervation in reducing the slope of dose-response curves for (—)-noradrenaline. BICKERTON (1963) showed dose-response curves for noradrenaline determined on isolated strips of the cat's spleen; from the illustrations it is

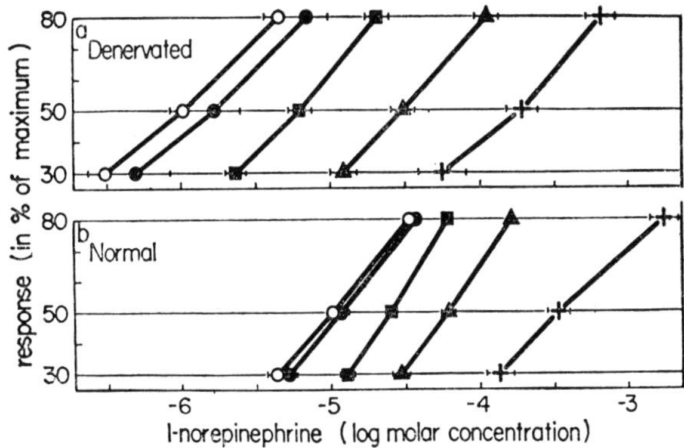

Fig. 6. The effect of phentolamine on dose-response curves for (—)-noradrenaline obtained on denervated (a) and normal (b) isolated nictitating membranes; Krebs' solution, 37 °C. Ordinates: magnitude of response (in percent of maximum). Abscissae: log molar concentration of (—)-noradrenaline. Shown are means (with S.E. as bars) of ED30, ED50 and ED80. Open circles, control; solid circles, 0.01; solid squares, 0.1; solid triangles, 1; and +, 10 μg/ml of phentolamine added 15 min earlier. Note striking dissimilarities in sensitivity and in slopes of dose-response curves between normal and denervated membranes. Taken from LANGER and TRENDELENBURG (1969) with permission of the publishers

evident that an α-receptor antagonist, tolazoline, caused an increase in the slope of the curves. On the isolated guinea-pig trachea, an antagonism by propranolol of the β-receptor stimulating effects of noradrenaline and adrenaline caused an increase in the slopes of dose-response curves; the increase was not observed in the presence of cocaine (CHAHL and O'DONNELL, 1967); similar observations with isolated atria were reported by BLINKS (1967). On kitten papillary muscle as well as on isolated guinea-pig atria, shifts by pronethalol of dose-response curves for (—)-noradrenaline were accompanied by increases in their slopes (Figs. 3B and 4 of KOCH-WESER, 1964). On the other hand, the phenomenon was not observed on isolated rabbit aortic strips where phentolamine leads to a parallel shift of dose-response curves for noradrenaline (URQUILLA et al., 1970). This is to be expected for a tissue which has a very large neuro-muscular distance (see section III).

b) The Apparent Potency of Competitive Antagonists

Under the conditions enumerated, there are not only changes in the slopes of dose-response curves but the magnitude of the shifts of dose-response curves is smaller for normal than for denervated muscles (LANGER and TRENDELENBURG, 1969). Again, this phenomenon is not seen when the agonist is not taken up (acetylcholine: LANGER and TRENDELENBURG, 1969; methoxamine: TRENDELENBURG et al., 1970). The pattern of a competitive antagonism between noradrenaline and phentolamine is observed only for denervated muscles (or muscles exposed to cocaine); for innervated muscles the pattern is seemingly inconsistent with a competitive interaction. This curious paradox is explained by the model mentioned in section VIa: since saturation of neuronal uptake leads to a disproportionality between increases in the bath concentration and in the concentration of noradrenaline at the receptors, and since the proportionality is maintained for phentolamine, the pattern typical for a competitive antagonist cannot be observed.

On the isolated guinea-pig trachea, CHAHL and O'DONNELL (1967) likewise observed that propranolol causes a smaller shift of the dose-response curve for noradrenaline in the absence than in the presence of cocaine (1.68 versus 2.45 log units); interestingly enough, this was not observed for isoprenaline (2.34 versus 2.16 log units), an amine which is not taken up by adrenergic nerves. Similar observations were reported by FURCHGOTT (1967) and BLINKS (1967), who emphasized the need for exclusion of the uptake mechanism in experiments designed to determine the antagonistic potency of α-receptor or β-receptor antagonists.

c) Stereospecificity of Cocaine Supersensitivity

Cocaine-induced supersensitivity to levorotatory isomers of sympathomimetic amines is greater than that to the corresponding dextrorotatory isomers (TRENDELENBURG, 1965; SEIDEHAMEL et al., 1966). This is also true for the effects of the isomers of noradrenaline on rabbit hearts, although there is no stereospecificity of the neuronal uptake mechanism (DRASKÓCZY and TRENDELENBURG, 1968). This apparent paradox is resolved by the fact that pharmacologically effective concentrations of the highly potent (—)-isomer are too low to saturate the uptake mechanism; hence, block of uptake by cocaine is very effective. The potency of the (+)-isomer, on the other hand, is so low that saturation of uptake occurs with pharmacologically effective concentrations; therefore, block by cocaine of the already ineffective uptake mechanism fails to cause any appreciable change in the concentration of the (+)-isomer at the receptors.

This explanation is also valid for the nictitating membrane of the cat: the sensitizing effect of cocaine is stereospecific (TRENDELENBURG, 1965; SEIDEHAMEL et al., 1966), while the neuronal amine uptake is not (GRAEFE and TRENDELENBURG, 1970). However, it remains possible that stereospecificity of the sensitizing action of cocaine can occur in other organs because of a different mechanism of action. If neuronal uptake is stereospecific, cocaine should fail to potentiate the effects of (+)-isomers because of their low rate of uptake. While neuronal uptake in rabbit hearts lacks stereospecificity (DRASKÓCZY and TRENDELENBURG, 1968), that of rat hearts is stereoselective (IVERSEN, 1963). This difference cannot be attributed to differences in methods, since JARROTT and IVERSEN (personal communication) repeated their experiments (in rats and guinea-pigs) with the method used by DRASKÓCZY and TRENDELENBURG (1968) (perfusion with 20 ng/ml of noradrenaline and determination of arterio-venous differences). They confirmed that the uptake of rat hearts is stereospecific, while that of guinea-pig hearts lacks stereospecificity.

d) The Magnitude of Decentralization Supersensitivity

Decentralization was found to cause a nonspecific (postjunctional) supersensitivity whose magnitude was very similar for a large variety of sympathomimetic amines (TRENDELENBURG et al., 1962; TRENDELENBURG, 1963). However, careful quantitative comparisons revealed a certain degree of stereospecificity (SEIDEHAMEL et al., 1966; LANGER et al., 1967b). Since this type of supersensitivity is due to postjunctional changes, equieffective concentrations at the receptors are lower after decentralization than normally. Hence, if the normal ED50 causes partial saturation of uptake, the degree of saturation is reduced after decentralization. The (+)-isomers of noradrenaline and adrenaline have a low potency, and the decrease in saturation of uptake permits a more effective removal of the isomer from the vicinity of the receptors; or in other words, part of the increase in sensitivity (induced by decentralization) is counteracted by the increased effectiveness of the uptake mechanism. For the more potent (—)-isomers, on the other hand, the counteracting influence should be less pronounced, since their ED50s cause very little saturation of the uptake mechanism of normal preparations. Hence, stereospecificity of decentralization supersensitivity seems to have its origin in the saturability of the neuronal uptake mechanism (LANGER and TRENDELENBURG, 1969).

e) Conclusions

The discussion serves to illustrate that saturation of neuronal uptake can adequately account for a variety of phenomena which otherwise do not fit the uptake theory (i.e., changes in slopes of dose-response curves; apparent deviations from the pattern expected for competitive antagonists of adrenoceptors; stereospecificity of some effects of cocaine; stereospecificity of decentralization supersensitivity). In order to assess the importance of neuronal uptake for the concentration of a sympathomimetic amine at the receptors of effector organs, the following points should be considered:

1. The functional state of the uptake mechanism (i.e., whether there is a cytoplasmic accumulation of the amine as discussed in section V),
2. the rate of neuronal uptake of the amine under study,
3. the relation between the K_m and the concentration used experimentally (i.e., the degree, if any, of the saturation of uptake), and
4. the morphology of the adrenergic innervation (i.e., its density, the neuromuscular distance and the homogeneity or asymmetry of the innervation).

These factors may well account for most species and organ differences. For instance, it is likely that the discussed changes in the concentration gradient from the medium to the receptors are of minor importance for organs with a high sensitivity to noradrenaline, since pharmacologically effective concentrations neither saturate the neuronal uptake nor exhaust the intraneuronal mechanisms of inactivation. However, for organs with a very low sensitivity to noradrenaline, the influence of these two mechanisms may well be pronounced, since pharmacologically effective concentrations are likely to saturate neuronal uptake and/or exhaust the intraneuronal mechanisms of inactivation. The same argument applies to studies of amines of differing potencies.

VII. The Role of Extraneuronal Uptake

In recent years convincing evidence for extraneuronal uptake of noradrenaline and other amines has been obtained (rat heart: IVERSEN, 1965; EISENFELD et al., 1967a, 1967b; SIMMONDS and GILLIS, 1968; LIGHTMAN and IVERSEN, 1969; CLARKE et al., 1969; vascular smooth muscle: GILLESPIE and HAMILTON, 1967; AVAKIAN and GILLESPIE, 1968; salivary glands: HAMBERGER et al., 1967; guinea-pig trachea: FOSTER, 1968, 1969; nictitating membrane: DRASKÓCZY and TRENDELENBURG, 1970). While extraneuronal uptake of amines may influence the concentration of these amines at the receptors under certain experimental conditions, the physiological and pharmacological importance of this uptake mechanism is not yet fully understood.

The first description of what eventually turned out to be extraneuronal uptake was made by IVERSEN (1965) who termed it uptake$_2$. He believed it to be a second type of intraneuronal uptake. This view has been revised recently (LIGHTMAN and IVERSEN, 1969). IVERSEN (1965) characterized uptake$_2$ as occurring only at high concentrations of noradrenaline or adrenaline; the recent study of LIGHTMAN and IVERSEN (1969) showed that the earlier conclusion was due to the fact that extraneuronal accumulation is inversely related to enzymic metabolism; extraneuronal uptake (or uptake$_2$) can be demonstrated with low bath concentrations of noradrenaline if the metabolizing enzymes (MAO and COMT) are blocked.

Extraneuronal accumulation differs from the intraneuronal one in the following respects. While cocaine blocks neuronal uptake, it does not affect extraneuronal accumulation (IVERSEN, 1965; EISENFELD et al., 1967a; SIMMONDS and GILLIS, 1968; DRASKÓCZY and TRENDELENBURG, 1970). Pretreatment with reserpine prevents intraneuronal storage but does not influence extraneuronal accumulation of noradrenaline (GILLESPIE et al., 1970; DRASKÓCZY and TRENDELENBURG, 1970). While metanephrine and normetanephrine have no effect on neuronal uptake, they are inhibitors of extraneuronal accumulation (IVERSEN, 1965; FOSTER, 1968; GILLESPIE et al., 1970; DRASKÓCZY and TRENDELENBURG, 1970). Phenoxybenzamine blocks both neuronal and extraneuronal accumulation (EISENFELD et al., 1967a; FOSTER, 1968; LIGHTMAN and IVERSEN, 1969; GILLESPIE et al., 1970; DRASKÓCZY and TRENDELENBURG, 1970). Block of MAO causes a small, block of COMT a pronounced, increase in extraneuronal accumulation; the latter procedure has no effect on neuronal uptake (DRASKÓCZY and TRENDELENBURG, 1970).

Structural requirements for the two mechanisms of accumulation differ: relative rates for neuronal accumulation are noradrenaline > adrenaline > isoprenaline; for extraneuronal accumulation they are reversed (DRASKÓCZY and TRENDELENBURG, 1970).

Extraneuronal uptake is not uniform for all tissues. GILLESPIE et al. (1970) exposed the cat spleen to noradrenaline (either by perfusion with the amine or by *in vitro* incubation of slices) and then assessed the catecholamine fluorescence (Falck method). Fluorescence appeared in arterial smooth muscle and endothelial cells after an exposure to 10 μg/ml of noradrenaline, in collagen and in reticular cells after 100 μg/ml. No fluorescence was observed in the red pulp, in lymphoid tissue and in phagocytic cells of ellipsoids; the perimeter, but not the interior, of the smooth muscle cells of the capsule-trabecula-vein system became fluorescent. In addition to these differences in the localization of extraneuronally retained noradrenaline, it was found that phenoxybenzamine, normetanephrine and cooling to 15°C prevented the appearance of fluorescence in arterial smooth muscle but not in collagen. Moreover, GILLESPIE and MUIR (1970) observed very pronounced species and organ differences for the extraneuronal accumulation of noradrenaline. All these results indicate that extraneuronal uptake may consist of a variety of mechanisms whose localization, sensitivity to drugs etc. is subject to great organ and species variability. Hence, it is very difficult to assess the importance of extraneuronal uptake for the physiology or pharmacology of organs.

In certain preparations (rabbit duodenum (STAFFORD, 1963); guinea-pig trachea (FOSTER, 1967)) phenoxybenzamine has been found to potentiate the effects of isoprenaline. Since there is no neuronal uptake of this amine, it is tempting to ascribe the phenoxybenzamine-induced supersensitivity towards isoprenaline to a block of extraneuronal uptake. However, a further effect of phenoxybenzamine may be responsible, namely its ability to prevent the O-methylation of catecholamines without inhibiting the enzyme (EISENFELD et al., 1967a; LANGER, 1968; IVERSEN and LANGER, 1969; LANGER, 1970). Since O-methylation is the most important pathway of metabolism of isoprenaline, it cannot yet be decided whether the potentiating effect of phenoxybenzamine is due to block of extraneuronal uptake or to prevention of O-methylation. This combination of two effects of phenoxybenzamine is very interesting, since it suggests a very close relationship between COMT and the extraneuronal binding sites.

There are at least three different models that might account for the close relation between COMT and extraneuronal accumulation. EISENFELD et al. (1967a) suggested that extraneuronal binding sites and COMT are located in one compartment, access to which is gained by a phenoxybenzamine-sensitive mechanism. This model accounts for the ability of phenoxybenzamine to prevent not only extraneuronal accumulation but also O-methylation of noradrenaline. Second, COMT generates a concentration gradient for noradrenaline in denervated muscles (see section VIII); block of the enzyme may well increase the concentration of noradrenaline at the sites of extraneuronal uptake and thus increase extraneuronal accumulation. While this model accounts for the increase in extraneuronal accumulation by block of COMT, it cannot account for the ability of phenoxybenzamine to prevent O-methylation of noradrenaline. A third interpretation for the increase in extraneuronal accumulation after block of COMT has to be considered: since normetanephrine and metanephrine are selective inhibitors of extraneuronal accumulation, a competition between catecholamines and their O-methylated metabolites for extraneuronal accumulation is possible, especially since SIMMONDS and GILLIS (1968) found a rapid extraneuronal accumulation of normetanephrine. Through abolition of this competition, block of COMT would thus increase the extraneuronal accumulation of catecholamines. Further studies are required to elucidate the mechanism of these interactions.

Inhibition of extraneuronal uptake of noradrenaline in the isolated rat heart was observed by IVERSEN and SALT (1970) for various corticosteroids. KAUMANN (1971) then showed that hydrocortisone is able to influence the sensitivity of the isolated cat papillary muscle to isoprenaline and noradrenaline. For isoprenaline (which is not taken up by adrenergic nerves) this effect is seen without cocaine, but for noradrenaline it is seen only when neuronal uptake is blocked. These results are qualitatively and quantitatively similar to those obtained in the same preparation with block of COMT (see section VIII).

Another aspect of extraneuronal uptake was revealed by the experiments of AVAKIAN and GILLESPIE (1968). After an exposure of vascular smooth muscle to high concentrations of noradrenaline, a pronounced catecholamine fluorescence of the muscle fibers was observed; pronounced extraneuronal accumulation had occurred. After termination of the exposure to noradrenaline, the catecholamine fluorescence declined very slowly and the vascular smooth muscle remained contracted for a prolonged period of time. As already observed by IVERSEN (1965), extraneuronal accumulation is a transient phenomenon. The results of AVAKIAN and GILLESPIE (1968) as well as our own findings with isolated nictitating membranes (DRASKÓCZY and TRENDELENBURG, 1970) indicate that at least some of the noradrenaline which, after termination of the exposure to noradrenaline, is gradually lost from extraneuronal binding sites, may reach the receptors of the effector organ. Hence, under these conditions, a shift of the amine from one compartment (extraneuronal retention) to another (vicinity of the receptors) is highly likely, since relaxation of the muscles is then greatly slowed.

This likely shift of noradrenaline is of interest in connection with the results reported by KALSNER and NICKERSON (1968, 1969a). After a steady response of rabbit aortic strips to noradrenaline had been observed, the muscles were immersed in mineral oil; the subsequent slow relaxation of the muscle was taken as a measure of the inactivation (by enzyme action and by neuronal uptake) of noradrenaline, since diffusion out of the tissue was prevented by the surrounding oil. The rate of relaxation was greatly decreased by block of COMT and/or MAO, while block of neuronal uptake by cocaine had little effect. Therefore, the authors concluded that neuronal uptake is not important for the removal of noradrenaline from the biophase, while COMT and MAO are.

An alternative explanation is offered by the results mentioned above. Since block of COMT and/or MAO greatly increases the extraneuronal accumulation of noradrenaline (LIGHTMAN and IVERSEN, 1969; DRASKÓCZY and TRENDELENBURG, 1970), the proposed shift of noradrenaline from sites of extraneuronal retention to the receptors should involve much greater amounts of the amine than when the enzymes are intact. According to this view, there may not exist the causal relation between rate of inactivation and rate of relaxation postulated by KALSNER and NICKERSON (1968, 1969a). It is equally possible that rate of relaxation is strongly influenced by the postulated shift of noradrenaline from the sites of extraneuronal retention to the receptors. Or in other words, rate of relaxation may be slow because of a long-lasting refilling of the biophase from the sites of extraneuronal retention. These considerations are of importance, since KALSNER and NICKERSON (1968, 1969a, 1969b) deny the importance of neuronal uptake for the maintenance of the concentration at the receptors. The proposed alternative explanation for the observed results shows that the assumptions made by KALSNER and NICKERSON require confirmation.

VIII. The Role of Catechol O-methyl Transferase

Determination of the activity of COMT in homogenized tissue does not necessarily provide a measure of the functional importance of this enzyme in the intact organ. For instance, LANGER (1970) obtained pronounced O-methylation of exogenous ($\pm$)-noradrenaline-H^3 in the isolated nictitating membrane, while hardly any O-methylation occurred in the isolated vas deferens of the rat under identical conditions. However, determinations of enzyme activity in homogenized tissues gave similar values for both organs (IVERSEN et al., 1968). Thus, the biological importance of the enzyme must be determined in intact systems.

Earlier studies did not provide support for the view that COMT exerts an appreciable influence on the concentration of noradrenaline at the receptors. Block of COMT failed to produce an unequivocal increase in the sensitivity of various organs to noradrenaline (blood pressure and heart: LEMBECK and RESCH, 1960; WYLIE et al., 1960; CROUT, 1961; KRONEBERG et al., 1961; IZQUIERDO and KAUMANN, 1963; nictitating membrane *in vivo*: LEMBECK and RESCH, 1960; isolated guinea-pig trachea: FOSTER, 1967; isolated atria: GILES and MILLER, 1967). The effects of isoprenaline, on the other hand, seemed to be potentiated by block of COMT (KONZETT, 1962; IZQUIERDO and KAUMANN, 1963; FOSTER, 1967; GILES and MILLER, 1967; KAUMANN, 1970). According to GILES and MILLER (1967), block of COMT causes a small degree of supersensitivity to adrenaline. A survey of the literature thus indicates that the likelihood of a potentiating effect of block of COMT is inversely proportional to the rate of neuronal uptake of sympathomimetic amines. Or in other words, COMT influences the concentration of sympathomimetic amines at the receptors only if neuronal uptake is of little importance.

Kaumann (1970) recently demonstrated on isolated cat papillary muscles that neuronal uptake determines whether or not block of COMT causes supersensitivity to catecholamines. While the effects of isoprenaline (which is not taken up by adrenergic nerves) are potentiated by block of COMT irrespective of the absence or presence of cocaine, those of noradrenaline and adrenaline are enhanced by block of COMT only in the presence of cocaine. However, block of COMT becomes ineffective again if the cocaine-induced increase in sensitivity is reversed by the additional presence of propranolol. Thus, the sensitivity of the tissue rather than the neuronal uptake mechanism seems to be of importance for the sensitizing effect of block of COMT.

Experiments with isolated nictitating membranes (Trendelenburg et al., 1971) support this view. Briefly, the following observations were made: 1. while block of COMT causes a pronounced supersensitivity to the beta-effects of isoprenaline (for which the sensitivity of the preparation is high), it fails to affect the alpha-effects of this amine (for which the sensitivity is very low); 2. block of COMT does not increase the sensitivity of normal muscles to noradrenaline or adrenaline, but that of the already supersensitive denervated muscle is increased 5-fold (noradrenaline) or 10-fold (adrenaline); 3. block of COMT causes supersensitivity to noradrenaline when neuronal uptake is blocked by cocaine; 4. if the high sensitivity of the denervated muscle to noradrenaline is reduced by phentolamine to that of the normal muscle, block of COMT fails to induce supersensitivity (this effect cannot be attributed to a prevention by phentolamine of the O-methylation of noradrenaline (Eisenfeld et al., 1967b), since Langer (1970) found no change in the O-methylation of this amine in isolated nictitating membranes exposed to 100 μg/ml of phentolamine); 5. block of COMT does not potentiate the effects of dopamine on either normal or denervated muscles (which have a low sensitivity to this amine).

These results reveal a striking relationship between the potency of the catecholamine and the degree of supersensitivity induced by block of COMT: if the ED50 is below 10^{-6}M, block of COMT results in supersensitivity; if it is higher, block of COMT has no effect (Trendelenburg et al., 1971).

It has not been possible to pinpoint the mechanism responsible for this relationship. Saturation of either COMT or extraneuronal uptake (a mechanism that seems to be in series with the enzyme, see Section VII) is very unlikely, since their Km values are considerably higher than 10^{-6}M. Moreover, the relation between the bath concentration of noradrenaline-H^3 and the total production of O-methylated metabolites-H^3 by denervated nictitating membranes was linear over the range from 10^{-7} to 10^{-4}M noradrenaline-H^3 (Trendelenburg et al., 1971). Finally, the block of COMT by the inhibitor used in these experiments (U-0521, 3′,4′-dihydroxy-2-methyl propiophenone) was as pronounced at 10^{-7} as at 10^{-5}M noradrenaline-H^3. These results do not provide an explanation for the observed relationship between potency of catecholamines and degree of supersensitivity induced by U-0521. One may speculate that the presence of two O-methylating enzymes could explain the experimental observations. If the main bulk of the O-methylated metabolites is produced by a COMT of high activity which cannot influence the concentration of catecholamines at the receptors, a second, more easily saturable COMT of low activity may be located in close proximity of the biophase. It is of interest that Jarrott (1971) has described a pre- and a postsynaptic COMT with different affinities to substrates. Though a presynaptic COMT cannot be present in denervated muscles, it is possible that postsynaptic COMT is not homogenous. Further studies must resolve this problem.

Experiments with cat and rat splenic strips also showed that block of COMT caused supersensitivity to noradrenaline and adrenaline only when uptake was blocked by cocaine (TRENDELENBURG et al., 1971). On rabbit aortic strips, on the other hand, block of COMT has this effect without any impairment of neuronal uptake (LEVIN and FURCHGOTT, 1970).

Conclusions. Under favourable conditions (i.e., when the sensitivity of the tissue to catecholamines is very high), block of COMT is able to cause substantial increases in the sensitivity to catecholamines. Apparently, COMT is then able to generate a concentration gradient from the medium to the receptors. However, this does not seem to occur when catecholamines have to be administered in high concentrations (i.e., when the sensitivity of the tissue is low); the reason for this phenomenon remains obscure.

IX. The Role of Monoamine Oxidase

As a mitochondrial enzyme, MAO is located not only in adrenergic neurones but also in the other cells of effector organs. For instance, in the rat submaxillary gland only one quarter to one third of the total MAO activity resides in adrenergic nerve endings, about 60% in the secretory cells (ALMGREN et al., 1966), whereas about half of the MAO activity of the nictitating membrane is intraneuronal and half is extraneuronal (JARROTT and LANGER, 1971).

The importance of intraneuronal MAO for neuronal net uptake has been discussed above (section V). Block of the intraneuronal MAO reduces net uptake by adrenergic nerves whenever the vesicular stores are filled to capacity.

Intraneuronal MAO also plays an important role in determining responses to indirectly acting sympathomimetic amines. The potentiation by block of MAO of responses to those amines which are substrates of the enzyme, is well established (SCHMITT and GONNARD, 1955; FURCHGOTT et al., 1955; BALZER and HOLTZ, 1956; VARAGIC, 1958; FREY, 1963) and is mainly due to the preservation of the indirectly acting amine within the nerve endings. In addition, block of MAO seems to prevent the deamination of the endogenous noradrenaline displaced from the storage sites by indirectly acting amines. This proposal is based on the observation that block of MAO increases responses to those indirectly acting amines which are not substrates of the enzyme (e.g., (+)-amphetamine and mephentermine) (SMITH 1966; ANTONACCIO and SMITH, 1969; PLUCHINO, 1972).

While there is good evidence to implicate intraneuronal MAO as a factor influencing the concentration of noradrenaline at the receptors, there is no convincing evidence that extraneuronal MAO plays such a role. For instance, block of MAO fails to increase the sensitivity of the isolated denervated nictitating membrane to either noradrenaline or phenylephrine (TRENDELENBURG, 1971). In vascular smooth muscle (which has a large neuromuscular distance, see section III) block of MAO also has very little (if any) effect on the sensitivity to noradrenaline (GRIESEMER et al., 1953; FURCHGOTT et al., 1955; KALSNER and NICKERSON, 1968, 1969a). Again, this agrees with the view that if extraneuronal MAO plays any role, it seems to be of minor importance.

X. The Concentration of Transmitter at the Receptors after its Release from Adrenergic Nerves

Nearly all the evidence discussed in preceding sections was related to exogenous noradrenaline. Thus, it remains to discuss the factors influencing the concentration of the transmitter at the receptors of effector organs after its release from nerve terminals. The interpretation of the evidence is complicated by the fact that the release of the transmitter involves additional possible sites of action for the various drugs which are in use as experimental tools. For instance, cocaine not only blocks neuronal uptake; as a potent local anaesthetic it may be able to reduce the release of the transmitter by nerve stimulation (HUKOVIĆ and MUSCHOLL, 1962). Field stimulation of isolated nictitating membranes which had been incubated with (±)-noradrenaline-H^3 (to label the stores) releases noradrenaline-H^3 as well as labeled metabolites. In the presence of 0.3 μg/ml of cocaine, the output of total radioactivity is more than doubled; however, in the presence of 3 μg/ml of cocaine, output is hardly greater than normal (LANGER, 1970). Apparently, the local anaesthetic action of high concentrations of cocaine masks the increase in output which is achieved by the impairment of neuronal uptake.

Even more complicated is the situation after the administration of phenoxybenzamine. This agent is known to increase the overflow of released transmitter into the venous effluent of perfused organs (spleen: BROWN and GILLESPIE, 1957) or into the medium surrounding an isolated nictitating membrane (LANGER, 1970). This phenomenon may be due to a combination of several effects: on the nictitating membrane phenoxybenzamine impairs neuronal uptake as well as extraneuronal accumulation (DRASKÓCZY and TRENDELENBURG, 1970), and it prevents the O-methylation of the released transmitter (LANGER, 1970). Each of these effects may contribute to the eventual increase in amount of noradrenaline recovered from either the venous effluent or the surrounding medium. Moreover, since phenoxybenzamine is more effective than cocaine in increasing the output of transmitter (LANGER, 1970), the possibility that phenoxybenzamine influences the release mechanism cannot be exlcuded.

There is good evidence that cocaine increases responses of the nictitating membrane to nerve stimulation *in vivo* (TRENDELENBURG, 1959; HAEFELY et al., 1964). The increase in response is most pronounced when single shocks are applied, and least with high rates of stimulation. In agreement with this finding, it was observed that cocaine increases the output of transmitter in the isolated preparation when the rate of stimulation is low (4/sec) but not when it is high (25/sec) (LANGER, 1970). Cocaine increases the sensitivity of the *in vivo* nictitating membrane to single shocks of preganglionic stimulation by a factor of 20—30. Apparently, less than 5% of the released transmitter reaches the vicinity of the receptors in the absence of cocaine; more than 95% is recaptured by the nerve endings (HAEFELY et al., 1964). For higher frequencies of stimulation the percentage of recaptured transmitter drops considerably (in the absence of cocaine). As a consequence, the overflow of transmitter (per shock) into the venous effluent increases with increasing rates of stimulation (BROWN and GILLESPIE, 1957). Apparently, the importance of neuronal uptake for recapture of the released transmitter is inversely related to the frequency of stimulation.

While it is conceivable that extraneuronal uptake also plays a role, there is no evidence in support of this view. It has been mentioned in section VII that extraneuronally accumulated noradrenaline may be able to reach the region of the receptors after leaving the extraneuronal storage sites; it is not known whether the release of transmitter from nerve endings can a) lead to an extraneuronal accumulation, and b) to a shift from the sites of accumulation to the receptors.

There is very little evidence pertinent to the influence of COMT on the concentration of transmitter at the receptors. Determinations of metabolites cannot solve this question, since the pronounced O-methylation of released noradrenaline (LANGER, 1970) may well occur *after* the transmitter has left the biophase. More relevant are studies of responses of effector organs to nerve stimulation before and after block of COMT. Block of COMT by pyrogallol caused a small potentiation of the responses of the isolated guinea-pig vas deferens to postganglionic sympathetic nerve stimulation and prolonged the junction potential recorded intracellularly. The effect of cocaine was similar, and the effects of cocaine and pyrogallol were additive. Block of MAO, on the other hand, failed to influence the junction potential (BELL, 1967). Apparently, both reuptake and COMT are involved in the inactivation of released noradrenaline; however, other factors such as diffusion, must be involved as well. Experiments with tyramine also shed some light on this problem. The O-methylated metabolites of noradrenaline account for about 50% of the radioactivity released by tyramine from the isolated nictitating membrane (LANGER, 1970). In spite of this high percentage of O-methylated metabolites, block of COMT causes not more than a very small increase in the sensitivity of this tissue to tyramine and mephentermine (TRENDELENBURG et al., 1971). Hence, the influence of COMT on the concentration of transmitter (released by indirectly acting amines) at the receptors must be rather small.

There are no reports to indicate that block of MAO causes any substantial potentiation of responses of effector organs to nerve stimulation. Hence, the role of MAO is probably minor.

Conclusions. While there is convincing evidence that recapture by adrenergic nerve endings is able to influence the concentration of the released transmitter at the receptors (especially at low rates of stimulation), the role of the other mechanisms remains to be determined. The available incomplete evidence indicates that these other mechanisms (extraneuronal uptake, COMT and MAO) play a minor role, if any.

XI. Supersensitivity versus Additive Effects

This review has shown that a considerable body of evidence is based on sensitivity studies, i.e., on the recording of responses under a variety of conditions. Before an increase in response is interpreted as potentiation or supersensitivity, additional evidence should be obtained to ensure that it is justified to use these terms. They should be reserved for nearly parallel shifts of dose-response curves. In experiments with single test doses (rather than with determinations of full dose-response curves), additive effects can easily be mistaken for potentiation. Additive effects are present when the agent under study causes an effect which is similar to that of noradrenaline (through activation of either adrenoceptors or other receptors); this increases responses to subsequent injections of noradrenaline by simple addition of effects. In that case, dose-response curves are convergent rather than parallel. For various examples of additive effects, the reader is referred to LANGER and TRENDELENBURG (1966), LANGER (1966b), LANGER et al. (1967b) and DRASKÓCZY and TRENDELENBURG (1968).

To illustrate the importance of this distinction, one example may be quoted. On the basis of experiments with normetanephrine and metanephrine, BACQ and RENSON (1961) concluded that the O-methylated metabolites potentiate the effects of noradrenaline and adrenaline. However, repetition of this work with full dose-response curves for noradrenaline revealed that the O-methylated metabolites are weak agonists whose effects are additive to those of the amines (LANGER et al., 1967a). Thus, the O-methylated metabolites do not induce supersensitivity to the amines. A very strict use of the nomenclature as well as the determination of full dose-response curves would greatly help to prevent confusion in a field which already provides more than enough complexities.

XII. Conclusions

The evidence discussed in this review is, on the whole, consistent with the view that neuronal uptake generates a concentration gradient for sympathomimetic amines from the medium to the region of the receptors. This is the basis of the uptake theory of denervation or cocaine supersensitivity. However, it has to be recognized that a variety of factors are able to modify either the importance of neuronal uptake or directly the concentration of amines at the receptors.

The importance of neuronal uptake is determined by:

1. the rate of neuronal uptake of the amine under study. It is determined by at least three factors: a) the maximal rate of transmembranal uptake which is characteristic for each amine; b) the saturation characteristics of the uptake mechanism; c) the intraneuronal fate of the amine, since an accumulation in the cytoplasm can reduce the net rate of transmembranal uptake. The pharmacological importance of the last two factors is a function of the sensitivity of the tissue to the amine under study; both saturation of uptake and intraneuronal accumulation in the axoplasm are observed only when the bath concentration of the amine exceeds a certain minimum value. Hence, the sensitivity of the tissue determines whether or not a pharmacologically effective concentration of an amine causes either saturation of the transmembranal uptake mechanism or an intraneuronal accumulation in the axoplasm or both. Thus, in addition to the well known cocaine-like drugs which impair the uptake mechanism by a direct effect, there is a variety of drugs and procedures which are able to exert an indirect effect on the rate of transmembranal uptake. The concentration gradient (from the medium to the receptors) existing for the ED50 of an amine can be altered by changes in sensitivity (e.g., decentralization supersensitivity or block of receptors) or by an impairment of the intraneuronal mechanisms for deamination and vesicular storage.

2. the morphology of the system (i.e., by the density of innervation, the neuromuscular distance and the symmetry or asymmetry of innervation).

COMT can influence the concentration of exogenous sympathomimetic amines at the receptors whenever this enzyme plays a substantial role in the metabolism of the amines. This is the case when the amine under study is a good substrate and is neither taken up intraneuronally nor deaminated (e.g., isoprenaline). The significance of COMT is restricted when the amine under study is taken up intraneuronally at a high rate (e.g., noradrenaline in innervated tissues) and when the neuromuscular distance is short. The importance of COMT seems to be limited when the bath concentrations of catecholamines are high. Thus, again, the importance of COMT of denervated tissues is a function of the sensitivity of the tissue.

The physiological and pharmacological role of extraneuronal uptake remains to be defined. However, since extraneuronal uptake is a transient phenomenon, the possibility has to be entertained that there might be, under certain experimental conditions, a shift of noradrenaline from extraneuronal sites of retention to the receptors.

Because of pronounced differences in rates of uptake, in morphology of the system, in the activity of the enzymes, in the sensitivity of organs, the relative importance of the various factors enumerated above should greatly differ from organ to organ and from amine to amine. Hence, it is not surprising that a survey of this field brings together seemingly contradictory evidence. On the contrary, it is impressive how much of the evidence can be adequately accounted for by the uptake theory if the various limiting factors are taken into consideration.

Most of what was thought to be contradictory evidence became compatible with the uptake theory, when the importance of the morphology of the adrenergic system as well as the importance of saturation of neuronal uptake was established. Further progress was made when it was established that cocaine, in addition to impairing neuronal uptake, can exert postjunctional effects. Thus, it can be stated that a considerable body of evidence is compatible with the uptake theory on which this discussion was based.

References

Acheson, G.H.: The topographical anatomy of the smooth muscle of the cat's nictitating membrane. Anat. Rec. **71**, 297—311 (1938).

Almgren, O., Andén, N.-E., Jonason, J., Norberg, K.-A., Olson, L.: Cellular localization of monoamine oxidase in rat salivary glands. Acta physiol. scand. **67**, 21—26 (1966).

Andén, N.-E., Corrodi, H., Ettles, M., Gustafsson, E., Persson, H.: Selective uptake of some catecholamines by the isolated heart and its inhibition by cocaine and phenoxybenzamine. Acta pharmacol. (Kbh.) **21**, 247—259 (1964).

Antonaccio, M.J., Smith, C.B.: Effects of chronic pretreatment with pargyline upon responses of the atrial pacemaker and of left atrial strips of guinea pigs to tyramine, mephentermine, d-amphetamine and adrenergic nerve stimulation. J. Pharmacol. exp. Ther. **170**, 97—107 (1969).

Avakian, O.V., Gillespie, J.S.: Uptake of noradrenaline by adrenergic nerves, smooth muscle and connective tissue in isolated perfused arteries and its correlation with the vasoconstrictor response. Brit. J. Pharmacol. **32**, 168—184 (1968).

Bacq, Z.M., Renson, J.: Actions et importance physiologique de la métanephrine et de la normétanephrine. Arch. int. Pharmacodyn. **130**, 385—402 (1961).

Balzer, H., Holtz, P.: Beeinflussung der Wirkung biogener Amine durch Hemmung der Aminoxydase. Naunyn-Schmiedeberg's Arch. Pharmak. exp. Path. **227**, 547—558 (1956).

Bell, C.: Effects of cocaine and of monoamine oxidase and catechol-O-methyl transferase inhibitors on transmission to the guinea-pig vas deferens. Brit. J. Pharmacol. **31**, 276—289 (1967).

Bennet, M.R., Rogers, D.C.: A study of the innervation of the taenia coli. J. Cell Biol. **33**, 573—596 (1967).

Bevan, J.A., Verity, M.A.: Sympathetic nerve-free vascular muscle. J. Pharmacol. exp. Ther. **157**, 117—124 (1967).

Bhagat, B., Bovell, G., Robinson, I.M.: Influence of cocaine on the uptake of H^3-norepinephrine and on the responses of isolated guinea-pig atria to sympathomimetic amines. J. Pharmacol. exp. Ther. **155**, 472—478 (1967).

Bickerton, R.K.: The response of isolated strips of cat spleen to sympathomimetic drugs and their antagonists. J. Pharmacol. exp. Ther. **142**, 99—110 (1963).

Birmingham, A.T.: Sympathetic denervation of the smooth muscle of the vas deferens. J. Physiol. (Lond.) **206**, 645—661 (1970).

Blinks, J.R.: Evaluation of the cardiac effects of several beta adrenergic blocking agents. Ann. N.Y. Acad. Sci. **139**, 673—685 (1967).

Bonaccorsi, A., Jespersen, J., Garattini, S.: The influence of desipramine on the sensitivity and accumulation of noradrenaline in the isolated tail artery of the rat. Europ. J. Pharmacol. **9**, 124—127 (1970).

Brimijoin, S., Pluchino, S., Trendelenburg, U.: On the mechanism of supersensitivity to norepinephrine in the denervated cat spleen. J. Pharmacol. exp. Ther. **175**, 503—513 (1970).

Brody, M.J.: Cardiovascular responses following immunological sympathectomy. Circulat. Res. **15**, 161—167 (1964).

Brown, G.L., Gillespie, J.S.: The output of sympathetic transmitter from the spleen of the cat. J. Physiol. (Lond.) **138**, 81—102 (1957).

Burford, H., Leick, J., Walaszek, E.J.: Modification of the effects of biogenic amines on the heart by iproniazid. Arch. int. Pharmacodyn. **128**, 39—50 (1960).

Cervoni, P., Reit, E., McCullough, J.: Studies on the decentralized nictitating membrane of the cat. II. Uptake and retention of norepinephrine and epinephrine. J. Pharmacol. exp. Ther. **175**, 649—663 (1970).

Chahl, L.A., O'Donnell, S.R.: The interaction of cocaine and propranolol with catecholamines on guinea pig trachea. Europ. J. Pharmacol. **2**, 77—82 (1967).

Clarke, D.E., Jones, C.J., Linley, P.A.: Histochemical fluorescence studies on noradrenaline accumulation by uptake in the isolated rat heart. Brit. J. Pharmacol. **37**, 1—9 (1969).

CROUT, J.R.: Effect of inhibiting both catechol-O-methyl transferase and monoamine oxidase on cardiovascular responses to norepinephrine. Proc. Soc. exp. Biol. (N.Y.) **108**, 482—484 (1961).
DE LA LANDE, I.S., FREWIN, D., WATERSON, J.G.: The influence of sympathetic innervation on vascular sensitivity to noradrenaline. Brit. J. Pharmacol. **31**, 82—93 (1967).
— JELLETT, L.B.: Relationship between the roles of monoamine oxidase and sympathetic nerves in the vasoconstrictor response of the rabbit ear artery to noradrenaline. J. Pharmacol. exp. Ther. (in press) (1971).
— WATERSON, J.G.: Site of action of cocaine on the perfused artery. Nature (Lond.) **214**, 313—314 (1967).
DRASKÓCZY, P.R., TRENDELENBURG, U.: The uptake of l- and d-norepinephrine by the isolated perfused rabbit heart in relation to the stereospecificity of the sensitizing action of cocaine. J. Pharmacol. exp. Ther. **159**, 66—73 (1968).
— — Intraneuronal and extraneuronal accumulation of sympathomimetic amines in the isolated nictitating membrane of the cat. J. Pharmacol. exp. Ther. **174**, 290—306 (1970).
EHINGER, B., FALCK, B., SPORRONG, B.: Adrenergic fibers to the heart and to peripheral vessels. Bibl. anat. (Basel) **8**, 35—45 (1967).
EISENFELD, A.J., AXELROD, J., KRAKOFF, L.: Inhibition of the extraneuronal accumulation and metabolism of norepinephrine by adrenergic blocking agents. J. Pharmacol. exp. Ther. **156**, 107—113 (1967a).
— LANDSBERG, L., AXELROD, J.: Effect of drugs on the accumulation and metabolism of extraneuronal norepinephrine in the rat heart. J. Pharmacol. exp. Ther. **158**, 378—385 (1967b).
EMMELIN, N.: Supersensitivity following "pharmacological denervation". Pharmacol. Rev. **13**, 17—38 (1961).
ESTERHUIZEN, A.C., GRAHAM, J.D.P., LEVER, J.D., SPRIGGS, T.L.B.: Catecholamine and acetylcholinesterase distribution in relation to noradrenaline release. An enzyme histochemical and autoradiographic study on the innervation of the cat nictitating membrane. Brit. J. Pharmacol. **32**, 46—56 (1968).
FLECKENSTEIN, A., BASS, H.: Zum Mechanismus der Wirkungsverstärkung und Wirkungsabschwächung sympathomimetischer Amine durch Cocain und andere Pharmaka. I. Die Sensibilisierung der Katzen-Nickhaut für Sympathomimetica der Brenzkatechin-Reihe. Naunyn-Schmiedeberg's Arch. exp. Path. Pharmak. **220**, 143—156 (1953).
— BURN, J.H.: The effect of denervation on the action of sympathomimetic amines on the nictitating membrane. Brit. J. Pharmacol. **8**, 69—78 (1953).
— STÖCKLE, D.: Zum Mechanismus der Wirkungsverstärkung und Wirkungsabschwächung sympathomimetischer Amine durch Cocaine und andere Pharmaka. II. Die Hemmung der Neuro-Sympathomimetica durch Cocain. Naunyn-Schmiedeberg's Arch. exp. Path. Pharmak. **224**, 401—415 (1955).
FLEMING, W.W., TRENDELENBURG, U.: Development of supersensitivity to norepinephrine after pretreatment with reserpine. J. Pharmacol. exp. Ther. **133**, 41—51 (1961).
FOSTER, R.W.: The potentiation of the responses to noradrenaline and isoprenaline of the guinea-pig isolated tracheal chain preparation by desipramine, cocaine, phentolamine, phenoxybenzamine, guanethidine, metanephrine and cooling. Brit. J. Pharmacol. **31**, 466—482 (1967).
— A correlation between inhibition of the uptake of ^{3}H from (±)-^{3}H-noradrenaline and potentiation of the responses to (—)-noradrenaline in the guinea-pig isolated trachea. Brit. J. Pharmacol. **33**, 357—367 (1968).
— An uptake of radioactivity from (±)-^{3}H-isoproterenol and its inhibition by drugs which potentiate the responses to (—)-isoproterenol in the guinea-pig isolated trachea. Brit. J. Pharmacol. **35**, 418—427 (1969).
FREY, H.H.: Monoamine oxidase inhibition and sensitivity of nictitating membrane to noradrenaline. Acta pharmacol. (Kbh.) **20**, 90—96 (1963).
FURCHGOTT, R.F.: The pharmacological differentiation of adrenergic receptors. Ann. N.Y. Acad. Sci. **139**, 553—570 (1967).
— KIRPEKAR, S.M., RIEKER, M., SCHWAB, A.: Actions and interactions of norepinephrine, tyramine and cocaine on aortic strips of rabbit and left atria of guinea pig and cat. J. Pharmacol. exp. Ther. **142**, 39—58 (1963).
— SANCHEZ-GARCIA, P.: Effects of inhibition of monoamine oxidase on the actions and interactions of norepinephrine, tyramine and other drugs on guinea-pig left atrium. J. Pharmacol. exp. Ther. **163**, 98—122 (1968).
— WEINSTEIN, HUEBL, H., BOZORGMEHRI, P., MENSENDIEK, R.: Effect of inhibition of monoamine oxidase on response of rabbit aortic strips to sympathomimetic amines. Fed. Proc. **14**, 341—342 (1955).
FURNESS, J.B.: The excitatory input to a single smooth muscle cell. Pflügers Arch. **314**, 1—13 (1970).

GILES, R.E., MILLER, J.W.: Studies on the potentiation of the inotropic actions of certain catecholamines by U-0521 (3′,4′-dihydroxy-α-methyl propiophenone). J. Pharmacol. exp. Ther. **157**, 55—61 (1967).
GILLESPIE, J.S., HAMILTON, D.N.H.: A possible active transport of noradrenaline into arterial smooth muscle cells. J. Physiol. (Lond.) **192**, 30P (1967).
— — HOSIE, R.J.A.: The extraneuronal uptake and localization of noradrenaline in the cat spleen and the effect on this of some drugs, of cold and of denervation. J. Physiol. (Lond.) **206**, 563—590 (1970).
— MUIR, T.C.: Species and tissue variation in extraneuronal and neuronal accumulation of noradrenaline. J. Physiol. (Lond.) **206**, 591—604 (1970).
GOVIER, W.C., SUGRUE, M.F., SHORE, P.S.: On the inability to produce supersensitivity to catecholamines in intestinal smooth muscle. J. Pharmacol. exp. Ther. **165**, 71—77 (1969).
GRAEFE, K.H., BÖNISCH, H., TRENDELENBURG, U.: Time-dependent changes in neuronal net uptake of noradrenaline after pretreatment with pargyline and/or reserpine. Naunyn-Schmiedeberg's Arch. Pharmak. **271**, 1—28 (1971).
— TRENDELENBURG, U.: The effect of cocaine on uptake of and sensitivity to noradrenaline in isolated nictitating membranes before and after storage in the cold. Naunyn-Schmiedeberg's Arch. Pharmak. **267**, 383—398 (1970).
GREEN, III, R.D., FLEMING, W.W.: Agonist-antagonist interactions in the normal and supersensitive nictitating membrane of the spinal cat. J. Pharmacol. exp. Ther. **156**, 207—214 (1967).
— — Analysis of supersensitivity in the isolated spleen of the cat. J. Pharmacol. exp. Ther. **162**, 254—262 (1968).
GRIESEMER, E.C., BARSKY, J., DRAGSTEDT, C.A., WELLS, A.J., ZELLER, E.A.: Potentiating effect of iproniazid on the pharmacological action of sympathomimetic amines. Proc. Soc. exp. Biol. (N.Y.) **84**, 699—701 (1953).
HAEFELY, W., HÜRLIMANN, A., THOENEN, H.: A quantitative study of the effect of cocaine on the response of the cat nictitating membrane to nerve stimulation and to injected noradrenaline. Brit. J. Pharmacol. **22**, 5—21 (1964).
HAEUSLER, G., HAEFELY, W., THOENEN, H.: Chemical sympathectomy of the cat with 6-hydroxydopamine. J. Pharmacol. exp. Ther. **170**, 50—61 (1969).
HAMBERGER, B., NORBERG, K.-A., OLSON, L.: Extraneuronal binding of catecholamines and 3,4-dihydroxyphenylalanine (dopa) in salivary glands. Acta physiol. scand. **69**, 1—12 (1967).
HARDMAN, J.G., MAYER, S.E., CLARK, B.: Cocaine potentiation of the cardiac inotropic and phosphorylase responses to catecholamines as related to the uptake of H^3-catecholamines. J. Pharmacol. exp. Ther. **150**, 341—348 (1965).
HEBB, C.O., KONZETT, H.: Vaso- and bronchodilator effects of N-isopropylnorepinephrine in isolated perfused dog lungs. J. Pharmacol. exp. Ther. **96**, 228—237 (1949).
HERTTING, G.: The fate of ^{3}H-isoproterenol in the rat. Biochem. Pharmacol. **13**, 1119—1128 (1964).
— SUKO, J., WIDHALM, S., HARBICH, I.: Über den Mechanismus der Potenzierung der Katecholaminwirkung nach chronisch postganglionärer sympathischer Denervierung. Naunyn-Schmiedeberg's Arch. Pharmak. exp. Path. **256**, 40—45 (1967).
HOLLANDS, B.C.S., VANOV, S.: Localization of catechol amines in visceral organs and ganglia of the rat, guinea-pig and rabbit. Brit. J. Pharmacol. **25**, 307—316 (1965).
HOLMAN, M.E.: Electrophysiology of vascular smooth muscle. Ergebn. Physiol. **61**, 137—177 (1969).
HUKOVIĆ, S., MUSCHOLL, E.: Die Noradrenalin-Abgabe aus dem isolierten Kaninchenherzen bei sympathischer Nervenreizung und ihre pharmakologische Beeinflussung. Naunyn-Schmiedeberg's Arch. exp. Path. Pharmak. **244**, 81—96 (1962).
INNES, I.R., KOSTERLITZ, H.W.: The effects of preganglionic and postganglionic denervation on the responses of the nictitating membrane to sympathomimetic substances. J. Physiol. (Lond.) **124**, 25—43 (1954).
IVERSEN, L.L.: The uptake of noradrenaline by the isolated perfused rat heart. Brit. J. Pharmacol. **21**, 523—537 (1963).
— The uptake of catechol amines at high perfusion concentrations in the rat isolated heart: a novel catechol amine uptake process. Brit. J. Pharmacol. **25**, 18—33 (1965).
— The uptake and storage of noradrenaline in sympathetic nerves. Cambridge: University Press 1967.
— LANGER, S.Z.: Effects of phenoxybenzamine on the uptake and metabolism of noradrenaline in the rat heart and vas deferens. Brit. J. Pharmacol. **37**, 627—637 (1969).
— SALT, P.J.: Inhibition of catecholamine uptake by steroids in the isolated rat heart. Brit. J. Pharmacol. **40**, 528—530 (1970).
IZQUIERDO, J.A., KAUMANN, A.J.: Effect of pyrogallol on the duration of the cardiovascular action of catecholamines. Arch. int. Pharmacodyn. **144**, 437—445 (1963).

JARROTT, B.: Occurrence and properties of catechol-O-methyl transferase in adrenergic neurons. J. Neurochem. **18**, 17—27 (1971).
— LANGER, S.Z.: Changes in monoamine oxidase and catechol-O-methyl transferase activities after denervation of the nictitating membrane of the cat. J. Physiol. (Lond.) **212**, 549—559 (1971).
KALSNER, S., NICKERSON, M.: Disposition of phenylephrine in vascular tissue, determined by the oil-immersion technique. J. Pharmacol. exp. Ther. **163**, 1—10 (1968).
— — Disposition of norepinephrine and epinephrine in vascular tissue, determined by the technique of oil immersion. J. Pharmacol. exp. Ther. **165**, 152—165 (1969a).
— — Mechanism of cocaine potentiation of responses to amines. Brit. J. Pharmacol. **35**, 428—439 (1969b).
KASUYA, Y., GOTO, K.: The mechanism of supersensitivity to norepinephrine induced by cocaine in rat isolated vas deferens. Europ. J. Pharmacol. **4**, 355—362 (1968).
KAUMANN, A.J.: Adrenergic receptors in heart muscle: relations among factors influencing the sensitivity of the cat papillary muscle to catecholamines. J. Pharmacol. exp. Ther. **173**, 383—398 (1970).
— Potentiation of (—)isoproterenol and (—)norepinephrine by hydrocortisone in cat heart muscle. Acta cient. venez. **22**, R-37 (1971).
KOCH-WESER, J.: Direct and *beta* adrenergic receptor blocking actions of nethalide on isolated heart muscle. J. Pharmacol. exp. Ther. **146**, 318—326 (1964).
KONZETT, H.: Verstärkung der Wirkung von Isopropylnoradrenalin durch Pyrogallol. Arch. int. Pharmacodyn. **139**, 558—563 (1962).
KRONEBERG, G., SCHLOSSMANN, K., HABERLAND, G.: O-Methyltransferase-Hemmung *in vitro* und Adrenalin-Noradrenalin-Sensibilisierung *in vivo*. Naunyn-Schmiedeberg's Arch. exp. Path. Pharmak. **241**, 522 (1961).
KUKOVETZ, W.R., LEMBECK, F.: Untersuchungen über die adrenalinpotenzierende Wirkung von Cocain und Denervierung. Naunyn-Schmiedeberg's Arch. exp. Path. Pharmak. **242**, 467—479 (1962).
LANGER, S.Z.: The degeneration contraction of the nictitating membrane in the unanesthetized cat. J. Pharmacol. exp. Ther. **151**, 66—72 (1966a).
— Presence of tone in the denervated and in the decentralized nictitating membrane of the spinal cat and its influence on determinations of supersensitivity. J. Pharmacol. exp. Ther. **154**, 14—34 (1966b).
— The effects of phenoxybenzamine on metabolism of ^{3}H-noradrenaline released from the isolated nictitating membrane. Brit. J. Pharmacol. **34**, 222P—223P (1968).
— The metabolism of H^3-noradrenaline released by electrical stimulation from the isolated nictitating membrane of the cat and from the vas deferens of the rat. J. Physiol. (Lond.) **208**, 515—546 (1970).
— BOGAERT, M.G., DE SCHAEPDRYVER, A.F.: Influence of metanephrine on responses of the nictitating membrane of the pithed cat to sympathomimetic amines. J. Pharmacol. exp. Ther. **157**, 517—523 (1967a).
— DRASKÓCZY, P.R., TRENDELENBURG, U.: Time course of the development of supersensitivity to various amines in the nictitating membrane of the pithed cat after denervation or decentralization. J. Pharmacol. exp. Ther. **157**, 255—273 (1967b).
— TRENDELENBURG, U.: The onset of denervation supersensitivity. J. Pharmacol. exp. Ther. **151**, 73—86 (1966).
— — Decrease in effectiveness of phenoxybenzamine after chronic denervation and chronic decentralization of the nictitating membrane of the pithed cat. J. Pharmacol. exp. Ther. **163**, 290—299 (1968).
— — The effect of a saturable uptake mechanism on the slopes of dose-response curves for sympathomimetic amines and on the shifts of dose-response curves produced by a competitive antagonist. J. Pharmacol. exp. Ther. **167**, 117—142 (1969).
LEMBECK, F., RESCH, H.: Die Potenzierung der Adrenalinwirkung durch Cocain und Pyrogallol. Naunyn-Schmiedeberg's Arch. exp. Path. Pharmak. **240**, 210—217 (1960).
LEVIN, J.A., FURCHGOTT, R.F.: Interactions between potentiating agents of adrenergic amines in rabbit aortic strips. J. Pharmacol. exp. Ther. **172**, 320—331 (1970).
LIGHTMAN, S.L., IVERSEN, L.L.: The role of uptake$_2$ in the extraneuronal metabolism of catecholamines in the isolated rat heart. Brit. J. Pharmacol. **37**, 638—649 (1969).
LINDMAR, R., MUSCHOLL, E.: Die Wirkung von Pharmaka auf die Elimination von Noradrenalin aus der Perfusionsflüssigkeit und die Noradrenalinaufnahme in das isolierte Herz. Naunyn-Schmiedeberg's Arch. exp. Path. Pharmak. **247**, 469—492 (1964).
LÖFFELHOLZ, K., LINDMAR, R., MUSCHOLL, E.: Analysis of wash-out of noradrenaline from the perfused rabbit heart after infusion of noradrenaline. Naunyn-Schmiedeberg's Arch. Pharmak. **270**, R87 (1971).

MAXWELL, R.A., PLUMMER, A.J., POVALSKI, H., SCHNEIDER, F., COOMBS, H.: A comparison of some of the cardiovascular actions of methylphenidate and cocaine. J. Pharmacol. exp. Ther. **126**, 250—257 (1959).
— WASTILA, W.B., ECKHARDT, S.B.: Some factors determining the response of rabbit aortic strips to dl-norepinephrine-7-H^3 hydrochloride and the influence of cocaine, guanethidine and methylphenidate on these factors. J. Pharmacol. exp. Ther. **151**, 253—261 (1966).
MCNEILL, J.H., BRODY, T.M.: The effect of various drug pretreatments on amine-induced phosphorylase activation and amine uptake. J. Pharmacol. exp. Ther. **162**, 121—133 (1968).
— — The effect of d- and l-norepinephrine on rat cardiac phosphorylase activation. J. Pharmacol. exp. Ther. **165**, 97—101 (1969).
MERRILLEES, N.C.R., BURNSTOCK, G., HOLMAN, M.E.: Correlation of fine structure and physiology of the innervation of smooth muscle in the guinea pig vas deferens. J. Cell Biol. **19**, 529—550 (1963).
MUSCHOLL, E.: Effect of cocaine and related drugs on the uptake of noradrenaline by heart and spleen. Brit. J. Pharmacol. **16**, 352—359 (1961).
PICK, J.: Fine structure of nerve terminals in the human gut. Anat. Rec. **159**, 131—138 (1967).
PLUCHINO, S.: Direct and indirect effects of 5-hydroxytryptamine and tyramine on cat smooth muscle. Naunyn-Schmiedebergs Arch. Pharmak. **272**, 189—224 (1972).
— TRENDELENBURG, U.: The influence of denervation and of decentralization on the *alpha* and *beta* effects of isoproterenol on the nictitating membrane of the pithed cat. J. Pharmacol. exp. Ther. **163**, 257—265 (1968).
— VAN ORDEN, L.S., III., DRASKÓCZY, P.R., LANGER, S.Z., TRENDELENBURG, U.: The effect of beta-TM10 on the pharmacological, biochemical and morphological changes induced by denervation of the nictitating membrane of the cat. J. Pharmacol. exp. Ther. **172**, 77—90 (1970).
REIFFENSTEIN, R.J.: Effects of cocaine on the rate of contraction to noradrenaline in the cat spleen strip: mode of action of cocaine. Brit. J. Pharmacol. **32**, 591—597 (1968).
ROSS, S.B., RENYI, A.L.: Uptake of some tritiated sympathomimetic amines by mouse brain cortex slices *in vitro*. Acta pharmacol. (Kbh.) **24**, 297—309 (1966).
SCHMITT, H., GONNARD, P.: Modifications par un inhibiteur de l'aminoxydase, l'iproniazide, des effets de quelques amines sympathicomimétiques sur la membrane nictitante du chat. Arch. int. Pharmacodyn. **108**, 74—83 (1956).
SCHÜMANN, H.J., GÜTHER, W.: Untersuchungen zum Wirkungsmechanismus von Angiotensin am isolierten Aortenpräparat und am Blutdruck von Ratten und Meerschweinchen. Naunyn-Schmiedeberg's Arch. Pharmak. exp. Path. **256**, 169—182 (1967).
SEIDEHAMEL, R.J., PATIL, P.N., TYE, A., LAPIDUS, J.B.: The effects of norepinephrine isomers on various supersensitivities of the cat nictitating membrane. J. Pharmacol. exp. Ther. **153**, 81—89 (1966).
SIMMONDS, M.A., GILLIS, C.N.: Uptake of normetanephrine and norepinephrine by cocaine-treated rat heart. J. Pharmacol. exp. Ther. **159**, 283—289 (1968).
SMITH, C.B.: The role of monoaminoxidase in the intraneuronal metabolism of norepinephrine released by indirectly-acting sympathomimetic amines or by adrenergic nerve stimulation. J. Pharmacol. exp. Ther. **151**, 207—220 (1966).
— TRENDELENBURG, U., LANGER, S.Z., TSAI, T.H.: The relation of retention of norepinephrine-H^3 to the norepinephrine content of the nictitating membrane of the spinal cat during development of denervation supersensitivity. J. Pharmacol. exp. Ther. **151**, 87—94 (1966).
SOMLYO, A.V., WOO, C.Y., SOMLYO, A.P.: Responses of nerve free vessels to vasoactive amines and polypeptides. Amer. J. Physiol. **208**, 748—753 (1965).
STAFFORD, A.: Potentiation of some catecholamines by phenoxybenzamine, guanethidine and cocaine. Brit. J. Pharmacol. **21**, 361—367 (1963).
STJÄRNE, L., VON EULER, U.S.: Stereospecificity of amine uptake mechanism in nerve granules. J. Pharmacol. exp. Ther. **150**, 335—340 (1965).
THOENEN, H., TRANZER, J.P.: Chemical sympathectomy by selective destruction of adrenergic nerve endings with 6-hydroxydopamine. Naunyn-Schmiedeberg's Arch. Pharmak. exp. Path. **261**, 271—288 (1968).
TRENDELENBURG, U.: The supersensitivity caused by cocaine. J. Pharmacol. exp. Ther. **125**, 55—65 (1959).
— The action of acetylcholine on the nicitating membrane of the spinal cat. J. Pharmacol. exp. Ther. **135**, 39—44 (1962).
— Supersensitivity and subsensitivity to sympathomimetic amines. Pharmacol. Rev. **15**, 225—276 (1963).
— Supersensitivity by cocaine to dextrorotatory isomers of norepinephrine and epinephrine. J. Pharmacol. exp. Ther. **148**, 329—338 (1965).

TRENDELENBURG, U.: Mechanisms of supersensitivity and subsensitivity to sympathomimetic amines. Pharmacol. Rev. **18**, 629—640 (1966a).

— Supersensitivity to norepinephrine induced by continuous nerve stimulation. J. Pharmacol. exp. Ther. **151**, 95—102 (1966b).

— The effect of cocaine on the pacemaker of isolated guinea-pig atria. J. Pharmacol. exp. Ther. **161**, 222—231 (1968).

— Supersensitivity of the isolated nictitating membrane of the cat to sympathomimetic amines after impairment of the intraneuronal mechanisms of inactivation. Naunyn-Schmiedeberg's Arch. Pharmak. **271**, 29—58 (1971).

— DRASKÓCZY, P.R.: The effect of intraneuronal inactivation on the transmembranal uptake of l- and d-norepinephrine. J. Pharmacol. exp. Ther. **175**, 521—524 (1970).

— — PLUCHINO, S.: The density of adrenergic innervation of the cat's nictitating membrane as a factor influencing the sensitivity of the isolated preparation to l-norepinephrine. J. Pharmacol. exp. Ther. **166**, 14—25 (1969).

— HÖHN, D., GRAEFE, K.H., PLUCHINO, S.: The influence of block of catechol-O-methyl transferase on the sensitivity of isolated organs to catecholamines. Naunyn-Schmiedeberg's Arch. Pharmak. **271**, 59—92 (1971).

— MAXWELL, R.A., PLUCHINO, S.: Methoxamine as a tool to assess the importance of intraneuronal uptake of l-norepinephrine in the cat's nictitating membrane. J. Pharmacol. exp. Ther. **172**, 91—99 (1970).

— MUSKUS, A., FLEMING, W.W., GOMEZ ALONSO DE LA SIERRA, B.: Effect of cocaine, denervation and decentralization on the response of the nictitating membrane to various sympathomimetic amines. J. Pharmacol. exp. Ther. **138**, 181—193 (1962).

— WEINER, N.: Sensitivity of the nictitating membrane after various procedures and agents. J. Pharmacol. exp. Ther. **136**, 152—161 (1962).

TSAI, T.H.: Time course of contraction of the isolated nictitating membrane of the cat in response to l-norepinephrine. Fed. Proc. **27**, 709 (1968).

URQUILLA, P.R., STITZEL, R.E., FLEMING, W.W.: The antagonism of phentolamine against exogenously administered and endogenously released norepinephrine in rabbit aortic strips. J. Pharmacol. exp. Ther. **172**, 310—319 (1970).

URSILLO, R.C., JACOBSON, J.: Potentiation of norepinephrine in the isolated vas deferens of the rat by some CNS stimulants and antidepressants. J. Pharmacol. exp. Ther. **148**, 246—251 (1965).

VAN ORDEN, L.S., III, BENSCH, K.G., LANGER, S.Z., TRENDELENBURG, U.: Histochemical and fine structural aspects of the onset of denervervation supersensitivity in the nictitating membrane of the spinal cat. J. Pharmacol. exp. Ther. **157**, 274—283 (1967).

VARAGIĆ, V.: The effect of isoniazide and isopropylisoniazide on the responses of the nictitating membrane of the cat to intraarterial adrenaline, noradrenaline and tyramine and to preganglionic sympathetic stimulation. Arch. int. Pharmacodyn. **114**, 426—434 (1958).

VARMA, D.R.: Effect of sympathetic denervation on the alpha receptors of the cat nictitating membrane. J. Pharmacol. exp. Ther. **153**, 48—61 (1966).

— MCCULLOUGH, H.N.: Dissociation of the supersensitivity to norepinephrine caused by cocaine from inhibition of H^3-norepinephrine uptake in cold-stored smooth muscle. J. Pharmacol. exp. Ther. **166**, 26—34 (1969).

VERITY, M.A.: Morphologic studies of vascular neuroeffector apparatus. Proc. Symp. Physiol. Pharmacol. Vasc. Neuroeffector Systems, Interlaken 1969, pp. 2—12. Basel: Karger 1971.

— BEVAN, J.A.: Fine structural study of the terminal effector plexus, neuromuscular and intermuscular relationships in the pulmonary artery. J. Anat. (Lond.) **103**, 49—63 (1968).

WAGNER, K., TRENDELENBURG, U.: Development of degeneration contraction and supersensitivity in the cat's nictitating membrane after 6-hydroxydopamine. Naunyn-Schmiedeberg's Arch. Pharmak. **270**, 215—236 (1971).

WAUD, D.R.: A quantitative model for the effect of a saturable uptake on the slope of the dose-response curve. J. Pharmacol. exp. Ther. **167**, 140—142 (1969).

WESTFALL, D.P., FLEMING, W.W.: The sensitivity of the guinea-pig pacemaker to norepinephrine and calcium after pretreatment with reserpine. J. Pharmacol. exp. Ther. **164**, 259—269 (1968).

WYLIE, D.W., ARCHER, S., ARNOLD, A.: Augmentation of pharmacological properties of catecholamines by O-methyl transferase inhibitors. J. Pharmacol. exp. Ther. **130**, 239 to 244 (1960).

ZAIMIS, E.: The immunosympathectomized animal: a valuable tool in physiological and pharmacological research. J. Physiol. (Lond.) **177**, 35—36P (1965).

Chapter 17

Interrelationships between Adrenergic and Cholinergic Mechanisms

H. W. KOSTERLITZ and G. M. LEES

With 23 Figures

A. Effects of Acetylcholine on Adrenergic Nerve Terminals

I. Introduction

After LOEWI (1921) had shown that impulse transmission from the autonomic nerves to the effector organ may be mediated by chemical agents, the classical theory of humoral transmission was developed; it was assumed that, with few exceptions, the fibres of the sympathetic outflow were adrenergic and those of the parasympathetic outflow cholinergic. This assumption was based on experiments in mammals; only little information was available on the transmitters in the autonomic nervous system of non-mammalian vertebrates. BURNSTOCK (1969) has summarized the position as follows: The primitive sympathetic excitatory supply to the viscera of fish and amphibia is predominantly cholinergic. There are various proportions of adrenergic and cholinergic fibres in sympathetic trunks in reptiles and birds while in mammals most, and sometimes all, of the fibres in sympathetic trunks are adrenergic.

Thus, there has been an overall trend from the cholinergic to adrenergic sympathetic control of visceral and vascular systems; cholinergic sympathetic post-ganglionic neurones are represented in much greater numbers in lower vertebrates.

II. Presence of Cholinergic Fibres in Mammalian Sympathetic Nerves

In 1959, BURN and RAND reviewed the literature and arrived at the conclusion that many sympathetic nerves contained also cholinergic fibres; this evidence was obtained either from the depression of the responses to nerve stimulation by atropine or hyoscine, in animals with noradrenaline stores depleted by reserpine, or from the release of acetylcholine after nerve stimulation. Thus, there are cholinergic fibres from the superior ganglion to the buccal mucous membrane of the cat and dog (EULER and GADDUM, 1931). The presence of cholinergic fibres was indicated by results of stimulation of the hypogastric nerve to the uterus of the dog (SHERIF, 1935), of the sympathetic nerves to the vessels of the muscles of the hindlimb of the dog and cat (BÜLBRING and BURN, 1935; FOLKOW et al., 1948a; LEADERS, 1965) and to the heart of the dog and cat (FOLKOW et al., 1948b) and of the rabbit (HUKOVIĆ, 1959). Similar findings were also obtained for the nerves to the spleen (BURN and RAND, 1960; BRANDON and RAND, 1961; LEADERS and DAYRIT, 1965), the nerves to the skin vessels of the rabbit ear (BURN and RAND,

1960; HOLTON and RAND, 1962), the nerves to the intestine of the rabbit (GILLESPIE and MACKENNA, 1961) and the nerves to the pilomotor muscles of the cat (WOLNER, 1965). The dilator muscle of the cat iris also contains both adrenergic and cholinergic fibres (EHINGER et al., 1968).

As far as the nictitating membrane of the cat is concerned, the evidence is controversial. BURN and RAND (1960) found that, in cats pretreated with reserpine, stimulation of the postganglionic fibres causes a small contraction which is abolished by atropine. On the other hand, GARDINER and THOMPSON (1961) could not obtain evidence for cholinergic transmission in the isolated preparation of the nictitating membrane which has specific receptors for acetylcholine (THOMPSON, 1958). The results obtained on the vas deferens of the guinea-pig are difficult to interpret because of the presence of ganglion cells in the nerve. BIRMINGHAM and WILSON (1962) and BURN and WEETMAN (1963) found that hyoscine causes a small reduction of the contraction due to stimulation of the hypogastric nerve or transmural stimulation but BURNSTOCK and HOLMAN (1964) could not demonstrate any effect of atropine on the junction potentials elicited by stimulation of the hypogastric nerve.

III. Cholinergic Link Hypothesis

The cholinergic link hypothesis states that, when the nerve impulse reaches the adrenergic nerve terminal, there is a release of acetylcholine which, by activation of nicotinic receptors, facilitates the entry of calcium ions; these, in turn, release noradrenaline from its store (BURN and RAND, 1959, 1965; BURN, 1961, 1963, 1966, 1967). The evidence for and against this hypothesis was reviewed by FERRY (1966). The experimental data on the relationship between cholinomimetic agents and release of noradrenaline from sympathetic nerve endings were recently analyzed by MUSCHOLL (1970).

A great deal of the evidence was obtained from the responses of effector organs innervated by adrenergic neurones excited either by nicotinic drugs or by electrical stimulation of the nerves. Since there is always the possibility that the excitable membrane of the smooth muscle has cholinoceptors in addition to adrenoceptors, the following conditions have to be fulfilled for support of the cholinergic link hypothesis: The responses must not be inhibited by atropine or hyoscine. They must be abolished by postganglionic denervation of the sympathetic supply, by reserpine, by such adrenergic neurone blocking agents as bretylium or guanethidine, or by α- or β-adrenoceptive blocking drugs. They should be reduced by hexamethonium, hemicholinium and botulinum toxin and enhanced by anticholinesterases.

However, because of the possible multiple sites of action of drugs on the excitable membrane of the nerve fibres, the structures involved in the release and re-uptake processes and the excitable structures of the effector organs, reliable evidence can be obtained only from measurement of noradrenaline release. It is also of importance to study the time course of the output of noradrenaline released by acetylcholine on the one hand and by electrical nerve stimulation on the other hand. Evidence has to be obtained that the circumstances in which acetylcholine or nicotine cause a release of noradrenaline, demonstrated either directly by measurement of the output or indirectly by the responses of the effector organs, are compatible with the conditions under which stimulation of adrenergic nerves causes release of transmitter. Finally, it will have to be decided whether any acetylcholine that causes release of noradrenaline has its origin in the adrenergic fibres themselves or in cholinergic fibres running in close proximity to the adrenergic nerve terminals.

1. Effects of Acetylcholine and Nicotine on Sympathetically Innervated Effector Organs

When BURN and RAND (1959) proposed the hypothesis of a cholinergic link, it was already well established that the noradrenaline-like effect of acetylcholine or nicotine was not suppressed by atropine. For instance, KOTTEGODA (1953b) had shown that, in the perfused rabbit ear, acetylcholine causes vasodilation which is converted to vasoconstriction by atropine. The vasoconstrictor effect is blocked by hexamethonium. Pretreatment with reserpine abolishes this vasoconstrictor effect of acetylcholine or nicotine (BURN, 1963). Similarly, in the presence of atropine, acetylcholine, nicotine and tetramethylammonium cause a positive inotropic effect on the heart which is blocked by hexamethonium or (+)-tubocurarine (HOFFMANN et al., 1945; KOTTEGODA, 1953a; LEE and SHIDEMAN, 1959), and by pretreatment with reserpine or by postganglionic denervation (CABRERA et al., 1966a). Injection of nicotine or of large doses of acetylcholine causes a contraction of the dog spleen which is not abolished by atropine but reduced by pretreatment with reserpine; hexamethonium abolishes the effect of acetylcholine and nicotine without affecting the response of the effector organ to nerve stimulation (DALY and SCOTT, 1961). Similar results were obtained on the perfused spleen of the cat (BRANDON and RAND, 1961); the effect of acetylcholine, in contrast to that of nerve stimulation, is abolished by hexamethonium (BLAKELEY et al., 1963). The acetylcholine-induced contraction of the pilomotor muscles in the skin of the cat's tail is not depressed by atropine in concentrations which abolish muscarinic effects (COON and ROTHMAN, 1940). *In vitro*, nicotine causes a contraction of the pilomotor muscles; hexamethonium blocks this effect without affecting the response to electrical stimulation (HELLMANN, 1963).

Such a noradrenaline-like effect of acetylcholine is not seen at all adrenergic junctions. For instance, in the isolated nictitating membrane of the cat, acetylcholine causes a contraction which is abolished by atropine but unaffected by hexamethonium; on the other hand, the contractor response due to nicotine is abolished by hexamethonium but only a little depressed by atropine (THOMPSON, 1958). Moreover, when nicotine is added to the organ bath in concentrations which cause autoinhibition, the response to stimulation of the nerves to the nictitating membrane is as large as that obtained before the addition of nicotine (THOMPSON, J.W., personal communication).

2. Effects of Acetylcholine on the Responses to Electrical Stimulation of Sympathetic Nerves

BRÜCKE (1935) first demonstrated that large doses of acetylcholine can abolish the effects of sympathetic stimulation of the pilomotor muscles of the tail of the cat. These observations were confirmed by COON and ROTHMAN (1940) and by BURN and RAND (1960).

BURN and RAND (1960) also observed that large doses of acetylcholine blocked the vasoconstrictor effect due to stimulation of the sympathetic fibres to the rabbit ear. In the isolated perfused mesenteric artery (22° C) of the rat, low concentrations (0.05 ng/ml) of acetylcholine enhance the responses to electrical stimulation (7 Hz); however, when the concentration is raised to 5 ng/ml, acetylcholine has a depressant effect on the responses to nerve stimulation (MALIK and LING, 1969a). At the same time, the response to noradrenaline is somewhat reduced. This blockade is overcome by increasing the Ca^{2+} concentration of the perfusion fluid or by adding dexamphetamine (0.4 μg/ml). Atropine (0.1 μg/ml) abolishes the blocking action of 5 ng/ml of acetylcholine and reduces by 50% the action of 50 ng/ml of acetylcholine.

The blocking effects of acetylcholine on the responses to nerve stimulation could be in favour of the cholinergic link hypothesis (BURN, 1963) but could also be explained by the fact that acetylcholine blocks conduction in C fibres (ARMETT and RITCHIE, 1960).

3. Effects of Hemicholinium on the Responses to Stimulation of Sympathetic Nerves

BRANDON and RAND (1961) found that, in the saline-perfused cat spleen, pretreatment with hemicholinium reduced the contractions of the spleen on stimulation of the splenic nerves at 50 Hz; addition of choline restored the responses. FERRY (1966) suggested that this effect of hemicholinium might be due to alterations in the responses of the spleen and not to interference with the release of noradrenaline which, unfortunately, was not measured. In the dog, hemicholinium does not prevent the contractile response of the perfused isolated spleen although cholinergic transmission, as measured by the acetylcholine content of splenic effluent, is greatly reduced (LEADERS and DAYRIT, 1965).

There is no evidence of any effect of hemicholinium on the responses of the nictitating membrane of the cat to stimulation of the postganglionic nerve although the effects of stimulation of the preganglionic trunk fail rapidly (BIRKS and MACINTOSH, 1961). Similarly, hemicholinium is without effect on the responses of the isolated innervated preparation of the nictitating membrane to nerve stimulation (GARDINER and THOMPSON, 1961).

The responses of isolated cat atria to sympathetic nerve stimulation can be prevented by exposure to hemicholinium for 4—5 hr and then restored by choline (CHANG and RAND, 1960); similar findings were obtained for the rabbit ear and the rabbit colon. The inhibitory effect of stimulation of the sympathetic nerves to the guinea-pig colon was prevented by hemicholinium in about two-thirds of the experiments (RAND and RIDEHALGH, 1965) whereas in the Finkleman preparation of the rabbit ileum hemicholinium was without effect (BENTLEY, 1962).

BURN (1966) pointed out that some of the negative results may have been due to insufficient duration of exposure (less than 3 hr) to hemicholinium. However, in experiments on rabbit isolated atria and vagina the responses to stimulation of the parasympathetic innervation are blocked 20—30 min after addition of hemicholinium (CHANG and RAND, 1960). Moreover, in spontaneously beating rabbit sinoatrial node-right atrium preparations, in which stimulation of intranodal autonomic fibres causes a decrease in the heart frequency followed by an increase, hemicholinium (200 μg/ml) has a different effect on the two phases of the response (APPEL and VINCENZI, 1970). It abolishes the negative chronotropic response without affecting the positive chronotropic response. On the other hand, bretylium (5 μg/ml) suppresses the positive chronotropic response and decreases the negative chronotropic response only a little. Hemicholinium does not inhibit the block of the positive chronotropic effect of bretylium.

The effect of hemicholinium on noradrenaline release has not been studied.

4. Effects of Sympathetic Denervation on Choline Acetyltransferase Content

There is evidence that, although parasympathetic denervation causes a fall in choline acetyltransferase content, sympathetic denervation does not cause a reduction in this enzyme in the salivary glands of the cat (NORDENFELDT, 1963, 1965).

5. Effects of Botulinum Toxin on the Response to Stimulation of Sympathetic Nerves

Botulinum toxin blocks the release of acetylcholine from the motor nerves of skeletal muscle (BURGEN et al., 1949) and from autonomic preganglionic nerves (AMBACHE, 1951). AMBACHE (1951) found that adrenergic nerves to the dilator muscle of the pupil and the nictitating membrane are resistant to botulinum toxin but RAND and WHALER (1965) and WESTWOOD and WHALER (1968) produced evidence for the view that postganglionic transmission in the vas deferens can be blocked by the toxin. No determinations of noradrenaline release have been made.

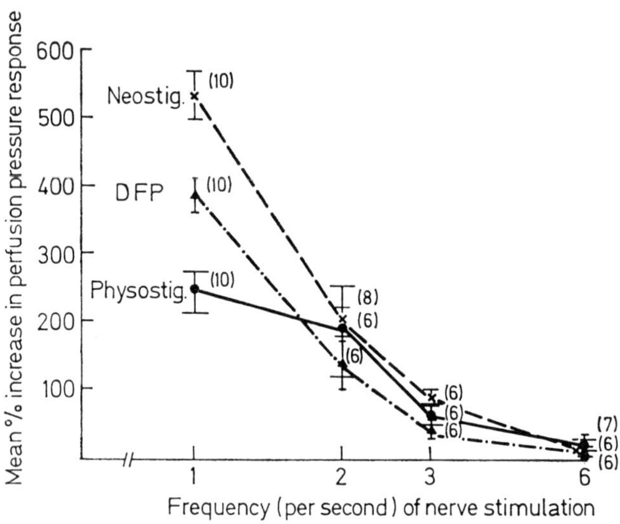

Fig. 1. Effect of the infusion of physostigmine, neostigmine and diisopropylfluorophosphate (DFP) on the responses of perfused mesenteric arteries of rat to sympathetic nerve stimulation at different frequencies. The mesenteric arteries were perfused with Tyrode's solution at a rate of 25 ml/min at 30°C. The perivascular nerves were stimulated with biphasic rectangular pulses (20 V; 1 msec) at different frequencies every 4 min for 20—40 sec. After recording four to six control responses to stimulation, physostigmine (6 μg/ml), neostigmine (2 μg/ml) or DFP (2 μg/ml) was infused for periods of 20—25 min and further responses recorded. Solid circles, effect of physostigmine; crosses, effect of neostigmine; triangles, effect of DFP. Ordinate: mean increase in response expressed as percentage of the control responses; abscissa: frequency (Hz) of nerve stimulation. The number in parentheses indicates the number of preparations perfused and the vertical bars S.E. of the mean. By courtesy of J.H. BURN

6. Effects of Anticholinesterases on the Responses to Stimulation of Sympathetic Nerves and on Release of Noradrenaline

The results obtained with anticholinesterases on the responses of the nictitating membrane of the cat are somewhat equivocal. The difficulty arises from the fact that it is not possible to exclude actions other than inhibition of cholinesterase. BURN et al. (1963) found that physostigmine increased the contraction of the nictitating membrane evoked by submaximal stimulation of the postganglionic nerves and that this increase was only partly prevented by atropine. BOWMAN et al. (1964) obtained variable results but the most consistent effect of large doses of physostigmine was a depression and prolongation of the contractions. In 10 out of 15 experiments they found an increase in the contractor responses. MIRKIN and CERVONI (1962) found no potentiation by physostigmine. In intact cats and in the isolated nerve-smooth preparation of the nictitating membrane, physostigmine, neostigmine and tetraethylpyrophosphate caused a reduction in the response to nerve stimulation, probably by a direct depression of the smooth muscle; at the same time, contractions due to acetylcholine were slightly potentiated (GARDINER et al., 1962).

Physostigmine has no effect on transmission in the innervated mesenteric artery preparation of the rat (McGREGOR, 1965) or in the recurrent cardiac nerve-pulmonary artery preparation stimulated at frequencies of 2—100 Hz (BEVAN and SU, 1964). On the other hand, BURN and MALIK (1970) showed that physostigmine, neostigmine or diisopropylfluorophosphate increases the responses of the innervated mesenteric artery preparation at low frequencies of stimulation, the maximum effect being obtained at 1 Hz but only a negligible effect at 6 Hz (Fig. 1). In the rabbit isolated heart perfused with McEwen's solution containing atropine and choline, the positive chronotropic effect caused by stimulation of the stellate ganglion is increased by physostigmine and neostigmine; this effect is also more marked at low than at high frequencies of stimulation (HUKOVIĆ, 1966). This experimental procedure, however, does not exclude stimulation of preganglionic fibres.

In the saline-perfused isolated spleen of the cat, THOENEN et al. (1966) investigated the actions of physostigmine, neostigmine, diisopropylfluorophosphate and sarin on the responses of the volume of the spleen and its vascular resistance either to stimulation of the splenic nerves or to injected acetylcholine. Whereas the effects of acetylcholine on the responses were increased by anticholinesterases, the effects of nerve stimulation (2—6 Hz) were unaffected. Only high concentrations of physostigmine (100 μg/ml) increased the responses to nerve stimulation but the output of noradrenaline in the splenic effluent evoked by nerve stimulation was not increased by low or high concentrations of physostigmine. These findings on noradrenaline output confirm earlier observations by BLAKELEY et al. (1963).

7. Effects of Acetylcholine and Other Cholinominetic Compounds on the Release of Noradrenaline

As stated earlier, the measurement of the release of noradrenaline is likely to give more information on the mode of action of acetylcholine than the responses of the effector organs. BRANDON and BOYD (1962) showed that noradrenaline appears in the venous effluent from the spleen of the cat after close-arterial injection of acetylcholine, an observation which was confirmed by BLAKELEY et al. (1963). The latter authors also showed that the release of noradrenaline by injection of large amounts of acetylcholine is prevented by hexamethonium which, however, does not affect the motor responses of the splenic blood vessels to nerve stimulation and has no effect on the output of noradrenaline after nerve stimulation. These two different effects of hexamethonium appear not to be compatible with the view that the nerve impulse liberates acetylcholine which, in turn, releases noradrenaline. It is quite possible, however, that, in view of the low lipid solubility of hexamethonium, only exogenous acetylcholine is blocked whereas acetylcholine liberated within the nerve terminal remains unaffected (BURN and FROEDE, 1963). On the other hand, pempidine, which penetrates membranes readily, has an effect similar to that of hexamethonium (HERTTING and WIDHALM, 1965). BURN and GIBBONS (1964a) suggested another explanation for this discrepancy, namely that hexamethonium prevents the sympathomimetic effect of acetylcholine not by blocking cholinoceptors but by preventing access of acetylcholine to them.

Most of the recent investigations on the action of cholinomimetic agents have been on the rabbit isolated heart. RICHARDSON and WOOD (1959) were the first to show that acetylcholine causes a release of noradrenaline; a similar finding was obtained by LINDMAR and MUSCHOLL (1961) on the perfused rabbit heart with the nicotinic stimulant drug, dimethylphenylpiperazinium, the action of which is prevented by hexamethonium. It was found later (LINDMAR et al., 1968) that high concentrations of acetylcholine increase the resting output of noradrenaline only a little but that this output is greatly enhanced by the presence of atropine (1 ng—1 μg/ml). In contrast, the large output of noradrenaline induced by dimethylphenylpiperazinium is not affected by moderate concentrations of atropine (1 μg/ml); higher concentrations of atropine depress the noradrenaline

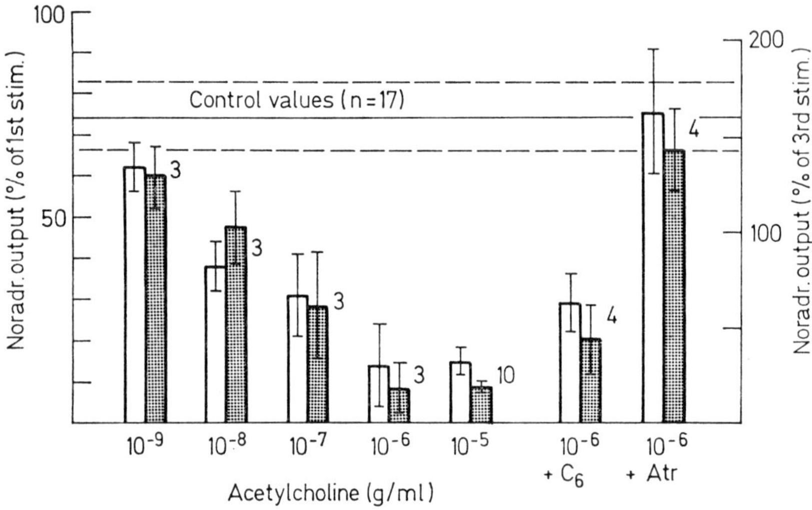

Fig. 2. Effect of acetylcholine on the noradrenaline output of the rabbit heart evoked by sympathetic nerve stimulation. The columns indicate noradrenaline output evoked during the second period of stimulation (in the presence of acetylcholine) as percentage of the two control values (without acetylcholine) obtained in the first period (ordinate at left margin, open columns) and in the third period (ordinate at right margin, shaded columns). The scale of the ordinate at the right margin was adapted in such a way that the two control values lay on one horizontal line at the top of the graph. The lower broken line indicates the S.E. of the control value corresponding to the left ordinate, the upper broken line shows the S.E. of the control value corresponding to the right ordinate. Vertical bars at the tops of the columns indicate S.E. of the mean and the figures beside the columns indicate the number of experiments. C_6, hexamethonium (3 μg/ml) *atr*, atropine (1 μg/ml) present throughout the experiment. Reproduced, with permission, from LÖFFELHOLZ and MUSCHOLL (1969)

release after acetylcholine or dimethylphenylpiperazinium. The noradrenaline release caused by dimethylphenylpiperazinium is depressed by acetylcholine, pilocarpine and methacholine; this inhibitory action of metacholine is reversed by atropine. LINDMAR et al. (1968) concluded from these findings that the peripheral adrenergic nerve fibres contain inhibitory muscarinic receptors in addition to nicotinic receptors mediating noradrenaline release. Because the muscarinic receptors are excited by much lower concentrations of acetylcholine than the nicotinic receptors, a substantial noradrenaline release is produced by acetylcholine only if its muscarinic action is blocked.

The inhibitory effects of the muscarinic drugs (RAND and VARMA, 1970a, b), acetylcholine, methacholine, muscarine, McN-A-343 (4-(m-chlorophenylcarbamoyloxy)-2-butynyltrimethylammonium chloride) on the vasoconstrictor responses of the rabbit perfused ear artery to sympathetic nerve stimulation at low frequencies can be explained by a depression of noradrenaline release.

In recent experiments, LÖFFELHOLZ and MUSCHOLL (1969) showed that, in the perfused heart of the rabbit, the reduction by acetylcholine of the noradrenaline release evoked by stimulation of the sympathetic nerves is dose-dependent for a range of 1 ng to 1 μg/ml (Fig. 2), whereas a concentration of 100 μg/ml or more is required to cause a release of noradrenaline. While the inhibitory action of low concentrations of acetylcholine is blocked by atropine and is not affected by hexamethonium, the excitatory action of the higher concentrations of acetylcholine is blocked by hexamethonium. These findings confirm the earlier obser-

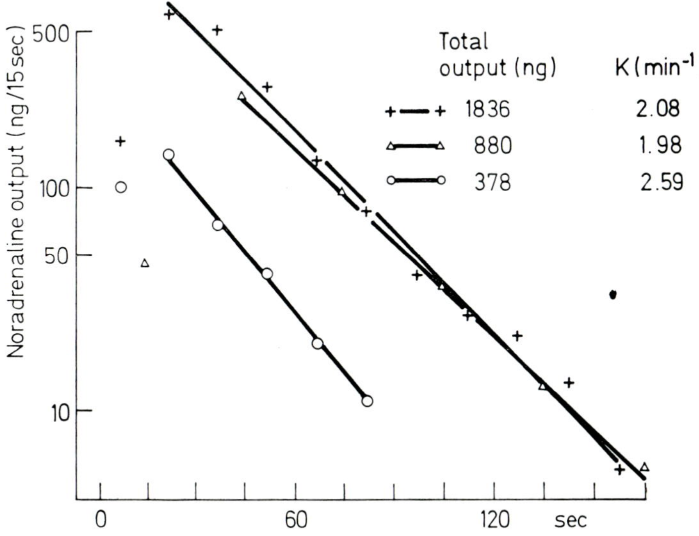

Fig. 3. Time-course of noradrenaline output during constant infusion of nicotinic drugs into isolated rabbit hearts. Ordinate, noradrenaline output (ng/15 sec; logarithmic scale). Abscissa, time (sec; linear scale) after start of infusion of dimethylphenylpiperazinium (3.1×10^{-5}M, triangles), or of acetylcholine (2.1×10^{-4}M) in the presence of atropine (crosses), or absence of atropine (circles). The perfusate samples were collected in periods of 15 sec (acetylcholine), or of 30 sec (dimethylphenylpiperazinium). In all experiments the outputs were expressed as ng/15 sec. K is the rate constant. For the calculation of the regression lines the first noradrenaline output was disregarded. Reproduced, with permission, from LÖFFELHOLZ (1970a)

vations that the inhibitory effect of acetylcholine on noradrenaline release is mediated by muscarinic receptors. This view obtains further support from the observation that dimethylphenylpiperazinium (1 μg/ml) has no inhibitory effect on noradrenaline release. Dimethylphenylpiperazinium (10 μg/ml) causes release of noradrenaline but does not affect the output of noradrenaline due to nerve stimulation if it is applied 3 min before nerve stimulation since it has only a brief action.

LÖFFELHOLZ (1967) showed that, when the isolated heart of the rabbit is perfused with acetylcholine at a constant concentration (100 μg/ml) for 10 min, an increased output of noradrenaline is observed only during the first 2 min of the perfusion. In a later investigation (LÖFFELHOLZ, 1970a), it was found that the dose-dependent activation of nicotinic receptors by acetylcholine, nicotine or dimethylphenylpiperazinium causes a release of noradrenaline which is terminated after 5—10 sec. Increases in heart rate in response to nicotine and dimethylphenylpiperazinium and increases in amplitude of contraction in response to acetylcholine plus atropine and to nicotine and dimethylphenylpiperazinium are related to the output of noradrenaline. The dose-response curves of the release of noradrenaline are parallel; the ED_{50} of dimethylphenylpiperazinium, nicotine and acetylcholine plus atropine are 2.1×10^{-5} M, 2.4×10^{-5} M and 1.1×10^{-4} M, respectively. During infusion of nicotinic drugs, the noradrenaline output rises to its maximum within 30 sec and then declines exponentially (Fig. 3). The rate constant (1.98—2.59/min) is not significantly different from the rate constant of the slow phase of washout after an infusion of noradrenaline (1.98—2.95/min), a fact which

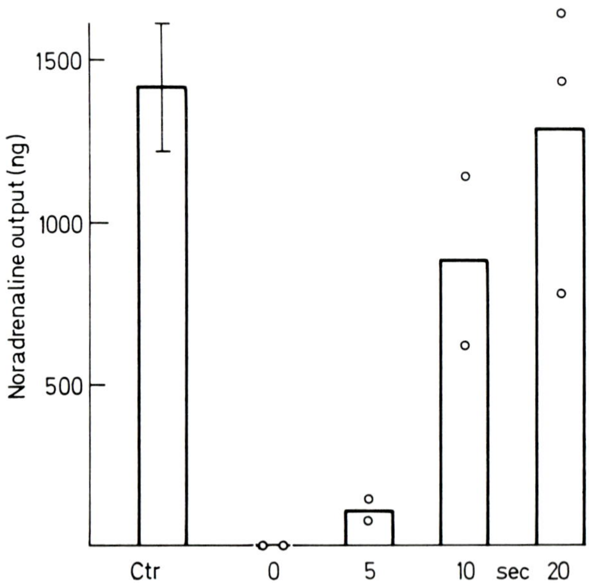

Fig. 4. Block by hexamethonium of acetylcholine-induced noradrenaline output. The columns indicate mean noradrenaline output (ng) evoked by acetylcholine (2.1×10^{-4} M) in the presence of atropine (1.4×10^{-6} M). Control (Ctr), noradrenaline output in the absence of hexamethonium (mean of 5 observations ± S.E.). The figures at the base of the columns indicate the time of addition (sec) of hexamethonium (1.1×10^{-5} M) after beginning of perfusion with acetylcholine. The vertical bar indicates S.E. of the mean; the individual figures are marked by open circles. Reproduced, with permission, from LÖFFELHOLZ (1970a)

indicates that release of noradrenaline takes place only during the first 30 sec of acetylcholine infusion. The facilitatory effect of atropine on noradrenaline release and the blocking effect of hexamethonium is observed only in the first 5—10 sec of an infusion of acetylcholine (Fig. 4). Moreover, pre-infusion with low concentrations of acetylcholine or nicotine blocks the noradrenaline output caused by a subsequent infusion of acetylcholine or nicotine in higher concentrations. Thus, nicotinic excitation causes a sudden and large release of noradrenaline which is rapidly terminated by autoinhibition.

Important for the physiological significance of these findings is the observation by LÖFFELHOLZ (1970b) that, when the nicotinic block or autoinhibition is established, release of noradrenaline evoked by electrical stimulation is not inhibited (Fig. 5). In contrast, activation of the muscarinic receptors by acetylcholine, methacholine or pilocarpine inhibits noradrenaline release caused either by nervous stimulation or drug stimulation of the nicotinic receptors (LINDMAR et al., 1968; LÖFFELHOLZ and MUSCHOLL, 1969). In the presence of atropine,

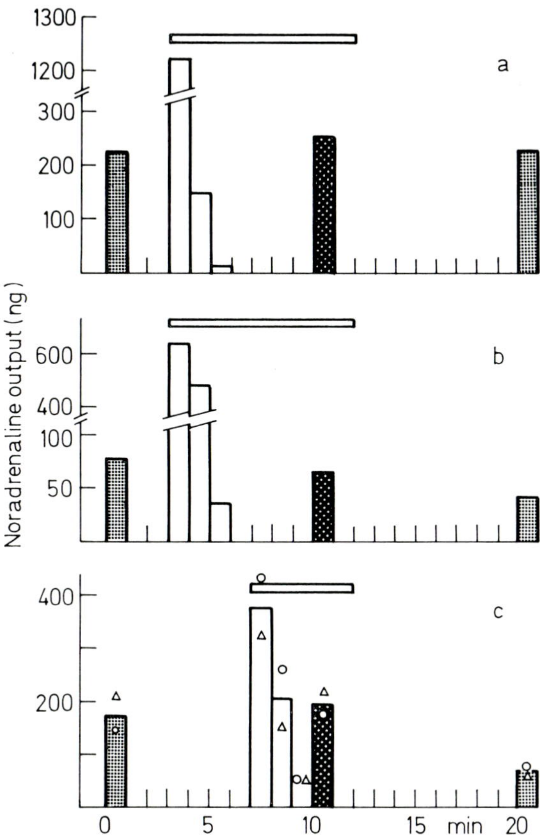

Fig. 5a—c. Effect of acetylcholine (in the presence of atropine), nicotine, or dimethylphenylpiperazinium on the noradrenaline output evoked by sympathetic nerve stimulation. Ordinate, output of noradrenaline (ng). Abscissa, time-course of experiment (min). Columns indicate output of noradrenaline obtained by single experiments (a and b), or by calculating the mean of 2 observations (c), each marked by a different symbol. The horizontal bars indicate infusion of the nicotinic drugs: acetylcholine (2.1×10^{-4}M) (a), nicotine (4×10^{-5}M) (b) and dimethylphenylpiperazinium (3.1×10^{-5}M) (c). Hatched columns, noradrenaline output evoked by standard stimulation of postganglionic nerves in the absence of a nicotinic drug. In a, atropine (1.4×10^{-6}M) present throughout the experiment. Stippled columns, noradrenaline output evoked by nerve stimulation in the presence of acetylcholine plus atropine, nicotine, or dimethylphenylpiperazinium. Open columns, drug-induced output of noradrenaline. Reproduced, with permission, from LÖFFELHOLZ (1970b)

acetylcholine facilitates neurogenic noradrenaline release for more than 1 min but less than 4 min (Fig. 6) (LÖFFELHOLZ, 1970b). This evidence suggests that postganglionic sympathetic transmission does not involve excitation of nicotinic receptors. The block of these receptors which occurs very readily resembles the non-depolarizing block observed in autonomic ganglia.

8. Effects of Dimethylphenylpiperazinium on the Responses to Stimulation of Sympathetic Nerves and on the Release of Noradrenaline

In their experiments on the release of noradrenaline from the perfused rabbit heart by cholinomimetic agents, MUSCHOLL and his colleagues (LINDMAR and MUSCHOLL, 1961; LINDMAR et al., 1968; LÖFFELHOLZ and MUSCHOLL, 1969; LÖFFELHOLZ, 1970a, b; MUSCHOLL, 1970) used acetylcholine in the presence of atropine, nicotine or dimethylphenylpiperazinium as nicotinic stimulating agents. It is therefore of importance that dimethylphenylpiperazinium may have actions other than the excitation of nicotinic receptors. For instance, the positive chronotropic and inotropic actions caused by nicotine and dimethylphenylpiperazinium on guinea-pig and rat isolated atria in the presence of atropine are abolished by pretreatment with reserpine; hexamethonium antagonizes the effect of nicotine but not that of dimethylphenylpiperazinium (LINDMAR, 1962). These findings were confirmed for the guinea-pig atria by BHAGAT (1966); BHAGAT et al. (1967b) showed that hexamethonium interferes with the nicotine-induced release of tritiated noradrenaline from guinea-pig isolated atria but does not affect the release caused by dimethylphenylpiperazinium or tyramine. Tritiated noradrenaline stored extraneuronally in guinea-pig isolated atria is partly released by dimethylphenylpiperazinium and tyramine but not by nicotine (BHAGAT et al., 1967a).

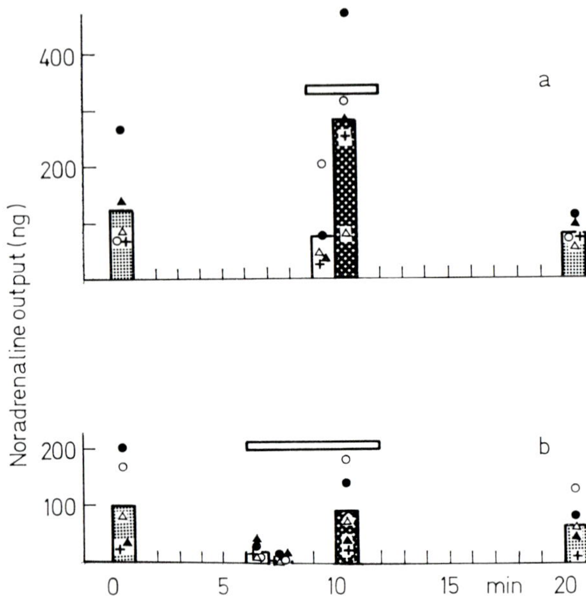

Fig. 6a and b. Facilitation by acetylcholine in the presence of atropine of the noradrenaline output evoked by sympathetic nerve stimulation. Ordinate, output of noradrenaline (ng). Abscissa, time course of experiment (min). Horizontal bars indicate infusion of acetylcholine (5.5×10^{-5} M) and columns the mean output of noradrenaline (ng); the individual results are marked by symbols. Atropine (1.4×10^{-6} M) was present throughout the experiments. Note facilitation of noradrenaline output evoked by nerve stimulation after 1 min (a) but not after 4 min (b) of infusion of acetylcholine. Columns as in Fig. 5. Reproduced, with permission, from LÖFFELHOLZ (1970b)

While this effect of dimethylphenylpiperazinium on guinea-pig and rat atria is tyramine-like rather than nicotine-like, pharmacological analysis has shown that the action on the perfused rabbit heart is nicotinic and not tyramine-like (LINDMAR and MUSCHOLL, 1961). Moreover, the time course of noradrenaline release by dimethylphenylpiperazinium is similar to that caused by acetylcholine in the presence of atropine and different from that induced by tyramine which, in contrast to the transient release by dimethylphenylpiperazinium, causes a constant release of noradrenaline throughout the infusion of tyramine (LINDMAR et al., 1967).

Another action of dimethylphenylpiperazinium which may complicate interpretation, is its bretylium-like effect. BIRMINGHAM and WILSON (1965) found that, in the Finkleman preparation of the small intestine of the guinea-pig and rabbit, dimethylphenylpiperazinium (0.2—5.0 μg/ml) depresses the inhibitory effects of sympathetic nerve stimulation but does not reduce the inhibitory action of noradrenaline. This effect is readily reversed by dopamine or dexamphetamine but not by washing; it is therefore similar to that of bretylium and guanethidine.

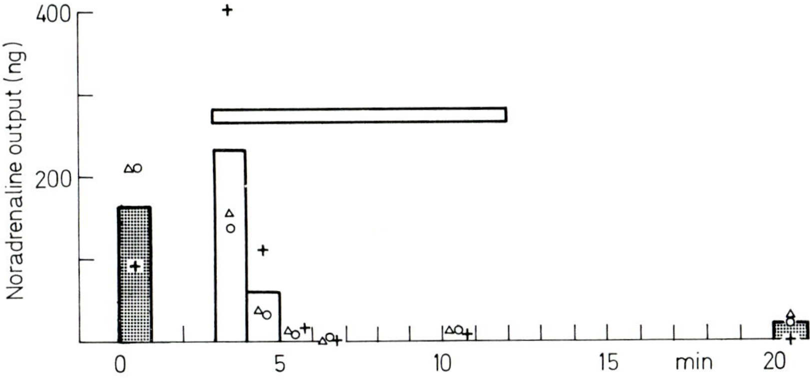

Fig. 7. Late occurring block by dimethylphenylpiperazinium of the noradrenaline output evoked by sympathetic nerve stimulation. Ordinate, output of noradrenaline (ng). Abscissa, time course of experiment (min). Horizontal bar indicates infusion of dimethylphenylpiperazinium (3.1×10^{-5}M) and the columns the mean output of noradrenaline (ng); the individual results are marked by symbols. Sympathetic nerve stimulation during 1st, 11th and 21st min. Reproduced, with permission, from LÖFFELHOLZ (1970b)

This finding was confirmed for the rat mesenteric artery by MALIK and LING (1969b) who also showed that the block induced by dimethylphenylpiperazinium (0.3 μg/ml) is reversed by increasing the calcium concentration or by adding dexamphetamine. This block is produced only after an infusion lasting for 16—40 min; when dimethylphenylpiperazinium is infused for periods of 3 min, it enhances the vasoconstriction due to nerve stimulation, probably by its nicotinic stimulant action.

The nicotinic effect and the bretylium-like action of dimethylphenylpiperazinium can be separated. The nicotinic effect on the rabbit heart is antagonized by hexamethonium (LINDMAR and MUSCHOLL, 1961) whereas the neurone-blocking effect in the rat mesenteric artery (MALIK and LING, 1969b) or the rabbit pulmonary artery (NEDERGAARD and BEVAN, 1969) is not affected by hexamethonium. The contractor response of the rabbit pulmonary artery to postganglionic sympathetic stimulation is not blocked by hexamethonium, mecamylamine or nicotine. LÖFFELHOLZ (1970b) has shown that in the early phase (4 min) of infusion of dimethylphenylpiperazinium, when a nicotinic block has occurred by autoinhibition, nerve stimulation still causes release of noradrenaline (Fig. 5) but at a later stage (8 min) noradrenaline is no longer released by nerve stimulation (Fig. 7). In contrast, when the block of nicotinic receptors is produced by acetylcholine, the release of noradrenaline by nerve stimulation remains unaffected (Fig. 5A). BIRMINGHAM and WILSON (1965) also stressed that the stimulating and blocking effects of dimethylphenylpiperazinium on ganglionic transmission occur sooner than its adrenergic neurone-blocking action.

9. Effects of Adrenergic Neurone Blocking Agents on the Responses of Sympathetic Neuroeffectors to Acetylcholine or Nerve Stimulation and on the Release of Noradrenaline

BURN (1961) put forward the hypothesis that bretylium acts as an adrenergic neurone blocking agent because it interacts with the acetylcholine liberated at the cholinergic link and thus prevents it from releasing noradrenaline. BURN and GIBBONS (1964b) later showed that, in the rabbit isolated ileum, hexamethonium prevents the blocking effect of bretylium on the inhibitory response to stimulation of the periarterial nerves; they interpreted this observation to mean that hexamethonium prevents the entry of bretylium into sympathetic fibres and probably prevents the action of acetylcholine in the same way.

Whereas hexamethonium blocks the responses of the spleen, rabbit heart, rabbit ileum and other sympathetic neuroeffectors to acetylcholine but not to stimulation of the postganglionic sympathetic nerves, bretylium can block both types of responses (BRANDON and RAND, 1961; BURN and GIBBONS, 1964b; HUKOVIĆ, 1960). The contraction of the pilomotor muscles of the cat tail, caused by high concentrations of acetylcholine, is blocked by hexamethonium which, however, does not affect the contraction induced by electrical stimulation of the postganglionic nerve supply. On the other hand, bretylium blocks the response to nerve stimulation without affecting the acetylcholine-induced contraction (WOLNER, 1965). Bretylium blocks the release of noradrenaline by acetylcholine and by nerve stimulation in the isolated perfused heart and, less regularly, in the isolated perfused spleen of the cat (HAEUSLER et al., 1969b; KRAUSS et al., 1970). Guanethidine prevents the release of noradrenaline in the isolated perfused heart of the rabbit by dimethylphenylpiperazinium (LINDMAR and MUSCHOLL, 1961) and nerve stimulation (HUKOVIĆ and MUSCHOLL, 1962).

In view of these findings, it is important for the elucidation of the mechanism by which acetylcholine acts to review more fully the evidence which may explain the actions of bretylium and guanethidine. According to FERRY (1963), acetylcholine acts upon the membrane of the nerve fibre of the spleen at or near the termination to cause a gradual depolarization. When this reaches a certain level, an all-or-none nerve impulse is set up and propagated both peripherally and centrally along the nerve fibre. By using the collision technique of DOUGLAS and RITCHIE (1957) it was shown that close-arterial injection of acetylcholine causes antidromic activation of 33—50% of the splenic C fibres. The invasion of the nerve terminal causes the release of the transmitter. Similar observations were made by CABRERA et al. (1966b) on the cat heart. These authors found that orthodromically conducted action potentials in cardiac nerves are reduced in size when acetylcholine or nicotine is injected into the left atrium, an observation which indicates the generation of antidromically conducted action potentials. The antidromic discharges are depressed by (+)-tubocurarine, bretylium, guanethidine and local anaesthetics.

HAEUSLER et al. (1968b) investigated the effects of acetylcholine, dimethylphenylpiperazinium and KCl on the cat isolated heart. Infusion of acetylcholine (50—80 μg/ml) induces asynchronous antidromically-conducted action potentials in the cardiac nerves and a release of noradrenaline. An increase in the concentration of acetylcholine or addition of atropine (Fig. 8) shortens the duration of the antidromic discharge but increases the amount of noradrenaline released. At very low concentrations, dimethylphenylpiperazinium causes continuous firing but at higher concentrations the antidromic discharges are restricted to the first few seconds of infusion. Since after destruction of the sympathetic nerve terminals by 6-hydroxydopamine (THOENEN and TRANZER, 1968) acetylcholine no longer evokes an antidromic discharge, it is assumed that these action potentials may

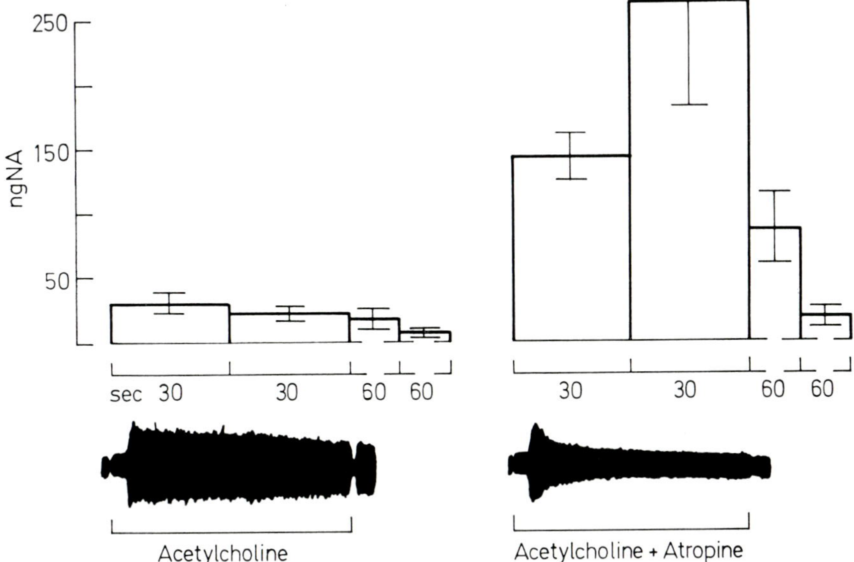

Fig. 8. Antidromic discharges induced by one-minute infusions of acetylcholine (50—80 μg/ml) in the absence and presence of atropine (1 μg/ml). The coronary perfusate collected during the infusion was fractionated in 30-sec samples. In addition, the amount of noradrenaline was estimated in two one-minute samples following the infusion of acetylcholine. Note that an appreciable amount of noradrenaline is liberated during that period of infusion of acetylcholine in which no asynchronous discharges can be recorded. Reproduced, with permission, from HAEUSLER et al. (1968b)

originate from the nerve terminals. Potassium chloride (>50 mM) induces very brief firing and a dose-dependent release of noradrenaline. It is concluded that the action potentials induced by acetylcholine or dimethylphenylpiperazinium contribute only little to the release of noradrenaline by these drugs. In this connection it should be remembered, however, that in the rabbit perfused heart, the actual release of noradrenaline by acetylcholine, nicotine or dimethylphenylpiperazinium is confined to the first 5—10 sec of the infusion of the drug (LÖFFELHOLZ, 1970a).

HERTTING and WIDHALM (1965) found that, in the perfused isolated spleen of the cat, atropine (8 μg/ml) and pempidine (0.2 μg/ml) inhibit the contraction of the spleen and the release of H^3-noradrenaline caused by acetylcholine or dimethylphenylpiperazinium but not the effects of electrical stimulation of the splenic nerve. On the other hand, bretylium (2.5—10 μg/ml) blocks only the effects of nerve stimulation but not those due to acetylcholine or dimethylphenylpiperazinium. A higher concentration of bretylium (50 μg/ml) is necessary to decrease the effects of acetylcholine or dimethylphenylpiperazinium. Similar results were obtained by FISCHER et al. (1966) who also showed that H^3-bretylium is taken up by the heart and spleen of the cat and released by nerve stimulation but not by acetylcholine, a fact which indicates that bretylium is not taken up by the noradrenaline storage sites.

These observations were re-examined by DAVEY et al. (1968) on the spleen *in situ*. Hexamethonium abolishes the antidromic excitation of the C fibres of the splenic nerve and the release of noradrenaline by close arterial injection of acetylcholine whereas the liberation of noradrenaline by electrical stimulation of the splenic nerve is unaffected. Low doses of bretylium (0.5—1 mg) depress the contractions and the noradrenaline release due to nerve stimulation much more than the contractions and release caused by acetylcholine. This differential action of bretylium is not seen with large doses (2—4 mg). Dexamphetamine partially restores the effects of both acetylcholine and nerve stimulation. It is of importance that the differential effect of bretylium is seen only with a stimulus frequency of 30 Hz and is absent at 10 Hz. The antidromic discharge of the C fibres is more resistant to bretylium than its noradrenaline-releasing effect. This may be explained by the fact that bretylium is more effective in blocking at high than low frequencies of stimulation. In this context it is of interest to note that the order of frequency of the antidromic discharge is estimated to be 5.4 spikes/sec. DAVEY et al. (1968) therefore hold the view that the conclusion reached by FISCHER et al. (1966) is probably incorrect, namely that bretylium blocks the nerve at a site proximal to the action of acetylcholine. Since acetylcholine, in the presence of bretylium in a concentration sufficient to prevent noradrenaline release, still causes antidromic discharge, bretylium prevents stimulus-transmitter release coupling without blocking conduction.

In a recent analysis of the action of bretylium, HAEUSLER et al. (1969b) arrived at the following conclusions: in the perfused heart of the cat, bretylium and tetracaine depress and, in sufficiently high concentrations, block acetylcholine-induced and KCl-induced antidromic discharges in the cardiac nerves. Acetylcholine-induced release of noradrenaline in the heart is somewhat more resistant to the action of bretylium than the acetylcholine-induced antidromic discharges in the cardiac nerve. In the sinus nerve of the perfused carotid sinus preparation, tetracaine is about 1,000 times more potent as a local anaesthetic than bretylium but in the cardiac nerves the two drugs are approximately equipotent. In the postganglionic sympathetic nerves to the heart and the spleen, the effect of bretylium develops slowly and has a long duration while the effect of tetracaine comes on rapidly and is rapidly washed out. It was concluded by HAEUSLER et al. (1969b) that bretylium, although a weak local anaesthetic, has a selective local anaesthetic action on the adrenergic nerve terminals because of its high accumulation in the endings (BOURA and GREEN, 1959, 1965; BOURA et al., 1960; EXLEY, 1960).

In view of the inhibitory effects of bretylium on the antidromic discharges induced by acetylcholine or KCl, HAEUSLER et al. (1969b) explain the blocking actions of bretylium on the effects of stimulation of adrenergic nerves by a stabilization of the membrane. There is no evidence that bretylium causes a local depolarization; the weak antinicotine action of bretylium (BOURA and GREEN, 1959; KOSTERLITZ and LEES, 1961; RAND and WILSON, 1967) is of minor importance because bretylium also blocks KCl-induced discharges. For an analysis of the effects of bretylium, it is important to remember that the anti-nicotine effect develops rapidly and is easily reversed by washing out of the drug, whereas the adrenergic neurone-blocking effect comes on more slowly and is not readily reversed.

An essentially similar mode of action has been described for guanethidine (HAEUSLER et al., 1968a; HAEUSLER et al., 1969a).

Recently, another view of the action of bretylium has received support (ABBS and ROBERTSON, 1970). It has been found that bretylium causes depletion of noradrenaline only in the supernatant fraction of a homogenate of cat spleen and that there is a good correlation of the depletion of this particular "store" with the adrenergic neurone-blocking action of bretylium. There are so far no data whether the blockade of acetylcholine-induced release of noradrenaline may be explained on a similar basis.

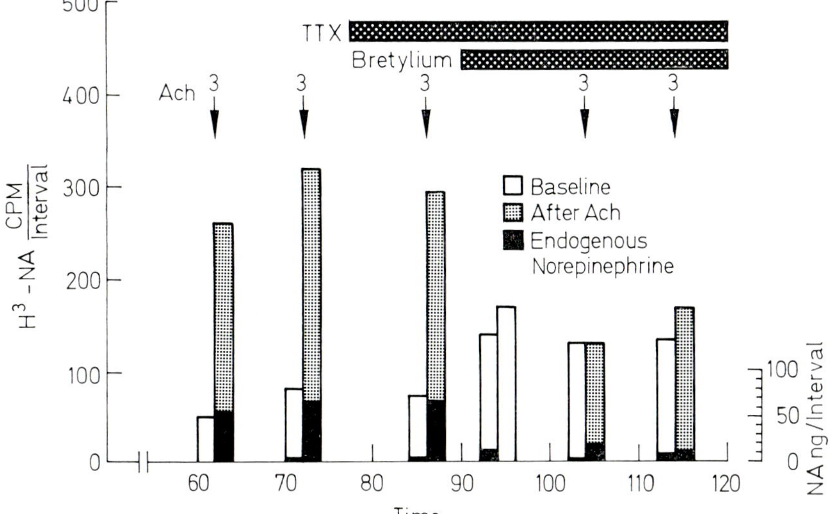

Fig. 9. Endogenous and H^3-noradrenaline present in the venous effluent of a perfused cat spleen. Release of H^3-noradrenaline (*NE*) by successive 3-mg doses of acetylcholine (*Ach*) are indicated as cross-hatched bars. Control efflux is shown in the immediately preceding sample. Scale on right indicates endogenous noradrenaline content of these samples (filled bars). Perfusion with tetrodotoxin (*TTX*) did not abolish the response to acetylcholine. Bretylium tosylate (50 μg/ml) perfused simultaneously with tetrodotoxin markedly reduced the release of labelled and unlabelled noradrenaline evoked by acetylcholine. Reproduced, with permission, from KRAUSS et al. (1970)

Since in the heart, tetrodotoxin (10^{-8}M) does not affect the release of noradrenaline by acetylcholine, it would appear that this release is not necessarily mediated by nervous conduction although the antidromic discharges are blocked (HAEUSLER et al., 1969c). Therefore, the changes in membrane potential by nicotinic agents may be of importance only in so far as they facilitate entry of Ca^{2+}.

In the isolated perfused spleen of the cat, tetrodotoxin (0.1 μg/ml) prevents the release of noradrenaline induced by stimulation of the splenic nerve; it also blocks the antidromic discharges produced by acetylcholine in the splenic nerve but does not abolish the noradrenaline release induced by acetylcholine (KRAUSS et al., 1970). When bretylium is injected rapidly in doses of 1—20 mg during continuous infusion of tetrodotoxin, it does not abolish the release of noradrenaline by acetylcholine. On the other hand, if bretylium (50 μg/ml) is perfused simultaneously with tetrodotoxin, the release of noradrenaline by acetylcholine is depressed (Fig. 9). This observation is in agreement with the findings of HAEUSLER et al. (1969b) that the action of bretylium develops slowly and increases during the course of a perfusion with bretylium.

From the results obtained with tetrodotoxin and bretylium on the rabbit heart and the cat spleen it is likely that the release of noradrenaline by acetylcholine may come about in two ways. Acetylcholine may set up action potentials in the sympathetic nerve fibre and thus release noradrenaline; this effect is blocked by tetrodotoxin or bretylium. The second type of action does not involve propagated action potentials in the nerve fibre since noradrenaline release still proceeds in the presence of tetrodotoxin; this effect is blocked by more prolonged exposure to bretylium. It is this second type of action of acetylcholine which may be the basis of the finding of BURN and GIBBONS (1964a) with regard to the importance of Ca^{2+} for noradrenaline release from postganglionic sympathetic nerve terminals; this observation will be considered later (p. 781).

IV. Morphological and Physiological Evidence for an Interaction between Cholinergic and Adrenergic Nerve Terminals

From the evidence presented so far, there is little doubt that acetylcholine can, by its nicotinic action, evoke release of noradrenaline from the adrenergic nerve terminal and, by its muscarinic action, reduce this release. If this relationship is due to a course of events as described by the cholinergic link hypothesis, then the adrenergic nerve terminals should contain stores of acetylcholine and of noradrenaline, both probably in the form of vesicles. If, however, cholinergic nerve terminals secrete acetylcholine which then acts on neighbouring noradrenaline-containing adrenergic terminals, there ought to be close apposition of cholinergic and adrenergic nerve terminals.

Two types of vesicles are found in adrenergic nerve terminals, large (type I) and small dense-core vesicles (types II and III, GRILLO and PALAY, 1962). The small granular vesicles are characteristic of central and peripheral adrenergic neurones and represent the main storage sites (HÖKFELT, 1968). There is evidence from observations on the iris and vas deferens of the cat that both types of vesicles contain noradrenaline (TRANZER and THOENEN, 1968). In the spleen, only large vesicles are present in axons but small and large vesicles are seen in the nerve terminals. The main splenic artery has both a cholinergic and an adrenergic supply but only adrenergic fibres are found in the spleen; acetylcholinesterase present in the spleen is confined to non-nervous structures (FILLENZ, 1970).

No unequivocal evidence has ever been obtained for the simultaneous presence of noradrenaline- and acetylcholine-containing vesicles in one and the same terminal. Large dense-core vesicles may be present in cholinergic nerves (GRILLO, 1966; CLEMENTI et al., 1966) but these vesicles do not lose their core after pretreatment of the animals with reserpine (CLEMENTI et al., 1966; FARRELL, 1968). On the other hand, THOENEN et al. (1966) found fibres containing adrenergic vesicles and fibres containing cholinergic vesicles in close apposition (Fig. 10).

Quite recently, EHINGER et al. (1970b) have identified adrenergic vesicles in the nerve terminals in the rat iris and heart by a highly specific method in which the tissues of animals pretreated with 5-hydroxydopamine are fixed with glutaraldehyde and post-fixed with osmium tetroxide (TRANZER and THOENEN, 1967). This technique makes the recognition of adrenergic and cholinergic vesicles much easier. Frequently, the terminal axon bundles contain structures having the characteristics of an axon varicosity, i.e. numerous synaptic vesicles and mitochondria. Usually, the individual axons are isolated from each other by the Schwann cell but not infrequently a varicosity containing adrenergic vesicles lies in close apposition to another preterminal axon or an axon varicosity containing

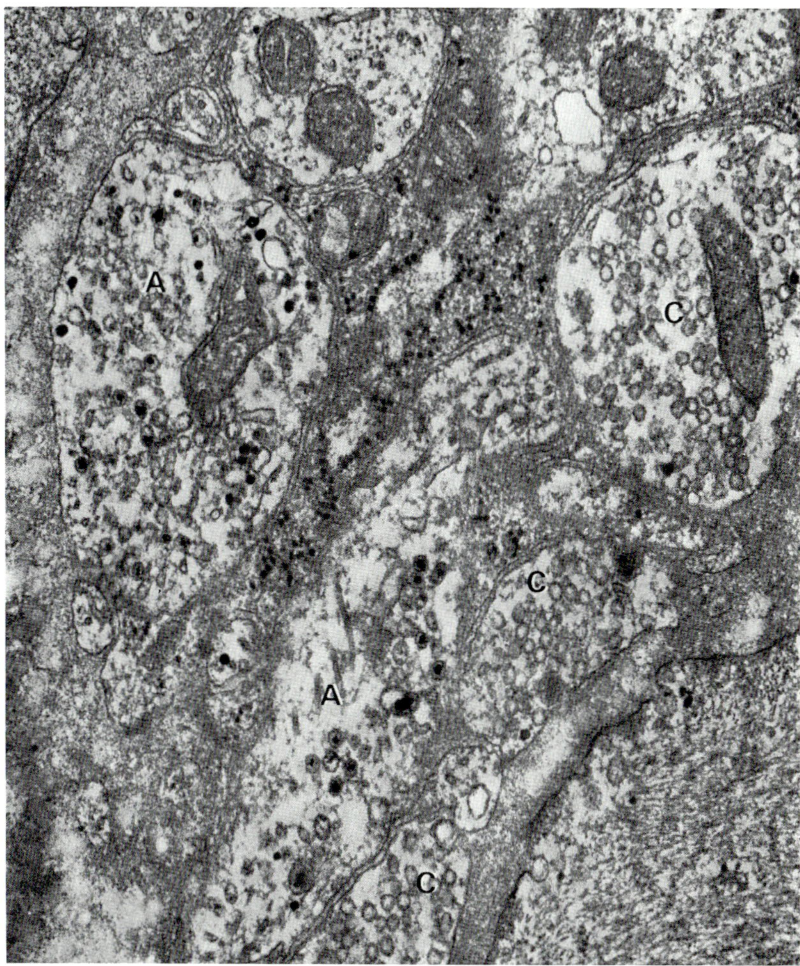

Fig. 10. Electron micrograph. Autonomic nerves of the guinea-pig vas deferens. Magnification: ×50,000. *A*: Adrenergic fibres: *C*: cholinergic fibres. Reproduced, with permission, from THOENEN et al. (1966)

cholinergic vesicles, the distance between the two membranes being of the order of 250 Å. The varicosities contain dense-core vesicles of about 400 Å diameter but larger vesicles of about 800 Å are present in addition to 1000 Å vesicles. No membrane specialization of the type of a truly synaptic structure has been observed in either the iris or the heart but sometimes a slight increase in membrane density has been found between the varicosity containing the adrenergic vesicles and those containing the cholinergic vesicles (Fig. 11).

By staining for cholinesterase and preparing electron autoradiographs for noradrenaline, ESTERHUIZEN et al. (1968) showed for the cat nictitating membrane and GRAHAM et al. (1968) for the arterioles of the cat pancreas that there is no morphological evidence for the simultaneous presence of acetylcholine and noradrenaline stores in one and the same nerve terminal. Cholinergic and adrenergic nerve terminals are closely associated with each other, often being enclosed by the same Schwann cell.

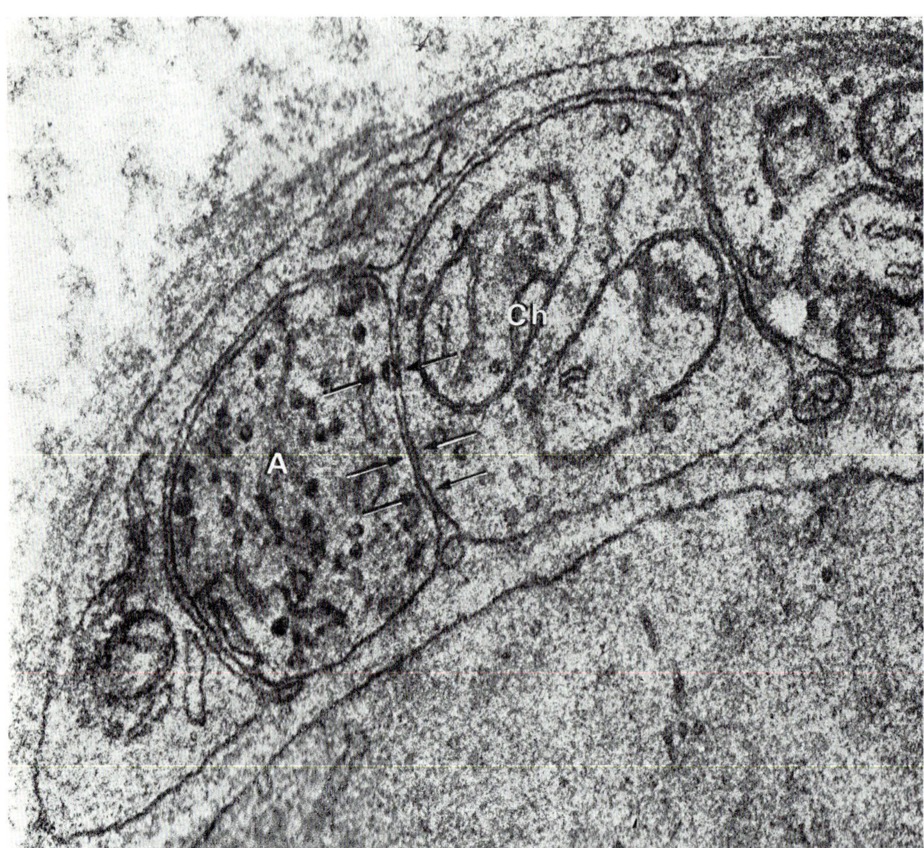

Fig. 11. Electron micrograph. Normal rat atrium. $KMnO_4$. At the close apposition between the cholinergic (*Ch*) and the adrenergic (*A*) varicosities, there is a slight thickening of the membranes. Cleft between varicosities indicated by arrows. Magnification: ×60,000. Reproduced, with permission, from EHINGER et al. (1970a)

Evidence for a close relationship between adrenergic and cholinergic mechanisms has also been obtained by WATERSON et al. (1970) for the central ear artery of the rabbit. By means of a "direct colouring" thiocholine technique for cholinesterase they found discrete heavy deposits of stain near the border between media and adventitia, i.e. near the site of the adrenergic nerve terminals. Treatment with inhibitors showed that the enzyme was preponderantly butyrylcholinesterase with some acetylcholinesterase being also present. Postganglionic denervation by removal of the superior cervical ganglion caused loss of staining except for a few discrete areas near the media. These findings cannot be used as support for the cholinergic link hypothesis since there is no evidence as to the relationship of the cholinesterase to adrenergic nerve terminals.

In the pineal glands of adult albino rats nerve nets showing catecholamine fluorescence and a positive acetylcholinesterase reaction form identical patterns (Eränkö et al., 1970). Bilateral extirpation of the superior cervical ganglia leads to disappearance of the fluorescence and the cholinesterase reaction from the nerve fibres. The results of electron microscopic observations are somewhat equivocal as far as the important question of the site of acetylcholinesterase is concerned. In formaldehyde-fixed specimens the enzyme is found on the axons in the membrane whereas after fixation with glutaraldehyde the enzyme is observed in the form of a chain of fine granules situated outside the axon membrane, between it and the neighbouring Schwann cell membrane.

Ehinger et al. (1970a) showed that, in the cat iris, removal of the ciliary ganglion leads to a loss of at least 95% of the acetylcholine content of the iris whereas removal of the superior cervical ganglion causes no significant change. Therefore, if adrenergic terminals contain any acetylcholine, it is less than what is detectable with present methods, i.e. less than 6% of the acetylcholine content of cholinergic neurones. From these findings and the electron micrographic evidence for axo-axonal synapses, the authors conclude that there is more reason to presume interactions between adrenergic and cholinergic nerve terminals than a cholinergic mechanism in the adrenergic terminals themselves.

Further support for the view that there is interaction between cholinergic and adrenergic nerve terminals was obtained by Löffelholz and Muscholl (1970). They determined the output of noradrenaline from perfused rabbit atria in the presence of dexamphetamine and found that stimulation of the right postganglionic sympathetic fibres increased the output more than does simultaneous stimulation of the sympathetic and vagus nerves. They concluded that the decrease in output found when the vagus was stimulated was due to peripheral cholinergic inhibition of noradrenaline release.

V. The Role of Ca^{2+} for the Noradrenaline-Releasing Effect of Acetylcholine on Adrenergic Nerve Terminals

Burn and Gibbons (1964a, 1965) showed that the inhibitory responses of the rabbit ileum to stimulation of the periarterial nerves are greater at high than at low concentrations of Ca^{2+}. Similarly, the increase in heart rate of rabbit isolated atria by acetylcholine (50 μg/ml) in the presence of atropine (1 μg/ml) is greater at high than at low concentrations of Ca^{2+}. The block by guanethidine is overcome by an increase of $[Ca^{2+}]$ (Burn and Welsh, 1967). In the rabbit ileum, an increase in Ca^{2+} concentrations from 2.2—6.6 mM overcomes the block by guanethidine (1 μg/ml) of the inhibitory responses to stimulation of the periarterial nerves; this effect is more pronounced when the nerves are stimulated at 5 Hz than at 80 Hz (Fig. 12) (Burn and Gibbons, 1965). Similar results were obtained on the mesenteric arteries of the rat (Malik and Ling, 1969a). This effect of Ca^{2+} in overcoming the guanethidine block may be due to an improvement in noradrenaline release, due to a physiological antagonism and not due to a true antagonism of the action of guanethidine, which probably interferes with the access of Ca^{2+} to its site of action in the adrenergic nerve ending (Wilson, 1970).

This important role of Ca^{2+} for the release mechanism of noradrenaline has been confirmed by direct measurement of the output of noradrenaline by the perfused spleen of the cat after nerve stimulation (Kirpekar and Misu, 1967) or depolarization by KCl (Kirpekar and Wakade, 1968). Similar findings were obtained for the isolated heart of the rabbit (Huković and Muscholl, 1962) and the cat colon (Boullin, 1967). In the perfused isolated heart of the rabbit, the release of noradrenaline by acetylcholine in the presence of atropine is also dependent on the Ca^{2+} concentration of the perfusion fluid (LÖFFELHOLZ, 1967). Lowering of $[Ca^{2+}]$ decreases and raising of $[Ca^{2+}]$ increases noradrenaline release by acetylcholine. The resting output of noradrenaline, however, is not affected by

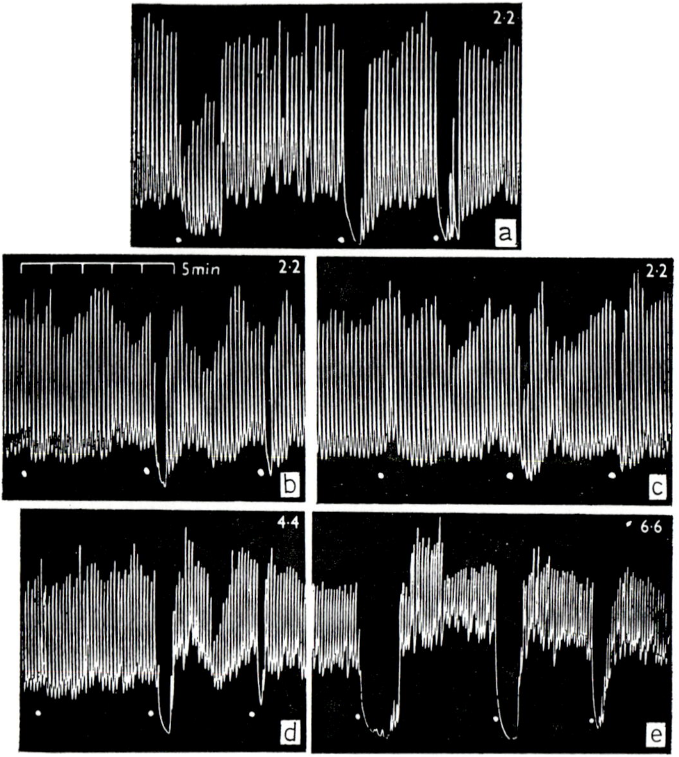

Fig. 12a—e. Rabbit ileum showing inhibitory responses to stimulation with 400 shocks at 5, 20 and 80 Hz. Top panel shows control responses. Middle panel shows responses after the addition of guanethidine (1 μg/ml). In the bottom panel, the calcium concentration was raised to 4.4 mM (on the left) and to 6.6 mM (on the right). Note the reversal of the block caused by guanethidine, particularly for the frequency of 5 Hz. Reproduced, with permission, from BURN and GIBBONS (1965)

changes in $[Ca^{2+}]$. Lowering of $[Na^{+}]$ to 50 mM or less increases noradrenaline output after acetylcholine (LÖFFELHOLZ, 1967) or after depolarization by KCl (KIRPEKAR and WAKADE, 1968) but not after nerve stimulation because conduction is affected (KIRPEKAR and MISU, 1967).

VI. Conclusions

The suggestion made by BURN and RAND (1959) that a cholinergic link essential for the release of noradrenaline exists in the adrenergic nerve terminals has stimulated a great deal of research designed either to confirm or disprove the hypothesis. When the evidence presented in this chapter is considered, it becomes quite clear that acetylcholine can either promote or inhibit release from the adrenergic nerve terminals. It is a much more difficult matter to assess the physiological significance of this phenomenon. The evidence available at present is overwhelmingly in favour of the view that there may be functional interaction between adrenergic and cholinergic nerve terminals (cf. MUSCHOLL, 1970). This interaction may result in a modulation of noradrenaline release by acetylcholine from cholinergic terminals as well as a modulation of acetylcholine release by noradrenaline from adrenergic terminals. This effect would be inhibitory rather than facilitatory.

Although these conclusions are backed by present evidence, the possibility of a cholinergic link in the mechanisms leading to noradrenaline release cannot be excluded until it becomes possible to visualize acetylcholine in nerve terminals. Such a technique would decide the crucial question of whether or not acetylcholine and noradrenaline occur in one and the same nerve terminal.

B. Effects of Catecholamines on Cholinergic Nerve Terminals

I. Effects on Transmission in Autonomic Ganglia

1. Introduction

The frequent reviews of the effects of catecholamines on ganglionic transmission (TRENDELENBURG, 1961, 1967; CURTIS, 1963; WEIR and MCLENNAN, 1963; NORBERG and SJÖQVIST, 1966; VOLLE, 1966; TAUC, 1967) reflect the increasing importance of this topic with regard to the concept of modulation of the action of transmitter substances at synapses by physiologically occurring substances.

The first unequivocal demonstration of an action of a catecholamine on ganglionic transmission was provided by MARRAZZI (1939), who showed that "small" doses (5—250 μg) of adrenaline, injected intravenously, depressed reversibly transmission through the cat superior cervical ganglion, transmission being measured as the height of the postganglionic action potentials in response to stimulation of the preganglionic nerves. With respect to the rates of release of adrenaline from the adrenal medulla under conditions of maximal reflex stimulation of the glands, as little as 1 μg of adrenaline or noradrenaline injected intravenously into a cat of average size should be regarded as a very large dose (FOLKOW 1955). However, that the observations by MARRAZZI (1939, 1947) might indeed be of physiological significance is suggested by the occurrence of an inhibition of transmission during endogenous release of catecholamines by splanchnic nerve stimulation. These findings have been confirmed for the cat (BÜLBRING, 1944; LUNDBERG, 1952; MATTHEWS, 1956; PARDO et al., 1963; WEIR and MCLENNAN, 1963; MCISAAC, 1966; CAIRNCROSS et al., 1967) and the rabbit (ECCLES and LIBET, 1961). In this action adrenaline is about four to ten times more potent than noradrenaline (LUNDBERG, 1952; PARDO et al., 1963). However, facilitation of transmission may occur in the presence of adrenaline when smaller doses (0.01 to 0.1 μg) are used (BÜLBRING and BURN, 1942; BÜLBRING, 1944; MATTHEWS, 1956). In the dog, facilitation of transmission has been observed in prevertebral ganglia and the adrenal medulla (MALMÉJAC, 1955).

Since it was thought that there were chromaffin cells in certain mammalian and amphibian autonomic ganglia (SMIRNOW, 1890; KOHN, 1903; IWANOW, 1932; STÖHR, 1939; GLEES, unpublished findings cited by BÜLBRING, 1944), the issue to be decided was whether or not the catecholamine could be released from such cells and thus would facilitate or inhibit transmission under physiological conditions. LISSÁK (1939) and BÜLBRING (1944) demonstrated an adrenaline-like substance in the effluent of perfused ganglia when the preganglionic nerves were stimulated.

In view of reports that chromaffin cells of prevertebral sympathetic ganglia were innervated by preganglionic nerves (SMIRNOW, 1890; STÖHR, 1939), it was tempting to speculate that these cells were the source of the adrenaline-like substance. At the time, however, there was no unequivocal evidence for the presence of chromaffin cells in cervical sympathetic ganglia. The possibility that the substance had come from adrenergic nerve terminals in vascular smooth muscle in the ganglion could be dismissed because there was little or no reduction in flow during prolonged stimulation of the preganglionic nerves (BÜLBRING, 1944). Another likely source was the adrenergic sympathetic ganglion cell itself because noradrenaline is released from these cells on antidromic stimulation (LISSÁK, 1939; REINERT, 1963). REINERT concluded from his results in normal, decentralized and reserpine-treated ganglia *in situ* that the noradrenaline released on orthodromic stimulation did not play a physiological role. This was also the view of LUNDBERG (1952) and of WEIR and MCLENNAN (1963).

ECCLES and LIBET (1961) used the rabbit superior cervical ganglion as a model to analyse pharmacologically the compound ganglionic potentials recorded extracellularly. On the basis of their results, they proposed that the origin of the inhibitory postsynaptic potential (IPSP) was as follows: acetylcholine released by stimulation of the preganglionic nerves acts not only on nicotinic receptors on the postjunctional neuronal membrane to initiate the permeability changes responsible for the excitatory potential (EPSP) but also on muscarinic receptors on catecholamine-containing cells close to the postganglionic neurone. The chromaffin cells thus excited release catecholamines, which cause a hyperpolarization of the neurone.

Following this lead, the research effort of the last decade has been concerned principally with answering these questions: 1. are there indeed catecholamine-containing cells in cervical and other sympathetic ganglia? 2. if so, do they have a physiological role? 3. how do the catecholamines released locally or elsewhere in the body inhibit and facilitate ganglionic transmission?

2. Intraganglionic Location of Catecholamine-containing Structures

a) Electron Microscopic Evidence

The possibility of cells interposed between the preganglionic nerve terminals and the postganglionic neurones has been debated for 80 years. Since some pericellular plexuses still remained after chronic decentralization (i.e. division of preganglionic nerves) of the superior cervical ganglion of the cat and rabbit, LAWRENTJEW (1924) concluded that these fibres were from intraganglionic cells, not necessarily identifiable with the principal postganglionic neurones. From a similar more recent investigation on rabbit superior cervical ganglia, SAMUEL (1953) thought that the evidence was not in itself sufficiently convincing to warrant the conclusion that there were neurones other than the principal ones. In the last 4 years, however, there have been several reports which establish that in

Fig. 13a—e. Electron micrograph. Synaptic connections of a small, vesicle-containing cell in a rat superior cervical ganglion. a synapse (E) between soma of a small cell and a spine-like projection arising from a process containing neuro-tubules (n) and ribosomes (R). Detail of synaptic region is shown in b. Fixation by a mixture of formaldehyde and glutaraldehyde, perfused through ganglion *in situ* for 30 min. Osmium postfixation. c small cell with a synapse (A), which is afferent with respect to it, at one pole of the soma and another synapse (E), which is efferent, at the opposite pole. Both the afferent terminal profile, shown in detail in d, and the postjunctional profile (Pr), shown in detail in e, deeply indent the body of the cell and are partly covered by vesicle-free extensions of its cytoplasm. Fixation by immersion in a mixture of formaldehyde and glutaraldehyde; osmium postfixation. Reproduced, with permission, from MATTHEWS and RAISMAN (1969)

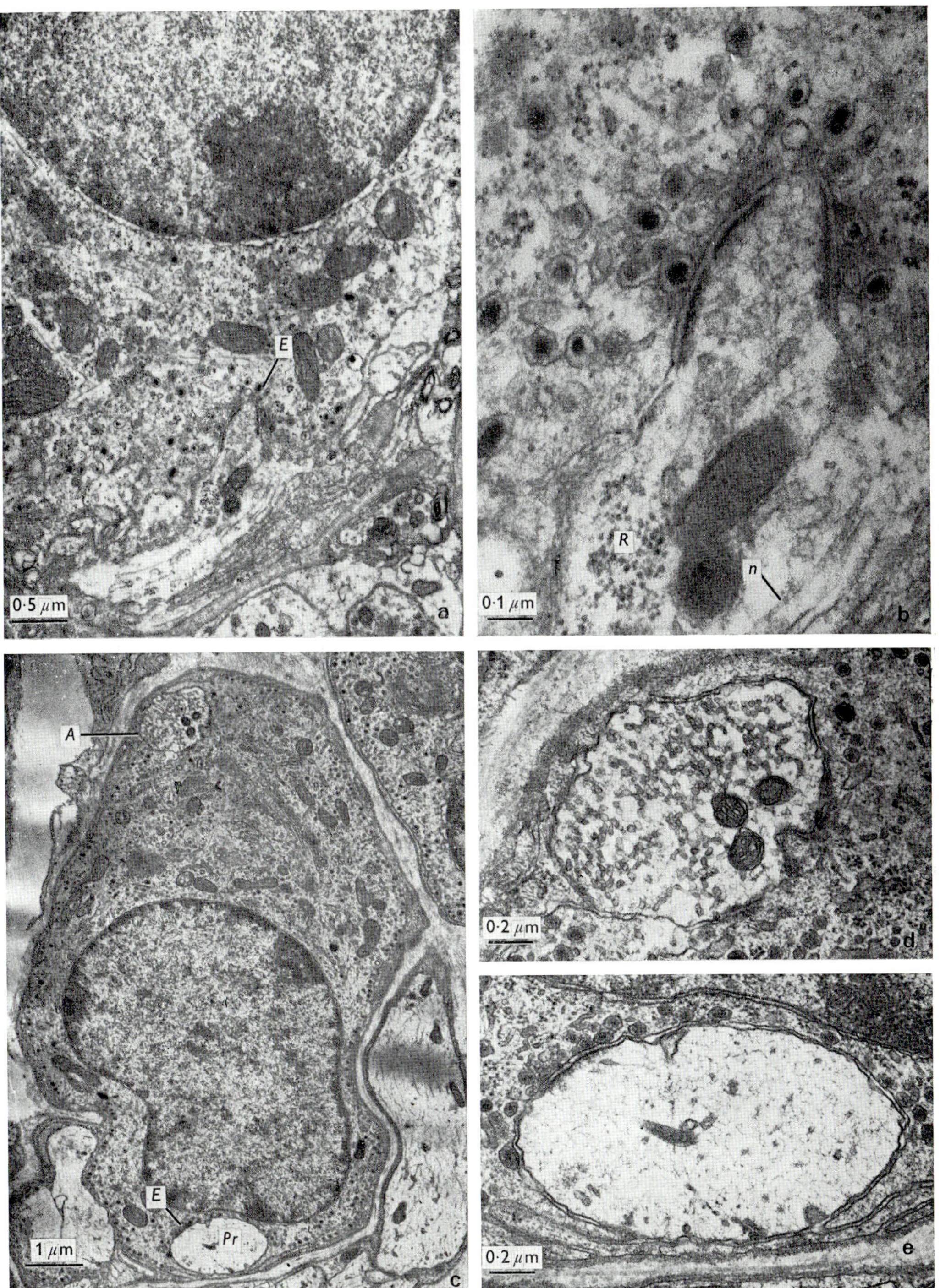

Fig. 13a—e

the superior cervical ganglion of the rat there are clusters of 2—5 cells that are smaller than the average principal postganglionic neurone and have morphological features in common with both neurones and chromaffin cells (GRILLO, 1966; WILLIAMS, 1967; SIEGRIST et al., 1968; MATTHEWS and RAISMAN, 1968, 1969; WILLIAMS and PALAY, 1969; VAN ORDEN et al., 1970). Similar observations have also been made in the inferior mesenteric ganglion of the rat (ELFVIN, 1968; VAN ORDEN et al., 1970). Terminals of preganglionic nerves are found to form junctions which are afferent in respect of these small cells, often in indentations of the body of the small cell; the junctions are often in pairs and at one pole of the cell (MATTHEWS and RAISMAN, 1969) (Fig. 13). In this latter respect, the junctions are unlike those upon the principal postganglionic neurones in rat ganglia which are predominantly axo-dendritic (TAXI, 1965). What is of fundamental importance, however, is the additional observation that these small cells in their turn make contact with processes, presumed to be dendrites, from the principal postganglionic neurones (WILLIAMS, 1967; SIEGRIST et al., 1968; WILLIAMS and PALAY, 1969; MATTHEWS and RAISMAN, 1969; MATTHEWS and NASH, 1970). These contacts meet all the criteria necessary for their identification as junctions with efferent polarity in respect of the small cell. The criteria are as follows: clustering of vesicles on the prejunctional side, a localized increase in electron density of the postjunctional membrane and an increase in the distance between pre- and postjunctional membranes. However, these efferent junctions are unusual in that they are found on both the processes of the small cells and the cell body. It is the presence of afferent and efferent junctions in one and the same cell that makes it likely that these cells function as interneurones (Fig. 13).

Clarification is required of the relationship, if any, between the afferent innervation of any one small cell and the afferent innervation of the principal postganglionic neurone with which the small cell makes contact. These cells are distributed very sparsely and form a very small proportion of the total number of "ganglion" cells; there is thus the possibility that their function as interneurones is restricted to only a fraction of the total population of principal postganglionic neurones in a ganglion. Clearly, the numbers of small cells as well as their distribution are important factors. From a detailed study of one rat superior cervical ganglion, MATTHEWS and RAISMAN (1969) found that small cells lay within 500 μm of any principal postganglionic neurone, which they showed to have a dendritic field of radius about 150 μm. The processes of small cells have been found by fluorescence microscopy to be up to 40 μm in length (NORBERG et al., 1966; CSILLIK et al., 1967). MATTHEWS and RAISMAN concluded that, even if the processes of the small cells do not extend far beyond the limits of the cluster, the cells would still be capable of coming into contact with a large proportion of principal postganglionic neurones. Since there is insufficient information about the intraganglionic location of any of the neurones whose axons innervate the various effector cells, the proposal that transmission to particular effectors is modified or inhibited by the small cells acting as interneurones cannot be tested at present.

A further point of interest regarding these cells is their close proximity to fenestrated blood capillaries but the functional significance of this observation is not immediately apparent. A local endocrine role has been tentatively suggested (SIEGRIST et al., 1968). The identification of similar cells in other ganglia and ganglia of other species is keenly awaited.

b) Histochemical Evidence

All but the cholinergic sympathetic ganglion cells (SJÖQVIST, 1963) show specific fluorescence of varying intensity (FALCK, 1962; ERÄNKÖ and HÄRKÖNEN,

1963). HAMBERGER and NORBERG (1963) further showed that, in some prevertebral ganglia of the rat and the inferior mesenteric ganglia of the cat, there is a system of adrenergic nerve terminals not ending near blood vessels but close to nerve cell bodies. Similar observations (HAMBERGER et al., 1965; HOLLANDS and VANOV, 1965; CSILLIK et al., 1967) were also made in rat and rabbit superior cervical ganglia, stellate ganglia of rat and cat, coeliac and inferior mesenteric ganglia of rabbit as well as cat. Adrenergic terminals in cat superior cervical ganglia have been identified (JACOBOWITZ and WOODWARD, 1968) and are considered to be axon collaterals from the adrenergic principal postganglionic neurones. The possibility of the fluorescent terminals being from "interneurones" has also been discussed (NORBERG and SJÖQVIST, 1966; CSILLIK et al., 1967).

Parasympathetic ganglia have also been shown to have a system of adrenergic nerve terminals surrounding the ganglion cells. This observation has been made rarely in ciliary ganglia of the cat, cebus monkey, squirrel monkey, cynomolgus monkey, marmoset, pig, goat and dog (HAMBERGER et al., 1965; EHINGER and FALCK, 1970) but commonly round intramural ganglion cells of the urinary bladder of the cat (HAMBERGER and NORBERG, 1965a) and intracardiac ganglion cells of mice, rats, guinea-pigs and cats (JACOBOWITZ, 1967). The intramural nerve plexuses of small and large intestine have a similar system of adrenergic nerve terminals round neuronal somata (NORBERG, 1964; HAMBERGER and NORBERG, 1965b; HOLLANDS and VANOV, 1965; JACOBOWITZ, 1965). See also p. 796.

Small, intensely-fluorescent catecholamine-containing cells have been described in sympathetic ganglia (NORBERG and HAMBERGER, 1964; HÄRKÖNEN, 1964; HAMBERGER et al., 1965; NORBERG et al., 1966) and have been equated tentatively with the small, vesicle-containing "interneurone" already discussed (GRILLO, 1966; SIEGRIST et al., 1968; MATTHEWS and RAISMAN, 1969; TAXI et al., 1969). From the results of a simultaneous investigation of catecholamine content of ganglia and fluorescent and electron microscopic appearance of the cells under various conditions, VAN ORDEN et al. (1970) concluded that the small, intensely-fluorescent, chromaffin-like "interneurones" may account for as much as 30% of the total noradrenaline content of the rat ganglion. Within these small cells there appear to be two stores of noradrenaline which show different rates of turnover and different sensitivities to amine-depleting drugs (TAXI et al., 1969; VAN ORDEN et al., 1970). Unfortunately, too little information is available at present to comment on their physiological significance.

In a recent study, BJÖRKLUND et al. (1970) determined the nature and amount of catecholamines in cervical and thoracic sympathetic ganglia of cats and pigs and found that noradrenaline and dopamine are present but not adrenaline. In two feline ganglia, the mean content of dopamine was 0.15 μg/g and in eleven porcine ganglia 0.24 μg/g; the noradrenaline contents were 1.3 μg/g and 1.56 μg/g, respectively. The values for the contents of dopamine agree well with those obtained by LAVERTY and SHARMAN (1965) for superior and inferior cervical and stellate ganglia of the dog, cat, rabbit, sheep and goat. On the other hand, the noradrenaline contents of cat ganglia determined by BJÖRKLUND et al. (1970) are much smaller than those obtained by other workers; MUSCHOLL and VOGT (1958) found 3.5 μg/g, COSTA et al. (1961) 7 μg/g, KIRPEKAR et al. (1962) 6.8 μg/g, REINERT (1963) 8.2 μg/g and LAVERTY and SHARMAN (1965) 2.8—5.3 μg/g. All authors are agreed, however, that there are only minute amounts of adrenaline in sympathetic ganglia, except in the prevertebral ganglia of rabbit and cat (MUSCHOLL and VOGT, 1958). BJÖRKLUND et al. (1970) have suggested that the dopamine is mainly located in the small intensely fluorescent cell.

3. Mode of Action of Catecholamines on Ganglionic Transmission

Until recently, attempts to clarify the site of action of catecholamines in ganglia were unsuccessful. It has been uncertain whether the inhibition of transmission is due to a change in the amount of acetylcholine released, a change in the resting membrane potential of the postganglionic neurone or a change in the sensitivity of the receptors to acetylcholine.

Lundberg (1952) concluded that the very small changes in the demarcation potential of the cat superior cervical ganglion could not account for the inhibition of transmission by adrenaline; he postulated that the mechanism was reduction in either acetylcholine output or sensitivity of the receptors. Paton and Thompson (1953) showed that adrenaline (1 μg, injected intraarterially) reduced by 50% the stimulated release of acetylcholine from the Locke-perfused superior cervical ganglion of the cat. Birks and MacIntosh (1961) confirmed their result in a single experiment in which they perfused the ganglion with a constant concentration of adrenaline (50 ng/ml), the reduction in output being about 50%. However, Birks and MacIntosh found in some other preparations that adrenaline (10 ng/ml) caused a reversible increase in acetylcholine output. Paton and Thompson (1953) observed that adrenaline depresses the stimulant effect of acetylcholine injected into the circulation of ganglia perfused with Locke solution not containing physostigmine but this finding is in disagreement with the observations of several workers (for references, Volle, 1966). The effects of nicotine-like and muscarine-like drugs injected into the circulation of the ganglion of the anaesthetized cat are complex and require involved explanations (Volle, 1966).

With regard to the possibility that the catecholamines exert their effect through a change in resting membrane potential of the postganglionic neurone, De Groat and Volle (1966a, b) correlated the facilitation and inhibition of transmission in the cat superior cervical ganglion with depolarization and hyperpolarization, respectively. It was found that isoprenaline consistently reduced the demarcation potential and facilitated transmission, an effect blocked by β-adrenoceptor blocking agents, whereas noradrenaline always increased the potential and inhibited transmission by an action on α-adrenoceptors; adrenaline exhibited both actions. In contrast, Paton and Thompson (1953) noted that the reduction by adrenaline of the compound ganglionic action potential was not accompanied by a change in resting potential of the ganglion.

Kobayashi and Libet (1968, 1970) and Libet and Kobayashi (1969) have investigated the effects of catecholamines on membrane resting potentials and their putative role in the production of the slow inhibitory postsynaptic potential (IPSP) evoked by orthodromic stimulation in the isolated superior cervical ganglion of the rabbit. They found that changes in resting potential were elicited by adrenaline, noradrenaline and isoprenaline only when a monoamine oxidase inhibitor, e.g. harmine or pargyline, was added to the bathing fluid. Furthermore, for consistent changes in potential, it was necessary to use very high concentrations of the amines. Although even after removal of the connective tissue capsule only the most superficial cells are impaled with microelectrodes, diffusional and enzymatic barriers may prevent catecholamines in the bathing fluid from reaching the ganglion cells (Kobayashi and Libet, 1970). It was found in one cell that adrenaline (100 μg/ml) caused a hyperpolarization of 4 mV. In another cell, adrenaline (1 μg/ml) produced no change. In two cells, isoprenaline (100 μg/ml) in the presence of harmine (5 μg/ml) did not change the resting potential. Noradrenaline, on the other hand, in eight out of twelve cells, caused hyperpolarization (2—8 mV) when the concentration was high (10—50 μg/ml) and when harmine

(5 μg/ml) present. A consistent observation was that the membrane resistance was not decreased during the hyperpolarization induced by noradrenaline and during the IPSP. The authors concluded that both these hyperpolarizations are produced by a mechanism other than the generation of membrane currents due to ions moving down their electrochemical gradients and that, therefore, the IPSP is induced by noradrenaline. In amphibian sympathetic ganglia, the IPSP recorded extracellularly is inhibited by ouabain (1 μM) and metabolic inhibitors (NISHI and KOKETSU, 1967) and for these and other reasons is due to the activity of an electrogenic sodium pump (NISHI and KOKETSU, 1968; KOKETSU, 1969). Whereas in the rabbit ganglion cells the electrogenic sodium pump is readily inhibited by ouabain (1—10 μM) (KOSTERLITZ et al., 1968, 1970a), the IPSP and the hyperpolarization induced by noradrenaline are reduced only by higher concentrations of ouabain (10—50 μM) and of metabolic inhibitors; moreover, these agents depress all postjunctional potentials (KOBAYASHI and LIBET, 1968; LIBET and KOBAYASHI, 1969). On the available evidence, however, it would be premature to state that an electrogenic sodium pump is not involved in the production of the IPSP of rabbit ganglion cells.

Contrary to what they observed in isolated ganglia, KOBAYASHI and LIBET (1970) found that, *in vivo*, adrenaline causes a depolarization which precedes the hyperpolarization. In view of this difference between the results obtained by the two methods of recording, it is unfortunate that the authors did not investigate the effect of harmine on the magnitude of the change in potential in response to close-arterial or intravenous injections of adrenaline.

With regard to the evidence that changes in resting potential account for the facilitatory and inhibitory effects of the catecholamines, important further observations have been made by CHRIST and NISHI (1969, 1971 and personal communication). These authors investigated the effects of catecholamines, especially adrenaline, on pre- and postjunctional events, which were recorded from isolated superior cervical ganglia of rabbits either intracellularly with microelectrodes or extracellularly by the sucrose-gap technique. They found that adrenaline (10^{-6} to 10^{-3} M) blocked initiation of postjunctional action potentials and decreased the amplitude of excitatory postsynaptic potentials (EPSPs) (Fig. 14a). Adrenaline did not hyperpolarize the postjunctional membrane nor did it change the electrical properties of the membrane, including the threshold for initiation of a ganglionic action potential by direct stimulation of the cell. Depolarizations by acetylcholine applied by iontophoresis or by addition to the bathing fluid were not altered by adrenaline (Fig. 14b). Noradrenaline (10^{-5} M) depressed the amplitude of EPSPs in each of three cells tested; isoprenaline (10^{-5} M) was effective in only one of three cells tested. In a single cell, all three amines were applied and the order of effectiveness was found to be adrenaline, noradrenaline and isoprenaline.

A prejunctional mechanism of action was suggested by the findings that the frequency of miniature EPSPs was reduced by adrenaline as were the quantal contents of EPSPs evoked in media with a low [Ca^{2+}] / [Mg^{2+}] ratio (Fig. 15). The prejunctional mechanism was further analysed by testing for changes in polarization of the prejunctional terminal membrane in the presence of adrenaline. The technique used was based on that described by HUBBARD and SCHMIDT (1963); the stimulating electrode, which is a NaCl-filled microelectrode of low resistance is manoeuvred into a position so close to the very end of a prejunctional terminal that the latency of excitation of the postjunctional membrane is minimal and of the same order as the junctional delay. When the electrode is in such a position, an increase in the current strength beyond that necessary for excitation of the preganglionic nerve terminals results in direct stimulation of the ganglion body.

Adrenaline (10^{-5}M) did not change the current threshold of the terminals, even when the EPSP was greatly depressed. From another kind of experiment, it was found that adrenaline diminished the stores of transmitter readily available for release; for this purpose, the technique of ELMQVIST and QUASTEL (1965) was

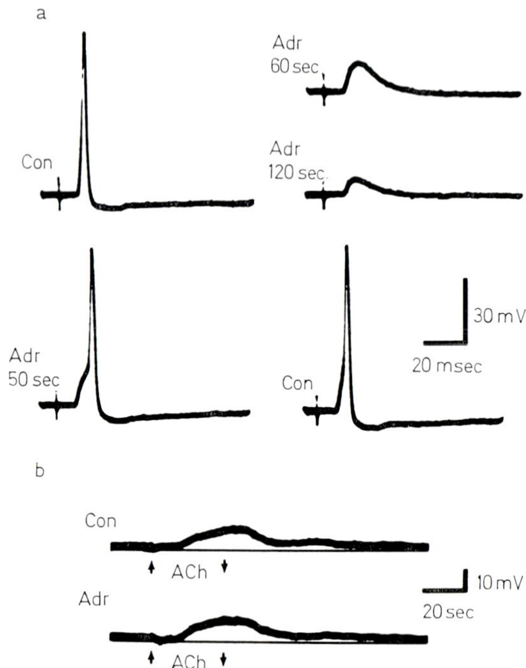

Fig. 14. a Effect of adrenaline on the response of a ganglion cell to an orthodromic stimulus. *Con*, control recording in Krebs solution before (upper left) and 4 min after (lower right) addition of adrenaline to the bathing fluid. *Adr*, recordings 50, 60 and 120 sec after beginning of exposure to adrenaline (10^{-5}M). Intracellular recording. b Effect of adrenaline on response of a ganglion cell to acetylcholine (ACh). *Con*, control. *Adr*, 3 min after beginning of exposure to adrenaline (10^{-5}M). Acetylcholine was present in the bathing fluid for the period indicated by the arrows. Intracellular recording. Reproduced, with permission, from CHRIST and NISHI (1969)

employed. The prejunctional effect of adrenaline was not reduced by the β-adrenoceptor blocking agents, propranolol (30 μM) and dichloroisoprenaline (10 μM), but was abolished by phenoxybenzamine (10 μM) and dihydroergotamine (10 μM). The adrenoceptor blocking drugs were used in concentrations which did not change the EPSP. On the basis of the results of CHRIST and NISHI (1969, 1970) it is not possible to suggest a mechanism for facilitation of transmission because there was no detectable augmentation of EPSPs even in the presence of α-adrenoceptor blocking agents.

In the rabbit superior cervical ganglion, the compound ganglionic potentials evoked by orthodromic stimulation and recorded extracellularly in the presence of a ganglion blocking agent, consist of an initial negative potential (EPSP) followed by a slowly-developing positive potential (IPSP) and an even slower negative potential (slow EPSP) (ECCLES, 1952). Since dibenamine markedly depressed the IPSP, ECCLES and LIBET (1961) concluded that a catecholamine, acting on α-adrenoceptors, is the chemical mediator of the IPSP. However, as already pointed out by TAUC (1967), they also found that the α-adrenoceptor blocking drugs, ergotamine and dihydroergotamine, did not depress the IPSP. Further, dibenamine, which is known to have potent atropine-like activity, reduced also the size of the slow EPSP and atropine, itself, was found to abolish

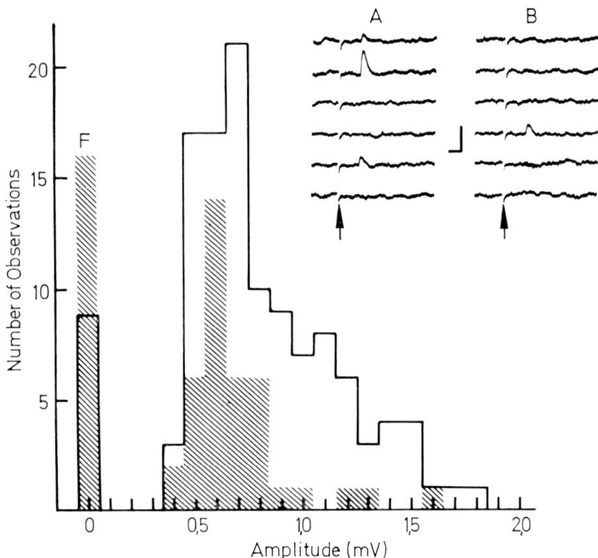

Fig. 15. Superior cervical ganglion of the rabbit. Effect of adrenaline on EPSPs. Histogram of amplitudes of EPSPs recorded in modified Ringer solution containing 0.5 mM $CaCl_2$ and 5.5 mM $MgCl_2$. Ordinate, number of observations. Abscissa, amplitude of EPSPs (mV). Clear areas, controls; shaded areas, adrenaline (10^{-5}M). Number of failures (*F*) in control period was 89 and, in the presence of adrenaline, 161. Inset, records of EPSPs before (*A*) and during (*B*) exposure to adrenaline; orthodromic stimulation at arrow. Calibration signals, 2 mV and 10 msec. Reproduced, with permission, from CHRIST and NISHI (1971)

the IPSP as well as the slow EPSP. Another point to be considered is that there was no facilitation of transmission when the IPSP was depressed by dibenamine. A report that pretreatment of an animal with reserpine results in facilitation of ganglionic transmission (COSTA et al., 1961) has not been confirmed (WEIR and McLENNAN, 1963; REINERT, 1963). Further, despite a report that adrenergic neurone blocking drugs may cause facilitation of transmission (FARMER et al., 1966), it cannot be stated with certainty that removal of catecholamines or blockade of their release or action leads to a facilitation of ganglionic transmission.

In conclusion, it has been found in rabbit ganglia that low concentrations of adrenaline readily and reversibly inhibit ganglionic transmission, probably mainly by an action on the prejunctional terminals which diminishes the readily-available stores of transmitter. This may be the mechanism of the depressant action on ganglionic transmission of adrenaline which has been released into the circulation. However, in view of the evidence against the presence of significant amounts of adrenaline in cervical sympathetic ganglia of many species it is unlikely that adrenaline is the humoral agent released within these ganglia and responsible for effects on transmission. It would be important to evaluate the significance of the presence of adrenaline in prevertebral sympathetic ganglia. Furthermore, the possibility of species variation should be kept in mind. With regard to the intraganglionic release of a substance responsible for the slow hyperpolarization of ganglion cells (IPSP), noradrenaline or dopamine would seem to more likely candidates than adrenaline.

II. Effects of Catecholamines on the Output of Acetylcholine in the Small and Large Intestines

In the guinea-pig isolated ileum, the peristaltic reflex is inhibited by concentrations of adrenaline and noradrenaline which are lower than those required to depress the response of the longitudinal muscle of the ileum to acetylcholine added to the bath fluid (MCDOUGAL and WEST, 1952, 1954; KOSTERLITZ and ROBINSON, 1957). In the myenteric plexus-longitudinal muscle preparation, the contractions

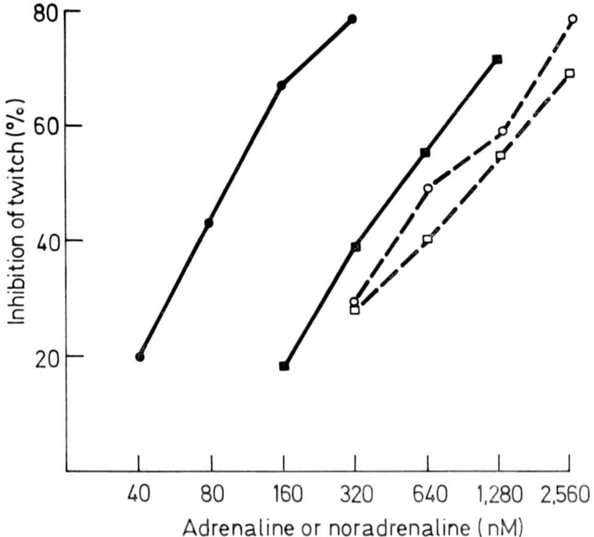

Fig. 16. Effects of phenoxybenzamine on the depression by catecholamines of the responses of the plexus-longitudinal muscle preparation to electrical stimulation at 0.1 Hz. Exposure to phenoxybenzamine (3×10^{-6}M) for 20 min in the presence of acetylcholine (1.5×10^{-4}M), added before phenoxybenzamine to protect the acetylcholine receptors; this procedure resulted in a reduction of the twitch height by 50%. Adrenaline, before (●) and after (○) exposure to phenoxybenzamine, noradrenaline before (■) and after (□) exposure to phenoxybenzamine. Reproduced, with permission, from KOSTERLITZ et al. (1970b)

of the muscle evoked by field stimulation are more easily depressed by adrenaline than by noradrenaline, while isoprenaline is of even less effect. Phenoxybenzamine is a more potent antagonist of the inhibitory action of adrenaline than of the action of noradrenaline (Fig. 16). Propranolol has very little antagonist action on the effect of adrenaline; it is more potent against the effect of noradrenaline and even more so against that of isoprenaline (KOSTERLITZ et al., 1970b). The observation that adrenaline is more potent than noradrenaline in activating α-receptors is not confined to the guinea-pig ileum; similar evidence has been obtained for the isolated terminal colon of the guinea-pig (BEANI et al., 1969) and the isolated small intestine of the rabbit (BOWMAN and HALL, 1970).

In the guinea-pig ileum, the β-receptors are on the smooth muscle fibres of the longitudinal muscle and there is no certain evidence for α-receptors on the muscle

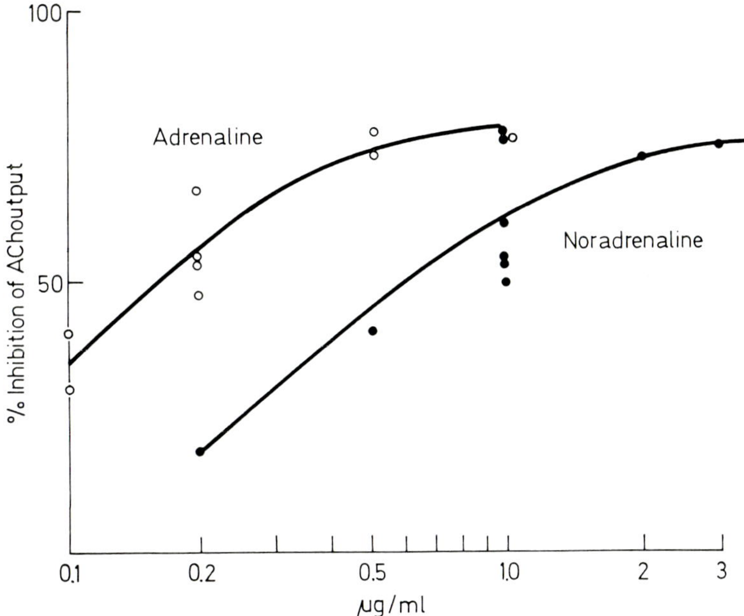

Fig. 17. Dose-response curve of inhibitory effect of adrenaline and noradrenaline on acetylcholine output induced by stimulation at 20/min. Ordinate, % inhibition; abscissa, concentration of amine. Number of shocks: 100 for adrenaline, 60 for noradrenaline. The drugs were given 5 sec before stimulation began. Potency ration of adrenaline to noradrenaline approximately 4. Reproduced, with permission, from PATON and VIZI (1969)

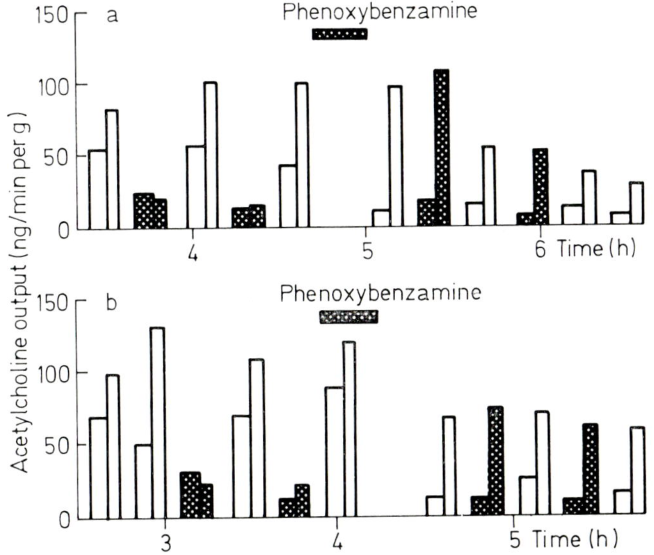

Fig. 18a and b. Effects of adrenaline (a) and noradrenaline (b) on the release of acetylcholine from the myenteric plexus-longitudinal muscle preparation. Abscissa, time (hr) since setting up preparation; ordinate, output of acetylcholine (ng/min per g tissue). The first of each pair of columns shows the spontaneous output and the second the output evoked by electrical stimulation (20/min). Clear columns, controls; black columns, during exposure to (a) adrenaline (6.4×10^{-7} M) or (b) noradrenaline (3.2×10^{-6} M). Horizontal bars, exposure to phenoxybenzamine (3×10^{-6} M). Reproduced, with permission, from KOSTERLITZ et al. (1970b)

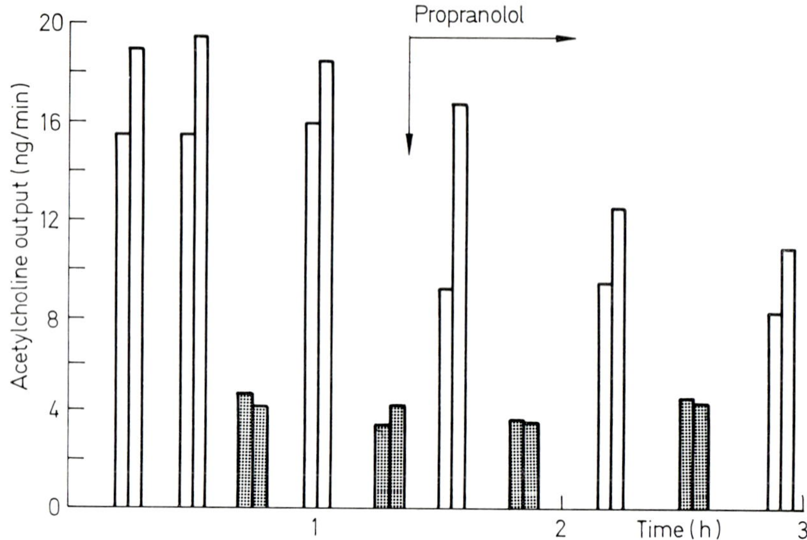

Fig. 19. Absence of an effect of propranolol on the depression by adrenaline of the release of acetylcholine from a segment of ileum. Abscissa, time (hr) since the beginning of the acetylcholine assays; ordinate, acetylcholine output (ng/min). The first of each pair of columns shows the spontaneous output and the second the output evoked by electrical stimulation (20/min). Clear columns, controls; black columns, during exposure to adrenaline (2.8×10^{-7}M). From the arrow until the end of the experiment propranolol (8.5×10^{-7}M) was present. Reproduced, with permission, from KOSTERLITZ et al. (1970b)

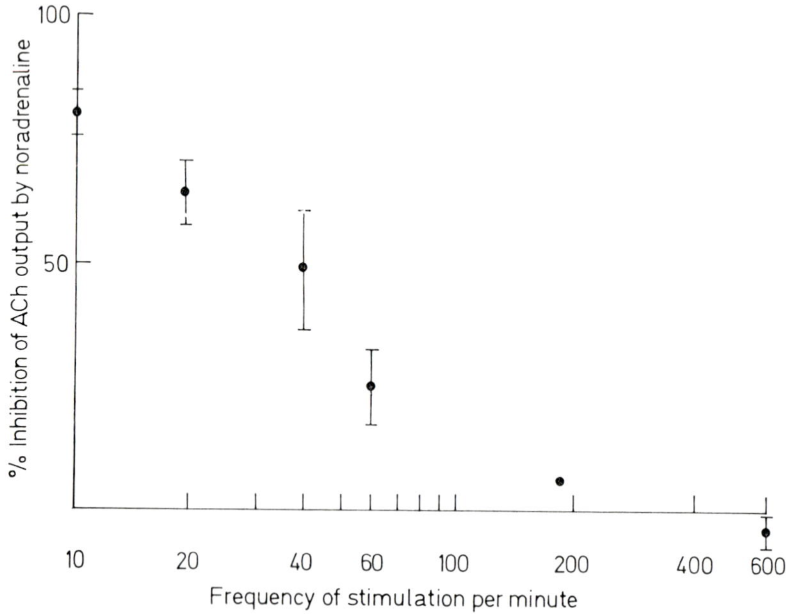

Fig. 20. Inhibition by noradrenaline, 1 µg/ml, of acetylcholine output induced by stimulation at various frequencies. Noradrenaline was given 5 sec before stimulation began. Number of shocks at 10/min, 50; at 20/min, 60; at 40/min, 200; at 60/min, 180; at 180/min 180; at 600/min, 600. Reproduced, with permission, from PATON and VIZI (1969)

(KOSTERLITZ et al., 1970b) but, in the guinea-pig taenia coli and the rabbit small intestine, α-receptors are also situated on the smooth muscle cells (JENKINSON and MORTON, 1967; BÜLBRING and TOMITA, 1969; BOWMAN and HALL, 1970).

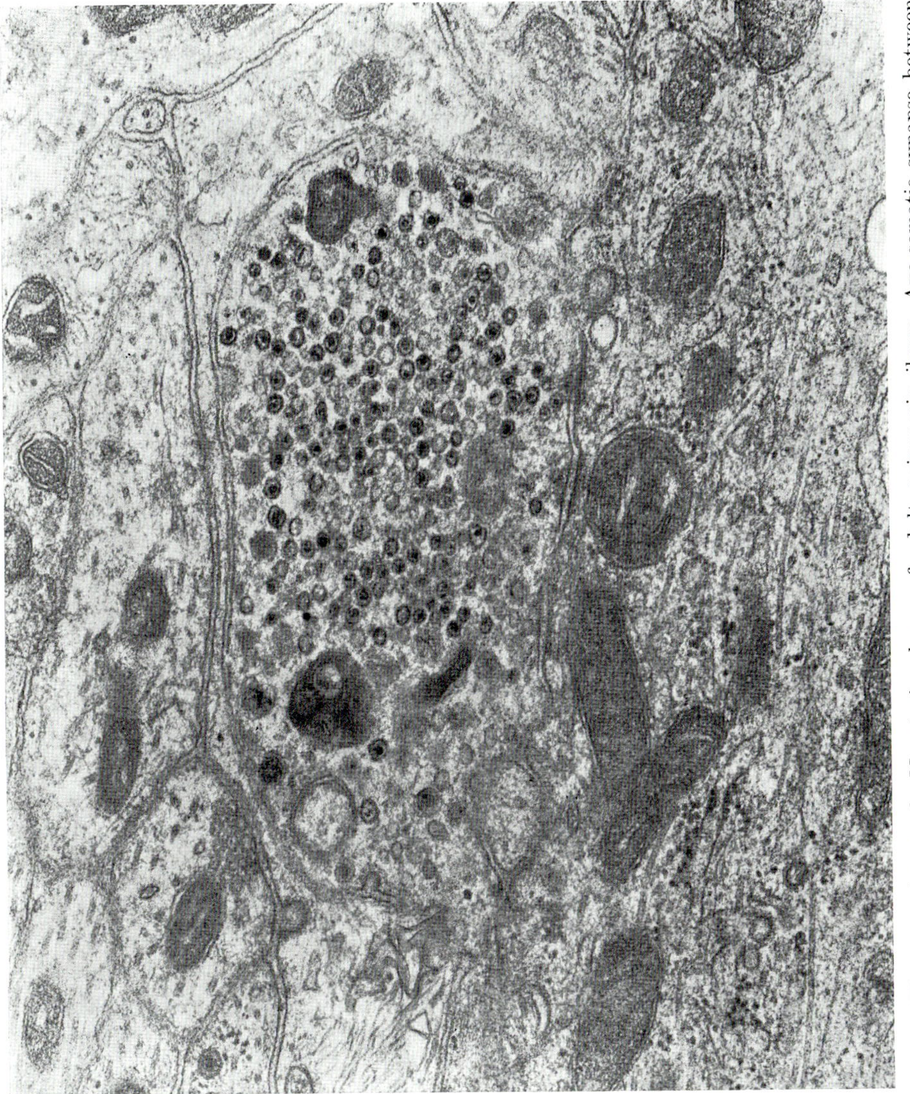

Fig. 21. Electron micrograph. Myenteric plexus of adult guinea-pig ileum. Axo-somatic synapse between adrenergic axon with small dense-cored vesicles and ganglion cell. Glutaraldehyde fixation, osmium post-fixation, uranyl acetate and lead citrate stain. Magnification, $\times$ 50,000. By courtesy of G. GABELLA

The view that, in the guinea-pig ileum, the receptors in the myenteric plexus are α-receptors is supported by the analysis of the actions of catecholamines on the release of acetylcholine induced by electrical stimulation of the plexus (WATT, 1966; COWIE et al., 1968; KOSTERLITZ and COWIE, 1968; VIZI, 1968; PATON and VIZI, 1969; KOSTERLITZ et al., 1970b). In agreement with the observations on the mechanical responses, adrenaline was found to be more potent in reducing acetylcholine output than noradrenaline (Fig. 17). The inhibitory effects of adrenaline and noradrenaline on acetylcholine output are antagonised by phenoxybenzamine but are unaffected by propranolol (Figs. 18 and 19). For an interpretation of the actions of the catecholamines it may be important that they are better inhibitors of acetylcholine release at low (0.1 Hz) than at high (1—10 Hz) frequencies of stimulation; this has been shown for adrenaline by COWIE et al. (1968) and for noradrenaline (Fig. 20) by VIZI (1968) and PATON and VIZI (1969). These findings are strong evidence for the view that the α-receptors are on the myenteric plexus, particularly since the whole of the output of acetylcholine induced by electrical stimulation originates from nervous tissue (PATON and ZAR, 1968).

Since, in the guinea-pig ileum, axons of the ganglion cells of the myenteric plexus are very short and do not penetrate into the longitudinal muscle layer (PATON and ZAR, 1968; GABELLA, 1970), the adrenergic nerve terminals which surround the ganglion cells of the plexus (NORBERG, 1964; HAMBERGER et al., 1965; JACOBOWITZ, 1965), are likely to have a considerable modulating effect on the output of acetylcholine induced by electrical field stimulation of the isolated myenteric plexus preparation or by physiological stimuli in the intact animal. Recent electron microscopic investigations have shown close contact of adrenergic boutons with dendrites and cell bodies of intrinsic nerve cells of the large intestine of several species (BAUMGARTEN et al., 1970). In the guinea-pig ileum, GABELLA (1971) has been able to demonstrate synaptic structures mainly of an axosomatic nature (Fig. 21).

These findings may be the morphological and physiological bases for the well-known facts that catecholamines originating either in the adrenal medulla or within the intestinal wall have a powerful inhibitory influence on intestinal motility (cf. KOSTERLITZ, 1968).

III. Effects on Transmission at the Neuromuscular Junction

1. Introduction

In mammalian skeletal muscle, the tension developed in response to single stimuli and during an incomplete tetanus may be altered by adrenaline and noradrenaline, the qualitative effects being dependent on several factors. The most important of these are a) the type of muscles, i.e. fast- or slow-contracting b) species from which it was taken c) the condition of the muscle d) stimulation to which it was previously subjected and e) the method used to induce contraction (BOWMAN and NOTT, 1969).

2. Direct Effects on Muscle

The maximal twitch tension of non-fatigued, fast-contracting muscles of the cat, rabbit, guinea-pig, rat and dog is increased by adrenaline, noradrenaline and isoprenaline (OLIVER and SCHÄFER, 1895; GRUBER, 1922a, b; BROWN et al., 1950; GOFFART, 1952a; MONTAGU, 1955; BOWMAN and ZAIMIS, 1958; BOWMAN et al., 1962, 1969; JURNA and RUMMEL, 1962; BLECKMAN et al., 1963; JURNA et al., 1963; BOWMAN and RAPER, 1967). In contrast, the maximal twitch tension of slow-contracting muscles of these species is diminished by these agents (Fig. 22). The two muscles also differ in their response to a tetanus following administration of adrenaline; the degree of fusion is increased in the fast-contracting muscle, tibialis anterior (Fig. 22c) but is diminished in the slow-contracting muscle, soleus (Fig. 22d). The explanation of these opposite responses to adrenaline lies in the observation that adrenaline slows the rate of decay of the active state of fast-contracting muscles but hastens the decline of the active state of slow-contracting muscles (JURNA and RUMMEL, 1962; BLECKMAN et al., 1963; JURNA et al., 1963), thus appearing to prolong or shorten the active state, as suggested by GOFFART and RITCHIE (1952) and SHAPIRO (1961). These effects of catecholamines are still observed in directly-stimulated muscles in which transmission has been blocked and also in chronically denervated muscles (GRUBER, 1922a; BROWN et al., 1950; GOFFART, 1952a; GOFFART and RITCHIE, 1952; BOWMAN and ZAIMIS, 1958; BOWMAN et al., 1962).

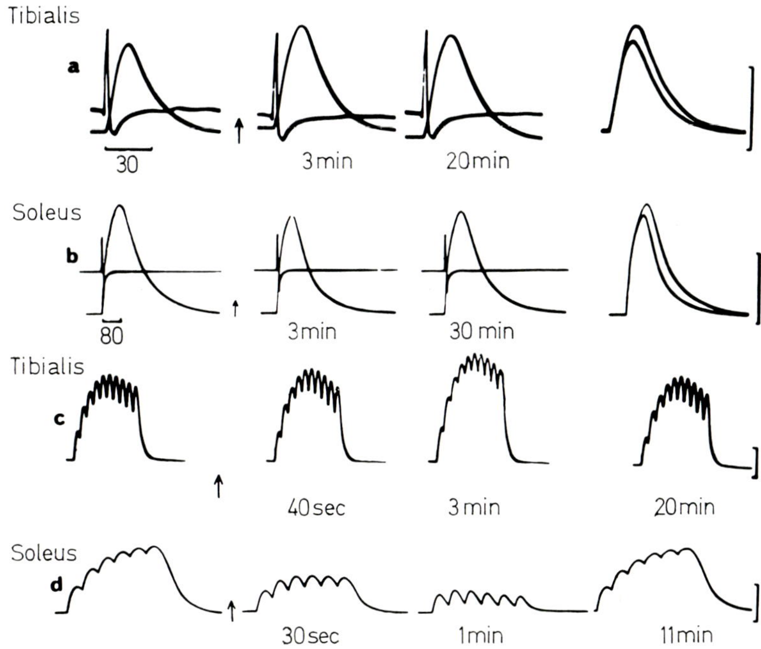

Fig. 22. Direct effects of adrenaline on fast- and slow-contracting muscle. *a*, rabbit, urethane anaesthesia; *b*, *c*, and *d*, cat, chloralose anaesthesia. In each experiment, contractions were elicited by stimulation of motor nerve at 0.1 Hz, but only representative contractions are shown. The first record in each row is one of a series of identical control responses. Adrenaline (10 μg/kg in *a*, 1 μg/kg in *b*, 8 μg/kg in *c* and 2 μg/kg in *d*) was injected intravenously at the arrows. Subsequent contractions were recorded at the times shown. In *a* and *b*, maximal twitches and compound muscle action potentials were elicited. The last records in *a* and *b* show the first two twitches superimposed. In *c* and *d*, incomplete tetani were elicited (40 Hz for 0.25 sec in *c*, and 6 Hz for 1 sec in *d*). Note that adrenaline augments the contractions of the fast-contracting muscle (tibialis anterior, *a* and *c*) but depresses those of the slow-contracting muscle (soleus, *b* and *d*). Time calibrations, msec. Tension calibrations on the right, 0.5 kg. Annals of The New York Academy of Sciences, volume 139, article 3, figure 1, page 742, W.C. BOWMAN and C. RAPER © The New York Academy of Sciences, 1967; reprinted by permission

The effects of adrenaline, noradrenaline and isoprenaline on fast- and slow-contracting muscles, stimulated directly, are not blocked by the α-adrenoceptor blocking agents dibenamine, phenoxybenzamine, phentolamine, ergotamine, ergotoxine, tolazoline and 933F (BROWN et al., 1950; GOFFART, 1952a; BOWMAN and ZAIMIS, 1958; BOWMAN et al., 1962); they are abolished by dichloroisoprenaline, pronethalol and propranolol (BOWMAN et al., 1962; BOWMAN and RAPER, 1967; BOWMAN and NOTT, 1970). Thus the direct effects of the catecholamines on mammalian muscles of different types is mediated by β-adrenoceptors. These findings have been extended to include muscles of normal human subjects and patients with Parkinson's disease (OWEN and MARSDEN, 1965; MARSDEN et al., 1967; MARSDEN and MEADOWS, 1968).

Changes in twitch tension of mammalian muscle after administration of catecholamines are rarely accompanied by changes in size of compound muscle action potentials (BOWMAN et al., 1962). BROWN et al. (1948, 1950) found that with adrenaline the duration, but not the amplitude, of the muscle action potential was increased in fast-contracting muscles. The reason for this observation was thought to be the result of the increase in demarcation potential recorded in the presence of adrenaline. Their observations on the change in demarcation potential have been confirmed by BOWMAN and RAPER (1966) who also found that the membrane of cat soleus muscle responds in the same manner. The mechanism of hyperpolarization awaits clarification although the characteristics of an electrogenic sodium pump described by DOCKRY et al. (1966) for rat extensor digitorum and soleus muscles are compatible with the observations made in cat soleus muscle. Thus, the origin of the increased demarcation potential may be similar to the adrenaline-induced hyperpolarization of smooth muscle cells of guinea-pig taenia (BUEDING and BÜLBRING, 1967). It seems unlikely that, in skeletal muscle, increases in intracellular K^+ concentration (GOFFART and PERRY, 1951) are primarily responsible for the hyperpolarization by adrenaline. This hyperpolarization is probably not responsible for changes in twitch tension in normal muscles exposed to catecholamines (BOWMAN and NOTT, 1969); changes in blood flow cannot account for the differences between the performances of fast- and slow-contracting muscles (BOWMAN and ZAIMIS, 1958).

3. Effects on Neuromuscular Transmission

Adrenaline and noradrenaline can be shown to affect neuromuscular transmission when this is depressed by drugs e.g. curarines; their effect, which can be either a reduction or enhancement of the degree of blockade (Fig. 23), is likewise not due to changes in local blood flow (BOWMAN and RAPER, 1966). Qualitatively, the response is the same in the two types of muscle and the sensitivities are similar whereas, to the direct action of the amines, slow-contracting muscle fibres are much more sensitive (BOWMAN and ZAIMIS, 1958; BOWMAN et al., 1962; BOWMAN and RAPER, 1967) and, as discussed above, the responses are dissimilar. Furthermore, the effects on neuromuscular transmission are not prevented by β-adrenoceptor blocking drugs; isoprenaline, which is the most potent compound with respect to the direct action, does not reduce the degree of block by (+)-tubocurarine and may even enhance it (BOWMAN and RAPER, 1966). Isoprenaline is also only slightly effective in relieving fatigue (BOWMAN and NOTT, 1969).

In partially curarized muscles, the compound muscle action potential increases in amplitude during facilitation of transmission produced by adrenaline, a phenomenon probably due to recruitment of previously blocked units (BOWMAN et al., 1962). However, NAESS and SIRNES (1953) found that the facilitation declines in a few minutes and gives way to a longer lasting depression of transmission, an observation which was confirmed by BOWMAN and RAPER (1966) (Fig. 23). This depression is associated with a reduced sensitivity of muscle to acetylcholine delivered by close-arterial injection (BOWMAN and RAPER, 1966) and a hyperpolarization of the muscle (BROWN et al., 1950; BOWMAN and RAPER, 1966). Curiously, the acetylcholine-induced contractions are depressed by adrenaline, noradrenaline and isoprenaline even at a time when transmission is facilitated. Adrenaline and isoprenaline also reduce the depolarization produced by decamethonium (BOWMAN and RAPER, 1966, 1967). These various actions could be explained by the hyperpolarization of the muscle membrane provided that the hyperpolarization is uniformly distributed over the cell membrane, including the end plate area, and is sufficiently large, being often of the order of 3 mV or less (BROWN et al., 1950; BOWMAN and RAPER, 1966). Neither of these possibilities has

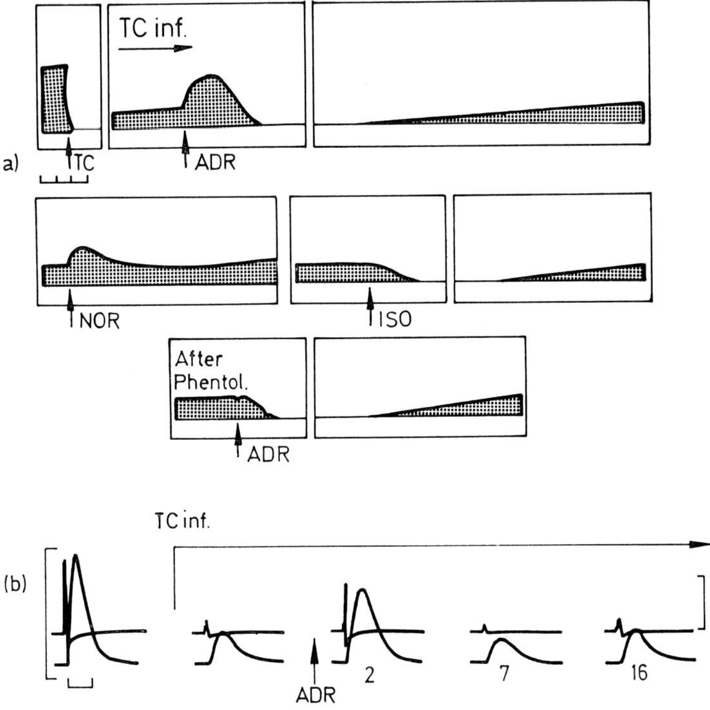

Fig. 23. Facilitation and inhibition of neuromuscular transmission by catecholamines. (*a*) Maximal twitches of a tibialis anterior muscle elicited by stimulation of the motor nerve at 1 Hz. At *TC*, a single intravenous injection of (+)-tubocurarine (0.3 mg/kg) was given. During recovery from this dose, an intravenous infusion of (+)-tubocurarine (*TC INF*) was started and was adjusted to give a constant degree of partial block. At *ADR*, *NOR* and *ISO*, 10 μg/kg of adrenaline, noradrenaline and isoprenaline were injected intravenously. After *Phentol.*, the second response to adrenaline recorded after the intravenous injection of phentolamine (2 m/kg). The gaps in the records of responses to adrenaline and isoprenaline each correspond to 10 min. Time calibration in minutes. (*b*) As for (*a*) but twitches and compound muscle action potentials were recorded on an oscilloscope. In this experiment, the dose of adrenaline (*ADR*) was again 10 μg/kg intravenously. Responses are shown at 2, 7 and 16 min after injection of adrenaline. Note that the changes in twitch tension are accompanied by corresponding changes in the amplitude of the compound action potentials. Calibrations: tension on left, 1 kg; time below, 30 msec; action potential on right, 20 mV. Reproduced, with permission, from BOWMAN and RAPER (1966)

been examined nor have results been reported of definitive experiments to test for a change in threshold for initiation of muscle action potentials during the hyperpolarization induced by adrenaline. However, in this connection it should be mentioned that the threshold for excitation of muscles, stimulated either directly or indirectly, has usually been found to be raised by adrenaline (OBRÉ, 1923;

Krnjević and Miledi, 1958b) or unchanged (Luco, 1939); reduction in threshold is only rarely found (Gruber, 1914).

Other more complex actions of catecholamines at the neuromuscular junction are potentiation of the twitch tension recorded from muscles treated with neostigmine (Naess and Sirnes, 1954; Bowman and Raper, 1966, 1967) and augmentation of repetitive firing produced by anticholinesterases (Blaber and Bowman, 1963). This latter effect is prevented by benzoquinonium (Bowman, 1958; Blaber and Bowman, 1962; Christ and Blaber, 1968), which also inhibits the prejunctional facilitatory actions of catechol and phenol acting on different receptors from those of the catecholamines (Blaber and Gallagher, 1971).

It should be noted in passing that the anticurare action of adrenaline in partially-curarized muscles is very susceptible to changes in extracellular K^+ and Ca^{2+} concentrations (Goffart and Brown, 1947; Goffart, 1949, 1952b and Montagu, 1955), findings which may account for the difficulty sometimes experienced in observing this effect in isolated muscles (Brown et al., 1948).

In non-fatigued fully curarized amphibian and avian muscle, the effects of catecholamines on directly-stimulated muscle are lacking (Corkill, and Tiegs, 1933; Brown et al., 1950; Hutter and Lowenstein, 1955; Raper and Bowman, 1968). A facilitatory action on transmission in partially curarized preparations is, however, observed and, as in mammalian muscles, is mediated by α-adrenoceptors (Jenkinson et al., 1968; Raper and Bowman, 1968). The amines do not cause changes in demarcation potential in frog muscle (Brown et al., 1950; Hutter and Lowenstein, 1955) but they hyperpolarize avian muscles (Raper and Bowman, 1968) and by this means potentiate blockade by tubocurarine.

In muscles fatigued by indirect stimulation, depression of neuromuscular transmission, which is partly the cause of the reduction in twitch tension, can be relieved by stimulation of the lumbar sympathetic chain (Orbeli, 1923; Corkill and Tiegs, 1933; Bowman and Nott, 1969), splanchnic nerves (Cannon and Nice, 1911, 1913) or the infusion of adrenaline, noradrenaline and, to a lesser extent, of isoprenaline (Dessy and Grandis, 1904; Cannon and Nice, 1911, 1913; Gruber, 1924; Burn, 1945; Shapiro, 1961; Bowman and Nott, 1969). The degree of relief obtained is in part dependent on the frequency of stimulation of the sympathetic nerves; for example, in fast-contracting muscles 1 Hz is more effective than 0.1 Hz (Bowman and Raper, 1966). At higher stimulus frequencies, however, twitch tension is either not further increased, as in the frog (Hutter and Lowenstein, 1955) or depressed, as in mammals, due to prolonged vasoconstriction (Brown et al., 1948). In the frog, facilitation of transmission by noradrenaline is abolished by phentolamine (Jenkinson et al., 1968). At mammalian neuromuscular junctions, however, such facilitation is reduced but not abolished by α-adrenoceptor blocking compounds, namely ergotoxine (Luco, 1939; Bülbring and Burn, 1940) and phenoxybenzamine and phentolamine (Bowman and Nott, 1969); the remaining effects, which are probably directly on the muscle fibres, are abolished by β-adrenoceptor blocking drugs. These findings are in keeping with the more complex nature of fatigue of mammalian muscle which has an important post-junctional component (Merton, 1956; Krnjević and Miledi, 1958a; Eberstein and Sandow, 1963).

4. Electrophysiological Analysis of Junctional Effects

There have been few attempts to use microelectrode techniques for the analysis of the site and mechanism of action of catecholamines and related substances at the neuromuscular junction. HUTTER and LOWENSTEIN (1955) found that in fast-contracting muscles of frogs, when transmission was blocked by (+)-tubocurarine, both adrenaline (0.05—1 μg/ml) and noradrenaline (0.1—10 μg/ml) increased the amplitude of end-plate potentials (EPPs) without altering the resting membrane potential. Since depolarization induced by acetylcholine added to the bathing solution was greater in the presence of noradrenaline, they thought that the amines were acting only postjunctionally, namely by increasing the sensitivity of the receptors to acetylcholine. More recently, JENKINSON et al. (1968) investigated the effect of noradrenaline (10^{-5}M) in fast-contracting muscles of frogs in which neuromuscular transmission was blocked by excessive concentrations of Mg^{2+}. Although they, too, observed an increase in amplitude of EPPs, they found that there was no concurrent change in amplitude of miniature EPPs nor increased depolarizations by acetylcholine applied iontophoretically close to the site of recording. Further evidence in favour of a prejunctional site of action of noradrenaline was obtained with the findings that the frequency of miniature EPPs was increased and the variance of the amplitudes of successive EPPs was reduced, as would be expected if there was an increased release of acetylcholine. They were able to confirm the results of HUTTER and LOWENSTEIN that the depolarization in response to acetylcholine added to the bathing solution was enhanced by noradrenaline. In the discussion of their results, JENKINSON et al. mention that the prejunctional action of noradrenaline was not blocked by pronethalol but was abolished by phentolamine, findings which are in keeping with the view that the prejunctional effects of catecholamines are mediated by α-adrenoceptors.

KRNJEVIĆ and MILEDI (1958b) investigated the effects of adrenaline on neuromuscular transmission in rat muscle both *in situ* (gracilis) and *in vitro* (diaphragm) when transmission was depressed by (+)-tubocurarine, excess Mg^{2+} or fatigue. Since, under these circumstances, there was an increase in the amplitude of EPPs, more transmitter may have been liberated in the presence of adrenaline. In confirmation of this view, they found in the diaphragm that there was no increase in the amplitude of miniature EPPs or of the depolarization due to acetylcholine applied iontophoretically to the end-plate; also, adrenaline regularly caused an increase in the frequency of miniature EPPs. Noradrenaline was tested in one preparation and was found to increase the frequency of miniature EPPs. There was no appreciable change in the postjunctional membrane resting potential but there was decreased excitability of isolated muscle fibres when stimulated at low frequencies in the presence of adrenaline (0.5—3 μg/ml). Since, however, adrenaline usually relieved the intermittent prejunctional failure of conduction associated with rapid tetanic stimulation (25 Hz), KRNJEVIĆ and MILEDI (1958b) concluded that the observed action of adrenaline would depend on whether facilitatory prejunctional or inhibitory postjunctional effects were predominant.

Recently, KUBA (1970) re-investigated the effects of catecholamines on junctional transmission in the rat isolated diaphragm when transmission was depressed by a reduced [Ca^{2+}] / [Mg^{2+}] ratio or by (+)-tubocurarine. Adrenaline (5 μg/ml) and isoprenaline (5 μg/ml) increased the resting membrane potential by 3—4 mV; noradrenaline (5 μg/ml) had little effect. Noradrenaline increased the frequency of miniature EPPs without increasing their amplitude, whereas isoprenaline increased the amplitude but not the frequency of miniature EPPs; adrenaline increased both frequency and amplitude. Noradrenaline and adrenaline augmented the extracellularly recorded end plate current but had no effect on the action current of the nerve terminal, on the synaptic delay, or on the duration of the end plate current. Isoprenaline had no effect on any of these parameters. The actions of noradrenaline and adrenaline on the end plate current were abolished by phentolamine (2 μg/ml) but were unaffected by pronethalol (2 μg/ml). Unlike noradrenaline, adrenaline and isoprenaline increased the input resistance of the membrane, thus increasing the amplitude of the EPP for the same amount of current flowing through the end plate membrane; this action was blocked by pronethalol but not by phentolamine. The amplitude of the potential elicited by iontophoretic application of acetylcholine was increased by adrenaline and isoprenaline but not by noradrenaline. It is therefore concluded that noradrenaline acts on the prejunctional terminal increasing the amount of transmitter released and that isoprenaline acts on the postjunctional membrane enhancing the input resistance; adrenaline has both pre- and post-junctional actions. In confirmation of previous findings, the prejunctional effect is mediated by an α-adrenoceptor and the postjunctional effect by a β-adrenoceptor.

The finding of an increase in frequency of miniature EPPs in the presence of the amines suggests that there is a prejunctional depolarization. However, such an explanation cannot account for the simulatenous occurrence of an increase in amplitude of EPPs because it has been established that, when the membrane potential of prejunctional terminals is altered, there is an inverse relationship between the resultant changes in frequency of miniature EPPs and amplitude of EPPs (DEL CASTILLO and KATZ, 1954; LILEY, 1956). Since the amplitude of miniature EPPs is not changed, the increase in amplitude of EPPs must be due to an increase in the quantal content but, paradoxically, increases in quantal content are usually the result of hyperpolarization of prejunctional terminals (HUBBARD and SCHMIDT, 1961; HUBBARD and WILLIS, 1962). One explanation for the simulatenous increase in frequency of miniature EPPs and increase in quantal content of EPPs may be that the site of hyperpolarization of the prejunctional terminal membrane is not the same as the site of depolarization (BOWMAN and NOTT, 1969). Alternatively, if noradrenaline and adrenaline increased the probability of release of acetylcholine, an increase in both frequency of miniature EPPs and quantal content of EPPs would be observed. In an investigation of the effects of catechol on fast-contracting muscle of the cat, it was found that there was an increase in frequency of miniature EPPs and amplitude of EPPs (GALLAGHER and BLABER, 1970 and personal communication). Further analysis showed that these effects were due to a common cause, namely an increase in the probability of release of acetylcholine. Since, however, catechol acts on receptors which are different from those for adrenaline and noradrenaline, the explanation for the mechanism of action prejunctionally of the catecholamines must remain uncertain.

Since the innervation of piscine red muscle is typical of slow muscle (NISHIHARA, 1966, 1967), it is of interest to know how this junction is affected by catecholamines. HIDAKA and KURIYAMA (1969) found marked differences between the effects of adrenaline and noradrenaline: a) noradrenaline (0.01—5 μg/ml) hyperpolarizes the muscle by up to 11 mV; b) adrenaline (0.01—5 μg/ml) unlike noradrenaline, increases input resistance of the membrane; c) noradrenaline raises the frequency of miniature excitatory junction potentials (EJPs) but does not alter their amplitude whereas adrenaline scarcely affects the frequency but considerably increases the amplitude of miniature EJPs; d) the amplitude of EJPs is more markedly increased by adrenaline than by noradrenaline, the increased input resistance being the principal factor responsible for the action of adrenaline. Correspondingly, the current associated with EJPs was increased by noradrenaline but not by adrenaline. Thus, these authors concluded that adrenaline acted mainly postjunctionally and noradrenaline only prejunctionally.

References

Abbs, E.T., Robertson, M.I.: Selective depletion of noradrenaline: a proposed mechanism of the adrenergic neurone-blocking action of bretylium. Brit. J. Pharmacol. **38**, 776—791 (1970).

Ambache, N.: A further study of the action of Clostridium botulinum toxin on different types of autonomic nerve fibre. J. Physiol. (Lond.) **113**, 1—17 (1951).

Appel, W.C., Vincenzi, F.F.: Effects of hemicholinium and bretylium on the release of autonomic transmitters in the isolated sino-atrial node. Brit. J. Pharmacol. **40**, 268—274 (1970).

Armett, C., Ritchie, J.M.: The action of acetylcholine in mammalian non-myelinated fibres and its prevention by an anticholinesterase. J. Physiol. (Lond.) **152**, 141—158 (1960).

Baumgarten, H.G., Holstein, A.F., Owman, Ch.: Auerbach's plexus of mammals and man: electron microscopic identification of three different types of neuronal processes in myenteric ganglia of the large intestine from rhesus monkeys, guinea-pigs and man. Z. Zellforsch. **106**, 376—397 (1970).

Beani, L., Bianchi, C., Crema, A.: The effect of catecholamines and sympathetic stimulation on the release of acetylcholine from the guinea-pig colon. Brit. J. Pharmacol. **36**, 1—17 (1969).

Bentley, G.A.: Studies on sympathetic mechanisms in isolated intestinal and vas deferens preparations. Brit. J. Pharmacol. **19**, 85—98 (1962).

Bevan, J.A., Su, C.: The sympathetic mechanism in the isolated pulmonary artery of the rabbit. Brit. J. Pharmacol. **22**, 176—182 (1964).

Bhagat, B.: Response of isolated guinea-pig atria to various ganglion-stimulating agents. J. Pharmacol. exp. Ther. **154**, 264—270 (1966).

— Bovell, G., Robinson, I.M.: Influence of cocaine on the uptake of H^3-norepinephrine and on the responses of isolated guinea-pig atria to sympathomimetic amines. J. Pharmacol. exp. Ther. **159**, 472—478 (1967a).

— Robinson, I.M., West, W.L.: Mechanism of sympathomimetic responses of isolated guinea-pig atria to nicotine and dimethylphenylpiperazinium iodide. Brit. J. Pharmacol. **30**, 470—477 (1967b).

Birks, R., MacIntosh, F.C.: Acetylcholine metabolism of a sympathetic ganglion. Canad. J. Biochem. **39**, 787—827 (1961).

Birmingham, A.T., Wilson, A.B.: Preganglionic and postganglionic stimulation of the guinea-pig isolated vas deferens preparation. Brit. J. Pharmacol. **21**, 569—580 (1962).

— — An analysis of the blocking action of dimethylphenylpiperazinium iodide on the inhibition of isolated small intestine produced by stimulation of the sympathetic nerves. Brit. J. Pharmacol. **24**, 375—386 (1965).

Björklund, A., Cegrell, L., Falck, B., Ritzen, M., Rosengren, E.: Dopamine-containing cells in sympathetic ganglia. Acta physiol. scand. **78**, 334—338 (1970).

Blaber, L.C., Bowman, W.C.: The interaction between benzoquinonium and anticholinesterases in skeletal muscle. Arch. int. Pharmacodyn. **138**, 90—104 (1962).

— — The effects of some drugs on the repetitive discharges produced in nerve and muscle by anticholinesterases. Int. J. Neuropharmacol. **2**, 1—16 (1963).

— Gallagher, J.P.: The facilitatory effects of catechol and phenol at the neuromuscular junction of the cat. Neuropharmacol. **10**, 153—159 (1971).

Blakeley, A.G.H., Brown, G.L., Ferry, C.B.: Pharmacological experiments on the release of the sympathetic transmitter. J. Physiol. (Lond.) **167**, 505—514 (1963).

Bleckman, I., Jurna, I., Rummel, W.: Vergleichende Untersuchungen von Methoden zur Bestimmung der Plateaudauer des aktiven Zustandes am Warmblütermuskel. Pflügers Arch. ges. Physiol. **277**, 422—433 (1963).

Boullin, D.J.: The action of extracellular cations on the release of the sympathetic transmitter from peripheral nerves. J. Physiol. (Lond.) **189**, 85—99 (1967).

Boura, A.L.A., Copp, F.C., Duncombe, W.G., Green, A.F., McCoubrey, A.: The selective accumulation of bretylium in sympathetic ganglia and their postganglionic nerves. Brit. J. Pharmacol. **15**, 265—270 (1960).

— Green, A.F.: The actions of bretylium: adrenergic blocking and other effects. Brit. J. Pharmacol. **14**, 538—548 (1959).

— — Adrenergic neurone blocking agents. Ann. Rev. Pharmacol. **5**, 183—212 (1965).

Bowman, W.C.: The neuromuscular blocking action of benzoquinonium chloride in the cat and the hen. Brit. J. Pharmacol. **13**, 521—530 (1958).

— Callingham, B.A., Cuthbert, A.W.: The effects of physostigmine on the mechanical and electrical responses of the cat nictitating membrane. Brit. J. Pharmacol. **22**, 558—576 (1964).

Bowman, W.C., Goldberg, A.A.J., Raper, C.: A comparison between the effects of a tetanus and the effects of sympathomimetic amines on fast- and slow-contracting mammalian muscles. Brit. J. Pharmacol. **19**, 464—484 (1962).

— — — Post-tetanic and drug-induced repetitive firing in the soleus muscle of the cat. Brit. J. Pharmacol. **35**, 62—78 (1969).

— Hall, M.T.: Inhibition of rabbit intestine mediated by α- and β-adrenoceptive receptors. Brit. J. Pharmacol. **38**, 399—415 (1970).

— Nott, M.W.: Actions of sympathomimetic amines and their antagonists on skeletal muscle. Pharmacol. Rev. **21**, 27—72 (1969).

— — Actions of some sympathomimetic bronchodilator and beta-adrenoceptor blocking drugs on contractions of the cat soleus muscle. Brit. J. Pharmacol. **38**, 37—49 (1970).

— Raper, C.: Effects of sympathomimetic amines on neuromuscular transmission. Brit. J. Pharmacol. **27**, 313—331 (1966).

— — Adrenotropic receptors in skeletal muscle. Ann. N.Y. Acad. Sci. **139**, 741—753 (1967).

— Zaimis, E.: The effects of adrenaline, noradrenaline and isoprenaline on skeletal muscle contractions in the cat. J. Physiol. (Lond.) **144**, 92—107 (1958).

Brandon, K.W., Boyd, H.: Release of noradrenaline from the spleen of the cat by acetylcholine. Nature (Lond.) **192**, 880—881 (1962).

— Rand, M.J.: Acetylcholine and the sympathetic innervation of the spleen. J. Physiol. (Lond.) **157**, 18—32 (1961).

Brown, G.L., Bülbring, E., Burns, B.D.: The action of adrenaline on mammalian skeletal muscle. J. Physiol. (Lond.) **107**, 115—128 (1948).

— Goffart, M., Vianna Dias, M.: The effects of adrenaline and of sympathetic stimulation on the demarcation potential of mammalian skeletal muscle. J. Physiol. (Lond.) **111**, 184—194 (1950).

Brücke, F.T. v.: Über die Wirkung von Acetylcholin auf die Pilomotoren. Klin. Wschr. **14**, 7—9 (1935).

Bueding, E., Bülbring, E.: Relationship between energy metabolism of intestinal smooth muscle and the physiological actions of epinephrine. Ann. N.Y. Acad. Sci. **139**, 758—761 (1967).

Bülbring, E.: The action of adrenaline on transmission in the superior cervical ganglion. J. Physiol. (Lond.) **103**, 55—67 (1944).

— Burn, J.H.: The sympathetic dilator fibres in the muscles of the cat and dog. J. Physiol. (Lond.) **83**, 483—501 (1935).

— — The effect of sympathomimetic and other substances on the contraction of skeletal muscle. J. Pharmacol. exp. Ther. **68**, 150—172 (1940).

— — An action of adrenaline on transmission in sympathetic ganglia, which may play a part in shock. J. Physiol. (Lond.) **101**, 289—303 (1942).

— Tomita, T.: Suppression of spontaneous spike generation by catecholamines in the smooth muscle of the guinea-pig taenia coli. Proc. roy. Soc. B. **172**, 103—119 (1969).

Burgen, A.S. V., Dickens, F., Zatman, L.J.: The action of botulinum toxin on the neuromuscular junction. J. Physiol. (Lond.) **109**, 10—24 (1949).

Burn, J.H.: The relation of adrenaline to acetylcholine in the nervous system. Physiol. Rev. **25**, 377—394 (1945).

— A new view of adrenergic nerve fibres, explaining the action of reserpine, bretylium and guanethidine. Brit. med. J. **1**, 1623—1627 (1961).

— The release of norepinephrine from the sympathetic postganglionic fiber. Bull. Johns Hopk. Hosp. **112**, 167—182 (1963).

— Adrenergic transmission .A. Introductory remarks. Pharmacol. Rev. **18**, 459—470 (1966).

— Release of noradrenaline from the sympathetic postganglionic fibre. Brit. med. J. **2**, 197—201 (1967).

— Froede, H.: The action of substances which block sympathetic postganglionic nervous transmission. Brit. J. Pharmacol. **20**, 378—387 (1963).

— Gibbons, W.R.: The part played by calcium in determining the response to stimulation of sympathetic postganglionic fibres. Brit. J. Pharmacol. **22**, 540—548 (1964a).

— — The sympathetic postganglionic fibre and the block by bretylium; the block prevented by hexamethoinum and imitated by mecamylamine. Brit. J. Pharmacol. **22**, 549—557 (1964b).

— — The release of noradrenaline from sympathetic fibres in relation to calcium concentrations. J. Physiol. (Lond.) **181**, 214—223 (1965).

— Malik, K.U.: Effect of anticholinesterases on the responses to stimulation of adrenergic fibres. J. Physiol. (Lond.) **208**, 82—83P (1970).

— Rand, M.J.: Sympathetic postganglionic mechanism. Nature (Lond.) **184**, 163—165 (1959)

— — Sympathetic postganglionic cholinergic fibres. Brit. J. Pharmacol. **15**, 56—66 (1960).

— — Acetylcholine in adrenergic transmission. Ann. Rev. Pharmacol. **5**, 163—182 (1965).

BURN, J.H., RAND, M.J., WIEN, R.: The adrenergic mechanism in the nictitating membrane. Brit. J. Pharmacol. **20**, 83—94 (1963).
— WEETMAN, D.F.: The effect of eserine on the response of the vas deferens to hypogastric nerve stimulation. Brit. J. Pharmacol. **20**, 74—82 (1963).
— WELSH, F.: The effect of calcium in removing the blocking action of bretylium and guanethidine. Brit. J. Pharmacol. **31**, 74—81 (1967).
BURNSTOCK, G.: Evolution of the autonomic innervation of visceral and cardiovascular systems in vertebrates. Pharmacol. Rev. **21**, 247—322 (1969).
— HOLMAN, M.E.: An electrophysiological investigation of the actions of some autonomic blocking drugs on transmission in the guinea-pig vas deferens. Brit. J. Pharmacol. **23**, 600—612 (1964).
CABRERA, R., COHEN, A., MIDDLETON, S., UTANO, L., VIVEROS, H.: The immediate source of noradrenaline released in the heart by acetylcholine. Brit. J. Pharmacol. **27**, 46—50 (1966a).
— TORRANCE, R.W., VIVEROS, H.: The action of acetylcholine and other drugs upon the terminal parts of the postganglionic sympathetic fibre. Brit. J. Pharmacol. **27**, 51—63 (1966b).
CAIRNCROSS, K.D., MCCULLOCH, M.W., STORY, D.F., TRINKER, F.: Modification of synaptic transmission in the superior cervical ganglion by epinephrine, norepinephrine and nortriptyline. Int. J. Neuropharmacol. **6**, 293—300 (1967).
CANNON, W.B., NICE, L.B.: The effect of splanchnic stimulation on muscular fatigue. Amer. J. Physiol. **29**, 24—25 (1911).
— — The effect of adrenalin secretion on muscular fatigue. Amer. J. Physiol. **32**, 44—60 (1913).
CHANG, V., RAND, M.J.: Transmission failure in sympathetic nerves produced by hemicholinium. Brit. J. Pharmacol. **15**, 588—600 (1960).
CHRIST, D.D., BLABER, L.C.: The actions of benzoquinonium in the isolated cat tenuissimus muscle. J. Pharmacol. exp. Ther. **160**, 159—165 (1968).
— NISHI, S.: Presynaptic action of epinephrine on sympathetic ganglia. Life Sci. **8**, 1235—1238 (1969).
— — Site of adrenaline blockade in the superior cervical ganglion of the rabbit. J. Physiol. (Lond.) **213**, 107—117 (1971).
CLEMENTI, F., MANTEGAZZA, P., BOTTURI, M.: A pharmacologic and morphologic study on the nature of the dense-core granules present in the presynaptic endings of sympathetic ganglia. Int. J. Neuropharmacol. **5**, 281—285 (1966).
COON, J.M., ROTHMAN, S.: The nature of the pilomotor responses to acetylcholine; some observations on the pharmacodynamics of the skin. J. Pharmacol. exp. Ther. **68**, 301—311 (1940).
CORKILL, A.B., TIEGS, O.W.: The effect of sympathetic nerve stimulation on the power of contraction of skeletal muscle. J. Physiol. (Lond.) **78**, 161—185 (1933).
COSTA, E., REVZIN, A.M., KUNTZMAN, R., SPECTOR, S., BRODIE, B.B.: Role for ganglionic norepinephrine in sympathetic synaptic transmission. Science **133**, 1822—1823 (1961).
COWIE, A.L., KOSTERLITZ, H.W., WATT, A.J.: Mode of action of morphine-like drugs on autonomic neuroeffectors. Nature (Lond.) **220**, 1040—1042 (1968).
CSILLIK, B., KÁLMÁN, G., KNYIHÁR, E.: Adrenergic nerve endings in the feline cervical superius ganglion. Experientia (Basel) **23**, 477—478 (1967).
CURTIS, D.R.: The pharmacology of central and peripheral inhibition. Pharmacol. Rev. **15**, 333—364 (1963).
DALY, B. DE B., SCOTT, M.J.: The effects of acetylcholine on the volume and vascular resistance of the dog's spleen. J. Physiol. (Lond.) **156**, 246—259 (1961).
DAVEY, M.J., HAYDEN, M.L., SCHOLFIELD, P.C.: The effects of bretylium on C fibre excitation and noradrenaline release by acetylcholine and electrical stimulation. Brit. J. Pharmacol. **34**, 377—387 (1968).
DE GROAT, W.C., VOLLE, R.L.: The actions of the catecholamines on transmission in the superior cervical ganglion of the cat. J. Pharmacol. exp. Ther. **154**, 1—13 (1966a).
— — Interactions between the catecholamines and ganglionic stimulating agents in sympathetic ganglia. J. Pharmacol. exp. Ther. **154**, 200—215 (1966b).
DEL CASTILLO, J., KATZ, B.: Changes in end-plate activity produced by pre-synaptic polarization. J. Physiol. (Lond.) **124**, 586—604 (1954).
DESSY, S., GRANDIS, V,: Contribution à l'étude de la fatigue. Action de l'adrénaline sur la fonction du muscle. Arch. ital. Biol. **41**, 225—233 (1904).
DOCKRY, M., KERNAN, R.P., TANGNEY, A.: Active transport of sodium and potassium in mammalian skeletal muscle and its modification by nerve and by cholinergic and adrenergic agents. J. Physiol. (Lond.) **186**, 187—200 (1966).

DOUGLAS, W. W., RITCHIE, J. M.: A technique for recording functional activity in specific groups of medullated and non-medullated fibres in whole nerve trunks. J. Physiol. (Lond.) **138**, 19—30 (1957).

EBERSTEIN, A., SANDOW, A.: Fatigue mechanisms in muscle fibres. In: *The Effect of Use and Disuse on Neuromuscular Functions*. Ed. by E. GUTMAN and P. HNÍK, pp. 515—526. Amsterdam: Elsevier Publishing Co. 1963.

ECCLES, R. M.: Responses of isolated curarized sympathetic ganglia. J. Physiol. (Lond.) **117**, 196—217 (1952).

— LIBET, B.: Origin and blockade of the synaptic responses of curarized sympathetic ganglia. J. Physiol. (Lond.) **157**, 484—503 (1961).

EHINGER, B., FALCK, B.: Uptake of some catecholamines and their precursors into neurons of the rat ciliary ganglion. Acta physiol. scand. **78**, 132—141 (1970).

— — PERSSON, H.: Function of cholinergic nerve fibres in the cat iris dilator. Acta physiol. scand. **72**, 139—147 (1968).

— — — ROSENGREN, A.-M., SPORRONG, B.: Acetylcholine in adrenergic terminals of the cat iris. J. Physiol. (Lond.) **209**, 557—565 (1970a).

— — SPORRONG, B.: Possible axo-axonal synapses between adrenergic and cholinergic nerve terminals. Z. Zellforsch. **107**, 508—521 (1970b).

ELFVIN, L.-G.: A new granule-containing nerve cell in the inferior mesenteric ganglion of the rabbit. J. Ultrastruct. Res. **22**, 37—44 (1968).

ELMQVIST, D., QUASTEL, D. M. J.: A quantitative study of end-plate potentials in isolated human muscles. J. Physiol. (Lond.) **178**, 505—529 (1965).

ERÄNKÖ, O., HÄRKÖNEN, M.: Histochemical demonstration of fluorogenic amines in the cytoplasm of sympathetic ganglion cells of the rat. Acta physiol. scand. **58**, 285—286 (1963).

— RECHARDT, L., ERÄNKÖ, L., CUNNINGHAM, A.: Light and electron microscopic histochemical observations on cholinesterase-containing sympathetic nerve fibres in the pineal body of the rat. Histochem. J. **2**, 479—489 (1970).

ESTERHUIZEN, A. C., GRAHAM, J. D. P., LEVER, J. D., SPRIGGS, T. L. B.: Catecholamine and acetylcholinesterase distribution in relation to noradrenaline release. An enzyme histochemical and autoradiographic study on the innervation of the cat nictitating membrane. Brit. J. Pharmacol. **32**, 46—56 (1968).

EULER, U. S. VON, GADDUM, J. H.: Pseudomotor contractures after degeneration of the facial nerve. J. Physiol. (Lond.) **73**, 54—66 (1931).

EXLEY, K. A.: The persistence of adrenergic nerve conduction after TM 10 or bretylium in the cat. In: *Adrenergic Mechanisms*, Ciba Foundation. Ed. by J. R. VANE, G. E. W. WOLSTENHOLME and M. O'CONNOR, pp. 158—161. London: Churchill 1960.

FALCK, B.: Observations on the possibilities of the cellular localization of mono-amines by a fluorescence method. Acta physiol. scand. **56**, Suppl. 197 (1962).

FARMER, J. B., RAND, M. J., WILSON, J.: Facilitation of ganglionic transmission by some adrenergic neurone blocking drugs. Int. J. Neuropharmacol. **5**, 241—246 (1966).

FARRELL, K. E.: Fine structures of nerve fibres in smooth muscle of the vas deferens in normal and reserpinized rats. Nature (Lond.) **217**, 279—280 (1968).

FERRY, C. B.: The sympathomimetic effect of acetylcholine on the spleen of the cat. J. Physiol. (Lond.) **167**, 487—504 (1963).

— Cholinergic link hypothesis in adrenergic neuroeffector transmission. Physiol. Rev. **46**, 420—456 (1966).

FILLENZ, M.: The innervation of the cat spleen. Proc. roy. Soc. B. **174**, 459—468 (1970).

FISCHER, J. E., WEISE, V. K., KOPIN, I. J.: Interactions of bretylium and acetylcholine at sympathetic nerve endings. J. Pharmacol. exp. Ther. **153**, 523—529 (1966).

FOLKOW, B.: Nervous control of the blood vessels. Physiol. Rev. **35**, 629—663 (1955).

— HAEGER, K., UVNÄS, B.: Cholinergic vasodilator nerves in the sympathetic outflow to the muscles of the hind limbs of the cat. Acta physiol. scand. **15**, 401—411 (1948a).

— — — Cholinergic fibres in the sympathetic outflow to the heart in the dog and cat. Acta physiol. scand. **15**, 421—426 (1948b).

GABELLA, G.: Electron microscopical examination of the junction between the myenteric plexus and the longitudinal muscle of the guinea-pig ileum. Brit. J. Pharmacol. **40**, 588P (1970).

— Synapses of adrenergic fibres. Experientia (Basel) **27**, 280—281 (1971).

GALLAGHER, J. P., BLABER, L. C.: Action of catechol on the isolated tenuissimus muscle of the cat. Pharmacologist **12**, 301 (1970).

GARDINER, J. E., HELLMANN, K., THOMPSON, J. W.: The nature of the innervation of the smooth muscle, Harderian gland and blood vessels of the cat's nictitating membrane. J. Physiol. (Lond.) **163**, 436—456 (1962).

— THOMPSON, J. W.: Lack of evidence for a cholinergic mechanism in sympathetic transmission. Nature (Lond.) **191**, 86 (1961).

GILLESPIE, J.S., MACKENNA, B.R.: The inhibitory action of the sympathetic nerves on the smooth muscle of the rabbit gut, its reversal by reserpine and restoration by catecholamines and DOPA. J. Physiol. (Lond.) **156**, 17—34 (1961).

GOFFART, M.: Calcium et action potentiatrice de quelques amines sympathicomimétiques sur la contraction du muscle strié non fatigué de mammifère. Experientia (Basel) **5**, 332—333 (1949).

— Recherches relatives à l'action de l'adrénaline sur le muscle strié de mammifère. I. Potentiation par l'adrénaline de la contraction maximale du muscle non fatigué. Arch. int. Physiol. **60**, 318—349 (1952a).

— Recherches relative à l'action de l'adrénaline sur le muscle strié de mammifère. II. Influence de l'équilibre ionique sur les effets musculaires de l'adrénaline. Arch. int. Physiol. **60**, 350—366 (1952b).

— BROWN, G.L.: Relation entre le potassium du milieu extracellulaire et l'action de l'adrénaline sur le muscle strié non fatigué du rat. C.R. Soc. Biol. (Paris) **141**, 958—959 (1947).

— PERRY, W.L.M.: The action of adrenaline on the rate of loss of potassium ions from unfatigued striated muscle. J. Physiol. (Lond.) **112**, 95—101 (1951).

— RITCHIE, J.M.: The effect of adrenaline on the contraction of mammalian skeletal muscle. J. Physiol. (Lond.) **116**, 357—371 (1952).

GRAHAM, J.D.P., LEVER, J.D., SPRIGGS, T.L.B.: An examination of adrenergic axons around pancreatic arterioles of the cat for the presence of acetylcholinesterase by high resolution autoradiographic and histochemical methods. Brit. J. Pharmacol. **33**, 15—20 (1968).

GRILLO, M.: Electron-microscopy of sympathetic tissue. Pharmacol. Rev. **18**, 387—399 (1966).

— PALAY, S.L.: Granule-containing vesicles in the autonomic nervous system. In: *V. Intern. Congr. Electron Microscopy*. Ed. by S.S. BREESE, vol. 2, p. U-1. New York: Academic Press 1962.

GRUBER, C.M.: Studies in fatigue III. The fatigue threshold as affected by adrenalin and by increased arterial pressure. Amer. J. Physiol. **33**, 335—355 (1914).

— Studies in fatigue XI. The effects of intravenous injections of massive doses of adrenalin upon skeletal muscle at rest and undergoing fatigue. Amer. J. Physiol. **61**, 475—492 (1922a.

— Studies in fatigue XII. The effect of adrenal secretion on non-fatigued and fatigued skeletal muscle. Amer. J. Physiol. **62**, 438—441 (1922b).

— The effect of adrenalin on the duration of the latent, the contraction and the relaxation periods of skeletal muscle at rest and undergoing fatigue. J. Pharmacol. exp. Ther. **23**, 335—351 (1924).

HAEUSLER, G., HAEFELY, W., HUERLIMANN, A.: Zum Mechanismus der adrenerg blockierenden Wirkung von Bretylium und Guanethidin. Naunyn-Schmiedeberg's Arch. Pharmak. **264**, 241—243 (1969a).

— — — On the mechanism of the adrenergic nerve blocking action of bretylium. Naunyn-Schmiedeberg's Arch. Pharmak. **265**, 260—277 (1969b).

— — THOENEN, H., HUERLIMANN, A.: Durch Acetylcholin hervorgerufene antidrome Aktivität im kardialen Sympathicus und Noradrenalinfreisetzung unter Guanethidin. Helv. physiol. pharmacol. Acta **26**, CR 352—354 (1968a).

— THOENEN, H., HAEFELY, W., HUERLIMANN, A.: Electrical events in cardiac adrenergic nerves and noradrenaline release from the heart induced by acetylcholine and KCl. Naunyn-Schmiedeberg's Arch. Pharmak. exp. Path. **261**, 389—411 (1968b).

— — — — Elektrosekretorische Koppelung bei der Noradrenalinfreisetzung aus adrenergen Nervenfasern durch nicotinartig wirkende Substanzen. Naunyn-Schmiedeberg's Arch. Pharmak. exp. Path. **263**, 217—218 (1969c).

HAMBERGER, B., NORBERG, K.-A.: Monoamines in sympathetic ganglia studied with fluorescence microscopy. Experientia (Basel) **19**, 580—581 (1963).

— — Adrenergic synaptic terminals and nerve cells in bladder ganglia of the cat. Int. J. Neuropharmacol. **4**, 41—45 (1965a).

— — Studies on some systems of adrenergic synaptic terminals in the abdominal ganglia of the cat. Acta physiol. scand. **65**, 235—242 (1965b).

— — UNGERSTEDT, U.: Adrenergic synaptic terminals in autonomic ganglia. Acta physiol. scand. **64**, 285—286 (1965).

HÄRKÖNEN, M.: Carboxylic esterases, oxidative enzymes and catecholamines in the superior cervical ganglion of the rat and the effect of pre- and post-ganglionic nerve division. Acta physiol. scand. **63**, Suppl. 237 (1964).

HELLMANN, K.: The isolated pilomotor muscles as an *in vitro* preparation. J. Physiol. (Lond.) **169**, 603—620 (1963).

HERTTING, G., WIDHALM, S.: Über den Mechanismus der Noradrenalin-Freisetzung aus sympathischen Nervenendigungen. Naunyn-Schmiedeberg's Arch. exp. Path. Pharmak, **250**, 257—258 (1965).

Hidaka, T., Kuriyama, H.: Effects of catecholamines on the cholinergic neuromuscular transmission in the fish red muscle. J. Physiol. (Lond.) **201**, 61—71 (1969).
Hökfelt, T.: *In vitro* studies on central and peripheral monoamine neurons at the ultrastructural level. Z. Zellforsch. **91**, 1—74 (1968).
Hoffmann, F., Hoffmann, E.J., Middleton, S., Talesnik, J.: The stimulating effect of acetylcholine on the mammalian heart and the liberation of an epinephrine-like substance from the isolated heart. Amer. J. Physiol. **144**, 189—198 (1945).
Hollands, B.C.S., Vanov, S.: Localization of catechol amines in visceral organs and ganglia of the rat, guinea-pig and rabbit. Brit. J. Pharmacol. **25**, 307—316 (1965).
Holton, P., Rand, M.J.: Sympathetic vasodilatation in the rabbit ear. Brit. J. Pharmacol. **19**, 513—526 (1962).
Hubbard, J.I., Schmidt, R.F.: Stimulation of motor nerve terminals. Nature (Lond.) **191**, 1103—1104 (1961).
— — An electrophysiological investigation of mammalian motor nerve terminals. J. Physiol. (Lond.) **166**, 145—167 (1963).
— Willis, W.D.: Hyperpolarization of mammalian motor nerve terminals. J. Physiol. (Lond.) **163**, 115—137 (1962).
Huković, S.: Isolated rabbit atria with sympathetic nerve supply. Brit. J. Pharmacol. **14**, 372—376 (1959).
— The action of sympathetic blocking agents on isolated and innervated atria and vessels. Brit. J. Pharmacol. **15**, 117—121 (1960).
— The effect of anticholinesterases on the increase in rate of the isolated heart in response to sympathetic stimulation. Brit. J. Pharmacol. **28**, 273—281 (1966).
— Muscholl, E.: Die Noradrenalin-Abgabe aus dem isolierten Kaninchenherzen bei sympathischer Nervenreizung und ihre pharmakologische Beeinflussung. Naunyn-Schmiedeberg's Arch. Pharmak. exp. Path. **244**, 81—96 (1962).
Hutter, O.F., Lowenstein, W.R.: Nature of neuromuscular facilitation by sympathetic stimulation in the frog. J. Physiol. (Lond.) **130**, 559—571 (1955).
Iwanow, G.: Das chromaffine und interrenale System des Menschen. Z. ges. Anat. **29**, 87—280 (1932).
Jacobowitz, D.: Histochemical studies of the autonomic innervation of the gut. J. Pharmacol. exp. Ther. **149**, 358—364 (1965).
— Histochemical studies of the relationship of chromaffin cells and adrenergic nerve fibres to the cardiac ganglia of several species. J. Pharmacol. exp. Ther. **158**, 227—240 (1967).
— Woodward, J.K.: Adrenergic neurons in the cat superior cervical ganglion and cervical sympathetic nerve trunk. A histochemical study. J. Pharmacol. exp. Ther. **162**, 213—226 (1968).
Jenkinson, D.H., Morton, I.K.M.: The role of α- and β-adrenergic receptors in some actions of catecholamines on intestinal smooth muscle. J. Physiol. (Lond.) **188**, 387—402 (1967).
— Stamenović, B.A., Whitaker, B.D.L.: The effect of noradrenaline on the end-plate potentials in twitch fibres of the frog. J. Physiol. (Lond.) **195**, 743—754 (1968).
Jurna, I., Rummel, W.: Die Wirkung von Adrenalin und Noradrenalin auf die Spannungsentwicklung vom Soleus und Tibialis anterior der Katze. Pflügers Arch. ges. Physiol. **275**, 137—151 (1962).
— — Schäfer, H.: Die abfallende Phase des aktiven Zustandes des Tibialis anterior, Gastrocnemius und Soleus der Katze und ihre Beeinflussung durch Dehnung und Sympathicomimetica. Pflügers Arch. ges. Physiol. **277**, 513—522 (1963).
Kirpekar, S.M., Cervoni, P., Furchgott, R.F.: Catecholamine content of the cat nictitating membrane following procedures sensitizing it to norepinephrine. J. Pharmacol. exp. Ther. **135**, 180—190 (1962).
— Misu, Y.: Release of noradrenaline by splenic nerve stimulation and its dependence on calcium. J. Physiol. (Lond.) **188**, 219—234 (1967).
— Wakade, A.R.: Release of noradrenaline from the cat spleen by potassium. J. Physiol. (Lond.) **194**, 595—608 (1968).
Kobayashi, H., Libet, B.: Generation of slow postsynaptic potentials without increases in ionic conductance. Proc. nat. Acad. Sci. (Wash.) **60**, 1304—1311 (1968).
— — Actions of noradrenaline and acetylcholine in sympathetic ganglion cells. J. Physiol. (Lond.) **208**, 353—372 (1970).
Kohn, A.: Die Paraganglien. Arch. mikr. Anat. **62**, 263—365 (1903).
Koketsu, K.: Cholinergic synaptic potentials and the underlying ionic mechanisms. Fed. Proc. **28**, 101—112 (1969).
Kosterlitz, H.W.: Intrinsic and extrinsic nervous control of motility of the stomach and the intestines. In: *Handbook of Physiology*, section 6, *Alimentary Canal*, volume IV, *Motility*. Ed. by C.F. Code and W. Heidel, pp. 2147—2171. Washington: American Physiological Society 1968.

KOSTERLITZ, H.W., COWIE, A.L.: Some aspects of transmission at the nerve-smooth muscle junction in the longitudinal muscle of the guinea-pig ileum. Amer. J. dig. Dis., N.S., **13**, 415—417 (1968).
— LEES, G.M.: Action of bretylium on the isolated guinea-pig ileum. Brit. J. Pharmacol. **17**, 82—86 (1961).
— — WALLIS, D.I.: Resting and action potentials recorded by the sucrose-gap method in the superior cervical ganglion of the rabbit. J. Physiol. (Lond.) **195**, 39—53 (1968).
— — — Further evidence for an electrogenic sodium pump in a mammalian sympathetic ganglion. Brit. J. Pharmacol. **38**, 464—465P (1970a).
— LYDON, R.J., WATT, A.J.: The effects of adrenaline, noradrenaline and isoprenaline on inhibitory α- and β-adrenoceptors in the longitudinal muscle of the guinea-pig ileum. Brit. J. Pharmacol. **39**, 398—413 (1970b).
— ROBINSON, J.A.: Inhibition of the peristalic reflex of the isolated guinea-pig ileum. J. Physiol. (Lond.) **136**, 249—262 (1957).
KOTTEGODA, S.R.: Stimulation of isolated rabbit auricles by substances which stimulate ganglia. Brit. J. Pharmacol. **8**, 83—86 (1953a).
— The action of nicotine and acetylcholine on the vessels of the rabbit ear. Brit. J. Pharmacol. **8**, 156—161 (1953b).
KRAUSS, K.R., CARPENTER, D.O., KOPIN, I.J.: Acetylcholine-induced release of norepinephrine in the presence of tetrodotoxin. J. Pharmacol. exp. Ther. **173**, 416—421 (1970).
KRNJEVIĆ, K., MILEDI, R.: Failure of neuromuscular propagation in rats. J. Physiol. (Lond.) **140**, 440—461 (1958a).
— — Some effects produced by adrenaline upon neuromuscular propagation in rats. J. Physiol. (Lond.) **141**, 291—304 (1958b).
KUBA, K.: Effects of catecholamines on the neuromuscular junction in the rat diaphragm. J. Physiol. (Lond.) **211**, 551—570 (1970).
LAVERTY, R., SHARMAN, D.F.: The estimation of small quantities of 3,4-dihydroxyphenylethylamine in tissues. Brit. J. Pharmacol. **24**, 538—548 (1965).
LAWRENTJEW, B.J.: Zur Morphologie des Ganglion cervical. super. Anat. Anz. **58**, 529—539 (1924).
LEADERS, F.E.: Separation of adrenergic and cholinergic fibres in sympathetic nerves to the hind limb of the dog by hemicholinium (HC-3). J. Pharmacol. exp. Ther. **148**, 238—246 (1965).
— DAYRIT, C.: The cholinergic component in the sympathetic innervation to the spleen. J. Pharmacol. exp. Ther. **147**, 145—152 (1965).
LEE, W.C., SHIDEMAN, F.E.: Mechanism of the positive inotropic response to certain ganglionic stimulants. J. Pharmacol. exp. Ther. **126**, 239—249 (1959).
LIBET, B., KOBAYASHI, H.: Generation of adrenergic and cholinergic potentials in sympathetic ganglion cells. Science **164**, 1530—1532 (1969).
LILEY, A.W.: The effects of presynaptic polarization on the spontaneous activity at the mammalian neuromuscular junction. J. Physiol. (Lond.) **134**, 427—443 (1956).
LINDMAR, R.: Die Wirkung von 1,1-Dimethyl-4-Phenyl-Piperazinium-Jodid am isolierten Vorhof im Vergleich zur Tyramin- und Nicotinwirkung. Naunyn-Schmiedeberg's Arch. Pharmak. exp. Path. **242**, 458—466 (1962).
— LÖFFELHOLZ, K., MUSCHOLL, E.: Unterschiede zwischen Tyramin und Dimethylphenylpiperazin in der Ca^{++}-Abhängigkeit und im zeitlichen Verlauf der Noradrenalin-Freisetzung am isolierten Kaninchenherzen. Experientia (Basel) **23**, 933—934 (1967).
— — — A muscarinic mechanism inhibiting the release of noradrenaline from peripheral adrenergic nerve fibres by nicotinic agents. Brit. J. Pharmacol. **32**, 280—294 (1968).
— MUSCHOLL, E.: Die Wirkung von Cocain, Guanethidin, Reserpin, Hexamethonium, Tetracain und Psicain auf die Noradrenalin-Freisetzung aus dem Herzen. Naunyn-Schmiedeberg's Arch. Pharmak. exp. Path. **242**, 214—227 (1961).
LISSÁK, K.: Liberation of acetylcholine and adrenaline by stimulating isolated nerves. Amer. J. Physiol. **127**, 263—271 (1939).
LOEWI, O.: Über humorale Übertragbarkeit der Herznervenwirkung. Pflügers Arch. ges. Physiol. **189**, 239—242 (1921).
LÖFFELHOLZ, K.: Untersuchungen über die Noradrenalin-Freisetzung durch Acetylcholin am perfundierten Kaninchenherzen. Naunyn-Schmiedeberg's Arch. Pharmak. exp. Path. **258**, 108—122 (1967).
— Autoinhibition of nicotinic release of noradrenaline from postganglionic sympathetic fibres. Naunyn-Schmiedeberg's Arch. Pharmak. **267**, 49—63 (1970a).
— Nicotinic drugs and postganglionic sympathetic transmission. Naunyn-Schmiedeberg's Arch. Pharmak. **267**, 64—73 (1970b).
— MUSCHOLL, E.: A muscarinic inhibition of the noradrenaline release evoked by postganglionic sympathetic nerve stimulation. Naunyn-Schmiedeberg's Arch. Pharmak. **265**, 1—15 (1969).

Löffelholz, K., Muscholl, E.: Inhibition by parasympathetic nerve stimulation of the release of the adrenergic transmitter. Naunyn-Schmiedeberg's Arch. Pharmak. **267**, 181—184 (1970).
Luco, J.V.: The defatiguing effect of adrenaline. Amer. J. Physiol. **125**, 196—204 (1939).
Lundberg, A.: Adrenaline and transmission in the sympathetic ganglion of the cat. Acta physiol. scand. **26**, 252—263 (1952).
Malik, K.U., Ling, G.M.: Modification by acetylcholine of the response of rat mesenteric arteries to sympathetic stimulation. Circulat. Res. **25**, 1—9 (1969a).
— — The effect of 1,1-dimethyl-4-phenylpiperazinium on the response of the mesenteric arteries to sympathetic nerve stimulation. J. Pharm. Pharmacol. **21**, 514—519 (1969b).
Malméjac, J.: Action of adrenaline on synaptic transmission and on adrenal medullary secretion. J. Physiol. (Lond.) **130**, 497—512 (1955).
Marrazzi, A.S.: Electrical studies on the pharmacology of autonomic synapses. II. The action of a sympathomimetic drug (epinephrine) on sympathetic ganglia. J. Pharmacol. exp. Ther. **65**, 395—404 (1939).
— Marrazzi, R.N.: Further localization and analysis of adrenergic synaptic inhibition. J. Neurophysiol. **10**, 167—178 (1947).
Marsden, C.D., Foley, T.H., Owen, D.A.L., McAllister, R.G.: Peripheral β-adrenergic receptors concerned with tremor. Clin. Sci. (Lond.) **33**, 53—65 (1967).
— Meadows, J.C.: The effect of adrenaline on the contraction of human muscle — one mechanism whereby adrenaline increases the amplitude of physiological tremor. J. Physiol. (Lond.) **194**, 70P (1968).
Matthews, M.R., Nash, J.R.G.: An efferent synapse from a small granule-containing cell to a principal neurone in the superior cervical ganglion. J. Physiol. (Lond.) **210**, 11—14P (1970).
— Raisman, G.: Two cell types in the superior cervical ganglion of the rat. J. Anat. (Lond.) **103**, 397—398 (1968).
— — The ultrastructure and somatic efferent synapses of small granule-containing cells in the superior cervical ganglion. J. Anat. (Lond.) **105**, 225—282 (1969).
Matthews, R.J.: The effect of epinephrine, levarterenol and dl-isoproterenol on transmission in the superior cervical ganglion of the cat. J. Pharmacol. exp. Ther. **116**, 433—443 (1956).
McDougal, M.D., West, G.B.: The action of isoprenaline on intestinal muscle. Arch. int. Pharmacodyn. **90**, 86—92 (1952).
— — The inhibition of the peristalic reflex by sympathomimetic amines. Brit. J. Pharmacol. **9**, 131—137 (1954).
McGregor, D.D.: The effect of sympathetic nerve stimulation on vasoconstrictor responses in perfused mesenteric blood vessels of the rat. J. Physiol. (Lond.) **177**, 21—30 (1965).
McIsaac, R.J.: Ganglion blocking properties of epinephrine and related amines. Int. J. Neuropharmacol. **5**, 15—26 (1966).
Merton, P.A.: Problems of muscular fatigue. Brit. med. Bull. **12**, 219—221 (1956).
Mirkin, B.L., Cervoni, P.: The adrenergic nature of neurohumoral transmission in the cat nictitating membrane following treatment with reserpine. J. Pharmacol. exp. Ther. **138**, 301—308 (1962).
Montagu, K.A.: On the mechanism of action of adrenaline in skeletal nerve-muscle. J. Physiol. (Lond.) **128**, 619—628 (1955).
Muscholl, E.: Cholinomimetic drugs and release of the adrenergic transmitter. In: *New aspects of storage and release mechanisms of catecholamines*. Ed. by H.J. Schümann and G. Kroneberg, pp. 168—186. Berlin-Heidelberg-New York: Springer 1970.
— Vogt, M.: The action of reserpine on the peripheral sympathetic system. J. Physiol. (Lond.) **141**, 132—155 (1958).
Naess, K., Sirnes, T.B.: A synergistic effect of adrenaline and d-tubocurarine on the neuromuscular transmission. Acta physiol. scand. **29**, 293—306 (1953).
— — An antagonistic effect between neostigmine and adrenaline on the striated muscle. Acta pharmacol. (Kbh.) **10**, 14—29 (1954).
Nedergaard, O.A., Bevan, J.A.: Effects of nicotine, dimethylphenylpiperazinium and cholinergic blocking agents at adrenergic nerve endings of the rabbit pulmonary artery. J. Pharmacol. exp. Ther. **168**, 127—136 (1969).
Nishi, S., Koketsu, K.: Origin of ganglionic inhibitory postsynaptic potential. Life Sci. **6**, 2049—2055 (1967).
— — Analysis of slow inhibitory post-synaptic potential of bullfrog sympathetic ganglion. J. Neurophysiol. **31**, 717—728 (1968).
Nishihara, H.: Some observations on the relationship between structure and function in fish red and white muscles. Proc. 6th Int. Congr. Electron Microsc. 693—694 (1966).
— Studies on the fine structure of red and white fin muscles of the fish (Carassius auratus). Arch. histol. jap. **28**, 425—447 (1967).

NORBERG, K.-A.: Adrenergic innervation of the intestinal wall studied by fluorescence microscopy. Int. J. Neuropharmacol. **3**, 379—382 (1964).

— HAMBERGER, B.: The sympathetic adrenergic neuron: Some characteristics revealed by histochemical studies on the intraneuronal distribution of the transmitter. Acta physiol. scand. **63**, Suppl. 238 (1964).

— RITZÉN, M., UNGERSTEDT, U.: Histochemical studies on a special catecholamine-containing cell type in sympathetic ganglia. Acta physiol. scand. **67**, 260—270 (1966).

— SJÖQVIST, F.: New possibilities for adrenergic modulation of ganglionic transmission. Pharmacol. Rev. **18**, 743—751 (1966).

NORDENFELDT, I.: Choline acetylase in normal and denervated salivary gland. Quart. J. exp. Physiol. **48**, 67—79 (1963).

— Choline acetylase in salivary glands of the cat after sympathetic denervation. Quart. J. exp. Physiol. **50**, 57—64 (1965).

OBRÉ, A.: Action de l'adrénaline et de l'extrait surrénal sur la fatigue musculaire. C.R Soc. Biol. (Paris) **88**, 585—588 (1923).

OLIVER, G., SCHÄFER, E.A.: The physiological effect of extracts of the suprarenal capsules. J. Physiol. (Lond.) **18**, 230—276 (1895).

ORBELI, L.A.: Die sympathische Innervation der Skelettmuskeln. Bull. Inst. sci. Leshaft. **6**, 194—197 (1923).

OWEN, D.A.L., MARSDEN, C.D.: Effect of adrenergic β-blockade on Parkinsonian tremor. Lancet ii, 1259—1262 (1965).

PARDO, E.G., CATO, J., GIJÓN, E., ALONSO- DE FLORIDA, F.: Influence of several adrenergic drugs on synaptic transmission through the superior cervical and the ciliary ganglion of the cat. J. Pharmacol. exp. Ther. **139**, 296—303 (1963).

PATON, W.D.M., THOMPSON, J.W.: The mechanism of action of adrenaline on the superior cervical ganglion of the cat. Proc. XIX Int. Physiol. Congr. Montreal, 664—665 (1953).

— VIZI, E.S.: The inhibitory action of noradrenaline and adrenaline on acetylcholine output by guinea-pig ileum longitudinal muscle strip. Brit. J. Pharmacol. **35**, 10—28 (1969).

— ZAR, M.A.: The origin of acetylcholine released from guinea-pig intestine and longitudinal muscle strip. J. Physiol. (Lond.) **194**, 13—33 (1968).

RAND, M.J., RIDEHALGH, A.: Actions of hemicholinium and triethylcholine on the responses of guinea-pig colon to stimulation of autonomic nerves. J. Pharm. Pharmacol. **17**, 144—156 (1965).

— VARMA, B.: The effects of cholinomimetic drugs on responses to sympathetic nerve stimulation and noradrenaline in the rabbit ear artery. Brit. J. Pharmacol. **38**, 758—770 (1970a).

— — Effects of McN-A-343 on responses induced by sympathetic nerve stimulation in the rabbit isolated ear artery. Brit. J. Pharmacol. **40**, 158—159P (1970b).

— WHALER, B.C.: Impairment of sympathetic transmission by botulinum toxin. Nature (Lond.) **206**, 588—591 (1965).

— WILSON, J.: The actions of some adrenergic neurone blocking drugs at cholinergic junctions. Europ. J. Pharmacol. **1**, 210—221 (1967).

RAPER, C., BOWMAN, W.C.: Effects of catecholamines on the gastrocnemius muscle of the domestic fowl. Europ. J. Pharmacol. **4**, 309—316 (1968).

REINERT, H.: Role and origin of noradrenaline in the superior cervical ganglion. J. Physiol. (Lond.) **167**, 18—29 (1963).

RICHARDSON, J.A., WOOD, E.F.: Release of norepinephrine from the isolated heart. Proc. Soc. exp. Biol. (N.Y.) **100**, 149—151 (1959).

SAMUEL, E.P.: Chromidial studies on the superior cervical ganglion of the rabbit. a) Caudally projected postganglionic axons, b) Intercalary "commissural" neurons. J. comp. Neurol. **98**, 93—111 (1953).

SHAPIRO, H.: Epinephrine and the latency of muscular contraction. J. cell. comp. Physiol. **58**, 35—47 (1961).

SHERIF, M.A.F.: The chemical transmitter of the sympathetic nerve to the uterus. J. Physiol. (Lond.) **85**, 298—308 (1935).

SIEGRIST, G., DOLIVO, M., DUNANT, Y., FOROGLOU-KERAMEUS, C., RIBAUPIERRE, FR. DE, ROUILLER, CH.: Ultrastructure and function of the chromaffin cells in the superior cervical ganglion of the rat. J. Ultrastruct. Res. **25**, 381—407 (1968).

SJÖQVIST, F.: The correlation between the occurrence and localization of acetylcholinesterase-rich cell bodies in the stellate ganglion and the outflow of cholinergic sweat secretory fibres to the fore paw of the cat. Acta physiol. scand. **57**, 339—351 (1963).

SMIRNOW, A.: Die Struktur der Nervenzellen im Sympatheticus der Amphibien. Arch. mikr. Anat. **35**, 407—424 (1890).

STÖHR, P.: Über „Nebenzellen" und deren Innervation in Ganglien des vegetativen Nervensystems, zugleich ein Beitrag zur Synapsenfrage. Z. Zellforsch. **29**, 569—612 (1939).

Tauc, L.: Transmission in invertebrate and vertebrate ganglia. Physiol. Rev. **47**, 521—593 (1967).

Taxi, J.: Contribution à l'étude des connexions des neurones moteurs du système nerveux autonome. Ann. Sci. nat. Zool. **7**, 413—674 (1965).

— Gautron, J., L'Hermite, P.: Données ultrastructures sur une éventuelle modulation adrénergique de l'activité du ganglion cervical supérieur du rat. C. R. Acad. Sci. (Paris) **269**, 1281—1284 (1969).

Thoenen, H., Tranzer, J.P.: Chemical sympathectomy by selective destruction of adrenergic nerve endings with 6-hydroxydopamine. Naunyn-Schmiedeberg's Arch. Pharmak. exp. Path. **261**, 271—288 (1968).

— — Hürlimann, A., Haefely, W.: Untersuchungen zur Frage eines cholinergischen Gliedes in der postganglionären sympathischen Transmission. Helv. Physiol. Acta **24**, 229—246 (1966).

Thompson, J.W.: Studies on the responses of the isolated nictitating membrane of the cat. J. Physiol. (Lond.) **141**, 46—72 (1958).

Tranzer, J.P., Thoenen, H.: Electronmicroscopic localization of 5-hydroxydopamine (3,4,5-trihydroxyphenylethylamine, a new "false" sympathetic transmitter. Experientia (Basel) **23**, 743 (1967).

— — Various types of amine-storing vesicles in peripheral adrenergic nerve terminals. Experientia (Basel) **24**, 484—486 (1968).

Trendelenburg, U.: Pharmacology of autonomic ganglia. Ann. Rev. Pharmacol. **1**, 219 to 238 (1961).

— Some aspects of the pharmacology of autonomic ganglion cells. Ergebn. Physiol. **59**, 1—85 (1967).

Van Orden, III, L.S., Burke, J.B., Geyer, M., Lodoen, F.V.: Localization of depletion-sensitive and depletion-resistant norepinephrine storage sites in autonomic ganglia. J. Pharmacol. exp. Ther. **174**, 56—71 (1970).

Vizi, E.S.: The inhibitory action of noradrenaline and adrenaline on release of acetylcholine from guinea-pig ileum longitudinal strips. Naunyn-Schmiedeberg's Arch. Pharmak. exp. Path. **259**, 199—200 (1968).

Volle, R.L.: Modification by drugs of synaptic mechanisms in autonomic ganglia. Pharmacol. Rev. **18**, 839—869 (1966).

Waterson, J.G., Hume, W.R., de la Lande, I.S.: The distribution of cholinesterase in the rabbit ear artery. J. Histochem. Cytochem. **18**, 211—216 (1970).

Watt, A.J.: Inhibitory mechanisms in guinea-pig isolated ileum. Aberdeen: Ph. D. thesis, Univ. 1966.

Weir, M.C.L., McLennan, H.: The action of catecholamines in sympathetic ganglia. Canad. J. Biochem. **41**, 2627—2636 (1963).

Westwood, D.A., Whaler, B.C.: Postganglionic paralysis of the guinea-pig hypogastric nerve — vas deferens preparation by *Clostridium botulinum* type D toxin. Brit. J. Pharmacol. **33**, 21—31 (1968).

Williams, T.H.: Electronmicroscopic evidence for an autonomic interneurone. Nature (Lond.) **214**, 309—310 (1967).

— Palay, S.L.: Ultrastructure of the small neurons in the superior cervical ganglion. Brain Res. **15**, 17—34 (1969).

Wilson, J.: The effects of calcium on adrenergic neuron blockade. J. Pharm. Pharmacol. **22**, 561—567 (1970).

Wolner, E.: Versuche über die Innervation der Pilomotoren. Naunyn-Schmiedeberg's Arch. Pharmak. exp. Path. **250**, 437—450 (1965).

Chapter 18

Surgical, Immunological and Chemical Sympathectomy

Their Application in the Investigation of the Physiology and Pharmacology of the Sympathetic Nervous System

H. THOENEN

With 8 Figures

I. Introduction

One of the oldest and most commonly used procedures in biological research to elucidate the physiological significance of an organ is its destruction or functional elimination. This principle has found wide application in the investigation of the physiological role of endocrine glands, in the characterization of the coordinative and regulatory function of different centres and tracts of the central nervous system and also in the study of the peripheral nervous system. Particularly for the sympathetic nervous system this procedure has proved to be most important in the elucidation of its general homeostatic function (CANNON et al., 1929; SAWYER et al., 1933; CANNON and ROSENBLUETH, 1937) and in the more detailed investigations concerning the sites of synthesis, storage and enzymatic degradation of the adrenergic transmitter (VON EULER and PURKHOLD, 1951; GOODALL, 1951; BURN et al., 1954; CROUT and COOPER, 1962; ANDÉN et al., 1964; WALTMAN and SEARS, 1964; HERTTING, 1965; KLINGMAN, 1965; POTTER et al., 1965; IVERSEN et al., 1966, 1968; SEDVALL and KOPIN, 1967; MUELLER et al., 1969; NAGATSU et al., 1969). Moreover, denervation experiments have been of crucial importance in detecting that uptake into the adrenergic nerve terminals is generally the main mechanism by which exogenously administered or neurally liberated noradrenaline is inactivated (HERTTING et al., 1961a; HERTTING and SCHIEFTHALER, 1964; HERTTING, 1965; POTTER et al., 1965) and that the activity of the adrenergic neurons beyond their actual effect have also "trophic" actions on the effector organs (BURN, 1952; TRENDELENBURG and WEINER, 1962; FLEMING, 1963; TRENDELENBURG, 1963a, b).

In their classical experiments, CANNON and coworkers (1929, 1937) removed the para- and prevertebral ganglia of adult cats stepwise within a 6-month period and made the crucial observation that the presence of the sympathetic nervous system is not an absolute requisite for existence and that these animals do not essentially differ from controls under laboratory conditions. However, they are unable to regulate body temperature and blood pressure.

The experiments of CANNON and coworkers (1929, 1937) not only elucidated the important homeostatic role of the sympathetic nervous system but they also clearly demonstrated that to achieve general sympathectomy by surgery is extremely cumbrous, time-consuming and virtually impracticable in smaller animals. The difficulties in the surgical procedure for general sympathectomy and for the denervation of organs with a complex and not easily accessible innervation explain the great interest taken in other methods, which bring about the destruction or prevent the development and differentiation of the sympathetic nervous system. In the last decade two such procedures have become available: Immunosympathectomy (COHEN, 1960; LEVI-MONTALCINI and BOOKER, 1960) and chemical sympathectomy with 6-hydroxydopamine (TRANZER and THOENEN, 1967a, 1968a; THOENEN and TRANZER, 1968). The term chemical sympathectomy has also been used for the action of drugs, which abolish the effect of sympathetic nerve stimulation either by interfering with the storage mechanism or by liberating the adrenergic transmitter (MUSCHOLL, 1959; STERN et al., 1964; MAICKEL et al., 1967), but within the context of this article the term chemical sympathectomy will be confined to the effect of drugs which lead to a selective destruction of the adrenergic nerve terminals.

Immunosympathectomy (LEVI-MONTALCINI and ANGELETTI, 1962; CARPI and OLIVERIO, 1964; ZAIMIS, 1965; KLINGMAN, 1965; IVERSEN et al., 1966) and chemical sympathectomy (THOENEN et al., 1968; CLARKE and JONES, 1969; CLARKE et al., 1969; HAEUSLER et al., 1971; MOLINOFF and AXELROD, 1969; MUELLER et al., 1969; FINCH and LEACH, 1970) have proved to be very useful tools in the investigation of the physiology and pharmacology of the sympathetic nervous system. These two methods complete the armature of drugs which interfere with the different steps of synthesis of the adrenergic transmitter (SOURKES, 1954; LOVENBERG et al., 1963; BURKARD et al., 1964; GOLDSTEIN et al., 1964; UDENFRIEND et al., 1965), its storage (HOLZBAUER and VOGT, 1956; CARLSSON et al., 1957; PLETSCHER et al., 1962) or liberation by nerve impulses (BOURA and GREEN, 1959; HERTTING et al., 1962; HUKOVIĆ and MUSCHOLL, 1962), its inactivation (AXELROD and LAROCHE, 1959; BACQ et al., 1959; ZELLER, 1959; PLETSCHER et al., 1960; BELLEAU and BURBA, 1961; HERTTING et al., 1961b; MUSCHOLL, 1961; IVERSEN, 1965) and its effect on the effector organs (AHLQUIST, 1948; NICKERSON, 1949; MORAN and PERKINS, 1958; POWELL and SLATER, 1958; FURCHGOTT, 1959; BIEL and LUM, 1966).

It is the purpose of the present article to review the different possibilities of sympathectomy, to delineate the advantages and drawbacks of the different procedures and to depict their application in the investigation of the physiology and pharmacology of the sympathetic nervous system.

II. Surgical Sympathectomy

The term *surgical sympathectomy* will here refer to the transection of postganglionic sympathetic nerves or the removal of the corresponding ganglia, whereas the term *decentralization* will be used for the transection of preganglionic nerves. Both procedures interrupt the flow of nerve impulses from the autonomic centres in the central nervous system to the peripheral effector organs. However, while decentralization produces a degeneration only of the preganglionic cholinergic fibres (LAWRENTJEW, 1925; HILLARP, 1946; DE CASTRO, 1950; QUILLIAM and TAMARIN, 1967), leaving the terminal adrenergic neurons intact (REHN, 1958; BROWN et al., 1961; KIRPEKAR et al., 1962; FISCHER and SNYDER, 1965), surgical sympathectomy results in a degeneration of peripheral adrenergic nerves (LAWRENTJEW and BOROWSKAJA, 1935; MALMFORS and SACHS, 1965; VAN ORDEN et al., 1967; WEINER et al., 1967), which is accompanied by a progressive decrease in the noradrenaline content of sympathetically innervated organs (KIRPEKAR et al.,

1962; SMITH et al., 1966). This effect of sympathetic denervation has been observed in a wide variety of species and organs (VON EULER and PURKHOLD, 1951; GOODALL, 1951; GOODALL and KIRSHNER, 1956; COOPER et al., 1961, 1962; COOPER and SJOERDSMA, 1962; SIDMAN et al., 1962; BENMILOUD and VON EULER, 1963; POTTER et al., 1965; HERTTING, 1965; BIRMINGHAM, 1967, 1968).

Whether the noradrenaline content of a sympathetically innervated organ can be diminished to virtually non-measurable values by surgical denervation depends on the topography of the innervation of the particular organ. The iris, salivary gland and nictitating membrane of various species are almost exclusively innervated by fibres originating from the superior cervical ganglion, and the removal of the latter leads to a severe decrease in the noradrenaline content of these organs (VON EULER and PURKHOLD, 1951; KIRPEKAR et al., 1962; BENMILOUD and VON EULER, 1963; SMITH et al., 1966; HAEUSLER et al., 1969). In contrast, the technically much more difficult cervico-thoracic ganglionectomy leads only to an incomplete denervation of the heart of the dog, sheep and cat (GOODALL and KIRSHNER, 1956; HERTTING and SCHIEFTHALER, 1964). In the latter species, for instance, the removal of the right and left stellate ganglia results in a reduction of the noradrenaline content of the heart to 15—30% only (HERTTING and SCHIEFTHALER, 1964). To achieve a degree of denervation comparable to that in the nictitating membrane, iris or salivary gland after extirpation of the superior cervical ganglion, a regional neural ablation (COOPER et al., 1961), a homotransplantation (WEGMANN et al., 1962) or an autotransplantation (COOPER et al., 1962; POTTER et al., 1965; COOPER, 1966) of the heart has to be performed.

In various species the noradrenaline content of the vas deferens and the accessory male genital glands is not reduced by cutting the hypogastric nerve, which carries mainly preganglionic fibres to ganglia located very close to or even in the wall of the aforementioned organs (for references see SJÖSTRAND, 1965). Therefore, the terminal postganglionic adrenergic fibres innervating their smooth muscles and glands are very short. By stripping the mesenteric attachment from the guinea-pig and rat vas deferens, BIRMINGHAM (1967, 1968) achieved a very effective sympathetic denervation, documented by a reduction of the noradrenaline content to less than 5% and a virtually complete disappearance of the usually dense network of varicose nerve terminals visualized by the fluorescence microscopic method of FALCK and coworkers (FALCK, 1962; FALCK et al., 1962). The value of this method of denervation is somewhat affected by the danger that stripping of the vas can also sever its vascular supply (HAEUSLER, personal communication; IVERSEN, personal communication).

The disappearance of noradrenaline from sympathetically innervated organs after severing the supplying postganglionic nerves has provided strong, yet indirect, evidence that peripheral organs do not themselves store noradrenaline, but contain it only by virtue of their adrenergic innervation. This conclusion had already been drawn by CANNON and LISSÁK (1939) at a time when adrenaline was still thought to be the physiological adrenergic transmitter in mammals.

This indirect evidence for an intraneuronal localization of the adrenergic neurotransmitter was substantiated more than two decades later by fluorescence microscopy (FALCK, 1962; MALMFORS and SACHS, 1965) and by electron microscopy (WOLFE et al., 1962; RICHARDSON, 1964; VAN ORDEN et al., 1966; TRANZER and THOENEN, 1967b, c), techniques which allow a more direct study at the cellular and subcellular localization of transmitter substances.

Denervation experiments provided not only decisive evidence for the intraneuronal localization of the adrenergic transmitter, noradrenaline, but they were also of primary importance in the study of the uptake of noradrenaline into sympathetic nerve endings as the main mechanism of its biological inactivation. The initial observation of RAAB and coworkers (1947, 1953, 1955) that the catecholamine content of the cat and dog heart increases after administration of large doses of adrenaline and noradrenaline, was confirmed in various organs of the rat not only after administration of large (STRÖMBLAD and NICKERSON, 1961; BHAGAT, 1963), but also of much smaller doses (MUSCHOLL, 1960, 1961) of noradrenaline. Experiments with tritiated noradrenaline revealed that the uptake is greatest in organs with a rich sympathetic innervation and that there is a good correlation between the amount of H^3-noradrenaline taken up and the endogenous noradrenaline content, if regional differences in the blood supply to various organs are taken into account (WHITBY et al., 1961; WURTMAN et al., 1964; KOPIN et al., 1965). Uptake of noradrenaline is severely impaired (HERTTING et al., 1961a; STRÖMBLAD and NICKERSON, 1961; HERTTING and SCHIEFTHALER, 1964; FISCHER et al., 1965; POTTER et al., 1965; JONASON, 1969) after surgical denervation of various organs in different species, thus indicating that intact adrenergic nerve terminals are required for this important mechanism of noradrenaline inactivation.

In addition to an extreme reduction in the endogenous noradrenaline content and a severe impairment of uptake and retention of injected noradrenaline, the degeneration of the postganglionic adrenergic nerve fibres is also accompanied by changes in the activity of enzymes involved in the synthesis and metabolic degradation of noradrenaline. Tyrosine hydroxylase, the rate-limiting enzyme in the synthesis of noradrenaline (LEVITT et al., 1965), disappears completely from organs deprived of their adrenergic innervation (SEDVALL and KOPIN, 1967; NAGATSU et al., 1969). Similarly, the β-hydroxylation of phenylethylamines is greatly reduced in surgically denervated tissues (FISCHER et al., 1964) as well as after immunological (IVERSEN et al., 1966) and chemical sympathectomy (MOLINOFF, personal communication). The activity of the aromatic L-amino acid decarboxylase is also markedly reduced in part of the surgically (ANDÉN et al., 1964) or immunologically denervated (KLINGMAN, 1965; IVERSEN et al., 1966) organs, but the association of the activity of this enzyme with intact adrenergic nerves is not as strict as that of tyrosine hydroxylase and dopamine β-hydroxylase. Similar observations have been reported for MAO. In organs with a dense sympathetic innervation such as the iris, vas deferens and nictitating membrane, destruction of adrenergic nerves is accompanied by a reduction of MAO-activity of 30—50% (BURN and ROBINSON, 1953; BURN et al., 1954; WALTMAN and SEARS, 1964; IVERSEN et al., 1968; CERVONI, 1969). In other organs only an insignificant reduction, if any at all, has been observed (STRÖMBLAD, 1956; HÅKANSON and OWMAN, 1965; POTTER et al., 1965; IVERSEN et al., 1966). Although COMT, the second enzyme involved in the metabolic degradation of catecholamines, has been reported present in sympathetic neurons (AXELROD et al., 1959a, b), its main activity results from extraneuronal sources (CROUT and COOPER, 1962; POTTER et al., 1965; IVERSEN et al., 1966, 1968; JONASON, 1969).

The time-course of the decrease in the noradrenaline content of sympathetically innervated organs after removal of the supplying ganglia or transection of the postganglionic fibres varies considerably from organ to organ and from species to species. In the submaxillary gland of the rat the noradrenaline content is reduced by 40% 12 hr after extirpation of the superior cervical ganglion and to non-measurable values after 24 hr (BENMILOUD and VON EULER, 1963). Similar results have been reported very recently by HENNEMANN and TRENDELENBURG (1970). In contrast, the noradrenaline content of the cat nictitating membrane is still normal 22—24 hr after removal of the superior cervical ganglion; the rapid decline to virtually non-measurable values occurs within the following 12—24 hr

(KIRPEKAR et al., 1962; SMITH et al., 1966). An even longer interval between removal of the ganglia and decline in the noradrenaline content of the innervated organ was observed in the cat spleen. There is no decrease in the splenic noradrenaline content up to 48 hr after removal of the superior celiac ganglion and a sharp drop to minimum values occurs in the following 48 hr (BRIMIJOIN, personal communication).

It is not clear what accounts for the differences in the time interval between transection of the postganglionic nerves and the beginning of the decline in noradrenaline content in the innervated organ. It could depend on the distance between the nerve terminals and the site at which the nerve trunk is severed.

In a series of very careful and extensive experiments, TRENDELENBURG and coworkers studied the time-course of functional (TRENDELENBURG and WEINER, 1962; TRENDELENBURG, 1963a, b; LANGER and TRENDELENBURG, 1966; LANGER et al., 1967; TRENDELENBURG et al., 1969), biochemical (SMITH et al., 1966; LANGER et al., 1967; TRENDELENBURG et al., 1969) and morphological (VAN ORDEN et al., 1967; WEINER et al., 1967) changes in the cat nictitating membrane after removal of the superior cervical ganglion. Immediately after the excision of the ganglion, the nictitating membrane relaxes. However, after about 22 hr a transient contraction appears, which lasts for 10—14 hr (LANGER, 1966); this is accompanied by a linear decline in the endogenous noradrenaline content, which reaches a very low level on termination of the contraction (SMITH et al., 1966). Almost parallel to the occurrence of this transient contraction, the nictitating membrane shows a rapidly developing supersensitivity to noradrenaline, accompanied by an impaired uptake of intravenously injected H^3-noradrenaline (LANGER and TRENDELENBURG, 1966; SMITH et al., 1966). The relationships between decline in the noradrenaline content of the nictitating membrane, changes in the uptake of H^3-noradrenaline, supersensitivity to intravenously injected noradrenaline and time-course of the transient contraction are summarized in Fig. 1.

The transient contraction of the nictitating membrane — for which the term degeneration contraction has been coined (LANGER, 1966) — appears to be the result of a leakage of noradrenaline from degenerating adrenergic nerve terminals. This view is in accordance with the observation that pretreatment with reserpine or administration of α-adrenergic blockers prevents this contraction (LANGER, 1966).

The functional and biochemical evidence for a rapid degeneration of the adrenergic nerve terminals in the nictitating membrane during the second day after denervation is further substantiated by electronmicroscopic investigations (VAN ORDEN et al., 1967). The ultramorphological correlate of the decline in the endogenous noradrenaline content is a reduction in the proportion of granulated vesicles in adrenergic nerve terminals. The degree of electronmicroscopically recognizable degenerative changes in adrenergic nerve endings correlates well with the impaired uptake of H^3-noradrenaline (SMITH et al., 1966; VAN ORDEN et al., 1967).

Observations corresponding to the degeneration contraction of the nictitating membrane of the cat have been reported for other organs and species such as the iris and supraorbital smooth muscle of the rat (MALMFORS and SACHS, 1965; LUNDBERG, 1969), the iris and ear arteries of the rabbit (SEARS and BÁRÁNY, 1960; SEARS and GILLIS, 1967; BÁRÁNY and TREISTER, in press) and the salivary gland of the cat (COATS and EMMELIN, 1962).

The degeneration contraction of blood vessels is most probably of considerable importance in transplantation surgery. It seems that about 24 hr after transplantation of human kidneys, very often a critical period with impaired renal functions occurs which can be linked to a degeneration contraction of renal blood vessels, since pre-transplantation perfusion of the kidney with phenoxybenzamine has a favourable effect (TRENDELENBURG and LUNDBERG, personal communication).

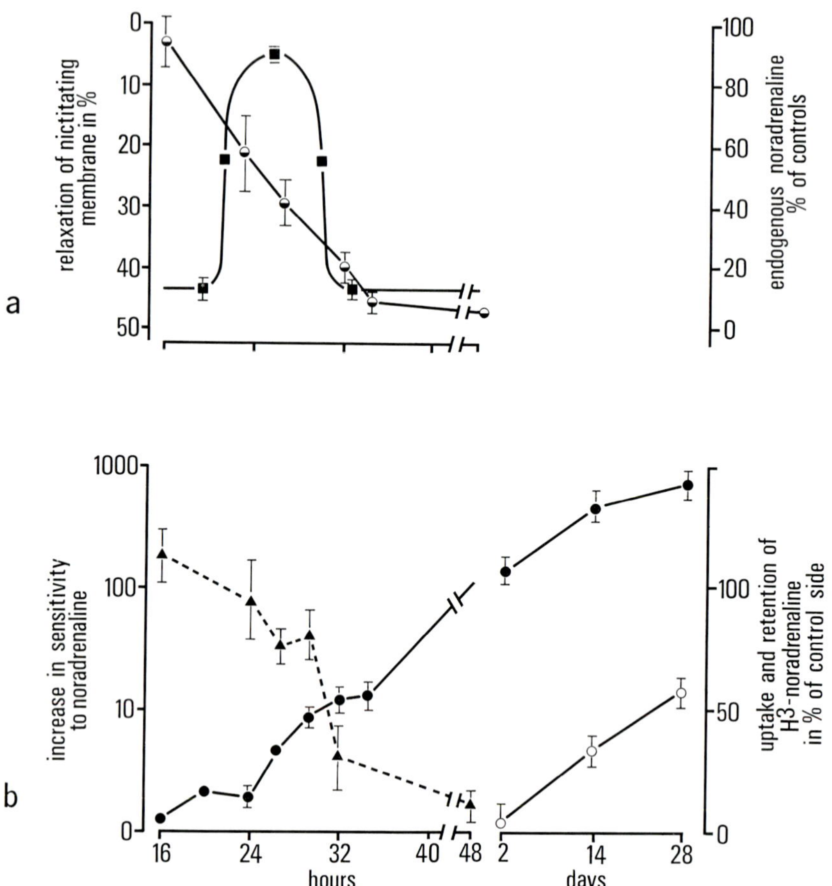

Fig. 1a and b. Effects of denervation and decentralization of the nictitating membrane of the cat. a Time course of changes in tonus (■—■) (degeneration contraction) and endogenous noradrenaline content (◒—◒) after removal of the superior cervical ganglion. b Development of supersensitivity to noradrenaline after denervation (●—●) and decentralization (○—○). Changes uptake of H^3-noradrenaline (▲---▲) after denervation. (According to LANGER, 1966; SMITH et al., 1966; LANGER et al., 1967)

III. Immunosympathectomy

In 1948, BUEKER reported on the abundant sensory innervation of pieces of mouse sarcoma implanted into chick embryos. The sensory ganglia providing these fibres were hypertrophic and hyperplastic. The growth-promoting effect was also evident in sensory ganglia remote from the implant and even more impressive in sympathetic ganglia (LEVI-MONTALCINI and HAMBURGER, 1951). This stimulation of nerve growth could also be seen in experiments (LEVI-MONTALCINI et al., 1954), in which sensory and sympathetic ganglia of chick embryos were incubated *in vitro* in semi-solid media, together with sarcoma tissue. The development of a dense fibrillar halo of nerve fibres from ganglia, adjacent to the fragments of mouse sarcoma, but absent in controls and in the presence of other tumors, was taken as evidence for the release of a specific growth-promoting substance. In the course of this work, additional and even higher nerve growth activity was discovered in extracts of snake venom glands (Levi-Montalcini and Cohen, 1956; Cohen, 1959) and in submaxillary glands of male mice (Levi-Montalcini, 1958; Cohen, 1960). These extracts revealed the same nerve growth-promoting effect that had been seen in sarcoma tissue and that elicited the characteristic nerve fibre halo in incubated sensory and sympathetic ganglia of chick embryos (Fig. 2).

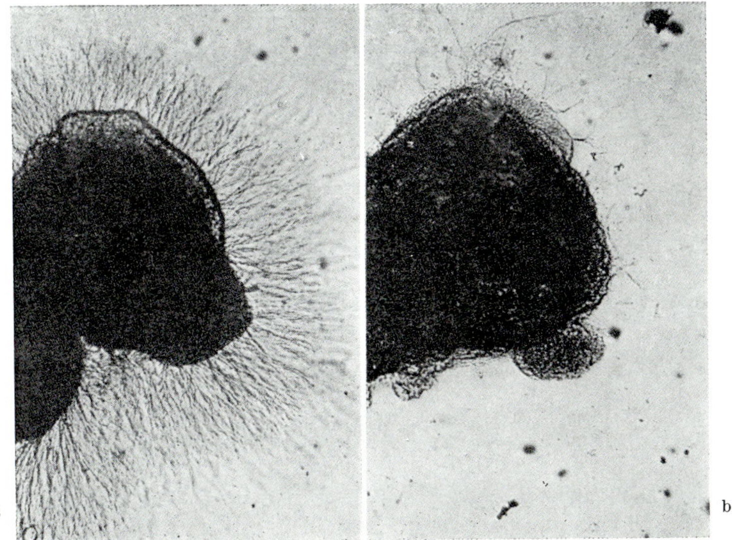

Fig. 2a and b. The effect of nerve growth factor on the outgrowth of nerve fibres from 14-day chick embryo sympathetic ganglia. a Ganglion incubated 20 hr with nerve growth factor. b Control ganglion, incubated 20 hr in the same medium but without nerve growth factor. (From Crain et al., 1964)

The availability of larger quantities of this growth-promoting factor(s) enabled an efficient purification and a more accurate biological and chemical characterization (Cohen, 1959, 1960; Schenkein and Bueker, 1962, 1964; Levi-Montalcini et al., 1965; Salvi et al., 1965; Angeletti et al., 1967; Varon et al., 1967a, b; Levi-Montalcini and Angeletti, 1968). The nerve growth-promoting substance has been identified as a protein (Cohen, 1958, 1959), but it is not yet clear to what extent the factors isolated from various sources differ and whether the differences in the molecular weights result from differences in the aggregation of identical or similar subunits (Levi-Montalcini and Angeletti, 1968).

A new aspect arose with the discovery that a specific antiserum to the mouse salivary nerve growth factor could be prepared which destroys the sympathetic ganglia of newborn animals (Levi-Montalcini and Booker, 1960; Levi-Montalcini and Cohen, 1960). The antiserum was first produced by Cohen (1960), who injected the purified nerve growth protein into rabbits together with Freund's adjuvant. Daily injections of antiserum to newborn mice for a period of 2—5 days result in permanent destruction of the paravertebral and part of the prevertebral ganglia. The destructive effect is already visible macroscopically due to a drastic reduction in size of the sympathetic ganglia (Fig. 3). In the paravertebral ganglia the number of neuronal cells is reduced by 90—95%, whereas in the prevertebral ganglia the reduction is generally somewhat less and amounts to 85—90% (LEVI-MONTALCINI and BOOKER, 1960). The peripheral sympathetic ganglia innervating the male and female sex organs are resistant to the antiserum (VOGT, 1964; LEVI-MONTALCINI and ANGELETTI, 1966) and they also fail to respond to the nerve growth factor (LEVI-MONTALCINI, 1966, 1967). The explanation for the differences in the susceptibility of different sympathetic ganglia to the antiserum is probably that the sympathetic neurons are particularly sensitive to the antiserum at a critical stage in their development. If the antiserum is administered either before the neurons have entered this stage of rapid proliferation and differentiation or after their development is completed, they may remain unaffected (VOGT, 1964; HAMBERGER et al., 1965; IVERSEN et al., 1966). This assumption is supported by the

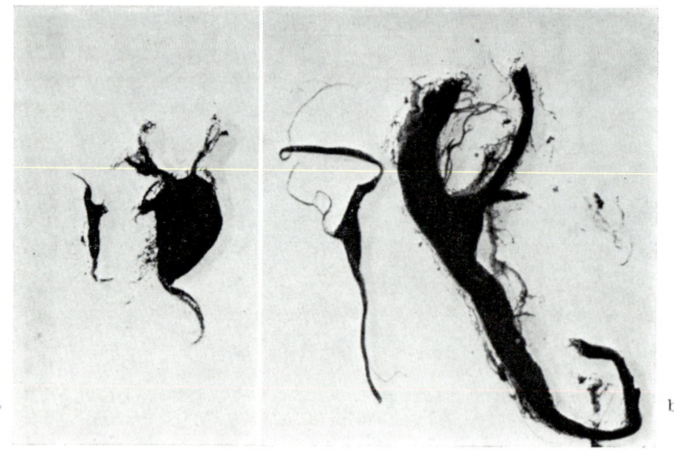

Fig. 3a and b. Effect of antiserum to nerve growth factor on sympathetic ganglia. Whole mounts of superior cervical ganglia of mice (a) and rats (b). In both figures the ganglia of immunosympathectomized animals are to the left, the control ganglia to the right. (From LEVI-MONTALCINI and ANGELETTI, 1966)

observation of GLOWINSKI et al. (1964) that the ability of the rat heart to accumulate H^3-noradrenaline is incomplete at birth and develops very rapidly between the first and second postnatal week. It can therefore be assumed that the sympathetic innervation of the rat heart is in rapid development at this time and particularly susceptible to the antiserum during this stage.

The effect of the antiserum is not limited to mice and rats, the two species most extensively studied, but is also present in young rabbits and kittens (LEVI-MONTALCINI and ANGELETTI, 1966).

The action of the antiserum is much less drastic in adult than in newborn animals. Repeated injection of adult mice with antiserum over several weeks results in only a moderate atrophy of the sympathetic ganglia (LEVI-MONTALCINI and BOOKER, 1960; LEVI-MONTALCINI and ANGELETTI, 1966).

In newborn animals regressive changes in the sympathetic nerve cells are detectable by light microscopy as early as 12 hr after the first injection of antiserum (LEVI-MONTALCINI and ANGELETTI, 1966, 1968). In superior cervical ganglia of mice the mitotic activity is very high from birth up to the 9th day. In ganglia of animals pretreated with antiserum, mitotic figures are rare and, if present, atypical. At the same time the process of differentiation, which is very active in control animals, breaks down completely and an increasing number of disintegrating neuroblasts is visible, surrounded by macrophages invading the necrotic cells (LEVI-MONTALCINI and ANGELETTI, 1966, 1968). Electronmicroscopic studies (SABATINI et al., 1965) of the same ganglion revealed morphological changes just 2 hr after the injection of the antiserum. The changes consist of a folding of the nuclear membrane and condensation of chromatin to form amorphous masses. Although mitochondrial alterations are also seen at this early stage, the nucleus of the sympathetic cells appears to be the primary target of the antiserum (LEVI-MONTALCINI and ANGELETTI, 1968).

Immunosympathectomized rats show a good general state of health, like cats deprived of the main part of their sympathetic nervous system by surgery (CANNON and ROSENBLUETH, 1937). They reveal no changes in their gross behaviour, show normal activity, eat, drink and clean themselves and even breed normally (BRODY, 1964; ZAIMIS, 1965; ZAIMIS et al., 1965; LEVI-MONTALCINI and ANGELETTI, 1966). The only features which distinguish them from controls on gross inspection are a narrow palpebral fissure, miosis and enophthalmus (VOGT, 1964; ZAIMIS, 1965; ZAIMIS et al., 1965). Their body temperature does not differ significantly from that of untreated animals under normal laboratory conditions, but like surgically denervated cats (CANNON and ROSENBLUETH, 1937), they show a deficient adaptability to changes in environmental temperature, above all after adrenal demedullation (LEVI-MONTALCINI and ANGELETTI, 1966). The heart rate is very similar to that of controls, and the blood pressure is slightly but significantly lower (ZAIMIS, 1965; ZAIMIS et al., 1965). The response to electrical stimulation of the cervical (ZAIMIS, 1965) and lumbar (BRODY, 1964) sympathetic trunk is, as is to be expected, abolished in immunosympathectomized rats.

There are regional differences not only in the degree to which the sympathetic ganglia are affected by the antiserum, but there are also corresponding differences in the reduction of the noradrenaline content of sympathetically innervated organs (LEVI-MONTALCINI and ANGELETTI, 1962; ZAIMIS et al., 1965; IVERSEN et al., 1966). In both rats and mice the catecholamine content of the heart, spleen and submaxillary gland is reduced to less than 10% of normal. In other organs such as the small intestine, liver, kidney, lungs and uterus the reduction only amounts to 15—50% and no significant reduction at all is found in the adrenal glands, vas deferens and brain (LEVI-MONTALCINI and ANGELETTI, 1962; KLINGMAN, 1965; ZAIMIS et al., 1965; IVERSEN et al., 1966). The reduction in the catecholamine content is parallelled by a decrease in the number of fluorescent fibres (HAMBERGER et al., 1965) and by a diminished uptake and retention of intravenously injected H^3-noradrenaline (IVERSEN, 1965, IVERSEN et al., 1966; ZAIMIS, 1965; SJÖQVIST et al., 1965, 1967). The amount of H^3-noradrenaline, taken up by the vas deferens of immunosympathectomized rats and mice is increased (IVERSEN et al., 1966; SJÖQVIST et al., 1967). This could be explained by the increased and prolonged elevation of H^3-noradrenaline blood levels resulting from the lack of uptake by the denervated organs which diverts a larger portion of the circulating amine to organs not affected by immunosympathectomy.

The alterations in the uptake of H^3-noradrenaline by various tissues of immunosympathectomized rats and mice are accompanied by changes in the metabolism of the noradrenaline administered. In both species there is a relative increase in the proportion of tritiated metabolites to unchanged noradrenaline (IVERSEN et al., 1966; SJÖQVIST et al., 1967). The metabolites mainly consist of

H^3-normetanephrine and both deaminated and O-methylated products. These findings agree with observations on H^3-noradrenaline metabolism in surgically denervated hearts of the dog (POTTER et al., 1965). In both conditions the uptake of noradrenaline is markedly diminished and the relative amounts of O-methylated metabolites are increased. Normally the uptake of noradrenaline into the adrenergic nerve terminals is the main mechanism of inactivation and the extraneuronal O-methylation is of minor importance (IVERSEN, 1967). However, in denervated organs inactivation by uptake is abolished and O-methylation, together with oxidative deamination, becomes the predominant mechanism of inactivation (POTTER et al., 1965; IVERSEN et al., 1966). The assumption that the enzyme COMT is mainly located extraneuronally is supported by the observation that neither surgical denervation nor immunosympathectomy produce a significant reduction in the activity of this enzyme in various peripheral sympathetically innervated organs of different species (CROUT and COOPER, 1962; POTTER et al., 1965; IVERSEN et al., 1966, 1968).

Results on the effect of immunosympathectomy on MAO activity are contradictory. LEVI-MONTALCINI and ANGELETTI (1962) reported a decrease in enzyme activity of 50—70% in various organs of the mouse and the rat, such as the heart, spleen, intestine and salivary gland. In contrast, IVERSEN et al. (1966) could not find a consistent change in the heart, intestine and liver of immunosympathectomized rats and they only observed a statistically significant reduction of 30% in the salivary gland. It seems that in many organs, the main part of the MAO content is located extraneuronally, and only in organs with a particularly dense adrenergic innervation, such as the iris, nictitating membrane, vas deferens and pineal gland is a relatively high proportion of the total enzyme content located in the sympathetic nerves (WALTMAN and SEARS, 1964; SNYDER et al., 1965b; IVERSEN et al., 1968; CERVONI, 1969).

Of the enzymes involved in the synthesis of the physiological transmitter, noradrenaline, only the changes in DOPA decarboxylase activity have been studied after immunosympathectomy. In rats there occurs a marked decrease in the activity of this enzyme in all peripheral organs so far investigated (KLINGMAN, 1965; IVERSEN et al., 1966). This suggests that a substantial proportion of DOPA decarboxylase is associated with adrenergic neurons, although this association does not seem to be as absolute as for tyrosine hydroxylase (SEDVALL and KOPIN, 1967; MUELLER et al., 1969; NAGATSU et al., 1969) and dopamine-β-hydroxylase (MOLINOFF, personal communication). The activity of these enzymes disappears virtually completely after surgical or chemical sympathectomy.

It is interesting to note that in immunosympathectomized mice the 5-hydroxytryptamine content of the intestine increases (IVERSEN et al., 1966; THOMPSON and CAMPBELL, 1966). However, the fact that this increase is restricted to the stomach and small intestine and is absent in the colon and appendix (THOMPSON and CAMPBELL, 1966) suggests that there is a relationship between the rise in the 5-hydroxytryptamine content of an organ and the susceptibility to the nerve growth antiserum of the sympathetic ganglia which supply this organ with adrenergic nerves. This assumption is supported by the recent observation of KLINGMAN (1969) that also in various organs of the rat there is a close correlation between the rise in their 5-hydroxytryptamine content and the extent of their immunological denervation. Furthermore, surgical denervation of the rat submaxillary gland also leads to a rise in the 5-hydroxytryptamine content (KLINGMAN and KLINGMAN, 1969).

The biological findings correlate well with the histochemical observation of HAMBERGER et al. (1965) that there is an increase in both the intensity of fluorescence and the number of 5-hydroxytryptamine containing mast cells in the small intestine of immunosympathectomized rats.

The mechanism of the increase in the 5-hydroxytryptamine content of organs deprived of their sympathetic innervation is not yet clear. Studies concerning the influence of sympathetic innervation or, more directly, of noradrenaline, the adrenergic neurohumoral transmitter, on the metabolism of 5-hydroxytryptamine have so far only been performed in the pineal gland. The observation of SNYDER et al. (1965a) that surgical denervation of the pineal gland produces a marked elevation of its 5-hydroxytryptophan decarboxylase activity is compatible with an increased synthesis of 5-hydroxytryptamine, although the catalytic activity of this enzyme is not rate-limiting in the synthesis of 5-hydroxytryptamine. On the other hand AXELROD et al. (1969) and WURTMAN et al. (1969) observed in organ cultures of rat pineal glands that noradrenaline increases the synthesis of 5-hydroxytryptamine and melatonin by way of an increased transport of the metabolic precursor tryptophan through the cell membrane of the pinealocytes.

IV. Chemical Sympathectomy

In 1959, SENOH and coworkers reported that 6-hydroxydopamine (3,4,6-trihydroxyphenylethylamine) might be formed from dopamine as a product of autoxidation and as a metabolite of dopamine (SENOH and WITKOP, 1959; SENOH et al., 1959a, 1959b). The quantitative aspects, physiological importance and site of this aberrant metabolic pathway have not been clarified so far.

Pharmacological studies with 6-hydroxydopamine revealed that this amine produces an efficient and very long lasting noradrenaline depletion of the peripheral sympathetically innervated organs of various species (PORTER et al., 1963; STONE et al., 1963; LAVERTY et al., 1965). Originally it was suggested that 6-hydroxydopamine might damage the amine storage sites of the adrenergic nerve terminals (PORTER et al., 1963; LAVERTY et al., 1965) or act as a "false transmitter" with an extremely long biological half-life (PORTER et al., 1965), resulting from a high affinity to the storage sites. However, recent electronmicroscopic studies have shown that high doses of 6-hydroxydopamine cause a selective destruction of adrenergic nerve terminals (TRANZER and THOENEN, 1967a, 1968a). These studies offer a reasonable explanation for the long-lasting noradrenaline depletion.

The peculiar properties of 6-hydroxydopamine were detected in the course of studies designed to localize at the ultramorphological level trihydroxyphenylethylamines which act as false adrenergic transmitters. 5-Hydroxydopamine, the chemical isomer of 6-hydroxydopamine, is a potent depletor of peripheral stores of noradrenaline in various species (THOENEN et al., 1967a, b; TRANZER et al., 1969). It is accumulated in sympathetically innervated organs and liberated as a false adrenergic transmitter, together with its β-hydroxylated and/or O-methylated metabolites (THOENEN et al., 1967b). After administration of 5-hydroxydopamine or its metabolic precursor 5-hydroxydopa in doses capable of reducing the noradrenaline content of sympathetically innervated organs to less than 10% of that of controls, all the vesicles of the adrenergic nerve endings are filled with a dense osmiophilic material (Fig. 4) which represents the ultramorphological localization of the false transmitter, 5-hydroxydopamine, and possibly also of its metabolites (TRANZER and THOENEN, 1967a, b).

The electronmicroscopic changes produced by 6-hydroxydopamine are completely different (TRANZER and THOENEN, 1967a, 1968a; TRANZER et al., 1969). Two to 3 days after administration of 6-hydroxydopamine in doses which cause a reduction of the noradrenaline content similar to that after 5-hydroxydopamine, the adrenergic nerve terminals are in various stages of degeneration (Fig. 5). Some of the nerves still show recognizable and characteristic ultramorphological structures, whereas others are completely lysed and can only be recognized by their localization between smooth muscle cells and the surrounding Schwann cells.

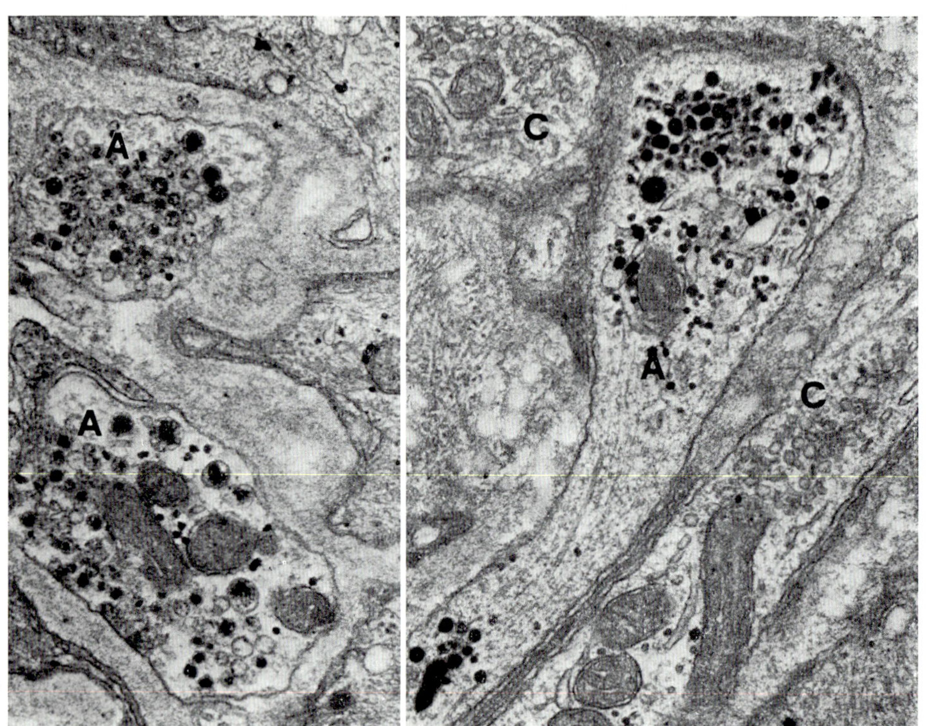

Fig. 4a and b. Ultramorphological localization of 5-hydroxydopamine in the cat iris. a Iris of an untreated cat; b Iris of a cat pretreated with 5-hydroxydopamine (noradrenaline content reduced to less than 10% of control values). A = adrenergic nerve terminals; C = cholinergic nerve terminals. (From TRANZER and THOENEN, 1967b and 1968b)

In many instances the Schwann cells seem to engulf the damaged nerve terminals, and the plasma membranes of the nerves are hardly discernible from those of the Schwann cells. The degeneration changes are strictly confined to the adrenergic nerve terminals. The surrounding Schwann cells, the smooth muscle cells and particularly the cholinergic nerve endings remain completely intact. The difference between the effect on cholinergic and adrenergic nerve terminals is very impressive in the vas deferens and the iris, where the two kinds of autonomic nerve endings are located in very close proximity to one another. The adrenergic nerve terminals undergo severe degenerative alterations and finally disappear, after about 10 days. The cholinergic nerve endings appear unchanged at any time of observation. In sympathetic ganglia of the cat, the cell bodies corresponding to the destroyed

Fig. 5a and b. Effect of 6-hydroxydopamine on adrenergic nerve endings in the cat iris (a) and the rat heart (b). 24—48 hr after administration of 6-hydroxydopamine the adrenergic (A) nerve endings are in various stages of degeneration. Cholinergic (C) nerve terminals do not show any signs of morphological alterations. (From TRANZER and THOENEN, 1968a; THOENEN and TRANZER, 1968)

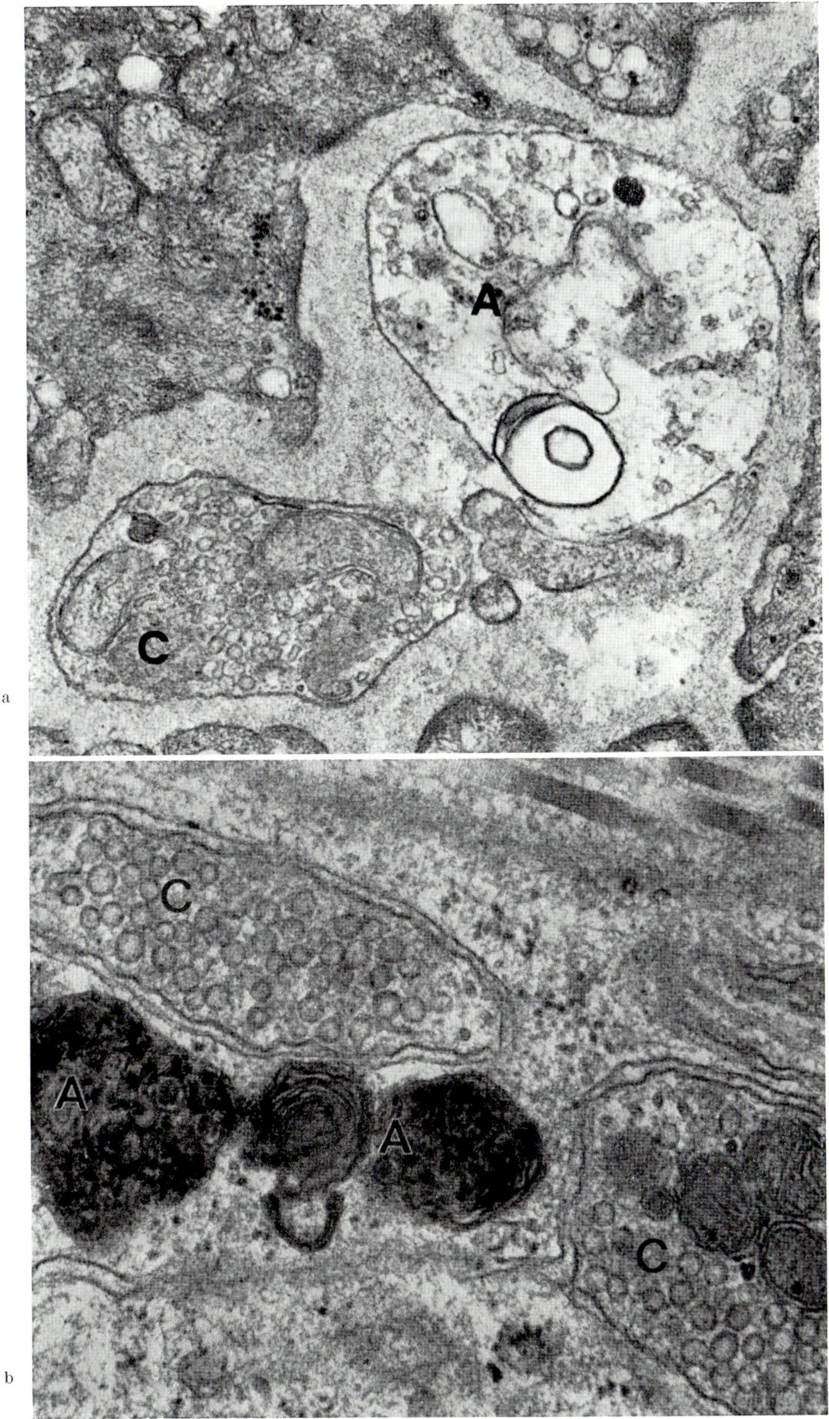

Fig. 5a and b

nerve terminals show no ultramorphological alteration (TRANZER and THOENEN, 1968a, TRANZER et al., 1969). This corresponds to the fluorescence microscopic observations which show that in rats, after treatment with 6-hydroxydopamine, the network of adrenergic nerve terminals in the iris disappears, whereas the fluorescence of more proximal axons persists or even increases (MALMFORS and SACHS, 1968). This increase in fluorescence could indicate that the noradrenaline storage granules produced by the undamaged cell body are transported down the axon (DAHLSTRÖM and HÄGGENDAL, 1966) and pile up in the "amputation stump", as after ligation of sympathetic nerves (KAPELLER and MAYOR, 1967, 1969; GEFFEN and OSTBERG, 1969).

The biochemical correlates to these ultramorphological and fluorescence microscopic findings after treatment with 6-hydroxydopamine are the long-lasting depletion of noradrenaline (PORTER et al., 1963; LAVERTY et al., 1965; THOENEN et al., 1968; THOENEN and TRANZER, 1968) and the very marked reduction in tyrosine hydroxylase (MUELLER et al., 1969) and dopamine-β-hydroxylase activity in sympathetically innervated organs (MOLINOFF, personal communication). These latter findings are consistent with the view that the two enzymes are selectively located within adrenergic neurons and thus corroborate observations, already discussed, that were obtained after surgical denervation or after immunosympathectomy.

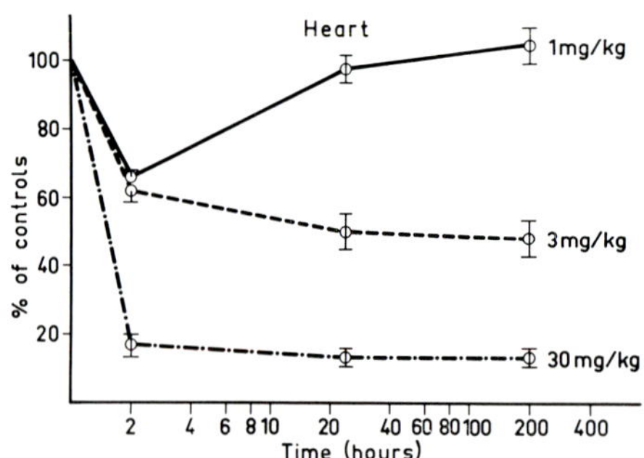

Fig. 6. The effect of single doses of 6-hydroxydopamine on the noradrenaline content of the rat heart. 6-Hydroxydopamine was given i.v. The noradrenaline content is expressed in % of that at controls. (From THOENEN and TRANZER, 1968)

The time-course of noradrenaline depletion of the rat heart after administration of a single dose of 6-hydroxydopamine makes it very probable that a critical dose of the latter is necessary for producing the characteristic long-lasting noradrenaline depletion (THOENEN and TRANZER, 1968). The intravenous administration of 1 mg/kg of 6-hydroxydopamine produces only a transient decrease in the noradrenaline content of the rat heart, and control levels are reached again after 24 hr (Fig. 6). However, 3 mg/kg cause a depletion which shows no tendency to recovery up to 1 week. Similar results are obtained in the rat spleen, but a long-lasting depletion occurs only after 30 mg/kg, implying that the critical dose varies from organ to organ.

The assumption that the destruction of adrenergic nerve terminals depends on the uptake of a critical amount of 6-hydroxydopamine is further supported by experiments showing that 30 min after intravenous administration of H^3-6-hydroxydopamine the quantity of H^3-amines retained in the rat heart corresponds to the dose injected. However, after 2 hr and even more strikingly after 24 hr, the amount of H^3-amines retained is inversely related to the dose initially administered (Fig. 7). It therefore seems that in low doses H^3-6-hydroxydopamine is taken up and stored in adrenergic nerve endings and can be liberated as a false adrenergic transmitter, as has been shown in the isolated perfused spleen of the cat (THOENEN and TRANZER, 1968). Higher doses of 6-hydroxydopamine, on the other hand, lead to a destruction of the adrenergic nerve terminals and thus to a destruction of the storage sites.

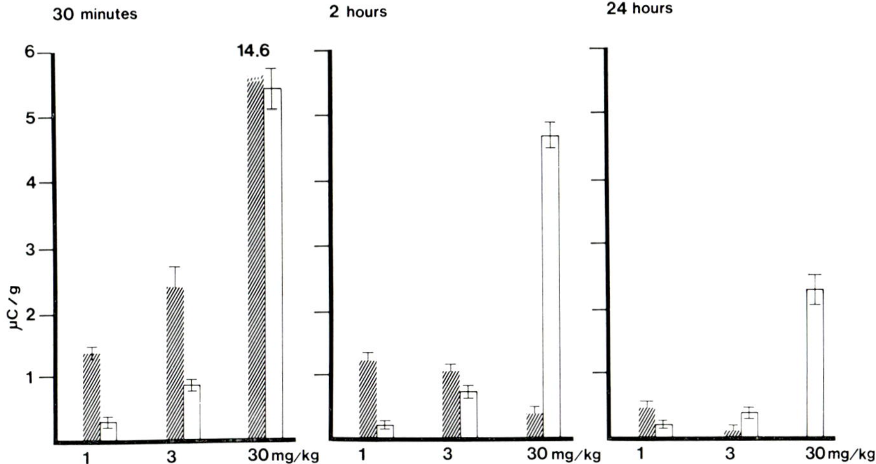

Fig. 7. Uptake and retention of H^3-6-hydroxydopamine in the rat heart. The animals were injected with 1, 3 or 30 mg/kg of H^3-6-hydroxydopamine i.v. and sacrificed 30 min, 2 hr or 24 hr later. The radioactivity present in the supernatant of hearts homogenized in 0.4 N perchloric acid was separated into acidic and basic (amine) fractions on DOWEX 50 WX 4 columns. Open columns = acidic and neutral fraction; shaded columns = amine fraction

That the uptake of 6-hydroxydopamine into the adrenergic nerve terminals is a prerequisite for its specific action can be deduced from the fact that imipramine and related drugs, which are known to interfere with the membrane transport of phenylethylamines into the adrenergic nerve endings (HERTTING et al., 1961b; AXELROD et al., 1962; THOENEN et al., 1964), abolish the noradrenaline depletion brought about by 6-hydroxydopamine in mice (STONE et al., 1964) and prevent the disappearance of the terminal network of adrenergic nerves in the rat iris (MALMFORS and SACHS, 1968). However, the uptake of 6-hydroxydopamine into the storage vesicles of adrenergic nerve endings is not necessary for its destructive effect, since pretreatment with reserpine prevents neither the ultramorphological changes of adrenergic nerve endings (RICHARDS, personal communication) nor the reduction of tyrosine hydroxylase (THOENEN et al., 1970) in sympathetically innervated organs.

Among the various treatment schedules designed to achieve the most complete destruction of adrenergic nerve terminals, the following procedure proved to be optimal in both rats and cats (THOENEN and TRANZER, 1968; HAEUSLER et al., 1968, 1969). Two doses of 6-hydroxydopamine (rats 50 mg/kg, cats 20 mg/kg) are given intravenously within 24 hr; two further doses (rats 100 mg/kg, cats 50 mg/kg) are given a week later. One week after the last dose of 6-hydroxydopamine, the noradrenaline content is reduced to 7% of normal in the rat heart, to 5% in the spleen but only to 19% in the vas deferens. The catecholamine content of the adrenals is not reduced at all. In accordance with the findings in immunosympathectomized rats (IVERSEN et al., 1966) the uptake and retention of H^3-noradrenaline are greatly reduced. In general the reduction in noradrenaline uptake by different organs parallels the reduction in their endogenous noradrenaline. There is also a relative increase of the O-methylated and/or deaminated metabolites of noradrenaline (THOENEN and TRANZER, 1968).

Two weeks after the last injection of 6-hydroxydopamine in rats there is no or at most an insignificant trend to recovery, whereas after 4 weeks there is a consistent rise of the noradrenaline content in all organs studied, reaching a level of 50% of normal in the vas deferens and of 34% in the rat heart (THOENEN and TRANZER, 1968).

Similar results were obtained after analogous treatment of cats with 6-hydroxydopamine (THOENEN and TRANZER, 1968; HAEUSLER et al., 1968, 1969). The noradrenaline content, one week after the last dose of 6-hydroxydopamine, was reduced to about 3% in the heart, spleen and iris and to 8% in the nictitating membrane. Three months after the last dose of 6-hydroxydopamine the noradrenaline content in all organs studied reached or very closely approached the pre-injection levels (TRANZER and THOENEN, 1968a; HAEUSLER et al., 1968, 1969); this is accompanied by the (re)appearance of newly formed adrenergic nerve endings (TRANZER and THOENEN, 1968a; TRANZER et al., 1969).

After chemical sympathectomy, the response of the isolated perfused cat heart to sympathetic nerve stimulation and to tyramine is completely abolished and that of the nictitating membrane greatly reduced (HAEUSLER et al., 1968, 1969). Similarly, in chemically sympathectomized rats the response of the blood pressure to tyramine and to electrical stimulation of the sympathetic nerves by the method of GILLESPIE and MUIR (1967) is markedly reduced (FINCH and LEACH, 1970).

After systemic administration of 6-hydroxydopamine, the noradrenaline content of the rat brain is not affected (THOENEN, unpublished results); this is probably due to the poor penetration of 6-hydroxydopamine through the blood-brain barrier. However, direct injection into the brain (UNGERSTEDT, 1968) or intraventricular administration (BLOOM et al., 1969; BURKARD et al., 1969; URETSKY and IVERSEN, 1969, 1970) results in a long-lasting reduction of the cerebral noradrenaline and dopamine content, whereas 5-hydroxytryptamine (BURKARD et al., 1969; URETSKY and IVERSEN, 1970) and γ-aminobutyric acid (URETSKY and IVERSEN, 1970) are not significantly diminished. After intraventricular injection of 3 doses of 250 μg of 6-hydroxydopamine, the noradrenaline content of the rat brain is reduced to 9% (URETSKY and IVERSEN, 1970). The catecholamine depletion is accompanied by a marked reduction in tyrosine hydroxylase and DOPA decarboxylase activity in hypothalamus and striatum (URETSKY and IVERSEN, 1970), areas which are rich in nerve terminals containing noradrenaline and dopamine (DAHLSTRÖM and FUXE, 1965). The diminished activity of these enzymes corresponds to their reduction in peripheral organs after surgical denervation (ANDÉN et al., 1964; SEDVALL and KOPIN, 1967) or immunosympathectomy (KLINGMAN, 1965; IVERSEN et al., 1966). In contrast to findings in peripheral organs there is no evidence of any recovery for a period of up to 75 days (URETSKY and IVERSEN, 1970). This could be taken to indicate that in the brain not only the nerve terminals, but also the cell bodies are damaged. Thus the question arises whether there is a major difference between the susceptibility of peripheral and central adrenergic cell bodies to 6-hydroxydopamine or whether these findings only reflect the concentrations of 6-hydroxydopamine reached in the brain after intraventricular or intracerebral administration, concentrations which are most probably higher than those reached in peripheral ganglia after intravenous injection[1].

As after intravenous administration, the gross behaviour of animals injected intraventricularly with 6-hydroxydopamine is not changed. At least they show a normal motor activity (BURKARD et al., 1969) and are able to maintain a normal control over their food and water intake (URETSKY and IVERSEN, 1970). It remains to be established whether changes in behaviour are completely absent or whether they can only be detected in more sophisticated studies.

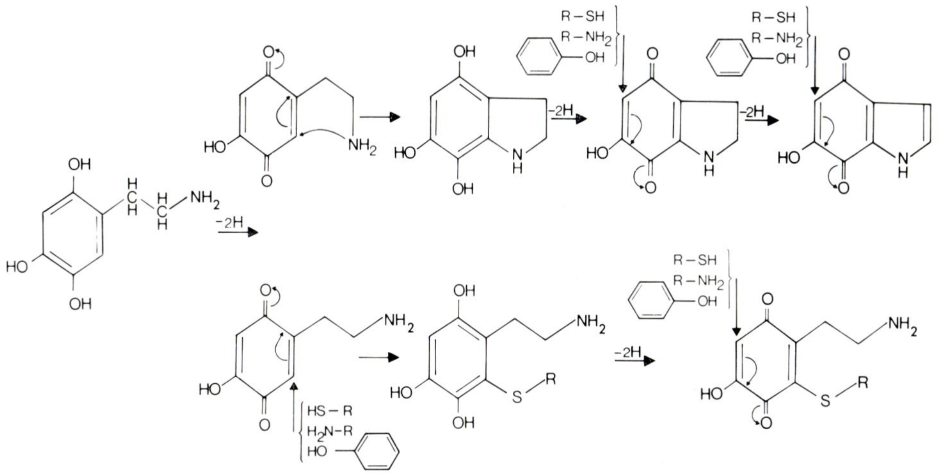

Fig. 8. Hypothetical mechanism of action of 6-hydroxydopamine. 6-Hydroxydopamine is oxidized to a para-quinone derivative which can undergo further transformation to an indoline, then indole derivative. Both the original para-quinone derivative and the indole derivative can form covalent bindings with nucleophilic groups of biological macromolecules

As to the mechanism of the destruction of adrenergic neurons, two properties of 6-hydroxydopamine seem to be of essential importance: a) the efficient accumulation of 6-hydroxydopamine in adrenergic neurons and b) the extreme susceptibility of this amine to non-enzymatic oxidation. Trihydroxyphenols with the structural features of 6-hydroxydopamine are easily oxidized to para-quinones which can be transformed to indolines and indoles or polymerized to melanin-like macromolecules (THOENEN et al., 1970; SANER and THOENEN, 1971). Both quinones and their melanin-like polymers can undergo covalent binding with a wide variety of nucleophilic groups such as SH, NH_2 and phenolic OH (Fig. 8). These covalent bindings may well account for irreversible alterations of various biological structures which are rich in these nucleophilic groups. This assumption is supported by the observation that 24 hr after intravenous administration of 30 mg/kg H^3-6-hydroxydopamine to rats, about 30% of the total radioactivity present in the rat heart is not extractable with 0.4 N perchloric acid when a procedure is used which allows the extraction of the total radioactivity after administration of H^3-noradrenaline (THOENEN and TRANZER, 1968). That both

[1] After this manuscript had been terminated, ANGELETTI and LEVI-MONTALCINI (Proc. N.A.S. **65**, 114—121, 1970) reported that treatment of newborn mice and rats resulted in severe damage of the cell bodies of peripheral sympathetic ganglia. This implies that the ganglia of newborn animals are not only more susceptible to the nerve growth antiserum but also to 6-hydroxydopamine.

extractable and non-extractable radioactivity mainly originate from sympathetic nerve endings can be concluded from the fact that in rats previously sympathectomized with non-labelled 6-hydroxydopamine, the total radioactivity retained in the heart is markedly reduced but the ratio between extractable and non-extractable radioactivity remains the same.

It seems that the electrophilic attack of the oxidation products of 6-hydroxydopamine on biological macromolecules is rather non-specific and that the high selectivity of the site of destruction is due to the efficient accumulation of 6-hydroxydopamine in adrenergic neurons.

V. Comparison between Surgical, Immunological, and Chemical Sympathectomy

In the preceding sections it has been shown that sympathectomy had, and still has, an important place in the investigation of the general homeostatic function of the sympathetic nervous system, in the elucidation of the sites of synthesis and storage of the adrenergic transmitter and in the cellular localization of the enzymes involved in its metabolic degradation. Denervation experiments also played a crucial role in the demonstration of the importance of uptake and re-uptake of adrenergic transmitter substances into the nerve terminals as the usually most important mechanism for the termination of the transmitter action on the effector organs.

Surgical denervation is still the method of choice for experiments designed to study the effect of deprivation from sympathetic innervation in single organs or groups of organs, possibly in comparison with an intact contralateral innervation. However, this is only possible if organs are innervated from single, easily accessible ganglia, as for instance the iris, salivary gland and nictitating membrane, which are exclusively innervated from the superior cervical ganglion. But even under these optimal conditions, incomplete denervation can occur as a result of anatomical variations, such as the location of groups of ganglionic cells within the "postganglionic" nerve trunk (LAWRENTJEW and BOROWSKAJA, 1935). The risk of incomplete denervation can be diminished by removing as large a piece as possible of the postganglionic nerve, together with the corresponding ganglia. Surgical denervation of the heart, an organ with a more complex and less easily accessible innervation, represents considerable technical difficulties, and complete denervation can only be achieved by autotransplantation (POTTER et al., 1965; COOPER, 1966). This, however, is a method which as yet has only been performed in larger animals and for obvious reasons in a limited number of animals. For a general sympathetic denervation the surgical procedure is even more cumbrous and time-consuming, as was very impressively demonstrated by the experiments of CANNON et al. (1929). It took more than 6 months stepwise to denervate adult cats, but this procedure is obviously not suitable for smaller animals and for experiments which require a larger number of animals. Here the other 2 methods are preferable, although both immunosympathectomy and chemical sympathectomy have their limitations. Both methods leave the adrenal medulla uninjured (HAMBERGER et al., 1965; KLINGMAN, 1965; IVERSEN et al., 1966; THOENEN and TRANZER, 1968; MUELLER et al., 1969), and in several other organs the denervation is incomplete (VOGT, 1964; ZAIMIS et al., 1965; KLINGMAN, 1965; LEVI-MONTALCINI and ANGELETTI, 1966, 1968) or even absent (KLINGMAN, 1965; IVERSEN et al., 1966). However, in other organs with a complex and not easily accessible innervation, the destruction of adrenergic nerves (HAMBERGER et al., 1965; KLINGMAN, 1965; ZAIMIS et al., 1965; IVERSEN et al., 1966; LEVI-MONTALCINI and ANGELETTI,

1966, 1968) or nerve endings respectively (THOENEN and TRANZER, 1968; TRANZER and THOENEN, 1968a; HAEUSLER et al., 1968, 1969) is virtually complete. Of particular interest is the denervation of the heart, a favourite organ for the study of intra- and extraneuronal uptake and metabolism of noradrenaline and related phenylethylamines (for references see IVERSEN, 1967). In this field, immunosympathectomy and chemical sympathectomy provide very useful new experimental approaches.

The limitation of the efficiency of immunosympathectomy most probably depends on the fact that sympathetic ganglia are particularly sensitive at a critical stage of their development and that this period of sensitivity is not the same for all ganglia (IVERSEN et al., 1966; LEVI-MONTALCINI and ANGELETTI, 1966). In some ganglia the period of highest susceptibility is before, in others immediately after birth. Therefore, the highest degree of immunosympathectomy can be achieved by combined pre- and postnatal administration of the antiserum (IVERSEN et al., 1966; LEVI-MONTALCINI and ANGELETTI, 1966; KLINGMAN and KLINGMAN, 1967). However, the adrenergic neurons in the central nervous system, the adrenal medulla and the vas deferens have been resistant to the antiserum at any stage of their development investigated so far. The ganglia of the vas deferens also do not respond to the nerve growth factor (LEVI-MONTALCINI, 1966, 1967). The resistance of the central adrenergic neurons to the antiserum may not so much result from a lack of susceptibility, but rather from a poor penetration of the antiserum through the blood-brain barrier.

In contrast to immunosympathectomy, which leads to a destruction of the whole adrenergic neuron (LEVI-MONTALCINI and BOOKER, 1960), chemical sympathectomy with 6-hydroxydopamine only affects its peripheral part (TRANZER and THOENEN, 1967a, 1968a; MALMFORS and SACHS, 1968). At least this seems to be the case after systemic application in the periphery. However, after intracerebral or intraventricular administration there is some evidence that the cell bodies of the central adrenergic neurons are also damaged (UNGERSTEDT, 1968; URETSKY and IVERSEN, 1970).

Considerable differences in the degree of denervation of different organs are also found after administration of 6-hydroxydopamine (THOENEN and TRANZER, 1968; HAEUSLER et al., 1969), most probably resulting from differences in the blood supply, with respect to both organ mass and especially their noradrenaline content which reflects the density of the adrenergic innervation. The denser the sympathetic innervation of an organ, the smaller is the share of 6-hydroxydopamine, delivered by the blood stream, to each single nerve ending. In this context, the recent observation by HAEUSLER et al. (1971) is remarkable in that the adrenergic nerves of the rat mesenteric vessels are poorly affected by 6-hydroxydopamine. Their noradrenaline content is only reduced to 50% of normal after administration of doses of 6-hydroxydopamine, which achieve a reduction to less than 10% in heart and spleen. This poor effect on the adrenergic nerves of blood vessels, which has been confirmed by several other authors (DEVINE, 1969; LAVERTY and PHELAN, 1969), may be due to their particular localization. These nerves are mainly found in the adventitiomedial junction (LEVER and ESTERHUIZEN, 1961; FUXE and SEDVALL, 1965) and the intima and media may represent a diffusion barrier between the vascular lumen and the nerve terminals in the adventitia; the blood supply to the adventitia by vasa vasorum (WOLINSKY and GLAGOV, 1967) is negligible in rats. In contrast, intraarterial infusion of relatively small doses of 6-hydroxydopamine into the femoral artery of the dog leads to a virtually complete denervation of the femoral artery and vein (HAEUSLER and GEROLD, personal communication). In this species vasa vasorum are well developed.

In the periphery both immunosympathectomy and chemical sympathectomy lead to an extensive destruction of the adrenergic nervous system. Neither of the two methods achieves a complete sympathectomy, and both methods have their own particular pattern of differences in the susceptibility of the adrenergic neurons of different organs. For immunosympathectomy the animals have to be treated with nerve growth antiserum pre- and/or postnatally, whereas chemical sympathectomy can be achieved at any age. However, administration of 6-hydroxydopamine leads only to a temporary denervation, i.e. a destruction of the adrenergic nerve endings, which regenerate from the undamaged proximal part of the neuron. Thus two methods of peripheral, non-surgical denervation are available. Immunosympathectomy implies a permanent destruction of the adrenergic neurons involved, whereas chemical sympathectomy with 6-hydroxydopamine is reversible.

The selective destruction of adrenergic and dopaminergic nerve endings and possibly also cell bodies in the central nervous system by local administration of 6-hydroxydopamine opens new possibilities for the investigation of the central nervous system.

In contrast to surgical denervation, chemical sympathectomy leaves the cholinergic fibres within the sympathetic nerves intact (TRANZER and THOENEN, 1968a). This peculiar selectivity of the 6-hydroxydopamine effect might be of interest in studies designed to investigate the function of cholinergic fibres within sympathetic nerves. It is not known whether the nerve growth antiserum displays a similar selectivity or whether the cholinergic neurons within the sympathetic ganglia are also destroyed.

VI. Compensatory Mechanism

The changes in the reactivity of the effector organs after removal of their nerve supply have been the object of investigation for more than a century. In 1855, BUDGE reported a phenomenon, occurring after sympathetic denervation, which later became known as "paradoxical pupillary dilatation" (LANGENDORFF, 1900). Experiments of ANDERSON (1904), MELTZER (1904), MELTZER and AUER (1904), and ELLIOTT (1905) revealed that the paradoxical reactions of the denervated iris and nictitating membrane of the cat are due to a supersensitivity of the denervated smooth muscle to circulating catecholamines.

Since then a vast amount of experimental data and explanatory hypotheses have been reported. They have been reviewed periodically both extensively and competently (CANNON and ROSENBLUETH, 1937, 1949; BURN, 1956; TRENDELENBURG, 1963b) and therefore only a brief survey on the more recent work is given. The main attention will be focussed on the phenomenon of denervation supersensitivity developing in smooth muscles, especially the nictitating membrane of the cat.

The careful studies of TRENDELENBURG and coworkers (TRENDELENBURG et al., 1962; TRENDELENBURG, 1963a, b), of FLEMING (1963) and GREEN and FLEMING (1967) provided convincing evidence that the supersensitivity to noradrenaline developing in the nictitating membrane after cutting the postganglionic sympathetic nerves is composed of two qualitatively and quantitatively different types of supersensitivity. One component is very similar to the increased sensitivity occurring after decentralization, and seems to develop whenever the influence of centrally originating impulses on the effector organ is abolished (TRENDELENBURG and WEINER, 1962). The second component remarkably resembles the supersensitivity occurring after administration of cocaine (FLECKEN-

STEIN and BASS, 1953; INNES and KOSTERLITZ, 1954; TRENDELENBURG, 1959; HAEFELY et al., 1964). This cocaine-like component develops very rapidly and is completed by the second day after removal of the superior cervical ganglion (TRENDELENBURG, 1963a), and is specific for noradrenaline and related phenylethylamines (TRENDELENBURG et al., 1962; TRENDELENBURG, 1963b). In contrast, the decentralization component of supersensitivity reaches its maximum not earlier than 2 weeks after removal of the superior cervical ganglion (TRENDELENBURG and WEINER, 1962; TRENDELENBURG et al., 1962), and more recent experiments revealed that even a further increase of up to one month takes place (LANGER et al., 1967). Furthermore, the decentralization component is nonspecific and an increased sensitivity to various agents such as acetylcholine, barium and potassium has been reported (TRENDELENBURG and WEINER, 1962; FLEMING, 1963; TRENDELENBURG, 1963b; SCHMIDT and FLEMING, 1964; MORRISON and FLEMING, 1967). It seems therefore that the effect of denervation is equal to the combined effects of cocaine and of decentralization. This interpretation is substantiated by the observation that cocaine does not produce any substantial increase in sensitivity to noradrenaline in the denervated nictitating membrane (HAEUSLER et al., 1969) and that long-term treatment with reserpine, chlorisondamine and choline 2:6-xylylether (TM_{10}), drugs which interfere with the transmission of sympathetic nerve impulses to the effector organs by different mechanisms, cause a decentralization type of supersensitivity (FLEMING and TRENDELENBURG, 1961; TRENDELENBURG and WEINER, 1962).

In the cocaine-like component of denervation supersensitivity a prejunctional mechanism is generally believed to be involved (TRENDELENBURG et al., 1962; TRENDELENBURG, 1963a, b; SMITH et al., 1966; VAN ORDEN et al., 1967). The destruction of adrenergic neurons, or their terminals, by the different methods of sympathectomy abolishes the mechanism mainly responsible for the inactivation of noradrenaline, i.e. its uptake into the adrenergic nerve terminals (HERTTING et al., 1961a, b; MUSCHOLL, 1961; TRENDELENBURG, 1963b). In the presence of a normal innervation, and consequently of a normal uptake capacity, noradrenaline is removed from the neighbourhood of the receptors. The efficiency of this removal determines to a large extent the sensitivity of an effector organ to noradrenaline. The rate and extent of this removal is determined by factors such as diffusion and convection, but mainly by the density of the adrenergic innervation. This is impressively documented by recent observations of TRENDELENBURG et al. (1969), which have shown that the densely innervated medial smooth muscle of the cat nictitating membrane is less sensitive to noradrenaline than the inferior smooth muscle and that this difference disappears after denervation. Moreover, not only the density of the adrenergic innervation but also the topography seems to be of importance, since in arteries in which the adrenergic nerves are mainly located in the adventitia (LEVER and ESTERHUIZEN, 1961; FUXE and SEDVALL, 1965) sympathetic denervation leads to a much higher increase in sensitivity to noradrenaline when it is administered to the outside of the artery, rather than into its lumen (DE LA LANDE et al., 1967).

In general, the rapidly developing denervation supersensitivity seems to be caused by the destruction of the adrenergic nerve endings and is restricted to the physiological transmitter noradrenaline and other mainly directly acting phenylethylamines (TRENDELENBURG et al., 1962; TRENDELENBURG, 1963b), those which are inactivated by uptake into the adrenergic nerve endings. Removal of this mechanism of inactivation by destruction of the nerve endings offers a reasonable explanation for the rapidly developing component of the denervation supersensitivity.

In contrast, the mechanism of the slowly developing decentralization component is poorly understood. It seems that its development depends on alterations in the effector organs. In general it is of moderate intensity and it is nonspecific (TRENDELENBURG and WEINER, 1962; FLEMING, 1963; SCHMIDT and FLEMING, 1964; MORRISON and FLEMING, 1967). Isoproterenol, which is not taken up by adrenergic nerves (HERTTING, 1964), shows only the decentralization component of denervation supersensitivity (PLUCHINO, 1967; PLUCHINO and TRENDELENBURG, 1968). This, however, is restricted to its α-adrenergic excitatory action, whereas no indication of an increase in the β-adrenergic inhibitory action could be detected (SMITH, 1963; PLUCHINO and TRENDELENBURG, 1968). The nonspecific, decentralization-type, component of supersensitivity seems to be directed to excitatory agents only. However, in the spleen (HERTTING et al., 1967; GREEN and FLEMING, 1968), the heart and the blood vessels (DEMPSEY and COOPER, 1968; HAEUSLER et al., 1971), organs where catecholamines have an excitatory effect, the increase in sensitivity after denervation seems to be entirely due to the absence of noradrenaline inactivation by uptake into the nerve endings, and no indication for a nonspecific decentralization component of supersensitivity has been detected.

The lack of specificity of the decentralization supersensitivity makes it unlikely that it can be due to an increase in the number of receptors or an expansion of their area of distribution, alterations which are responsible for the increased sensitivity of denervated skeletal muscles to acetylcholine (AXELSSON and THESLEFF, 1959; MILEDI, 1960). The changes involved in the development of decentralization supersensitivity seem to be localized beyond the level of receptors at a site where the response to the excitation of various kinds of receptors converges on a common pathway. The site and nature of these changes are unknown, and this is the reason why they develop in some organs but not in others. The situation becomes even more complex if one considers the recent observation of TSAI et al. (1968) that the nonspecific decentralization supersensitivity is absent in the isolated nictitating membrane, implying that the factors responsible for this type of supersensitivity are rather labile or have to be complemented by a blood-borne factor. This assumption is supported by the finding of VOGT (1965) that there are considerable differences in the sensitivity of the receptors to angiotensin, bradykinin and histamine when the adrenal medulla of the dog is either perfused with blood or with Locke's solution.

Teleologically the supersensitivity to the transmitter can be considered as a compensatory mechanism, which helps to maintain the homeostasis of autonomic functions after destruction of a great part of the sympathetic nervous system by surgical denervation, immunosympathectomy or chemical sympathectomy. The denervated organs no longer receive nerve impulses which normally control their activity, but they may still take part in some general reaction of the organism by their increased reactivity to circulating catecholamines.

Both chemical and immunosympathectomy leave the adrenal medulla unaffected. It seems that this organ takes over — at least partially — the function of the destroyed sympathetic nervous system, by an augmented delivery of catecholamines into the circulation, in response to an increased reflex activity of the splanchnic nerves. The enhanced splanchnic activity increases the turnover and synthesis of adrenal catecholamines (IVERSEN et al., 1966; MUELLER et al., 1969), which is accompanied by an induction of tyrosine hydroxylase (MUELLER et al., 1969; THOENEN et al., 1970), the enzyme catalyzing the rate-limiting step in the synthesis of catecholamines.

VII. Concluding Remarks

Sympathetic denervation was, and still is, an important method for the investigation of the physiology and pharmacology of the sympathetic nervous system. Sympathectomy has played a crucial role in the elucidation of the general homeostatic function of the sympathetic nervous system and in the localization of the cellular sites of synthesis, storage and enzymatic degradation of the adrenergic transmitter noradrenaline. Furthermore, denervation experiments have been useful in demonstrating the role of uptake and re-uptake of adrenergic transmitter substances into the nerve endings as the most important mechanisms for terminating the transmitter action on the effector organs.

Surgical denervation is still the method of choice for the denervation of organs which are supplied by sympathetic fibres from single, easily accessible ganglia. However, for denervation of organs with a more complex innervation or for general sympathectomy the surgical procedure is too cumbrous, time-consuming and in smaller animals virtually impracticable. Two other methods, immunosympathectomy and chemical sympathectomy, which became available within the last decade, seem to be preferable. Although these two methods result in a more general effect on the sympathetic nervous system, they have also their limitations and drawbacks. Thus, sympathetic ganglia are sensitive to the nerve growth antiserum only at a critical stage of their development and this period of sensitivity is not identical for all ganglia. Consequently, the highest degree of immunosympathectomy can be achieved by combined pre- and postnatal administration of the antiserum. However, the adrenal medulla, the adrenergic neurons in the central nervous system and those innervating the vas deferens are resistant to the antiserum at any stage of their development studied so far.

In contrast to immunosympathectomy, which leads to a destruction of the whole neuron, chemical sympathectomy affects mainly the adrenergic nerve terminals. The differences in the degree of denervation of different organs after administration of 6-hydroxydopamine is probably due to differences in blood supply, both with respect to organ mass and particularly with respect to their noradrenaline content which reflects the density of the adrenergic innervation.

Neither immunosympathectomy nor systemic administration of 6-hydroxydopamine affect the adrenergic neurons in the central nervous system. Whether the resistance of the central adrenergic neurons to immunosympathectomy is due to their lack of susceptibility to the antiserum or to poor penetration of the antiserum across the blood-brain barrier is not known. 6-Hydroxydopamine, however, given by intraventricular or intracerebral injection, selectively destroys central adrenergic neurons, thus opening new possibilities in the investigation of the central nervous system.

References

Ahlquist, R.P.: A study of adrenotropic receptors. Amer. J. Physiol. **153**, 586—600 (1948).

Andén, N.E., Magnusson, T., Rosengren, E.: On the presence of dihydroxyphenylalanine decarboxylase in nerves. Experientia (Basel) **20**, 328—329 (1964).

Anderson, H.K.: The paralysis of involuntary muscle, with special reference to the occurrence of paradoxical contraction. Part I. Paradoxical pupil-dilatation and other ocular phenomena caused by lesions of the cervical sympathetic tract. J. Physiol. (Lond.) **30**, 290—310 (1904).

Angeletti, P., Calissano, P., Chen, J.S., Levi-Montalcini, R.: Multiple molecular forms of the nerve growth factor. Biochim. biophys. Acta (Amst.) **147**, 180—182 (1967).

Axelrod, J., Albers, W., Clemente, C.D.: Distribution of catechol-O-methyl transferase in the nervous system and other tissues. J. Neurochem. **5**, 68—72 (1959a).

AXELROD, J., HERTTING, G., POTTER, L.: Effect of drugs on the uptake and release of H^3-norepinephrine in the rat heart. Nature (Lond.) **194**, 297 (1962).
— LAROCHE, M.J.: Inhibitor of O-methylation of epinephrine and norepinephrine in vitro and in vivo. Science **130**, 800 (1959).
— SHEIN, H.M., WURTMAN, R.J.: Stimulation of C^{14}-melatonin synthesis from C^{14}-tryptophan by noradrenaline in rat pineal in organ culture. Proc. nat. Acad. Sci. (Wash.) **62**, 544—549 (1969).
— WEIL-MALHERBE, H., TOMCHICK, R.: The physiological disposition of H^3-epinephrine and its metabolite metanephrine. J. Pharmacol. exp. Ther. **127**, 251—256 (1959b).
AXELSSON, J., THESLEFF, S.: A study of supersensitivity in denervated mammalian skeletal muscle. J. Physiol. (Lond.) **147**, 178—193 (1959).
BACQ, Z.M., GOSSELIN, L., DRESSE, A., RENSON, J.: Inhibition of O-methyl-transferase by catechol and sensitization to epinephrine. Science **130**, 453—454 (1959).
BÁRÁNY, E.H., TREISTER, G.: Time relations of degeneration mydriasis and degeneration vasoconstriction in the rabbit ear after sympathetic denervation. Effect of bretylium. Acta physiol. scand. (in press).
BELLEAU, B., BURBA, J.: Tropolones: a unique class of potent non-competitive inhibitors of S-adenosylmethionine-catechol methyltransferase. Biochim. biophys. Acta (Amst.) **54**, 195—196 (1961).
BENMILOUD, M., EULER, U.S. v.: Effects of bretylium, reserpine, guanethidine and sympathetic denervation on the noradrenaline content of the rat submaxillary gland. Acta physiol. scand. **59**, 34—42 (1963).
BHAGAT, B.: Effect of noradrenaline injection on the catecholamine content of the rat heart. Arch. int. Pharmacodyn. **146**, 47—55 (1963).
BIEL, J.H., LUM, B.K.B.: The β-adrenergic blocking agents. Pharmacology and structure-activity relationships. Fortschr. Arzneimittelforsch. **10**, 46—89 (1966).
BIRMINGHAM, A.T.: Denervation of the vas deferens of the guinea-pig. J. Physiol. (Lond.) **190**, 16P—17P (1967).
— Post-ganglionic denervation of the rat vas deferens. J. Physiol. (Lond.) **197**, 37P—38P (1968).
BLOOM, F., GROPPETTI, A., REVUELTA, A., COSTA, E.: Biochemical and fine structural effects of 6-hydroxydopamine on rat central nervous system after intracisternal injection. 4th Int. Congr. Pharmac. Abstr. 218—219 (1969).
BOURA, A.L.A., GREEN, A.F.: The actions of bretylium: adrenergic neurone blocking and other effects. Brit. J. Pharmacol. **14**, 536—548 (1959).
BRODY, M.J.: Cardiovascular responses following immunological sympathectomy. Circulat. Res. **15**, 161—167 (1964).
BROWN, G.L., DAVIES, B.M., FERRY, C.B.: The effect of neuronal rest on the output of sympathetic transmitter from the spleen. J. Physiol. (Lond.) **159**, 365—380 (1961).
BUDGE, J.L.: Über die Bewegung der Iris; für Physiologen und Ärzte. Braunschweig: Vieweg 1855.
BUEKER, E.D.: Implantation of tumors in the hind limb field of the embryonic chick and developmental response of the lumbosacral nervous system. Anat. Rec. **102**, 369—390 (1948).
BURKARD, W.P., GEY, K.F., PLETSCHER, A.: Inhibition of decarboxylase of aromatic amino acids by 2,3,4-trihydroxybenzylhydrazine and its seryl derivatives. Arch. Biochem. **107**, 187—196 (1964).
— JALFRE, M., BLUM, J.: Effect of 6-hydroxydopamine on behaviour and cerebral amine in rats. Experientia (Basel) **25**, 1295—1296 (1969).
BURN, J.H.: Practical pharmacology. Oxford: Blackwell 1952.
— Functions of autonomic transmitters. Baltimore: The Williams and Wilkins Co. 1956.
— PHILPOT, F.J., TRENDELENBURG, U. v.: Effect of denervation on enzymes in iris and blood vessels. Brit. J. Pharmacol. **9**, 423—428 (1954).
— ROBINSON, J.: Hypersensitivity of the denervated nictitating membrane and amine oxidase. J. Physiol. (Lond.) **120**, 224—229 (1953).
CANNON, W.B., LISSÁK, K.: Evidence for adrenaline in adrenergic neurones. Amer. J. Physiol. **125**, 765—777 (1939).
— NEWTON, H.F., BRIGHT, E.M., MENKIN, V., MOORE, R.M.: Some aspects of the physiology of animals surviving complete exclusion of sympathetic nerve impulses. Amer. J. Physiol. **89**, 84—107 (1929).
— ROSENBLUETH, A.: Autonomic neuro-effector systems. New York: The MacMillan Co. 1937.
— — The supersensitivity of denervated structures. A law of denervation. New York: The MacMillan Co. 1949.
CARLSSON, A., ROSENGREN, E., BERTLER, A., NILSSON, J.: The effect of reserpine on the metabolism of catecholamines. In: S. GARATTINI and V. GHETTI: Psychotropic drugs, pp. 363—372. Amsterdam: Elsevier 1957.

CARPI, A., OLIVERIO, A.: Urinary excretion of catecholamines in the immunosympathectomized rat — Balance phenomena between the adrenergic and the noradrenergic system. Int. J. Neuropharmacol. **3**, 427—431 (1964).

CERVONI, P.: Monoamine oxidase activity of the cat nictitating membrane and superior cervical ganglion under various experimental conditions. Biochem. Pharmacol. **18**, 1427—1433 (1969).

CLARKE, D.E., JONES, C.J.: Are adrenergic nerves required for uptake$_2$ in the isolated perfused rat heart? Europ. J. Pharmacol. **7**, 121—124 (1969).

— — LINLEY, P.A.: Histochemical fluorescence studies on noradrenaline accumulation by uptake$_2$ in the isolated rat heart. Brit. J. Pharmacol. **34**, 1—9 (1969).

COATS, D.A., EMMELIN, N.: The short-term effects of sympathetic ganglionectomy on the cat's salivary secretion. J. Physiol. (Lond.) **162**, 282—288 (1962).

COHEN, S.: A nerve growth-promoting protein. In: W.D. MCELROY and B. GLASS: Basis of development, pp. 665—667. Baltimore: Johns Hopkins Press 1958.

— Purification and metabolic effects of a nerve growth-promoting protein from snake venom. J. biol. Chem. **234**, 1129—1137 (1959).

— Purification of a nerve-growth promoting protein from the mouse salivary gland and its neuro-cytotoxic antiserum. Proc. nat. Acad. Sci. (Wash.) **46**, 302—311 (1960).

COOPER, T.: Surgical sympathectomy and adrenergic function. Pharmacol. Rev. **18**, 611—618 (1966).

— GILBERT, J.W., BLOODWELL, R.D., CROUT, J.R.: Chronic extrinsic cardiac denervation by regional neural ablation: Description of the operation, verification of the denervation and its effects on myocardial catecholamines. Circulat. Res. **9**, 275—281 (1961).

— SJOERDSMA, A.: Depletion of splenic norepinephrine in rat by celiac ganglionectomy. Proc. Soc. exp. Biol. (N.Y.) **109**, 538—539 (1962).

— WILLMAN, V.L., JELLINEK, M., HANLON, C.R.: Heart autotransplantation: Effect on myocardial catecholamines and histamine. Science **138**, 40—41 (1962).

CRAIN, S.M., BENITZ, H., VATTER, A.E.: Some cytologic effects of salivary nerve-growth factor on tissue cultures of peripheral ganglia. Ann. N.Y. Acad. Sci. **118**, 206—231 (1964).

CROUT, J.R., COOPER, T.: Myocardial catechol-O-methyl transferase activity after chronic cardiac denervation. Nature (Lond.) **194**, 387 (1962).

DAHLSTRÖM, A., FUXE, K.: Evidence for the existence of monoamine neurons in the central nervous system. Acta physiol. scand. **64**, Suppl. 247 (1965).

— HÄGGENDAL, J.: Studies on the transport and lifespan of amine storage granules in a peripheral adrenergic neuron system. Acta physiol. scand. **67**, 278—288 (1966).

DE CASTRO, F.: Die normale Histologie des peripheren vegetativen Nervensystems. Das Synapsen-Problem: Anatomisch-experimentelle Untersuchungen. Verh. dtsch. path. Ges. **34**, 1—52 (1950).

DE LA LANDE, I.S., FREWIN, D., WATERSON, J.G.: The influence of sympathetic innervation on vascular sensitivity to noradrenaline. Brit. J. Pharmacol. **31**, 82—93 (1967).

DEMPSEY, P.J., COOPER, T.: Supersensitivity of the chronically denervated feline heart. Amer. J. Physiol. **215**, 1245—1249 (1968).

DEVINE, C.E.: The fine structure of vascular axons after treatment with 6-hydroxydopamine. Proc. Univ. Otago med. Sch. **47**, 4—6 (1969).

ELLIOTT, T.R.: The action of adrenaline. J. Physiol. (Lond.) **32**, 401—467 (1905).

EULER, U.S. v., PURKHOLD, A.: Effect of sympathetic denervation on the noradrenaline and adrenaline content of the spleen, kidney, and salivary glands in the sheep. Acta physiol. scand. **24**, 212—217 (1951).

FALCK, B.: Observations on the possibilities of the cellular localization of monoamines by a fluorescence method. Acta physiol. scand. **56**, Suppl. 197 (1962).

— HILLARP, N.-Å., THIEME, G., TORP, A.: Fluorescence of catecholamines and related compounds condensed with formaldehyde. J. Histochem. Cytochem. **10**, 348—354 (1962).

FINCH, L., LEACH, G.D.H.: A comparison of the effects of 6-hydroxydopamine immunosympathectomy and reserpine on the cardiovascular reactivity in the rat. J. Pharm. Pharmacol. **22**, 354—360 (1970).

FISCHER, J.E., KOPIN, I.J., AXELROD, J.: Evidence for extraneuronal binding of norepinephrine. J. Pharmacol. exp. Ther. **147**, 181—185 (1965).

— MUSACCHIO, J., KOPIN, I.J., AXELROD, J.: Effects of denervation on the uptake and β-hydroxylation of tyramine in the rat salivary gland. Life Sci. **3**, 413—419 (1964).

— SNYDER, S.: Disposition of norepinephrine-H^3 in sympathetic ganglia. J. Pharmacol. exp. Ther. **150**, 190—195 (1965).

FLECKENSTEIN, A., BASS, H.: Zum Mechanismus der Wirkungsverstärkung und Wirkungsabschwächung sympathomimetischer Amine durch Cocain und andere Pharmaka. I. Mitteilung: Die Sensibilisierung der Katzen-Nickhaut für Sympathomimetica der Brenzkatechin-Reihe. Naunyn-Schmiedeberg's Arch. exp. Path. Pharmak. **220**, 143—156 (1953).

FLEMING, W. W.: A comparative study of supersensitivity to norepinephrine and acetylcholine produced by denervation, decentralization and reserpine. J. Pharmacol. exp. Ther. **141**, 173—179 (1963).

— TRENDELENBURG, U.: The development of supersensitivity to norepinephrine after pretreatment with reserpine. J. Pharmacol. exp. Ther. **133**, 41—51 (1961).

FURCHGOTT, R. F.: The receptors for epinephrine and norepinephrine (adrenergic receptors). Pharmacol. Rev. **11**, 429—441 (1959).

FUXE, K., SEDVALL, G.: The distribution of adrenergic nerve fibres to the blood vessels in skeletal muscle. Acta physiol. scand. **64**, 75—86 (1965).

GEFFEN, L. B., OSTBERG, A.: Distribution of granular vesicles in normal and constricted sympathetic neurones. J. Physiol. (Lond.) **204**, 583—592 (1969).

GILLESPIE, J. S., MUIR, T. C.: A method of stimulating the complete sympathetic outflow from the spinal cord to blood vessels in the pithed rat. Brit. J. Pharmacol. **30**, 78—87 (1967).

GLOWINSKI, J., AXELROD, J., KOPIN, I. J., WURTMAN, R. J.: Physiological disposition of H^3-norepinephrine in the developing rat. J. Pharmacol. exp. Ther. **146**, 48—53 (1964).

GOLDSTEIN, M., ANAGNOSTE, B., LAUBER, E., MCKEREGHAN, M. R.: Inhibition of dopamine-β-hydroxylase by disulfiram. Life Sci. **3**, 763—767 (1964).

GOODALL, MC. C.: Studies of adrenaline and noradrenaline in mammalian heart and suprarenals. Acta physiol. scand. **24**, Suppl. 85 (1951).

— KIRSHNER, N.: Effect of cervico-thoracic ganglionectomy on the adrenaline and noradrenaline content of the mammalian heart. J. clin. Invest. **35**, 649—656 (1956).

GREEN III, R. D., FLEMING, W. W.: Agonist-antagonist interactions in the normal and supersensitive nictitating membrane of the spinal cat. J. Pharmacol. exp. Ther. **156**, 207—214 (1967).

— — Analysis of supersensitivity in the isolated spleen of the cat. J. Pharmacol. exp. Ther. **162**, 254—262 (1968).

HAEFELY, W., HUERLIMANN, A., THOENEN, H.: A quantitative study of the effect of cocaine on the response of the cat nictitating membrane to nerve stimulation and to injected noradrenaline. Brit. J. Pharmacol. **22**, 5—21 (1964).

HAEUSLER, G., HAEFELY, W., HUERLIMANN, A.: Effect of surgical and chemical adrenergic denervation on vascular responses. Proc. Symp. Physiol. Pharmacol. Vasc. Neuroeffector System, Interlaken 1969, pp. 141—159. Basel: Karger 1971.

— — THOENEN, H.: Chemical sympathectomy of the cat with 6-hydroxydopamine. J. Pharmacol. exp. Ther. **170**, 50—61 (1969).

— THOENEN, H., HAEFELY, W.: Chemische Sympathektomie der Katze mit 6-Hydroxydopamin: Veränderungen von Sympathicusreizeffekten und Noradrenalinempfindlichkeit. Helv. physiol. pharmacol. Acta **26**, CR 223—225 (1968).

HÅKANSON, R., OWMAN, CH.: Effect of denervation and enzyme inhibition on DOPA decarboxylase and monoamine oxidase activities of rat pineal gland. J. Neurochem. **12**, 417—429 (1965).

HAMBERGER, B., LEVI-MONTALCINI, R., NORBERG, K. A., SJÖQVIST, F.: Monoamines in immunosympathectomized rats. Int. J. Neuropharmacol. **4**, 91—95 (1965).

HENNEMANN, H.-M., TRENDELENBURG, U.: Effect of the adrenergic neurone blocker β-TM_{10}, on the depletion of noradrenaline induced by denervation or reserpine. Naunyn-Schmiedeberg's Arch. Pharmak. **265**, 363—371 (1970).

HERTTING, G.: The fate of ^3H-iso-proterenol in the rat. Biochem. Pharmacol. **13**, 1119—1128 (1964).

— Effect of drugs and sympathetic denervation on noradrenaline uptake and binding in animal tissues. In: G. B. KOELLE, W. W. DOUGLAS, and A. CARLSSON: Pharmacology of cholinergic and adrenergic transmission, pp. 277—288. Oxford: Pergamon Press 1965.

— AXELROD, J., KOPIN, I. J., WHITBY, L. G.: Lack of uptake of catecholamines after chronic denervation of sympathetic nerves. Nature (Lond.) **189**, 66 (1961a).

— — PATRICK, R. W.: Actions of bretylium and guanethidine on the uptake and release of ^3H-noradrenaline. Brit. J. Pharmacol. **18**, 161—166 (1962).

— — WHITBY, L. G.: Effect of drugs on the uptake and metabolism of ^3H-norepinephrine. J. Pharmacol. exp. Ther. **134**, 146—153 (1961b).

— SCHIEFTHALER, T.: The effect of stellate ganglion excision on the catecholamine content and the uptake of H^3-norepinephrine in the heart of the cat. Int. J. Neuropharmacol. **3**, 65—69 (1964).

— SUKO, J., WIDHALM, S., HARBICH, I.: Über den Mechanismus der Potenzierung der Katecholaminwirkung nach chronisch postganglionärer sympathischer Denervierung. Naunyn-Schmiedeberg's Arch. Pharmak. exp. Path. **256**, 40—54 (1967).

HILLARP, N.-Å.: Structure of the synapse and the peripheral innervation apparatus of the autonomic nervous system. Acta anat. (Basel) **2**, Suppl. IV (1946).

Holzbauer, M., Vogt, M.: Depression by reserpine of the noradrenaline concentration in the hypothalamus of the cat. J. Neurochem. **1**, 8—11 (1956).

Huković, S., Muscholl, E.: Die Noradrenalin-Abgabe aus dem isolierten Kaninchenherzen bei sympathischer Nervenreizung und ihre pharmakologische Beeinflussung. Naunyn-Schmiedeberg's Arch. exp. Path. Pharmak. **244**, 81—96 (1962).

Innes, I.R., Kosterlitz, H.W.: The effects of preganglionic and postganglionic denervation on the responses of the nictitating membrane to sympathomimetic substances. J. Physiol. (Lond.) **124**, 25—43 (1954).

Iversen, L.L.: The inhibition of noradrenaline uptake by drugs. In: N.J. Harper and A.B. Simmonds: Advances Drug Res. **2**, pp. 1—46. London: Academic Press 1965.

— The uptake and storage of noradrenaline in sympathetic nerves. Cambridge: University Press 1967.

— Glowinski, J., Axelrod, J.: The physiologic disposition and metabolism of norepinephrine in immunosympathectomized animals. J. Pharmacol. exp. Ther. **151**, 273—284 (1966).

— Jarrott, B., Langer, S.Z.: Monoamine oxidase and catechol-O-methyl transferase activities in cat nictitating membrane and rat and guinea pig vas deferens after sympathectomy. Brit. J. Pharmacol. **34**, 693P—694P (1968).

Jonason, J.: Metabolism of dopamine and noradrenaline in normal atrophied and postganglionically sympathectomized rat salivary glands in vitro. Acta physiol. scand. **76**, 299—311 (1969).

Kapeller, K., Mayor, D.: The accumulation of noradrenaline in constricted sympathetic nerves as studied by fluorescence and electron microscopy. Proc. roy. Soc. B. **167**, 282—292 (1967).

— — An electron microscopic study of the early changes proximal to a constriction in sympathetic nerves. Proc. roy. Soc. B. **172**, 39—51 (1969).

Kirpekar, S.M., Cervoni, P., Furchgott, R.F.: Catecholamine content of the cat nictitating membrane following procedures sensitizing it to norepinephrine. J. Pharmacol. exp. Ther. **135**, 180—190 (1962).

Klingman, G.I.: Catecholamine levels and dopa-decarboxylase activity in peripheral organs and adrenergic tissues in the rat after immunosympathectomy. J. Pharmacol. (Lond.) **148**, 14—21 (1965).

— 5-Hydroxytryptamine levels in peripheral organs of immunosympathectomized rats. Biochem. Pharmacol. **18**, 2061—2067 (1969).

— Klingman, J.D.: Catecholamines in peripheral tissues of mice and cell counts of sympathetic ganglia after the prenatal and postnatal administration of the nerve growth factor antiserum. Int. J. Neuropharmacol. **6**, 501—508 (1967).

— — Effect of sympathetic denervation on the 5-hydroxytryptamine levels of the submaxillary glands of rats. Biochem. Pharmacol. **18**, 2069—2074 (1969).

Kopin, I.J., Gordon, E.K., Horst, W.D.: Studies of uptake of l-norepinephrine-^{14}C. Biochem. Pharmacol. **14**, 753—759 (1965).

Langendorff, O.: Zur Deutung der „paradoxen" Pupillenerweiterung. Klin. Mbl. Augenheilk. **38**, 823—827 (1900).

Langer, S.Z.: The degeneration contraction of the nictitating membrane in the unanesthetized cat. J. Pharmacol. exp. Ther. **151**, 66—72 (1966).

— Draskóczy, P.R., Trendelenburg, U.: Time course of the development of supersensitivity to various amines in the nictitating membrane of the pithed cat after denervation or decentralization. J. Pharmacol. exp. Ther. **157**, 255—273 (1967).

— Trendelenburg, U.: The onset of denervation supersensitivity. J. Pharmacol. exp. Ther. **151**, 73—86 (1966).

Laverty, R., Phelan, E.L.: Effects of 6-hydroxydopamine on noradrenaline storage and uptake in the rat. Proc. Univ. Otago med. Sch. **47**, 18—19 (1969).

— Sharman, D.F., Vogt, M.: Action of 2,4,5-trihydroxyphenylethylamine on the storage and release of noradrenaline. Brit. J. Pharmacol. **24**, 549—560 (1965).

Lawrentjew, B.I.: Über die Erscheinung der Degeneration und Regeneration im sympathischen Nervensystem. Z. mikr.-anat. Forsch. **2**, 201—223 (1925).

— Borowskaja, A.J.: Die Degeneration der postganglionären Fasern des autonomen Nervensystems und deren Endigungen. Z. Zellforsch. Abt. Histochem. **23**, 761—796 (1935).

Lever, J.D., Esterhuizen, A.C.: Fine structure of the arteriolar nerves in the guinea pig pancreas. Nature (Lond.) **192**, 566—567 (1961).

Levi-Montalcini, R.: Chemical stimulation of nerve growth. In: W.D. McElroy and B. Glass: Chemical basis of development, pp. 646—664. Baltimore: Johns Hopkins Press 1958.

Levi-Montalcini, R.: The nerve growth factor: its mode of action on sensory and sympathetic nerve cells. Harvey Lect. **60**, 217—259 (1966).
— Differentiation and growth control mechanisms in the nervous systems. In: E. Hagen, W. Wechsler, and P. Zilliken: Experimental biology and medicine. Morphological and biochemical aspects of cytodifferentiation, vol. 1, pp. 170—182. Basel: Karger 1967.
— Angeletti, P.U.: Noradrenaline and monoaminoxidase content in immunosympathectomized animals. Int. J. Neuropharmacol. **1**, 161—164 (1962).
— — Immunosympathectomy. Pharmacol. Rev. **18**, 619—628 (1966).
— — Nerve growth factor. Physiol. Rev. **48**, 534—569 (1968).
— Booker, B.: Destruction of sympathetic ganglia in mammals by antiserum to a nerve-growth protein. Proc. nat. Acad. Sci. (Wash.) **42**, 384—391 (1960).
— Cohen, S.: In vitro and in vivo effects of a nerve growth-stimulating agent isolated from snake venom. Proc. nat. Acad. Sci. (Wash.) **42**, 695—699 (1956).
— — Effects of the extract of the mouse submaxillary salivary glands on the sympathetic system of mammals. Ann. N.Y. Acad. Sci. **85**, 324—341 (1960).
— Hamburger, V.: Selective growth stimulating effects of mouse sarcoma on the sensory and sympathetic nervous system of the chick embryo. J. exp. Zool. **116**, 321—361 (1951).
— Meyer, H., Hamburger, V.: In vitro experiments on the effects of mouse sarcomas 180 and 37 on the spinal and sympathetic ganglia of the chick embryo. Cancer Res. **14**, 49—57 (1954).
— Tentori, L., Vivaldi, G., Angeletti, P.U., Marini-Bettolo, G.B.: Composizione in amino acidi del fattore di crescita del sistema nervoso (NGF). Gazz. chim. ital. **95**, 333—337 (1965).
Levitt, M., Spector, S., Sjoerdsma, A., Udenfriend, S.: Elucidation of the rate-limiting step in norepinephrine biosynthesis in the perfused guinea-pig heart. J. Pharmacol. exp. Ther. **148**, 1—8 (1965).
Lovenberg, W., Barchas, J., Weissbach, H., Udenfriend, S.: Characteristics of the inhibition of aromatic L-amino acid decarboxylase by α-methylamino acids. Arch. Biochem. **103**, 9—14 (1963).
Lundberg, D.: Adrenergic neuron blockers and transmitter release after sympathetic denervation studied in the conscious rat. Acta physiol. scand. **75**, 415—426 (1969).
Maickel, R.P., Matussek, N., Stern, D.N., Brodie, B.B.: The sympathetic nervous system as a homeostatic mechanism. I. Absolute need for sympathetic nervous function in body temperature maintenance of cold-exposed rats. J. Pharmacol. exp. Ther. **157**, 103—110 (1967).
Malmfors, T., Sachs, C.: Direct studies on the disappearance of the transmitter and changes in the uptake-storage mechanisms of degenerating adrenergic nerves. Acta physiol. scand. **64**, 211—223 (1965).
— — Degeneration of adrenergic nerves produced by 6-hydroxydopamine. Europ. J. Pharmacol. **3**, 89—92 (1968).
Meltzer, S.J.: Studies on the "paradoxical" pupil-dilatation caused by adrenaline. II. — On the influence of subcutaneous injections of adrenaline upon the eyes of cats after removal of the superior cervical ganglion. Amer. J. Physiol. **11**, 37—51 (1904).
— Auer, C.M.: Studies on the "paradoxical" pupil-dilatation caused by adrenaline. I. — The effect of subcutaneous injections and instillations of adrenaline upon the pupils of rabbits. Amer. J. Physiol. **11**, 28—36 (1904).
Miledi, R.: The acetylcholine sensitivity of frog muscle fibres after complete or partial denervation. J. Physiol. (Lond.) **151**, 1—23 (1960).
Molinoff, P., Axelrod, J.: Octopamine: normal occurrence in sympathetic nerves of rats. Science **164**, 428—429 (1969).
Moran, N.C., Perkins, M.E.: Adrenergic blockade of the mammalian heart by a dichloro analogue of isoproterenol. J. Pharmacol. exp. Ther. **124**, 223—237 (1958).
Morrison, J.M., Jr., Fleming, W.W.: The non specific supersensitivity of the cat nictitating membrane. Pharmacologist **9**, 234 (1967).
Mueller, R.A., Thoenen, H., Axelrod, J.: Adrenal tyrosine hydroxylase: compensatory increase in activity after chemical sympathectomy. Science **163**, 468—469 (1969).
Muscholl, E.: Über den Wirkungsmechanismus von Reserpin. Klin. Wschr. **37**, 217—226 (1959).
— Die Hemmung der Noradrenalin-Aufnahme des Herzens durch Reserpin und die Wirkung von Tyramin. Naunyn-Schmiedeberg's Arch. exp. Path. Pharmak. **240**, 234—241 (1960).
— Effect of cocaine and related drugs on the uptake of noradrenaline by heart and spleen. Brit. J. Pharmacol. **16**, 352—359 (1961).
Nagatsu, T., Rust, L.A., DeQuattro, V.: The activity of tyrosine hydroxylase and related enzymes of catecholamine biosynthesis and metabolism in dog kidney — effects of denervation. Biochem. Pharmacol. **18**, 1441—1446 (1969).

Nickerson, M.: The pharmacology of adrenergic blockade. Pharmacol. Rev. **1**, 27—101 (1949).

Pletscher, A., Brossi, A., Gey, K.F.: Benzoquinolizine derivatives, a new class of monoamine decreasing drugs with psychotropic action. Int. Rev. Neurobiol. **6**, 275—306 (1962).

— Gey, K.F., Zeller, P.: Monoaminoxydase-Hemmer. In: E. Jucker: Fortschr. Arzneimittelforsch. **2**, 417—590 (1960).

Pluchino, S.: α- and β-effects of isoproterenol (ISO) on the cat's nictitating membrane. Pharmacologist **9**, 248 (1967).

— Trendelenburg, U.: The influence of denervation and of decentralization on the alpha and beta effects of isoproterenol on the nictitating membrane of the pithed cat. J. Pharmacol. exp. Ther. **163**, 257—265 (1968).

Porter, C.C., Totaro, J.A., Burcin, A.: The relationship between radioactivity and norepinephrine concentrations in the brains and hearts of mice following administration of labeled methyldopa or 6-hydroxydopamine. J. Pharmacol. exp. Ther. **150**, 17—22 (1965).

— — Stone, C.A.: Effect of 6-hydroxydopamine and some other compounds on the concentration of norepinephrine in the hearts of mice. J. Pharmacol. exp. Ther. **140**, 308—316 (1963).

Potter, L.T., Cooper, T., Willman, V.L., Wolfe, D.E.: Synthesis, binding, release, and metabolism of norepinephrine in normal and transplanted dog hearts. Circulat. Res. **16**, 468—481 (1965).

Powell, C.E., Slater, I.H.: Blocking of inhibitory adrenergic receptors by a dichloro analog of isoproterenol. J. Pharmacol. exp. Ther. **122**, 480—488 (1958).

Quilliam, J.P., Tamarin, D.L.: Ultrastructural changes in the superior cervical ganglion of the rat following preganglionic denervation. J. Physiol. (Lond.) **189**, 13P—15P (1967).

Raab, W., Gigee, W.: Die Katecholamine des Herzens. Naunyn-Schmiedeberg's Arch. exp. Path. Pharmak. **219**, 248—262 (1953).

— — Specific avidity of heart muscle to absorb and store epinephrine and norepinephrine. Circulat. Res. **3**, 553—558 (1955).

— Humphreys, R.J.: Drug action upon myocardial epinephrine-sympathin concentration and heart rate (nitroglycerine, papaverine, priscol, dibenamine-hydrochloride). J. Pharmacol. exp. Ther. **89**, 64—76 (1947).

Rehn, N.O.: Effect of decentralisation on the content of catechol amines in the spleen and kidney of the cat. Acta physiol. scand. **42**, 309—312 (1958).

Richardson, K.C.: The fine structure of the albino rabbit iris with special reference to the identification of adrenergic and cholinergic nerves and nerve endings in its intrinsic muscles. Amer. J. Anat. **114**, 173—184 (1964).

Sabatini, M.T., DeIraldi, A.P., de Robertis, E.: Early effects of antiserum against the nerve growth factor on fine structure of sympathetic neurons. J. exp. Neurol. **12**, 370—383 (1965).

Salvi, M.L., Angeletti, P.U., Frati, L.: Frazionamento delle proteine solubili della ghiandola sottomascellare del topo: localizzazione di alcune componenti biologicamente attive. Il Farmaco **20**, 12—21 (1965).

Saner, A., Thoenen, H.: Model experiments on the molecular mechanism of action of 6-hydroxydopamine. Molec. Pharmacol. **7**, 147—154 (1971).

Sawyer, M.E., Mac, K., Schlossberg, T.: Studies of homeostasis in normal, sympathectomized and ergotaminized animals. Amer. J. Physiol. **104**, 172—203 (1933).

Schenkein, I., Bueker, E.D.: Dialyzable cofactor in nerve growth promoting protein from mouse salivary glands. Science **137**, 433—434 (1962).

— — The nerve growth factor as two essential components. Ann. N.Y. Acad. Sci. **118**, 171—182 (1964).

Schmidt, J.L., Fleming, W.W.: Supersensitivity to barium in the denervated nictitating membrane of the spinal cat. Proc. Soc. exp. Biol. (N.Y.) **117**, 302—303 (1964).

Sears, M.L., Bárány, E.H.: Outflow resistance and adrenergic mechanisms. Arch. Ophthal. **64**, 839—848 (1960).

— Gillis, C.N.: Mydriasis and the increase in outflow of the aqueous humor from the rabbit eye after cervical ganglionectomy in relation to the release of norepinephrine from the iris. Biochem. Pharmacol. **16**, 777—782 (1967).

Sedvall, G.C., Kopin, I.J.: Influence of sympathetic denervation and nerve impulse activity of tyrosine hydroxylase in the rat submaxillary gland. Biochem. Pharmacol. **16**, 39—46 (1967).

Senoh, S., Creveling, C.R., Udenfriend, S., Witkop, B.: Chemical, enzymatic and metabolic studies on the mechanism of oxydation of dopamine. J. Amer. chem. Soc. **81**, 6236 to 6240 (1959a).

SENOH, S., WITKOP, B.: Non-enzymatic conversions of dopamine to norepinephrine and trihydroxyphenethylamines. J. Amer. chem. Soc. **81**, 6222—6231 (1959).

— — CREVELING, C.R., UDENFRIEND, S.: 2,4,5-Trihydroxyphenethylamine, a new metabolite of 3,4-dihydroxyphenethylamine. J. Amer. chem. Soc. **81**, 1768—1769 (1959).

SIDMAN, R.L., PERKINS, M., WEINER, N.: Noradrenaline and adrenaline content of adipose tissue. Nature (Lond.) **193**, 36—37 (1962).

SJÖQVIST, F., TAYLOR, P.W., JR., TITUS, E.: The effect of immunosympathectomy on the retention and metabolism of noradrenaline. Acta physiol. scand. **69**, 13—22 (1967).

— TITUS, E., MICHAELSON, I.A., TAYLOR, JR., P.W., RICHARDSON, K.C.: Uptake and metabolism of d, l-norepinephrine-7-H^3 in tissues of immunosympathectomized mice and rats. Life Sci. **4**, 1125—1133 (1965).

SJÖSTRAND, N.O.: The adrenergic innervation of the vas deferens and the accessory male genital glands. Acta physiol. scand. **65**, Suppl. 257, 1—82 (1965).

SMITH, C.B.: Relaxation of the nictitating membrane of the spinal cat by sympathomimetic amines. J. Pharmacol. exp. Ther. **142**, 163—170 (1963).

— TRENDELENBURG, U., LANGER, S.Z., TSAI, T.H.: The relation of retention of norepinephrine-H^3 to the norepinephrine content of the nictitating membrane of the spinal cat during development of denervation supersensitivity. J. Pharmacol. exp. Ther. **151**, 87—94 (1966).

SNIPES, R.L., THOENEN, H., TRANZER, J.P.: Fine structural localization of exogenous 5-HT in vesicles of adrenergic nerve terminals. Experientia (Basel) **24**, 1026—1027 (1968).

SNYDER, S.H., AXELROD, J., WURTMAN, R.J., FISCHER, J.E.: Control of 5-hydroxytryptophan decarboxylase activity in the rat pineal gland by sympathetic nerves. J. Pharmacol. exp. Ther. **147**, 371—375 (1965a).

— FISCHER, J., AXELROD, J.: Evidence for the presence of monoamine oxidase in sympathetic nerve endings. Biochem. Pharmacol. **14**, 363—365 (1965b).

SOURKES, T.L.: Inhibition of dihydroxyphenylalanine decarboxylase by derivatives of phenylalanine. Arch. Biochem. **51**, 444—456 (1954).

STERN, D.N., MALING, H.M., ALTLAND, P.D., BRODIE, B.B.: Exhaustion and metabolic changes during exercise in adrenalectomized and chemically sympathectomized rats. Pharmacologist **6**, 185 (1964).

STONE, C.A., PORTER, C.C., STAVORSKI, J.M., LUDDEN, C.T., TOTARO, J.A.: Antagonism of certain effects of catecholamine-depleting agents by antidepressant and related drugs. J. Pharmacol. exp. Ther. **144**, 196—204 (1964).

— STAVORSKI, J.M., LUDDEN, C.T., WENGER, H.C., ROSS, C.A., TOTARO, J.A., PORTER, C.C.: Comparison of some pharmacologic effects of certain 6-substituted dopamine derivatives with reserpine, guanethidine and metaraminol. J. Pharmacol. exp. Ther. **142**, 147—156 (1963).

STRÖMBLAD, B.C.R.: Supersensitivity and amine oxidase activity in denervated salivary glands. Acta physiol. scand. **36**, 137—153 (1956).

— NICKERSON, M.: Accumulation of epinephrine and norepinephrine by some rat tissues. J. Pharmacol. exp. Ther. **134**, 154—159 (1961).

THOENEN, H., HAEFELY, W., GEY, K.F., HÜRLIMANN, A.: Die Wirkung der Vorbehandlung mit 5-Hydroxy-DOPA auf die postganglionäre sympathische Transmission der Katze. Naunyn-Schmiedeberg's Arch. Pharmak. exp. Path. **257**, 342—343 (1967a).

— — — — Diminished effect of sympathetic nerve stimulation in cats pretreated with 5-hydroxydopa; formation and liberation of false adrenergic transmitters. Naunyn-Schmiedeberg's Arch. Pharmak. exp. Path. **259**, 17—33 (1967b).

— HUERLIMANN, A., HAEFELY, W.: Mode of action of imipramine and 5-(3'methylaminopropyliden)-dibenzo[a,e]cyclohepta[1,3,5]trien hydrochloride (Ro 4—6011), a new antidepressant drug, on peripheral adrenergic mechanisms. J. Pharmacol. exp. Ther. **144**, 405—414 (1964).

— — — Mechanism of amphetamine accumulation in the isolated perfused heart of the rat. J. Pharm. Pharmacol. **20**, 1—11 (1968).

— TRANZER, J.P.: Chemical sympathectomy by selective destruction of adrenergic nerve endings with 6-hydroxydopamine. Naunyn-Schmiedeberg's Arch. Pharmak. exp. Path. **261**, 271—288 (1968).

— — HAEUSLER, G.: Chemical sympathectomy with 6-hydroxydopamine. In: New aspects of storage and release mechanisms of catecholamines. Berlin-Heidelberg-New York: Springer 1970.

THOMPSON, J.H., CAMPBELL, L.B.: Bowel 5-hydroxytryptamine in the immunosympathectomised mouse. J. Pharm. Pharmacol. **18**, 753—755 (1966).

TRANZER, J.P., THOENEN, H.: Ultramorphologische Veränderungen der sympathischen Nervenendigungen der Katze nach Vorbehandlung mit 5- und 6-Hydroxy-Dopamin. Naunyn-Schmiedeberg's Arch. Pharmak. exp. Path. **257**, 343—344 (1967a).

— — Electronmicroscopic localization of 5-hydroxydopamine (3,4,5-trihydroxy-phenylethylamine), a new 'false' sympathetic transmitter. Experientia (Basel) **23**, 743—745 (1967b).

— — Significance of 'empty vesicles' in postganglionic sympathetic nerve terminals. Experientia (Basel) **23**, 123—124 (1967c).

— — An electron microscopic study of selective, acute degeneration of sympathetic nerve terminals after administration of 6-hydroxydopamine. Experientia (Basel) **24**, 155—156 (1968a).

— — Various types of amine-storing vesicles in peripheral adrenergic nerve terminal. Experientia (Basel) **24**, 484—486 (1968b).

— — SNIPES, R.L., RICHARDS, J.G.: Recent developments on the ultrastructural aspect of adrenergic nerve endings in various experimental conditions. Progr. Brain Res. **31**, 33—46 (1969).

TRENDELENBURG, U.: The supersensitivity caused by cocaine. J. Pharmacol. exp. Ther. **125**, 55—63 (1959).

— Time course of changes in sensitivity after denervation of the nictitating membrane of the spinal cat. J. Pharmacol. exp. Ther. **142**, 335—342 (1963a).

— Supersensitivity and subsensitivity to sympathomimetic amines. Pharmacol. Rev. **15**, 225—276 (1963b).

— DRASKÓCZY, P.R., PLUCHINO, S.: The density of adrenergic innervation of the cats nictitating membrane as a factor influencing the sensitivity of the isolated preparation to l-norepinephrine. J. Pharmacol. exp. Ther. **166**, 14—25 (1969).

— MUSKUS, A., FLEMING, W.W., GOMEZ ALONSO DE LA SIERRA, B.: Effect of cocaine, denervation and decentralization on the response of the nictitating membrane to various sympathomimetic amines. J. Pharmacol. exp. Ther. **138**, 181—193 (1962).

— WEINER, N.: Sensitivity of the nictitating membrane after various procedures and agents. J. Pharmacol. exp. Ther. **136**, 152—161 (1962).

TSAI, T.H., DENHAM, S., MCGRATH, W.R.: Sensitivity of the isolated nictitating membrane of the cat to norepinephrine and acetylcholine after various procedures and agents. J. Pharmacol. exp. Ther. **164**, 146—157 (1968).

UDENFRIEND, S., ZALTZMAN-NIRENBERG, P., NAGATSU, T.: Inhibitors of purified beef adrenal tyrosine hydroxylase. Biochem. Pharmacol. **14**, 837—845 (1965).

UNGERSTEDT, U.: 6-Hydroxydopamine induced degeneration of central monoamine neurons. Europ. J. Pharmacol. **5**, 107—110 (1968).

URETSKY, N.J., IVERSEN, L.L.: Effects of 6-hydroxydopamine on noradrenaline-containing neurones in the rat brain. Nature (Lond.) **221**, 557—559 (1969).

— — Effects of 6-hydroxydopamine on catecholamine containing neurones in the rat brain. J. Neurochem. **17**, 269—278 (1970).

VAN ORDEN, L.S., III, BENSCH, K.G., LANGER, S.Z., TRENDELENBURG, U.: Histochemical and fine structural aspects of the onset of denervation supersensitivity in the nictitating membrane of the spinal cat. J. Pharmacol. exp. Ther. **157**, 274—283 (1967).

— BLOOM, F.E., BARRNETT, R.J., GIARMAN, N.J.: Histochemical and functional relationships of catecholamines in adrenergic nerve endings: I. Participation of granular vesicles. J. Pharmacol. exp. Ther. **154**, 185—199 (1966).

VARON, S., NOMURA, J., SHOOTER, E.M.: Subunit structure of a high-molecular-weight form of the nerve growth factor from mouse submaxillary gland. Proc. nat. Acad. Sci. (Wash.) **57**, 1782—1789 (1967a).

— — — The isolation of the mouse nerve growth factor protein in a high molecular weight form. Biochemistry **6**, 2202—2209 (1967b).

VOGT, M.: Sources of noradrenaline in the 'immunosympathectomized' rat. Nature (Lond.) **204**, 1315—1316 (1964).

— Release of medullary amines from the isolated perfused adrenal gland of the dog. Brit. J. Pharmacol. **24**, 561—565 (1965).

WALTMAN, S., SEARS, M.: Catechol-O-methyl transferase and monoamine oxidase activity in the ocular tissues of albino rabbits. Invest. Ophthal. **3**, 601—605 (1964).

WEGMANN, A., CHIBA, C., CHRYSOHOU, A., BING, J.R.: Catecholamines in homologous heart grafts. Proc. Soc. exp. Biol. (N.Y.) **109**, 543—545 (1962).

WEINER, N., LANGER, S.Z., TRENDELENBURG, U.: Demonstration by the histochemical fluorescence method of the prolonged disappearance of catecholamines from the denervated nictitating membrane of the cat. J. Pharmacol. exp. Ther. **157**, 284—289 (1967).

WHITBY, L.G., AXELROD, J., WEIL-MALHERBE, H.: The fate of H^3-norepinephrine in animals. J. Pharmacol. exp. Ther. **132**, 193—201 (1961).
WOLFE, D.E., POTTER, L.T., RICHARDSON, K.C., AXELROD, J.: Localizing tritiated norepinephrine in sympathetic axons by electon microscopic autoradiography. Science **138**, 440—442 (1962).
WOLINSKY, H., GLAGOV, S.: Nature and species differences in the medial distribution of aortic vasa vasorum in mammals. Circulat. Res. **20**, 409—421 (1967).
WURTMAN, R.J., KOPIN, I.J., HORST, D., FISCHER, J.E.: Epinephrine and organ blood flow: effects of hyperthyroidism, cocaine, and sympathetic denervation. Amer. J. Physiol. **207**, 1247—1250 (1964).
— SHEIN, H.M., AXELROD, J., LAREN, F.: Incorporation of ^{14}C-tryptophan into ^{14}C-protein by cultured rat pineals: Stimulation by l-norepinephrine. Proc. nat. Acad. Sci. (Wash.) **62**, 749—755 (1969).
ZAIMIS, E.: The immunosympathectomized animal: a valuable tool in physiological and pharmacological research. J. Physiol. (Lond.) **177**, 35P—37P (1965).
— BERK, L., CALLINGHAM, B.: Morphological, biochemical, and functional changes in the sympathetic nervous system of rats treated with nerve growth factor-antiserum. Nature (Lond.) **206**, 1220—1222 (1965).
ZELLER, E.A.: Amine oxidase inhibitors. Ann. N.Y. Acad. Sci. **80**, 551—1045 (1959).

Chapter 19

Catecholamine Synthesis and Metabolism in Man: Clinical Implications (With Special Reference to Parkinsonism)

MERTON SANDLER

With 9 Figures

I. Introduction

The accompanying chapters in this volume attest to the growth and complexity of catecholamine studies in recent years and provide some pointer to the correspondingly large literature associated with this field of research. Running parallel to these fundamental contributions and associated with what is probably an even larger number of publications, is that area of "applied" catecholamine study dealing with the clinical implications of this knowledge (FRANZEN and EYSELL, 1969). Thus there has been vast research effort concerning the role of monoamines in psychiatric disease, particularly in the pathogenesis of depressive illness (e. g. COLE and WITTENBORN, 1966) and of schizophrenia (e.g. SMYTHIES, 1963) and the drugs which have been used to treat them (e. g. CLARK and DEL GIUDICE, 1970); the tumours secreting catecholamines, phaeochromocytoma and neuroblastoma-ganglioneuroma, have provided much information on amine disposition (e. g. SANDLER and RUTHVEN, 1972); the genetically determined diseases such as familial dysautonomia (e. g. GITLOW et al., 1970), phenylketonuria (e. g. LYMAN, 1963) and tyrosinosis (e. g. GJESSING, 1966) have overtones relating to catecholamine metabolism as does the study of such disparate clinical problems as essential hypertension (e. g. MENDLOWITZ et al., 1970) and morphine addiction (e. g. GUNNE, 1963). Above all, it is in the study of Parkinson's disease (CALNE, 1970; BARBEAU and MCDOWELL, 1970) that "biochemical investment" has yielded the most handsome "clinical dividend" (UDENFRIEND, 1969). To attempt to evaluate each of these topics exhaustively would occupy considerably more space than is available to the writer in this volume. It has therefore seemed most valuable to tackle in depth a single topic, parkinsonism, and its relationship to the major and minor pathways of catecholamine biosynthesis and metabolism, whilst not omitting to point out, where relevant, the implications of this knowledge in the study of other disorders of monoamine metabolism.

Over the ten-year period 1957—1967, recognition of the central role of these pathways in the pathogenesis and therapy of parkinsonism gradually gathered way. There are a number of important milestones in the journey. BLASCHKO (1957) first suggested that dopamine might be rather more than a precursor of noradrenaline and that it might have some regulating functions of its own. Two years later CARLSSON (1959) proposed that it might, in its own right, act as a neurotransmitter in the central nervous system, a view which has been amply supported by subsequent evidence (see HORNYKIEWICZ, 1966). It is perhaps invidious to attempt to rank individual links in any chain of events but it must be recognised that without the penetrating observation of EHRINGER and HORNYKIEWICZ (1960) of a gross depletion of striatal dopamine in affected subjects, subsequent therapeutic developments would not have been possible. This finding led to a trial of L-DOPA, at first using relatively small dosage (BIRKMAYER and HORNYKIEWICZ, 1961; BARBEAU, 1961), with modest improvement and later by heavy, prolonged oral treatment (COTZIAS et al., 1967) with dramatic clinic benefit.

II. Parkinsonism

The disease bears the eponym of a London physician and reformer, James PARKINSON who published the definitive description of its clinical features (PARKINSON, 1817). The typical "pill-rolling" tremor, rigidity, mask-like facies, poverty of movement (hypokinesia) and characteristic posture and gait of the advanced case are easily recognised.

1. Anatomical Considerations

a) Man

Widespread degenerative changes are usually but not invariably present in the basal ganglia of the brain (STERN, 1966). PAKKENBERG and BRODY (1965) noted a reduction of neurones by 59% in the basal ganglia of parkinsonian patients compared with a control population. SABUNCU (1969) was unable to quantify the pallidal lesion however. The observations of HUBERT and VAN ROSSUM (1969) raise the interesting possibility that *formes frustes* of parkinsonism might exist: they described two depressed patients in whom neuropathological changes of idiopathic parkinsonism were demonstrated at autopsy who had failed to manifest clinically any of the stigmata of the disease with the possible exception of the depression itself, a common accompaniment of parkinsonism (MJÖNES, 1949). In retrospect, it might have been instructive to estimate homovanillic acid, the major metabolite of dopamine, in the cerebrospinal fluid of these patients. As will be discussed later (p. 859), there is a characteristic decrease in concentration of this compound in parkinsonian compared with normal subjects, presumably stemming from its impaired production; the distinction may be sharpened by the prior administration of probenecid (OLSSON and ROOS, 1968) which blocks the transport of the acid out of the nervous system. MENDELL et al. (1970) have noted a patient with L-DOPA-responsive progressive supranuclear palsy with low homovanillic acid in the cerebrospinal fluid which indicates that a proportion of affected subjects may be parkinsonian variants. In fact, it seems likely that many of the non-parkinsonian subjects who respond to L-DOPA, such as the retarded depressive patients of GOODWIN et al. (1970a, b) fall into a similar category and have a relative dopamine deficiency; and taking this particular group as an example, there appears to be a tendency for cerebrospinal fluid homovanillic acid concentration to be lower in depression (BOWERS et al., 1969). ROOS and SJÖSTROM (1969) were unable to detect any increase in homovanillic acid in the cerebrospinal fluid in some depressive subjects after the administration of probenecid.

b) Animal Models

It has been known for many years that placing a lesion in the tegmental area of the upper brain stem of monkeys results in various motor disturbances including hypokinesia, hypotonicity and postural tremor (WARD et al., 1948). Indeed similar parkinsonian signs have been observed in human patients with midbrain lesions (Kremer et al., 1947). Because Poirier (1960) was able to show that monkeys and cats with these tegmental lesions showed a substantial loss of dopamine-containing cells in the substantia nigra (Andén et al., 1964; Dahlström and Fuxe, 1964), the preparation in monkey, cat and rat has been regarded as a useful model for human parkinsonism and used extensively in the investigation of alterations in monoamine localization and metabolism (e. g. Poirier and Sourkes, 1965; Goldstein et al., 1966; Sourkes and Poirier, 1966; Goldstein et al., 1967; Poirier et al., 1967; Sharman et al., 1967; Faull and Laverty, 1969; Sourkes et al., 1969; Goldstein et al., 1970b; Lancaster et al., 1970). The fact that a second lesion in the ventrolateral thalamic area of the monkey immediately relieves the tremor (Battista et al., 1969), in a somewhat similar manner to the effect produced by the operation for human parkinsonism (Hassler and Riechert, 1954), appears to make the model even more apt. A correlative study of the implications of these recent neuroanatomical and neurochemical findings concerning the nigrostriatal pathway in the cat and monkey has recently been carried out (Bédard et al., 1969).

2. Aetiological Factors

a) Idiopathic

The commonest variant of parkinsonism is the idiopathic form ("paralysis agitans"). It results from degenerative changes in the basal ganglia and, characteristically, develops insidiously at about 50—60 years of age. The rare progressive degenerative disease of the central nervous system, parkinsonism dementia of Guam (Brody et al., 1970), is also of unknown aetiology.

b) Postencephalitic

An epidemic of encephalitis lethargica, presumably of viral origin, followed the First World War: fresh cases of this disease have apparently not been seen for about forty years. Signs of parkinsonism of a pattern somewhat different to the idiopathic form made their appearance in affected individuals at varying intervals after the acute infection. In this connexion, it is of interest that intracerebral inoculation of mice with *Herpes simplex* virus gives rise, prior to death, to a hyperactive state similar to that associated with high dosage of L-DOPA and indeed, at this time, the brains of affected animals contain a high concentration of homovanillic acid, indicative of an excessive production of dopamine (Lycke and Roos, 1968). Treatment with a tyrosine hydroxylase inhibitor prevents the homovanillic acid over-production, hyperactivity and death, which all supervene when the inhibitor is withdrawn (Lycke and Roos, 1969). To what extent this experimental situation has any relevance to postencephalitic parkinsonism cannot be established at present.

c) Arteriosclerotic

In this variant, which may sometimes be difficult to distinguish from idiopathic paralysis agitans, neuronal degeneration derives from vascular causes. The patients are characteristically elderly and, apart from their extrapyramidal disease, may have signs of diffuse cerebral disease such as dementia and pyramidal tract lesions.

d) Toxic

Manganese intoxication (Mena et al., 1967) is a well-known but uncommon cause of a parkinsonian syndrome. There is an associated decrease in brain dopamine (BERNHEIMER et al., 1969). This pattern can be mimicked in the monkey by administration of manganese compounds (e. g. NEFF et al., 1969).

Carbon monoxide poisoning may give rise to diffuse cerebral damage and produce a variety of neurological sequelae including extrapyramidal signs (GARLAND and PEARCE, 1967) although such an end-result appears to be rare (SMITH and BRANDON, 1970).

SANDLER et al. (1970a) have recently drawn attention to a possible association between alkaptonuria and parkinsonism and have suggested that the three patients involved may have been examples of a new syndrome, striatonigral ochronosis.

Parkinsonism is a well-documented side-effect of a variety of tranquilizing drugs (HAASE and JANSSEN, 1965) including reserpine, the phenothiazines and haloperidol. These effects may also be produced in the experimental animal e. g. by reserpine in the chimpanzee (MÜLLER-CALGAN and SOMMER, 1968). It is even possible for the drug to give rise to toxic effects in the foetus when administered to a pregnant subject — phenothiazines have provoked neonatal extrapyramidal signs (TAMER et al., 1969). It is of interest in this connexion that it might be relatively simple to provoke parkinsonism at this period of life for the concentration of dopamine in the brain is low in newborn infants although noradrenaline level is normal (EHRINGER and HORNYKIEWICZ, 1960).

3. Biochemical Considerations

The main pathway of catecholamine biosynthesis (Fig. 1) was first adumbrated by BLASCHKO (1939) in an elegant inductive exercise. Reasoning only from the properties of the then recently discovered (HOLTZ et al., 1938) enzyme, L-DOPA decarboxylase, he inferred that the metabolic route from L-tyrosine must travel via L-DOPA to a "non-N-methylated amine"; neither tyrosine nor N-methyldopa, a theoretical precursor of epinine (N-methyldopamine) are substrates for the enzyme. There was no evidence at that time pointing to the stage at which the hydroxyl group is introduced to the side-chain.

Our knowledge of catecholamine disposition stems from the seminal observations of ARMSTRONG and his colleagues (ARMSTRONG, MCMILLAN and SHAW, 1959) who identified 4-hydroxy-3-methoxymandelic acid, found in high concentration in the urine of patients with phaeochromocytoma, as the major metabolite of adrenaline and noradrenaline. This compound and many others derive from the competing and complementary actions of two enzymes COMT and MAO which both utilize the catecholamines as substrates (Fig. 2). These pathways form the subject of an exhaustive review (SANDLER and RUTHVEN, 1969).

The plan to be followed in the present chapter will be to consider, step by step, the main stages in these metabolic pathways in relation to their status in Parkinson's disease, which will be considered in depth as an example of the complex changes which may occur in human disease. These and other degradation routes will later be further discussed in the light of new knowledge arising from the L-DOPA therapy of parkinsonism and related topics.

a) Tyrosine Hydroxylase

The first and probably rate-limiting (UDENFRIEND, 1966) step in the biosynthetic pathway, tyrosine hydroxylase, was characterized quite recently (NAGATSU et al., 1964). Its Km is such that it is normally more or less saturated in relation to its substrate (PETERS et al., 1968) i. e. the plasma concentration is

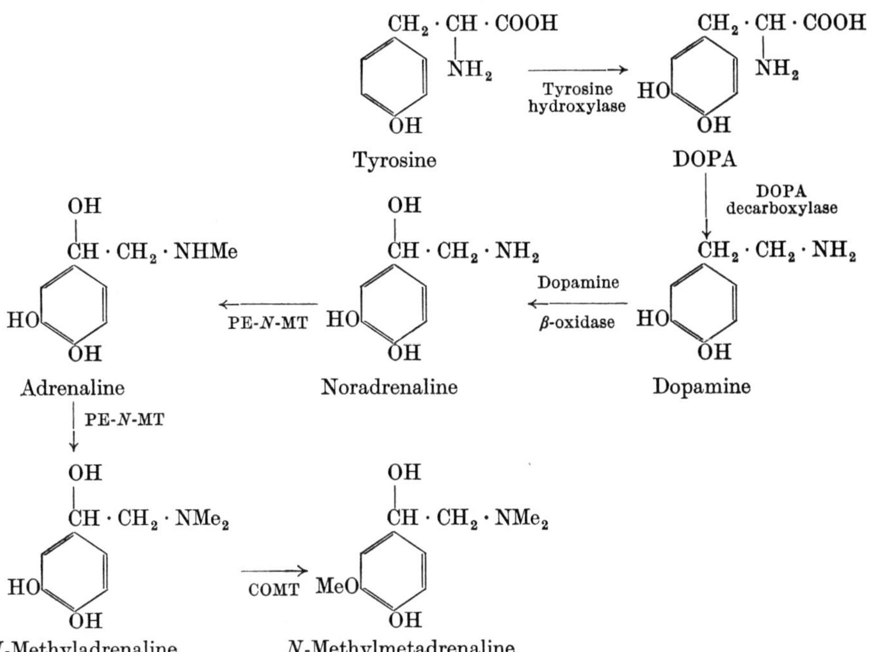

Fig. 1. Biosynthesis of the catecholamines (PE-N-MT = phenylethanolamine N-methyltransferase) (from SANDLER, M., Schweiz. med. Wschr., **100**, 526—531 [1970], Schwabe & Co., Basel)

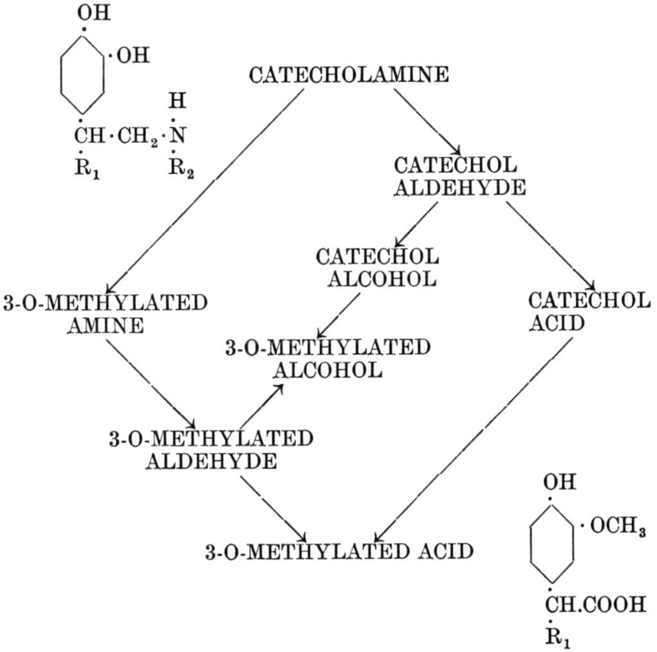

Fig. 2. General scheme of catecholamine metabolism: dopamine pathway —R_1 = H,R_2 = H; noradrenaline pathway — R_1 = OH, R_2 = H; adrenaline pathway — R_1 = OH, R_2 — Me. (from SANDLER, M., Schweiz. med. Wschr., **100**, 526—531 [1970], Schwabe & Co., Basel)

similar to the Km (UDENFRIEND, 1966). Thus the reaction cannot be driven and it probably follows that parkinsonism cannot be effectively treated by feeding an excess of L-tyrosine (CALNE and SANDLER, 1970). Nor therefore is treatment with the pteridine cofactor of the enzyme (KAUFMAN, 1966), as suggested by STOCK (1969) and KUEHL et al. (1969), with encouragement by COTZIAS (1969), likely to be of much therapeutic assistance.

Comparatively little attention has been paid to this enzyme in human parkinsonism although the animal model of the disease produced by a ventromedial tegmental lesion is characterized by a decreased ability of the striatum on the same side to convert tyrosine to DOPA (GOLDSTEIN et al., 1966). The suggestion has been made however (BRUCK et al., 1964; WATT, 1967; BRAHAM et al., 1969) that a defect of tyrosine hydroxylase might exist in Parkinson's disease although supporting evidence is scanty. If tyrosine transported into the cell prior to hydroxylation were to build up because of such a defect, its further metabolism might be diverted into more minor pathways. In their search for the identity of the notorious "pink spot" (FRIEDHOFF and VAN WINKLE, 1962), the putative causative agent (or its close relative) of schizophrenia, BOULTON and his colleagues (BOULTON et al., 1967) noted an increase in urinary free tyramine output in parkinsonian patients, a finding confirmed by SMITH and KELLOW (1969). An excess of tryptamine has also been claimed (KUEHL et al., 1968). Such evidence of increased amine production might have prepared the ground for some explanation of the pathogenesis of parkinsonism based on the ability of tyramine to deplete dopamine stores: COLLINS and WEST (1968) noted an efflux of labelled dopamine from a gut preparation perfused with tyramine; BONHAM CARTER et al. (1970) detected an increase in urinary homovanillic acid, the major metabolite of dopamine, after intravenous injection of tyramine into human volunteers; GOLDSTEIN et al. (1970a) observed that unchanged ^{3}H-tyramine accumulates in the striatum of the experimental animal after intraventricular injection, perhaps displacing endogenous dopamine from its binding sites. Whilst monoamines are unlikely, even in the presence of a suitable concentration gradient from the blood stream, to cross the blood-brain barrier in appreciable concentration (WEIL-MALHERBE et al., 1959), such a conjectural explanation of the aetiology of parkinsonism might have envisaged a train of events occurring insidiously, over a period of many years. The normal human gut (LEVINE and SJOERDSMA, 1962), and supporting it the liver (DAVISON, 1958), appear to carry sufficient MAO to inactivate a large dietary excess of tyramine, assisted by a sulphate conjugation mechanism (SMITH et al., 1970). Even so, a heavy oral tyramine load results in an impressive overspill into the urine (HORWITZ et al., 1964), presumably from the blood stream. It is of interest that there is at least one clinical condition, tyramine-sensitive migraine (HANINGTON, 1967), characterized by a defect in tyramine conjugation (SMITH et al., 1971; YOUDIM et al., 1971) where evidence of a release of catecholamines from storage sites has been observed after oral tyramine challenge (SANDLER et al., 1970b). An explanation for migrainous headache has been invoked in terms of such catecholamine release (HANINGTON and HARPER, 1968) and indeed ENGELMAN et al. (1968) described one migrainous subject who obtained relief after the administration of α-methyl-tyrosine, which blocks tyrosine hydroxylation (UDENFRIEND et al., 1965) and hence catecholamine production. A meaningful association has yet to be observed between migraine and parkinsonism however.

A defect in MAO activity, presumably local, has been noted in the small intestinal mucosa of patients with malabsorption syndromes (CHALLACOMBE et al., 1971). Such clinical states appear to be characterized by stagnation of gut contents so that an excess of biologically active monoamines is likely to be produced by the action of gut flora on amino acid residues (HAVERBACK et al., 1960). Indeed, it would seem that a major proportion of urinary tyramine derives from this source (PERRY et al., 1966) although such a view is disputed by DE QUATTRO and SJOERDSMA (1967) who postulate a tissue origin.

Urinary tyramine output does in fact provide some index of *in vivo* MAO status (SJOERDSMA, 1961) and it thus seems possible that if an increase in parkinsonism can be proved, it represents some degree of enzyme deficit (SANDLER, 1970c). Although SANDLER et al. (1969b) obtained some preliminary data indicating that a decrease in blood platelet MAO is present in the postencephalitic disease, these results must be treated as tentative, for it was not possible to withdraw other antiparkinsonian drugs at the time of observation.

The tyrosine absorption data of BRAHAM et al. (1969) in parkinsonism, probably point to some degree of delayed intestinal absorption, although the findings of MONTPLAISIR and BARBEAU (1969) are not in full agreement. BONHAM CARTER et al. (1971) whilst providing further data in parkinsonian subjects compatible with some degree of malabsorption have not been able to confirm the original observation (BOULTON et al., 1967; SMITH and KELLOW, 1969) of an increase in urinary free tyramine. They did observe, however, that an oral tyramine load led to an increase in *conjugated* tyramine excretion, spread over a longer period of time. Whilst these data are difficult to interpret, especially in the absence of evidence about MAO status in parkinsonism, it seems possible that a compensatory increase in conjugation machinery might have taken place to deal with an amine excess produced by gut stagnation. What appears to be needed of course is not so much a knowledge of urinary concentrations which are a composite of many different factors but direct measurements of tyramine in human parkinsonian and control brains similar to those which have recently been carried out with success in rat brain (BOULTON et al., 1970).

If there is a *prima facie* case for a further clinical trial of α-methyl-tyrosine in migraine, the drug has proved its usefulness in the treatment of inoperable malignant phaeochromocytoma, to limit the vast over-production of catecholamines (e. g. SJOERDSMA et al., 1965; JONES et al., 1968). One such patient was of particular interest in the present context (JONES et al., 1968). Whilst the drug was able to contain the catecholamine over-production, a distressing complication supervened, the onset of a whole body tremor which necessitated withdrawing the treatment. It is probably relevant that BIRKMAYER (1969a) showed that α-methyl-tyrosine makes parkinsonian tremor worse. BÉDARD et al. (1970) were able to produce a tremor in experimental animals by treating them with α-methyl-tyrosine, an effect which they could neutralize by L-DOPA administration.

Apart from competitively inhibiting tyrosine hydroxylase, α-methyl-tyrosine also inhibits tyrosine transaminase (SPECTOR et al., 1965) although the mechanism is not as obvious. Reserpine similarly inhibits cerebral tyrosine transaminase and it seems plausible that such a decrease in activity derives from a low concentration of amine (GIBB and WEBB, 1969). The catecholamines, and DOPA, appear to increase tyrosine transaminase activity, at least in rat liver (BARTHOLINI et al., 1970a), an observation which will be seen, later in this essay, to have certain implications for the DOPA treatment of parkinsonism (p. 876). This enzyme has a very high Km - approx. 3.0×10^{-3} (WURTMAN and LARIN, 1968; GEORGE and GABAY, 1968). It is thus capable of transaminating tyrosine at a rate about one hundred times greater than that at which tyrosine is hydroxylated to dopa. It seems likely that tyrosine transaminase acts as a shunt mechanism for available tyrosine, so regulating catecholamine production (GIBB and WEBB, 1969).

b) DOPA

Sixty years ago FUNK (1911) devised the first synthesis of DOPA which was identified in high concentration from biological sources 2 years later, in the broad bean, *Vicia faba* (GUGGENHEIM, 1913; TORQUATI, 1913); about 25 g of L-DOPA may be extracted from a kilogram of beans (SEALOCK, 1949). DOPA has also been found in a number of other plants (e. g. FENG et al., 1961; ANDREWS and PRIDHAM, 1967) and also in fungi (SIH et al., 1969).

In the animal kingdom, MEDES (1932) detected the amino-acid in the urine of a patient with a unique disease pattern which she termed tyrosinosis. DOPA was first identified from "normal" animal sources in the adrenal gland of the thyroidectomized sheep (GOODALL, 1950). It is of interest therefore that ARAKAWA et al. (1963) have detected it in appreciable concentration in the urine of a new-born infant with hyperpigmentation whose mother was being treated with antithyroid drugs. Perhaps the effect of thyroid hormones on the enzymes of DOPA synthesis or disposition is worthy of further study.

Another unexplained syndrome associated with excess urinary DOPA excretion was recorded in two undersized boys who presented with hirsuties and a large appetite (COPPS et al., 1963).

DOPA has been detected in increased amounts in the urine of patients with certain tumours including melanoma (SCOTT, 1962), malignant phaeochromocytoma (ANTON et al., 1967), neuroblastoma (VON STUDNITZ, 1960) and the related ganglioneuroma (SMELLIE and SANDLER, 1961; GJESSING, 1968). The L-DOPA utilized in the brain for catecholamine biosynthesis is presumably elaborated *in situ*, although transport mechanisms have been described (YOSHIDA et al., 1963) which are likely to assume importance during the L-DOPA treatment of parkinsonism. SHAH et al. (1968) have pointed out that other amino acids such as tryptophan and methionine are likely to compete with L-DOPA for uptake.

c) L-DOPA Decarboxylase

As noted earlier, our knowledge of the major catecholamine biosynthetic pathway was conjointly made possible by the identification of L-DOPA decarboxylase *in vitro* by HOLTZ et al. (1938) together with other important observations on its properties by BLASCHKO (1939). This information was soon consolidated *in vivo* when intravenous DOPA in man was shown to give rise to large amounts of urinary dopamine (HOLTZ et al., 1942a). It is a matter for conjecture whether BLASCHKO's pathway would have received such ready acceptance had it been appreciated at the time that another of the theoretical precursors of noradrenaline, *threo*-dihydroxyphenylserine, is a substrate of the enzyme (BLASCHKO et al., 1950; WERLE and SELL, 1955) albeit a poorer one than DOPA. This amino acid is decarboxylated directly to noradrenaline (BLASCHKO et al., 1950)

$$(HO)_2C_6H_3\text{—}CH(OH)CH(NH_2)\text{—}COOH \rightarrow (HO)_2C_6H_3\text{—}CH(OH)CH_2NH_2$$

Fig. 3. Decarboxylation of dihydroxyphenylserine to form noradrenaline

(Fig. 3) without the intermediate formation of dopamine. *In vivo*, it gives rise to an increase in urinary noradrenaline both in the experimental animal (SCHMITERLÖW, 1951) and in man (GUNNE and LIDVALL, 1966). This alternative pathway was first put forward by ROSENMUND and DORNSAFT (1919); experimental proof for its existence could not be obtained in a carefully designed *in vitro* investigation by KIRSHNER (1957). Nor could dihydroxyphenylserine be found in phaeochromocytoma tumour tissue after thorough search (GELINAS et al., 1959). Thus the route has tended to be discounted in recent years. The fact that L-DOPA administration in the experimental animal, whilst provoking a large increase in brain dopamine, fails to affect the concentration of noradrenaline significantly (BARTHOLINI and PLETSCHER, 1968; BUTCHER and ENGEL, 1969; EVERETT and BORCHERDING, 1970) and that a noradrenaline buildup is not merely prevented by dopamine occupying its binding sites (BUTCHER et al., 1970) should alert us to the possibility of some other biosynthetic route to noradrenaline operating, perhaps even that from dihydroxylphenylserine, which is as good a substrate for L-DOPA decarboxylase as another amino acid with an undisputed *in vivo* role, L-5-HTP.

After much early doubt, the enzymes which decarboxylate L-5-HTP and L-DOPA in the mammal are now known to be identical (LOVENBERG et al., 1962). L-DOPA decarboxylase is widespread in animal tissues where activity tends to decrease with age (GEY et al., 1965). Activity has been detected in insects (SEKERIS and KARLSON, 1966) and bacteria (BLASCHKO, 1950) although these enzymes differ in certain physicochemical characteristics. Why particularly high concentrations are present in mammalian liver and kidney, without possessing any apparent function, is a finding as puzzling today as it was to BLASCHKO (1959) 13 years ago.

With the rise of interest in parkinsonism in recent years, the enzyme is once more being studied intensively after a relative decline in interest. Thus CHRISTENSON et al. (1970) have achieved a preparation from hog kidney of high purity. COULSON et al. (1969) have been able to demonstrate a number of different isoenzymes; an enzyme variant in kidney possesses a pH optimum of 7.5 rather than the more usual value of about 9 (CRAWFORD and BURKHALTER, 1970). One interpretation of the rather complex data of POIRIER et al. (1968) which concern the differential *in vivo* effect of harmaline on DOPA and 5-HTP decarboxylation in the experimental animal would be in terms of differing inhibition of more than one isoenzyme. Although differences in the substrate specificity of the isoenzymes have yet to be demonstrated, it would seem sensible to search for them in decarboxylase-containing tissues specialized for the production of a particular amine. Thus the decarboxylase of carcinoid tumor tissue (LANGEMANN, 1956; LANGEMANN et al., 1962), which is responsible for the production of relatively large amounts of 5-hydroxytryptamine (for reviews see KÄHLER and HEILMEYER, 1961; STACEY, 1966; SANDLER, 1968) may be well worth comparing with that (LANGEMANN et al., 1962) in catecholamine-secreting (for reviews see GJESSING, 1968; SANDLER and RUTHVEN, 1972) tumours. With this line of argument, it might be expected that striatal decarboxylase consists of, or includes, an isoenzyme with high specificity for L-DOPA. Because of certain difficulties inherent in the nature of the enzyme, however, testing this hypothesis as far as human striatal decarboxylase is concerned is not likely to prove an easy experiment.

Some interesting information has lately emerged about the properties of the human enzyme. Human tissues tend to have lower activity than other species (VOGEL et al., 1970a). VOGEL et al. (1970b) have recently carried out a careful reinvestigation of the characteristics of human liver decarboxylase. Whilst they were able to confirm an earlier observation (HARTMAN et al., 1955; FELLMAN, 1956; DAVISON and SANDLER, 1958) that enzyme activity is inhibited by phenylpyruvic acid they also showed that there is great individual variation in sensitivity to it. Whether this finding indicates the presence of pharmacogenetic variations in the multiple enzyme forms is an open question. The concentrations of phenylpyruvic acid which may sometimes be inhibitory are of the same order as those present in phenylketonuria where decreased plasma levels of catecholamines (WEIL-MALHERBE, 1955) and 5-hydroxytryptamine (PARE et al., 1957) and, in fact, of *in vivo* decarboxylase activity (PARE et al., 1958) are observed; it is tempting to suggest that the individual variation in sensitivity of L-DOPA decarboxylase to phenylpyruvic acid may provide the basis of an explanation for the wide variation in intelligence noted in affected children (PARE et al., 1959; KNOX, 1966) for which there has not so far been any convincing explanation.

The status of human brain DOPA decarboxylase has been controversial. BERNHEIMER and HORNYKIEWICZ (1962) were able to detect the presence of low concentrations but failed to note any difference between normal and parkinsonian brains. A succession of workers then attempted to estimate the enzyme in human brain specimens obtained at autopsy (LANGEMANN and ACKERMANN, 1961; ROBINS et al., 1967; METZEL et al., 1969; VOGEL et al., 1969, 1970a) but were unable to detect more than trace activity. It was thus suggested (ROBINS et al., 1967) that decarboxylation rather than tyrosine hydroxylation might be the rate-limiting step in the human brain. METZEL et al. (1969) did claim to find activity in biopsy samples of brain however with some decrease in material from parkinsonian patients compared with that from control subjects with unrelated neurological conditions. Very recently LLOYD and HORNYKIEWICZ (1970a) appear to have overcome the technical difficulties involved in the assay and have confirmed (LLOYD and HORNYKIEWICZ, 1970b; HORNYKIEWICZ, 1970b) that there is a decrease in striatal decarboxylase activity in parkinsonism. With such modified technique, it might be instructive to measure brain L-DOPA decarboxylase in human essential hypertension. YAMORI et al. (1970) demonstrated low activity, together with decreased noradrenaline concentration in the lower brain stem and hypothalamus of genetically hypertensive rats.

d) Dopamine

Dopamine, which was first synthesized by BARGER and DALE (1910), is widely distributed in nature as reviewed by WELSH (p. 79), and by HOLZBAUER and SHARMAN (p. 110).

Over the past decade evidence has gradually mounted confirming the concept of an independent role for dopamine (BLASCHKO, 1957) in animal physiology. There are sound theoretical reasons for believing that separate receptors for dopamine and noradrenaline exist (KIER and TRUITT, 1970). In fact, good evidence for the former has been obtained, at least in the mammalian kidney (McNAY et al., 1965). These receptors are selectively blocked by drugs such as haloperidol (VAN ROSSUM, 1966; YEH et al., 1969) and chlorpromazine (GOLDBERG and YEH, 1969) which are widely employed in clinical practice and possess a profound central action. Indeed, it is precisely from indirect evidence concerning the action of this type of drug (e. g. UNGERSTEDT et al., 1969; ANDÉN et al., 1970a; SNYDER et al., 1970) that the present concept of central dopamine receptors arises. Such receptors may also be stimulated by other compounds such as dexamphetamine (COOLS and VAN ROSSUM, 1970) and by apomorphine (ERNST, 1965, 1969; BUTCHER et al., 1969; ANDÉN et al., 1967, 1970a; FEKETE and KURTI, 1970). Apomorphine will be discussed again in relation to the therapy of parkinsonism (p. 863). Blocking central dopamine receptors with bulbocapnine (ERNST, 1969; TSENG and WALASZEK, 1970) produces an extreme Parkinson-like catatonic response in the experimental animal. The phenothiazines and drugs with similar action are also well-known to produce parkinsonian side-effects (BERNHEIMER and HORNYKIEWICZ,

1965a; HORNYKIEWICZ, 1966); by blocking the dopamine receptor in the experimental animal they appear to provoke an increase in dopamine turnover (e. g. ANDÉN et al., 1964b; LAVERTY and SHARMAN, 1965; O'KEEFE et al., 1970) as a consequence of release from feedback inhibition (DA PRADA and PLETSCHER, 1966). They appear to have a similar action in man, giving rise to an increased homovanillic acid output (BOZZI et al., 1965). Conversely, stimulating the dopamine receptor with apomorphine decreases dopamine turnover in the animal brain (ROOS, 1969).

In contrast with the parkinsonian syndrome produced by drugs such as haloperidol, other forms of the disease are probably characterized by a decreased dopamine turnover, a report to the contrary by BARBEAU and TROMBITAS (1969) notwithstanding; the climate of opinion is that these changes derive from damage to the cells in which the synthesis is carried out rather than from a specific defect in the actual biosynthetic pathway of dopamine production (VOGT, 1970). Nevertheless, there is some puzzling evidence concerning parkinsonism as a systemic disease (BARBEAU, 1969a, b) which is difficult to fit into the procrustean frame of such a cell damage hypothesis. BARBEAU et al. (1961, 1962) noted a decreased urinary dopamine output in affected subjects, an observation which has since, with one opposing voice (SMITH and KELLOW, 1969) been confirmed (BISCHOFF and TORRES, 1962; WEIL-MALHERBE and VAN BUREN, 1969). Although ŠIMEK (1968) believed the contrary, there does not appear to be any significant decrease in output of homovanillic acid (GREER and WILLIAMS, 1963; CALNE et al., 1969a) or of other acidic or alcoholic catecholamine metabolites (CALNE et al., 1969a) in parkinsonian compared with normal subjects. A rise in dopamine output after thalamotomy (WESTLAKE and TEW, 1966) has been disputed (SCHNIEDEN and WILLIAMS, 1970).

A reduction in urinary dopamine is not specific to parkinsonism. WEIL-MALHERBE and VAN BUREN (1969) drew attention to the possibility of this phenomenon being an effect of chronic drug treatment but this interpretation cannot account for an increased output recorded in mania which returns to normal during lithium treatment (MESSIHA et al., 1970). WEIL-MALHERBE and VAN BUREN (1969) noted an even greater reduction in dopamine output when their patients were on a milk diet. Such a diet is probably alkaline, however, and SANDLER et al. (1967) have shown that free dopamine excretion, which probably occurs by a renal tubular mechanism (RENNICK, 1968), is highly dependent on urinary pH, being facilitated in an acid urine and retarded in an alkaline one. The studies of GOODALL and ALTON (1969) do not make the picture any clearer; these workers administered labelled dopamine to parkinsonian patients and noted a tendency to a diminished excretion of "noradrenaline series" metabolites and an increase of "dopamine series" metabolites, compared with control subjects. They had previously recorded a similar tendency in an earlier study on patients with orthostatic hypotension (GOODALL et al., 1968); it is of interest that patients with parkinsonism tend to have a low blood pressure which may therefore be the primary factor in the pathway shift noted by GOODALL and ALTON (1969). Indeed, patients with parkinsonism plus extreme postural hypotension and other features characteristic of autonomic deficit are sometimes observed, the so-called Shy-Drager syndrome (SHY and DRAGER, 1960).

It might even be possible to quantify the degree of pheripheral adrenergic system deficit in parkinsonism and allied disorders in the forseeable future for WEINSHILBOUM and AXELROD (1970) have recently developed what appears to be a sensitive assay procedure for dopamine β-hydroxylase in human and rat serum, although full details are not yet available. Evidence is mounting (see chapter 13 in this volume, by SMITH and WINKLER) to suggest that this enzyme is liberated together with transmitter noradrenaline and chromogranin, in a concentration directly related to the degree of nervous activity.

In the central nervous system, parkinsonism is characterised by a virtual absence of dopamine from the striatum (EHRINGER and HORNYKIEWICZ, 1960; BERNHEIMER et al., 1963, 1965; BERNHEIMER and HORNYKIEWICZ, 1964, 1965b, 1966) and substantia nigra (HORNYKIEWICZ, 1963) accompanied by a decreased concentration of homovanillic acid (BERNHEIMER, 1964; GOTTFRIES et al., 1969) in striatum, pallidum and substantia nigra (BERNHEIMER and HORNYKIEWICZ, 1964, 1965b). The ratio of dopamine to homovanillic acid is shifted, however, in favour of the latter, in the parkinsonian striatum so that the homovanillic acid deficiency is less severe than that of dopamine. It seems likely that striatal dopamine still remaining is being turned over faster than in normal brain, as a compensatory measure (HORNYKIEWICZ, 1970b).

Although the concentration of hypothalamic noradrenaline (EHRINGER and HORNYKIEWICZ, 1960; BERNHEIMER et al., 1963) and of brain 5-hydroxytryptamine (BERNHEIMER et al., 1961) are also decreased, the reduction is not of the same order of magnitude as that of dopamine. Moreover, whereas these values return to normal after MAO inhibition, striatal dopamine deficiency is uninfluenced (BERNHEIMER and HORNYKIEWICZ, 1963; BERNHEIMER et al., 1963). A particularly important patient was recorded by BAROLIN et al. (1964), who had hemiparkinsonism; striatal dopamine concentration was markedly reduced in one side of the brain only. It is probably relevant that lesions in the experimental animal leading to Parkinson-like morphological changes in the substantia nigra produce a fall in dopamine concentration in the side of the striatum to which they are connected (e. g. POIRIER and SOURKES, 1965; FAULL and LAVERTY, 1969).

Despite the suggestion (METZEL et al., 1969) that brain dopamine tends to disappear after death, the work of JOYCE (1962) in both experimental animals and man would appear to indicate that, provided the brain is left in the skull and removed just prior to chemical extraction and assay, the data so obtained are likely to be valid. The experience of other workers tends to confirm this view (PARE et al., 1969).

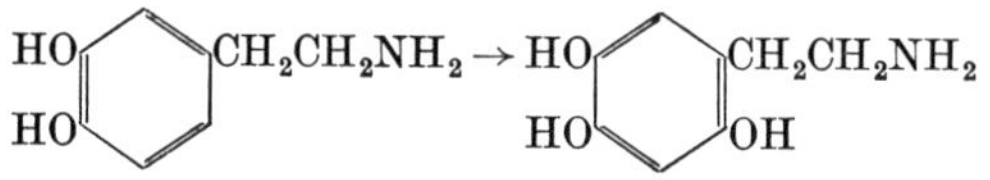

HO, HO C_6H_3 $CH_2CH_2NH_2$ → HO, HO, OH C_6H_2 $CH_2CH_2NH_2$

Fig. 4. Hydroxylation of dopamine to form 6-hydroxydopamine

What possible biochemical factors might conceivably be involved in the pathogenesis of a disease characterized by severe striato-nigral dopamine depletion and cell destruction, accompanied by some degree of autonomic nervous system deficit? SANDLER (1970b) has tentatively suggested that 6-hydroxydopamine (Fig. 4), or a compound similar to it, might be generated endogenously in patients with idiopathic parkinsonism, causing neuronal degeneration in areas of high dopamine concentration. SENOH et al. (1959b) showed that administration of dopamine to rabbits resulted in the autoxidative formation of 6-hydroxydopamine. This amine can produce a "chemical sympathectomy" either temporarily or permanently depending on the age of the experimental animal (for review, see THOENEN, p. 823). In addition intraventricular administration can give rise to a "central sympathectomy", being taken up by and producing destruction of catecholamine-containing neurones within the brain (see THOENEN,

p. 813). It seems, however, that noradrenaline-containing neurones are more sensitive to the action of intraventricular 6-hydroxydopamine than those which contain dopamine (Groppetti et al., 1969), although to what extent this is a matter of access is difficult to decide.

With the sensitive mass spectrometric techniques at present being developed it might be worth looking for 6-hydroxydopamine or its metabolites (Daly et al., 1965) in specimens of brain or urine from parkinsonian subjects.

e) Melanin Formation

One neuropathological manifestation of parkinsonism which has attracted much attention is a decrease in melanin containing granules in the cells of the substantia nigra (e. g. Hassler, 1938; Pakkenberg and Brody, 1965). The difference is quantitative: there is no alteration in the ultrastructural appearance of the granule itself (Roy and Wolman, 1969). The pigment appears to be a true melanin (van Woert et al., 1967; Maeda and Wegman, 1969), probably derived from dopamine (Vander Wende and Spoerlein, 1963): its formation may be inhibited by 5-hydroxytryptamine (Vander Wende and Johnson, 1970). The suggestion that neuromelanin is concerned in the regulation of catecholamine synthesis in the pigmented brain stem nuclei (Marsden, 1965) is probably fallacious (Hornykiewicz, 1966). There have been attempts to link the features of parkinsonism with the associated pigment deficit (Cotzias et al., 1964; Cotzias, 1966), culminating in an unsuccessful therapeutic trial of melanocyte-stimulating hormone (Cotzias et al., 1967). Birkmayer (1970) has claimed that the substantia nigra of parkinsonian patients who fail to respond to L-DOPA contains no melanin, a pointer presumably, to the severity of the anatomical defect.

f) Catechol O-methyltransferase

COMT has been identified and intensively studied by Axelrod and his group (for reviews, see Axelrod, 1959, 1966). Although it preferentially O-methylates the *meta*-hydroxyl group of 3,4-dihydroxy catechols (Masri et al., 1962), it has some action on the *para*-hydroxyl group both *in vitro* (Senoh et al., 1959a; Masri et al., 1964; Creveling et al., 1970) and *in vivo* (Daly et al., 1960). Despite the failure of von Studnitz (1967) to detect evidence of 4-O-methylation in the urine of patients with catecholamine-secreting tumours, it has become obvious that small amounts of 4-O-methylated compounds, produced endogenously, are excreted in human urine. Matthieu and Revol (1970) claim that as much as

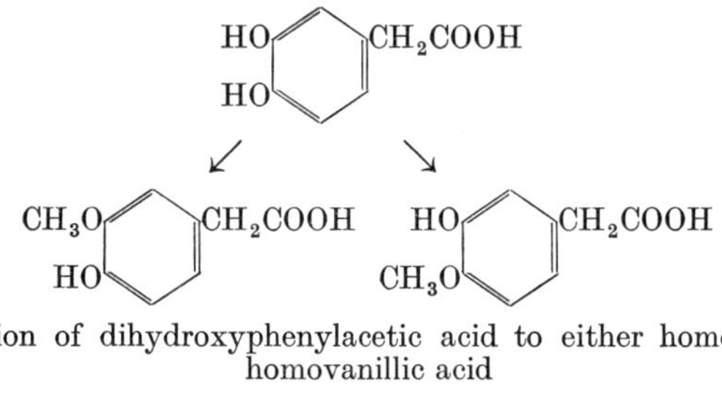

HO, HO, CH_2COOH

↙ ↘

CH_3O, HO, CH_2COOH HO, CH_3O, CH_2COOH

Fig. 5. O-Methylation of dihydroxyphenylacetic acid to either homovanillic acid or *iso*-homovanillic acid

10—20% of urinary homovanillic acid is composed of its geometrical isomer, *iso*-homovanillic acid (Fig. 5). The latter reacts more intensively with diazo reagent however and the authors may not have taken this fact into account; work in progress in the writer's laboratory indicates that a few percent of the normal homovanillic acid output in man is likely to be composed of *iso*-homovanillic acid and rather less in the rat (GOODWIN, et al. 1971). The failure of DACRE et al. (1968) to find evidence of 4-O-methylation after the administration of labelled dihydroxyphenyl acetic acid to rats must be attributed to the insensitivity of their method.

It seems that isoenzymes of COMT exist (ANDERSON and D'IORIO, 1968). To what extent they vary in their action, and in particular, whether one variant tends to act on the 4-position more than another, although this seems to be unlikely, must be decided on the basis of future observation. These studies may be relevant to the pathogenesis of parkinsonism; ERNST (1962), foreshadowed by EPSTEIN et al. (1932) thirty years earlier, showed that administration of 4-methoxy compounds provokes a "hyperkinetic rigid syndrome" reminiscent of human parkinsonism and raised the possibility that agents of this type might contribute to the disease in man. GOODWIN et al. (1971) have obtained preliminary evidence, however, to indicate that parkinsonian patients do not have a higher urinary output of *iso*-homovanillic acid than control subjects.

As has been stated, COMT carries out O-methylation either at the 3-position or at the 4-position of a catechol. From the known characteristics of the enzyme, it does not appear to act on both hydroxyl groups of the *same* molecule. If 3,4-dimethoxyphenylethylamine, the most persistent of the "pink spots" (for reviews see PUSHPATHADAM and BARBEAU, 1969; SANDLER and RUTHVEN, 1969), which also exerts an akinetic action in the experimental animal (BARBEAU et al., 1965) is excreted in significant amounts in parkinsonism (BARBEAU et al., 1963), and does turn out to be synthesized endogenously, the enzymic mechanism responsible for the double O-methylation would be of some little interest.

DOPA itself is a good substrate for COMT (AXELROD and TOMCHICK, 1958). 3-O-Methyl DOPA (Fig. 6) was first detected by VON STUDNITZ (1961) in the urine of patients with neural tumours producing an excess of DOPA. The amino acid, which has not been detected in urine from normal subjects, is an important metabolite of DOPA administered therapeutically in parkinsonian patients (see p. 876).

g) Monoamine Oxidase

The study of MAO and its recently characterized isoenzymes is another area of the field of biologically active monoamine research in which there has been a recent upsurge of interest (for review, see SANDLER et al., 1971a). Dopamine is known to be an excellent substrate of the brain enzyme (WEINER, 1960). It is of interest that one of the isoenzymes of human brain, termed MAO_4, has a particular affinity for dopamine and whilst there was great variation in the different brain areas examined, the highest specific activity of this isoenzyme towards dopamine as substrate was found in the basal ganglia (COLLINS et al., 1970b).

BERNHEIMER and HORNYKIEWICZ (1962) were unable to detect any abnormality of MAO in the brains of parkinsonian patients. METZEL et al. (1969), however, found an increase in activity in samples obtained at brain biopsy compared with control material, although their data do not appear to have been published in full. If such an increase were confirmed, it might conceivably be an important factor in the pathogenesis of the disease. Further observations on parkinsonian material, with particular reference to the status of MAO_4, are urgently needed.

h) Conjoint Pathway Metabolites (Fig. 2)

There appears to be little information concerning the relative production of 3-O-methylated amines in parkinsonian compared with normal subjects. Little difference exists however between the two groups with respect to urinary output of acids and alcohols deriving from catecholamine degradation, whether of the "dopamine series" or the β-hydroxylated "noradrenaline series" (CALNE et al., 1969a). Thus the known biochemical changes in dopamine metabolism within the parkinsonian brain are presumably relatively circumscribed; the metabolite

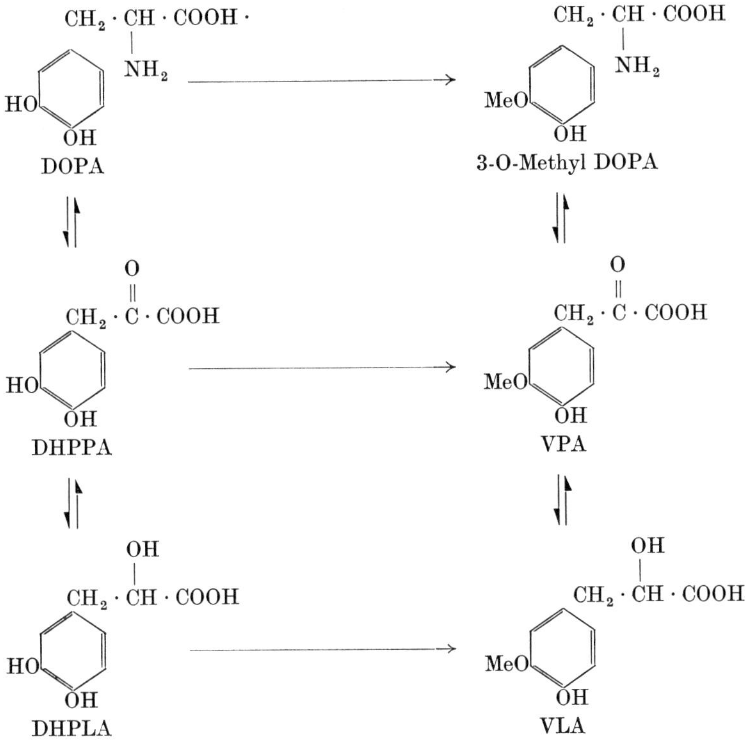
CH2 · CH · COOH ·
NH2
HO
OH
DOPA
CH2 · CH · COOH
NH2
MeO
OH
3-O-Methyl DOPA
O
CH2 · C · COOH
HO
OH
DHPPA
O
CH2 · C · COOH
MeO
OH
VPA
OH
CH2 · CH · COOH
HO
OH
DHPLA
OH
CH2 · CH · COOH
MeO
OH
VLA

Fig. 6. Transamination pathways of L-DOPA. (DHPPA = dihydroxyphenylpyruvic acid; DHPLA = dihydroxyphenyllactic acid; VPA = 4-hydroxy-3-methoxyphenylpyruvic acid; VLA = 4-hydroxy-3-methoxyphenyllactic acid) (reproduced from Schweiz. med. Wschr., **100**, 526—531 [1970], by permission of the Editor)

contribution from the central nervous system forms a sufficiently small proportion of the total pool to leave it unaltered. The cerebrospinal fluid, however, which bathes the central nervous system, appears to reflect these biochemical changes more faithfully (MOIR et al., 1970). Opinions to the contrary (GOODWIN et al., 1970a, b; LAVERTY and TAYLOR, 1969) have all been based on evidence obtained under abnormal conditions, during treatment with high DOPA dosage.

Because of methodological limitations, it is possible to measure relatively few catecholamine metabolites in the cerebrospinal fluid. However, the major end-product of dopamine metabolism, homovanillic acid, can be assayed relatively simply and a significant decrease has been noted consistently in parkinsonian patients (ANDÉN et al., 1963a; BERNHEIMER et al., 1966; GULDBERG et al., 1967; JOHANSSON and ROOS, 1967; PULLAR et al., 1969; PAPESCHI et al., 1970; VAN WOERT and BOWERS, 1970). A similar decrease, compared with non-parkinsonian control subjects, is present in ventricular fluid from affected patients, although the total concentrations are higher in both groups (GULDBERG et al., 1967). Probenecid, which blocks the transport of acids out of the cerebrospinal fluid

(GULDBERG et al., 1966; WERDINIUS, 1967) causes a rise in homovanillic acid concentration in normal subjects; however the level remains low in parkinsonism (OLSSON and ROOS, 1968). An approach of this style offers a useful diagnostic test (TAMARKIN et al., 1970) which may be needed to sharpen the distinction between parkinsonian and other groups: even leaving aside probable parkinsonian variants such as parkinsonism dementia of Guam (BRODY et al., 1970) or some cases of progressive supranuclear palsy (MENDELL et al., 1970) where low cerebrospinal fluid values have been noted, decreased concentrations of homovanillic acid have also been reported in some dementias (GOTTFRIES et al., 1969), depression (BOWERS et al., 1969) and in acute inflammatory conditions (BAROLIN and HORNYKIEWICZ, 1967). Although the concentration normally rises in patients treated with haloperidol or phenothiazines, those who develop parkinsonism in response to drug treatment shown significantly lower values (CHASE et al., 1970). Low values have been observed in animal models of parkinsonism produced by appropriate surgical lesions in the midbrain (SOURKES et al., 1969).

III. L-DOPA Treatment of Parkinsonism

1. Response of Different Clinical Subgroups

a) Idiopathic Parkinsonism

The management of Parkinson's disease has recently been transformed by the advent of oral L-DOPA treatment. Whilst its potentialities have only been widely appreciated since the important paper of COTZIAS et al. (1967), this therapeutic approach has in fact been practised since 1961, when two separate groups independently reported on its usefulness. BIRKMAYER and HORNYKIEWICZ (1961) noted a transitory improvement in akinesia after intravenous administration of L-DOPA to affected patients, whilst BARBEAU (1961) observed a similar effect after oral treatment. In this early phase the drug was used mostly by the intravenous route and experience was gained at a number of centres. Whilst some (FEHLING, 1966; RINNE and SONNINEN, 1968b) thought it of questionable value, BIRKMAYER and HORNYKIEWICZ (1964) were able to confirm their original observations in a larger series and their findings were mirrored by others (see BARBEAU, 1969b). Oral DOPA therapy has had a rather more chequered history. Despite the original promise (BARBEAU et al., 1962) doubts were soon cast on its effectiveness (GREER and WILLIAMS, 1963; MCGEER and ZELDOWICZ, 1964). There is an interesting postscript to the therapeutic failure of MCGEER and ZELDOWICZ (1964) trial. In an earlier attempt at the treatment of drug induced parkinsonism, following optimistic claims by DEGKWITZ et al. (1960), MCGEER et al. (1961) gave affected patients relatively vast doses of DL-DOPA, supplementing it with large amounts of pyridoxine. Although pyridoxal phosphate is a cofactor of DOPA decarboxylase (HOLTZ and PALM, 1964), so that the treatment is a rational one, it is now known that pyridoxine effectively neutralises the therapeutic effect of L-DOPA in Parkinsonism (this phenomena is discussed further below, p. 867). It may be that MCGEER and ZELDOWICZ (1964) treated their parkinsonian patients with a similar supplement — although this is not stated in their paper.

The present phase was heralded by the report of COTZIAS et al. (1967) that gradually increasing (COTZIAS et al., 1969b; JENKINS, 1970) doses of oral DL-DOPA administered for long periods of time give rise to improvement ranging from slight to apparently complete recovery. DL-DOPA, which was on occasion employed by other workers (HOFMANN and RYAN, 1970; RAO, 1970), has generally been abandoned, for several of the original patients of COTZIAS et al. (1967)

developed transient granulocytopenia; the tendency has been noted even with L-DOPA (COTZIAS, 1968; RINNE et al., 1970b), as has thrombocytopenia (STEG, 1969); but in general L-DOPA is a far more potent therapeutic agent than any previously available and there is a remarkable consistency in the degree of benefit achieved at different centres (e. g. COTZIAS et al., 1969b; BARBEAU, 1969b; YAHR et al., 1969 McDOWELL et al., 1970;). Hypokinesia is the clinical feature which responds best. The major side effects of this treatment, including nausea and vomiting, adventitious movements, hypotension and psychiatric disturbances will be discussed below in greater detail; but certain other general effects should be noted. These include an occasional positive Coombs test, with haemolysis (COTZIAS and PAPAVASILIOU, 1969a), as may sometimes be seen during α-methyldopa administration (WORLLEDGE et al., 1966); death from thromboembolic phenomena has been mentioned just frequently enough to arouse suspicion (GREEN, 1970; MONES et al., 1970; STELLAR et al., 1970; YAHR, 1970c). Profuse sweating is sometimes observed (McGEER et al., 1961; CALNE et al., 1969b) not unlike phaeochromocytoma, a catecholamine-secreting tumour (HERMANN and MORNEX, 1964), and is occasionally extreme (GREEN, 1970): McGEER et al. (1961) remarked on the occurrence of black sweat in some of their patients on very high dosage, presumably deriving from catechol oxidation products. This phenomenon is reminiscent of what is sometimes seen in the 5-hydroxyindole-secreting carcinoid disease (ANLYAN et al., 1960). Certain long-term side-effects are just beginning to be observed, supervening after something well over a year of treatment (BARBEAU, 1970b; SACKS et al., 1970b), including akinesia, stupor, withdrawal symptoms, never observed after cessation of short-term treatment where improvement may even persist for many months (MAWDSLEY, 1970; RAO, 1970), and accelerated adverse reactions after readministration. The whole pattern of these late effects is suggestive of the gradual supervention of organic damage to the central nervous system and must inevitably raise the question once more (see p. 856) of possible contamination of the drug with, or the endogenous generation of, traces of 6-hydroxydopamine (SANDLER, 1970b).

b) Postencephalitic Parkinsonism

Compared with idiopathic parkinsonism, the L-DOPA treatment of postencephalitic parkinsonism is not as successful (KRASNER and CORNELIUS, 1970), although useful improvement may still be achieved (HUNTER et al., 1970e). The patients only tolerate comparatively low dosage (CALNE et al., 1969b; MARKHAM, 1970) and there is a high incidence of side-effects including psychiatric (CELESIA and BARR, 1970), respiratory (SACKS et al., 1970a) and ocular; after some alleviation in the short-term, prolonged oculogyric crises of unusual intensity ("supercrises") develop (SACKS and KOHL, 1970b); indeed, even intravenous iproniazid, an MAO inhibitor, will make oculogyric crises worse (BIRKMAYER and HORNYKIEWICZ, 1961).

c) Drug-induced Parkinsonism

In general, this form of treatment has met with little success (FLEMING et al., 1970). Although BRUNO and BRUNO (1966) may have seen some response, HIPPIUS and LOGEMANN (1970) noted an increase in extrapyramidal signs.

d) Manganism

COTZIAS and his colleagues (COTZIAS et al., 1969a; MENA et al., 1970) reported a good therapeutic response in 5 out of 6 hypertonic and 2 dystonic cases. One hypotonic case, made worse by L-DOPA, responded dramatically to 5-HTP.

e) Miscellaneous Diseases

α) Depression. There appears to be a real improvement in a small number of retarded depressives (e. g. INGVARSSON, 1965a; MATUSSEK et al., 1970; GOODWIN et al., 1970a, b) despite early reports to the contrary (PARE and SANDLER, 1959; KLERMAN et al., 1963). As cerebrospinal fluid homovanillic acid concentration appears to be decreased in some cases of depression (BOWERS et al., 1969), it would be of interest to ascertain whether the subjects who respond best have the lowest concentration in this location. Depression is likely to be an end-result of a variety of metabolic derangements; one of these may be dopamine deficiency (GOODWIN et al., 1970a, b), so that a therapeutic test with L-DOPA may well prove helpful in the classification of depressive illness.

β) Progressive supranuclear palsy. Some patients appear to have reponded; others have proved refractory (see MENDELL et al., 1970). As mentioned earlier (p. 846), the finding of a low cerebrospinal fluid homovanillic acid concentration in one patient (MENDELL et al., 1970) raises the question of possible overlap with parkinsonism.

γ) Head injury. There have been three reports of dramatic improvement after DOPA administration to patients with posttraumatic coma (BETTAG and HOLBACH, 1969; BRICCOLO and DALLE ORE, 1970; GERSTENBRAND, 1970). Further investigation is obviously needed.

δ) Migraine. ANTUNES et al. (1970) report the case of a parkinsonian patient and YAHR (1970b) and McDOWELL (1970) have each treated another whose coincidental migraine was relieved complete by L-DOPA.

ε) Asthma. Both INGVARSSON (1965b) and BARBEAU (1970b) consider L-DOPA to be helpful, although the coincidental asthma of one drug-induced parkinsonian patient reported by FLEMING et al. (1970) became worse on treatment.

ζ) Wilson's disease. The patient of BARBEAU and FRIESEN (1970) was improved but that of MORGAN et al. (1970a) was unaffected.

η) Torsion dystonias. This complex group of neurological conditions, presumably arising from disorders of the basal ganglia, has recently been intensively studied in relation to response to L-DOPA. Some representatives of the group are benefitted, whilst others are refractory (e. g. COLEMAN and BARNET, 1969; BARBEAU, 1970a). As AXELROD (1970) remarked, "There must be some difference between patients who respond and those who don't". Such a difference has not yet been identified.

ϑ) Hepatic coma. High acute dosage of L-DOPA produced a striking though temporary improvement in level of consciousness in these patient (PARKES et al., 1970a). There is some indication that patients with hepatic cirrhosis may only tolerate a low dose of L-DOPA (SCHWARZ and FAHN, 1970).

ν) Miscellaneous. Dementias deteriorate (VAN WOERT et al., 1970), as does schizophrenia (TOBIAS, 1970; YARYURA-TOBIAS et al., 1970). Amyotrophic lateral sclerosis does not respond (LIEBERMAN and PEDERSEN, 1970; MONES et al., 1970); nor do Huntington's chorea, encephalitis, pseudobulbar palsy, cerebral palsy or posterior fossa tumour (MONES et al., 1970).

2. L-DOPA plus Peripheral Decarboxylase Inhibitor

Certain effective DOPA decarboxylase inhibitors, e. g. the hydrazine derivatives Ro 4-4602 (BURKARD et al., 1962) and MK 485 (PORTER et al., 1962) fail to cross the blood-brain barrier. They consequently inhibit "peripheral" concentrations of the enzyme which normally decarboxylate by far the greater proportion of ingested L-DOPA. Central nervous system activity is left relatively intact, however (SCHECKEL et al., 1965; BARTHOLINI and PLETSCHER, 1968, 1969; TISSOT et al., 1969a). Thus these agents possess a DOPA-sparing action so that a considerably smaller dose is required for the same therapeutic effect (BIRKMAYER, 1969b). As a consequence, and for reasons which are not fully understood, the incidence and intensity of side-effects such as nausea and vomiting, and adventitious movements, tend to be reduced (SIEGFRIED, 1970; KRAYENBÜHL and SIEGFRIED, 1970). Whether these decarboxylase inhibitors, despite their limited penetration into the brain, gain access to and prevent the generation of dopamine in some unidentified vomiting centre (LOTTI and PORTER, 1970) has yet to be decided. Despite certain toxic effects occasionally noted in experimental animals (e. g. LAMMERS and VAN ROSSUM, 1968; CHRUSCIEL, 1969; THEISS and SCHÄRER, 1970), the combination of these inhibitors with DOPA is likely to be the treatment of choice in the future, to judge from clinical reports so far available (e. g. BIRKMAYER, 1969b; SIEGFRIED, 1970; KRAYENBÜHL and SIEGFRIED, 1970).

3. Major Side-effects of L-DOPA Treatment

a) Nausea and Vomiting

It is assumed if not actually stated in most studies reviewed here that the toxic actions of dopa therapy derive from the generation of dopamine (CARLSSON, 1970) often at adventitious sites in the central nervous system (KOPIN, 1970). There is, indeed, much indirect evidence to suggest that some intrinsic property of the dopamine molecule itself is responsible for nausea and vomiting during L-DOPA therapy. Thus, apomorphine, which bears a structural similarity to dopamine and also stimulates the vomiting centre, is known to act on dopaminergic receptors both centrally (e. g. ERNST, 1965b, 1969b; FEKETE and KURTI, 1970) and peripherally (GOLDBERG et al., 1968). This drug potentiates the suppressive action of L-DOPA on tremor in the lesioned monkey (GOLDSTEIN et al., 1970b) and, perhaps the most telling point of all, it possesses a beneficial effect in human parkinsonism (SCHWAB et al., 1951; BRAHAM et al., 1970; COTZIAS et al., 1970).

Nausea and vomiting is found not only in patients with Parkinson's disease on L-DOPA but is also observed when normal subjects ingest the drug (ANSEL and MARKHAM, 1970). It is an effect quite dissociated from the therapeutic action for it gradually becomes less severe over a period of time, although there is no falling off of benefit; as noted above, its severity may be attenuated by the coincident administration of peripheral decarboxylase inhibitors.

b) Hypotension

Hypertension is rather uncommon in parkinsonian patients (HUNTER et al., 1970b). They tend as a group to be hypotensive, perhaps from some degree of autonomic nervous system deficit (MCDOWELL, 1970; p. 855). L-DOPA therapy may result in an exaggeration of this tendency in some affected subjects (e. g. CALNE et al., 1970; MARKHAM et al., 1970). The effects are rarely serious however and tend to become less severe with time.

The mechanism of production of this side-effect is not immediately obvious. Dopamine infusion in man is unequivocably pressor (HORWITZ et al., 1960). Preventing dopamine degradation by treatment with MAO inhibitors prior to L-DOPA administration may result in a massive rise in blood pressure (see HUNTER et al., 1970a). Against this background, there is probably little force in the "false transmitter" argument put forward by Burn (1970) that hypotension after L-DOPA therapy may derive from an excess of dopamine displacing noradrenaline in sympathetic fibres where, after the passage of a nerve impulse, it exerts a smaller vasoconstrictor action. Henning and Rubenson (1970) have been able to demonstrate a central hypotensive effect of L-DOPA in the experimental animal similar to that of α-methyldopa (Henning, 1969) whilst Watanabe et al. (1970) found in man that peripheral decarboxylase inhibition enhances the hypotensive effect of L-DOPA. On balance, therefore, it would seem that an explanation based on a central action of the drug must be considered the most plausible. Nevertheless, there is no absence of other candidates for the role of hypotensive agent during L-DOPA therapy. Barbeau et al. (1969), for instance, noted a decrease in plasma renin concentration in parkinsonian subjects, although neither Fotino and Blaufox (1970) nor Michelakis and Robertson (1970) agree with their finding that this tendency is exaggerated by L-DOPA treatment. There is one other, at present theoretical, mechanism of great interest, the possibility of hypotensive Schiff's bases being formed *in vivo* after L-DOPA administration.

More than thirty years ago, Holtz et al. (1938) incubated dopamine with an MAO preparation and noted its transformation into a compound which lowers cat blood pressure. They at first suspected that the responsible agent was the immediate product of oxidative deamination, 3,4-dihydroxyphenylacetaldehyde (Holtz, 1966). The intermediate aldehydes of the biologically active monoamines were shown, much later, to be without apparent pharmacological action, however (Renson et al., 1964). When Holtz et al. (1964) resumed their experiments, they were in fact able to show that epinine (N-methyldopamine), an even better substrate for MAO than dopamine (Wiseman-Distler et al., 1965), which gives rise to the same aldehyde by oxidative deamination, did not provoke a depressor response after similar incubation. The compound responsible for the hypotensive effect was later identified as tetrahydropapaveroline, a hypotensive Schiff's base (Laidlaw, 1910) formed from the condensation of dopamine with its aldehyde. Davis and her colleagues (Davis et al., 1970; Walsh et al., 1970; Yamanaka et al., 1970) have studied this problem more recently and were able to show in experiments *in vitro* that ethanol facilitates the formation of tetrahydropapaveroline, or of the related compound, salsolinol. They suggested that generation of these alkaloids might conceivably be the basis for alcohol addiction, a view shared by Cohen and Collins (1970). Trace amounts only of tetrahydropapaveroline could be detected in the liver in *in vivo* experiments (Halushka and Hoffmann, 1968). It should obviously be sought in the urine of patients during L-DOPA treatment, especially after ethanol ingestion.

c) Adventitious Movements

Almost as soon as high dosage regimens for L-DOPA were embarked upon, it was noted (Cotzias et al., 1967) that after a period of a few weeks to a few months had elapsed, abnormal involuntary movements developed. It soon became apparent that they are the main factor limiting the usefulness of the treatment. These movement disorders have been the subject of careful study by a number of authors (e. g. Sigwald and Raymondeaud, 1970; Yahr, 1970a, c). They are presumably caused by some vicarious action of dopamine generated within the brain, for Cotzias et al. (1970) observed similar movements in parkinsonian patients treated with apomorphine, which for the purposes of discussion may be considered a dopamine analogue (see p. 863). It seems likely however that there is some characteristic of the parkinsonian state which predisposes to the onset of these movements. ANSEL and MARKHAM (1970) failed to observe them in four adult volunteers who ingested increasing amounts of L-DOPA, up to a maximum of 3—5 g, for a period of up to one month. Nor did MENA et al. (1970) observe these movements in their Chilean manganese miners, despite a full therapeutic response to L-DOPA. The patients of VAN WOERT et al. (1970), who were treated with L-DOPA for dementia, similarly did not get any involuntary movements. On the other hand, GOODWIN et al. (1970a, b) noted mild involuntary movements in their L-DOPA-treated depressive subjects, whilst LIEBERMAN and PEDERSEN'S (1970) patients with amyotrophic lateral sclerosis were badly troubled by them. In this connexion, it is of interest that LUSE et al. (1970) were unable to produce adventitious movements experimentally by treating normal monkeys with L-DOPA, but severe muscular contractions supervened with L-DOPA treatment after the substantia nigra had been damaged with sodium azide.

A number of factors may modify these involuntary movements. Decarboxylase inhibition apparently leads to fewer and less severe movements (SIEGFRIED, 1970). Previous thalamotomy tends to protect against them (HUGHES et al., 1971). JAMESON (1970) has claimed that he can achieve a dissociation of the antidystonic and antiparkinsonian effects of pyridoxine by the use of small doses (10 mg) intravenously.

CALNE et al. (1969b) have drawn attention to the restlessness which accompanies the abnormal movements, whilst "stereotype" behaviour has also been observed (ANDÉN et al., 1970d), very reminiscent of one particular manifestation of dexamphetamine toxicity. COOLS and VAN ROSSUM (1970) have pointed out that dopamine and amphetamine both elicit a similar type of stereotype behaviour which may be antagonised by haloperidol. Intraventricular amphetamine, indeed, may produce a very similar pattern of stereotype behaviour in rats ("mock-fighting") (EVETTS et al., 1970) to that reported by LAMMERS and VAN ROSSUM (1968) after the administration of L-DOPA plus a peripheral decarboxylase inhibitor. Thus both agents may stimulate central dopaminergic receptors. Amine uptake mechanisms in the striatum appear to possess little stereospecificity, so that (—)-amphetamine is almost as effective as the (+)-isomer in provoking compulsive gnawing behaviour, the characteristic response of the rat to dopaminergic receptor stimulation (COYLE and SNYDER, 1969; TAYLOR and SNYDER, 1970).

Haloperidol appears to be the treatment of choice for a rare disease in man which may stem from overstimulation of central dopaminergic receptors, Gilles de la Tourettes disease (SNYDER et al., 1970). Affected patients manifest with coprolalia, sudden explosive cries and tics, which appear to be reminiscent of certain types of toxic reaction to L-DOPA overdosage e. g. compulsory and obscene swearing (MAWDSLEY, 1970), "incontinent nostalgia" (SACKS and KOHL, 1970a).

d) Psychiatric Aspects

The most detailed study to date of psychiatric aspects of L-DOPA treatment comes from McDOWELL (1970) who analysed 365 patients. Depression may be evident (CHERINGTON, 1970; DAMASIO et al., 1970; JENKINS and GROH, 1970a) which may often usefully be countered with imipramine without recurrence of parkinsonism (JENKINS and GROH, 1970b). The most common untoward reaction however was delirium which tends to supervene in elderly arteriosclerotic subjects, who posses some degree of dementia (CELESIA and BARR, 1970; STELLAR et al., 1970; SACKS et al., 1970c). McDOWELL (1970) records that the "state closely resembles an acute drug intoxication or a toxic delirium". It is perhaps interesting at this point to recall that certain DOPA metabolites are potentially hallucinogenic; both SMYTHIES et al. (1967) and SHULGIN et al. (1969) have indicated that O-methylation at the 4-position (see p. 857) gives rise to compounds which possess this property most powerfully. Although preliminary studies of the production of 4-O-methylated compounds after L-DOPA administration have taken place (O'GORMAN et al., 1970; GOODWIN et al., 1971), it might be instructive to compare the degree of 4-O-methylation in parkinsonian patients who get delirium on L-DOPA with those who do not.

e) Sexual Aspects

One facet of treatment with L-DOPA which became notorious, receiving much publicity in the lay press, is its putative aphrodisiac effect. Well-authenticated confirmatory reports in the scientific literature were tardy in arriving, and it was first suggested (e. g. CALNE and SANDLER, 1970) that effects of this type were merely a by-product of increased physical well-being. VAN WOERT et al. (1970) however noted the case of an 88-year old female patient with senile dementia without physical impairment in whom treatment with L-DOPA was followed by an intense preoccupation with sex. It is not a common side-effect in parkinsonism: MONES et al. (1970) noted 3 patients with increased sexual awareness in a series of 152. The number of recorded cases is now growing fairly rapidly (BARBEAU, 1969b; ANDÉN et al., 1970d; GREER, 1970; HUGHES et al., 1971; MAWDSLEY, 1970; SACHS and KOHL, 1970a; YARYURA-TOBIAS et al., 1970).

Experimental evidence does exist pointing to the importance of dopamine in sexual function (HYYPPÄ et al., 1970). It can be restored by apomorphine, which acts on dopamine receptors (see p. 863), after suppression by tetrabenazine (BUTCHER et al., 1969), which possesses an amine-liberating action somewhat similar to reserpine (CARLSSON, 1966). FUXE and his colleagues (e. g. FUXE et al., 1969) have studied a tubero-infundibular dopaminergic neurone system which appears to play a role in the regulation of gonadotrophin secretion, whilst KAMBERI and his colleagues (e.g. KAMBERI et al., 1969) were able to show that dopamine discharges a luteinizing-hormone releasing factor from the rat hypothalamus. It is perhaps just worth looking for an effect on the production or discharge of exophthalmos-producing substance, for ANDÉN et al. (1970d) noted eyelid retraction in most of their patients being treated with L-DOPA.

Apart from its actions in the central nervous system, dopamine may play some more local role in the male genital system. Thus, it is the predominant amine in the penis and may well take part in the train of events leading to penile erection (PENTTILÄ and VARTIAINEN, 1964). Two psychiatric patients who were given L-DOPA subsequently had a normal erection and orgasm; however there was non-emission of semen (HÄLLSTRÖM and PERSSON, 1970). The four patients with increased libido recorded by BARBEAU (1969b) were unable to sustain their erection and had premature orgasm. In the prostate of the dog, there are dopamine-containing cells, but their role is unknown (BJÖRKLUND and CEGRELL, 1970).

If, on balance, dopamine appears to promote sexual activity, 5-hydroxytryptamine inhibits it and the two monoamines are likely to have opposing actions. TAGLIAMONTE et al. (1969) showed that administration of *p*-chlorophenylalanine, a blocker of 5-hydroxyindole production (KOE and WEISSMAN, 1968), to male rats, provokes a considerable increase in sexual activity. *p*-Chlorophenylalanine does not appear to have any effect on sexual receptivity in the female rat however; its action seems to be confined to provoking increased mounting activity between male rats (SEGAL and WHALEN, 1970). There seems to be no evidence for it possessing any aphrodisiac effect in man (SJOERDSMA et al., 1970).

f) Drug Incompatibilities

i *Pyridoxine.* Pyridoxal phosphate (vitamin B 6) is a coenzyme for L-DOPA decarboxylase and also many other decarboxylases and transaminases (for review, see HOLTZ and PALM, 1964). It might have thus been reasonable to assume that it would enhance any therapeutic action possessed by DOPA, and as mentioned earlier (p. 860), it was administered together with DOPA in the early trial of McGEER et al. (1961). DUVOISIN et al. (1969) subsequently showed, however, that pyridoxine effectively neutralizes the therapeutic action of L-DOPA, an observation which has subsequently been confirmed (BOUDIN et al., 1970; HUNTER et al., 1970b). The mechanism of this interaction remains unclear. DUVOISIN et al. speculated that pyridoxine might so enhance the activity of peripheral decarboxylase that insufficient L-DOPA is available to cross into the central nervous system. Although this explanation appears unlikely, the experiment to disprove it, to determine whether pyridoxine counters the therapeutic effect of an L-DOPA-peripheral decarboxylase inhibitor combination, does not yet appear to have been performed*. A more likely explanation perhaps is the formation of a Schiff's base (CALNE and SANDLER, 1970). SCHOTT and CLARK (1952) showed that pyridoxal phosphate cyclizes non-enzymatically with DOPA or dopamine to form a tetrahydroisoquinoline; in the process, dopamine loses its pharmacological activity (HOLTZ and WESTERMANN, 1957). The one drawback to such a explanation is that reversal of the therapeutic action may occur after extremely small doses: JAMESON (1970), for example, began to observe a return of parkinsonian tremor after only 10 mg of pyridoxine had been given intravenously. This amount, which might easily be present in proprietary vitamin preparations (against which, patients should be warned) would scarcely be sufficient to reverse the effect of, say, 6 g of L-DOPA.

There is a further possibility. DOPA decarboxylase is sensitive to certain aromatic keto-acids including phenylpyruvic acid (HARTMAN et al., 1955; FELLMAN, 1956; DAVISON and SANDLER, 1958; VOGEL et al., 1970b) (p. 853) and more importantly for the present argument, dihydroxyphenylpyruvic acid (GEY and MESSIHA, 1964). DOPA transaminase (CAMMARATA and COHEN, 1950) which is active in brain (see SEMBA and CIVEN, 1970) can generate dihydroxyphenylpyruvic acid from L-DOPA, employing α-oxoglutaric acid as receptor (FONNUM and LARSEN, 1965). In the rat heart, at least, DOPA transaminase remains constant with age whereas DOPA decarboxylase undergoes a considerable decrease (GEY et al., 1965). Compared with DOPA decarboxylation, the DOPA transaminase reaction is very susceptible to a pyridoxine deficiency state (SOURKES and MISSALA, 1969). It seems possible that the converse may apply and that it is equally strongly potentiated by high concentrations of pyridoxine. Parkinsonian patients are usually elderly and, in any case, the reponsible pathological process is now known to leave them with a tenuous supply of cerebral DOPA decarboxylase (LLOYD and HORNYKIEWICZ, 1970b). It thus seems possible that pyridoxine overtreatment brings about excessive formation of dihydroxyphenylpyruvic acid which prevents dopamine being formed from administered L-DOPA.

There springs to mind yet a further explanation (SANDLER, 1971) which appears to account for some of the major inconsistencies and in many ways,

* Note added in proof: Although experiments along these lines have now been reported from two centres (COTZIAS, G.C., PAPAVASILIOU, P.: Blocking the negative effects of pyridoxine on patients receiving levodopa. J. Amer. med. Ass. **215**, 1504 (1971); YAHR, M.D., DUVOISIN, R.C.: Pyridoxine, levodopa, and L-α-methyldopa hydrazine regimen in parkinsonism. J. Amer. med. Ass. **216**, 2141 (1971)), the decarboxylase inhibitors employed would, as hydrazines, have formed Schiff's bases with pyridoxal. Thus, interpretation is difficult.

possesses the most far-reaching implications. One surprising finding in this field of research is how such an exiguous supply of DOPA decarboxylase (see p. 854), which is even further reduced in the parkinsonian striatum (LLOYD and HORNYKIEWICZ, 1970b), can supply therapeutically useful concentrations of dopamine. Invoking vicarious decarboxylation of DOPA at, for example, 5-hydroxytryptamine-producing sites raises the further problem of transport to the dopamine-deficient zone. Even more paradoxical is the fact that, whilst pyridoxine counters the beneficial effect of administered L-DOPA in parkinsonian patients, large amounts of pyridoxine may be given in safety to untreated subjects and far from interfering with their restricted endogenous supply of dopamine, may even be beneficial (see HOLTZ and PALM, 1964). It seems to the writer that the crucial observation, which may provide the key to all these problems, is that of VOGEL (1969) who described the non-enzymatic decarboxylation of L-DOPA, noting amongst other properties that it is *inhibited* by pyridoxal phosphate and also by a small dialysable molecule in fresh human liver homogenate (VOGEL et al., 1970b). Thus it may well be that such non-enzymatic decarboxylation of L-DOPA contributes to, or is even wholly responsible for the generation of dopamine in the parkinsonian striatum.

Two approaches to test the validity of this hypothesis suggest themselves:

a) the more important experiment would be to administer to parkinsonian patients a DOPA decarboxylase inhibitor which *crosses* the blood-brain barrier (BARTHOLINI and PLETSCHER, 1969) in order to inhibit intracerebral decarboxylase and note whether L-DOPA therapy is still beneficial.

β) After brain lesions have been placed in certain animal parkinsonian models, acute treatment with L-DOPA fails to bring about an increase in the lowered concentration of striatal dopamine (POIRIER et al., 1967). It might be informative to treat such animals *chronically* with oral L-DOPA to see if, in the absence of decarboxylase (LANCASTER et al., 1970), a delayed rise in dopamine level occurs. It might also be important to identify the nature of the tissue inhibitor, for its action may help to explain the variations between the response of different parkinsonian patients to L-DOPA.

BRAHAM (1970) has argued that if pyridoxine excess is harmful to parkinsonian patients on L-DOPA therapy, a deficiency may be therapeutic. He therefore treated his patients with isoniazid, which forms a Schiff's base with pyridoxal phosphate (HOLTZ, 1959). Whilst his patients suffered neither benefit nor ill-effect, for the pyridoxal-isoniazid compound probably continues to have coenzyme activity (PALM, 1958), the approach may not be without its dangers: GOLDEN et al. (1970) described a patient on L-DOPA treatment who also presented with evidence of a pyridoxine deficiency state.

ii *Monoamine oxidase inhibitors*. HOLZER and HORNYKIEWICZ (1959) showed that the MAO inhibitors iproniazid and harmine increase the dopamine content of rabbit brain. Harmine had, in fact, previously been used in the treatment of parkinsonism (BEHRINGER and WILMANNS, 1929) although the beneficial effect claimed for it may not have stemmed from its MAO inhibitory ability; the related compound, harmalol, which has a similar therapeutic effect (COOPER and GUNN, 1931), is not a MAO inhibitor. Iproniazid and other MAO inhibitors have been carefully considered for the treatment of parkinsonism. Whilst they may, by themselves, give rise to modest improvement (ROSEN, 1969), their use is not associated with any rise in brain dopamine (BERNHEIMER et al., 1963). It therefore seemed more reasonable to treat affected subjects with a DOPA-MAO inhibitor combination. A number of groups who carried out such a trial noted beneficial results (e. g. BIRKMAYER and HORNYKIEWICZ, 1961, 1962; MCGEER et al., 1961;

BARBEAU et al., 1962) although marginal benefit only was recorded by others (HIRSCHMANN and MAYER, 1964).

Both McGEER et al. (1961) and BARBEAU et al. (1962) observed that the combination of drugs brought about a large increase in blood pressure, a finding in accord with that of HORWITZ et al. (1960) who noted that the pressor effect of intravenous dopamine in man was markedly potentiated by MAO inhibition. Since these early observations, the hypertensive action of DOPA plus MAO inhibitor has repeatedly been recorded (see HUNTER et al., 1970a). MONES et al. (1970) attempted to make use of this hypertensive response in the treatment of a patient with Shy-Drager syndrome whose existing orthostatic hypotension was exacerbated by L-DOPA alone; however, the rise in blood pressure so obtained was fluctuating and uncontrolled and the treatment had to be abandoned. Whilst no deaths have so far been recorded, it would seem safest to avoid conjoint L-DOPA-MAO inhibitor therapy, with one proviso: a precedent already exists for preferential inhibition of particular MAO isoenzymes (JOHNSTON, 1968). If a specific inhibitor of human brain MAO_4 (COLLINS et al., 1970b) were to be synthesized, it might play a useful adjuvant role to L-DOPA, in the treatment of parkinsonism.

iii *Miscellaneous.* SCHWARZ and FAHN (1970) noted that chlordiazepoxide countered the beneficial effect of L-DOPA in one patient, and HUNTER et al. (1970b) reported that other benzodiazepines may occasionally bring about deterioration. HUNTER and his colleagues, who carried out a careful study of possible interactions of a wide range of common drugs, found that guanethidine dosage had to be reduced in one patient with the uncommon combination of hypertension and parkinsonism; one subject had an increase in postural hypotension when imipramine was added to his L-DOPA treatment. There were no contraindications to chlorpromazine, although trifluoperazine another phenothiazine, has repeatedly been noted by others to attenuate the antiparkinsonian effect of L-DOPA (BARBEAU, 1969b; JENKINS, 1970; YAHR, 1970a). As might be expected, haloperidol, even in small doses, also antagonizes this effect (JENKINS, 1970).

IV. Other Treatments of Parkinsonism in Relation to Catecholamine Metabolism

a) Surgery

The long-term benefits of stereotactic surgery for parkinsonism have, in general, failed to confirm all the initial enthusiastic claims. There may be a place for it in the treatment of patients where tremor and rigidity predominate but L-DOPA is the treatment of choice for akinetic subjects (KRAYENBÜHL and SIEGFRIED, 1970). L-DOPA, in fact, often provides useful relief even after surgery (WYCIS et al., 1970) but the response does not appear to be as good in treated patients (KLAWANS et al., 1969; STELLAR et al., 1970). The present philosophy of treatment seems to be, try L-DOPA first and surgery on its failures (e. g. WYCIS et al., 1970). One possible advantage of previous surgery is that it may protect against L-DOPA-induced involuntary movements (MAWDSLEY, 1970; HUGHES et al., 1971).

b) Amantadine

SCHWAB et al. (1969) reported that the antiviral drug, amantadine, is an effective antiparkinsonian agent and the consensus of opinion confirms that it gives rise to some modest improvement (e. g. HUNTER et al., 1970c; PARKES et al., 1970b). SCHWAB (1970) has also claimed that the effect of amantadine and L-DOPA is additive. More critical experimentation, however, appears to indicate that there is little additional benefit to be obtained by using the drug combination (GODWIN-AUSTEN et al., 1970; HUNTER et al., 1970d) although the combination may occasionally be helpful in subjects who are unable to tolerate more than a small amount of L-DOPA (GODWIN-AUSTEN et al., 1970).

Although amantidine is usually considered an easily tolerated, relatively non-toxic drug, SHEALY et al. (1970) reported the appearance of livedo reticularis, a pronounced mottling of the skin, in more than half the female (but not the male) patients they treated. Because of the possible association of this condition with the collagenoses, a sharp eye should be kept on patients undergoing long-term treatment with the drug.

Whilst the mechanism of action of amantadine is unknown, there are indications that dopamine may be implicated. Thus, GRELAK et al. (1970a, b) have shown in dogs that it releases dopamine and other catecholamines from neuronal storage sites. It is just conceivable that the antiviral action of the drug may play some part in its therapeutic action in view of experimental findings of LYCKE and ROOS (1968) pointing to increased dopamine synthesis following induction of a virus encephalitis.

c) Anticholinergic Drugs

The paradox exists that while much of the experimental and clinical work in the parkinsonian field in recent years has centred on dopamine and its role in the central nervous system, anticholinergic drugs have formed the basis of anti-parkinsonian therapy for many years. Theoretical constructs have therefore been erected postulating the existence of a balance between the activity of acetylcholine and dopamine in the striatum in the normal state: in parkinsonism, a disequilibrium in the direction of cholinergic dominance has been postulated (BARBEAU, 1962, 1970b). Drugs such as reserpine which deplete the brain of dopamine or increase the concentration of acetylcholine as does physostigmine, exacerbate parkinsonism (BIRKMAYER and HORNYKIEWICZ, 1964; DUVOISIN, 1967). Conversely, L-DOPA and atropine are beneficial.

Recently, COYLE and SNYDER (1969) have suggested an alternative mechanism of action for the anticholinergic agents. In studies on isolated synaptosomes, they produced evidence to indicate that these drugs inhibit reuptake of dopamine at nerve endings, so that higher concentrations persist in the region of the synapse. Evidence to confirm this view has been produced by another group (FUXE et al., 1970) whose work provides a rationale for the continuation of anticholinergic drug therapy in patients under treatment with L-DOPA. In a study of structure activity-relationships of compounds which inhibit catecholamine uptake in the central nervous system, HORN et al. (1970) noted that presence of a tropine nucleus tends to favour selective action at dopaminergic sites.

V. L-DOPA Treatment: Metabolic Pathway Considerations

The metabolic degradation of orally administered L-DOPA in man is qualitatively similar to that of the endogenous substance (see SANDLER and RUTHVEN, 1969; p. 852 *et seq*) but there are a number of quantitive differences which will be discussed below. As L-DOPA is administered in relatively enormous dosage in parkinsonian patients, it is practicable to study minor metabolic pathways (Fig. 7) which are not normally accessible to study.

1. Compartmental Factors

Absorption of L-DOPA depends to some extent on the rate of gastric emptying, for appreciable metabolic degradation appears to take place in the gastrointestinal wall, rather faster in the stomach than in the small intestine (RIVERA-CALIMLIM et al., 1970c). High gastric acidity slows emptying whilst alkali promotes

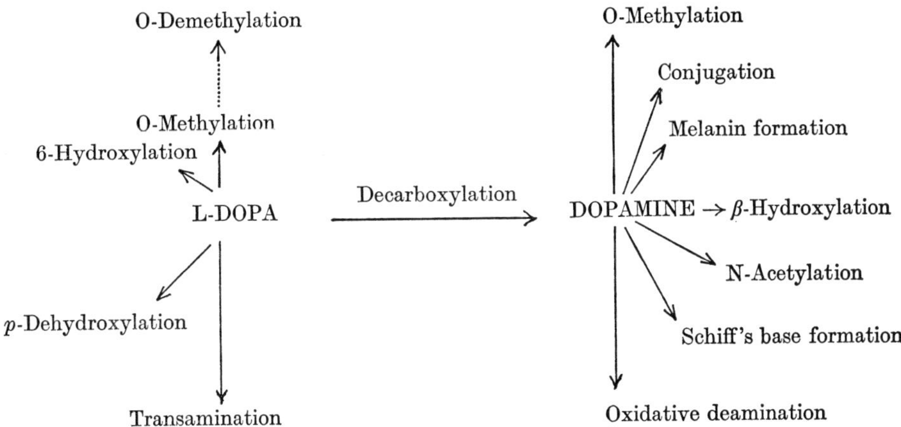

Fig. 7. Major and quantitively minor metabolic transformations of L-DOPA and dopamine

it (RIVERA-CALIMLIM et al., 1970a). In the small intestine, absorption is faster than in the stomach. These considerations were particularly meaningful in a parkinsonian patient described by RIVERA-CALIMLIM et al. (1970b) who appeared to be refractory to L-DOPA. He had a comparatively low absorption rate to judge from plasma levels of administered ^{14}C-DOPA. Neutralization of his highly acid gastric contents facilitated gastric emptying and hence, absorption from the small bowel; he then showed a good therapeutic response, which was accompanied by higher plasma levels of ^{14}C-DOPA after a similar dose to that used before alkali treatment.

Peak plasma concentration of L-DOPA occurs at about 2 hours after administration, when approximately 0.5% of the administered dose is present in the plasma. Negligible values are recorded after about 10 hours (MORGAN et al., 1970b; PEASTON and BIANCHINE, 1970; TYCE et al., 1970a, b). Circulating levels are raised after the administration of a peripheral decarboxylase inhibitor so that a higher concentration is available to cross into the brain (GOODWIN et al., 1970b). After L-DOPA alone, some can be demonstrated in the white blood cells (MANGER and BESSIS, 1969) and variable amounts are absorbed by many others tissues; an initial high uptake has been noted in the pancreas of the mouse (ROSELL et al., 1963; ALM et al., 1969) and it is of interest that in the pregnant mouse, there was similar uptake in maternal and foetal pancreas (ROSELL et al., 1963). Thus in one species at least, L-DOPA passes freely across the placental barrier where it is not impeded by DOPA decarboxylase. Presumably the pregnant parkinsonian female, if such a case were to arise, would present no barrier to the passage of L-DOPA to the foetus similarly, for a minute activity only of this enzyme is present in the human placenta (CONTRACTOR et al., 1971). Higher activity has been detected in other species, however (PEPEU and GIARMAN, 1962).

Whether the blood-testis barrier for L-DOPA (Kormano, 1967) is due to DOPA decarboxylase is not yet known. However, there is a wealth of evidence to show that the blood-brain barrier for L-DOPA derives largely from the presence of high concentrations of this enzyme in brain capillaries (see Bertler et al., 1966). So-called peripheral decarboxylase inhibitors inactivate the enzyme in areas outside the central nervous system but also inhibit it in the brain capillaries. Enzyme within the brain itself is spared and is thus able to decarboxylate the raised blood levels of L-DOPA which are presented to it (Constantinidis et al., 1969).

2. Brain Dopamine

Despite relatively vast dosage, experimental observations indicate that comparatively small concentrations of L-DOPA enter the brain (Rose et al., 1970). Nevertheless they are sufficient to produce an increase in brain dopamine (Strömberg, 1970) with maximum concentration being reached in about one hour (van Rossum et al., 1969). Newly formed dopamine is taken up not only in normal dopamine binding sites but in those usually occupied by 5-hydroxytryptamine as well (Ng et al., 1970).

Hornykiewicz (1970b) has constructed a tight argument to prove that dopamine is responsible for the therapeutic benefit obtained from L-DOPA administration in parkinsonian patients. Perhaps his strongest point is that intravenous L-DOPA produces a temporary alleviation of akinesia. Most of the evidence he adduced, which has been noted earlier in this chapter, is indirect; whilst it points strongly to dopamine being the most important factor, there are certain anomalous findings, noted below, which point to the possibility of some contribution from other active metabolites.

Direct evidence of dopamine generation within the human brain after oral L-DOPA is in fact minimal. Yahr (1970c) has described the single case of a parkinsonian patient who died during L-DOPA therapy on whom biochemical measurements were carried out: compared with the minute concentrations of dopamine normally detected in parkinsonian brains, a value approaching normal was obtained; homovanillic acid concentration was somewhat greater than normal. Further confirmation of these measurements is urgently needed. Apart from this isolated case, pertinent direct observations in man have been confined to cerebrospinal fluid and, of more questionable relevance, to platelets.

Many different groups have now measured cerebrospinal fluid homovanillic acid and noted an increase after L-DOPA treatment (e. g. Pullar et al., 1969; Andén et al., 1970d; Rinne and Sonninen, 1970; van Woert and Bowers, 1970); this increase was comparatively smaller in parkinsonian subjects compared with that following similar dosage in normal controls (Rinne and Sonninen, 1970). Some have claimed to find a degree of correlation between the extent of this rise and the therapeutic response (Pullar et al., 1969; Klawans et al., 1969). Goodwin et al. (1970b) noted a moderate increase only of homovanillic acid concentration in cerebrospinal fluid in subjects on a peripheral DOPA-decarboxylase inhibitor regime compared with those taking L-DOPA alone. They suggested, therefore, in agreement with the views of Taylor and Laverty (1969), that their findings provide strong evidence in favour of an extraneuronal origin, probably the brain capillaries, for the greater portion of the increase. On balance, however, whilst this argument is convincing, it seems likely that the endogenously produced compound, present in reduced concentration in the untreated parkinsonian, derives from DOPA metabolism within the brain (Moir et al., 1970; p. 859). A marginal rise only in dihydroxyphenylacetic acid concentration was observed (PULLAR et al., 1969); production of this compound may to some extent be independent of homovanillic acid formation (MURPHY et al., 1969).

The presence of dopamine itself has not been reported in the cerebrospinal fluid, presumably because its concentration is too low to be recorded by available methods. Catecholamines have difficulty in traversing lipid barriers into the brain (p. 850), at least in the adult, although they can cross the blood-brain barrier to some extent in the newborn chick (KEY and MARLEY, 1962) and rat (LOIZOU, 1970). Even so, dopamine does not pass through as well as noradrenaline (MARLEY and STEPHENSON, 1970). Certain compounds, such as ethanol (HANIG et al., 1970) or, to a lesser extent, dimethyl sulphoxide (HANIG et al., 1970; DE LA TORRE, 1970) which possess both aqueous and lipid solubility, modify the blood-brain barrier and may apparently assist the transport of dopamine into the brain. This is one therapeutic avenue to explore in the future. Another has been proposed by PINDER (1970): he suggested that the dopamine molecule might be altered to increase its lipid solubility whilst yet preserving its ability to activate dopaminergic receptors in the brain. A precedent for this type of compound exists in apomorphine (p. 863), although a possible danger is that endogenous production of dopamine might be inhibited by the suppression of tyrosine hydroxylase activity (GOLDSTEIN et al., 1970c). As L-DOPA itself appears to inhibit this enzyme (DAIRMAN and UDENFRIEND, 1970), the consequences are not likely to be serious.

The blood platelets are even more remote from the brain. The suggestion has been made, however, that they might provide a model system for brain uptake mechanisms (ABRAMS and SOLOMON, 1969). This concept can, of course, only be the roughest of approximations, as the brain is not a homogeneous organ and its uptake mechanisms are known to vary from area to area (SNYDER and COYLE, 1969). Nevertheless, it provides a not unhelpful framework for a number of observations of interest.

Human platelets take up dopamine (BOULLIN and O'BRIEN, 1970; SOLOMON et al., 1970) into the 5-hydroxytryptamine storage organelles (DA PRADA and PLETSCHER, 1969). Many compounds inhibit this uptake including 5-hydroxytryptamine and also drugs active at the dopamine receptor such as apomorphine and haloperidol (SOLOMON et al., 1970). Although the finding is disputed by LEON et al. (1970), BOULLIN and O'BRIEN (1970) noted a facilitated dopamine transport process in parkinsonian platelets: they also observed a greater efflux of dopamine from the loaded platelet. Thus, there may be some diminution of dopamine binding in the parkinsonian platelet perhaps not unlike a similar defect in the striatal neurone.

This type of observation is probably marginal to the main problem of whether dopamine is the main agonist in the L-DOPA treatment of parkinsonism. Whilst HORNYKIEWICZ (1970b) remains convinced of this, he has indeed not ruled out the possibility of some other metabolite playing a subsidiary role (HORNYKIEWICZ, 1970a), although he was unable to nominate a suitable candidate.

There are several anomalous findings which do not fit completely with the thesis that dopamine alone is responsible for clinical improvement after L-DOPA: the time course of the therapeutic response is slow (CALNE et al., 1969b; COTZIAS et al., 1969b); increasing benefit may occur over a period of many months and indeed, YAHR (1970c) carries on treatment for 1 year before admitting failure in an individual patient. However, indirect evidence indicates that dopamine generation in the central nervous system is rapid (PLETSCHER et al., 1967). Another inconsistency is that the response to L-DOPA does not cease immediately after withdrawal of the drug but may linger for a considerably period (MAWDSLEY, 1970; RAO, 1970). Thus the possibility of some minor metabolite unconnected with the main route of DOPA degradation has been invoked, acting in concert with dopamine in bringing about the clinical response (CALNE et al., 1969a; SANDLER et al., 1969a; SANDLER, 1970b; CALNE and SANDLER, 1970; SOURKES, 1970). Careful and detailed attention to minor pathways of DOPA metabolism (Fig. 7) revealed by the high dosage of the drug employed may thus be of more than theoretical interest.

3. Urinary Metabolite Pattern (Fig. 2)

Up to about 1% of ingested L-DOPA is excreted unchanged in the urine (COTZIAS et al., 1969b; ANDÉN et al., 1970d; GOODWIN et al., 1970b). Approximately two-thirds of a single dose, which is rapidly absorbed from the alimentary tract, is excreted in the urine as degradation products within 8 hours (PEASTON and BIANCHINE, 1970) and 85% at 48 hours (MORGAN et al., 1970b). A proportion, variously estimated as about 35% (CALNE et al., 1969a), 30% (GOODWIN et al., 1970b), 25% (TYCE et al., 1970b; O'GORMAN et al., 1970) and about 20% (ANDÉN et al., 1970d) of the ingested dose is excreted as homovanillic acid; its urinary concentration tends to be directly proportional to dose (COTZIAS et al., 1969b). Some delay in homovanillic acid excretion may occasionally occur in postencephalitic parkinsonism (SOURKES et al., 1965). Otherwise, findings in patients under treatment (CALNE et al., 1969a) are not too dissimilar from those following L-DOPA administration to normal subjects (SHAW et al., 1957; SOURKES et al., 1965). About as much dihydroxyphenylacetic acid is excreted as homovanillic acid (CALNE et al., 1969a; O'GORMAN et al., 1970) and its output shows a tendency to rise with increasing dose (CALNE et al., 1969a), presumably from a relative deficiency of methionine to provide methyl groups for its conversion to homovanillic acid (WURTMAN et al., 1970a, b). Inhibition of COMT, which carries out this 0-methylation step, enhances the ability of L-DOPA to relieve tremor in lesioned monkeys (GOLDSTEIN et al., 1970b). Such a combination thus seems worthy of trial in human parkinsonism (BRAHAM, 1970; WURTMAN et al., 1970a, b).

Children with dopamine-secreting tumours may sometimes put out as much homovanillic acid as parkinsonian patients under treatment with L-DOPA. Dihydroxyphenylacetic acid excretion, on the other hand, although greater than normal, forms a proportionally smaller part of the total metabolite output (VON STUDNITZ, 1960; SOURKES et al., 1963). Such a finding implies that the site of metabolic degradation of this endogenously secreted dopamine differs from that of dopamine generated from exogenously administered L-DOPA.

CALNE et al. (1969a) noted other points of difference from dopamine-secreting tumours; there was a tendency for a proportionally even smaller output of the complementary alcohol to homovanillic acid, 4-hydroxy-3-methoxyphenylethanol (GOLDSTEIN et al., 1961) to be observed after L-DOPA ingestion then in tumour patients (RUTHVEN et al., 1969). This finding agrees with the impression of TAYLOR and LAVERTY (1969) that more endogenous dopamine is reduced to its corresponding alcohol than exogenous.

A further important difference concerns degree of β-hydroxylation of the side chain. Apart from the "dopamine-series" metabolites, patients with dopamine-secreting tumours almost invariably have a large output of the β-hydroxylated "noradrenaline-series" metabolites, with a relatively large contribution from the reduction product of the intermediate aldehyde, 4-hydroxy-3-methoxyphenylglycol. Oral L-DOPA treatment however results in a marginal rise only in urinary 4-hydroxy-3-methoxymandelic acid output (CALNE et al., 1969a; TYCE et al., 1970b) and perhaps even a decrease after acute dosage (O'GORMAN et al., 1970). MCGEER et al. (1961) noted a "somewhat increased concentration" in the urine after oral DOPA. As with the "dopamine-series", CALNE et al. (1969a) found a proportionately greater decrease in the "noradrenaline-series" alcohol, 4-hydroxy-3-methoxyphenylglycol. In the light of these differences, it seems likely that further metabolism of dopamine involving β-hydroxylation takes place largely within the tumour tissue of affected subjects (SANDLER and RUTHVEN, 1966), where perhaps the inhibition of dopamine β-hydroxylase by L-DOPA (MOLINOFF, 1970), one possible explanation of a puzzling finding, is prevented by suitable compartmental barriers.

As with its metabolites, GUNNE and LIDVALL (1966) failed to find an increase in urinary noradrenaline itself after L-DOPA infusion although large amounts of dopamine were excreted: the finding of COLEMAN and BARNET (1969) of an increased noradrenaline output after intravenous L-DOPA in a child with dystonia is at variance with the general pattern and is difficult to explain. There is no increase, for instance, in brain noradrenaline in the experimental animal after L-DOPA administration (BARTHOLINI and PLETSCHER, 1968; BUTCHER and ENGEL, 1969; EVERETT and BORCHERDING, 1970). In view of these findings, treating a parkinsonian patient on L-DOPA therapy with a dopamine β-hydroxylase inhibitor (BRAHAM, 1970; SERRANO, 1970) probably has little to recommend it; this conclusion has especial force in view of the finding of THOENEN et al. (1967) who noted that disulfiram, a dopamine β-hydroxylase inhibitor, decreases noradrenaline concentration without giving rise to a compensatory increase in dopamine.

Urinary dopamine output itself is greatly increased after ingestion of L-DOPA. Estimates of output vary from 3% of the dose (GOODWIN et al., 1970b) to considerably more (ANDÉN et al., 1970d), whilst COTZIAS et al. (1969b) suggest that output rises with increasing dose of the drug. This finding presumably stems to some extent from direct renal decarboxylation of DOPA by decarboxylase located in the capillaries of the kidney (CONSTANTINIDIS et al., 1969), a phenomenon which has been recognized for many years (HOLTZ et al., 1942). Measuring the output of free dopamine in the urine should be a useful index of decarboxylase activity and hence of the efficacy of decarboxylase-inhibiting drugs. After intravenous DOPA administration, RINNE and SONNINEN (1970) noted a reduced conversion to dopamine in patients with postencephalitic parkinsonism, a finding which suggests that more careful inquiry might be pursued into the decarboxylase status of patients in this sub-group.

About half the urinary dopamine, during L-DOPA treatment, is excreted as free amine and the rest in conjugated form (ANDÉN et al., 1970d). This finding appears to be a pointer to the degree of dopamine generated by DOPA decarboxylation in the gut, for ingested monoamines, in contrast with those administered parenterally, are characteristically conjugated to an appreciable extent (see MORGAN et al., 1969).

4. N-Acetylation: Possible Enterohepatic Circulation

TYCE (1970) in perfusion experiments on isolated rat liver, noted significant concentrations of N-acetyldopamine and its O-methylated metabolite in the bile, although GOODWIN (1971) was unable to detect these compounds in the urine of parkinsonian subjects during L-DOPA treatment. This finding is in contrast with their occasional presence in urine from patients with catecholamine-secreting tumours (SEKERIS and HERRLICH, 1963; HANSON and VON STUDNITZ, 1965). It seems possible, therefore, that if these compounds are produced in the human liver and excreted into the bile, they are reabsorbed from the gut and perhaps further metabolised. Less than 2% of radioactivity from a dose of labelled L-DOPA is excreted in the stool (MORGAN et al., 1970b; PEASTON and BIANCHINE, 1970). It would seem important to subject to analysis samples of bile from patients being treated with this drug.

In insects, N-acetyldopamine plays an important role as cuticle sclerotizing agent (see SEKERIS and KARLSON, 1966). It is just conceivable that it may, in man, contribute to melanogenesis.

5. The Role of Transamination

Mention has already been made (p. 851) of the observation of BARTHOLINI et al. (1970a) that catecholamines and DOPA activate the tyrosine transaminase of rat liver. They observed, in consequence, a decrease in plasma tyrosine and it is interesting, therefore, that VAN WOERT and BOWERS (1970) have noted a reduction in circulating tyrosine level in parkinsonian patients under treatment with L-DOPA. BARTHOLINI et al. (1970a) also found further *in vivo* evidence of facilitated transamination in their experimental animals, an increase in the urinary output of *p*-hydroxyphenylpyruvic acid. This observation provides an experimental counterpart to a clinical observation of CALNE et al. (1969a) who during L-DOPA treatment, detected an increased urinary output of *p*-hydroxyphenyllactic acid, the immediate reduction product (WEBER and ZANNONI, 1966) of *p*-hydroxyphenylpyruvic acid. Thus L-DOPA therapy seems to facilitate transamination. Untreated parkinsonian patients, in any event, tend to have an increased urinary output of *p*-hydroxyphenylpyruvic acid (HONOS et al., 1970), a non-specific manifestation perhaps, of connective tissue changes associated with long-standing disease (McCANN et al., 1967).

CALNE et al. (1969a) also found increased amounts of 4-hydroxy-3-methoxyphenyllactic acid, once again the immediate reduction product of the corresponding pyruvate (Fig. 6), in the urine of patients during L-DOPA treatment. They noted that approximately 1% of the dose was converted to the transamination product, although rather less was found by O'GORMAN et al. (1970) in acute feeding experiments. SMITH (1967) noted a small excretion of the pyruvate after acute DOPA ingestion. Thus the degradation of L-DOPA by transamination (see p. 867) is a relatively minor metabolic pathway. Conversion of 3,4-dihydroxyphenylpyruvic acid to L-DOPA, presumably by the same enzyme, appears to take place with greater facility (POGRUND et al., 1961; GEY, 1965). The metabolism of L-DOPA by this route is likely to achieve greater importance after peripheral decarboxylase inhibition, although to the reviewer's knowledge, relevant measurements have not so far been carried out.

6. The Special Properties of 3-O-methylDOPA

During a recent investigation in normal subjects, involving the ingestion of single high doses of L-DOPA, whilst the major urinary acidic metabolites, homovanillic acid and dihydroxyphenylacetic acid, showed peak urinary excretion soon after the dose was administered, maximal output of 4-hydroxy-3-methoxyphenyllactic acid was not achieved until the 6—9 hours post-ingestion urine sample (KAROUM et al., 1971). A likely explanation of this finding is that it predominantly represents the further metabolism of 3-O-methylDOPA. This compound is formed from L-DOPA in the tissues and disappears extremely slowly (PLETSCHER et al., 1967; BARTHOLINI and PLETSCHER, 1968; KURUMA et al., 1970): its biological half-life is much longer than that of L-DOPA, 12—13 hours compared with about 0.5 hour (BARTHOLINI and PLETSCHER, 1968). It is eliminated poorly and metabolized slowly. Its slow metabolism, in turn, seems to be a consequence of 3-O-methylDOPA being a poor substrate for DOPA decarboxylase (Ferrini and Glässer, 1964), although the finding of homovanillic acid as a metabolite (Bartholini et al., 1970b) indicates that decarboxylation at some stage does take place. Bartholini et al. (1970b) also identified the transamination product (Fig. 6), 4-hydroxy-3-methoxyphenyllactic acid, as a major metabolite of 3-O-methyl-DOPA; its delayed appearance in human urine after oral DOPA (Karoum et al., 1971) is consistent with an origin, in part at least, from this source.

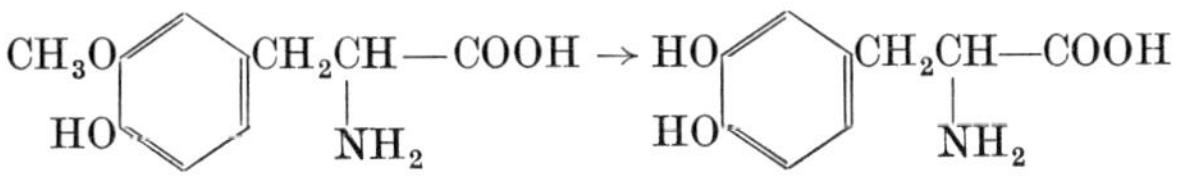

CH_3O, HO–C_6H_3–$CH_2CH(NH_2)$–COOH → HO, HO–C_6H_3–$CH_2CH(NH_2)$–COOH

Fig. 8. Demethylation of O-methyl DOPA to regenerate DOPA

Very recently, Bartholini et al. (1970c) presented evidence to show that 3-O-methylDOPA may be demethylated *in vivo*, DOPA being slowly regenerated (Fig. 8). No information is yet available about the site of this transformation*. The urinary homovanillic acid noted after administration of 3-O-methylDOPA may thus stem from this source. The observation is likely to have important consequences: 3-O-methylDOPA penetrates readily into the tissues of the body, including the brain; some preliminary observations by Tissot (1970), in fact, suggest that it can be used successfully instead of L-DOPA in the treatment of parkinsonism, presumably providing a depot supply of L-DOPA to be slowly released in the brain. This early report also mentioned that such a treatment appears to be relatively free from side-effects. Further information is awaited with interest**.

7. p-Dehydroxylation: the Role of Gut Flora

Calne et al. (1969a) found an increased excretion of *m*-hydroxyphenylacetic acid in parkinsonian patients during treatment with L-DOPA; this compound had previously been found in the urine of experimental animals after feeding them with DOPA (DeEds et al., 1957). Whilst it is possible that trace *m*-hydroxylation of phenylalanine, in addition to *p*-hydroxylation, is carried out by phenylalanine hydroxylase (Coulson et al., 1968), it seems clear that the excretion of *m*-hydroxylated compounds after DOPA administration is the result of bacterial *p*-dehydroxylation (Scheline, 1968). Thus, a suspension of human (Booth and Williams, 1963a) or animal (Booth and Williams, 1963a, b) faeces can bring about this change in a variety of phenolic acids *in vitro*; conversely *p*-dehydroxylation of caffeic acid does not occur in germ-free rats (Scheline and Midtvedt, 1970) whilst neomycin suppresses the production of *m*-hydroxylated acids from dietary (Asatoor et al., 1967) or orally administered catechol acids in man (Shaw et al., 1961) or experimental animal (Dacre and Williams, 1968; Dacre

* Note added in proof: Recent work indicates that such demethylation, at least in the rat, occurs solely by the action of gut flora (Chalmers, J.P., Davies, D.S., Draffan, G.H., Reid, J.L., Thorgeirsson, S.S.: Demethylation of 3-O-methyldopa. Brit. J. Pharmacol. **43**, 455P—456P (1971)).

** Note added in proof: Latest evidence would suggest that the treatment has not fulfilled its original promise (De Ajuriaguerra, J., Gauthier, G., Geissbuhler, F., Simona, B., Constantinidis, J., Yanniotis, G., Krassoievitch, M., Eisenring, J.-J., Tissot, R.: Thérapeutique substitutive des syndromes de Parkinson. Résultats insuffisants de l'administration de la 3-O-méthyldopa. Presse méd. **79**, 1396 (1971)).

et al., 1968). The increased urinary output of *m*-hydroxyphenylacetic acid during L-DOPA therapy can similarly be suppressed by neomycin (SANDLER et al., 1969a). Although DEEDS et al. (1957) assumed that the increased production of this acid which they observed derived from *p*-dehydroxylation of dihydroxyphenylacetic acid, and indeed, much of the experimental work quoted above has employed a catechol acid as substrate, SANDLER et al. (1971b) have recently shown that dehydroxylation may take place at an earlier metabolic stage. They detected increased amounts of metatyramine in the urine of patients taking L-DOPA and observed that its production could be suppressed with neomycin. Thus, *p*-dehydroxylation must have occurred either at the dopamine stage or, more likely, by the transformation of L-DOPA itself, to form metatyrosine (Fig. 9).

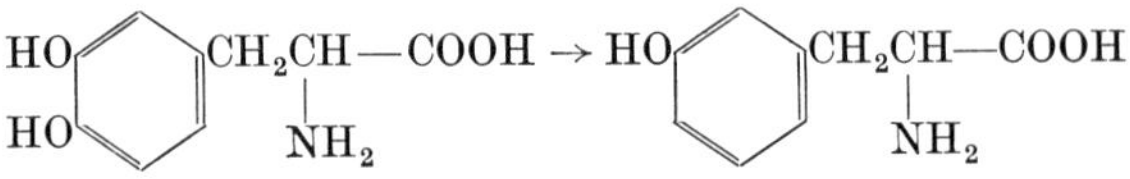

HO, HO (ring) $CH_2CH(NH_2)$—COOH → HO (ring) $CH_2CH(NH_2)$—COOH

Fig. 9. *p*-Dehydroxylation of L-DOPA

Attention has earlier been drawn to the fact that certain features of the clinical response to L-DOPA are difficult to explain by assuming that the active agent is dopamine alone; it was suggested that certain minor metabolites might contribute to the therapeutic action (p. 873). In this connexion, metatyrosine is of great interest, for it possesses pharmacological properties which make it worthy of further study. Its excitation effect in experimental animals (MITOMA et al., 1957; BLASCHKO and CHRUSCIEL, 1960) presumably stems from its ability to cross the blood-brain barrier to be converted rapidly to metatyramine (ANDÉN et al., 1970b). It is an excellent substrate for DOPA decarboxylase (BLASCHKO et al., 1949; FERRINI and GLÄSSER, 1964). One action of metatyrosine which may be of particular importance in the context of the present discussion is its ability to protect dopamine stores in the brain against depletion by reserpine (CARLSSON and LINDQVIST, 1967; ANDÉN et al., 1970c). Although the build-up of dopamine noted by CARLSSON and LINDQVIST after metatyrosine administration is open to another interpretation, that the former may derive synthetically from the latter, it has not been possible to confirm in the author's laboratory (GOODWIN, 1971) the claim of SOURKES et al. (1961) that a proportion of administered metatyrosine in the rat is actually coverted to dopamine; metatyrosine is not, in any case a substrate for tyrosine hydroxylase (NAGATSU et al., 1964b). It may be relevant that another *m*-hydroxylated amine, metaraminol, provides protection against the nerve degeneration action of 6-hydroxydopamine (BENNETT et al., 1970). If idiopathic parkinsonism derives from the action of some unknown, perhaps endogenously formed, reserpine or 6-hydroxydopamine-like substance (see p. 856), as is just conceivable, it follows that metatyrosine may have a synergistic role to play in maintaining the levels of dopamine accumulated from L-DOPA during the treatment of parkinsonism.

Apart from its ability to protect monoamine stores from depletion, metatyrosine possesses, in common with other potentially active metabolites synthesized by gut flora from inactive compounds (SMITH, 1971), one further characteristic: its production, to gauge from metatyramine (SANDLER et al., 1971b) and *m*-hydroxyphenylacetic acid (SANDLER et al., 1969a) generation, is likely to be extremely variable, corresponding with the presence of appropriate gut flora in a particular individual. If the bacterial production of cyclohexylamine from cyclamate (SMITH, 1971) may be quoted as a precedent, this ability may later be acquired during chronic ingestion of substrate for the bacterial enzyme, in this case L-DOPA.

Translated into terms of clinical practice, the response to oral L-DOPA in parkinsonism varies considerably from patient to patient (e. g. YAHR, 1970c). Some patients respond rapidly, others may only obtain benefit after many weeks, whilst another group may fail to respond altogether. Whilst such unpredictability may derive from an inability to build up an effective local concentration of dopamine, for a variety of possible reasons including defective enzymatic or non-enzymatic (see p. 868) striatal decarboxylation, it might equally stem from a capricious production of metatyrosine, insufficient on occasions to provide enough metatyramine to *maintain* adequate striatal dopamine levels.

If this hypothesis were correct, it follows that there should be a correlation between production of *m*-hydroxylated metabolites and clinical response to L-DOPA in parkinsonian patients: this possibility has yet to be investigated. There would be another important consequence: L-DOPA therapy, supplemented by oral metatyrosine, should achieve better clinical results than L-DOPA alone. Very early in the present phase of parkinsonian studies BARBEAU et al. (1962) gave oral metatyrosine to affected patients and briefly recorded a degree of improvement, although not on the scale of that achieved by DOPA. Similarly BIRKMAYER and HORNYKIEWICZ (1964) gave intravenous metatyrosine to a few parkinsonian subjects but were deterred from further study by a marked hypertensive response, presumably from the metatyramine generated in the process (POGRUND et al., 1961). The author and his colleagues have just begun a trial of oral metatyrosine in parkinsonism.

8. Interrelationships with 5-Hydroxytryptamine

5-Hydroxytryptamine concentrations tend to be low in the brain of the parkinsonian patient (BERNHEIMER et al., 1961). The level increases after MAO inhibitors have been given, in contrast with dopamine, which remains unaltered (BERNHEIMER et al., 1963). When L-DOPA is administered to the experimental animal, there is a decrease in cerebral 5-hydroxytryptamine (BARTHOLINI et al., 1968; BUTCHER and ENGEL, 1969; EVERETT and BORCHERDING, 1970). The most likely cause seems to be a displacement of 5-hydroxytryptamine from its storage sites by the large excess of dopamine (KOPIN, 1970), for NG et al. (1970) have demonstrated that L-DOPA, by virtue of the dopamine synthesized from it, displaces the tritiated amine from brain slices. Presumably it displaces other monoamines indiscriminately; it might be worth, for instance, examining the effects of L-DOPA on octopamine concentration in brain (MOLINOFF and AXELROD, 1969). There are, however, at least two other possible explanations; competition of L-DOPA for amino acid transport (GERSTENBRAND and GRUNDIG, 1970) with the precursor of 5-hydroxytryptamine, 5-HTP; and inhibition of tryptophan hydroxylase by L-DOPA or dopamine (JÉQUIER et al., 1969), so that 5-HTP production is inhibited. Neither mechanism would account for the decreased 5-hydroxytryptamine concentration noted in the blood platelets of parkinsonian subjects after L-DOPA treatment (BOULLIN and O'BRIEN, 1970), where uptake competition with dopamine (SOLOMON et al., 1970) presumably exists.

Apart from measuring 5-hydroxytryptamine concentration in platelets, assessment of 5-hydroxyindole metabolism in patients on L-DOPA therapy has been confined to an examination of 5-hydroxyindoleacetic acid, the major metabolite of 5-hydroxytryptamine, in the cerebrospinal fluid and urine. It tends to be reduced in concentration in the former (VAN WOERT and BOWERS, 1970).

An early claim that 5-hydroxyindoleacetic acid output is decreased in parkinsonism (BARBEAU and JASMIN, 1961) has been disputed by RESNICK et al. (1962). These workers were also unable to detect any difference in urinary 5-hydroxyindole metabolite output between parkinsonian and normal subjects after intravenous 5-HTP injection. After L-DOPA therapy, there appears to be a decrease in 5-hydroxyindoleacetic acid excretion (TYCE et al., 1970). In general, therefore, it seems likely that a decreased concentration of 5-hydroxytryptamine is present in the brains of parkinsonian subjects, stemming partially from displacement by dopamine and partially from inhibition of production.

It does not seem possible in the present state of our knowledge to identify any specific consequence of this deficit, even though SONNEVILLE (1968) claims that in certain anatomical sites, dopamine acts by releasing 5-hydroxytryptamine from its binding sites. SCHECKEL et al. (1969) considered that 5-hydroxytryptamine is necessary for the stimulant action L-DOPA possesses when given in combination with a peripheral decarboxylase inhibitor in the rat, for it could be prevented by the tryptophan hydroxylase inhibitor, *p*-chlorophenylalanine and restored with 5-HTP. An important observation was made by GOLDSTEIN et al. (1969), who noted that 5-HTP protects against the tremor produced by harmaline in the "lesioned" monkey. The findings in this parkinsonian model seemed to fit in well with the statement added as a postscript to the classical paper of BIRKMAYER and HORNYKIEWICZ (1961) that intravenous 5-HTP "seems to alleviate certain deficits of the parkinsonian syndrome". Dramatic clinical improvement had also been effected by oral 5-HTP in one patient with manganese parkinsonism, whose condition had deteriorated during L-DOPA therapy (MENA et al., 1970). However, indifferent results were obtained with 5-HTP in parkinsonian subjects by COTZIAS et al. (1968) and this report was followed by COLEMAN and BARNET'S (1969) description of a child with a dystonic syndrome who deteriorated on 5-HTP but responded to L-DOPA. Very recently, CHASE (1970) demonstrated quite unequivocally that L-5-HTP, given in combination with a peripheral decarboxylase inhibitor to increase its effective central concentration, brought about a sharp deterioration in four parkinsonian patients. Deterioration was similarly observed (HUNTER and STERN, 1971) in one parkinsonian patient being treated with large amounts of L-tryptophan, which on theoretical grounds, are likely to give rise to an increased formation of 5-hydroxyindoles (PETERS et al., 1968). It would seem that the harmaline tremor in the experimental preparation of GOLDSTEIN et al. (1969e) is not a good model of the parkinsonian situation. Why the patient of MENA et al. (1970), who differed from the DOPA-responsive subjects studied by these authors by being hypotonic, improved on 5-HTP therapy can only be decided in the future on the basis of careful clinical observation.

VI. Some Further Problems

The author is well aware that many other problems in this research area remain to be resolved. What is the nature of the unknown brain metabolite noted by SCHECKEL et al. (1969) in their imaginative paper and how are we to interpret the many puzzling drug interactions they describe? Why does tolbutamide promote the production in the guinea pig of *m*-hydroxyphenylacetic acid from a number of related compounds including dopamine (SMITH et al., 1964)? What is the effect of dietary constituents, e. g. coffee, which contains a fairly powerful decarboxylase inhibitor, caffeic acid (HARTMAN et al., 1955), on the response to L-DOPA? What of the effect of glucocorticoids on dopamine metabolism (KORDUBA et al., 1970)? Is there a place for γ-hydroxybutyric acid, which gives rise to an increased concentration of striatal dopamine (GESSA et al., 1966) in the treatment of parkinsonism? Are there any clinical consequences of the ability of L-DOPA to potentiate endometrial MAO (COLLINS et al., 1970a)? The L-DOPA treatment of parkinsonism, which has completely changed the outlook of the disease, accustoms us to be on the watch for answers of potential clinical usefulness to even the most academic of questions.

References

ABRAMS, W.B., SOLOMON, H.M.: The human platelet as a pharmacologic model for the adrenergic neuron. Clin. Pharmacol. Ther. **10**, 702—709 (1969).

ALM, P., EHINGER, B., FALCK, B.: Histochemical studies on the metabolism of L-DOPA and some related substances in the exocrine pancreas. Acta physiol. scand. **76**, 106—120 (1969).

ANAGNOSTE, B., GOLDSTEIN, M.: The metabolism of tyramine-H^3 in different regions of the CNS. Life Sci. **6**, 1535—1540 (1967).

ANDÉN, N.E., BUTCHER, S.G., CORRODI, H., FUXE, K., UNGERSTEDT, U.: Receptor activity and turnover of dopamine and noradrenaline after neuroleptics. Europ. J. Pharmacol. **11**, 303—314 (1970a).

— — ENGEL, J.: Central dopamine and noradrenaline receptor activity of the amines formed from *m*-tyrosine, *a*-methyl-*m*-tyrosine and *a*-methyldopa. J. Pharm. Pharmacol. **22**, 548—550 (1970b).

— — FUXE, K.: Protection of the neostriatal dopamine stores against reserpine by local treatment with metatyramine. Acta pharmacol. (Kbh.) **28**, 39—48 (1970c).

— CARLSSON, A., DAHLSTROM, A., FUXE, K., HILLARP, N.-A., LARSSON, K.: Demonstration and mapping out of nigro-neostriatal dopamine neurons. Life Sci. **3**, 523—530 (1964a).

— — KERSTELL, J., MAGNUSSON, T., OLSSON, R., ROOS, B.E., STEEN, B., STEG, G., SVANBORG, A., THIEME, G., WERDINIUS, B.: Oral L-dopa treatment of parkinsonism. Acta med. scand. **187**, 247—255 (1970d).

— ROOS, B.-E., WERDINIUS, B.: On the occurrence of homovanillic acid and 3-methoxy-4-hydroxymandelic acid in human cerebrospinal fluid. Experientia (Basel) **19**, 359—360 (1963a).

— — — Effects of chlorpromazine, haloperidol and reserpine on the levels of phenolic acids in rabbit corpus striatum. Life Sci. **3**, 149—158 (1964b).

ANDERSON, P.J., D'IORIO, A.: Purification and properties of catechol-*O*-methyltransferase. Biochem. Pharmacol. **17**, 1943—1949 (1968).

ANDREWS, R.S., PRIDHAM, J.B.: Melanins from DOPA-containing plants. Phytochemistry **6**, 13—18 (1967).

ANLYAN, W.G., HARGROVE, M.D., JR., RUFFIN, J.M., WALLACE, D.K., WEAVER, W.T., KIRSHNER, N.: Metastasizing bronchial adenoma. Occurrence in patient with the functioning carcinoid syndrome. J. Amer. med. Ass. **174**, 415—417 (1960).

ANSEL, R.D., MARKHAM, C.H.: Effects of L-dopa in normal humans. In: L-Dopa and Parkinsonism, pp. 69—72, edit. A. BARBEAU and F.H. MCDOWELL. Philadelphia: Davis 1970.

ANTON, A.H., GREER, M., SAYRE, D.F., WILLIAMS, C.M.: Dihydroxyphenylalanine secretion in a malignant pheochromocytoma. Amer. J. Med. **42**, 469—475 (1967).

ANTUNES, J.L., MACEDO, C., DAMASIO, A.R.: Levodopa and migraine Lancet **ii**, 928 (1970).

ARAKAWA, T., WADA, Y., TADA, K., ITO, H.: Hyperpigmentation of the skin with DOPA-uria of a newborn. (A peculiar sign of an infant born of a thyrotoxic mother treated with methimazole.) Tohoku J. exp. Med. **80**, 329—337 (1963).

ARMSTRONG, M.D., MCMILLAN, A., SHAW, K.N.F.: 3-Methoxy-4-hydroxy-D-mandelic acid, a urinary metabolite of norepinephrine. Biochim. biophys. Acta (Amst.) **25**, 422—423 (1957).

ASATOOR, A.M., CHAMBERLAIN, M.J., EMMERSON, B.T., JOHNSON, J.R., LEVI, A.J., MILNE, M.D.: Metabolic effects of oral neomycin. Clin. Sci. **33**, 111—124 (1967).

AXELROD, J.: Metabolism of epinephrine and other sympathomimetic amines. Physiol. Rev. **39**, 751—776 (1959).

— Methylation reactions in the formation and metabolism of catecholamines and other biogenic amines. Pharmacol. Rev. **18**, 95—113 (1966).

— Discussion on paper of CHASE, T.N.: Neurology **20**, 130 (1970).

— TOMCHICK, R.: Enzymatic 0-methylation of epinephrine and other catechols. J. biol. Chem. **233**, 702—705 (1958).

BARBEAU, A.: Biochemistry of Parkinson's disease. Proc. 7th int. Congr. Neurol., Rome, Vol. 2, Societa Grafica Romana, Rome, p. 925 (1961).

Barbeau, A.: The pathogenesis of Parkinson's disease: a new hypothesis. Canad. med. Ass. J. **87**, 802—807 (1962).
— Parkinson's disease as a systemic disorder. In: Third Symposium on Parkinson's Disease, pp. 66—73, edit. F. J. Gillingham and I. M. L. Donaldson. Edinburgh: Livingstone 1969a.
— L-dopa therapy in Parkinson's disease: a critical review of nine years experience. Canad. med. Ass. J. **101**, 791—800 (1969b).
— Rationale for the use of L-dopa in the torsion dystonias. Neurology **20**, 96—102 (1970a).
— Functions of the striatum. A new proposal based on experience with L-DOPA in extrapyramidal disorders. Proc. 4th Bel-Air Symposium, Geneva (1970b) (in the press).
— De Groot, J.A., Joly, J.G., Raymond-Tremblay, D., Donaldson, J.: Urinary excretion of a 3-4, dimethoxyphenylethylamine-like substance in Parkinson's disease. Rev. canad. Biol. **22**, 469—472 (1963).
— Friesen, H.: Treatment of Wilson's disease with L-dopa after failure with penicillamine Lancet **i**, 1180—1181 (1970).
— Gillo-Joffroy, L., Boucher, R., Nowaczynski, W., Genest, J.: Renin-aldosterone system in Parkinson's disease. Science **165**, 291—292 (1969).
— Jasmin, G.: Dosage de l'acide 5-hydroxyindoleacétique urinaire dans la maladie de Parkinson. Rev. canad. Biol. **20**, 837—838 (1961).
— McDowell, F.H. edit: L-Dopa and Parkinsonism, pp. 1—433. Philadelphia: Davis 1970.
— Murphy, G.F., Sourkes, T.L.: Excretion of dopamine in diseases of the basal ganglia. Science **133**, 1706—1707 (1961).
— Singh, P., Gaudreau, P., Joubert, M.: Effect of 3,4-dimethoxyphenylethylamine injections on the concentration of catecholamines in the rat brain. Rev. canad. Biol. **24**, 229—232 (1965).
— Sourkes, T.L., Murphy, G.F.: Les catécholamines dans la maladie de Parkinson. In: Monoamines et système nerveux central, pp. 247—262, edit. J. de Ajuriaguerra. Genève: Georg 1962.
— Trombitas, S.: The metabolism of tritium labelled dopamine in parkinsonian patients. In: Progress in Neuro-genetics, pp. 352—356, edit. A. Barbeau and J.-R. Brunette, Int. Congr. Series 175. Amsterdam: Excerpta Med. Fndn. 1969.
Barger, G., Dale, H.H.: Chemical structure and sympathomimetic action of amines. J. Physiol. (Lond.) **41**, 19—59 (1910).
Barolin, G.S., Bernheimer, H., Hornykiewicz, O.: Seitenverschiedenes Verhalten des Dopamins (3-Hydroxytyramin) in Gehirn eines Falles von Hemiparkinsonismus. Schweiz. Arch. Neurol. Neurochir. Psychiat. **94**, 241—248 (1964).
— Hornykiewicz, O.: Zur diagnostischen Wertigkeit der Homovanillinsäure im Liquor cerebrospinalis. Wien. klin. Wschr. **79**, 815—818 (1967).
Bartholini, G., Da Prada, M., Pletscher, A.: Decrease of cerebral 5-hydroxytryptamine by 3,4-dihydroxyphenylalanine after inhibition of extracerebral decarboxylase. J. Pharm. Pharmacol. **20**, 228—229 (1968).
— Gey, K.F., Pletscher, A.: Enhancement of tyrosine transamination in vivo by catecholamines. Experientia (Basel) **26**, 980—981 (1970a).
— Kuruma, I., Pletscher, A.: Distribution and metabolism of L-3-0-methyldopa in rats. Brit. J. Pharmacol. **40**, 461—467 (1970b).
— Pletscher, A.: Cerebral accumulation and metabolism of C^{14}-dopa after selective inhibition of peripheral decarboxylase. J. Pharmacol. exp. Ther. **161**, 14—20 (1968).
— — Effect of various decarboxylase inhibitors on the cerebral metabolism of dihydroxyphenylalanine. J. Pharm. Pharmacol. **21**, 323—324 (1969).
— — Kuruma, I.: New approaches for enhancing the dopamine content in the basal ganglia. Proc. 4th Bel-Air Symposium, Geneva, 1970 (In the press).
Battista, A.F., Goldstein, M., Nakatani, S., Anagnoste, B.: The effects of ventrolateral thalamic lesions on tremor and the biosynthesis of dopamine in monkeys with lesions in the ventromedial tegmentum. J. Neurosurg. **31**, 164—171 (1969).
Bédard, P., Larochelle, L., Parent, A., Poirier, L.J.: The nigrostriatal pathway: a correlative study based on neuroanatomical and neurochemical criteria in the cat and the monkey. Exp. Neurol. **25**, 365—377 (1969).
— — Poirier, L.J., Sourkes, T.L.: Reversible effect of L-DOPA on tremor and catatonia induced by a-methyl-p-tyrosine. Canad. J. Physiol. Pharmacol. **48**, 82—84 (1970).
Behringer, K., Wilmanns, K.: Zur Harmin-Banisterin-Frage. Dtsch. med. Wschr. **55**, 2081—2086 (1929).
Bernheimer, H.: Distribution of homovanillic acid in the human brain. Nature (Lond.) **204**, 587—588 (1964).
— Birkmayer, W., Hornykiewicz, O.: Verteilung des 5-Hydroxytryptamins (Serotonin) im Gehirn des Menschen und sein Verhalten bei Patienten mit Parkinsonsyndrom. Klin. Wschr. **39**, 1056—1059 (1961).

Bernheimer, H., Birkmayer, W., Hornykiewicz, O.: Zur Biochemie des Parkinson-Syndroms des Menschen. Einfluß der Monoaminoxydase-Hemmer-Therapie auf die Konzentration des Dopamins, Noradrenalins und 5-Hydroxytryptamins im Gehirn. Klin. Wschr. **41**, 465—469 (1963).

— — — Homovanillinsäure im liquor cerebrospinalis: Untersuchungen beim Parkinson-Syndrom und anderen Erkrankungen des ZNS. Klin. Wschr. **78**, 417—419 (1966).

— — — Jellinger, K., Seitelberger, F.: Zur Differenzierung des Parkinson-Syndroms: Biochemisch-neurohistologische Vergleichsuntersuchungen. Proc. 8th int. Congr. Neurol., Vienna, Vol. 4, Pt. I, Wiener medizinischen Akademie, Wien, 1965, pp. 145—148.

— — — — — Paper presented at the 9th International Congress of Neurology, New York, 1969.

— Hornykiewicz, O.: Das Verhalten einiger Enzyme im Gehirn normaler und Parkinson-kranker Menschen. Arch. exp. Pathol. Pharmakol. **243**, 295 (1962).

— — Monoaminoxydase-Hemmer und Dopamin-, Noradrenalin- und 5-Hydroxytryptamin-Stoffwechsel im Gehirn Parkinson-kranker Menschen. Arch. exp. Pathol. Pharmakol. **245**, 52 (1963).

— — Das Verhalten des Dopamin-Metaboliten Homovanillinsäure im Gehirn von normalen und Parkinson-kranken Menschen. Arch. exp. Pathol. Pharmakol. **247**, 305—306 (1964).

— — Wirkung von Phenothiazinderivaten auf den Dopamin- (= 3-Hydroxytyramin) Stoffwechsel im Nucleus caudatus. Arch. exp. Pathol. Pharmakol. **251**, 135—136 (1965a).

— — Herabgesetzte Konzentration der Homovanillinsäure im Gehirn von Parkinson-kranken Menschen als Ausdruck der Störung des zentralen Dopaminstoffwechsels. Klin. Wschr. **43**, 711—715 (1965b).

— — Dopaminumsatz im Gehirn von normalen und parkinsonkranken Menschen. Wien. Z. Nervenheilk. **23**, 110—114 (1966).

Bertler, A., Falck, B., Owman, C., Rosengren, E.: The localization of monoaminergic blood-brain barrier mechanisms. Pharmacol. Rev. **18**, 369—385 (1966).

Bettag, W., Holbach, K.H.: Effect of L-dopa on different symptoms of Parkinson's disease. In: Third Symposium on Parkinson's Disease, pp. 181—184, edit. F.J. Gillingham and I.M.L. Donaldson. Edinburgh: Livingstone 1969.

Birkmayer, W.: Der α-Methyl-P-Tyrosin-Effekt bei extrapyramidalen Erkrankungen. Wien. klin. Wschr. **81**, 10—12 (1969a).

— Experimentelle Ergebnisse über die Kombinationsbehandlung des Parkinson-syndroms mit L-DOPA und einen Decarboxylasehemmer (Ro 4-4602). Wien. klin. Wschr. **81**, 677—679 (1969b).

— Failures in L-dopa therapy. In: L-Dopa and Parkinsonism, pp. 12—16, edit. A. Barbeau and F.H. McDowell. Philadelphia: Davis 1970a.

— Hornykiewicz, O.: Der L-3,4-Dioxyphenylalanin (= DOPA)-Effekt bei der Parkinson-Akinese. Wien. klin. Wschr. **73**, 787—788 (1961).

— — Der L-Dioxyphenylalanin (= DOPA)-Effekt beim Parkinson-Syndrom des Menschen: Zur Pathogenese und Behandlung der Parkinson-Akinese. Arch. Psychiat. Nervenkr. **203**, 560—574 (1962).

— — Weitere experimentelle Untersuchungen über L-DOPA beim Parkinson-Syndrom und Reserpin-Parkinsonismus. Arch. Psychiat. Nervenkr. **206**, 367—381 (1964).

Bischoff, F., Torres, A.: Determination of urine dopamine. Clin. Chem. **8**, 370—377 (1962).

Björklund, A., Cegrell, L.: Unpublished work quoted in: Björklund, A., Cegrell, L., Falck, B. and Ritzén, M. Dopamine-containing cells in sympathetic ganglia. Acta physiol. scand. **78**, 334—338 (1970).

Blaschko, H.: The specific action of *l*-DOPA decarboxylase. J. Physiol. (Lond.) **96**, 50P—51P (1939).

— Substrate specificity of amino-acid decarboxylases. Biochim. biophys. Acta (Amst.) **4**, 130—137 (1950).

— Metabolism and storage of biogenic amines. Experientia (Basel) **13**, 9—12 (1957).

— The development of current concepts of catecholamine formation. Pharmacol. Rev. **11**, 307—316 (1959).

— Burn, J.H., Langemann, H.: The formation of noradrenaline from dihydroxyphenylserine. Brit. J. Pharmacol. **5**, 431—437 (1950).

— Chrusciel, T.L.: The decarboxylation of amino acids related to tyrosine and their awakening action in reserpine-treated mice. J. Physiol. (Lond.) **151**, 272—284 (1960).

— Holton, P., Sloane Stanley, G.H.: Enzymic formation of pressor amines. J. Physiol. (Lond.) **108**, 427—439 (1949).

Bonham Carter, S., Hunter, K.R., Laurence, D.R., Sandler, M., Stern, G.M., Youdim, M.B.H.: In preparation (1971).

— Karoum, F., Sandler, M., Youdim, M.B.H.: The effect of tyramine on phenolic acid and alcohol excretion in man. Brit. J. Pharmacol. **39**, 202P—203P (1970).

BOOTH, A.N., WILLIAMS, R.T.: Dehydroxylation of catechol acids by intestinal contents. Biochem. J. **88**, 66P—67P (1963a).
— — Dehydroxylation of caffeic acid by rat and rabbit caecal contents and sheep rumen liquor. Nature (Lond.) **198**, 684—685 (1963b).
BOUDIN, G., CASTAIGNE, P., LHERMITTE, F., BECK, H., GUILLARD, A., MARTEAU, R., PÉPIN, B., ROUDOT, P., RAPHY, B.: Traitement des syndromes parkinsoniens par la L-dopa. A propos de 77 observations. Rev. Neurol. **122**, 89—102 (1970).
BOULLIN, D.J., O'BRIEN, R.A.: Accumulation of dopamine by blood platelets from normal subjects and parkinsonian patients under treatment with L-DOPA. Brit. J. Pharmacol. **39**, 779—788 (1970).
BOULTON, A.A., POLLITT, R.J., MAJER, J.R.: Identity of a urinary 'pink spot' in schizophrenia and Parkinson's disease. Nature (Lond.) **215**, 132—134 (1967).
— QUAN, L., MAJER, J.R.: Urinary excretion and cerebral distribution of *p*-tyramine. In: L-dopa and Parkinsonism, pp. 227—231, edit. A. BARBEAU and F.H. MCDOWELL. Philadelphia: Davis 1970.
BOWERS, M.B., JR., HENINGER, G.R., GERBODE, F.: Cerebrospinal fluid 5-hydroxyindoleacetic acid and homovanillic acid in psychiatric patients. Int. J. Neuropharmacol. **8**, 255—262 (1969).
BOZZI, R., BRUNO, A., ALLEGRANZA, A.: Urinary metabolites of some monoamines and clinical effects under reserpine and chlorpromazine. Brit. J. Psychiat. **111**, 176—182 (1965).
BRAHAM, J.: Adjuvants to L-dopa for Parkinsonism. Brit. med. J. **2**, 540 (1970).
— SAROVA-PINHAS, I., CRISPIN, M., GOLAN, R., LEVIN, N., SZEINBERG, A.: Oral phenylalanine and tyrosine tolerance tests in Parkinsonian patients. Brit. med. J. **2**, 552—555 (1969).
— — GOLDHAMMER, Y.: Apomorphine in Parkinsonian tremor. Brit. med. J. **3**, 768 (1970).
BRICOLO, A., DALLE ORE, G.: Prime esperienze nel trattamento con L-dopa degli comatose prolungati posttraumatici. Sist. nerv., Fasc. **2—3**, 175—180 (1970).
BRODY, J.A., CHASE, T.N., GORDON, E.K.: Depressed monoamine catabolite levels in cerebrospinal fluid of patients with Parkinsonism dementia of Guam. New Engl. J. Med. **282**, 947—950 (1970).
BRUCK, H., GERSTENBRAND, F., GRÜNDIG, E., TEUFLMAYR, R.: Über Ergebnisse von Liquoranalysen beim Parkinson-Syndrom. Acta neuropath. (Berl.) **3**, 638—644 (1964).
BRUNO, A., BRUNO, S.C.: Effects of L-DOPA on pharmacological Parkinsonism. Acta psychiat. scand. **42**, 264—271 (1966).
BURKARD, W.P., GEY, K.F., PLETSCHER, A.: A new inhibitor of decarboxylase of aromatic amino acids. Experientia (Basel) **18**, 411—412 (1962).
BURN, J.H.: Hypotension caused by L-dopa. Brit. med. J. **1**, 629 (1970).
BUTCHER, L.L., BUTCHER, S.G., LARSSON, K.: Effects of apomorphine, (+)-amphetamine, and nialamide on tetrabenazine-induced suppression of sexual behaviour in the male rat. Europ. J. Pharmacol. **7**, 283—288 (1969).
— ENGEL, J.: Behavioural and biochemical effects of L-DOPA after peripheral decarboxylase inhibition. Brain Res. **15**, 233—242 (1969).
CALNE, D.B.: Parkinsonism: physiology, pharmacology and treatment, pp. 1—136. London: Arnold 1970.
— BRENNAN, J., SPIERS, A.S.D., STERN, G.M.: Hypotension caused by L-dopa. Brit. med. J. **1**, 474—475 (1970).
— KAROUM, F., RUTHVEN, C.R.J., SANDLER, M.: The metabolism of orally administered L-DOPA in Parkinsonism. Brit. J. Pharmacol. **37**, 57—68 (1969a).
— SANDLER, M.: L-Dopa and Parkinsonism. Nature (Lond.) **226**, 21—24 (1970).
— SPIERS, A.S.D., STERN, G.M., LAURENCE, D.R., ARMITAGE, P.: L-Dopa in idiopathic Parkinsonism. Lancet **ii**, 973—976 (1969b).
— STERN, G.M., LAURENCE, D.R., SHARKEY, J., ARMITAGE, P.: L-dopa in postencephalitic Parkinsonism. Lancet **i**, 744—747 (1969b).
CAMMARATA, P.S., COHEN, P.P.: Scope of transamination reaction in animal tissues. J. biol. Chem. **187**, 439—452 (1950).
CARLSSON, A.: The occurrence distribution and physiological role of catecholamines in the nervous system. Pharmacol. Rev. **11**, 490—493 (1959).
— Drugs which block the storage of 5-hydroxytryptamine and related amines. In: Handbuch der experimentellen Pharmakologie, Vol. 19, 5-Hydroxytryptamine and Related Indolealkylamines, pp. 529—592, edit. V. ERSPAMER. Berlin: Springer 1966.
— Biochemical implications of dopa-induced actions on the central nervous system, with particular reference to abnormal movements. In: L-dopa and Parkinsonism, pp. 205—213, edit. A. BARBEAU and F.H. MCDOWELL. Philadelphia: Davis 1970.
— LINDQVIST, M.: Metatyrosine as a tool for selective protection of catecholamine stores against reserpine. Europ. J. Pharmacol. **2**, 187—192 (1967).

CELESIA, G.G., BARR, A.N.: Psychosis and other psychiatric manifestations of levodopa therapy. Arch. Neurol. **23**, 193—200 (1970).
CHALLACOMBE, D.N., SANDLER, M., SOUTHGATE, J.: Decreased duodenal monoamine oxidase activity in coeliac disease. Arch. Dis. Childh. **46**, 213—215 (1971).
CHASE, T.N.: 5-Hydroxytryptophan in Parkinsonism. Lancet **ii**, 1029—1030 (1970).
— SCHNUR, J.A., GORDON, E.K.: Cerebrospinal fluid monoamine catabolites in drug-induced extrapyramidial disorders. Neuropharmacology **9**, 265—268 (1970).
CHERINGTON, M.: Parkinsonism, L-dopa and mental depression. J. Amer. Geriat. Soc. **18**, 513—516 (1970).
CHRISTENSON, J.G., DAIRMAN, W., UDENFRIEND, S.: Preparation and properties of a homogenous aromatic *L*-amino acid decarboxylase from hog kidney. Arch. Biochem. Biophys. **141**, 356—367 (1970).
CHRUSCIEL, M.: Changes resembling lupus erythematosus after prolonged treatment with Ro-4-4602, a potent inhibitor of 5-HTP-decarboxylase in white rats. Europ. J. Pharmacol. **8**, 192—199 (1969).
CLARK, W.G., DEL GIUDICE, J.: Principles of psychopharmacology, pp. 1—814. New York: Academic Press 1970.
COHEN, G., COLLINS, M.: Alkaloids from catecholamines in adrenal tissue: possible role in alcoholism. Science **167**, 1749—1751 (1970).
COLE, J.O., WITTENBORN, J.R. (edit.): Pharmacology of depression, pp. 1—189. Springfield: Thomas 1966.
COLEMAN, M.P., BARNET, A.: L-Dopa reversal of muscular spasm, vomiting and insomnia in a patient with an atypical form of familial dystonia. Trans. Amer. neurol. Ass. **94**, 91—93 (1969).
COLLINS, G.G.S., PRYSE-DAVIES, J., SANDLER, M., SOUTHGATE, J.: Effect of pretreatment with oestradiol, progesterone and DOPA on monoamine oxidase activity in the rat. Nature (Lond.) **226**, 642—643 (1970a).
— SANDLER, M., WILLIAMS, E.D., YOUDIM, M.B.H.: Multiple forms of human brain mitochondrial monoamine oxidase. Nature (Lond.) **225**, 817—820 (1970b).
— WEST, G.B.: The release of 3-H-dopamine from the isolated rabbit ileum. Brit. J. Pharmacol. **34**, 514—522 (1968).
CONSTANTINIDIS, J., DE LA TORRE, J.C., TISSOT, R., GEISSBUHLER, F.: La barrière capillaire pour la dopa dans le cerveau et les différents organes. Psychopharmacologia (Berl.) **15**, 75—87 (1969).
CONTRACTOR, S.F., PANIGEL, M., SANDLER, M., SOUTHGATE, J.: In preparation (1971).
COOLS, A.R., VAN ROSSUM, J.M.: Caudal dopamine and stereotype behaviour of cats. Arch. int. Pharmacodyn. **187**, 163—173 (1970).
COOPER, H.A., GUNN, J.A.: Harmalol in the treatment of parkinsonism. Lancet **ii**, 901—902 (1931).
COPPS, S.G., GERRITSEN, T., SMITH, D.W., WAISMAN, H.A.: Urinary excretion of 3,4-dihydroxyphenylalanine (DOPA) in two children of short stature with malnutrition. J. Pediat. **62**, 208—216 (1963).
COTZIAS, G.C.: Manganese, melanins and the extrapyramidal system. J. Neurosurg. **24**, 170—175 (1966).
— L-DOPA for Parkinsonism. New Engl. J. Med. **278**, 630 (1968).
— 2-Amino-4-hydroxy-6,7-dimethyl-tetrahydropteridine in Parkinson's disease. J. Amer. med. Ass. **210**, 1594 (1969).
— MENA, I., PAPAVASILIOU, P.S.: Amelioration of the dystonia of chronic manganese poisoning by L-dopa. Neurology **19**, 284—285 (1969a).
— PAPAVASILIOU, P.S.: Autoimmunity in patients treated with levodopa. J. Amer. med. Ass. **207**, 1353 (1969a).
— — GELLENE, R.: Modification of Parkinsonism: chronic treatment with L-dopa. New Engl. J. Med. **280**, 337—345 (1969b).
— — FEHLING, C., KAUFMAN, B., MENA, I.: Similarities between neurologic effects of L-dopa and of apomorphine. New Engl. J. Med. **282**, 31—33 (1970).
— — GELLENE, R., ARONSON, R.B.: Parkinsonism and dopa. Trans. Ass. Amer. Phys. **81**, 171—182 (1968).
— — VAN WOERT, M.H., SAKAMOTO, A.: Melanogenesis and extrapyramidal diseases. Fed. Proc. **23**, 713—718 (1964).
— VAN WOERT, M.H., SCHIFFER, L.M.: Aromatic amino acids and modification of Parkinsonism. New Engl. J. Med. **276**, 374—379 (1967).
COULSON, W.F., BENDER, D.A., JEPSON, J.B.: Multiple electrophoresis peaks of rat liver decarboxylases for 3,4-dihydroxyphenylalanine and 5-hydroxytryptophan. Biochem. J. **115**, 63P (1969).
— HENSON, G., JEPSON, J.B.: The production of *m*-tyrosine from L-phenylalanine by rat liver preparations. Biochim. biophys. Acta (Amst.) **156**, 135—139 (1968).

COYLE, J.T., SNYDER, S.H.: Antiparkinsonian drugs: inhibition of dopamine uptake in the corpus striatum as a possible mechanism of action. Science **166**, 899—901 (1969).
CRAWFORD, J.A., BURKHALTER, A.: L-Aromatic amino acid decarboxylase of mouse kidney. Pharmacologist **12**, 205 (1970).
CREVELING, C.R., DALGARD, N., SHIMIZU, H., DALY, J.W.: Catechol 0-methyltransferase. III. *m*- and *p*-0-methylation of catecholamines and their metabolites. Molec. Pharmacol. **6**, 691—696 (1970).
DACRE, J.C., SCHELINE, R.R., WILLIAMS, R.T.: The role of the tissues and gutflora in the metabolism of [^{14}C] homoprotocatechuic acid in the rat and rabbit. J. Pharm. Pharmacol. **20**, 619—625 (1968).
— WILLIAMS, R.T.: The role of the tissues and gut microorganisms in the metabolism of [^{14}C] protocatechuic acid in the rat. Aromatic dehydroxylation. J. Pharm. Pharmacol. **20**, 610—618 (1968).
DAHLSTRÖM, A., FUXE, K.: Evidence for the existence of monoamine-containing neurons in the central nervous system. I. Demonstration of monoamines in the cell bodies of brain stem neurons. Acta physiol. scand. **62**, Suppl. 232, pp. 1—55 (1964).
DAIRMAN, W., UDENFRIEND, S.: The effect of L-dihydroxyphenylalanine administration on the level of adrenal tyrosine hydroxylase. Pharmacologist **12**, 269 (1970).
DALY, J.W., AXELROD, J., WITKOP, B.: Dynamic aspects of enzymatic 0-methylation and demethylation of catechols *in vitro* and *in vivo*. J. biol. Chem. **235**, 1155—1159 (1960).
— BENIGNI, J., MINNIS, R., KANAOKA, Y., WITKOP, B.: Synthesis and metabolism of 6-hydroxycatecholamines. Biochemistry **4**, 2513—2525 (1965).
DAMÁSIO, A.R., ANTUNES, J.L., MACEDO, C.: L-Dopa, parkinsonism and depression. Lancet **ii**, 611—612 (1970).
DA PRADA, M., PLETSCHER, A.: Acceleration of the cerebral dopamine turnover by chlorpromazine. Experientia (Basel) **22**, 465—466 (1966).
— — Differential uptake of biogenic amines by isolated 5-hydroxytryptamine organelles of blood platelets. Life Sci. **8**, 65—72 (1969).
DAVIS, V.E., WALSH, M.J., YAMANAKA, Y.: Augmentation of alkaloid formation from dopamine by alcohol and acetaldehyde *in vitro*. J. Pharmacol. exp. Ther. **174**, 401—412 (1970).
DAVISON, A.N.: Physiological role of monoamine oxidase. Physiol. Rev. **38**, 729—747 (1958).
— SANDLER, M.: Inhibition of 5-hydroxytryptophan decarboxylase by phenylalanine metabolites. Nature (Lond.) **181**, 186—187 (1958).
DEEDS, F., BOOTH, A.N., JONES, F.T.: Methylation and dehydroxylation of phenolic compounds by rats and rabbits. J. biol. Chem. **225**, 615—621 (1957).
DEGKWITZ, R., FROWEIN, R., KULENKAMPFF, C., MOHS, V.: Über die Wirkungen des L-Dopa beim Menschen und deren Beeinflussung durch Reserpin, Chlorpromazin, Iproniazid und Vitamin B_6. Klin. Wschr. **38**, 120—123 (1960).
DE LA TORRE, J.C.: Relative penetration of L-dopa and 5-HTP through the brain barrier using dimethyl sulfoxide. Experientia (Basel) **26**, 1117—1118 (1970).
DEQUATTRO, V.L., SJOERDSMA, A.: Origin of urinary tyramine and tryptamine. Clin. chim. Acta **16**, 227—233 (1967).
DUVOISIN, R.: Cholinergic — anticholinergic antagonism in parkinsonism. Arch. Neurol. **17**, 124—136 (1967).
DUVOISIN, R.C., YAHR, M.D., COTE, L.D.: Pyridoxine reversal of L-dopa effects in Parkinsonism. Trans. Amer. neurol. Ass. **94**, 81—82 (1969).
EHRINGER, H., HORNYKIEWICZ, O.: Verteilung von Noradrenalin und Dopamin (3-Hydroxytyramin) im Gehirn des Menschen und ihr Verhalten bei Erkrankungen des extrapyramidalen Systems. Klin. Wschr. **38**, 1236—1239 (1960).
EPSTEIN, D., GUNN, J.A., VIRDEN, C.J.: The action of some amines related to adrenaline. I. Methoxyphenylethylamines. J. Physiol. (Lond.) **76**, 224—246 (1932).
ERNST, A.M.: Phenomena of the hypokinetic rigid type caused by 0-methylation of dopamine in the *para*-position. Nature (Lond.) **193**, 178—179 (1962).
— Relation between the action of dopamine and apomorphine and their 0-methylated derivatives upon the CNS. Psychopharmacologia (Berl.) **7**, 391—399 (1965).
— The role of biogenic amines in the extra-pyramidal system. Acta physiol. pharmacol. neerl. **15**, 141—154 (1969).
EVERETT, G.M., BORCHERDING, J.W.: L-Dopa: effect on concentrations of dopamine, norepinephrine and serotonin in brains of mice. Science **168**, 849—850 (1970).
EVETTS, K.D., URETSKY, N.J., IVERSEN, L.L., IVERSEN, S.D.: Effects of 6-hydroxydopamine on CNS catecholamines, spontaneous motor activity and amphetamine induced hyperactivity in rats. Nature (Lond.) **225**, 961—962 (1970).
FAULL, R.L.M., LAVERTY, R.: Changes in dopamine levels in the corpus striatum following lesions in the substantia nigra. Exp. Neurol. **23**, 332—340 (1969).

FEHLING, C.: Treatment of Parkinson's syndrome with L-DOPA, a double blind study. Acta neurol. scand. **42**, 367—372 (1966).

FEKETE, M., KURTI, A.M.: On the dopaminergic nature of the gnawing compulsion induced by apomorphine in mice. J. Pharm. Pharmacol. **22**, 377—379 (1970).

FELLMAN, J.H.: Inhibition of DOPA decarboxylase by aromatic acids associated with phenylpyruvic oligophrenia. Proc. Soc. exp. Biol. (N.Y.) **93**, 413—414 (1956).

FERRINI, R., GLÄSSER, A.: *In vitro* decarboxylation of new phenylalanine derivatives. Biochem. Pharmacol. **13**, 798—801 (1964).

FLEMING, P., MAKAR, H., HUNTER, K.R.: Levodopa in drug-induced extrapyramidal disorders. Lancet **ii**, 1186 (1970).

FONNUM, F., LARSEN, K.: Purification and properties of dihydroxyphenylalanine transaminase from guinea pig brain. J. Neurochem. **12**, 589—598 (1965).

FOTINO, S., BLAUFOX, M.D.: Renin activity and catecholamine excretion in Parkinsonism. Clin. Res. **18**, 499 (1970).

FRANZEN, F., EYSELL, K.: Biologically active amines found in man. Their biochemistry, pharmacology and pathophysiological importance, pp. 1—244. Oxford: Pergamon 1969.

FRIEDHOFF, A.J., VAN WINKLE, E.: Isolation and characterization of a compound from the urine of schizophrenics. Nature (Lond.) **194**, 897—898 (1962).

FUNK, C.: Synthesis of *dl*—3: 4-dihydroxyphenylalanine. J. Chem. Soc. **99**, 554—557 (1911).

FUXE, K., GOLDSTEIN, M., LJUNGDAHL, A.: Antiparkinsonian drugs and central dopamine neurons. Life Sci. Pt. I **9**, 811—824 (1970).

— HÖKFELT, T., NILSSON, O.: Factors involved in the control of the activity of the tuberoinfundibular dopamine neurons during pregnancy and lactation. Neuroendocrinology **5**, 257—270 (1969).

GARLAND, H., PEARCE, J.: Neurological complications of carbon monoxide poisoning. Quart. J. Med. **36**, 445—455 (1967).

GELINAS, R., PELLERIN, J., D'IORIO, A.: Biochemical observations of a chromaffine tumour. Rev. canad. Biol. **16**, 445—450 (1957).

GEORGE, H., GABAY, S.: Brain aromatic aminotransferase. I. Purification and some properties of pig brain L-phenylalanine-2-oxoglutarate aminotransferase. Biochim. biophys. Acta (Amst.) **167**, 555—566 (1968).

GERSTENBRAND, F.: Failures of L-dopa treatment. In: L-Dopa and Parkinsonism, pp. 16—20, edit. A. BARBEAU and F.H. MCDOWELL. Philadelphia: Davis 1970.

— GRÜNDIG, E.: Amino acids after L-dopa. In: L-Dopa and Parkinsonism, pp. 246—249, edit. A. BARBEAU and F.H. MCDOWELL. Philadelphia: Davis 1970.

GESSA, G.L., VARGIU, L., CRABAI, F., BOERO, G.C., CABONI, F., CAMBA, R.: Selective increase of brain dopamine induced by gamma-hydroxybutyrate. Life Sci. **5**, 1921—1930 (1966).

GEY, K.F.: 4-Hydroxyphenylpyruvat und 3,4-Dihydroxyphenylpyruvat als Noradrenalin-Vorstufen. Helv. physiol. Acta **23**, C89 (1965).

— BURKARD, W.P., PLETSCHER, A.: Variation of the norepinephrine metabolism of the rat heart with age. Gerontologia (Basel) **11**, 1—11 (1965).

— MESSIHA, F.: Einfluß der DOPA-Transaminierung auf die DOPA-Decarboxylierung *in vitro*. Experientia (Basel) **20**, 498—499 (1964).

GIBB, J.W., WEBB, J.G.: The effects of reserpine, α-methyltyrosine, and L-3,4-dihydroxyphenylalanine on brain tyrosine transaminase. Proc. nat. Acad. Sci. (Wash.) **63**, 364—369 (1969).

GITLOW, S.E., BERTANI, L.M., WILK, E., LI, B.L., DZIEDZIC, S.: Excretion of catecholamine metabolites by children with familial dysautonomia. Pediatrics **46**, 513—522 (1970).

GJESSING, L.R. (edit.): Symposium on tyrosinosis, 1966, Universitetsforlaget, Oslo, pp. 1—132 (1966).

— Biochemistry of functional neural crest tumors. Advanc. clin. Chem. **11**, 82—131 (1968).

GODWIN-AUSTEN, R.B., FREARS, C.C., BERGMANN, S., PARKES, J.D., KNILL-JONES, R.P.: Combined treatment of Parkinsonism with L-dopa and amantadine. Lancet **ii**, 383—385 (1970).

GOLDBERG, L.I., SONNEVILLE, P.F., MCNAY, J.L.: An investigation of the structural requirements for dopamine-like renal vasodilation: phenylethylamines and apomorphine. J. Pharmacol. exp. Ther. **163**, 188—197 (1968).

— YEH, B.K.: Specific block of dopamine receptors in the renal vascular bed by chlorpromazine. Abstr. 4th int. Congr. Pharmacol. Basel, p. 359 (1969).

GOLDEN, R.L., MORTATI, F.S., SCHROETER, G.A.: Levodopa, pyridoxine and burning feet. J. Amer. med. Ass. **213**, 628 (1970).

GOLDSTEIN, M., ANAGNOSTE, B., OWEN, W.S., BATTISTA, A.F.: The effects of ventromedial tegmental lesions on the biosynthesis of catecholamines in the striatum. Life Sci. **5**, 2171—2176 (1966).

— — — — The effects of ventromedial tegmental lesions on the disposition of dopamine in the caudate nucleus of the monkey. Brain Res. **4**, 298—300 (1967).

GOLDSTEIN, M., ANAGNOSTE, B., YAMAMOTO, A., FELCH, W.C., JR.: Regional distribution and metabolism of H^3-tyramine in the rat brain. J. Pharmacol. exp. Ther. **171**, 196—204 (1970a).
— BATTISTA, A.F., NAKATANI, S., ANAGNOSTE, B.: Drug-induced relief of the tremor in monkeys with mesencephalic lesions. Nature (Lond.) **224**, 382—384 (1969e).
— — — — Drug-induced relief of experimental tremor in monkeys. Neurology **20**, 89—95 (1970b).
— FREEDMAN, L.S., BACKSTROM, T.: The inhibition of catecholamine biosynthesis by apomorphine. J. Pharm. Pharmacol. **22**, 715—717 (1970c).
— FRIEDHOFF, A.J., POMERANTZ, S., CONTRERA, J.F.: The formation of 3,4-dihydroxyphenylethanol and 3-methoxy-4-hydroxyphenylethanol from 3,4-dihydroxyphenylethylamine in the rat. J. biol. Chem. **236**, 1816—1821 (1961).
— FUXE, K., BATTISTA, A.F., BACKSTROM, T., NAKATANI, S.: The effects of antiparkinsonian drugs (AP) on striatal dopamine. Fed. Proc. **29**, 680 (1970d).
GOODALL, McC.: Dihydroxyphenylalanine and hydroxytyramine in mammalian suprarenals. Acta chem. scand. **4**, 550 (1950).
— ALTON, H.: Dopamine (3-hydroxytyramine) metabolism in parkinsonism. J. clin. Invest. **48**, 2300—2308 (1969).
— HARLAN, W.R., JR., ALTON, H.: Decreased noradrenaline (norepinephrine) synthesis in neurogenic orthostatic hypotension. Circulation **38**, 592—603 (1968).
GOODWIN, B.L.: In preparation (1971).
— KAROUM, F., RUTHVEN, C.R.J., SANDLER, M.: In preparation (1971).
GOODWIN, F.K., BRODIE, H.K.H., MURPHY, D.L., BUNNEY, W.E., JR.: Administration of a peripheral decarboxylase inhibitor with L-dopa to depressed patients. Lancet **i**, 908—911 (1970a).
— — — — L-Dopa, catecholamines and behaviour: a clinical and biochemical study in depressed patients. Paper presented at Annual Meeting, Society of Biological Psychiatry, San Francisco, May 9th (1970b).
GOTTFRIES, C.G., GOTTFRIES, I., ROOS, B.E.: Homovanillic acid and 5-hydroxyindoleacetic acid in the cerebrospinal fluid of patients with senile dementia, presenile dementia and parkinsonism. J. Neurochem. **16**, 1341—1345 (1969).
GREEN, J.: The treatment of parkinsonism with L-dopa and amantadine. J. Fla. med. Ass. **57**, 28—33 (1970).
GREER, M.: L-Dopa therapy in Parkinson's disease. J. Fla. med. Ass. **57**, 23—27 (1970).
— WILLIAMS, C.M.: Dopamine metabolism in Parkinson's disease. Neurology **13**, 73—76 (1963).
GRELAK, R.P., CLARK, R., STUMP, J.M., VERNIER, V.G.: Amantadine, rimantadine, catecholamine release and parkinsonism. Pharmacologist **12**, 235 (1970a).
— — — — Amantadine-dopamine interaction: possible mode of action in Parkinsonism. Science **169**, 203—204 (1970b).
GROPPETTI, A., ALGERI, S., BLOOM, F., COSTA, E., REVUELTA, A.: Central effects of intracisternal injections of 6-hydroxy dopamine (6-HDM). Pharmacologist **11**, 275 (1969).
GUGGENHEIM, M.: Dioxyphenylalanin, eine neue Aminosäure aus Vicia faba. Z. physiol. Chem. **88**, 276—284 (1913).
GULDBERG, H.C., ASHCROFT, G.W., CRAWFORD, T.B.B.: Concentrations of 5-hydroxyindolylacetic acid and homovanillic acid in the cerebrospinal fluid of the dog before and during treatment with probenecid. Life Sci. **5**, 1571—1575 (1966).
— TURNER, J.W., HANIEH, A., ASHCROFT, G.W., CRAWFORD, T.B.B., PERRY, W.L.M., GILLINGHAM, F.J.: On the occurrence of homovanillic acid and 5-hydroxyindol-3-ylacetic acid in the ventricular CSF of patients suffering from Parkinsonism. Confin. neurol. (Basel) **29**, 73—77 (1967).
GUNNE, L.: Catecholamines and 5-hydroxytryptamine in morphine tolerance and withdrawal. Acta physiol. scand. **58**, Suppl. 204, pp. 1—91 (1963).
GUNNE, L.-M., LIDVALL, H.-F.: The urinary output of catecholamines in narcolepsy under resting conditions and following administration of dopamine, dopa and dops. Scand. J. clin. Lab. Invest. **18**, 425—430 (1966).
HAASE, H.J., JANSSEN, P.A.J.: The action of neuroleptic drugs, pp. 1—174. Amsterdam: North-Holland 1965.
HÄLLSTRÖM, T., PERSSON, T.: L-Dopa and non-emission of semen. Lancet **i**, 1231—1232 (1970).
HALUSHKA, P.V., HOFFMANN, P.C.: Does tetrahydropapaveroline contribute to the cardiovascular actions of dopamine? Biochem. Pharmacol. **17**, 1873—1880 (1968).
HANIG, J.F., MORRISON, J.M., JR., KROP, S.: Dimethyl sulfoxide (DMSO) and ethanol (EtOH) induced alteration in the permeability of the blood-brain barrier (BBB) to parenteral catecholamines in the neonate chick. Pharmacologist **12**, 223 (1970).

HANINGTON, E.: Preliminary report on tyramine headache. Brit. med. J. **2**, 550—551 (1967).
— HARPER, A.M.: The role of tyramine in the aetiology of migraine and related studies on the cerebral and extracerebral circulations. Headache **78**, 84—97 (1968).
HANSON, A., VON STUDNITZ, W.: Demonstration of urinary N-acetyldopamine in patients with neuroblastoma. Clin. chim. Acta **11**, 384—385 (1965).
HARTMAN, W.J., AKAWIE, R.I., CLARK, W.G.: Competitive inhibition of 3,4-dihydroxyphenylalanine (DOPA) decarboxylase in vitro. J. biol. Chem. **216**, 507—529 (1955).
HASSLER, R.: Zur Pathologie der Paralysis agitans und des postenzephalitischen Parkinsonismus. J. Psychol. Neurol. (Lpz.) **48**, 387—476 (1938).
— RIECHERT, T.: Indikationen und Lokalisations-Methode der gezielten Hirnoperation. Nervenarzt **25**, 441—447 (1954).
HAVERBACK, B.J., DYCE, B., THOMAS, H.V.: Indole metabolism in the malabsorption syndrome. New Engl. J. Med. **262**, 754—757 (1960).
HENNING, M.: Studies on the mode of action of α-methyldopa. Acta physiol. scand. Suppl. **322**, 1—37 (1969).
— RUBENSON, A.: Central hypotensive effect of L-3, 4-dihydroxyphenylalanine in the rat. J. Pharm. Pharmacol. **22**, 553—560 (1970).
HERMANN, H., MORNEX, R.: Human tumours secreting catecholamines. Clinical and physiopathological study of the pheochromocytomas, pp. 1—207. Oxford: Pergamon 1964.
HIPPIUS, H., LOGEMANN, G.: Zur Wirkung von Dioxyphenylalanin (L-DOPA) auf extrapyramidalmotorische Hyperkinesen nach langfristiger neuroleptischer Therapie. Arzneimittel-Forsch. **20**, 894—896 (1970).
HIRSCHMANN, J., MAYER, K.: Zur Beeinflussung der Akinese und anderer extrapyramidalmotorischer Störungen mit L-Dopa (L-Dihydroxyphenylalanin). Dtsch. med. Wschr. **89**, 1877—1880 (1964).
HOFMANN, W.W., RYAN, R.L.: A controlled study of L-DOPA in Parkinson's disease. Calif. Med. **112**, 9—14 (1970).
HOLTZ, P.: Introductory remarks. Pharmacol. Rev. **18**, 85—88 (1966).
— CREDNER, K., KOEPP, W.: Die enzymatische Entstehung von Oxytyramin im Organismus und die physiologische Bedeutung der Dopadecarboxylase. Arch. exp. Pathol. Pharmakol. **200**, 356—388 (1942).
— HEISE, R., LÜDKE, K.: Fermentativer Abbau von L-Dioxyphenylalanin (Dopa) durch Niere. Arch. exp. Pathol. Pharmakol. **191**, 87—118 (1938).
— PALM, D.: Pharmacological aspects of vitamin B_6. Pharmacol. Rev. **16**, 113—178 (1964).
— STOCK, K., WESTERMANN, E.: Pharmakologie des Tetrahydropapaverolins und seine Entstehung aus Dopamin. Arch. exp. Pathol. Pharmakol. **248**, 387—405 (1964).
— WESTERMANN, E.: Hemmung der Glutaminsäuredecarboxylase des Gehirns durch Brenzcatechinderivate. Arch. exp. Pathol. Pharmakol. **231**, 311—332 (1957).
HOLZER, G., HORNYKIEWICZ, O.: Über den Dopamin-(Hydroxytyramin-) Stoffwechsel im Gehirn der Ratte. Arch. exp. Pathol. Pharmakol. **237**, 27—33 (1959).
HONOS, E., ERICSSON, A.D., MCCANN, D.S.: Parahydroxyphenylpyruvic acid excretion in parkinsonism. Life Sci. Part I, **9**, 159—166 (1970).
HORN, A.S., COYLE, J.T., SNYDER, S.H.: Inhibition of catecholamine (CA) uptake into rat brain synaptosomes by antiparkinsonian drugs: structure-activity relationships. Pharmacologist **12**, 295 (1970).
HORNYKIEWICZ, O.: Die topische Lokalisation und das Verhalten von Noradrenalin und Dopamin (3-Hydroxytyramin) in der Substantia nigra des normalen und Parkinsonkranken Menschen. Wien klin. Wschr. **75**, 309—312 (1963).
— Dopamine (3-hydroxytyramine) and brain function. Pharmacol. Rev. **18**, 925—964 (1966).
— How does L-dopa work in Parkinsonism? In: L-Dopa and Parkinsonism, pp. 393—399, edit. A. BARBEAU and F.H. MCDOWELL, Philadelphia: Davis 1970a.
— Histochemistry, biochemistry and pharmacology of brain catecholamines in extrapyramidal syndromes in man. Proc. 4th Bel-Air Symposium, Geneva, 1970b. In the press.
HORWITZ, D., GOLDBERG, L.I., SJOERDSMA, A.: Increased blood pressure responses to dopamine and norepinephrine produced by monoamine oxidase inhibitors in man. J. Lab. clin. Med. **56**, 747—753 (1960).
— LOVENBERG, W., ENGELMAN, K., SJOERDSMA, A.: Monoamine oxidase inhibitors, tyramine and cheese. J. Amer. med. Ass. **188**, 1108—1110 (1964).
HUBERT, J.W.A., VAN ROSSUM, J.G.: An abortive form of Parkinson's Disease? Psychiat. Neurol. Neurochir. (Amst.) **72**, 525—531 (1969).
HUGHES, R.C., POLGAR, J.G., WEIGHTMAN, D., WALTON, J.N.: L-Dopa in Parkinsonism and the influence of previous thalamotomy. Brit. med. J. **1**, 7—13 (1971).
HUNTER, K.R., BOAKES, A.J., LAURENCE, D.R., STERN, G.M.: Monoamine oxidase inhibitors and L-dopa. Brit. med. J. **3**, 388 (1970a).
— STERN, G.M.: Personal communication (1971).

HUNTER, K.R., STERN, G.M., LAURENCE, D.R.: Use of levodopa with other drugs. Lancet **ii**, 1283—1285 (1970b).
— — — ARMITAGE, P.: Amantadine in parkinsonism. Lancet **i**, 1127—1129 (1970c).
— — — — Combined treatment of parkinsonism with L-dopa and amantadine. Lancet **ii**, 566 (1970d).
— — SHARKEY, J.: Levodopa in postencephalitic parkinsonism. Lancet **ii**, 1366—1367 (1970e).
HYYPPÄ, M., RINNE, U.K., SONNINEN, V.: The activating effect of L-dopa treatment on sexual functions and its experimental background. Acta neurol. scand. **46**, Suppl. 43, 223 (1970).
INGVARSSON, C.G.: Orientierende klinische Versuche zur Wirkung des Dioxyphenylalanins (l-Dopa) bei endogener Depression. Arzneimittel-Forsch. **15**, 849—852 (1965a).
INGVARSSON, G.: L-Dopa och astmatisk bronkit. Nord. Med. **74**, 1166—1167 (1965b).
JAMESON, H.D.: Pyridoxine for levodopa-induced dystonia. J. Amer. med. Ass. **211**, 1700 (1970).
JENKINS, R.: Laevo-dopa for parkinsonism. Brit. med. J. **2**, 361—362 (1970).
JENKINS, R.B., GROH, R.H.: Psychic effects from levodopa. J. Amer. med. Ass. **212**, 2265 (1970a)·
— — Mental symptoms in parkinsonian patients treated with L-dopa. Lancet **ii**, 177—180 (1970b).
JÉQUIER, E., ROBINSON, D.S., LOVENBERG, W., SJOERDSMA, A.: Further studies on tryptophan hydroxylase in rat brainstem and beef pineal. Biochem. Pharmacol. **18**, 1071—1081 (1969).
JOHANSSON, B., ROOS, B.-E.: 5-Hydroxyindoleacetic and homovanillic acid levels in the cerebrospinal fluid of healthy volunteeers and patients with Parkinson's syndrome. Life Sci. **6**, 1449—1454 (1967).
JOHNSTON, J.P.: Some observations upon a new inhibitor of monoamine oxidase in brain tissue. Biochem. Pharmacol. **17**, 1285—1297 (1968).
JONES, N.F., WALKER, G., RUTHVEN, C.R.J., SANDLER, M.: *a*-Methyl-*p*-tyrosine in the management of phaeochromocytoma. Lancet **ii**, 1105—1110 (1968).
JOYCE, D.: Changes in the 5-hydroxytryptamine content of rat, rabbit and human brain after death. Brit. J. Pharmacol. **18**, 370—380 (1962).
KÄHLER, H.J., HEILMEYER, L.: Klinik und Pathophysiologie des Karzinoids und Karzinoidsyndroms unter besonderer Berücksichtigung der Pharmakologie des 5-Hydroxytryptamins. Ergebn. inn. Med. Kinderheilk. **16**, 292—559 (1961).
KAMBERI, I.A., MICAL, R.S., PORTER, J.C.: Luteinizing hormone-releasing activity in hypophysial stalk blood and elevation by dopamine. Science **166**, 388—390 (1969).
KAROUM, F., POLIAKOFF, S., RUTHVEN, C.R.J., SANDLER, M.: To be published (1971).
KAUFMAN, S.: Coenzymes and hydroxylases: ascorbate and dopamine-*β*-hydroxylase; tetrahydropteridines and phenylalanine and tyrosine hydroxylases. Pharmacol. Rev. **18**, 61—69 (1966).
KEY, B.J., MARLEY, E.: The effect of the sympathomimetic amines on behaviour and electrocortical activity of the chicken. Electroenceph. clin. Neurophysiol. **14**, 90—105 (1962).
KIER, L.B., TRUITT, E.B., JR.: The preferred conformation of dopamine from molecular orbital theory. J. Pharmacol. exp. Ther. **174**, 94—98 (1970).
KIRSHNER, N.: Pathway of noradrenaline formation from dopa. J. biol. Chem. **226**, 821—825 (1957).
KLAWANS, H.L., JR., GARVIN, J.S., SHEKELLE, R.B.: The effect of previous anti-parkinson surgery on L-dopa treatment. Presbyterian-St. Lukes Hosp. med. Bull. **8**, 115—117 (1969).
— WEINER, W.: L-Dopa and cerebrospinal fluid homovanillic acid in parkinsonism. Proc. 2nd int. Meeting int. Soc. Neurochem., Milan, p. 245 (1969).
KLERMAN, G.L., SCHILDKRAUT, J.J., HASENBUSH, L.L.: Clinical experiences with dihydroxyphenylalanine (dopa) in depression. J. psychiat. Res. **1**, 289—297 (1963).
KNOX, W.E.: Phenylketonuria. In: The Metabolic Basis of Inherited Disease, 2nd Edn., pp. 258—294, edit. J.B. STANBURY, J.B. WYNGAARDEN and D.S. FREDRICKSON. New York: McGraw-Hill 1966.
KOE, B.K., WEISSMAN, A.: The pharmacology of *para*-chlorophenylalanine, a selective depletor of serotonin stores. Advanc. Pharmacol. **6B**, 29—47 (1968).
KOPIN, I.J.: Catecholamines in blood pressure regulation. In: L-Dopa and Parkinsonism, pp. 277—280, edit. A. BARBEAU and F.H. MCDOWELL. Philadelphia: Davis 1970.
KORDUBA, C.A., VEALS, J., SYMCHOWICZ, S.: Effect of glucocorticoids on 14C-dopamine metabolism in rat brain. Pharmacologist **12**, 287 (1970).
KORMANO, M.: Distribution of injected L-3, 4-dihydroxyphenylalanine (L-dopa) in the adult rat testis and epididymis. Acta physiol. scand. **71**, 125—126 (1967).
KRASNER, N., CORNELIUS, J.M.: L-Dopa for postencephalitic Parkinsonism. Brit. med. J. **4**, 496 (1970).

KRAYENBÜHL, H., SIEGFRIED, J.: Treatment of Parkinson's disease: stereotaxic operation or L-DOPA. Neuro-chirugie **16**, 71—76 (1970).

KREMER, M., RUSSELL, W.R., SMYTH, G.E.: A mid-brain syndrome following head injury. J. Neurol. Neurosurg. Psychiat. **10**, 49—60 (1947).

KUEHL, F.A., JR., VANDENHEUVEL, W.J.A., ORMOND, R.E.: Urinary metabolites in Parkinson's disease. Nature (Lond.) **217**, 136—138 (1968).

KURUMA, I., BARTHOLINI, G., PLETSCHER, A.: L-Dopa induced accumulation of 3-0-methyldopa in brain and heart. Europ. J. Pharmacol. **10**, 189—192 (1970).

LAIDLAW, P.P.: The action of tetrahydropapaveroline hydrochloride. J. Physiol. (Lond.) **40**, 480—491 (1910).

LAMMERS, A.J.J.C., VAN ROSSUM, J.M.: Bizarre social behaviour in rats induced by a combination of a peripheral decarboxylase inhibitor and DOPA. Europ. J. Pharmacol. **5**, 103—106 (1968).

LANCASTER, G., LAROCHELLE, L., BÉDARD, P., MISSALA, K., SOURKES, T.L., POIRIER, L.J.: Effect of brain lesions and of harmaline on the DOPA decarboxylase activity in the striatum of the cat. J. neurol. Sci. **11**, 265—274 (1970).

LANGEMANN, H.: Bestimmungen von Fermentaktivitäten in Geweben eines Falls von metastasierenden Karzinoid. Arch. exp. Pathol. Pharmakol. **228**, 244—245 (1956).

— ACKERMANN, H.: Über die Aktivität der Aminosäuren-Decarboxylasen im Gehirn des Menschen. Helv. physiol. Acta **19**, 399—406 (1961).

— BONER, A., MÜLLER, P.B.: Aminosäurendecarboxylase in Phäochromocytom- und Karzinoidgewebe. Schweiz. med. Wschr. **92**, 27—34 (1962).

LAVERTY, R., SHARMAN, D.F.: Modification by drugs of the metabolism of 3,4-dihydroxyphenylethylamine, noradrenaline and 5-hydroxytryptamine in the brain. Brit. J. Pharmacol. **24**, 759—772 (1965).

LEON, A.S., SOLOMON, H.M., ROSS, I., GOLDEN, R.M., ABRAMS, W.B.: Cardiovascular activity of L-dopa. Clin. Res. **18**, 340 (1970).

LEVINE, R.J., SJOERDSMA, A.: Monoamine oxidase activity in human tissues and intestinal biopsy specimens. Proc. Soc. exp. Biol. (N.Y.) **109**, 225—227 (1962).

LIEBERMAN, A.N., PEDERSEN, B.: Levodopa and adventitious movements. Lancet **ii**, 985 (1970).

LLOYD, K., HORNYKIEWICZ, O.: Occurrence and distribution of L-DOPA decarboxylase in the human brain. Brain Res. **22**, 426—428 (1970a).

— — Parkinson's disease: activity of L-dopa decarboxylase in discrete brain regions. Science **170**, 1212—1213 (1970b).

LOIZOU, L.A.: Uptake of monoamines into central neurones and the blood-brain barrier in the infant rat. Brit. J. Pharmacol. **40**, 800—813 (1970).

LOTTI, V.J., PORTER, C.C.: Potentiation and inhibition of some central actions of L(—)-dopa by decarboxylase inhibitors. J. Pharmacol. exp. Ther. **172**, 406—415 (1970).

LOVENBERG, W., WEISSBACH, H., UDENFRIEND, S.: Aromatic L-amino acid decarboxylase. J. biol. Chem. **237**, 89—93 (1962).

LUSE, S.A., BLANK, W., METTLER, F.A.: L-DOPA and hyperkinesia. Fed. Proc. **29**, 512 (1970).

LYCKE, E., ROOS, B.-E.: Effect on the monoamine metabolism of the mouse brain by experimental *Herpes simplex* injection. Experientia (Basel) **24**, 687—689 (1968).

— — Some virological and biochemical aspects of the pathogenesis of Parkinson's disease. In: Third Symposium on Parkinson's Disease, pp. 16—19, edit. F.J. GILLINGHAM and I.M.L. DONALDSON. Edinburgh: Livingstone 1969.

LYMAN, F.L.: Phenylketonuria, Springfield: Thomas, 1963, pp. 1—318.

MCCANN, D.S., MITCHELL, J.G., KEECH, M.K., BOYLE, A.J.: Tyrosine metabolism in connective tissue disease. J. chron. Dis. **20**, 781—786 (1967).

MCDOWELL, F.H.: Changes in behavior and mentation. In: L-Dopa and Parkinsonism, pp. 321—325, edit. A. BARBEAU and F.H. MCDOWELL. Philadelphia: Davis 1970.

— LEE, J.E., SWIFT, T., SWEET, R.D., OGSBURY, J.S., KESSLER, J.T.: Treatment of Parkinson's syndrome with L-dihydroxyphenylalanine (levodopa). Ann. intern. Med. **72**, 29—35 (1970).

MCGEER, P.L., BOULDING, J.E., GIBSON, W.C., FOULKES, R.G.: Drug-induced extrapyramidal reactions. J. Amer. med. Ass. **177**, 665—670 (1961).

— ZELDOWICZ, L.R.: Administration of dihydroxyphenylalanine to parkinsonian patients. Canad. med. Ass. J. **90**, 463—466 (1964).

MCNAY, J.L., MCDONALD, R.H., GOLDBERG, L.I.: Direct renal vasodilation produced by dopamine in the dog. Circulat. Res. **16**, 510—517 (1965).

MAEDA, T., WEGMANN, R.: Infrared spectrometry of locus coeruleus and substantia nigra pigments in human brain. Brain Res. **14**, 673—681 (1969).

MANGER, W.M., BESSIS, M.: White cell uptake of L-dihydroxyphenylalanine (L-DOPA), catecholamines (CAs) and 5-hydroxytryptamine (5-HT). Pharmacologist **11**, 263 (1969).

MARKHAM, C.H.: Major treatment problems in L-dopa therapy in Parkinson's disease. In: L-Dopa and Parkinsonism, pp. 10—16, edit. A. BARBEAU and F.H. McDOWELL. Philadelphia: Davis 1970.
— TRECIOKAS, L., ANSEL, R.D.: Blood pressure in parkinsonian patients receiving L-dopa. In: L-Dopa and Parkinsonism, pp. 255—262, edit. A. BARBEAU and F.H. McDOWELL. Philadelphia: Davis 1970.
MARLEY, E., STEPHENSON, J.D.: Effects of catecholamines infused into the brain of young chickens. Brit. J. Pharmacol. **40**, 639—658 (1970).
MARSDEN, D.: Brain pigment and its relation to brain catecholamines. Lancet **ii**, 475—476 (1965).
MASRI, M.S., BOOTH, A.N., DEEDS, F.: 0-Methylation *in vitro* of dihydroxy- and trihydroxyphenolic compounds by liver slices. Biochim. biophys. Acta (Amst.) **65**, 495—500 (1962).
— ROBBINS, D.J., EMERSON, O.H., DEEDS, F.: Selective *para-* or *meta-*0-methylation with catechol 0-methyl transferase from rat liver. Nature (Lond.) **202**, 878—879 (1964).
MATTHIEU, P., REVOL, L.: Les métabolites 4-0-méthylés des catecholamines chez l'homme: identification chromatographique de l'acide 3-hydroxy, 4-méthoxyphénylacétique (acide homo-iso-vanillique, iso-HVA). Bull. Soc. Chim. biol. (Paris) **52**, 1039—1050 (1970).
MATUSSEK, N., BENKERT, O., SCHNEIDER, K., OTTEN, H., POHLMEIER, H.: L-Dopa plus decarboxylase inhibitor in depression. Lancet **ii**, 660—661 (1970).
MAWDSLEY, C.: Treatment of Parkinsonism with laevo-dopa. Brit. med. J. **1**, 331—337 (1970).
MEDES, G.: A new error of tyrosine metabolism: tyrosinosis. The intermediary metabolism of tyrosine and phenylalanine. Biochem. J. **26**, 917—940 (1932).
MENA, I., COURT, J., FUENZALIDA, S., PAPAVASILIOU, P.S., COTZIAS, G.C.: Modification of chronic manganese poisoning: treatment with L-dopa or 5-OH tryptophane. New Engl. J. Med. **282**, 5—10 (1970).
— MARIN, O., FUENZALIDA, S., COTZIAS, G.C.: Chronic manganese poisoning: clinical picture and manganese turnover. Neurology **17**, 128—136 (1967).
MENDELL, J.R., CHASE, T.N., ENGEL, W.K.: Modification by L-dopa of a case of progressive supranuclear palsy with evidence of defective cerebral dopamine metabolism. Lancet **i**, 593—594 (1970).
MENDLOWITZ, M., WOLF, R.L., GITLOW, S.E.: Catecholamine metabolism in essential hypertension. Amer. Heart J. **79**, 401—407 (1970).
MESSIHA, F.S., AGALLIANOS, D., CLOWER, C.: Dopamine excretion in affective states and following Li_2 CO_3 therapy. Nature (Lond.) **225**, 868—869 (1970).
METZEL, E., WEINMANN, D., RIECHERT, T.: A study of the enzymes of dopa metabolism in parkinsonism from biopsies of the basal ganglia. In: Third Symposium on Parkinson's Disease, pp. 47—50, edit. F.J. GILLINGHAM and I.M.L. DONALDSON. Edinburgh: Livingstone 1969.
MICHELAKIS, A.M., ROBERTSON, D.: Plasma renin activity and levodopa in Parkinsonism. J. Amer. med. Ass. **213**, 83—85 (1970).
MITOMA, C., POSNER, H.S., BOGDANSKI, D.F., UDENFRIEND, S.: Biochemical and pharmacological studies on o-tyrosine and its meta- and para-analogues; a suggestion concerning phenylketonuria. J. Pharmacol. exp. Ther. **120**, 188—194 (1957).
MJÖNES, H.: Paralysis agitans. A clinical and genetic study. Acta psychiat. neurol. scand. Suppl. **54**, pp. 1—195 (1949).
MOIR, A.T.B., ASHCROFT, G.W., CRAWFORD, T.B.B., ECCLESTON, D., GULDBERG, H.C.: Cerebral metabolites in cerebrospinal fluid as a biochemical approach to the brain. Brain **93**, 357—368 (1970).
MOLINOFF, P.B.: Personal communication (1970).
MOLINOFF, P., AXELROD, J.: Octopamine: normal occurrence in sympathetic nerves of rats. Science **164**, 428—429 (1969).
MONES, R.J., ELIZAN, T.S., SIEGEL, G.J.: Evaluation of L-dopa therapy in Parkinson's disease. N.Y. St. J. Med. **70**, 2309—2318 (1970).
MONTPLAISIR, J., BARBEAU, A.: Serum tyrosine in Parkinson's disease. In: Progress in Neurogenetics, pp. 331—335, edit. A. BARBEAU and J.R. BRUNETTE, International Congress Series No. 175. Amsterdam: Excerpta Medica Foundation 1969.
MORGAN, C.D., RUTHVEN, C.R.J., SANDLER, M.: The quantitative assessment of isoprenaline metabolism in man. Clin. chim. Acta **26**, 381—386 (1969).
MORGAN, J.P., PREZIOSI, T.J., BIANCHINE, J.R.: Ineffectiveness of L-dopa as supplement to penicillamine in a case of Wilson's disease. Lancet **ii**, 659 (1970a).
— SPIEGEL, H.E., HERSEY, R.M., CALIMLIM, L.R., BIANCHINE, J.R.: Metabolism of oral L-dopa in parkinsonian patients. Clin. Res. **18**, 342 (1970b).

Müller-Calgan, H., Sommer, S.: Das Reserpin-Parkinsonoid beim Schimpansen und seine Behandlung mit Fencamfamin. Arch. Pharmakol. exp. Path. **260**, 177 (1968).

Murphy, G.F., Robinson, D., Sharman, D.F.: The effect of tropolone on the formation of 3,4-dihydroxyphenylacetic acid and 4-hydroxy-3-methoxyphenylacetic acid in the brain of the mouse. Brit. J. Pharmacol. **36**, 107—115 (1969).

Nagatsu, T., Levitt, M., Udenfriend, S.: Tyrosine hydroxylase. The initial step in norepinephrine biosynthesis. J. biol. Chem. **239**, 2910—2917 (1964).

Neff, N.H., Barrett, R.E., Costa, E.: Selective depletion of caudate nucleus dopamine and serotonin during chronic manganese dioxide administration to squirrel monkeys. Experientia (Basel) **25**, 1140—1141 (1969).

Ng, K.Y., Chase, T.N., Colburn, R.W., Kopin, I.J.: L-Dopa-induced release of cerebral monoamines. Science **170**, 76—77 (1970).

O'Gorman, L.P., Borud, O., Khan, I.A., Gjessing, L.R.: The metabolism of L-3,4-dihydroxyphenylalanine in man. Clin. chim. Acta **29**, 111—119 (1970).

O'Keefe, R., Sharman, D.F., Vogt, M.: Effects of drugs used in psychoses on cerebral dopamine metabolism. Brit. J. Pharmacol. **38**, 287—304 (1970).

Olsson, R., Roos, B.-E.: Concentrations of 5-hydroxyindoleacetic acid and homovanillic acid in the cerebrospinal fluid after treatment with probenecid in patients with Parkinson's disease. Nature (Lond.) **219**, 502—503 (1968).

Pakkenberg, H., Brody, H.: The number of nerve cells in the substantia nigra in paralysis agitans. Acta neuropath. (Berl.) **5**, 320—324 (1965).

Palm, D.: Über die Hemmung der Dopa-Decarboxylase durch Isonicotinsäurehydrazid. Arch. exp. Pathol. Pharmakol. **234**, 206—209 (1958).

Papeschi, R., Molina-Negro, P., Sourkes, T.L., Hardy, J., Bertrand, C.: Concentration of homovanillic acid in the ventricular fluid of patients with Parkinson's disease and other dyskinesias. Neurology **20**, 991—995 (1970).

Pare, C.M.B., Sandler, M.: A clinical and biochemical study of a trial of iproniazid in the treatment of depression. J. Neurol. Neurosurg. Psychiat. **22**, 247—251 (1959).

— — Stacey, R.S.: 5-Hydroxytryptamine deficiency in phenylketonuria. Lancet **i**, 551—553 (1957).

— — — Decreased 5-hydroxytryptophan decarboxylase activity in phenylketonuria. Lancet **ii**, 1099—1101 (1958).

— — — The relationship between increased 5-hydroxyindole metabolism and mental defect in phenylketonuria. Arch. Dis. Childh. **34**, 422—423 (1959).

— Yeung, D.P.H., Price, K., Stacey, R.S.: 5-Hydroxytryptamine, noradrenaline and dopamine in brainstem, hypothalamus, and caudate nucleus of controls and of patients committing suicide by coal-gas poisoning. Lancet **ii**, 133—135 (1969).

Parkes, J.D., Sharpstone, P., Williams, R.: Levodopa in hepatic coma. Lancet **ii**, 1341—1343 (1970a).

— Zilkha, K.J., Calver, D.M., Knill-Jones, R.P.: Controlled trial of amantadine hydrochloride in Parkinson's disease. Lancet **i**, 259—262 (1970b).

Parkinson, J.: An essay on the shaking palsy, pp. 1—66. London: Sherwood, Neely and Jones 1817.

Peaston, M.J.T., Bianchine, J.R.: Metabolic studies and clinical observations during L-dopa treatment of Parkinson's disease. Brit. med. J. **1**, 400—403 (1970).

Penttilä, O., Vartiainen, A.: Acetylcholine, histamine, 5-hydroxytryptamine and catecholamine contents of mammalian penile and urethral tissue. Acta pharmacol. (Kbh.) **21**, 145—151 (1964).

Pepeu, G., Giarman, N.J.: Serotonin in the developing mammal. J. gen. Physiol. **45**, 575—583 (1962).

Perry, T.L., Hestrin, M., MacDougall, L., Hansen, S.: Urinary amines of intestinal bacterial origin. Clin. chim. Acta **14**, 116—123 (1966).

Peters, D.A.V., McGeer, P.L., McGeer, E.G.: The distribution of tryptophan hydroxylase in cat brain. J. Neurochem. **15**, 1431—1435 (1968).

Pinder, R.M.: Possible dopamine derivatives capable of crossing the blood-brain barrier in relation to parkinsonism. Nature (Lond.) 228—229 (1970).

Pletscher, A., Bartholini, G., Tissot, R.: Metabolic fate of L-(^{14}C) dopa in cerebrospinal fluid and blood plasma of humans. Brain Res. **4**, 106—109 (1967).

Pogrund, R.S., Drell, W., Clark, W.G.: Metabolism of 3-hydroxy- and 3,4-dihydroxyphenylpyruvic acids *in vivo*. J. Pharmacol. exp. Ther. **131**, 294—307 (1961).

Poirier, L.J.: Experimental and histological study of midbrain dyskinesias. J. Neurophysiol. **23**, 534—551 (1960).

— Singh, P., Boucher, R.: Opposite effect of harmaline on serotonin and on dopamine and its metabolites, homovanillic acid and norepinephrine, in the brain of the cat. Canad. J. Physiol. Pharmacol. **46**, 585—589 (1968).

POIRIER, L.J., SINGH, P., SOURKES, T.L., BOUCHER, R.: Effect of amine precursors on the concentration of striatal dopamine and serotonin in cats with and without unilateral brain stem lesions. Brain Res. **6**, 654—666 (1967).

— SOURKES, T.L.: Influence of the substantia nigra on the catecholamine content of the striatum. Brain **88**, 181—192 (1965).

PORTER, C.C., WATSON, L.S., TITUS, D.C., TOTARO, J.A., BYER, S.S.: Inhibition of dopa decarboxylase by the hydrazino analog of α-methyldopa. Biochem. Pharmacol. **11**, 1067—1077 (1962).

PULLAR, I.A., WEDDELL, J.M., HANIEH, A., AHMED, R., GILLINGHAM, F.J.: Changes in acid metabolites of dopamine and 5-hydroxytryptamine in lumbar CSF of patients treated with L-DOPA. Proc. 2nd int. Meeting int. Soc. Neurochem., Milan, pp. 328—329 (1969).

PUSHPATHADAM, J.J., BARBEAU, A.: The 'pink spot' and Parkinson's disease. In: Progress in Neurogenetics, pp. 413—417, edit. A. BARBEAU and J.R. BRUNETTE, International Congress Series No. 175. Amsterdam: Excerpta Medica Foundation 1969.

RAO, N.S.: Effects of withdrawing dopa in Parkinson's disease. Lancet **ii**, 470—471 (1970).

RENNICK, B.R.: Dopamine: renal tubular transport in the dog and plasma building studies. Amer. J. Physiol. **215**, 532—534 (1968).

RENSON, J., WEISSBACH, H., UDENFRIEND, S.: Studies on the biological activities of the aldehydes derived from norepinephrine, serotonin, tryptamine and histamine. J. Pharmacol. exp. Ther. **143**, 326—331 (1964).

RESNICK, R.H., GRAY, S.J., KOCH, J.P., TIMBERLAKE, W.H.: Serotonin metabolism in paralysis agitans. Proc. Soc. exp. Biol. (N.Y.) **110**, 77—79 (1962).

RINNE, U.K., SONNINEN, V.: Homovanillic acid of the cerebrospinal fluid in Parkinson's disease. Scand. J. clin. Lab. Invest. Suppl. 101, p. 22 (1968a).

— — A double blind study of l-dopa treatment in Parkinson's disease. Europ. Neurol. **1**, 180—191 (1968b).

— — Catecholamines in Parkinson's disease. Acta neurol. scand. **46**, Suppl. 43, 217 (1970).

RIVERA-CALIMLIM, L., DUJOVNE, C.A., MORGAN, J.P., LASAGNA, L., BIANCHINE, J.R.: L-Dopa absorption and metabolism by the human stomach. Pharmacologist **12**, 269 (1970a).

— — — — — L-Dopa treatment failure: explanation and correction. Brit. med. J. **4**, 93—94 (1970b).

— MORGAN, J.P., DUJOVNE, C.A., BIANCHINE, J.R., LASAGNA, L.: L-Dopa metabolism by rat gut *in vitro*. Clin. Res. **18**, 343 (1970c).

ROBINS, E., ROBINS, J.M., CRONINGER, A.B., MOSES, S.G., SPENCER, S.J., HUDGENS, R.W.: The low level of 5-hydroxytryptophan decarboxylase in human brain. Biochem. Med. **1**, 240 (1967).

ROOS, B.-E.: Decrease in homovanillic acid as evidence for dopamine receptor stimulation by apomorphine in the neostriatum of the rat. J. Pharm. Pharmacol. **21**, 263—264 (1969).

— SJÖSTRÖM, R.: 5-Hydroxyindoleacetic acid (and homovanillic acid) levels in the cerebrospinal fluid after probenecid application in patients with manic depressive psychosis. Pharmacol. Clin. **1**, 153—155 (1969).

ROSE, C.M., CHOU, C., WURTMAN, R.J.: The metabolism of ^{14}C-dopa in the whole mouse. Fed. Proc. **29**, 511 (1970).

ROSELL, S., SEDVALL, G., ULLBERG, S.: Distribution and fate of dihydroxyphenylalanine-2-^{14}C (DOPA) in mice. Biochem. Pharmacol. **12**, 265—269 (1963).

ROSEN, J.A.: The effect of a monoamine oxidase inhibitor on the bradykinesia of human parkinsonism. In: Progress in Neuro-genetics, **1**, pp. 346—351, edit. A. BARBEAU and J.R. BRUNETTE, Int. Congr. Series No. 175. Amsterdam: Excerpta Medica Foundation 1969.

ROSENMUND, K.W., DORNSAFT, H.: Über Oxy- und Dioxyphenylserin und die Muttersubstanz des Adrenalins. Ber. dtsch. chem. Ges. **52**, 1734—1749 (1919).

ROY, S., WOLMAN, L.: Ultrastructural observations in parkinsonism. J. Path. **99**, 39—44 (1969).

RUTHVEN, C.R.J., KAROUM, F., ANAH, C.O., CHAPMAN, J., SANDLER, M.: The study of catecholamine secreting tumours by gas-liquid chromatography. Enzym. biol. clin. **10**, 456 (1969).

SABUNCU, N.: Quantitative Untersuchungen am Pallidum beim Parkinson-Syndrom. Dtsch. Z. Nervenheilk. **196**, 40—48 (1969).

SACKS, O.W., KOHL, M.: Incontinent nostalgia induced by L-dopa. Lancet **i**, 1394 (1970a).

— — L-Dopa and oculogyric crises. Lancet **ii**, 215—216 (1970b).

— — SCHWARTZ, W.F., MESSELOFF, C.R.: Side-effects of L-dopa in postencephalitic parkinsonism. Lancet **i**, 1006 (1970a).

— MESSELOFF, C.R., SCHWARTZ, W.F.: Long-term levodopa in the severely disabled. J. Amer. med. Ass. **213**, 2270 (1970b).

SACKS, O.W., MESSELOFF, C.R., SCHWARTZ, W.F., GOLDFARB, A., KOHL, M.: Effects of L-dopa in patients with dementia. Lancet **i**, 1231 (1970c).

SANDLER, M.: The role of 5-hydroxyindoles in the carcinoid syndrome. Advanc. Pharmacol. **6B**, 127—142 (1968).

— Biosynthesis and metabolism of the catecholamines. Schweiz. med. Wschr. **100**, 526—531 (1970a).

— The role of minor pathways of dopa metabolism. In: L-Dopa and Parkinsonism, pp. 72—75, edit. A. BARBEAU and F.H. MCDOWELL. Philadelphia: Davis 1970b.

— Discussion remark. In: L-Dopa and Parkinsonism, p. 251, edit. A. BARBEAU and F.H. MCDOWELL, Philadelphia: Davis 1970c.

— In preparation (1971).

— COLLINS, G.G.S., YOUDIM, M.B.H.: Inhibition patterns of monoamine oxidase isoenzymes: clinical implications. In: Mechanisms of Toxicity, pp. 3—11, edit. W.N. ALDRIDGE. London: Macmillan 1971a.

— GOODWIN, B.L., RUTHVEN, C.R.J., CALNE, D.B.: *m*-Tyramine formation from L-dopa in man: therapeutic implications in Parkinsonism. Nature (Lond.) **229**, 414—415 (1971b).

— KAROUM, F., RUTHVEN, C.R.J.: Parkinsonism with alkaptonuria: a new syndrome? Lancet **ii**, 770 (1970a).

— — — CALNE, D.B.: *m*-Hydroxyphenylacetic acid formation from L-dopa in man: suppression by neomycin. Science **166**, 1417—1418 (1969a).

— — — SOUTHGATE, J., CALNE, D.B.: Metabolism of L-DOPA in Parkinsonism. Abstr. 4th int. Congr. Pharmacol., Basel, p. 81 (1969b).

— RUTHVEN, C.R.J.: 4-Hydroxy-3-methoxyphenylglycol and other compounds in neuroblastoma. In: Recent Results in Cancer Research. II. Neuroblastomas. Biochemical Studies, pp. 55—59, edit. C. BOHUON. Berlin: Springer 1966.

— — The biosynthesis and metabolism of the catecholamines. In: Progress in Medicinal Chemistry, edit. G.P. ELLIS and G.B. WEST, Vol. 6, pp. 200—265. London: Butterworth 1969.

— — Monoamine-secreting tumours. In: Tumours in Children, edit. A.E. CLAIREAUX. Springfield: Thomas 1972, in the press.

— — CAESAR, P.M.: Urinary pH and the excretion of biologically active amines and their acidic metabolites. Proc. 7th int. Congr. Biochem. Tokyo, 1967, p. 971.

— YOUDIM, M.B.H., SOUTHGATE, J., HANINGTON, E.: The role of tyramine in migraine: some possible biochemical mechanisms. In: Background to Migraine. 3rd Migraine Symposium, pp. 104—115, edit. A.L. COCHRANE. London: Heinemann 1970b.

SCHECKEL, C.L., BOFF, E., PAZERY, L.M.: Behavioral and biochemical effects of interacting 3,4-dihydroxyphenylalanine (DOPA) and an inhibitor of aromatic acid decarboxylase (Ro4-4602). Fed. Proc. **24**, 195 (1965).

— — — Hyperactive states related to the metabolism of norepinephrine and similar biochemicals. Ann. N.Y. Acad. Sci. **159**, 939—958 (1969).

SCHELINE, R.R.: Drug metabolism by intestinal microorganisms. J. pharm. Sci. **57**, 2021—2037 (1968a).

— MIDTVEDT, T.: Absence of dehydroxylation of caffeic acid in germ-free rats. Experientia (Basel) **26**, 1068—1069 (1970).

SCHMITERLÖW, C.G.: Formation *in vivo* of noradrenaline from 3,4-dihydroxyphenylserine (noradrenaline carboxylic acid). Brit. J. Pharmacol. **6**, 127—134 (1951).

SCHNIEDEN, H., WILLIAMS, T.: Effect of thalamotomy on urinary dopamine levels in patients with parkinsonism. Europ. Neurol. **3**, 290—292 (1970).

SCHOTT, H.F., CLARK, W.G.: DOPA decarboxylase inhibition through the interaction of coenzyme and substrate. J. biol. Chem. **196**, 449—462 (1952).

SCHWAB, R.S.: Combining L-dopa and amantadine hydrochloride (Symmetrel). In: L-Dopa and Parkinsonism, p. 58, edit. A. BARBEAU and F.H. MCDOWELL. Philadelphia: Davis 1970.

— AMADOR, L.V., LETTVIN, J.Y.: Apomorphine in Parkinson's disease. Trans. Amer. neurol. Ass. **76**, 251—253 (1951).

— ENGLAND, A.C., JR., POSKANZER, D.C., YOUNG, R.R.: Amantadine in Parkinson's disease. J. Amer. med. Ass. **208**, 1168—1170 (1969).

SCHWARZ, G.A., FAHN, S.: Newer medical treatments in parkinsonism. Med. Clin. N. Amer. **54**, 773—785 (1970).

SCOTT, J.A.: 3,4-Dihydroxyphenylalanine (dopa) excretion in patients with malignant melanoma. Lancet **ii**, 861—862 (1962).

SEALOCK, R.R.: β-3,4-Dihydroxyphenyl-L-alanine. Biochem. Prep. **1**, 25—33 (1949).

SEGAL, D.S., WHALEN, R.E.: Effect of chronic administration of p-chlorophenylalanine on sexual receptivity of the female rat. Psychopharmacologia (Berl.) **16**, 434—438 (1970).

SEKERIS, C.E., HERRLICH, P.: Nachweis von N-Acetyl-dopamin bei einem Fall von Phäochromocytom. Z. physiol. Chem. **331**, 289—291 (1963).

SEKERIS, C.E., KARLSON, P.: Biosynthesis of catecholamines in insects. Pharmacol. Rev. **18**, 89—94 (1966).

SEMBA, T., CIVEN, M.: Subcellular distribution of aromatic amino acid transaminases in rat brain. J. Neurochem. **17**, 795—800 (1970).

SENOH, S., DALY, J., AXELROD, J., WITKOP, B.: Enzymatic *p*-0-methylation by catechol-0-methyl transferase. J. Amer. chem. Soc. **81**, 6240—6245 (1959a).

— WITKOP, B., CREVELING, C.R., UDENFRIEND, S.: 2,4,5-Trihydroxyphenylethylamine, a new metabolite of 3,4-dihydroxyphenylethylamine. J. Amer. chem. Soc. **81**, 1768—1769 (1959b).

SERRANO, P.: Personal communication to SOURKES, T.L.: On the mode of action of L-dopa in Parkinson's disease. Biochem. Med. **3**, 321—325 (1970).

SHAH, N.S., KAMANO, A., GLISSON, S., CALLISON, D.: Studies on the uptake of radiolabeled DOPA, 5-HTP and tryptophan in rat tissues *in vivo*: effect of methionine, tryptophan and some keto acids. Int. J. Neuropharmacol. **7**, 75—86 (1968).

SHARMAN, D.F.: The effect of drugs on the metabolism of dopamine in the striatum. In: Third Symposium on Parkinson's Disease, pp. 24—26, edit. F.J. GILLINGHAM and I.M.L. DONALDSON. Edinburgh: Livingstone 1969.

— POIRIER, L.J., MURPHY, G.F., SOURKES, T.L.: Homovanillic acid and dihydroxyphenylacetic acid in the striatum of monkeys with brain lesions. Canad. J. Physiol. **45**, 57—62 (1967).

SHAW, K.N.F., GUTENSTEIN, M., JEPSON, J.B.: Intestinal flora and diet in relation to *m*-hydroxyphenyl acids of human urine. Proc. 5th int. Cong. Biochem. Moscow, Vol. 9, p. 427. Oxford: Pergamon 1961.

— MCMILLAN, A., ARMSTRONG, M.D.: The metabolism of 3,4-dihydroxyphenylalanine. J. biol. Chem. **226**, 255—266 (1957).

SHEALY, C.N., WEETH, J.B., MERCIER, D.: Livedo reticularis, parkinsonism and amantadine. J. Amer. med. Ass. **212**, 1522—1523 (1970).

SHULGIN, A.T., SARGENT, T., NARANJO, C.: Structure-activity relationships of one-ring psychotomimetics. Nature (Lond.) **221**, 537—541 (1969).

SHY, M., DRAGER, G.: A neurological syndrome associated with orthostatic hypotension. Arch. Neurol. **2**, 41—57 (1960).

SIEGFRIED, J.: Deux ans d'expérience avec la L-DOPA associée à un inhibiteur de la décarboxylase. Rev. Neurol. **122**, 243—248 (1970).

SIGWALD, J., RAYMONDEAUD, C.: Les movements abnormaux observés au cours du traitement de la maladie de Parkinson par la L-dopa. Rev. Neurol. **122**, 103—112 (1970).

SIH, C.J., FOSS, P., ROSAZZA, J., LEMBERGER, M.: Microbiological synthesis of L-3,4-dihydroxyphenylalanine. J. Amer. chem. Soc. **91**, 6204 (1969).

ŠIMEK, J.: Vylučovaní kyseliny 3-metoxy 4-hydroxyfenyloctové (homovanilové) u parkinsoniků. Čas. Lék. česk. **107**, 544—546 (1968).

SJOERDSMA, A.: Techniques for measuring monoamine oxidase inhibiting activity in man. J. Neuropsychiat. **2**, S159—S162 (1961).

— ENGELMAN, K., SPECTOR, S., UDENFRIEND, S.: Inhibition of catecholamine synthesis in man with alpha-methyl-tyrosine, an inhibitor of tyrosine hydroxylase. Lancet **ii**, 1092—1094 (1965).

— LOVENBERG, W., ENGELMAN, K., CARPENTER, W.T., JR., WYATT, R.J., GESSA, G.L.: Serotonin now: clinical implications of inhibiting its synthesis with *para*-chlorophenylalanine. Ann. intern. Med. **73**, 607—629 (1970).

SMELLIE, J.M., SANDLER, M.: Secreting intrathoracic ganglioneuroma. Proc. roy. Soc. Med. **54**, 327—329 (1961).

SMITH, A.A., FABRYKANT, M., KAPLAN, M., GAVITT, J.: Dehydroxylation of some catecholamines and their products. Biochim. biophys. Acta (Amst.) **86**, 429—437 (1964).

SMITH, I., KELLOW, A.H.: Aromatic amines and Parkinson's disease. Nature (Lond.) **221**, 1261 (1969).

— — HANINGTON, E.: Tyramine metabolism in dietary migraine. In: Background to Migraine. Third Migraine Symposium, p. 120—124, edit. A.L. COCHRANE. London: Heinemann 1970a.

— — MULLEN, P.E., HANINGTON, E.: Dietary migraine and tyramine metabolism. A possible inborn error of conjugation. Nature (Lond.) **230**, 246—248 (1971).

SMITH, J.S., BRANDON, S.: Acute carbon monoxide poisoning — 3 years' experience in a defined population. Postgrad. med. J. **46**, 65—70 (1970).

SMITH, P.: Metabolism of dihydroxyphenylalanine in human subjects. Nature (Lond.) **213**, 802—803 (1967).

SMITH, R.L.: The role of the gut flora in the conversion of inactive compounds to active metabolites. In: Mechanisms of Toxicity, edit. W.N. ALDRIDGE. London: Macmillan 1971, pp. 229—241.

SMYTHIES, J.R.: Schizophrenia: chemistry, metabolism and treatment, pp. 1—86. Springfield: Thomas 1963.
— JOHNSTON, V.S., BRADLEY, R.J., BENINGTON, F., MORIN, R.D., CLARK, L.C., JR.: Some new behaviour-disrupting amphetamines and their significance. Nature (Lond.) **216**, 128—129 (1967).
SNYDER, S.H., COYLE, J.T.: Regional differences in H^3-norepinephrine and H^3-dopamine uptake into rat brain homogenates. J. Pharmacol. exp. Ther. **165**, 78—86 (1969).
— TAYLOR, K.M., COYLE, J.T., MEYERHOFF, J.L.: The role of brain dopamine in behavioral regulation and the actions of psychotropic drugs. Amer. J. Psychiat. **127**, 199—207 (1970).
SOLOMON, H.M., SPIRT, N.M., ABRAMS, W.B.: The accumulation and metabolism of dopamine by the human platelet. Clin. Pharmacol. Ther. **11**, 838—845 (1970).
SONNEVILLE, P.F.: An indirect action of dopamine on the rat fundus strip mediated by 5-hydroxytryptamine. Europ. J. Pharmacol. **2**, 367—370 (1968).
SOURKES, T.L.: On the mode of action of L-dopa in Parkinson's disease. Biochem. Med. **3**, 321—325 (1970).
— DENTON, R.L., MURPHY, G.F., CHAVEZ, B., SAINT CYR, S.: The excretion of dihydroxyphenylalanine, dopamine, and dihydroxyphenylacetic acid in neuroblastoma. Pediatrics **31**, 660—668 (1963).
— MISSALA, K.: Metabolism of dihydroxyphenylalanine and tryptophan in pyridoxine-deficient rats. Ann. N.Y. Acad. Sci. **159**, 235—245 (1969).
— MURPHY, G.F., RABINOVITCH, A.: Conversion of DL-m-tyrosine to dopamine in the rat. Nature (Lond.) **189**, 577—578 (1961).
— PIVNICKI, D., BROWN, W.T., WISEMAN-DISTLER, M.H., MURPHY, G.F., SANKOFF, I., SAINT CYR, S.: A clinical and metabolic study of dopa (3,4-dihydroxyphenylalanine) and methyldopa in Huntington's chorea. Psychiat. et Neurol. (Basel) **149**, 7—27 (1965).
— POIRIER, L.J.: Amines of the striatum: relation to experimental tremor in the monkey. In: Biochemistry and Pharmacology of the Basal Ganglia, pp. 187—190, edit. E. COSTA, L.H. CÔTÉ and M.D. YAHR. Hewlett, N.Y.: Raven Press 1966.
— — SINGH, P.: Biochemical-histological-neurological models of Parkinson's disease. In: Third Symposium on Parkinson's Disease, pp. 54—60, edit. F.J. GILLINGHAM and I.M.L. DONALDSON. Edinburgh: Livingstone 1969.
SPECTOR, S., SJOERDSMA, A., UDENFRIEND, S.: Blockade of endogenous norepinephrine synthesis by α-methyl-tyrosine, an inhibitor of tyrosine hydroxylase. J. Pharmacol. exp. Ther. **147**, 86—95 (1965).
STACEY, R.S.: Clinical aspects of cerebral and extracerebral 5-hydroxytryptamine. In: Handbuch der experimentellen Pharmakologie, Vol. XIX, 5-Hydroxytryptamine and Related Indolealkylamines, pp. 744—786, edit. V. ERSPAMER. Berlin: Springer 1966.
STEG, G.: Side-effects during treatment with L-DOPA in Parkinsonism. Proc. 9th int. Congr. Neurol., N.Y., pp. 171—172 (1969).
STELLAR, S., MANDELL, S., WALTZ, J.M., COOPER, I.S.: L-Dopa in the treatment of Parkinsonism. A preliminary appraisal. J. Neurosurg. **32**, 275—280 (1970).
STERN, G.: The effect of lesions in the substantia nigra. Brain **89**, 449—478 (1966).
STOCK, R.: 2-Amino-4-hydroxy-6-7-dimethyl-tetrahydropteridine in Parkinson's disease. J. Amer. med. Ass. **210**, 1594 (1969).
TAGLIAMONTE, A., TAGLIAMONTE, P., GESSA, G.L., BRODIE, B.B.: Compulsive sexual activity induced by *p*-chlorophenylalanine in normal and pinealectomized male rats. Science **166**, 1433—1435 (1969).
TAMARKIN, N.R., GOODWIN, F.K., AXELROD, J.: Rapid elevation of biogenic amine metabolites in human CSF following probenecid. Life Sci. Pt. I. **9**, 1397—1408 (1970).
TAMER, A., MCKEY, R., ARIAS, D., WORLEY, L., FOGEL, B.J.: Phenothiazine Hinduced extrapyramidal dysfunction in the neonate. J. Pediat. **75**, 479—480 (1969).
TAYLOR, K.M., LAVERTY, R.: The metabolism of tritiated dopamine in regions of the rat brain *in vivo*. — II. The significance of the neutral metabolites of catecholamines. J. Neurochem. **16**, 1367—1376 (1969).
— SNYDER, S.H.: Amphetamine: differentiation by *d* and *l* isomers of behavior involving brain norepinephrine or dopamine. Science **168**, 1487—1489 (1970).
THEISS, E., SCHÄRER, K.: Toxicity of L-dopa and a decarboxylase inhibitor in animal experiments. Proc. 4th Bel-Air Symposium, Geneva, 1970, in the press.
THOENEN, H., HAEFELY, W., GEY, K.F., HUERLIMANN, A.: Quantitative aspects of the replacement of norepinephrine by dopamine as sympathetic transmitter after inhibition of dopamine-β-hydroxylase by disulfiram. J. Pharmacol. exp. Ther. **156**, 246—251 (1967).
TISSOT, R.: Communication to 4th Bel-Air Symposium, Geneva (1970).
— PLETSCHER, A., BARTHOLINI, G., CONSTANTINIDIS, J.: La barrière enzymatique pour la L-dopa au des capillaires du cerveau et son abolition. Proc. 2nd int. Meeting int. Soc. Neurochem. Milan, pp. 394—396 (1969c).

TOBIAS, J.A.Y.: Levodopa and schizophrenia. J. Amer. med. Ass. **211**, 1857 (1970).
TORQUATI, T.: Sulla presenza di una sostanza azotata nei germogli dei semi di "Vicia faba". Arch. Farmacol. sper. **15**, 213—223 (1913).
TSENG, L.F., WALASZEK, E.J.: Influence of alteration of catecholamine and serotonin levels on bulbocapnine-induced catatonia. Pharmacologist **12**, 198 (1970).
TYCE, G.M.: The metabolism of L-dihydroxyphenylalanine-^{14}C by isolated perfused rat liver. In: L-Dopa and Parkinsonism, pp. 86—88, edit. A. BARBEAU and F.H. MCDOWELL. Philadelphia: Davis 1970.
— MUENTER, M.D., OWEN, C.A., JR.: Dihydroxyphenylalanine (dopa) in plasma during dopa treatment of patients with Parkinson's disease. Mayo Clin. Proc. **45**, 438—443 (1970a).
— — — Metabolism of L-dihydroxyphenylalanine by patients with Parkinson's disease. Mayo Clin. Proc. **45**, 645—656 (1970b).
UDENFRIEND, S.: Tyrosine hydroxylase. Pharmacol. Rev. **18**, 43—51 (1966).
— Biochemical investment, clinical dividend. Hosp. Pract. **4**, 33—34 (1969).
— ZALTZMAN-NIRENBERG, P., NAGATSU, T.: Inhibitors of purified beef adrenal tyrosine hydroxylase. Biochem. Pharmacol. **14**, 837—845 (1965).
UNGERSTEDT, U., BUTCHER, L.L., BUTCHER, S.G., ANDÉN, N.-E., FUXE, K.: Direct chemical stimulation of dopaminergic mechanisms in the neostriatum of the rat. Brain Res. **14**, 461—471 (1969).
VANDER WENDE, C., JOHNSON, J.C.: Interaction of serotonin with the catecholamines. — I. Inhibition of dopamine and norepinephrine oxidation. Biochem. Pharmacol. **19**, 1991—2000 (1970).
— SPOERLEIN, M.T.: Oxidation of dopamine to melanin by an enzyme of rat brain. Life Sci. **2**, 386—392 (1963).
VAN ROSSUM, J.M.: The significance of dopamine-receptor blockade for the mechanism of action of neuroleptic drugs. Arch. int. Pharmocodyn. **160**, 492—494 (1966).
— WIJFFELS, C.C.B., RIJNTJES, N.V.M.: Autoradiography of ^{14}C-DOPA in gerbils. Europ. J. Pharmacol. **7**, 337—341 (1969).
VAN WOERT, M.H., BOWERS, M.B., JR.: The effect of L-dopa on monoamine metabolites in Parkinson's disease. Experientia (Basel) **26**, 161—163 (1970).
— HENINGER, G., RATHEY, V., BOWERS, M.B., JR.: L-Dopa in senile dementia. Lancet **i**, 573—574 (1970).
— PRASAD, K.N., BORG, D.C.: Spectroscopic studies of *substantia nigra* pigment in human subjects. J. Neurochem. **14**, 707—716 (1967).
VOGEL, W.H.: Non-enzymatic decarboxylation of dihydroxyphenylalanine. Naturwissenschaften **56**, 462 (1969).
— MCFARLAND, H., PRINCE, L.N.: Decarboxylation of 3,4-dihydroxyphenylalanine in various human adult and fetal tissues. Biochem. Pharmacol. **19**, 618—620 (1970a).
— ORFEI, V., CENTURY, B.: Activities of enzymes involved in the formation and destruction of biogenic amines in various areas of human brain. J. Pharmacol. exp. Ther. **165**, 196—203 (1969).
— SNYDER, R., HARE, T.A.: The enzymatic decarboxylation of DOPA in human liver homogenates. Proc. Soc. exp. Biol. (N. Y.) **134**, 477—481 (1970b).
VOGT, M.: Drug-induced changes in brain dopamine and their relation to Parkinsonism. Sci. Basis Med. pp. 276—291 (1970).
VON STUDNITZ, W.: Methodische und klinische Untersuchungen über die Ausscheidung der 3-Methoxy-4-Hydroxymandelsäure im Urin. Scand. J. clin. Lab. Invest. **12**, Suppl. 48, 1—58 (1960).
— Occurrence, isolation and identification of 3-methoxy-4-hydroxyphenylalanine. Clin. chim. Acta **6**, 526—530 (1961).
— Zur Frage des Vorkommens von 3-Hydroxy-4-methoxymandelsäure beim normalen und gesteigerten Katecholaminstoffwechsel. Klin. Wschr. **45**, 307—308 (1967).
WALSH, M.J., DAVIS, V.E., YAMANAKA, Y.: Tetrahydropapaveroline: an alkaloid metabolite of dopamine *in vitro*. J. Pharmacol. exp. Ther. **174**, 388—400 (1970).
WARD, A.A., JR., MCCULLOUGH, W.S., MAGOUN, H.W.: Production of an alternating tremor at rest in monkeys. J. Neurophysiol. **11**, 317—330 (1948).
WATANABE, A.M., CHASE, T.N., CARDON, P.V.: Effect of L-dopa alone and in combination with an extracerebral decarboxylase inhibitor on blood pressure and some cardiovascular reflexes. Clin. Pharmacol. Ther. **11**, 740—746 (1970).
WATT, J.: Dopa and Parkinsonism. Brit. med. J. **3**, 437 (1967).
WEBER, W.W., ZANNONI, V.G.: Reduction of phenylpyruvic acids to phenyllactic acids in mammalian tissues. J. biol. Chem. **241**, 1345—1349 (1966).
WEIL-MALHERBE, H.: The concentration of adrenaline in human plasma and its relation to mental activity. J. ment. Sci. **101**, 733—755 (1955).

WEIL-MALHERBE, H., AXELROD, J., TOMCHICK, R.: Blood-brain barrier for adrenaline. Science **129**, 1226—1227 (1959).
— VAN BUREN, J.M.: The excretion of dopamine and dopamine metabolites in Parkinson's disease and the effect of diet thereon. J. Lab. clin. Med. **74**, 305—318 (1969).
WEINER, N.: Substrate specificity of brain amine oxidase of several mammals. Arch. Biochem. Biophys. **91**, 182—188 (1960).
WEINSHILBOUM, R., AXELROD, J.: Dopamine-β-hydroxylase activity in human blood. Pharmacologist **12**, 214 (1970).
WERDINIUS, B.: Effect of probenecid on the levels of monoamine metabolites in the rat brain. Acta pharmacol. (Kbh.) **25**, 18—23 (1967).
WERLE, E., SELL, J.: Über die fermentative Decarboxylierung von Mono- und Dioxyphenylserin. Biochem. Z. **326**, 110—122 (1955).
WESTLAKE, R.J., TEW, J.M.: Urinary amines in patient undergoing thalamotomy for Parkinson's disease. Neurology **16**, 619—620 (1966).
WISEMAN-DISTLER, M.H., SOURKES, T.L., CARABIN, S.: Precursors of 3,4-dihydroxyphenylacetic acid and 4-hydroxy-3-methoxyphenylacetic acid in the rat. Clin. chim. Acta **12**, 335—339 (1965).
WORLLEDGE, S.M., CARSTAIRS, K.C., DACIE, J.V.: Autoimmune haemolytic anaemia associated with α-methyldopa therapy. Lancet **ii**, 135—139 (1966).
WURTMAN, R.J., CHOU, C., ROSE, C.: The fate of C^{14}-dihydroxyphenylalanine (C^{14}-dopa) in the whole mouse. J. Pharmacol. exp. Ther. **174**, 351—356 (1970a).
— LARIN, F.: A sensitive and specific isotopic assay for the estimation of tyrosine transaminase. Biochem. Pharmacol. **17**, 817—818 (1968).
— ROSE, C.M., MATTHYSSE, S., STEPHENSON, J., BALDESSARINI, R.: L-Dihydroxyphenylalanine: effect on S-adenosylmethionine in brain. Science **169**, 395—397 (1970b).
WYCIS, H.T., CUNNINGHAM, W., KELLETT, G., SPIEGEL, E.A.: L-Dopa in the treatment of post-surgical Parkinson patients. J. Neurosurg. **32**, 281—285 (1970).
YAHR, M.D.: Abnormal involuntary movements induced by dopa: clinical aspects. In: L-Dopa and Parkinsonism, pp. 101—108, edit. A. BARBEAU and F.H. MCDOWELL. Philadelphia: Davis 1970a.
— Psychiatric aspects of L-dopa treatment. In: L-Dopa and Parkinsonism, pp. 328—329, edit. A. BARBEAU and F.H. MCDOWELL. Philadelphia: Davis 1970b.
— Results of long-term administration of levodopa in parkinsonism. Proc. 4th Bel-Air Symposium, Geneva, 1970c, in the press.
— DUVOISIN, R.C., SCHEAR, M.J., BARRETT, R.E., HOEHN, M.M.: Treatment of Parkinsonism with levodopa. Arch. Neurol. **21**, 343—354 (1969).
YAMANAKA, Y., WALSH, M.J., DAVIS, V.E.: Salsolinol, an alkaloid derivative of dopamine formed *in vitro* during alcohol metabolism. Nature (Lond.) **227**, 1143—1144 (1970).
YAMORI, Y., LOVENBERG, W., SJOERDSMA, A.: Norepinephrine metabolism in brainstem of spontaneously hypertensive rats. Science **170**, 544—546 (1970).
YARYURA-TOBIAS, J.A., DIAMOND, B., MERLIS, S.: The action of L-dopa on schizophrenic patients. Curr. ther. Res. **12**, 528—531 (1970).
YEH, B.K., MCNAY, J.L., GOLDBERG, L.I.: Attenuation of dopamine renal and mesenteric vasodilation by haloperidol: evidence for a specific dopamine receptor. J. Pharmacol. exp. Ther. **168**, 303—309 (1969).
YOSHIDA, H., KANUKE, K., NAMBA, J.: Properties of a carrier system to transport L-dopa into brain slices. Nature (Lond.) **198**, 191—192 (1963).
YOUDIM, M.B.H., BONHAM CARTER, S., SANDLER, M., HANINGTON, E., WILKINSON, M.: A conjugation defect in tyramine-sensitive migraine. Nature (Lond.) **230**, 127—128 (1971).

Chapter 20

Phaeochromocytoma and Other Catecholamine-Producing Tumours

H. WINKLER and A.D. SMITH

With 1 Figure

I. Introduction

In a book entitled "Human tumours secreting catecholamines", which covers the literature up to 1961, HERMANN and MORNEX (1964) give 826 references. Since 1961, at least another 500 papers on these tumours have been published; it is, therefore, not our intention or inclination to give a comprehensive review of the subject. Our task is made easier because several books and reviews are available: HUME (1960), SACK and KOLL (1963), GIFFORD et al. (1964), COUPLAND (1965), KÄSER (1966a), CROUT (1966), STUDNITZ (1966), HOLTZ and PALM (1966), GJESSING (1968). This review will concentrate on the biochemistry and cell biology of the tumours in relation to the abilities of the tissue to synthesise, store and release the catecholamines. Many of the results merely describe for tumours what is already known for the normal tissues. Nevertheless, it is our belief that studies on the tumours may help to elucidate the fundamental mechanisms which control the functional relationship between the synthesis, storage and secretion of the catecholamines in normal tissues.

The chapter will be subdivided into three sections: The first section deals with phaeochromocytomas and phaeochromoblastomas; the second with neuroblastomas and ganglioneuromas; and the last with tumours of the carotid body and related structures, sometimes called chemodectomas (MULLIGAN, 1950). Phaeochromocytomas and the malignant phaeochromoblastomas are considered to arise from adrenal or extra-adrenal chromaffin tissue, whereas neuroblastomas are tumours arising from primitive sympathetic cells or the sympathoblast (GJESSING, 1968; KÄSER, 1966a; see also chapter by COUPLAND). Tumours of the extra-adrenal chromaffin tissue are sometimes called paragangliomas (see e. g. BRANTIGAN and KATESE, 1969); neuroblastomas which reveal a certain degree of maturation have been named ganglioneuroblastomas. Ganglioneuroma is a benign tumour of mature sympathetic cells.

II. Phaeochromocytomas and Phaeochromoblastomas

1. Occurence

Judging from the number of publications dealing with these tumours one would tend to think that phaeochromocytomas are quite frequent. However, this is not the case. Thus, only between 1.3 and 4.2 phaeochromocytomas were found per 100,000 new patient registrations (MILES, 1960; BELLAS, 1963; MOORHEAD et al., 1966). As many as 30—60% of these tumours were not found until autopsy, which emphasises the need for the wider use of diagnostic procedures (MILES, 1960; DE GRAEFF and HORAK, 1964; MOORHEAD et al., 1966; SCOTT et al., 1965; RIDDELL et al., 1963; KIRKENDALL et al., 1965).

If only hypertensive patients are considered, the frequency of these tumours appears to be much higher; thus, an incidence ranging from 0.12—0.7% has been reported (HUME, 1960; ROTH et al., 1960; PRIESTLEY et al., 1963; GREER et al., 1964; PERTSEMLIDIS et al., 1969). The variation in these figures probably depends very much on the selection of patients. Thus, 36 tumours were found among 4467 hypertensive patients by PRIESTLEY et al. (1963); but these hypertensive patients were already selected and represented only 15% of all hypertensives. Such a preselection of patients might explain the exceptionally high incidence of tumours, i. e. 2.2%, among hypertensive cases that was reported by GOODALL and STONE (1960).

Many studies have established that phaeochromocytomas which occur in close relations are inherited and are transmitted in a dominant fashion, but with variable degrees of penetrance. Ten families with such tumours were reviewed by CARMAN and BRASHEAR in 1960. Since then, additional cases have been reported; thus 12 families were reviewed by HERMANN and MORNEX (1964), 16 families by NOUROK (1964), 18 families by SCHIMKE and HARTMANN (1965) and 20 families by DONATH et al. (1965).

Phaeochromocytomas can occur together with other diseases in a frequency higher than can be attributed to chance. Thus, an association of phaeocromocytoma and neurofibromatosis has been noted. SCHLEGEL (1960), in a very complete review, compiled 45 cases from the literature and added two of his own. An association of phaeochromocytoma and cerebellar hemangioblastomas which represent part of the Hippel Lindau's syndrome has also been suggested (CHAPMAN and DIAZ-PEREZ, 1962; MULLHOLLAND et al., 1969; NIBBELINK et al., 1969).

The occurrence of phaeochromocytoma together with thyroid cancer is also quite well established. The cases of this syndrome, described in the literature, have been reviewed several times; 31 cases being the latest score (SIPPLE, 1961; WILLIAMS, 1965; SAPIRA et al., 1965; HUANG and MCLEISH. 1968; SLAROTINEK et al., 1968). In these patients the phaeochromocytomas are frequently bilateral and the thyroid cancer appears to be mainly of the otherwise rare medullary type (WILLIAMS, 1965). Furthermore, a familial occurence of this syndrome has been observed (NOUROK, 1964; WILLIAMS, 1965; SCHIMKE and HARTMANN, 1965; HUANG and MCLEISH, 1968).

In some patients this syndrome is associated with parathyroid adenomas (SAROSI and DOE, 1968; SCHIMKE et al., 1968) which may be, as suggested by SCHIMKE et al. (1968), a secondary response to excess calcitonin released from the thyroid carcinoma.

It is noteworthy that the cells of both types of tumour contain biogenic amines, i. e. catecholamines and serotonin, as demonstrated by histochemical and biochemical methods (FALCK et al., 1968). Secretion granules have been observed by electron microscopy both in the cells of the thyroid tumours and in the cells from the phaeochromocytoma (HUANG and MCLEISH, 1968; see also section II, 3, d). The anology between these two types of tumour (see LJUNGBERG et al., 1967) may reflect characteristics of the normal cells from which they originate. Thus, at least in animals, the chromaffin cells of adrenal medulla contain catecholamines and also traces of serotonin (SNYDER et al., 1965) in secretory granules, and the parafollicular cells contain serotonin in the secretion granules (JAIM-ETCHEVERRY and ZIEHER, 1968), which probably also contain the calcitonin (FOSTER, 1968).

2. Synthesis and Metabolism of Catecholamines in Tumours

a) Synthesis of Catecholamines

There is good evidence for the capacity of tumour tissue to synthesise noradrenaline and adrenaline from tyrosine, and the presence of the various enzymes necessary for the different steps in catecholamine synthesis has been demonstrated. The first step in the synthesis of these amines is the conversion of tyrosine to dopa, catalysed by tyrosine hydroxylase. GOLDSTEIN (1966) was unable to detect this enzyme in phaeochromocytoma tissue, but ROTH et al. (1968) could clearly demonstrate it. Under optimal conditions the tumour tissue synthesized 38 μg catecholamines/g tissue/hr, which is a relatively high value when compared with bovine medulla, where a rate of 1.4 μg/g tissue/hr has been reported (NAGATSU et al., 1964). The next step in the synthesis, i. e. the formation of dopamine by dopadecarboxylase, has been investigated by several authors (GÉLINAS et al., 1957; SJOERDSMA et al., 1958; HAGEN, 1962; LANGEMANN et al., 1963). The activity of this enzyme was found to be comparable to that in normal human or animal adrenal medulla (HAGEN, 1962; LANGEMANN et al., 1963). In quite a few tumours the activity was higher than that in normal human medulla (LANGEMANN et al., 1963).

Dopamine-β-hydroxylase was also studied by several authors (SJOERDSMA et al., 1958; BOHUON and GUÉRINOT, 1966; GOLDSTEIN, 1966; BOHUON and GUÉRINOT, 1968). In a quantitative study BOHUON and GUÉRINOT (1968) found in a tumour which had a relatively low concentration of catecholamines enzyme activity of about 1/3 of that of bovine adrenal medulla.

The formation of adrenaline from noradrenaline, catalysed by phenylethanolamine-N-methyltransferase is of special interest. It has often been pointed out (see below) that tumours contain a smaller proportion of adrenaline than is found in the normal medulla, or even no adrenaline at all. In 1957, VON EULER and STRÖM suggested (based on their studies of 35 phaeochromocytoma patients) that adrenaline is only produced and secreted by tumours arising from the adrenal medulla, whereas extraadrenal tumours secrete only noradrenaline. The localisation of these tumours might, therefore, be recognized preoperatively by the urinary excretion patterns of these hormones. However, VON EULER and STRÖM already found exceptions to this rule and this was confirmed in a study of 75 cases by CROUT and SJOERDSMA (1960). The latter authors reported that in 42% of the patients the amount of adrenaline in the urine was increased and that, in these patients, 95% of the tumours were in the adrenal region. When, on the other hand, only the amount of noradrenaline was increased, then 67% of the tumours were still found near the adrenal. Thus, the urinary excretion patterns are not an unequivocable guide to the location of the tumour. As might be expected, therefore, the relative adrenaline content of phaeochromocytoma tissue bears no strict correlation with the location of the tumour. Many extraadrenal tumours have been described where no adrenaline could be detected (VON EULER and STRÖM, 1957; SCHÜMANN, 1960; KENNEDY et al., 1961; HUNTER et al., 1963; HERMANN and MORNEX, 1964; BESSER and PFAU, 1968). A particularly illustrative case is the malignant tumour described by KENNEDY et al. (1961), where the primary tumour, near the adrenal, contained about 10% adrenaline, whereas a metastasis in the liver contained no adrenaline at all. On the other hand, extraadrenal tumours can contain a substantial proportion of adrenaline (HERMANN and MORNEX, 1964; SCHÜMANN, 1960; MIĆIĆ et al., 1962; FRIES and CHAMBERLIN, 1968; see also ENGELMANN and HAMMOND, 1968). The case described by MIĆIĆ et al. (1962) is in fact rather exceptional, since the tumour found in the urinary bladder contained 1.5 mg adrenaline and only 0.03 mg noradrenaline per g of tissue.

As already mentioned, the normal human adrenal medulla contains a relatively high proportion of adrenaline, i. e. about 85% of the total catecholamines (SHEPHERD and WEST, 1953), and so the question arises, why do tumours rarely contain such a large proportion of adrenaline? As early as 1951 it was suggested that the methylation of adrenaline in the medulla depends on the size and vicinity of the cortex (SHEPHERD and WEST, 1951; COUPLAND, 1953). More recently, it has been shown that the activity of phenylethanolamine-N-methyltransferase in the medulla depends on a high concentration of corticosteroids in adrenal blood (WURTMAN and AXELROD, 1966; MARGOLIS et al., 1966). Such a high concentration is normally present because the blood from the cortex is drained through the medulla. It is, therefore, easy to understand why tumours, especially extraadrenal ones, contain little adrenaline, since they will not be exposed to a high concentration of corticosteroids. Why, then, do occasional tumours contain high concentrations of adrenaline? An explanation has been offered by WURTMAN et al. (1968), who suggested that phenylethanolamine-N-methyltransferase in some tumours might be a non-inducible form of the enzyme, i. e. an enzyme whose synthesis is not controlled by corticosteroids. Such a non-inducible enzyme has already been found in frog tissues and recent studies have shown that the tumour enzyme has some properties in common with those of this non-inducible enzyme (GOLDSTEIN et al., 1969).

All the studies discussed above have demonstrated that tumour tissue can synthesise catecholamines, but we would like to present more quantitative data concerning the actual synthesising capacity, which would permit the calculation of the rate of turnover of the catecholamines present in the tumour. Earlier attempts to obtain an estimate of this turnover were based on the fact that about 3% of any dose of catecholamines infused is excreted unchanged in the urine. The urinary excretion of catecholamines in a patient was then used to calculate the total amount secreted by the tumour. The figure so obtained was related to the tumour content of catecholamines. In 1958, VON EULER found that in 14 cases 1 to 142% of the tumour catecholamine content was released per day. DE SCHAEPDRYVER (1959) described values ranging from 11.8 to 700% depending on whether or not the urinary catecholamines were determined during a crisis. From the data given by HERMAN and MORNEX (1964), values from 1.1 to 180% can be calculated (6 cases). There is no indication of a preferentially high turnover of either noradrenaline or adrenaline (DE SCHAEPDRYVER, 1959; VON EULER, 1958; HERMAN and MORNEX, 1964).

The urinary excretion of catecholamines relative to that of the metabolites can vary enormously in tumour patients (see below) and so the method of calculation used by all the authors quoted above is rather unreliable. More recently, the secretory capacity of these tumours was calculated from the urinary excretion of the sum of the catecholamines and their metabolites (CROUT and SJOERDSMA, 1964). In the 24 patients studied, turnovers ranging from 1.4 to 220% were found. Similarly, WINKLER and SMITH (1968) found turnovers of 0.4 to 95% in 5 patients, and ROSENTHAL, et al. (1966) described one case with the exceedingly high turnover of 768%. In this connection it would be useful to know the turnover in normal human adrenal medulla. This can be calculated from the urinary metanephrine, which disappears after adrenalectomy (COWARD et al., 1962). About 40% of a dose of adrenaline infused in the blood stream is excreted as metanephrine (LA BROSSE et al., 1961) and the normal urinary excretion of metanephrine ranges from 40—330 μg/24 hr (WEIL-MALHERBE and SMITH, 1966). The catecholamine content of the human adrenal medulla is about 6 mg (VON EULER et al., 1954). If we use these figures we find that from about 2.0—14.0% of the adrenaline content of the human adrenal gland is secreted per day, which is a figure of the same order as that found for the rat adrenal medulla by LEDUC (1961).

There is no doubt that many phaeochromocytomas possess an enormous capacity to synthesise catecholamines and one wonders how such a high rate of synthesis can occur in view of the high concentration of catecholamines in the tumour (see Table 1). As an explanation it has been suggested several times that some mechanism regulating the synthesis, e. g. a feed-back inhibition of tyrosine hydroxylase, might be disturbed (HILLARP et al., 1961; WINKLER and SMITH, 1968). It was, therefore, illuminating when ROTH et al., (1968) demonstrated that the activity of tyrosine hydroxylase in homogenates of tumour tissue was much less sensitive to inhibition by noradrenaline than was the enzyme from normal human adrenal medulla. It would be of interest to know whether this is a property of the enzyme itself or whether it is due to different amounts of co-factors in the tumour tissue, since the catecholamines inhibit the enzyme by competition with the pteridine co-factor (UDENFRIEND et al., 1965). The studies of NAGATSU et al. (1970) are consistent with the first possibility since they found that partly purified tyrosine hydroxylase of human phaeochromocytoma had a higher affinity for the pteridine co-factor, and was less sensitive to inhibition by noradrenaline, than was a similar preparation from bovine adrenal medulla. However, a definite answer requires a comparison of the properties of purified tyrosine hydroxylase from normal and tumour tissue of the same species.

In connection with the possibility, discussed below, that the tyrosine hydroxylase of tumours (which are not innervated) is different from that of normal tissue we should like to speculate that in normal tissue there are two forms of tyrosine hydroxylase: one form independent of nervous activity and relatively insensitive to inhibition by noradrenaline, and the other form which is more sensitive to noradrenaline and is induced by nervous activity. MUELLER et al. (1969) have demonstrated a marked rise in tyrosine hydroxylase activity in the adrenal medulla after several procedures which stimulate the nerve to the gland.

b) Metabolism of Catecholamines

The first evidence for the presence of MAO was given by BURGER and LANGEMAN (1956), who found a relatively low concentration in homogenates from tumours by a manometric technique. After incubation of tumour tissue with [^{14}C]-DOPA, labelled 3, 4-dihydroxymandelic acid has been isolated (GÉLINAS et al., 1957); this was presumably produced from noradrenaline by MAO. A more extensive study was performed by AMAR-COSTESEC et al. (1965), who measured this enzyme in several fragments of three tumours. In comparison with liver, kidney or neuroblastoma tissue a relatively low activity was found. COMT has also been detected in tumour tissue, but only after adding S-adenosylmethionine to the *in vitro* system (SJOERDSMA et al., 1958). It is clear that data concerning metabolising enzymes are scarce, which makes quantitative statements about the metabolism of catecholamines very difficult.

3. Storage of Catecholamines in Tumours

a) Tissue Content of Catecholamines and Metabolites

In 1929, Rabin extracted an adrenaline-like substance from a phaeochromocytoma (see also BLASCHKO, 1966) and 20 years later noradrenaline was demonstrated in tumour tissue (HOLTON, 1949). In the meantime, the catecholamine content of numerous tumours has been determined. HERMAN and MORNEX (1964, Fig. 39) compiled the data for 88 tumours from the literature; the catecholamine concentration in these tumours ranged from 0.076—50 mg/g tissue. Most of the tumours (77 out of 88) contained from 1—10 mg/g. Noradrenaline was usually the predominant amine, but one tumour contained 99% adrenaline. Other reviews of the literature include those by STRAUS and WURM (1960) and ROBINSON (1963). From the table compiled by the latter author it can be seen that the relative adrenaline content varied from 0—86%. A large series of 24 tumours was studied recently by one group of authors (CROUT and SJOERDSMA, 1964). The catecholamine concentration varied from 0.7—19.6 mg/g; adrenaline comprised 0—56% of the catecholamines. The total catecholamine content of one tumour, which weighed 850 g, reached the enormous value of 10.6 g. Normal human adrenal medulla has been reported to contain from 0.9—1.5 mg catecholamines per g of tissue (SCHÜMANN, 1960; BURGER and LANGEMANN, 1956; SHEPHERD and WEST, 1953). This is relatively low compared with the catecholamine concentration of the medulla of various animal species which ranges from 3.6—8.0 mg/g (WEST, 1953). This discrepancy may be due to difficulties in separating, in human glands, the cortical tissue completely from the medulla. In any case, it is quite clear that tumour tissue contains a high concentration of catecholamines, which indicates that the storage of amines is just as efficient as in the normal gland. Evidence concerning the mode of storage of the amines in tumours will be described below.

Various precursors and metabolites of catecholamines together with serotonin have also been reported to be present in tumours. Table 1 is an attempt to compile these results from the quantitative data given in the literature. There is no doubt that noradrenaline and adrenaline are the predominant amines, only in one case was dopamine the major amine (MCMILLAN, 1956). Dopamine and DOPA are present in

Table 1. *Content of various substances in phaeochromocytoma tissue. The figures give the concentration of each substance in μg/g tissue.* (VMA = vanillylmandelic acid, 5-HT = 5 hydroxytryptamine)

Authors	No. of cases	Nor-adrenaline	Adrenaline	Dopa	Dopamin	Meta-nephrines	VMA	5-HT
MCMILLAN (1956)	1	150	0	0	1970	—	—	0
WEIL-MALHERBE (1956)	2	722; 764	106; 115	8; 147	41; 494	—	—	—
SATO et al. (1962)	3	624—4250	66—5100	—	—	6.7—19.7	0.3—0.73	—
PAGE and JACOBY (1964)	2	1185; 1326	590; 5180	—	—	1.54; 2.3	0.57 (1)	—
DONATH et al. (1965)	2	2245; 5140	25; 76	—	3.4; 9.4	—	—	—
ROSENTHAL et al. (1966)	1	354	19	—	—	246	—	—
ZIEGLER et al. (1967)	18	100—10000	0 (4)—9514	—	0 (4)—37	—	—	0 (13)—1.8
ANTON et al. (1967)	2	1125; 1470	37; 150	<25	<25	15.5	<50	—
VOORHESS (1968)	4	367—6486	0 (1)—7221	—	0	—	<0.5	—
FALCK et al. (1968)	2	3500; 5600	1330; 1350	—	5; 12.7	—	—	0.3; 0.9
BOHUON (1968)	1	49	0	0.05	0.15	—	—	—
HINTERSBERGER et al. (1969)	4	41—7700		—	0 (2)—0.1	—	0	—

rather low concentration in a few tumours and have not even been detected in some tumours (Shepherd and West, 1953; Kennedy et al., 1961; Cabana et al., 1964).

Metabolites are only present in small amounts. N-methylmetanephrine (Itoh et al., 1962) and 3-methoxy-4-hydroxyphenylglycol — 5—10 μg/g tissue — (Kopin and Axelrod, 1960) have been demonstrated in tumours. The presence of homocysteine was reported by Biserte (1957).

b) Isolation of Chromaffin Granules from Phaeochromocytoma

When homogenates of normal adrenal medulla are subjected to differential centrifugation, then, depending on the efficiency of the homogenisation procedure, a variable proportion of the catecholamines is lost in the first sediment within unbroken cells. A large part of the catecholamines present in the remaining low speed supernatant can be sedimented in the large granule fraction, indicating that the amines are stored in particles.

The first differential centrifugation of homogenates from phaeochromocytoma tissue was performed by Burger and Langemann (1956). In this study on two tumours most of the catecholamines were found not to be sedimentable, but the authors considered the possibility that this finding was due to methodical difficulties. Since then, several studies on tumour tissue have demonstrated that a large part of the catecholamines is sedimentable. Thus, Gélinas et al. (1957) found that 50% of the catecholamines present in the low speed supernatant could be sedimented. In a subsequent study (Leduc and D'Iorio, 1960) a figure of 75% was obtained. Similar values were found in the three tumours studied by Schümann (1960), in two others described by Page and Jacoby (1964) and in one investigated by Stjärne et al. (1964). Recently, in a relatively large series of five tumours values ranging from 66—78% were reported (Blaschko et al., 1968). When adrenal medullae of ox, pig and horse were studied with exactly the same methods, 65—74% of the catecholamines present in the low speed sediment were found to be sedimentable (Winkler et al., 1967).

Thus it is justifiable to conclude that in normal adrenal medulla and in tumours of the same tissue most of the catecholamines are sedimentable and are, therefore, present in a particle. There remains, for both normal and tumour tissue, the still unresolved question whether the unbound fraction of catecholamines is an expression of a soluble cytoplasmic pool of catecholamines *in vivo* or whether it is due to leakage of catecholamines from particles during homogenisation and centrifugation (see chapter by Smith and Winkler).

The 'large granule' fraction obtained from normal adrenal medulla consists of mitochondria (Blaschko et al., 1957), lysosomes (Smith and Winkler, 1966), some contaminating microsomes (Smith and Winkler, 1968; Winkler, 1969) and the chromaffin granules, which contain the catecholamines. These granules, due to their high density, can be separated from the other cell particles by density gradient centrifugation. The first indication of a relatively high density of tumour granules was obtained by Leduc and D'Iorio (1960). They centrifuged the large granule fraction obtained from two homogenates over 1.5 M sucrose and found that 58% of the catecholamines were sedimented through this sucrose solution. In another study (Stjärne et al., 1964) no sediment of granules was obtained after centrifugation of the large granule fraction over 1.6 M sucrose, but there was a sediment when 1.2 M sucrose was used. However, in these experiments the centrifugal force applied was relatively low (50000 g for 60 min). A more detailed study of chromaffin granules in sucrose density gradients was undertaken by Blaschko et al. (1968), who studied five tumours. In separate experiments with two different tumours, the large granule fractions were resolved by centrifugation over density gradients ranging from 1.3—2.0 M sucrose. After centrifugation the gradients were cut; in the fractions so obtained enzymes and constituents typical for the different cell particles were determined. Mitochondria were found in the top fraction of the gradient and lysosomes in an intermediate position. Chromaffin granules sedimented to the bottom fractions of the gradient. Chromaffin granules from a tumour which contained mainly noradrenaline exhibited the highest density and were recovered in the bottom fraction of the gradient, where they had partly sedimented. It is already known from studies on chromaffin granules of the adrenal medulla of several species that noradrenaline-containing granules possess a higher density than those containing adrenaline (EADE, 1958; SCHÜMANN, 1957; WINKLER, 1969). The large granule fractions from three of the five tumours were centrifuged over 1.6 M sucrose according to the simplified gradient method of SMITH and WINKLER (1967). From 60—73% of the catecholamines sedimented to the bottom of the tube. The chromaffin granules thus obtained were contaminated by only small amounts of other cell organelles (WINKLER et al., 1967).

c) Properties of Chromaffin Granules from Phaeochromocytoma

The isolation of highly purified chromaffin granules has made it possible to investigate the composition of these organelles by biochemical techniques. From the differential and density gradient centrifugation experiments it can already be concluded that chromaffin granules from phaeochromocytoma are similar to normal granules as far as fragility, weight and density are concerned.

Are the other properties of the tumour granules, notably their ability to store amines, similar to those of normal chromaffin granules? This question is pertinent in view of repeated suggestions that the reason for the release of large amounts of catecholamines from phaeochromocytomas lies in an impaired storage capacity of the tissue. The first indication that tumour granules might be different from normal granules was provided by D'IORIO and collaborators (GÉLINAS et al., 1957; LEDUC and D'IORIO, 1960). These authors found that the molar ratios of catecholamines to ATP in the large granule fraction from two tumours were 8 and 12.6 respectively, which is significantly higher than the ratio of 5.3 found in granules from normal human adrenal medulla (SCHÜMANN, 1960). Ratios varying from 10.3—35.4 were found by SCHÜMANN (1960) in 3 tumours and by STJÄRNE et al. (1964) in one tumour. HILLARP et al. (1961) reported a ratio of catecholamines to ATP and metabolites of 16 for tumour tissue, but they did not isolate a large granule fraction. The values of the molar ratio catecholamine/ATP in the large granule fractions of the 6 tumours described by the above authors ranged from 8—35.4 (see Table 2). On the other hand, in the series of five tumours investigated by BLASCHKO et al. (1968) catecholamine/ATP ratios from 4.7—6.5 were obtained, which are essentially normal values. These ratios were obtained in highly purified chromaffin granules isolated by density gradient centrifugation, but there is no reason to suggest that this might be the cause of the discrepancies in the results. We can say at present that it appears that in some tumours there is a deficiency of ATP, whereas in others there is not. Further studies are necessary in order to show which of the catecholamine/ATP ratios is more representative of granules present in tumours.

Other properties of highly purified tumour granules are given in Table 2. For comparison, the composition of highly purified chromaffin granules of ox, horse and pig adrenals (WINKLER et al., 1967) are shown in a separate column. The catecholamine content (per mg protein-N) varies over a wide range but is similar to that in normal granules. The ability of tumour granules to store catecholamines is, therefore, just as good as that of normal granules.

Table 2. *Properties of chromaffin granules from phaeochromocytoma*

	Phaeochromocytoma	Adrenal Medulla (ox, horse and pig)
Catecholamine/ATP (molar ratio)	8—35 (6): [a, b, c, d] 4.7—6.5 (5)	5.3[a] (human)
μ mole catecholamine/mg protein-N	4.3—27.7 (5)	6.8—15.7
Cholesterol/lipid-P (molar ratio)	0.5 (1)	0.48—0.53
Lysolecithin % of total lipid-P	11.7—23.8 (3)	7.1—16.8
% soluble protein	63 (1)	57—74
% catecholamine released per hr at 37°	27—33 (2)	25—30

Most values included in this table are taken from Blaschko et al. (1968) and Winkler et al. (1967), some are taken from the puplications given below. The number of tumours investigated is indicated in parenthesis.

[a] Schümann (1960).
[b] Gélinas et al. (1957).
[c] Leduc and D'Iorio (1960).
[d] Stjärne et al. (1964).

As far as the lipids are concerned, tumour and normal granules are similar, both being characterised by a high cholesterol/lipid-P ratio and a high lysolecithin content.

A characteristic feature of adrenal chromaffin granules is their high content of water-soluble proteins, and this is also true for tumour granules. Further studies (Strieder et al., 1968) on these water-soluble proteins revealed that the tumour proteins gave an identical pattern in gel electrophoresis with granule proteins from normal human medulla. The amino-acid composition of the soluble proteins from tumour granules was similar to that of soluble proteins from granules of animal adrenals.

All these studies indicate that tumour granules are remarkably similar to those of normal adrenal medulla, with the exception of those granules which have a relatively low ATP-content. It is, therefore, not surprising that the rate of release of catecholamines from isolated granules, incubated at 37° in isotonic sucrose, is about the same as that from granules of normal adrenal: in 1 hour only 27 and 33 %, respectively, of the catecholamines were released (see Table 2). These results refer to granules relatively rich in ATP (Blaschko et al., 1968) and so it would be of interest to know the rate of release of catecholamines *in vitro* from those tumour granules which are deficient in ATP.

It was concluded from all these studies that the storage of catecholamines in tumours is normal (Winkler and Smith, 1968). One might, of course, argue that this is only true for the granules with a normal catecholamine/ATP ratio, but could be quite different for those containing a low content of ATP. However it has already been pointed out (Winkler and Smith, 1968) that even when the ATP content of the granules was relatively low, the tumours contained high concentrations of catecholamines most of which were present in chromaffin granules. The large granules isolated by SCHÜMANN (1960) were low in ATP and yet as rich or even richer in catecholamines than granules from normal adrenal medulla. In conclusion, we would like to reiterate that biochemical investigations have given no indication that the storage of catecholamines in tumours is in any way defective. The morphological findings of normal chromaffin granules in tumour tissues, which will be discussed in the next section, are consistent with this conclusion.

d) Electron-Microscopical Observations

We shall confine our discussion mainly to studies performed with the electron microscope since the site of storage of the catecholamines, the chromaffin granules, can only be seen at the ultrastructural level. The first electron micrographs of tumour tissue were published by KLEINSCHMIDT and SCHÜMANN (1961). Abundant chromaffin granules were demonstrated. The presence of chromaffin granules varying in size from 100—300 mμ in tumour cells has been confirmed by many subsequent studies (PAGE and JACOBY, 1964; BÄSSLER and HABIGHORST, 1964; COUPLAND, 1965; ROSENTHAL et al., 1966; HUANG and MCLEISH, 1968; BLASCHKO et al., 1968; LAUMONIER et al., 1968; RATZENHOFER et al., 1968; MISUGI et al., 1968; YOKOYAMA and TAKAYASU, 1969; BENEDECZKY and LAPIS, 1968; ALBORES-SAAVEDRA et al., 1969; GREENBERG et al., 1969). The granules exhibit a variable electron density depending on the fixative used (see below) and are limited by a *unit* membrane. In a few studies normal human adrenal medulla and phaeochromocytomas have been compared (BÄSSLER and HABIGHORST, 1964; BENEDECZKY and LAPIS, 1968; YOKOYAMA and TAKAYASU, 1969).

There appears to be some correlation between the catecholamine content of the tumours and the abundancy of chromaffin granules as seen by the electron microscope. This is illustrated by Fig. 1.

Several histochemical methods have been developed which allow a differentiation of noradrenaline- or adrenaline-containing granules at the level of the electron microscope (see chapter by COUPLAND). With some of these methods noradrenaline granules appear very electron-dense whereas adrenaline granules are of moderate density. In tumour tissue a correlation of the density of granules with the noradrenaline/adrenaline content was reported, but only in an abstract (TANNENBAUM et al., 1966). Adrenaline-rich tumours contained only moderately dense granules, noradrenaline-rich tumours only dense granules; noradrenaline/adrenaline tumours contained a mixture of both. There is no indication in this report whether dense and moderately dense granules were observed within the same cell. Such a phenomenon has been described for the tumours studied by BLASCHKO et al. (1968). This finding suggests that granules containing adrenaline or noradrenaline are present within the same cell. It is interesting that an indication for this was already obtained with the light microscope (GHISLANDI et al., 1955). These authors observed that potassium iodate, which produces a dark precipitate with noradrenaline, stained some cells very dark (noradrenaline cells) but also stained the rest of the cells moderately, whereas in normal medulla only the noradrenaline cells are stained. The presence of noradrenaline and adrenaline within one cell is in contrast to the situation in normal medulla of adult animals where the granules containing noradrenaline and adrenaline respectively are confined to separate cells. Only in the foetal rabbit is a mixture of granules observed within one cell (COUPLAND and WEAKLEY, 1968).

As to other cell structures in phaeochromocytoma, there is some evidence (LAUMONIER et al., 1968; RATZENHOFER et al., 1968; YOKOYAMA and TAKAYASU, 1969) that the Golgi region is the locus for the formation of chromaffin granules,

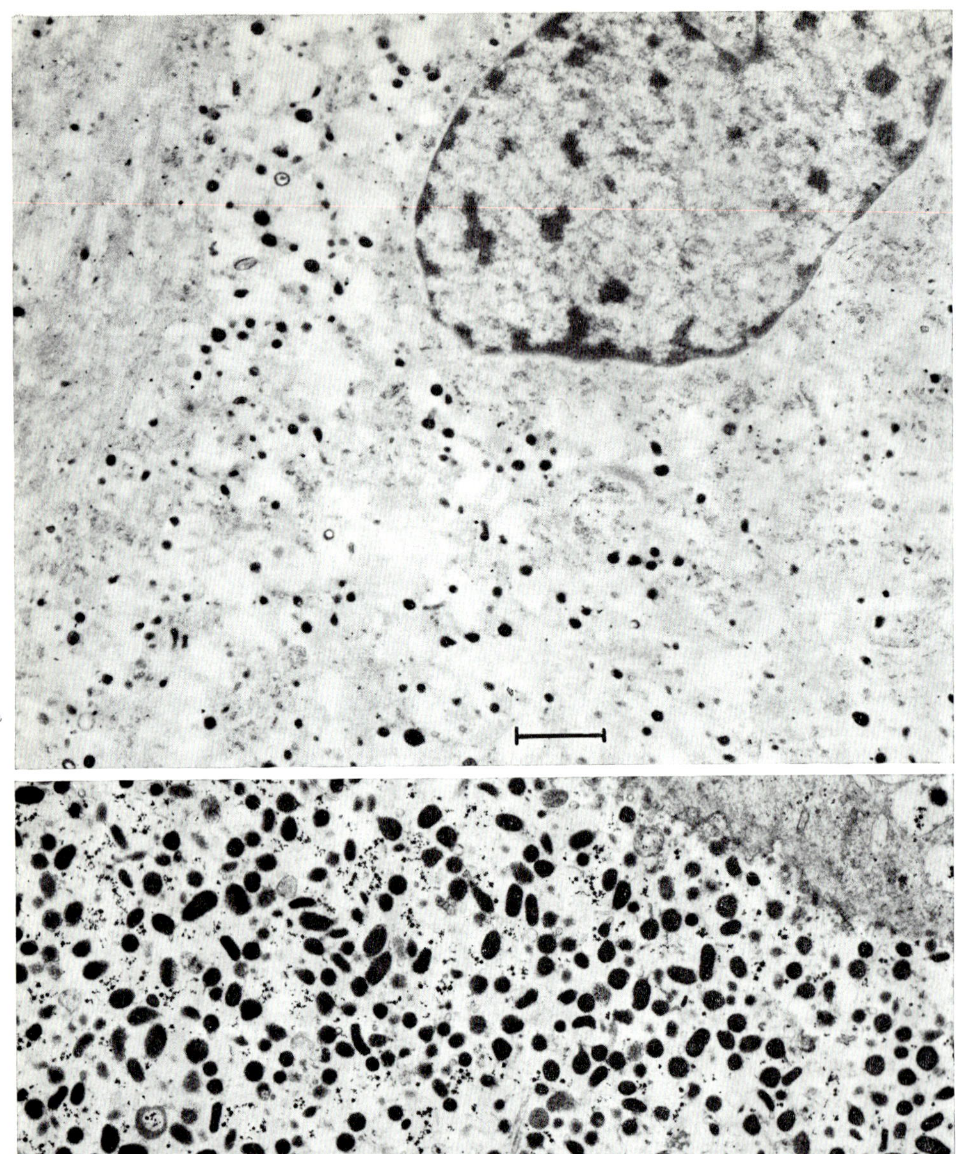

a

b

just as it is in normal tissue. Endoplasmic reticulum is relatively sparse in the cells containing many chromaffin granules, but in cells containing few chromaffin granules it can be more abundant (RATZENHOFER et al., 1968). There is no morphological indication that tumour cells are particularly rich in endoplasmic reticulum when compared with normal tissue (RATZENHOFER et al., 1968; BENEDECZKY and LAPIS, 1968; YOKOYAMA and TAKAYASU, 1969; GREENBERG et al., 1969).

Lysosomes were seen in tumour tissue by BLASCHKO et al. (1968) and RATZENHOFER et al. (1968). It is also quite likely that the so-called spheroid bodies of BÄSSLER and HABIGHORST (1964) are lysosomes. Lysosomal structures resembling autophagic vacuoles were described by BLASCHKO et al. (1968), RATZENHOFER et al. (1968) and YOKOYAMA and TAKAYASU (1969). It seems rather unlikely that autophagic vacuoles are characteristic of phaeochromocytoma, since they are also present in normal adrenal medulla (YOKOYAMA and TAKAYASU, 1969).

Finally, it has been clearly established by these morphological studies that tumour cells are not innervated (RATZENHOFER et al., 1968; BENEDECZKY and LAPIS, 1969). This has also been shown by histochemical methods which demonstrate acid phosphatase and cholinesterase in nerves (COUPLAND, 1965): the tumours are devoid of acid phosphatase-positive nerve fibres.

4. Release of Catecholamines from Phaeochromocytomas

The ability of tumour tissue to release catecholamines is revealed by the presence of large amounts of the amines or their metabolites in the blood plasma and urine of patients, and by the clinical consequences of a high level of circulating catecholamines. We shall give a short account of the biochemical studies on the nature of the substances released. Other aspects will be discussed in the chapter by SANDLER.

a) Clinical Biochemistry

α) Plasma Catecholamines: The clinical symptoms are a direct consequence of the presence of high levels of catecholamines (from about 5—4200 μg/l) in the plasma of phaeochromocytoma patients. This has been demonstrated in several biochemical studies, some of them dealing with large groups of patients (see review by ROBINSON, 1963; GOLDFIEN et al., 1961; PRIESTLEY et al., 1963; SHEPS et al., 1966). Exceptionally high levels of plasma catecholamines have been described, e. g. 360 μg/l (PRIESTLEY et al., 1963), 1070 μg/l (ANTON et al., 1967) and 4200 μg/l (ETSTEN and SHIMOSATO, 1965). It is interesting to compare these values with those found in the plasma of patients who died of adrenaline poisoning (LUND and MØLLER, 1958). In the three cases investigated the highest adrenaline level was found to be 91 μg/l. The noradrenaline present in plasma does not seem to enter the cerebrospinal fluid since despite a plasma catecholamine level of 50 μg/l, no noradrenaline was found in the cerebrospinal fluid (HARANATH et al., 1967).

An interesting diagnostic application of the determination of plasma catecholamines is provided by the method of blood sampling at different levels of the vena cava. This procedure, which allows in some cases an exact localisation of the tumour, was originally introduced by EULER et al. (1955) and has been repeatedly used since (CROUT and SJOERDSMA, 1960; VENDSALU, 1960; FAIVRE et al., 1962;

Fig. 1a and b. Comparison of catecholamine content of two tumours with the number of chromaffin granules. a Section from tumour II (BLASCHKO et al., 1968) which contained 1.2 mg catecholamines per g and gave a count of 178 chromaffin granules (mean of 4 sections). The scale represents 1 μ. b Section from tumour III which contained 6 mg catecholamines per g and gave a count of 740 chromaffin granules (mean of 6 sections). The scale represents 1 μ.

MAHAUX et al., 1963; MAHONEY et al., 1963; McGUIRE and FOX, 1964; DONATH et al., 1965; PEKKARINEN et al., 1967; HARRISON et al., 1967b; LAURSEN et al., 1967; ENGELMAN and HAMMOND, 1968). It has been noted (CROUT and SJOERDSMA, 1960) that various blood samples drawn from one point in the vena cava within a short period can contain quite variable amounts of catecholamines. Thus, the release of catecholamines from the tumour can vary considerably; this may be caused either by intermittent release from the tumour cell or by a variation in blood flow through the tumour (see below).

The venous sampling technique allows sampling of blood just above the site of drainage of the tumour and thus the secretory products of the tumour can be obtained before they have been diluted in the vascular system or before they become altered by the passage through various organs which, like the liver, contain a high concentration of enzymes that metabolise catecholamines. Such an approach enabled SUNDERMAN et al. (1965) to conclude that, at least in one patient, vanillylmandelic acid originated in the liver.

β) Urinary Catecholamines and Metabolites: The chance of diagnosing a phaeochromocytoma was improved considerably when ENGEL and EULER (1950) found that the urine of phaeochromocytoma patients contained increased amounts of catecholamines. Later it was discovered that there was also an increase in the urinary excretion of catecholamine metabolites, e. g. vanillylmandelic acid (ARMSTRONG et al., 1957), the metanephrines (LA BROSSE et al., 1958), 3-methoxy-4-hydroxyphenylglycol sulphate (AXELROD et al., 1959) and N-methylmetanephrine (ROBINSON and SMITH, 1962; ITOH et al., 1962; GJESSING, 1963a).

In several subsequent studies of large series of patients urinary catecholamines and/or their metabolites were determined (STUDNITZ, 1960; GITLOW et al., 1961; JACOBS et al., 1961; KELLEHER et al., 1964; SJOERDSMA et al., 1966; SHEPS et al., 1966; KÄSER, 1966b). These investigations have demonstrated the great reliability of biochemical procedures for the diagnosis of phaeochromocytoma. Thus, SJOERDSMA et al. (1966) found in 62 cases of proved phaeochromocytoma that vanillylmandelic acid was normal in only 3 cases, and metanephrines and total catecholamines in only 2 cases each. However, in no patient was the excretion of *all* these compounds normal.

The amounts of the catecholamines in relation to their main metabolites have also been evaluated. In the urine of normal patients the ratios of vanillylmandelic acid to the total catecholamines is about 100 (STUDNITZ, 1960; CROUT et al., 1961; SATO et al., 1962; GREEFF and STROBACH, 1966). In the urine of tumour patients this ratio varies considerably and values of 3 to 260 have been found or can be calculated from the literature. Nevertheless, there is a clear preponderance of low ratios, since the average of the values (±S.D.) from 108 patients is 33±45 (STUDNITZ, 1960; GITLOW et al., 1961; CROUT and SJOERDSMA, 1964; KELLEHER et al., 1964; ZIMON et al., 1966; SCHMID, 1966).

The ratio of the amount of metanephrines to total catecholamines ranges from about 10 to 20 in normal urine (CROUT et al., 1961; SATO et al., 1962) whereas in the urine of 63 tumour patients these ratios vary from 1 to 65 with a mean value (± S.D.) of 15±16 (SATO et al., 1962; CROUT and SJOERDSMA, 1964; KELLEHER et al., 1964; ZIMON et al., 1966). It is clear that there are great variations in the excretion patterns and their significance will be disscussed below.

γ) Biochemical Aspects of Malignancy: In some cases of phaeochromocytoma there has been an increase in the excretion of other metabolites of catecholamines. Special attention was paid to homovanillic acid, a metabolite of dopamine, since this compound may have diagnostic significance as far as the malignancy of the tumours is concerned. Such a possibility was suggested by McMILLAN (1956), who found that dopamine was the predominant amine (see Table 1) in the tissue of a malignant phaeochromocytoma. Subsequently, evidence for the secretion of dopamine from a malignant tumour was obtained by ROBINSON et al. (1964), who observed an increased urinary excretion of homovanillic acid and 3-methoxytyramine (methoxydopamine). In 48 cases of benign tumours these metabolites were excreted in normal amounts. The occurrence of such an excretion pattern in malignant phaeochromocytoma seems to be in agreement with the findings of several authors (SANKOFF and SOURKES, 1963; RUTHVEN and SANDLER; 1964; DONATH et al., 1965; BOHOUN and GUÉRINOT, 1966; STUDNITZ, 1966; ANTON et al., 1967; JONES et al., 1968). The last two groups of authors also found an increased excretion of DOPA. In addition, N-acetyldopamine (SEKERIS and HERRLICH, 1963), 3-methoxy-4-hydroxyphenylethylamine (GREER et al., 1968), dihydroxyphenylformaldehyde (HERRLICH and SEKERIS, 1963) and vanillic acid (STURM, 1963) have been demonstrated. One might also mention the rather unrelated fact that cystathionine is excreted in increased amounts (STUDNITZ, 1965a). Most of these excretion products are, as will be shown below, typical of consistently malignant tumours i. e. the neuroblastomas. However, there are also benign phaeochromocytomas which lead to an increased urinary excretion of dopamine and its metabolites. This was, for example, true for a "dopamine secreting" tumour described by RUTHVEN and SANDLER (1964), for two tumours reported by GJESSING (1964) and for one described by PAGE and JACOBY (1964). Furthermore, only one out of five patients with a malignant tumour was found by SATO and SJOERDSMA (1965) to excrete increased amounts of homovanillic acid and there was also no increase of urinary homovanillic acid in a malignant case mentioned by PERTSEMLIDIS et al. (1969). The correlation is, therefore, far from clear-cut; further studies are necessary, which, however, are not easily carried out since only less then 10% of all phaeochromocytomas are malignant (HERMAN and MORNEX, 1964). In 1964 WÜST et al. (1964) collected 81 cases of malignant phaeochromocytomas from the literature.

b) Mechanism of Release of Amines from Phaeochromocytoma

We shall start this section by reiterating that phaeochromocytomas are not under nervous control, as demonstrated by the morphological findings discussed above. This accounts for the absence of a significant increase in catecholamine excretion in two patients bearing a tumour upon the injection of insulin (HERMAN and MORNEX (1964), which causes the secretion of adrenal medullary hormones by a central mechanism. However, tumours are continuously or intermittently releasing amines and we have, therefore, to ask by what mechanism this is brought about.

It has been known for a long time that many different procedures can precipitate clinical symptoms, such as a hypertensive crisis, in tumour patients: manipulation of the tumour; lying in a particular position; bending; straining at stool; swallowing, in the case of an intrathoracic tumour; and micturition in cases with a tumour in the bladder (see COUPLAND, 1965). One might also add laughing, and a tight girdle (LANCE et al., 1958), and also work (EULER, 1958). A common characteristic of these procedures is that they can exert a mechanical influence on the tumour, which might lead to the expulsion of blood, enriched in catecholamines that was stagnating in sinusoidal spaces. Such sinusoidal spaces have been seen by the histologists in many tumours (see COUPLAND, 1965). A rich vascularisation of the tumours has also been demonstrated by angiography which is used as a diagnostic procedure for localising these tumours (PYLE, 1961; HOLSTI, 1962; ROSSI et al., 1966; MEANY and BUONOCORE, 1966).

α) Drug-induced Release of Catecholamines: The introduction, in 1964 by ENGELMAN and SJOREDSMA, of the tyramine test for phaeochromocytoma led to an entirely new concept of the mode of action of drugs which are used to provoke a release of catecholamines in phaeochromocytoma patients.

ENGELMAN and SJOERDSMA (1964) found that an intravenous injection of a small dose (1 mg) of tyramine led to a rise exceeding 20 mm Hg in the blood pressure of patients bearing a tumour. In a later report ENGELMAN et al. (1968) stated that 19 out of 26 patients with a tumour gave positive results, whereas only 3 out of 88 patients gave falsely positive results. Further reports on positive tyramine tests, but also on negative ones, have since been published (PONTASSE and GIFFORD, 1965; SHEPS and MAHER, 1966; SCHMID et al., 1966; THURM et al., 1966; STUDNITZ and LJUNGBERG, 1967; LOUIS and DOYLE, 1967; LIEBAU, 1968).

What is the explanation for the increased sensitivity of phaeochromocytoma patients to tyramine? Tyramine can release catecholamines directly from the adrenal medulla, as demonstrated in experiments with animals, but very high doses are necessary (HAAG et al., 1961; GARRETT et al., 1965; RUBIN and JAANUS, 1966; R. L. ROBINSON, 1966). The high doses may explain why some authors did not find an effect of tyramine in animals (STRÖMBLAD, 1960; STJÄRNE, 1961; WEINER et al., 1962). The high doses of tyramine which are required to cause a release of amines from normal chromaffin tissue make it very unlikely that 1 mg of tyramine given to patients could act on the tumour. In fact, ENGELMAN and SJOERDSMA (1964) observed that for a short time after removal of the tumour, patients, were still sensitive to tyramine and there was only a "gradual return to normal within the first postoperative week". Similarly, it has been reported that there is a slow return to normal in the amounts of catecholamines in the urine of patients after operation (EULER et al., 1955; SJOERDSMA, 1966). These findings suggest that there is an elevated store of catecholamines outside the tumour, and that tyramine releases catecholamines from this store and not from the tumour itself (ENGELMAN and SJOERDSMA, 1964).

The store of catecholamines not present in the tumour itself is likely to be in peripheral sympathetic neurons. It has been repeatedly demonstrated that infusions of noradrenaline can lead to an increase in the noradrenaline concentration in peripheral nerves (MUSCHOLL, 1960; STRÖMBLAD and NICKERSON, 1961). The plasma levels of catecholamines in phaeochromocytoma patients (see above) are very high; consequently one can assume that the neuronal stores of catecholamines are greater than normal in these patients. Small intravenous doses of tyramine are known to release noradrenaline from nerve endings; tyramine might, therefore, release abnormally large amounts of amines from the nerve terminals of phaeochromocytoma patients.

Two experiments which might settle the question of the mechanism of action of tyramine, have not been carried out. Firstly, there are no data available on the amine content of sympathetically innervated tissues in phaeochromocytoma patients; the amounts should be increased. Secondly, if tyramine releases catecholamines only from peripheral stores, then no massive increase of catecholamines should be seen in blood collected from the vena cava above the site of drainage of the tumour when the drug is administered.

Another drug, which has been used for the past 20 years for a provocative test of phaeochromocytoma, is histamine. Histamine was considered to act directly on the tumour tissue, since it will cause a release of catecholamines from the adrenal medulla of cats (TRENDELENBURG, 1954; STASZEWSKA-BARCZAK and VANE, 1965; POISNER and DOUGLAS, 1966) and oxen (GARRETT et al., 1965). However, in the dog, the direct action of histamine on the adrenal medulla is only demonstrable with large doses (STASZEWSKA-BARCZAK and VANE, 1965). One wonders whether the small doses (25—50 μg) of histamine used in the test for phaeochromocytoma could act directly on the tumour. It seems more likely that histamine acts through its most obvious effect, i. e. vasodilatation. Vasodilation in the splanchnic area could lead to an increased blood flow through the tumour, causing a discharge of blood rich in catecholamines. However, vasodilation would also evoke a reflex activation of the sympathetic system. Since the tumours are not innervated, they will not participate in the reflex. The reflex will be confined to the sympathetic neurons which probably contain an unusally high concentration of catecholamines. Accordingly, the rise in blood pressure induced by histamine in phaeochromocytoma may be due to release of catecholamine from the extra-tumoral store (ENGELMAN and SJOERDSMA, 1964).

A third drug which has been used in provocative tests for phaeochromocytoma is the hormone glucagon. The glucagon test, i. e. an i. v. injection of 0.5—1.0 mg of glucagon leading to a rise in blood pressure, was introduced in 1964 (LAWRENCE and FORLAND, 1964; LAWRENCE, 1967). It has been used repeatedly during the last few years, but the number of patients is still small; negative results have also been described (PONTASSE and GIFFORD, 1965; SHEPS and MAHER, 1968). An increased concentration of plasma catecholamines in patients following the administration of glucagon has been reported (CREMER et al., 1968; LEFEBVRE et al., 1968).

We would like to suggest that glucagon, like tyramine and histamine, causes a release of catecholamines from extra-tumoral stores. Glucagon, like the other two drugs, acts directly on the adrenal medulla only when applied in large doses (SCIAN et al., 1960; ATHOS et al., 1962; LEFEBVRE et al., 1968), whereas small doses cause in dog (MERILL et al., 1967) and in man (FERUGLIO et al., 1966) pronounced vasodilatation in the splanchnic area, which, LEFEBVRE et al. (1968) suggested, might lead to a reflex activation of the sympathetic nervous system. In tumour patients, the vasodilatation might increase the blood flow through the tumour and might also lead, via reflex activation of the sympathetic system, to a release of extratumoral stores of catecholamines.

Independent evidence for a reflex release of extra-tumoral stores of catecholamines comes from the work of HARRISON et al. (1967a), who found that raising a phaeochromocytoma patient from a horizontal position produced an increased urinary excretion of noradrenaline. Such a response, which was not seen when subjects without a tumour were tilted, may in part be due to mechanical factors causing blood pooled in the tumour to be expelled (see above) and in part to the reflex stimulation of the sympathetic nervous system. An activation of the sympathetic system might also be the cause of the hypertensive crises which occur in tumour patients during emotional upsets.

β) Cellular Mechanisms: So far, we have discussed the various procedures which can produce a release of catecholamines in tumour patients. However, it is well known that tumours continuously release catecholamines without any apparent stimulus. What is the mechanism of this release process? In the normal adrenal medulla acetylcholine, released by the nerve endings, initiates a chain of events culminating in the fusion of the membrane of the chromaffin granule with that of the cell, followed by the discharge of the total soluble constituents of the granules, i. e. protein, ATP and catecholamines (see chapter by SMITH and WINKLER). In a morphological study of a tumour (RATZENHOFER et al., 1968) pictures which might represent this process have been obtained. This kind of mechanism may, therefore, occur in tumour tissue.

However, it seems unlikely that the bulk of the catecholamines is released in this way, for the following reasons: First of all, the normal stimulus to these cells, acetylcholine, is lacking. Secondly, as already pointed out, the turnover of catecholamines in many tumours is much faster than normal and may reach about 100 times the normal rate. If the catecholamines are entirely secreted by exocytosis, the cell would not only have to synthesise the catecholamines and ATP, but also the proteins which are present in the granules. Such a high rate of protein synthesis requires a marked increase in the amount of endoplasmic reticulum. However, there is no morphological evidence for this (see above). It has, therefore, been suggested (Winkler and Smith, 1968) that the continuous release of catecholamines takes place by their diffusion through the cytoplasm and across the cell membrane. This happens because the cell is continuously synthesising far more catecholamines than can be accommodated in the chromaffin granules, which are filled to saturation. In other words, a dissociation of the synthetic ability of the cell from its storage capacity was postulated. One important experimental point in support of this hypothesis was the finding, mentioned before, that the enzyme tyrosine hydroxylase lacks the sensitivity to feed-back inhibition found in normal adrenal medulla (Roth et al., 1968; Nagatsu et al., 1970).

It is noteworthy that α-methyltyrosine, an inhibitor of tyrosine hydroxylase, reduces the blood pressure and urinary catecholamines of patients with phaeochromocytoma within a day. It does not have this effect, with the doses employed, in other hypertensive patients (Sjoerdsma et al., 1965; Jones et al., 1968; Amery et al., 1969). This suggests, but by no means proves, that the rate of release of catecholamines from the tumours is dependent upon the rate of biosynthesis and not upon the size of the store.

Further evidence consistent with the hypothesis that the bulk of the amines released bypasses the store, comes from the work of Crout and Sjoerdsma (1964). These authors distinguished two groups of tumours in a total of 75 patients. In one group, the tumour was small in weight and had a low content of catecholamines; in the second group the catecholamine content was high. In the first group the rate of turnover of the catecholamines was high and unmetabolised catecholamines were apparently released into the blood. This was deduced by comparing the ratio of vanillylmandelic acid to catecholamines in the urine which was, on average, about 10; this is very similar to the value found after an intravenous infusion of catecholamines. In the second group of tumours the rate of turnover of catecholamines was low, and the ratio of vanillylmandelic acid to catecholamines in the urine was high (about 90) suggesting that up to 90% of the catecholamines were already metabolised before they left the tumour. The same conclusion can be reached by considering the ratio of metanephrines to catecholamines in the urine: in the first group this ratio is 4, and in the second group it is 20. That catecholamines are metabolised within some tumours would fit quite well with the idea that in these tumours the catecholamines released are not protected by the granule membrane and secreted by exocytosis, but by-pass the storage site and diffuse out from the cell. In the first group described by Crout and Sjoerdsma, catecholamines are released more or less unmetabolised from the tumour. This could be accounted for if one assumes that secretion by exocytosis occurs in these tumours. However, as pointed out above, exocytosis is unlikely and the possibility should be considered that in these tumours there is a relative lack of metabolising enzymes and so the amines could diffuse across the cytoplasm and out of the cell without much degradation.

In any case, a study of the activity of metabolising enzymes in the two types of tumours should be performed, as suggested by Crout and Sjoerdsma (1964). Also, a search for the specific soluble proteins of the chromaffin granules in blood collected from the vena cava above the site of the drainage of the tumour should be undertaken. One would expect that, compared to the catecholamine released, only small amounts of the specific proteins (the chromogranins, including dopamine-β-hydroxylase) might be secreted.

III. Neuroblastomas and Ganglioneuromas

Neuroblastomas are tumours of the early childhood, about 50% of them occurring below the age of 3 years (e. g. BACHMANN, 1962; DE LORIMIER et al., 1969), whereas ganglioneuromas are usually detected at an older age. Neuroblastomas are relatively frequent tumours, representing about 10% of all childhood cancers (KOOP et al., 1955; MARSDEN, 1962).

Although a few cases of neuroblastoma in the same family have been reported — for instance, 3 out of 4 children in one family had tumours (CHATTEN and VOORHEES, 1967) —, in a survey of about 2000 cases and of the literature no convincing evidence of hereditary factors was found (MILLER et al., 1968).

1. Synthesis of Catecholamines in Tumours

There are only a few studies concerning the enzymes for catecholamine synthesis in neuroblastomas. Tyrosine hydroxylase has been studied by GOLDSTEIN (1966) and STUDNITZ (1965b). The latter author found that the activity of this enzyme was comparable to that in adrenal medulla. Dopamine-β-hydroxylase was not detected in these tumours by GOLDSTEIN (1966); however in a more detailed study this enzyme was demonstrated (BOHUON and GUÉRINOT, 1968). Dopadecarboxylase and phenylethanolamine-N-methyl transferase have apparently not been studied; their occurence is, however, suggested by the presence of dopamine and adrenaline in these tumours (see below). In a recent paper by IMASHUKU and LA BROSSE (1971) it was reported that tyrosine hydroxylase from neuroblastoma tissue is inhibited by catecholamines to the same extent as bovine adrenal tyrosine hydroxylase. This is in contrast to the results obtained with tyrosine hydroxylase from phaeochromocytoma tissue (see section II, 2a).

2. Metabolism of Catecholamines in Tumours

The addition of tritiated noradrenaline to tissue cultures of neuroblastoma led to the appearance of labelled 3-methoxy-4-hydroxyphenylglycol, normetanephrine and their sulphate conjugates (LA BROSSE et al., 1964), which makes it likely that these tumours contain MAO, COMT, aldehydereductase and sulphate conjugase. In later studies the same group of workers (AMAR-COSTESEC et al., 1965; BOHUON et al., 1966) obtained more quantitative data. The activities of MAO and COMT, which varied from tumour to tumour, were found to be comparable to those of liver. MAO activity was generally higher than in phaeochromocytoma. GOLDSTEIN et al. (1968) demonstrated MAO by incubating tumour tissue with labelled tyramine. The main metabolite formed was p-hydroxyphenylacetaldehyde. Histochemical evidence for the presence of MAO was produced by ANTHONY et al. (1965).

3. Storage of Catecholamines in Tumours

a) Tissue Content of Catecholamines and Metabolites

The first evidence for the presence of catecholamines in neuroblastomas was provided by MASON et al. (1957), who found an equivalent of 0.14 mg of pressor amines/g of tumour. This has been confirmed in many subsequent studies, some of which are compiled in Table 3. Additional values for noradrenaline and adrena-

Table 3: *Content of catecholamines and related compounds in tissue of neuroblastomas in μg/g tissue.* (VMA = vanillylmandelic acid, HVA = Homovanillic acid)

Authors	No. of cases	Noradrenaline	Adrenaline	Dopa	Dopamine	VMA	HVA
a) *Neuroblastoma:*							
PAGE and JACOBY (1964)	1	<1	0	—	1	0.56	—
GJESSING (1964)	3	6—25	10—78	—	6—40	—	—
GREER et al. (1965)	5	0.01—2.4	0.01—1.1	0.05—0.6	0.02—2.2	—	—
KÄSER (1966)	5	0.2—4	0 (3)—0.07	—	0.04—1	—	—
ANTON et al. (1967)	1	2.0	1.1	0,05	0.3	—	—
CAMERON et al. (1967)	1	557	151	—	10.5	—	—
BOHUON and GUÉRINOT (1968)	11	0.01—10	0 (1)—11	0 (3)—3	0 (6)—0.5	—	—
VOORHEES (1968)	10	0.13—276	0 (2)—3.3	—	0 (7)—1.3	0 (2)—0.5	0 (3)—2.0
SILVERMAN et al. (1964)	5	0.1—6.5		—	0.2—16.0	—	—
HINTERSBERGER et al. (1969)	4	0.34—11.6		—	0 (1)—6.4	2.9—3.6	0.8 (1)
b) *Ganglioneuroma:*							
GREENBERG and GARDNER (1960)	1	8.6	0.07	—	2.1	—	—
ROSENSTEIN and ENGELMAN (1963)	1	10.4	—	0.72	1.83	—	—
HINTERSBERGER et al. (1969)	2	6.3—30.0		—	0.8—12.4	—	0.1
ROSENTHAL et al. (1969)	1	95.0	0	—	3.0	—	—

line in single cases of neuroblastoma can be found in several papers (GRAHAM, 1959; SMITH et al., 1961; see also BELL, 1962; ANTHONY et al., 1965).

It is quite obvious that these tumours contain very small amounts of catecholamines when compared with those present in phaeochromocytoma. Metanephrine (4.1 μg/g) was found in a case of neuroblastoma (PAGE and JACOBY, 1964) and in a ganglioneuroma (4 μg/g) (ROSENTHAL et al., 1969), whereas GREENBERG and GARDNER (1960) could not detect it. The presence of 3-methoxy-4-hydroxyphenyl glycol has also been described (LA BROSSE et al., 1968). In a ganglioneuroma histamine in a concentration of 0.37 μg/g was detected (GREENBERG and GARDNER 1960). The presence of cystathionine was reported by GJESSING (1963c), who found 2.2—8 μg/g tissue. Homovanillic acid and dihydroxyphenylacetic acid were detected in neuroblastoma tissue by KÄSER et al. (1971). These authors point out that the tissue concentration of these metabolites relative to the catecholamine content is high which indicates that the catecholamines are already metabolised extensively within the neuroblastoma tissue.

b) Isolation of Storage Organelles

Apparently only two attempts have been made to study the subcellular distribution of catecholamines in these tumours. PAGE and JACOBY (1964) obtained a large granule fraction by differential centrifugation of a homogenate of neuroblastoma. This fraction contained 0.48 μg catecholamines/g original tissue (PAGE and JACOBY, 1964). Since the noradrenaline concentration in the homogenate is not given it cannot be stated how much of the noradrenaline was sedimentable. A large granule fraction from a ganglioneuroma contained 37 % of the noradrenaline present in the homogenate (ROSENTHAL et al., 1969). Further biochemical studies should be undertaken to obtain information on the properties of the catecholamine-containing particles in these tumours.

c) Microscopical Observations

Two problems arise when one attempts to evaluate the morphological findings. Firstly, there are no studies, with the exception of those of PAGE and JACOBY (1964) and GREENBERG et al. (1969), which attempt to correlate biochemical and morphological findings. Secondly, the uncertainty in the classifaction of these tumours is also present at the ultrastructural level. This is illustrated by the studies of LUSE (1964), who describes „synaptic structures occuring in neuroblastoma". This tumour, representing a metastasis of a ganglio-neuroblastoma, contained ganglionic structures which are clearly distinct from the undifferentiated neuroblastoma cells seen by MISUGI et al. (1968). The latter cells are characterized by a large nucleus occupying a major portion of the cell. The cytoplasmic organelles were scarce, and poorly developed Golgi lamella were only occasionally observed. One wonders whether such tumours can synthesise noradrenaline, if we consider that the enzyme dopamine-β-hydroxylase is localised within the storage granules in adrenal medulla, in peripheral sympathetic nerve and probably, therefore, also in neuroblastoma. Since these undifferentiated cells do not, apparently, contain storage granules how can they synthesise noradrenaline? It may well be that in these tumours some cells are further developed and that these cells are responsible for the formation of catecholamines, or that dopamine-β-hydroxylase can exist in these cells elsewhere than in storage granules. The lack of correlating biochemical studies, mentioned above, becomes apparent here.

In more differentiated tumour cells a rich spectrum of intracytoplasmic organelles was observed (LUSE, 1964; STALEY et al., 1967; MISUGI et al., 1968; ROSENTHAL et al., 1969; GREENBERG et al., 1969; BELTRAN et al., 1969). Of special interest for the present discussion are membrane-limited organelles which might be concerned with noradrenaline-storage. MISUGI et al. (1968), observed osmiophilic granules, about 100 mμ in size, in the cytoplasm, which seemed to originate in the Golgi Complex. In neurites of ganglionic cells, some of which made a synaptic like contact with other cells, dense core-granules about 100 mμ in size were observed, in addition to clear vesicles, 50—120 mμ in diameter. A differentiation of vesicles and granules according to their size was discussed by STALEY et al. (1967), by ROSENTHAL et al. (1969) and GREENBERG et al. (1969). They described spherical opaque granules, of about 140 mμ diameter, which were considered to correspond to type I granules (see GRILLO, 1966) found in sympathetic nerves (see chapter by BLOOM). Smaller granules were not (STALEY et al., 1967), or rarely seen (ROSENTHAL et al., 1969); however, empty vesicles of 60 mμ diameter were present. The possibility was considered that these vesicles represented the catecholamine storage organelles which might have lost their typical dense core appearance by prolonged fixation. It is known that the dense core of catecholamine storage vesicles in normal tissue is very sensitive to fixation procedures (TRANZER and THOENEN, 1967). In a central ganglioneuroma "secretory" granules, varying in size from 100—150 mμ were observed (ROBERTSON et al., 1964; see also GREENBERG et al., 1969).

4. Release of Catecholamines and Related Substances

In this section we shall discuss the great variety of compounds occuring in the urine of patients with neuroblastomas. Some of the substances released by the tumour are further metabolised in the various tissues of the body and, therefore, not all of the substances found in the urine originate directly from the tumour. The clinical symptomes caused by these substances are dealt with in the chapter by SANDLER.

In 1957, MASON et al. described a child with a functioning neuroblastoma who had an increased amount of catecholamines in the urine. Numerous studies, some in large series of patients, have confirmed this finding. The investigations have been extended to the various metabolites of catecholamines and to their precursors. Usually total catecholamines were determined and found to be excreted in increased amounts in a majority of patients (STICKLER and FLOCK, 1962; STUDNITZ et al., 1963; BELL, 1966; HINTERSBERGER and BARTHOLOMEW, 1969). In some cases noradrenaline and adrenaline have been determined separately and some workers found an insignificant rise in adrenaline (VOORHEES and GARDNER, 1962; SOURKES et al., 1963; KÄSER, 1966a, b; GREEF and STROBACH, 1966), whereas GREER et al. (1965) found it elevated in 9 out of 13 patients.

The main metabolite of noradrenaline and adrenaline, i. e. vanillylmandelic acid is also increased in the urine (VOORHEES and GARDNER, 1962; KONTRAS, 1962; YOUNG et al., 1963; STUDNITZ et al., 1963; GJESSING, 1963a; RUTHVEN and SANDLER, 1964; MCKENDRICK and EDWARDS, 1965; CLARK et al., 1965; GREER et al., 1965; R. ROBINSON, 1966; SCHWEISSGUTH, 1966; KÄSER, 1966b; BELL, 1966; HINTERSBERGER and BARTHOLOMEW, 1969). KÄSER et al. (1969) e. g. found an increased excretion of vanillylmandelic acid in 129 of 142 cases. When ratios of vanillylmandelic acid to catecholamines in urine are calculated from the two large series of STUDNITZ et al. (1963) and HINTERSBERGER and BARTHOLOMEW (1969), a wide range of values, i. e. from 25 to 3660 is obtained (mean value: 455 ± 720, $n = 55$). A comparison with the figures given for phaeochromocytoma reveals that the values for neuroblastomas have a larger variation and also a higher mean value indicating a more extensive metabolism of the various compounds within the tumour (see also below).

Metanephrines are also elevated in urine (STICKLER et al., 1960; VOORHEES and GARDNER, 1962; STUDNITZ et al., 1963; GJESSING, 1963a; CLARK et al., 1965; BELL, 1966; R. ROBINSON, 1966; GREER et al., 1968). However, no paramethylated compounds have been observed (STUDNITZ, 1967). As far as other metabolites of noradrenaline and adrenaline are concerned, urinary excretion of 3-methoxy-4-hydroxyphenylglycol (GJESSING, 1963a), vanillic acid (GJESSING, 1963a), and N-acetylnoradrenaline (HERRLICH and SEKERIS, 1964) has been reported.

It is a significant symptom of neuroblastoma that, in addition to an overproduction of noradrenaline and adrenaline, there is also an increase in the synthesis of the precursors dopamine and DOPA. Dopamine is found to be increased in many neuroblastoma patients (VOORHEES and GARDNER, 1962; STUDNITZ et al., 1963; SOURKES et al., 1963; GREER et al., 1968; HINTERSBERGER and BARTHOLOMEW, 1969) e. g. in 20 out of 21 cases as described by STUDNITZ et al. (1963). An increase has also been reported for the metabolites of dopamine, i. e. 3-methoxytyramine (GJESSING, 1963a; R. ROBINSON, 1966; GREER et al., 1969; STUDNITZ, 1968) and homovanillic acid (STUDNITZ et al., 1963; GJESSING, 1963a; RUTHVEN and SANDLER, 1964; GREER et al., 1965; CLARK et al., 1965; KÄSER, 1966a; BELL, 1966; R. ROBINSON, 1966; VOORHEES, 1968; HINTERSBERGER and BARTHOLOMEW, 1969). Other metabolites which can be derived from dopamine, but also from DOPA, have been found including 3-methoxy-4-hydroxyphenylethanol (GJESSING, 1963a), dihydroxyphenylacetic acid (STUDNITZ, 1960; WILLIAMS and LEONARD, 1963; SOURKES et al., 1963) and N-acetyldopamine (HANSON and STUDNITZ, 1965). In a few studies DOPA (STUDNITZ et al., 1963; PAGE and JACOBY, 1964; GREER et al., 1965) and its metabolites were studied and found to be increased in amount. These metabolites include 3-methoxy-4-hydroxyphenylalanine (STUDNITZ, 1961; GJESSING, 1963a) and dihydroxyphenylpyruvic acid (GJESSING and BORUD, 1965).

Other metabolites which were found in the urine of patients bearing a neuroblastoma include N-acetyltyramine (STUDNITZ and HANSON, 1967; HINTERSBERGER and BARTHOLOMEW, 1969) and tyramine (STUDNITZ et al., 1963; HINTERSBERGER and BARTHOLOMEW, 1969) which was found to be elevated in 5 of 21 cases (STUDNITZ et al., 1963). The urinary excretion of homoserine was reported by STUDNITZ (1965c) and that of cystathionine by GJESSING (1963b) and GEISER and EFRON (1968). This latter compound seems to be an indication of the malignancy of these tumours (see GJESSING, 1968), however, it is also present in various other diseases like hepatoma (GJESSING and MAURITZEN, 1965; SHAW et al., 1967), glycogen storage disease and congenital portal vein obstruction (SHAW et al., 1967). The common link among these diseases may be the interference with the liver by metastases, or other causes leading, perhaps, to a partial deficiency of pyridoxine in the liver, with the consequent accumulation of cystathionine (see HOPE, 1957).

The ganglioneuromas are also characterized by an increased excretion of the various compounds mentioned above (GREENBERG and GARDNER, 1960; KONTRAS, 1962; VOORHEES and GARDNER, 1962; SANKOFF and SOURKES, 1963; STUDNITZ et al., 1963; YOUNG et al., 1963; RUTHVEN and SANDLER, 1964; CLARK et al., 1965; GREER et al., 1965). However, it seems that negative findings are more frequent in these tumours, thus, KÄSER (1966b) found an increase in vanillylmandelic acid-excretion in only 2 out of 9 patients and an increased homovanillic acid excretion in 1 out of 6. Cystathionine is not excreted in increased amounts (GJESSING, 1963b, c).

A classification of neuroblastomas into four groups according to their urinary excretion patterns has been attempted by VOORHESS and GARDNER (1962) from their studies of 17 cases and by BELL (1966) from 26 cases. The largest group comprised patients who excreted increased amounts of noradrenaline, dopamine, metanephrines and vanillylmandelic acid. In the second group dopamine and noradrenaline were predominant, whereas the metabolites were not increased. This group, therefore, corresponds to those phaeochromocytomas where the vanillylmandelic acid/catecholamine ratio in urine is low. These phaeochromocytomas were considered (Crout and Sjoerdsma, 1964) to release unmetabolised catecholamines into the blood. A similar assumption can be made for this group of neuroblastomas. In group 3 the catecholamines were found to be normal, but the metabolites were increased. This group also has its analogue in the phaeochromocytoma patients, namely in those where considerable amounts of the catecholamines are metabolised *in situ*. A final group of neuroblastoma patients did not excrete increased amounts of noradrenaline, dopamine or vanillylmandelic acid. It may be that the study of additional metabolites might have also revealed an increased metabolism of catecholamines in this group. This view is supported by the extensive studies of Käser et al. (1969), who claim that all malignant sympathetic tumours lead to abnormal excretion of at least one of the catecholamine metabolites.

IV. Tumours of the Carotid Body and Related Structures

Several biogenic amines have been found in the carotid body: the carotid body of the cat, for example, contains noradrenaline (2 μg/g), dopamine (4.4 μg/g), adrenaline (0.9 μg/g) and 5-hydroxytryptamine (6.9 μg/g) (Chiocchio et al., 1967). There are very few biochemical studies on human carotid body, but noradrenaline has been identified by Karnauchow (1965) and by Pryse-Davies et al. (1964). The latter authors reported that the tissue contained 56 μg noradrenaline/g; adrenaline was not measured. Histochemical procedures have been applied to the human carotid body by Niemi and Ojala (1964), who found only a green fluorescence suggestive of noradrenaline, and by Hamberger et al. (1966), who observed in addition a yellow fluorescence characteristic of 5-hydroxytryptamine.

Three different types of cells have been identified in the carotid body of the cat by electron microscopic histochemistry (Chiocchio et al., 1967): the first cell type has typical noradrenaline-containing granules; the second, which is the most common, contains 5-hydroxytryptamine storage granules; and the third cell type has adrenaline-containing granules. These elegant histochemical procedures have not yet been applied to the human carotid body, the chief cells of which contain osmiophilic membrane limited granules of diameter 130 mμ (Grimley and Glenner, 1968).

Although tumours of the catecholamine-containing cells of the carotid body have been found, it is not known whether the 5-hydroxytryptamine-containing cells ever give rise to tumours. In the catecholamine-containing tumours, 5-hydroxytryptamine could be detected neither histochemically (Hamberger et al., 1967) nor biochemically (Berdal et al., 1962; Pryse-Davies et al., 1964; Grimley and Glenner, 1968).

The concentration of catecholamines in tumours of the carotid body and glomus jugulare (see Table 4) is sometimes of the same order as in normal tissue, ranging from 1.2—18.0 μg noradrenaline/g, but it is sometimes very much higher, ranging from 0.195 mg noradrenaline/g to 1.5 mg noradrenaline for carotid body tumours, and a concentration of 14.1 mg noradrenaline/g (Duke et al., 1964) was found in a glomus jugulare tumour. The high content of amines in some tumours may be because these tumours contain only one type of cell, whereas the carotid body contains many cell types.

Membrane-limited osmiophilic granules (100—200 mμ in diameter) are present in cells of carotid body tumours (GRIMLEY and GLENNER, 1967; TOKER, 1967; MACADAM, 1969) and in tumours of the glomus jugulare (GEJROT et al., 1963; BALOGH et al., 1966), which is consistent with the presence of amines in these tissues.

Table. 4. *Catecholamine concentration of tumours of the carotid body and glomus jugulare in μg noradrenaline and adrenaline /g tissue*

Authors	No. of cases	Nor-adrenaline	Adrenaline
LE COMPTE (1948)	1		8 (?)
BERDAL et al. (1963)	6	0 (5)—1.2	0 (5)—3.5
BERDAL et al. (1962)	1	550	33
GLENNER et al. (1962)	1	1500	0
PRYSE-DAVIES et al. (1964)	5	0 (1)—245	0
DUKE et al. (1965)	1	195	18
BALOGH et al. (1965)	7	up to 296	present
GRIMLEY and GLENNER (1967)	2	0; 2.6	—

It might be expected that those tumours which are rich in catecholamines would produce clinical symptomes, but no correlation has yet been established between catecholamine content and symptoms. In fact, there are many studies which reveal a lack of clinical symptomes in patients with tumours of the carotid body or glomus jugulare. Thus, FULLER et al. (1967) described 72 cases of tumours of the glomus jugulare, ten of which were associated with high blood pressure giving an incidence of 14%, which was said to be the same as that in the general population. However, in a few cases the functioning of the tumour has been established by an increased urinary excretion of catecholamines and catecholamine-metabolites (GLENNER et al., 1962; BERDAL et al., 1962; TIEDGE et al., 1964; DUKE et al., 1964; LEVIT et al., 1969) or by an increase in blood pressure following manipulation of the tumour (GLENNER et al., 1962; BERDAL et al., 1962, 1963; TIEDGE et al., 1964).

V. Conclusion

There is abundant information available on some aspects of phaeochromocytoma; for instance, as far as the catecholamine content, the mode of storage and the nature of the secretory products are concerned. However, the more complicated questions about the mechanism regulating synthesis and secretion of the amines are still largely unresolved. These are, in fact, the same questions which are at the moment much discussed for normal chromaffin tissue (see chapters by EULER, STJÄRNE and SMITH and WINKLER). It is not unreasonable to suggest that some of these fundamental problems will be better understood if we gain further insight into the nature of the disturbance in these functions in phaeochromocytoma. This will require a deepening of the biochemical analysis from the subcellular to the molecular level.

The other two types of tumours, i. e. neuroblastomas and tumours of the carotid body, have also been dealt with in numerous papers. However, the mode of storage and secretion of amines in these tumours has not yet been investigated in any detail. Further studies correlating biochemical and morphological observations might be rewarding and may also provide interesting comparisons with the normal tissues from which these tumours are derived.

References

Albores-Saavedra, J., Maldonado, M.C., Ibarra, J., Rodriguez, H.A.: Phaeochromocytoma of the urinary bladder. Cancer **23**, 1110—1118 (1969).

Amar-Costesec, A., Bohuon, C., Schweissguth, O.: Activité Mono Amine oxydase dans les tumeurs de le Crête Neurale. Europ. J. Cancer **1**, 225—231 (1965).

Amery, A., Moerman, E.J., Bossaert, H., de Schaepdryver, A.F.: α-Methyl-p-tyrosine in malignant pheochromocytoma. Pharmacol. Clin. **1**, 174—176 (1969).

Anthony, P.P., Coles, H.M.T., Pryse-Davies, J., Sinclair, L.: Biochemical, pharmacological and histochemical studies in neuroblastoma. Arch. Dis. Childh. **40**, 411—417 (1965).

Anton, A.H., Greer, M., Sayre, D.F., Williams, C.M.: Dihydroxyphenylalanine secretion in a malignant pheochromocytoma. Amer. J. Med. **42**, 469—475 (1967).

Armstrong, M.D., McMillan, A., Shaw, K.N.F.: 3-Methoxy-4-hydroxy-D-mandelic acid, a urinary metabolite of NE. Biochim. biophys. Acta (Amst.) **25**, 422—423 (1957).

Athos, W.J., McHugh, B.P., Fineberg, S.E., Hilton, J.G.: The effects of guanethidine on the adrenal medulla. J. Pharmacol. exp. Ther. **137**, 229—234 (1962).

Axelrod, J., Kopin, I.J., Mann, J.D.: 3-Methoxy-4-hydroxyphenylglycol sulfate, a new metabolite of epinephrine and norepinephrine. Biochim. biophys. Acta (Amst.) **36**, 576—577 (1959).

Bachmann, K.P.: Das Neuroblastoma sympathicum: Klinik und Prognose von 1030 Fällen. Z. Kinderheilk. **86**, 710—724 (1962).

Balogh, K., Draskóczy, P.R., Caulfield, J.B.: Norepinephrine in tumours of the jugular glomus. Amer. J. Path. **48**, 40a (1966).

Bässler, R., Habighorst, L.V.: Vergleichende licht- und elektronenmikroskopische Untersuchungen am Nebennierenmark und Phäochromocytom. Beitr. path. Anat. **130**, 446—488 (1964).

Bell, M.: The clinical chemistry of neuroblastomas. In: The clinical chemistry of monoamines, pp. 82—91. Ed. H. Varley and A.H. Gowenlock. Amsterdam: Elsevier 1962.

— Observations on the biochemical diagnosis of neuroblastoma. In: Neuroblastomas. Biochemical studies, pp. 42—51. Ed. C. Bohuon. Heidelberg: Springer 1966.

Beltran, G., Leiderman, E., Stuckey, W.J., Ferrans, V.J., Mogabgab, W.J.: Metastatic ganglioneuroblastoma. Cancer, Vol. **24**, 552—559 (1969).

Bellas, J.E.: Nonsurgical pheochromocytoma. J. Amer. med. Ass. **185**, 601—602 (1963).

Benedeczky, I., Lapis, K.: Vergleichende elektronenmikroskopische Untersuchungen an Nebennierenmark und Phäochromocytom des Menschen. Beitr. path. Anat. **137**, 403—438 (1968).

Berdal, P., Braaten, M., Cappelen, C., Mylius, E.A.: Glomus tumours s. nonchromaffin paragangliomas of the head and neck. Acta oto-laryng. (Stockh.) Suppl. **188**, 211—218 (1963).

— — — — Walaas, O.: Noradrenaline-adrenaline producing nonchromaffin paraganglioma. Acta med. scand. **172**, 249—257 (1962).

Besser, M.I.B., Pfau, A.: Pheochromocytoma of the urinary bladder. Brit. J. Urol. **40**, 245—247 (1968).

Biserte, G.: Présence d'homocystine dans les extraits des surrénales humaines. Bull. Soc. Chim. biol. (Paris) **39**, 549—557 (1957).

Blaschko, H.: Observations on chromaffin tissue. Med. College of Virginia Quarterly, **2**, 111—113 (1966).

— Hagen, J.M., Hagen, P.: Mitochondrial enzymes and chromaffin granules. J. Physiol. (Lond.) **139**, 316—322 (1957).

— Jerrome, D.W., Robb-Smith, A.H.T., Smith, A.D., Winkler, H.: Biochemical and morphological studies on catecholamine storage in human phaeochromocytoma. Clin. Sci. **34**, 453—465 (1968).

Bohuon, C.: Catecholamine metabolism in neuroblastoma. J. pediat. Surg. **3**, 114—118 (1968).

— Guérinot, F.: Dopamine-β-hydroxylase dans les tumeurs d'origine sympathique. Clin. chim. Acta. **14**, 414—416 (1966).

— — Dopamine-β-hydroxylase humaine et bovine, activité vis à vis de la dopamine et de la méthoxytyramine. Clin. chim. Acta **19**, 125—129 (1968).

— La Brosse, E.H., Assicot, M., Amar-Costesec, A.: Réflexion sur le dosage de la catéchol-0-méthyltransférase et de la monoamine oxydase dans les neuroblastomas. In: Neuroblastomas. Biochemical studies, pp. 16—22. Ed. C. Bohuon. Heidelberg: Springer 1966.

Brantigan, C.O., Katese, R.Y.: Clinical and pathologic features of paragangliomas of the organ of Zuckerkandl. Surgery **65**, 898—905 (1969).

BURGER, M., LANGEMAN, N.H.: Bestimmungen von Adrenalin und Noradrenalin sowie von Decarboxylaseaktivitäten in Zellfraktionen von Phäochromocytomen. Klin. Wschr. **34**, 941—944 (1956).

CABANA, B.E., PROKESCH, J.C., CHRISTIANSEN, G.S.: Study on the biogenesis of catecholamines in pheochromocytoma tissue culture. Arch. Biochem. Biophys. **106**, 123—130 (1964).

CAMERON, D.C., WARNER, H.A., SZABO, A.J.: Chronic diarrhea in an adult with hypokalemic nephropathy and ostemalacy due to a functioning ganglioneuroblastoma. Amer. med. Sci. **253**, 417—424 (1967).

CARMAN, C.T., BRASHEAR, R.E.: Pheochromocytoma as an inherited abnormality. Report of the tenth affected kindred and review of the literature. New. Engl. J. Med. **263**, 419—423 (1960).

CHAPMAN, R·C., DIAZ-PEREZ, R.: Pheochromocytoma associated with cerebellar hemangioblastoma. Familial ocurrence. J. Amer. med. Ass. **182**, 1014—1017 (1962).

CHATTEN, J., VOORHEES, M.L.: Familial neuroblastoma. Report of a kindred with multiple disorders, including neuroblastomas in four siblings. New Engl. J. Med. **277**, 1230—1236 (1967).

CHIOCCHIO, S.R., BISCARDI, A.M., TRAMEZZANI, J.H.: 5-Hydroxytryptamine in the carotid body of the cat. Science **158**, 790—791 (1967).

CLARK, A.C.L., MOORE, A.E., NIALL, M.: Metabolites of catecholamines in the urine of children with tumours of neural crest origin. Aust. pediat. J. **I**, 42—55 (1965).

COUPLAND, R.E.: On the morphology and adrenalin-noradrenaline content of chromaffin tissue. J. Endocr. **9**, 194—203 (1953).

— The natural history of the chromaffin cell, pp. 180—213. London: Longmans 1965.

— WEAKLEY, B.S.: Developing chromaffin tissue in the rabbit: an electron microscopic study. J. Anat. (Lond.) **102**, 425—455 (1968).

COWARD, R.F., SMITH, P., WILSON, O.S.: Urinary amines after adrenalectomy. Nature (Lond.) **193**, 1295—1296 (1962).

CREMER, G.M., MOLNAR, G.D., MOXNESS, K.E., SHEPS, S.G., MAHER, F.T., JONES, J.D.: Hormonal and biochemical response to glucagon administration in patients with pheochromocytoma and in control subjects. Mayo Clin. Proc. **43**, 161—176 (1968).

CROUT, J.R.: Pheochromocytoma. Pharmacol. Rev. **18**, 651—657 (1966).

— PISANO, J.J., SJOERDSMA, A.: Urinary excretion of catecholamines and their metabolites in pheochromocytoma. Amer. Heart. J. **61**, 375—381 (1961).

— SJOERDSMA, A.: Catecholamines in the localisation of pheochromocytoma. Circulation **22**, 516—525 (1960).

— — Turnover and metabolism of catecholamines in patients with pheochromocytoma. J. clin. Invest. **43**, 94—102 (1964).

DONATH, A., KÄSER, H., ROSS, B., ZIEGLER, W., OETLIKER, O., COLOMBO, J.P., BETTEX, M.: Le phéochromocytoma familial. Discussion de la malignité et du mode heréditaire à propos d'un cas chez l'enfant á secrétion particuliére. Helv. paediat. Acta **20**, 1—18 (1965).

DUKE, W.W., BOSHELL, B.R., SOTERES, P., CARR, J.H.: A norepinephrine-secreting glomus jugulare tumour presenting as a pheochromocytoma. Ann. intern. Med. **60**, 1040—1047 (1964).

— DONALD, J.M., BOSHELL, B.R.: A norepinephrine-secreting glomic tissue tumour (chemodectoma). J. Amer. med. Ass. **193**, 108—110 (1965).

EADE, N.R.: The distribution of the catecholamines in homogenates of the bovine adrenal medulla. J. Physiol. (Lond.) **141**, 183—192 (1958).

ENGEL, A., VON EULER, U.S.: Diagnostic value of increased urinary output of NA and A in pheochromocytoma. Lancet **II**, 387 (1950).

ENGELMAN, K., HAMMOND, W.G.: Adrenaline production by an intrathoracic pheochromocytoma. Lancet **I**, 609—611 (1968).

— HORWITZ, D., AMBROSE, J.M., SJOERDSMA, A.: Further evaluation of the tyramine test for pheochromocytoma. New Engl. J. Med. **278**, 705—709 (1968).

— SJOERDSMA, A.: A new test for pheochromocytoma: Pressor responsiveness to tyramine. J. Amer. med. Ass. **189**, 81—86 (1964).

ETSTEN, B.E., SHIMOSATO, S.: Halothane anesthesia and catecholamine levels in a patient with pheochromocytoma. Anesthesiology **26**, 688—691 (1965).

EULER, U.S. VON: Adrenal medullary and other chromaffin cell tumours. Ciba Found. Coll. on Endocr. **12**, 268—277 (1958).

— FRANKSSON, G., HELLSTRÖM, J.: Adrenaline and noradrenaline content of surgically removed human suprarenal glands. Acta physiol. scand. **31**, 6—8 (1954).

— GEMZELL, C.A., STRÖM, G., WESTMAN, A.: Report of a case of pheochromocytoma, with special regard to preoperative diagnostic problems. Acta med. scand. **153**, 127—136 (1955).

— STRÖM, G.: Present status of diagnosis and treatment of pheochromocytoma. Circulation **15**, 5—13 (1957).

Faivre, G., Sommelet, J., Gilgenkrantz, J.M., Cherrier, F., Masse, G.: Diagnostic topographique d'un phéochromocytoma par dosage étagé des catécholamines dans le système veineux cave. Bull. Mém. Soc. méd. Hôp. Paris **113**, 129—137 (1962).
Falck, B., Ljungberg, O., Rosengren, E.: On the occurence of monoamines and related substances in familial medullary thyroid carcinoma with pheochromocytoma. Acta path. microbiol. scand. **74**, 1—10 (1968).
Feruglio, F.S., Greco, F., Cesano, L., Colongo, P.G., Sardi, G., Ghiandussi, L.: The effects of glucagon on systemic and hepatosplanchnic haemodynamics and on net peripheral and heptatosplanchnic balance of glucose, lactic and pyruvic acid in norma subjects and cirrhotics. Clin. Sci. **30**, 43—50 (1966).
Foster, G.V.: Calcitonon (thyrocalcitonin). New Engl. J. Med. **279**, 349—360 (1968).
Fries, J.G., Chamberlin, J.A.: Extra-adrenal pheochromocytoma: Literature review and report of cervical pheochromocytoma. Surgery, St. Louis **63**, 268—279 (1968).
Fuller, A.M., Brown, H.A., Harrison, E.G., Siekert, R.G.: Chemodectomas of the glomus jugulare tumours. Laryngoscope (St. Louis) **77**, 218—238 (1967).
Garrett, J., Osswald, W., Rodrigues-Pereira, E., Guimarães, S.: Catecholamine release from the isolated perfused adrenal gland. Naunyn-Schmiedeberg's Arch. exp. Path. Pharmak. **250**, 325—336 (1965).
Geiser, C.F., Efron, M.L.: Cystathioninuria in patients with neuroblastoma or ganglioneuroblastoma: its correlation to vanilmandelic acid excretion and its values in diagnosis and therapy. Cancer **22**, 856—860 (1968).
Gejrot, T., Lagerlöf, B., Wersäll, J.: Tumours of the glomus jugulare, a light and electron microscopic study. Acta oto-laryng. (Stockh.) Suppl. **188**, 220—226 (1963).
Gélinas, R., Pellerin, J., D'Iorio, A.: Biochemical observations of a chromaffine tumour. Rev. canad. Biol. **16**, 445—450 (1957).
Ghislandi, E., Guidotti, G., Cavalca, L.: Physiomorphologische Betrachtungen über einen Fall von Phäochromocytom, histologisch untersucht mit der Methode von Hillarp-Hökfelt. Virchows. Arch. path. Anat. **327**, 92—111 (1955).
Gifford, R.W., Kvale, W.F., Maher, F.T., Roth, G.M., Priestley, J.T.: Clinical features, diagnosis and treatment of pheochromocytoma: a review of 76 cases. Proc. Staff Meeting Mayo Clin. **39**, 280—302 (1964).
Gitlow, S.E., Mendlowitz, M., Kruk, E., Khassis, S.: Diagnosis of pheochromocytoma by assay of catecholamine metabolites. Circulat. Res. **9**, 746—753 (1961).
Gjessing, L.R.: Studies of functional neural tumours: I. Urinary 3-methoxy-4-hydroxyphenyl metabolites. Scand. J. clin. Lab. Invest. **15**, 463—473 (1963a).
— Studies on functional neural tumours. II. Cystathioninuria. Scand. J. clin. Lab. Invest. **15**, 474—478 (1963b).
— Studies of functional neural tumours. III. Cystathionine in the tumours tissue. Scand. J. clin. Lab. Invest. **15**, 479—482 (1963c).
— Studies of functional neural tumours. VI. Biochemical diagnosis. Scand. J. clin. Lab. Invest. **16**, 661—669 (1964).
— Biochemistry of functional neural crest tumours. Advanc. clin. Chem. **11**, 81—131 (1968).
— Borud, O.: Studies of functional neural tumours. VII. Urinary excretion of phenolicpyruvic acids. Scand. J. clin. Lab. Invest. **17**, 80—84 (1965).
— Mauritzen, K.: Cystathioninuria in hepatoblastoma. Scand. J. clin. Lab. Invest. **17**, 513—514 (1965).
Glenner, G.G., Crout, J.R., Roberts, W.C.: A functional carotid body-like tumour secreting levarterenol. Arch. Path. **73**, 230—240 (1962).
Goldfien, A., Zileli, S., Goodman, D., Thorn, G.W.: The estimation of epinephrine and norepinephrine in human plasma. J. clin. Endocr. **21**, 281—295 (1961).
Goldstein, M.: Enzymes controlling the biosynthesis of catecholamines, In: Neuroblastomas. Biochemical studies, pp. 66—70. Ed. C. Bohuon. Heidelberg: Springer 1966.
— Anagnoste, B., Goldstein, M.N.: Tyramine-H^3: Deaminated metabolites in neuroblastoma tumours and in continuous cell line of a neuroblastoma. Science **160**, 767—768 (1968).
— Gang, H., Joh, T.H.: Subcellular distribution and properties of phenylethanolamine-N-methyl transferase (PNMT). Fed. Proc. **28**, 287 (1969).
Goodall, Mc C., Stone, C.: Adrenaline and Noradrenaline producing tumours of the adrenal medulla and sympathetic nerves. Ann. Surg. **151**, 391—398 (1960).
Graeff, J. de, Horak, B.J.V.: The incidence of pheochromocytoma in the Netherlands. Acta med. scand. **176**, 583—593 (1964).
Graham, J.D.P.: Pressor amines and neuroblastoma. Nature (Lond.) **183**, 1733—1734 (1959).
Greeff, K., Strobach, H.: Bestimmung der Katecholamine und Vanillinmandelsäureausscheidung zur Diagnose des Phäochromocytoms. Verh. dtsch. Ges. inn. Med. **72**, 637—640 (1966).

Greenberg, R.E., Gardner, L.I.: Catecholamine metabolism in a functional neural tumour. J. clin. Invest. **39**, 1729—1736 (1960).

— Rosenthal, I., Falk, G.S.: Electron microscopy of human tumours secreting catecholamines: correlation with biochemical data. J. Neuropath. exp. Neurol. **28**, 475—500 (1969).

Greer, M., Anton, A.H., Williams, C.M., Echevarria, R.A.: Tumours of neural crest origin. Arch. Neurol. **13**, 139—148 (1965).

— Sprinkle, T.J., Williams, C.M.: Determination of urinary 3-methoxytyramine, normetanephrine and metanephrine in pheochromocytoma and neuroblastoma by gas chromatography. Clin. chim. Acta. **21**, 247—253 (1968).

Greer, W.E.R., Robertson, W., Smithwick, R.H.: Pheochromocytoma: Diagnosis, operative experiences and clinical result. Amer. J. Surg. **107**, 192—201 (1964).

Grillo, M.A.: Electron microscopy of sympathetic tissues. Pharmacol. Rev. **18**, 387—399 (1966).

Grimley, P.M., Glenner, G.G.: Histology and ultrastructure of carotid body paragangliomas: Comparison with the normal gland. Cancer **20**, 1473—1488 (1967).

— — Ultrastructure of the human carotid body: A perspective on the mode of chemoreception. Circulation **37**, 648—665 (1968).

Haag, H.W., Philippu, A., Schümann, H.J.: Freisetzung von Brenzcatechinaminen aus der isoliert durchströmten Nebenniere durch Tyramin und β-Phenyläthylamine. Experientia (Basel) **17**, 187—188 (1961).

Hagen, P.: Oberservations on the substrate specifity of dopa decarboxylase from ox adrenal medulla, human pheochromocytoma and human argentaffinoma. Brit. J. Pharmacol. **18**, 175—182 (1962).

Hamberger, C.A., Hamberger, C.B., Wersäll, J., Wågermark, J.: Malignant catecholamine-producing tumour of the carotid body. Acta path. microbiol. scand. **69**, 489—492 (1967).

Hamberger, B., Ritzen, M., Wersäll, J.: Demonstration of catecholamines and 5-hydroxytryptamine in the human carotid body. J. Pharmacol. exp. Ther. **152**, 197—201 (1966).

Hanson, A., Studnitz, W.v.: Demonstration of urinary N-acetyldopamine in patients with neurblastoma. Clin. chim. Acta **11**, 384—385 (1965).

Haranath, P.S.R.K., Premalatha, K., Rao, N.R.: Estimation of catecholamines in cerebrospinal fluid, plasma and urine in a case of pheochromocytoma. Indian J. med. Sci. **21**, 176—177 (1967).

Harrison, T.S., Barlett, J.D., Seaton, J.F.: Exaggerated urinary norepinephrine response to tilt in pheochromocytoma. Diagnostic implications. New Engl. J. Med, **277**, 725—728 (1967a).

— Seaton, J.F., Cerny, J.C., Bookstein, J.J., Bartlett, J.D.: Localisation of pheochromocytoma by caval catheterisation. Arch. Surg. **95**, 339—343 (1967b).

Hermann, H., Mornex, R.: Human tumours secreting catecholamines. Oxford: Pergomon Press 1964.

Herrlich, P., Sekeris, C.E.: Vorkommen vom Protocatechualdehyd bei einem Fall von bösartigem Pheochromocytom. Biochim. biophys. Acta (Amst.) **78**, 750 (1963).

— — Identifizierung von N-acetyl-noradrenalin im Urin eines Patienten mit Neuroblastom. Hoppe-Seylers Z. physiol. Chem. **339**, 249—250 (1964).

Hillarp, N.Å., Lindqvist, M., Vendsalu, A.: Catecholamines and nucleotides in pheochromocytoma. Exp. Cell. Res. **22**, 40—44 (1961).

Hintersberger, H., Bartholomew, J.R.: Catecholamines and their acidic metabolites in urine and in tumour tissue in neuroblastoma, ganglioneuroma and pheochromocytoma. Clin. chim. Acta **23**, 169—175 (1969).

Holsti, L.R.: Pheochromocytoma demonstrated by aortography: Report of two cases. Acta radiol. **57**, 259—263 (1962).

Holton, P.: Noradrenaline in adrenal medullary tumours. Nature (Lond.) **163**, 217 (1949).

Holtz, P., Palm, D.: Brenzchatechinamine und andere sympathicomimetische Amine. Biosynthese und Inaktivierung, Freisetzung und Wirkung. Ergebn. Physiol. **58** (1966).

Hope, D.B.: L-cystathionine in the urine of pyridoxine deficient rats. Biochem. J. **66**, 486—489 (1957).

Huang, S.N., Mc Leish, W.A.: Pheochromocytoma and medullary carcinoma of thyroid. Cancer **21**, 302—311 (1968).

Hume, D.M.: Pheochromocytoma in the adult and in the child. Amer. J. Surg. **99**, 458—496 (1960).

Hunter, R.B., Marshall, P.B., Oram, F.J.: Catecholamine excretion in normal persons and in cases of pheochromocytoma. Quart. J. Med. **32**, 225—242 (1963).

Imashuku, S., La Brosse, E.H.: Tyrosine hydroxylase in neuroblastoma. Biochem. Med. **5**, 22—29 (1971).

ITOH, C., YOSHINAGA, K., SATO, T., ISHIDA, N., WADA, Y.: Presence of N-methylmetadrenaline in human urine and tumour tissue of pheochromocytoma. Nature (Lond.) **193**, 477—478 (1962).
JACOBS, L.S., SOBEL, C., HENRY, R.J.: Excretion of 3-methoxy-4-hydroxymandelic acid and catecholamines in patients with pheochromocytoma. J. clin. Endocr. **21**, 315—320 (1961).
JAIM-ETCHEVERRY, G., ZIEHER, L.M.: Cytochemical localization of monoamine stores in sheep thyroid gland at the electron microscope level. Experientia (Basel) **24**, 593—595 (1968).
JONES, N.F., WALKER, G., RUTHVEN, C.R.J., SANDLER, M.: α-Methyl-p-tyrosine in the management of phaeochromocytoma. Lancet **II**, 1105—1110 (1968).
KARNAUCHOW, P.N.: The carotid body: a pathologist's view. Canad. med. Ass. J. **92**, 1298—1302 (1965).
KÄSER, H.: Catecholamine-producing neural tumours other than pheochromocytoma. Pharmacol. Rev. **18**, 659—665 (1966a).
— Zur biochemischen Differentialdiagnose Katecholaminproduzierender Tumouren. Oncologia (Basel) **20**, Suppl., 52—59 (1966b).
— TÜRLER, K., BURRI, P.H.: Zum Katecholaminstoffwechsel im Gewebe maligner und benigner Tumoren des sympathischen Nervensystems. Schweiz. med. Wschr. **101**, 484—487 (1971).
— WAGNER, H.P., KÜFFER, F.: Maligne, sekretorisch anscheinend inaktive Sympathikustumoren im Kindesalter. Helv. paediat. Acta **24**, 128—135 (1969).
KELLEHER, J., WATTERS, G., ROBINSON, R., SMITH, P.: Chemical tests for pheochromocytoma. J. clin. Path. **17**, 399—404 (1964).
KENNEDY, J.S., SYMINGTON, T., WOODGER, B.A.: Chemical and histochemical observations in benign and malignant phaeochromocytoma. J. Path. Bact. **81**, 409—418 (1961).
KIRKENDALL, W.M., LIECHTY, R.D., CULP, D.A.: Diagnosis and treatment of patients with pheochromocytoma: Experience at University Hospitals from 1941—1964. Ann. intern. Med. **115**, 529—536 (1965).
KLEINSCHMIDT, A., SCHÜMANN, H.J.: Strukturuntersuchungen über die Adrenalin- und Noradrenalin speichernden Granula des Nebennierenmarkes. Naunyn-Schmiedeberg's Arch. exp. Path. Pharmak. **241**, 260—272 (1961).
KONTRAS, S.B.: Urinary excretion of 3-methoxy-4-hydroxymandelic acid in children with neuroblastoma. Cancer **15**, 978—986 (1962).
KOOP, C.E., KIESEWETTER, W.B., HORN, R.C.: Neuroblastoma in childhood. Survival after major surgical insult to the tumour. Surgery **38**, 272—278 (1955).
KOPIN, I.J., AXELROD, J.: Presence of 3-methoxy-4-hydroxyphenylglycol and metanephrine in pheochromocytoma tissue. Nature (Lond.) **185**, 788—790 (1960).
LA BROSSE, E.H., AXELROD, J., KOPIN, I.J., KETY, S.S.: Metabolism of 7-H^3-Epinephrine-bitartrate in normal young men. J. clin. Invest. **40**, 253—260 (1961).
— — SJOERDSMA, A.: Urinary excretion of normetanephrine by man. Fed. Proc. **17**, 386 (1958).
— BELEHRADEK, J., BARSKI, G., BOHUON, C., SCHWEISSGUTH, O.: Metabolic activity of neural crest tumours in tissues culture. Nature (Lond.) **203**, 195—196 (1964).
— SCHWEISSGUTH, O., BOHUON, C.: A biochemical study of neuroblastoma *in vivo* and *in vitro*. Biochem. Med. **2**, 12—25 (1968).
LANCE, E.M., CATE, W.R., LIDDLE, G.W., SCOTT, H.W.: Clinical experiences with pheochromocytoma. Surg. Gynec. Obstet. **106**, 25—37 (1958).
LANGEMANN, H., BONER, A., MÜLLER, P.B.: Aminosäurendecarboxylase im Phäochromocytom und Karzinoidgewebe. Schweiz. med. Wschr. **92**, 1621—1623 (1962).
LAUMONIER, R., MARCHE, C., MARCHE, J.: Étude ultrastructurale d'un phaeochromocytoma. Ann. Anat. path. **13**, 137—146 (1968).
LAURSEN, T., DAVIDSEN, G., HASNER, E.H., LINDBERG, J., SØRENSEN, B.: Determination of adrenaline and noradrenaline in human plasma in localisation of pheochromocytoma. Scand. J. clin. Lab. Invest. **19**, Suppl. 100, 137 (1967).
LAWRENCE, A.M.: Glucagon provocative test for pheochromocytoma. Ann. intern. Med. **66**, 1091—1096 (1967).
— FORLAND, M.: Glucagon provocative test for pheochromocytoma. J. Lab. clin. Med. **64**, 878 (1964).
LE COMPTE, P.M.: Tumours of the carotid body. Amer. J. Path. **24**, 305—321 (1948).
LEDUC, J.: Catecholamine production and release in exposure and acclimation to cold. Acta physiol. scand. **53**, Suppl. 183 (1961).
— D'IORIO, A.: Etudes biochimiques de deux cas de pheochromocytoma. Rev. canad. Biol. **19**, 34—52 (1960).

LEFEBVRE, P.J., CESSION-FOSSION, A.M., LUYCKX, A.S., LECOMTE, J.L., VAN CAUWENBERGE, H.S.: Interlationships glucagon-adrenergic system in experimental and clinical conditions. Arch. int. Pharmacodyn. **172**, 393—404 (1968).

LEVIT, S.A., SHEPS, S.G., ESPINOSA, R.E., REMINE, W.H., HARRISON, E.G.: Catecholamine-secreting paraganglioma of glomus-jugulare region resembling pheochromocytoma. N.E.J. Med. **281**, 805—811 (1969).

LIEBAU, H.: Blutdruckansprechbarkeit auf vasoaktive Substanzen und Blutdruckregulationsfähigkeit bei Patienten mit Phäochromocytom. Arch. Klin. Med. **215**, 219—228 (1968).

LJUNGBERG, O., CEDERQUIST, E., STUDNITZ, W. v.: Medullary thyroid carcinoma and phaeochromocytoma: a familial chromaffinomatosis. Brit. med. J. **I**, 279—281 (1967).

LORIMIER, A. DE, BRAGG, U., LINDEN, G.: Neurblastoma in Childhood. Amer. J. Dis. Child **118**, 441—450 (1969).

LOUIS, W.J., DOYLE, A.E.: The tyramine test for pheochromocytoma. Med. J. Aust. 1023 to 1026 (1967).

LUND, A., MØLLER, K.O.: Adrenaline concentration in the blood of human patients dying of adrenaline poisoning. Acta pharmacol. (Kbh.) **14**, 363—366 (1958).

LUSE, S.A.: Synaptic structures occuring in a neuroblastoma. Arch. Neurol. **11**, 185—190 (1964).

MACADAM, R.F.: The fine structure of a human carotid body tumour. J. Pathol. **99**, 101—104 (1969).

MAHAUX, J.E., SCHAEPDRYVER, A.F. DE, VERNIORY, A., ENDERLE, J., SMETS, W., REINHOLD, H., ROOD, M. DE, MEUNIER, A.: Phéochromocytome à symptômes pseudohyperthyroidiens. Localisation de la tumeur per rétropneumopéritoine et par dosage étagé des catecholamines dans la veine cave inférieure. Ann. Endocr. (Paris) **24**, 93—101 (1963).

MAHONEY, E.M., FRIEND, O.G., DEXTER, L., HARRISON, H.: Localisation of (adrenal and extra-adrenal) pheochromocytomas by vena caval blood sampling. Surg. Forum **14**, 495—496 (1963).

MARGOLIS, F.L., ROFFI, J., JOST, A.: Norepinephrine methylation in fetal rat adrenals. Science (N.Y.) **154**, 275—276 (1966).

MARDSEN, H.B.: Clinical and pathological features of neuroblastoma. In: The clinical chemistry of monoamines, pp. 71—87. Ed. H. VARLEY and A.H. GOWENLOCK. Amsterdam: Elsevier 1962.

MASON, G.A., HART-MERCER, J., MILLAR, E.J., STRANG, L.B.: Adrenaline secreting neuroblastoma in an infant. Lancet **II**, 322—325 (1957).

McGUIRE, L.B., FOX, L.M.: Recurrent pheochromocytoma with recognition of site of metastasis by means of venous catheterization. A case study. Ann. intern. Med. **60**, 125—130 (1964).

McKENDRICK, T., EDWARDS, R.W.H.: The excretion of 4-hydroxy-3-methoxy-mandelic acid by children. Arch. Dis. Childh. **40**, 418—425 (1965).

McMILLAN, M.: Identification of hydroxytyramine in a chromaffin tumour. Lancet **II**, 284 (1956).

MEANEY, T.F., BUONOCORE, E.: Selective arteriography as a localizing and provocative test in the diagnosis of pheochromocytoma. Radiology **87**, 209—314 (1966).

MERRILL, S., CHROJKA, V.E., BERKOWITZ, G.M., TEXTER, E.C.: The effects of glucagon on the superior mesenteric vascular bed. Fed. Proc. **21**, 200 (1967).

MIĆIĆ, R., KIČIČ, M., ADANJA, S.: Pheochromocytoma of urinary bladder. Acta endocr. (Kbh.) **39**, 1—12 (1962).

MILES, R.M.: Pheochromocytoma: A review of ten cases. Arch. Surg. **80**, 283—295 (1960).

MILLER, R.W., FRAUMENI, J.F., HILL, J.A.: Neuroblastoma: Epidemiologic approach to its origin. Amer. J. Dis. Child. **115**, 253—261 (1968).

MISUGI, K., MISUGI, N., NEWTON, W.A.: Fine structural study of neuroblastoma, ganglioneuroblastoma and pheochromocytoma. Arch. Path. **86**, 160—170 (1968).

MOORHEAD, E.L., CALDWELL, J.R., KELLY, A.R., MORALES, A.R.: The diagnosis of pheochromocytoma: Analysis of 26 cases. J. Amer. med. Ass. **196**, 1107—1113 (1966).

MUELLER, R.A., THOENEN, H., AXELROD, J.: Increase in tyrosine hydroxylase activity after reserpine administration. J. Pharmacol. exp. Ther. **169**, 74—79 (1969).

MULHOLLAND, S.G., ATUK, M.O., WALZAK, M.P.: Familial pheochromocytoma and cerebellar hemangioblastoma. J. Amer. med. Ass. **207**, 1709—1711 (1969).

MULLIGAN, R.M.: Chemodectoma in the dog. Amer. J. Path. **26**, 680—681 (1950).

MUSCHOLL, E.: Die Hemmung der Noradrenalin-Aufnahme des Herzens durch Reserpin und die Wirkung von Tyramin. Naunyn-Schmiedeberg's Arch. exp. Path. Pharmak. **240**, 234—241 (1960).

NAGATSU, T., ZAMAMOTO, T., NAGATSU, I.: Partial separation and properties of tyrosine hydroxylase from the human phaeochromocytome. Effect of norepinephrine. Biochim. biophys. Acta (Amst.) **198**, 210—218 (1970).

NAGATSU, T., LEVITT, M., UDENFRIEND, S.: Tyrosine Hydroxylase: The initial step in norepinephrine biosynthesis. J. biol. Chem. **239**, 2910—2917 (1964).
NIBBELINK, D.W., PETERS, B.H., MCCORMICK, W.F.: On the association of pheochromocytoma and cerebellar hemangioblastoma. Neurology (Minneap.) **19**, 455—460 (1969).
NIEMI, M., OJALA, K.: Cytochemical demonstration of catecholamines in the human carotid body. Nature (Lond.) **203**, 539—540 (1964).
NOUROK, D.S.: Familial pheochromocytoma and thyroid carcinoma. Ann. intern. Med. **60**, 1028—1040 (1964).
PAGE, L.B., JACOBY, G.A.: Catecholamine metabolism and storage granules in pheochromocytoma and neuroblastoma. Medicine (Baltimore) **43**, 379—386 (1964).
PEKKARINEN, A., SCHEININ, T.M., NANTÖ, V.: Localisation of pheochromocytoma by vena caval catheterisation of plasma catecholamines. Ann. Chir. Gynaec. Fenn. **56**, 419—423 (1967).
PERTSEMLIDIS, D., GITLOW, S.E., SIEGEL, W.C., KORK, A.E.: Pheochromocytoma, I. Specificity of Laboratory Diagnostic Tests, II. Safeguards during Operative Removal. Ann. Surg. **169**, 376—385 (1969).
POISNER, A.M., DOUGLAS, W.W.: The need for calcium in adreno-medullary secretion evoked by biogenic amines, polypeptides and muscarinic agents. Proc. Soc. exp. Biol. (N.Y.) **123**, 62—64 (1966).
PONTASSE, E.F., GIFFORD, R.W.: Pheochromocytoma: Diagnosis and treatment. Progr. cardiol. Dis. **8**, 235—252 (1965).
PRIESTLEY, J.T., KVALE, W.F., GIFFORD, R.W.: Pheochromocytoma: clinical aspects and surgical treatment. Arch. Surg. **86**, 778—790 (1963).
PRYSE-DAVIES, J., DAWSON, J.M.P., WESTBURY, G.: Some morphologic, histochemical and chemical observations on chemodectomas and the normal carotid body including a study of the chromaffin reaction and possible ganglion cell elements. Cancer **17**, 185—202 (1964).
PYLE, R.: Succesive, bilateral pheochromocytomas demostrated by aortography. Brit. J. Radiol. **34**, 668—670 (1961).
RABIN, C.B.: Chromaffin cell tumours of the suprarenal medulla (pheochromocytoma) A.M.A. Arch. Path. **7**, 228—244 (1929).
RATZENHOFER, M., AUBÖCK, L., MÜLLER, O.: Zur Kenntnis von Feinbau und Sekretionsmechanismus der Phäochromocytome. Beitr. path. Anat. **137**, 36—64 (1968).
RIDDELL, D.H., SCHULL, L.G., FRIST, T.F., BAKER, T.D.: Experience with pheochromocytoma in 21 patients: use of dichlorisoproterenol hydrochloride for cardiac arrhythmia. Ann. Surg. **157**, 980—988 (1963).
ROBERTSON, D.M., HENDRY, W.S., VOGEL, F.S.: Central ganglioneuroma: A case study using electron microscopy. J. Neuropath. **23**, 692—705 (1964).
ROBINSON, R.: The clinical chemistry of pheochromocytomas. In: The clinical chemistry of monoamines, pp. 63—70. Ed. H. VARLEY and A.H. GOWEMLOCK. Amsterdam: Elsevier 1963.
— Biochemical features of malignant tumours of sympathetic tissue. In: Neuroblastoma. Biochemical Studies, pp. 37—42. Ed. C. BOHUON. Heidelberg: Springer 1966.
— SMITH, P.: Urinary amines in pheaochromocytoma. Clin. Chim. Acta **7**, 29—33 (1962).
— — WHITTAKER, S.R.F.: Secretion of catecholamines in malignant phaeochromocytoma. Brit. med. J. **I**, 1422—1424 (1964).
ROBINSON, R. L.: Stimulation of release of CA from isolated adrenal glands by tyramine. J. Pharmacol. exp. Ther. **151**, 55—58 (1966).
ROSENSTEIN, B.J., ENGELMAN, K.: Diarrhea in a child with a catecholamine-secreting gangioneuroma. Case report and review of the literature. J. Pediat. **63**, 217—226 (1963).
ROSENTHAL, I.M., GREENBERG, R., GOLDSTEIN, R., KATHAN, R., CADKIN, L.: Catecholamine metabolism in a pheochromocytoma. Amer. J. Dis. Child. **112**, 389—395 (1966).
— — KATHAN, R., FALK, G.W., WONG, R.: Catecholamine metabolism of ganglioneuroma: correlation with electronmicrographs. Pediat. Res. **3**, 413—424 (1969).
ROSSI, P., KAUFMAN, L., RUZICKA, F.F., PANKE, W.: Angiographic localization of pheochromocytoma. Radiology **86**, 266—275 (1966).
ROTH, B.H., STJÄRNE, L., LEVINE, R.L., GIARMAN, N.J.: Abnormal regulation of catecholamine synthesis in pheochromocytoma. J. Lab. clin. Med. **3**, 397—403 (1968).
ROTH, G.M., FLOCK, E.V., KVALE, W.F., WAUGH, J.M., OGG, J.: Pharmacologic and chemical tests as an aid in the diagnosis of pheochromocytoma. Circulation **21**, 769—778 (1960).
RUBIN, R.P., JAANUS, S.D.: A study of the release of catecholamines from the adrenal medulla by indirectly acting sympathomimetic amines. Naunyn-Schmiedeberg's Arch. Pharmak. exp. Path. **254**, 125—137 (1966).
RUTHVEN, C.R.J., SANDLER, M.: Estimation of homovanillic acid in urine. Analyt. Biochem. **8**, 282—292 (1964).
SACK, H., KOLL, J.F.: Das Phäochromocytom. Ergebn. inn. Med. Kinderheilk. **19**, **446**—555 (1963).

SANKOFF, I., SOURKES, T.L.: Determination by thin-layer chromatography of urinary homovanillic acid in normal and disease states. Canad. J. Biochem. **41**, 1381—1388 (1963).

SAPIRA, J.P., ALTMAN, M., VANDYK, K., SHAPIRO, A.P.: Bilateral adrenal pheochromocytoma and medullary thyroid carcinoma. New Engl. J. Med. **273**, 140—143 (1965).

SAROSI, G., DOE, R.P.: Familial ocurrence of parathyroid adenomas, phaeochromocytoma and medullary carcinoma of the thyroid with amyloid stroma (Sipple's syndrom). Ann. intern. Med. **68**, 1305—1309 (1968).

SATO, T., ISHIDA, N., ITOH, C., WADA, Y., YOSHINAGA, K.: Studies on the metabolism of catecholamines in pheochromocytoma. Tohoku J. exp. Med. **76**, 313—318 (1962).

SATO, T.L., SJOERDSMA, A.: Urinary homovanillic acid in pheochromocytoma. Brit. med. J. **II**, 1472—1473 (1965).

SCHAEPDRYVER, A.F. DE: Fluorimetric estimation of A and NA in urine and blood and diagnosis of chromaffin cell tumours. Arch. int. Pharmacodyn. **121**, 489—499 (1959).

SCHIMKE, R.N., HARTMANN, W.H.: Familial amyloid-producing medullary thyroid carcinoma and pheochromocytoma. A distinct genetic entity. Ann. intern. Med. **63**, 1027—1039 (1965).

— — PROUT, T.E., RIMOIN, D.L.: Syndrome of bilateral pheochromocytoma, medullary thyroid carcinoma and multiple neuromas: A possible regulatory defect in the differentiation of chromaffin tissue. New Engl. J. Med. **279**, 1—7 (1968).

SCHLEGEL, G.G.: Neurofibromatose Recklinghausen und Phäochromocytom. Schweiz. med. Wschr. **90**, 31—39 (1960).

SCHMID, E.: Untersuchungen über Physiologie und Pathophysiologie des sympaticoadrenalen Systems durch Bestimmung der Vanillin-Mandelsäure-Ausscheidung im Harn mit Dünnschicht chromatographischer Technik. Arch. Kreisl.-Forsch. **49**, 83—116 (1966).

— BACHMANN, K., HEYNEN, H.P., GRAF, N., KRAUTHEIM, J.: Möglichkeiten und Grenzen der Phäochromocytom-Diagnostik mit dem Tyramintest. Z. Kreisl.-Forsch. **55**, 540—548 (1966).

SCHÜMANN, H.J.: The distrubtion of adrenaline and noradrenaline in chromaffine granules of the chicken. J. Physiol. (Lond.) **137**, 318—326 (1957).

— Hormon- und ATP-Gehalt des menschlichen Nebennierenmarkes und des Phäochromocytomgewebes. Klin. Wschr. **38**, 11—13 (1960).

SCHWEISSGUTH, O.: Intérêt pour le Pédiatre des Dosages d'acide vanillylmandélique dans les urines. In: Neuroblastoma. Biochemical studies, pp. 59—65. Ed. C. BOHUON. Heidelberg: Springer 1966.

SCIAN, L.F., WESTERMANN, C.D., VERDESCA, A.S., HILTON, J.G.: Adrenocortical and medullary effects of glucagon. Amer. J. Physiol. **199**, 867—870 (1960).

SCOTT, H.W., RIDELL, D.H., BROCKMAN, S.K.: Surgical management of pheochromocytoma. Surg. Gynec. Obstet. **120**, 707—724 (1965).

SEKERIS, C.E., HERRLICH, P.: Nachweis von N-acetyl-dopamin bei einem Fall von Phäochromocytom. Hoppe-Seylers Z. physiol. Chem. **331**, 289—291 (1963).

SHAW, K.N.F., LIEBERMAN, E., KOCH, R., DONNELL, G.N.: Cystathionuria. Amer. J. Dis. Child. **113**, 119 (1967).

SHEPHERD, D.M., WEST, G.B.: Noradrenaline and the suprarenal medulla. Brit. J. Pharmacol. **6**, 665—674 (1951).

— — Hydroxytyramine and the adrenal medulla. J. Physiol. (Lond.) **120**, 15—19 (1953).

SHEPS, S.G., MAHER, F.T.: Comparison of the histamine and tyramine hydrochloride tests in the diagnosis of pheochromocytoma. J. Amer. med. Ass. **195**, 265—267 (1966).

— — Histamine and glucagon tests in diagnosis of pheochromocytoma. J. Amer. med. Ass. **205**, 895—899 (1968).

— TYCE, G.M., FLOCK, E.V., MAHER, F.I.: Current experience in the diagnosis of pheochromocytoma. Circulation **34**, 473—483 (1966).

SILVERMAN, L., DAHLIN, D.C., TYCE, G.M., STICKLER, G.B.: Ganglionneuroblastoma. Studies of pathologic changes and content of catecholamine. Amer. J. clin. Path. **42**, 145—151 (1964).

SIPPLE, J.H.: The association of pheochromocytoma with carcinoma of the thyroid gland. Amer. J. Med. **31**, 163—166 (1961).

SJOERDSMA, A.: Pheochromocytoma as a model in clinical pharmacology. Proceeding of the 3rd International Pharmacological Meeting, Vol. **3**, 65—71 (1966).

— ENGELMAN, K., SPECTOR, S., UDENFRIEND, S.: Inhibition of catecholamine synthesis in man with a-methyltyrosine, an inhibitor of tyrosine hydroxylase. Lancet **II**, 1092—1094 (1965).

— — WALDMANN, T.A., COOPERMAN, L.K., HAMMOND, W.G.: Pheochromocytoma: Current concepts of diagnosis and treatment. Ann. intern. Med. **65**, 1302—1326 (1966).

— LEEPER, L.C., TERRY, L.L., UDENFRIEND. S.: Studies on the biogenesis and metabolism of NE in patients with pheochromocytoma. J. clin. Invest. **38**, 31—38 (1958).

Slarotinek, A., De la Lande, I.S., Head, R.: Medullary thyroid carcinomas with bilateral pheochromocytomas. Aust. J. Med. **17**, 320—326 (1968).
Smith, A.D., Winkler, H.: The localization of lysosomal enzymes in chromaffin tissue. J. Physiol. (Lond.) **182**, 179—188 (1966).
— — A simple method for the isolation of adrenal chromaffin granules on a large scale. Biochem. J. **103**, 480—482 (1967).
— — Lysosomal phospholipases A_1 and A_2 of bovine adrenal medulla. Biochem. J. **108**, 867—874 (1968).
Smith, R.A., Whitehead, T.P., Morris, L., Williams, H.P.: Functionally active intrathoracic neuroblastoma. Amer. J. Dis. Child. **36**, 82—89 (1961).
Snyder, S.H., Axelrod, J., Zweig, M.: A sensitive and specific fluorescence assay for tissue serotonin, Biochem. Pharmacol. **14**, 832—835 (1965).
Sourkes, T.L., Denton, R.L., Murphy, G.F., Chavez, B., Saint Cyr, S.: The excretion of dihydroxyphenylalanine, dopamine and dihydroxyphenylalanine, dopamine and dihydroxyphenylacetic acid in neuroblastoma. Pediatrics **31**, 660—668 (1963).
Staley, N.A., Polesky, H.F., Bensch, K.G.: Fine structural and biochemical studies on the malignant ganglioneuroma. J. Neuropath. **26**, 634—653 (1967).
Staszewska-Barczak, J., Vane, J.R.: The release of catechol amines from the adrenal medulla by histamine. Brit. J. Pharmacol. **25**, 728—742 (1965).
Stickler, G.B., Flock, E. v.: Neuroblastoma and ganglioneuroblastoma: Associated increased urinary excretion of catecholamines. Canad. Chemother. Rep. **16**, 439—442 (1962).
— Hallenbeck, G.A., Flock, E. v.: Ganglioneuroblastoma associated with increased excretion of catecholamines. Amer. J. Dis. Child. **100**, 634 (1960).
Stjärne, L.: Tyramine effects on catecholamine release from spleen and adrenals in the cat. Acta physiol. scand. **51**, 224—229 (1961).
— Euler, U.S. v., Lishajko, F.: Catecholamines and nucleotides in phaeochromocytoma. Biochem. Pharmacol. **13**, 809—818 (1964).
Straus, R., Wurm, M.: Catecholamines and the diagnosis of pheochromocytoma: a review and evaluation. Amer. J. clin. Path. **34**, 403—425 (1960).
Strieder, N., Ziegler, E., Winkler, H., Smith, A.D.: Some properties of the soluble proteins from chromaffin granules of different species. Biochem. Pharmacol. **17**, 1553—1556 (1968).
Strömblad, B.C.R.: Effect of denervation and of cocaine on the action of sympathomimetic amines. Brit. J. Pharmacol. **15**, 328—332 (1960).
Strömblad, C.R., Nickerson, M.: Accumulation of epinephrine and norepinephrine by some rat tissues. J. Pharmacol. exp. Ther. **134**, 154—159 (1961).
Studnitz, W. v.: Methodische und klinische Untersuchungen über die Ausscheidung der 3-Methoxy-4-Hydroxymandelsäure im Urin. Scand. J. clin. Lab. Invest. **12**, Suppl. 48 (1960).
— Occurence, isolation and identification of 3-methoxy-4-hydroxyphenylalanine. Clin. chim. Acta **6**, 526—530 (1961).
— Homoserine in urine of patients with neuroblastoma. Scand. J. clin. Lab. Invest. **17**, 558—564 (1965a).
— Tyrosine hydroxylase activity in human adrenals and tumours of the neural crest. Clin. chim. Acta **12**, 597—599 (1965b).
— Sulfur-containing amino acids in the urine of patients with tumours from sympathic nervous tissue. Scand. J. clin. Lab. Invest. **17**, Suppl. 86, 190 (1965c).
— Chemistry and Pharmacology of catecholamine secreting tumours. Pharmacol. Rev. **18**, 645—650 (1966).
— Zur Frage des Vorkommens von 3-Hydroxy-4-methoxymandelsäure beim normalen und gesteigerten Katecholaminstoffwechsel. Klin. Wschr. **45**, 307—308 (1967).
— Urinary excretion of methoxycatecholamines in neuroblastoma. Scand. J. clin. Lab. Invest. **21**, 333—336 (1968).
— Hanson, A.: Demonstration of urinary N-acetyltyramine in patients with neuroblastoma. Clin. chim. Acta **16**, 180—183 (1967).
— Käser, H., Sjoerdsma, A.: Spectrum of catecholamine biochemistry in patients with neuroblastoma. New Engl. J. Med. **269**, 232—235 (1963).
— Ljungberg, O.: Tyramine test and phaeochromocytoma. Acta med. scand. **182**, 341—344 (1967).
Sturm, A.: Erhöhtes Vorkommen, Bedeutung und Bestimmung der Vanillinsäure im Harn bei einem Phäochromoblastom. Dtsch. med. Wschr. **88**, 1000—1005 (1963).
Sunderman, C.R., Sunderman, F.W., Ballinger, W.F.: Measurements of serum vanilmandelic acid in a patient with pheochromocytoma. Amer. J. clin. Path. **43**, 122—129 (1965).
Tannenbaum, M., Spiro, D., Lattimer, J.K.: Norepinephrine and epinephrine secreting tumours of the adrenal medulla: An electron microscopic and biochemical study. Amer. J. Path. **48**, 48a (1966).

THURM, R.H., HEIDENBERG, W.J., HERRON, G.R., LAU, S.H.: Evaluation of the tyramine test in hypertensive patients and controls. J. Amer. med. Ass. **196**, 613—616 (1966).
TIEDGE, F., SCHEIFFARTH, F., SCHMID, E.: Über eine Sonderform von hormonal aktivem Tumor des Glomus jugulare-tympanicum. Z. Laringologie **43**, 271—273 (1964).
TOKER, C.: Ultrastructure of a chemodectoma. Cancer **20**, 271—280 (1967).
TRANZER, J.P., THOENEN, H.: Significance of "Empty Vesicles" in postganglionic sympathetic nerve terminals. Experientia (Basel) **23**, 123—124 (1967).
TRENDELENBURG, U.: The action of histamine and pilocarpine on the superior cervical ganglion and the adrenal glands of the cat. Brit. J. Pharmacol. **9**, 481—487 (1954).
UDENFRIEND, S., ZALTZMAN-NIRENBERG, P., NAGATSU, T.: Inhibitors of purified beef adrenal tyrosine hydroxylase. Biochem. Pharmacol. **14**, 837—845 (1965).
VENDSALU, A.: Studies on adrenaline and noradrenaline in human plasma. Acta physiol. scand. **49**, Suppl. 173 (1960).
VOORHEES, M.L.: The catecholamines in tumour and urine from patients with neuroblastoma, ganglioneuroblastoma and pheochromocytoma. J. pediat. Surg. **3**, 147—148 (1968).
— GARDNER, L.I.: Studies of catecholamine excretion by children with neural tumours. J. clin. Endocr. **22**, 126—133 (1962).
WEIL-MALHERBE, H.: Pheochromocytoma: Catechols in urine and tumour tissue Lancet **II**, 282—284 (1956).
— SMITH, E.R.B.: The estimation of metanephrine, normetanephrine and 3,4-dihydroxymandelic acid in urine. Pharmacol. Rev. **18**, 331—341 (1966).
WEINER, N., DRASKÓCZY, P.R., BURACK, W.R.: The ability of tyramine to liberate catecholamines *in vivo*. J. Pharmacol. exp. Ther. **137**, 47—55 (1962).
WEST, G.B.: The suprarenal glands of the hare and horse. J. Pharm. Pharmacol. **5**, 460—464 (1953).
WILLIAMS, C.M., LEONARD, R.H.: Microanalytical determination of dihydroxy aromatic acids by gas chromatography. Analyt. Biochem. **5**, 362—366 (1963).
WILLIAMS, E.D.: A review of 17 cases of carcinoma of the thyroid and pheochromocytoma. J. clin. Path. **18**, 288—292 (1965).
WINKLER, H.: Isolierung und Eigenschaften von Noradrenalin-speichernden Granula des Nebennierenmarkes. Arch. Pharmakol. exp. Path. **263**, 340—357 (1969).
— SMITH, A.D.: Catecholamines in pheochromocytoma. Lancet **I**, 793—795 (1968).
— ZIEGLER, E., STRIEDER, N.: Gewinnung und Eigenschaften der Katecholaminspeichernden Granula eines Phäochromocytoms. Klin. Wschr. **45**, 1238—1241 (1967).
WURTMAN, R.J., AXELROD, J.: Control of enzymatic sythesis of adrenaline in the adrenal medulla by adrenal cortical steroids. J. biol. Chem. **241**, 2301—2305 (1966).
— — VESELL, E.S., ROSS, G.T.: Species differences in inducibility of phenylethanolamine-N-methyl transferase. Endocrinology **82**, 584—590 (1968).
WÜST, G., KLUGE, A., BARKHOFF, E.R.: Zur Klinik und Morphologie maligner Tumoren des chromaffinen Systems. Oncologia (Basel) **18**, 101—119 (1964).
YOKOYAMA, M., TAKAYASU, H.: An electron microscopic study of the human adrenal medulla and pheochromocytoma. Urol. Intern. **24**, 79—95 (1969).
YOUNG, R.B., STEIKER, D.D., BONGIOVANNI, A.M., KOOP, G.E., EBERLEIN, W.R.: Urinary vanillmandelic acid (VMA) excretion: use of a single semiquantitative test. J. Pediat. **62**, 844—854 (1963).
ZIEGLER, W.H., LANGEMANN, H., MÜLLER, P.B.: Vergleichende Untersuchungen an Tumorgeweben von Phäochromocytom und Karzinoid. Schweiz. med. Wschr. **97**, 1731—1734 (1967).
ZIMON, R.P., SHEPS, S.G., HAZELRIG, C.G., SCHIRGER, A., OWEN, C.A.: In vitro blood cell uptake of radioactive norepinephrine: experience in pheochromocytoma and idiopathic orthostatic hypotension. Mayo Clin. Proc. **41**, 649—656 (1966).

Author Index

Page numbers in *italics* refer to the bibliography

Subject Index*

f = Reference to a figure or formula;
t = reference to a table.

* Prepared by H. Kilbinger, R. Lindmar, K. Löffelholz and E. Muscholl